Community Nutrition

Applying Epidemiology to Contemporary Practice

Second Edition

Gail C. Frank, DrPH, RD, CHES

Professor of Nutrition
California State University, Long Beach
Long Beach, CA

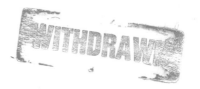

JONES AND BARTLETT PUBLISHERS

Sudbury, Massachusetts

BOSTON　　TORONTO　　LONDON　　SINGAPORE

World Headquarters

Jones and Bartlett Publishers	Jones and Bartlett Publishers	Jones and Bartlett
40 Tall Pine Drive	Canada	Publishers International
Sudbury, MA 01776	6339 Ormindale Way	Barb House, Barb Mews
978-443-5000	Mississauga, Ontario L5V 1J2	London W6 7PA
info@jbpub.com	Canada	United Kingdom
www.jbpub.com		

Jones and Bartlett's books and products are available through most bookstores and online booksellers. To contact Jones and Bartlett Publishers directly, call 800-832-0034, fax 978-443-8000, or visit our website www.jbpub.com.

Substantial discounts on bulk quantities of Jones and Bartlett's publications are available to corporations, professional associations, and other qualified organizations. For details and specific discount information, contact the special sales department at Jones and Bartlett via the above contact information or send an email to specialsales@jbpub.com.

This publication is designed to provide accurate and authoritative information in regard to the Subject Matter covered. It is sold with the understanding that the publisher is not engaged in rendering legal, accounting, or other professional service. If legal advice or other expert assistance is required, the service of a competent professional person should be sought.

Production Credits
Publisher: Michael Brown
Production Director: Amy Rose
Associate Production Editor: Rachel Rossi
Associate Editor: Katey Birtcher
Marketing Manager: Wendy Thayer
Manufacturing Buyer: Therese Connell
Composition: PrePressPMG
Cover Design: Kristin E. Ohlin
Cover Image: Copyright © Shutterstock
Printing and Binding: Malloy, Inc.
Cover Printing: Malloy, Inc.

Library of Congress Cataloging-in-Publication Data

Frank, Gail C.
Community nutrition : applying epidemiology to contemporary practice / Gail C. Frank. — 2nd ed.
    p. ; cm.
  Includes bibliographical references and index.
  ISBN-13: 978-0-7637-3062-8 (alk. paper)
  ISBN-10: 0-7637-3062-9 (alk. paper)
  1. Nutritionally induced diseases--Epidemiology. I. Title.
  [DNLM: 1. Nutrition–United States. 2. Community Health Services–United States. 3. Nutrition Assessment–United States. 4. Nutrition Disorders–United States. 5. Nutrition Policy–United States. QU 145 F828c 2007]
  RA645.N87F73 2007
  614.5'939–dc22

                              2006034285

6048

Printed in the United States of America

11 10 09 08 07 10 9 8 7 6 5 4 3 2 1

This book is dedicated to my Mom for her unwavering love and support.

Born on March 11, 1919
Passed to Heaven on November 25, 2006

CONTENTS

PREFACE

Inside the second edition of *Community Nutrition: Applying Epidemiology to Contemporary Practice,* students and faculty will find pages offering the latest rendering of community nutrition—one which will clarify their understanding of and approach for improving the quality of lives in U.S. communities. The latest research studies involving the major causes of morbidity and mortality among children, youth, men, and women are presented. Major programs funded by the U.S. Congress, as well as those made viable by local volunteer agencies, enrich the canvas.

As a text for either a one-semester upper division undergraduate or graduate level course, the text has three distinct parts that can stand alone or flow from Part I to Part III. Part I addresses nutrition in US communities and lays the groundwork for primary, secondary, and tertiary prevention. With five chapters, this section defines epidemiology and describes the progression of nutrition care from early public health initiatives to today's contemporary approach in multicultural and multiethnic communities.

National nutrition directives and guidelines for health promotion and disease prevention across the life cycle are discussed. "My Pyramid" replaces the "Food Guide Pyramid," which had a 20-year history as a major nutrition education tool. The new "2005 Dietary Guidelines for Americans" and "Healthy People in Healthy Communities 2010 Objectives" are presented and enrich each chapter thereafter.

The latest nutritional health claims and terms visible on our food labels and insight into how community nutrition professionals can strengthen their media skills are presented. Discussions about state and federal legislation to address community nutrition needs, sections on hunger and homelessness, and discussions about the needs of individuals at high nutritional risk, such as adults who are HIV+, are included in this section.

Part II focuses on primary prevention of disease by first addressing food-borne illness as a recurrent food safety and sanitation concern and then spans the life cycle with individual chapters on children, adults, and seniors. Detailed tables listing the daily recommended intakes (DRIs) and the latest Recommended Dietary Allowances by gender and age complement the science. Discussions include recently published data from the Women's Health Initiative clinical trial and expanded information on prostate cancer prevention for men. Decreasing chronic disease and reducing comorbidity of diseases are presented as viable themes for older adults.

Part III broadens the understanding and science base of specific chronic diseases and clarifies the role of eating behavior in disease development. Both secondary and tertiary prevention are presented. Individual chapters address coronary heart disease and the role of food as an intermediate substrate, as well as cancer risk and foods promoting its initiation. Obesity, hypertension, and diabetes are presented as single diseases demanding specific attention, but discussed as highly interrelated.

Osteoporosis, arthritis, alcoholism, and renal disease are presented for a comprehensive approach to nutritional well-being of all individuals. Incidence and prevalence rates are included for each chapter and popular diet and complementary approaches are discussed. The last chapter addresses community planning for health promotion and disease prevention and the role of self-management and behavioral change.

Learning objectives are listed at the beginning of each chapter and High Definition Nutrition sections showcase key terms and concepts useful to understanding content. "Info Lines" are within each chapter to encapsulate an important Web site, a significant research finding, or even an effective and creative community program. Relevant "Healthy People in Healthy Communities 2010" objectives are enumerated near the close of each chapter. Each chapter contains numerous figures, tables, and exhibits. Instructor and student resources, including appendices are available online at: http://nutrition.jbpub.com/book/community/2e/.

Students will remain contemporary in the 21st century if they assess their communities, determine the priorities, and then meet current needs of their target with the latest and most valid research available to them. This text is written to enrich and to excite community nutrition professionals, whether health educators, nurses, nutritionists, physical therapists, medical students, journalists, sociologists, behavioral psychologists, or epidemiologists, to name a few, and then to empower them to create their own canvas, to draft their own blueprint, and to build their own healthy community.

FOREWORD

Lisa Nicholson, PhD, RD

The goal of education is to prepare students for the future. But today that goal is more challenging than ever because of how rapidly the factors that influence community nutrition are changing. The future of the 21st-century nutrition professional will include continued growth in information technology; increasing complexity in both public health and medical care funding; a more nuanced understanding of preventive nutrition research; and managing the impact of the diversity of a global society. Effective education therefore needs to be centered around our students, giving them the tools to be flexible, lifelong learners. This *Community Nutrition* text creates a timely and very useful "toolbox" of skills and knowledge for the future community nutrition professional.

Community Nutrition is organized into three broad sections: Nutrition in the diverse communities of the United States; understanding nutrition-related primary prevention of disease; and an exploration of disease management and care of disease through nutrition. I refer to giving students a working toolbox for the future because in each section of the text the emphasis is on understanding how research and science affect nutrition recommendations. In a changing world, this approach can be used as new trends and research findings change the face of prevention and treatment in the United States.

In Part I, *Nutrition in US Communities*, the chapters focus on nutritional epidemiology in prevention and disease, our national nutrition policies and programs, and how the community nutrition professional functions in these environments. The foundation of the text is epidemiology. The methods and measures used in nutrition epidemiology are clearly and logically laid out. Providing our students with an understanding of the science on which much of our national nutrition policy is based is extremely important. Chapter 1 is a solid foundation for the text—clearly useful in an undergraduate community nutrition class. Using current study results to explain the research concepts is a particular strength of this text. Critical thinking is emphasized through the use of research to understand the science behind the new DRIs, food guidance systems, and labeling laws. Nutrigenomics is covered. The influence of food consumption research and disease monitoring on the creation of and influence on policy is clearly and logically laid out.

In addition, the skills needed for working in community nutrition, as well as various career options are covered in Part I. In my experience nutrition students who are not going on to become registered dietitians often wonder what jobs are available in nutrition without the RD. Chapter 3 describes a wide variety of approaches to working in the community. Approaches vary from research, to jobs in public community settings, to working with the media. Lots of very practical information and communication strategies are included. Another forward-looking aspect of this text is the emphasis on how technology is changing the spheres in which our students will be working. The author does an excellent job in broadening our use of the term *community* in sections on working with special groups, HIV, and ethnic minorities in a complex environment. The ethnic diversity section is especially strong.

Part II, *Primary Preventions of Disease,* uses the prevention model to look at specific populations and community nutrition. Chapter 6 covers the epidemiology of food-borne illness, which is missing in most of the other community nutrition texts currently available. Food-borne illness is also a relatively clear way for students to grasp many of the concepts involved in epidemiology. The text is up-to-date with HACCP, bioterrorism, "mad cow" disease, and hepatitis C information. In addition to the other information about healthy eating in early childhood is information about the world of child-care professionals. This is lacking in other texts. Of particular interest today is the thorough explanation of how childhood obesity tracks into adulthood. Chapter 8 on nutrition for school-age children provides excellent coverage of the many different environments surrounding child and adolescent issues. The text is nicely organized first around health issues and then around the child's environments such as the schools, home, and media. Coordinated school approaches to health are well covered. Health risk behaviors, including alcohol and supplement use, as well as eating disorders, are included.

The primary prevention issues of adult and older adults are covered using the latest research results. In addition to good coverage given to nutrition programs and delivery systems, the author's comprehensive and solid knowledge of nutrition research is well demonstrated in these chapters. The nutritional needs of adults, from pregnancy to men's health, are concise yet thorough. The description of the Women's Health Initiative (WHI) methods and study design will make this text very useful now and into the future. Understanding of the context of the WHI findings will be important as results continue to be published and affect future policy. The chapter on older adults provides good coverage and descriptions of the field of gerontology. The biology of aging gives a context to our current social programs and program delivery. Applications of the current research into aging are used to suggest directions for the future of care and prevention with elderly populations. Educators will appreciate the well-written section on minorities and aging.

In Part III, *Secondary and Tertiary Prevention—Managing Disease and Avoiding Complications,* the specific nutrition relationships with each of the major chronic diseases are each given a chapter. Chapter 11 on coronary heart disease provides an excellent, current review of the topic. This well-organized chapter covers the recent science and research findings, then moves into population versus medical approaches for treatment and prevention. Chapter 12, *Cancer,* first covers the cancer process, which provides a clearly organized context to understand how different diet patterns and specific food constituents affect or are affected by the different cancer stages. Study designs and data collection methods are addressed to explain some of the contradictions and uncertainties in the nutrition epidemiology of cancer. Chapter 13, *Diabetes Mellitus,* provides good coverage of the Diabetes Control and Complications Trial (DCCT) study that has given us so much data to work with in prevention of complications. The chapter also includes a section on eating disorders and insulin dependent diabetes mellitus (IDDM). Chapter 14, *Hypertension,* provides extensive coverage of the research literature associating nutrition, fitness, and hypertension. Results are very up-to-date. Many of the subcategories of hypertension relationships (i.e., in different ethnic or age groups) are addressed.

Also included in this third section of the book is the topic of obesity, as well as a final chapter on other debilitating diseases. The author takes an original approach to addressing the hot topic of obesity. She organizes the chapter around the parameters of qualitative and then quantitative measures of obesity. This organization allows her to cover a great many of the variables in the field of obesity. This is a very comprehensive chapter including both studies that are associated with developing obesity and studies regarding the health risks of excess weight. Levels of intervention efforts covered include what the individual can do (diet books and counseling methods) up through policy and environmental issues. This chapter does a great job reviewing a complex set of research studies. Ending the section on tertiary prevention by grouping osteoporosis, alcoholism, arthritis, and renal disease together into the context of debilitating diseases is an interesting and original approach. Chapter 16 picks up on some of the issues not previously covered. The section on calcium intake and studies relating to disease is very comprehensive. Including a section on arthritis and how anti-inflammatory diets may assist in symptom management is an asset to the text. Nutrition professionals will also appreciate the discussion of alcoholism and its nutrition implications.

The final chapter, *Preventing Single and Cluster Diseases,* brings the book full circle. Nutritional epidemiology is complicated by the multiple interrelationships between diseases, between eating patterns, and between the interactions of genetics with an environment. In essence, nutrition epidemiology can seem somewhat fuzzy without clear-cut results associated with clear-cut risks. This chapter puts the intrinsic difficulties associated with the complexity of studying nutrition and disease in populations into perspective.

As an educator, I found the structure of the text to be its primary strength. The learning objectives and the High Definition Nutrition section at the beginning of each chapter are well thought out and useful. The three-part organization of the text was an interesting, creative approach to community nutrition. The book starts out by explaining primary, secondary, and tertiary prevention. Then the book, as organized, uses Part II to address primary prevention approaches. Part III then covers secondary and tertiary approaches regarding nutrition and disease. This logical framework for the text allows the author to integrate policies and programs with what we know from the research on prevention and treatment. I really appreciate this organizational approach to handling such a multitude of information.

This book differs from other community nutrition texts with the strong emphasis on research as the framework for programs and policy. Understanding nutrition-related health issues is the backbone of this text. Effective interventions are based on understanding the factors associated with the origins of health and disease. In preparing students for the future, I see that they will have greater (indeed perhaps overwhelming) access to information. Under-standing how research works and how it affects policy and recommendations will help build the critical thinking skills needed to work in the complex and changing future.

Lisa Nicholson, PhD, RD
Associate Professor
Food Science and Nutrition Department
California Polytechnic State University
San Luis Obispo, CA

ABOUT THE AUTHOR

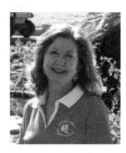

Dr. Gail Frank is a Professor of Nutrition and Director of an American Dietetic Association (ADA)-Accredited Dietetic Internship at California State University Long Beach. In addition to being a Certified Health Education Specialist (CHES), she trained as a chronic disease Epidemiologist at Tulane University, New Orleans. Gail served as a consultant for the USDA National Evaluation of the School Breakfast and School Lunch programs. For 16 years she investigated the heart disease risk factors of children while directing the dietary studies for Bogalusa Heart Study (BHS), and has since developed weight-loss, cholesterol, and diabetes interventions for both children and adults.

She was President of the New Orleans Dietetic Association and developed nutrition programs for the Diabetes Treatment Center at Tulane University Medical Center while serving as President-elect of the American Diabetes Association, New Orleans Chapter. She also held private contracts to train child-care providers about nutrition and food safety for young children, to develop education for Congregate Meal Programs, and to implement wellness programs.

Relocating to California in 1989, Gail developed "The Healthy Kids Club," which focuses on nutrition education and training of overweight youth, seniors, and school food service staff. She worked with private pediatricians to implement programs for the weight management of preschoolers and youth, and was Director of the California Department of Education's first contracted "Program Management Center for Child Nutrition."

Gail was Co-Principal Investigator for the Women's Health Initiative clinical trial at the University of California, Irvine, from 1994 to 2005. This program used motivational interviewing for increased adherence to low-fat eating. She is currently on the ADA Weight Management Certificate Program for Children and Youth. She is an active member of the Orange County American Academy of Pediatrics School Health Committee and recently joined the Editorial Board of *Obesity Management*.

Gail received the American Dietetic Association award for Excellence in Education and Research (1991), the ADA Outstanding Dietetic Internship Director for California (2003), and the California Dietetic Association Award for Excellence in Community Nutrition (2000). In addition to authoring nutrition textbooks, she has published over 100 articles in peer-review journals. She was Chair of the Board for the Long Beach American Heart Association, Chair of the Nutrition Task Force for the Long Beach American Cancer Society, Vice-Chair of the California Adolescent Nutrition and Fitness Board, and prior member of the KOCE-TV Health Programs Advisory Committee. Gail was a national media spokesperson for the American Dietetic Association for 19 years. Gail is a frequent speaker for national programs focusing on healthy eating, behavioral change, and program development for children and adults.

ACKNOWLEDGMENTS

This book would not have been written without the wonderful support and assistance of Marie Dufour, Karen Chan, Melissa Felix, Dorothy Cotton, Jennelle Koch, and Quyen Nguyen. Thank you so very much for honoring me with your time, skills, and love of community nutrition.

PART 1

NUTRITION IN US COMMUNITIES

CHAPTER ONE

EPIDEMIOLOGY—THE FOUNDATION OF COMMUNITY NUTRITION

Learning Objectives

- Define epidemiology, the traditional epidemiologic model to explore disease causation, various types of epidemiologic studies, and nutritional epidemiology.
- Track the early history of epidemiology.
- Identify the characteristics of a chronic disease.
- Describe a model for primary, secondary, and tertiary prevention of disease.
- Discuss the purpose of surveillance and monitoring in epidemiologic exploration.
- Describe various rates used to characterize or monitor health status of populations of people.

High Definition Nutrition

Meta-analysis—analysis that statistically integrates the *results* of individual studies.

Nutritional epidemiology—the study of eating behavior and how it influences the etiology, occurrence, prevention, and treatment of disease.

Pathway linking food and health—dietary component → food → food group → eating pattern → health/disease.

Sample size—the number of individuals surveyed.

The epidemiologic fabric was woven together largely from the numerical (quantitative) method, the development of a vital statistics system, the stimulus of a hygienic or public health movement, and the concept of comparative studies. It has now matured as a scientific discipline so that its study is necessary for a full understanding of the etiology of human and other diseases as well as their prevention and treatment.[1(p43)]

Epidemiology is the study of the occurrence and determinants of health events among people. It is a process to identify and to control health problems.[2] It uses biostatistics, statistical processes, and methods applied to the analysis of biological phenomena to describe and quantitate health events and the factors that place individuals at risk for health events. Epidemiology began as an approach to control communicable disease. The methods and principles have been applied with equal success to improve our understanding of chronic disease.[3]

Epidemiology is the basic science for public and community health. It characterizes the health status of a community and can influence public health policy. Baseline data are used as the foundation for program planning, which may involve treatment and monitoring an intervention or monitoring the effectiveness of a primary prevention or awareness campaign. The epidemiologic scope ranges from maternal and child health to adolescent school health, on one hand, and from health education in the managed-care setting to well-defined protocols to treat life-threatening disease among older adults, on the other hand. Epidemiology provides a canvas upon which health care paints the story of people in their daily lives.

The role of human behavior in health and illness has created a new generation of approaches to explore disease etiology and treatment.[4] Behavioral epidemiology assesses what people do and what they avoid. Nutritional epidemiology focuses on eating behavior and how that behavior influences health status, disease morbidity, and mortality. These approaches are in contrast to clinical medicine, which focuses on diagnosing and treating sick people. Community nutrition has reached a new level of functioning—one that complements what people choose to eat with programs and guidance about how to make healthy food choices for health promotion and disease prevention.

Epidemiology's Early History

Twentieth-century epidemiology is built on events that occurred over 200 years ago. In 1662, John Graunt, of England, quantified birth, death, and disease occurrence. He identified differences between men and women and differences between urban and rural locations. He also analyzed infant deaths and characterized seasonal variations. William Farr extended Graunt's contribution by collecting and analyzing mortality statistics for Great Britain. He developed the field of vital statistics and disease classifications and identified the effects of marital status and occupation on morbidity and mortality.

Noah Webster (1758–1843), who compiled the first American dictionary, studied epidemics of the New World. In *Epidemic and Pestilential Diseases*, he related specific events in the environment to influenza, yellow fever, and scarlet fever.

John Snow (1813–1858), an anesthesiologist, is called "the father of field epidemiology." In 1854, he studied cholera outbreaks in London; after determining where afflicted individuals lived and worked, he created a spot map. Snow hypothesized that water was a source of cholera infection and marked where water pumps were located. He linked cases to the water source. He noted that a number of cases occurred around the Broad Street pump. Further, he observed that individuals who did not contract cholera lived near a brewery,

Info Line

> Ralph Frerichs, DrPH, DVM, past chairman, department of
> epidemiology, University of California, Los Angeles, created an
> Internet site on John Snow, the famous 19th-century British
> epidemiologist. (http://www.ph.ucla.edu/epi/snow.html).

where they worked and received their water supply. To thwart the disease, the
handle of the Broad Street pump was removed and the source of the cholera
was stopped.

Snow studied another cholera outbreak and developed sequential steps
to investigate disease outbreaks. He provided the classical process of describing individuals with and without disease, establishing testable hypotheses,
and then testing the hypotheses with individuals matched on important characteristics. In effect, Snow used what we now call epidemiologic techniques
to identify water as a substrate for transmitting cholera and to evoke public
health action.[4]

Modern Epidemiology

By the 1900s, epidemiologic methods were extended to noninfectious diseases.
Since World War II, research methods and theoretical frameworks for epidemiologic exploration have flourished. Epidemiology has expanded to include health-related outcomes other than disease.[5] For example, behaviors,
knowledge, and attitudes of individuals and groups have been evaluated
as predisposing or antecedent to the occurrence of health events. This is
demonstrated in studies by Doll and Hill linking smoking to lung cancer.[6]
The Framingham Heart Study, spanning over 40 years, has observed the role
of men's personal and physiological characteristics on cardiovascular disease
morbidity and mortality.[7] The Bogalusa Heart Study (BHS), using an observational, natural history design, focuses on an entire community of school-age
children.[8] The Minnesota Heart Health Program, the Stanford Heart Disease Prevention Trials, and the North Karelia Study have multidimensional study designs.[9-11] The Multiple Risk Factor Intervention Trial was a major clinical trial
enrolling more than 50,000 men at clinical sites across the United States.[12]

Nutritional Epidemiology

James Lind conducted one of the first—if not *the* first—experimental trial of
a nutrition-based disease, scurvy, which was common on all long trips by
sea. On May 20, 1747, he set sail on the *Salisbury*. While at sea, 12 sailors
developed scurvy. Symptoms identical among the individuals were putrid
gums and weakness in their limbs. Their breakfast consisted of water and
sweetened gruel, and other meals consisted of fresh mutton broth or puddings
with a boiled sweet biscuit. Sometimes barley and raisins, rice and currants,

or sago and wine were served. Lind devised a modern intervention trial with 5 strategies:

1. Once a day, 2 patients received a quart of cider to gargle and then swallow on an empty stomach.
2. Two patients were given 2 spoons of vinegar, 3 times a day on an empty stomach, and had vinegar added to their cereals and other foods. They were also required to gargle with vinegar.
3. Two patients drank a half pint of sea water every day.
4. Two others received 2 oranges and 1 lemon every day on an empty stomach.
5. The final pair consumed a mixture consisting of nutmeg tree, garlic, mustard seed, and other herbs. They also drank barley water that was mixed with tamarind, and periodically they had a gentle enema.

The men who consumed oranges and lemons had the most rapid recovery and reported to duty after 6 days. Their bloody gums disappeared, and they appeared healthy before the ship reached land on June 16.

The result of this experiment was the identification of an effective therapeutic agent for treating a disorder and preventing its occurrence. The experiment resulted in a health policy in 1795 that required that limes or lime juice be included in the meals of all sailors. Thus, sailors were nicknamed "limeys."[1]

In 1923, Joseph Goldberger conducted what is considered a classic epidemiologic investigation that altered the belief that pellagra was an infectious disease. Goldberger observed that health care personnel attending patients with pellagra did not develop the disease. By studying individuals with and without the disease, he hypothesized and proved that diet initiated the disease.[13,14] Nicotinic acid was later determined to be the specific dietary deficiency causing pellagra among the patients.[5]

These classical studies and events laid the groundwork for nutritional epidemiology. Simply defined, nutritional epidemiology is the study of eating behavior and how it influences the etiology, occurrence, prevention, and treatment of disease. Nutritional epidemiology is the great-grandchild and hybrid of epidemiology, nutrition, and public health. The sequence of development might be envisioned as follows:

Public health → Epidemiology → Public health nutrition → Community nutrition → Nutritional epidemiology

Community nutrition is a contemporary and comprehensive discipline that encompasses, among other disciplines, public health nutrition. The beginning of public health nutrition can be traced to the early efforts of Ellen Richards and Mary Abel in home economics and public health in the late 1800s.[15,16] The US Children's Bureau was formed as a result of the first White House Conference on Children in 1909. Considered the mother of public health nutrition, the Children's Bureau initiated nutrition publications, led children's campaigns, and pioneered community-based programs.[17]

In 1917, the state of Massachusetts employed its first nutritionist and followed in 1922 to employ a second one.[18] Responsibilities involved development and distribution of nutrition pamphlets and professional education.

These early efforts complemented the work of Frances Stern and Lucy Gillett, who blended nutrition education into pediatricians' practices and special clinics.[19] A brief chronology of the development of nutrition positions, services, and departments at the state level is outlined in Table 1-1.

Public health nutrition has developed in the United States in response to numerous societal events and changes, including the following:

- infant mortality, access to health care
- epidemics of communicable disease
- poor hygiene and sanitation, malnutrition
- agriculture and food production
- economic depression, wars, civil rights
- aging of the population

TABLE 1–1 Chronology of the Early Development of Nutrition Positions and Services Within the United States

Year	Activity
1917	First public health nutritionist employed in Massachusetts.
1922	Second public health nutritionist employed in Massachusetts.
1936	11 nutrition positions established in 4 states.
1936	First nutrition consultant, Marjorie Heseltine, employed at the US Children's Bureau, which initiated a concerted effort to include nutrition services at the state level.
1938	First qualifications established for nutritionists in public health.
1939	39 nutrition positions existed in 24 states.
1945	45 state health departments had nutritionists.
1952	Association of State and Territorial Public Health Nutrition Directors was organized.
1969	> 300 nutrition positions in 53 Maternal and Infant Programs and 58 Children and Youth Programs.
1973	Nutrition programs for older patients began to establish nutrition staff positions at the state level.
1981	Guidelines for specialized services in prenatal care were developed and revised in 1992.
1995	US Congress appropriated $3.5 billion for the Special Supplemental Food Program for Women, Infant and Children (WIC), which included coverage of positions for nutritionists and nutrition aides.
2000	WIC was the primary funding source for the public health nutrition workforce as reported in the 1999–2000 Survey of the Public Health Nutrition Workforce conducted by the Association of State and Territorial Public Health Nutrition Directors (9,853 of 10,904 respondents stated WIC was their employer).
2002	April enrollment was 8,016,918 women, infants, and children with approximately one half infants.

Source: Data from Egan MC, Public health nutrition: a historic perspective. *J Am Diet Asso.* 1994; 94(3):298-304. Executive summary: 1999-2000 survey of the Public Health Nutrition Workforce. Washington, DC: Food & Nutrition Service, USDA; 2000; and Executive Summary—WIC participant and program characteristics. Washington, DC: Office of Analysis, Nutrition and Evaluation, Food & Nutrition Service, USDA; 2003.

- behavior-related problems, chronic diseases
- poverty, immigration
- preschool/after-school child care and school-based meals

As public health nutrition has evolved, professional practice standards and training qualifications have developed.[20] Assessing, screening, and monitoring individuals, groups, and communities have become more common. Indicators of effectiveness and efficiency have been identified and have set the stage for improved opportunities for research.[21,22]

Public health nutrition has developed in response to federal legislation, but the field has also led the charge to create new or to change old legislation. The WIC program demonstrates the arduous effort on the part of public health nutritionists to market the program to nonbelievers, to evaluate and enroll eligible women and children, to employ and train staff, and to testify and lobby for increased funding for prenatal and infant care to meet the needs of a growing target population.[17]

Today an environment exists in which chronic disease control has emerged as a priority. Public health nutrition provides a national resource base to address nutritional needs across the life cycle. The emerging field of nutritional epidemiology is enriched by this valuable resource base, yet it has its own identity. Eating behavior (rather than diet) and specific methods to collect data about eating behavior and its relation to wellness and disease are the essence of nutritional epidemiology. The process is dynamic. Nutritional epidemiology explores what people eat and how long they follow certain food patterns; how much people eat on the average and how their eating patterns change over time, as they age; why they choose the foods they eat; whether lifestyles, taste, economics, food availability, or some other factor has the greatest impact on health; and who eats what (for example, who avoids certain foods while eating other foods in excess). The methods used to investigate, monitor, or ensure adherence to an intervention not only follow the epidemiologic process and study designs but also address reliability, validity, and standardization. Conducting community nutrition programs to meet *Healthy People in Healthy Communities 2010* objectives presents the current challenge and the agenda for nutritional epidemiology.

The Territory of Epidemiology—Principles and Application

Epidemiologic methods are tools to explore disease occurrence, treatment, prevention, and cure. A traditional model explores the causes of infectious disease, using 3 components: an agent, a host, and an environment that is conducive to linking the first 2 components. This model does not differentiate among the strength of any of the 3 components. The environment influences agent, host, and the process that links the 2. Figure 1–1 illustrates this model.[1,5]

In the infectious disease model, an agent has historically been an infectious microorganism, bacterium, virus, parasite, or other microbe whose presence is required for disease occurrence. The agent alone may cause disease. In a noninfectious disease model, an agent may be a chemical or toxin, or a missing physical or behavioral factor. It might even be multifactorial. An example of a chemical factor is coal tar, which causes lung cancer.

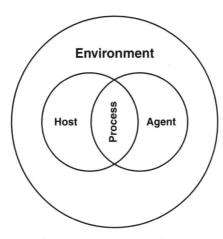

FIGURE 1–1 A conceptual model for the process by which host and agent interact within an environment

An example of a behavioral factor is a sedentary lifestyle, which promotes weight gain.

Host factors are personal characteristics that are influenced by the type, intensity, duration, and response of one's exposure to an etiologic agent. Age, ethnicity, sex, socioeconomic status, eating patterns, exercise behaviors, and lifestyle are examples. Some personal characteristics such as age, sex, and ethnicity are nonmodifiable, but some are modifiable. Characteristics that can be changed include nutritional status, leisure time activity, geographic location, and occupation. These modifiable host characteristics can be considered environmental factors.

Environmental factors are external factors that encompass an agent and a host. They may be exclusively physical, such as geology, climate, or living surroundings (e.g., an urban housing area in the southern United States). An environmental factor may have multiple levels, such as low, middle, and high socioeconomic status (SES). Low SES is often linked to crowding, poor sanitation, and reduced availability of health and social services. High SES may evoke excessive behaviors such as heavy drinking, overeating, and risk taking.

The required trio of agent, host, and environment interact to produce various health outcomes, including disease. Exploration of disease etiology demands an awareness of each component and a vigilance using epidemiologic methods.[5]

The *natural history* of a disease is the progression of a disease in an individual or group over time. No interventions occur, other than changes occurring naturally for all people. To document natural history, the individual's or group's exposure to environmental factors that place them at risk of diseases is assessed. As the individual or group is followed, morbidity and mortality are monitored. Outcomes are compared with host and environmental factors to estimate the effect each has on morbidity or mortality.[23] A model that shows the relationship between understanding of disease progression and level of intervention is presented in Figure 1–2.

UNDERSTANDING LEVEL

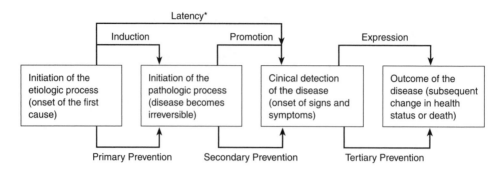

FIGURE 1–2   Levels of epidemiologic research: a conceptual elaboration.
Source: Adapted from Kleinbaum DG, Kupper LL. *Epidemiologic Research: Principles and Quantitative Methods solution manual.* New York, NY: Van Nostrand Reinhold; 1982:22. Used with permission.

Natural history is influenced by the genetic variability of individuals and their response to the environment. With an infectious disease, if a host is exposed to a causal agent frequently and with great intensity, disease will likely occur. For a chronic disease such as breast cancer, the critical factors causing the disease may include an initiating factor (such as not breastfeeding) and a promoter (such as dietary fat and low fiber intake) to cause an effect. Reduced exposure to the promoter at the early stage of development constitutes *primary prevention.*

Because chronic disease progression generally includes an asymptomatic period, individuals and groups are unaware of their exposure and the effect their behavior can have on the disease. This phase is called an incubation period for infectious disease and a latency period for chronic disease. The range of time for this phase varies greatly—from 2 to 4 hours for a food-borne illness such as salmonella poisoning, to as many as 20 to 40 years for arteriosclerosis. Even for one specific disease, the incubation period will vary as a result of environmental and host characteristics. For a chronic disease, positive eating or exercise habits may forestall the disease progression by years.

Another example is a nutritionally deprived older person who may demonstrate signs of degenerative diseases earlier than a nutritionally sound individual. Screening programs can identify risk factor levels as the individual ages and can alert health professionals to potential high-risk individuals or groups who require intervention. Early screening for chronic disease risk factors and an intervention focused on those factors may forestall the disease progression.

Once symptoms appear, the individual moves from a subclinical to a clinical disease phase. The clinical diagnosis documents this transition. Intervention at this point is termed *secondary prevention.* The outcome varies, and clinical disease may or may not progress. The disease expression may result in a single diagnosis sustained and treated for 20 years. Such is the case for a single, treatable diagnosis of hypercholesterolemia. On the other hand, comorbidity or multiple illnesses that include the initial diagnosis of hypercholesterolemia but later combine with obesity, diabetes, and hypertension may occur. Intervention to reduce the severity of the comorbidity and death is called *tertiary prevention.*

In primary, secondary, and tertiary prevention, the association of factors or variables is the basis of action. The association between 2 variables can be explored by statistical means. If the change (increase or decrease) of one variable parallels a change in a second variable, then an association may exist. A *positive association* occurs when 2 variables increase (e.g., as body weight increases, blood pressure increases). When one variable increases and a second decreases, an *inverse* or *negative association* occurs (e.g., as insulin level increases, blood sugar level decreases). Significance of association can be tested using a Pearson product moment correlation, for example. The statistical r value of 1 is perfect agreement; a value of 0 means no agreement.

Rarely are significant correlations of the magnitude of > 0.600 found when testing the association between a dietary component and a risk factor variable. In fact, it is more common to see significant correlation analysis at the $p < .05$ level of significance, at $r = 0.250$ to 0.400, depending on the sample size, or number of individuals surveyed.

Error can occur. Bias, which might be considered an error that occurs in unknown ways, can lead to overestimating or underestimating a characteristic, quality, or variable. An error or bias that can occur in the exploration of a disease is called *confounding*. A factor is considered a *confounding variable* if it is associated with both the health outcome and the risk factor being studied. Obesity and smoking are considered confounding variables in many studies.

Measurement of confounding variables increases one's precision when evaluating how variables relate and how they influence potential health outcome. When published research studies identify variables that are associated with health outcomes, these variables could then become potential confounders to be assessed in the next research study. The purpose is to explore further their true association or effect on the outcome.

Extreme *outliers* or unusual values can distort the statistical description of the data. To avoid this distortion, researchers often remove these values from the analysis, but the process is complicated by the ambiguity in defining the outliers. They can be unreasonable on the basis of biological fact, or they may represent measurement error from a human or equipment failure. Outliers can be defined statistically as significant deviations from a measure of central tendency of the distribution.

The easiest way to identify outliers is to examine bivariate scatterplots of the distribution of the data. The values that lie markedly outside the population are suspect. If the outliers are confirmed as errors, they can be removed from subsequent analyses. There are 2 concerns for nutrition or dietary variables: (1) outliers are often dismissed as errors to "clean" the data and increase the r value, which may be a mistake; and (2) the extreme values may be real, because individuals can make severe behavioral changes (for example, individuals can have fat intake less than 20% or more than 40% of total energy), which dramatically alters a mean value for a group or a correlation coefficient.

Surveillance or monitoring are processes used to assess community health. They allow an individual, agency, or research group to collect, analyze, interpret, and disseminate health data on a continuous basis.[24] Surveillance in public health is called "information for action,"[25] and it profiles a community's health status. Programs can later address the identified community health problems with prevention and control strategies. Sophisticated surveillance systems use computer technology, link data from several communities and states to provide a broader base of data, detect potential problems, and influence programs and policy. Surveillance data can guide policy makers to develop and to reassess interventions. Epidemiologic techniques are used to assess community health and to identify potential solutions to problems. Several types of studies are described next.

Types of Studies

Population or Community Health Assessment

This type of study assesses the health of the population or community. The type, cost, availability, and accessibility of services are studied. Health status—defined as disease risk factor levels, morbidity, and mortality—is measured. Public policy and program planning may stem from these assessments.

The Minnesota Community Prevention Program for Cardiovascular Diseases paired 6 Minnesota communities; one community provided an intensive educational program for cardiovascular risk factor reduction, and the other served as a comparison. A pair of medium-sized towns were studied initially, then a set of larger towns, and then suburban census tracts. This sequential, comparative design had the scientific advantage of control and repetition, and the practical value of economy and opportunity to improve as the program advanced.

Assessment of Individual Health Choices

Often, individuals unknowingly base decisions on epidemiologic data. For example, when an individual walks a minimum of 20 minutes 3 times a week, eats 5 fruits or vegetables a day, or trims the fat from a serving of meat, that person bases his or her knowledge and behavior on epidemiologic data linking these behaviors to health promotion. Today, epidemiologists may explore how leisure activities and eating behaviors influence chronic disease risk factors such as adiposity, serum total cholesterol, and blood pressure. The Stanford Three-Community Heart Disease Prevention Program used mass media campaigns and face-to-face instruction to change knowledge and improve attitudes and behaviors about cardiovascular risk factors. Significant change was noted and sustained for the intervention communities compared to the control community.[26]

Clinical Profile

Epidemiologists collaborate with clinicians to diagnose individuals and to classify them accurately into groups or communities with and without risk factors and with and without disease. The Pawtucket Heart Study demonstrates this type of approach. From 1981 to 1993, researchers completed biennial cardiovascular risk factor (CVRF) surveys in 2 cities, they randomly selected residents who were 18 to 64 years old. The purpose was to test the hypothesis that CVRF intensity or prevalence would decrease significantly in the city that provided multi-level education, screening, and counseling (regarding risk factor, behavior change, and community activation).[27] Small, but nonsignificant, positive differences were noted in the intervention community for blood cholesterol and blood pressure. A significant increase was seen for body-mass index in the comparison community. The predicted cardiovascular disease rates were 16% (significant) and 8% less in the intervention community than in the comparison community during and after the education. These findings suggest the need for sustained, consistent effort within the community, along with national directives and policies from the outside, to reinforce the importance of the intervention.[27]

Etiological Factor Exploration

Data from epidemiologic studies cannot prove a causal association between a factor and a disease. Data can identify risk factors of a disease that require further testing to prove a cause-and-effect relationship. The data can effect change in behavior, norms, and public policy. The Framingham Heart Study and the Bogalusa Heart Study are examples of adult and pediatric community assessments using cohorts and cross-sectional samples, respectively, to identify risk factors for cardiovascular disease.[7,8]

The Bogalusa Heart Study (BHS) is a community-based program that examines the distribution and secular trends of CVRF variables in youth, the interrelationships of the variables, and genetic and environmental determinants (such as dietary and biobehavioral factors). The investigation is a prospective survey with a mixed epidemiologic design to study the early natural history of atherosclerosis in a biracial pediatric population. Cross-sectional studies linked with longitudinal observations of specific age cohorts (groups whose members were all born in the same year) permit collection of data over an extended range of ages from birth to over 30 years of age, but within a short observational time period. The biracial population is 65% white and 35% black.[8]

The Framingham Heart Study began in 1948 as a survey of 2,366 men and 2,873 women 30 to 62 years old. Survivors of this original cohort have been monitored every 2 years for their risk factor status. Data from offspring and spouses of participants in the Framingham Heart Study showed that certain characteristics can aggregate in families and that these characteristics can be called *risk factors* for coronary heart disease (CHD). The study identified the major risk factors and established a database that provided rates for CHD separately for men, their children, and their grandchildren.

Community Nutrition Assessment

Assessing the initial awareness among community members about nutrition and then supporting community nutrition needs and services are essential if changes in behavior, norms, and public policy are to be evaluated. Table 1–2 presents a subjective data assessment grid that can be used to evaluate the knowledge of nutrition, perceived need for nutrition, and attitude of health-care professionals and other important community members. These data,

TABLE 1-2 A Community Nutrition Assessment Worksheet to Acquire Subjective Data About Nutrition Needs, Attitudes, and Knowledge— Possible Responses

Community Members	Perceived Nutrition Needs in the Community	+	0	−	Attitude Toward Nutrition Services +	0	−	Knowledge of Nutrition +	0	−
Clients/patients	Weight management	+				0			0	
Public	Weight management	+				0			0	
Media	Overeating, nutrition education for seniors	+				0			0	
Government officials	None						−			−
Agency administrators	None						−			−
Physicians/dentists	Lower fat and sugar	+			+			+		
Hospital administrators	Weight management	+				0			0	
Nurses	Work with teens, train diabetics, education about fat	+			+			+		
Health educators	Lifestyle	+			+			+		
Nutritionists/dietitians	Food selection	+			+			+		
Agency board members	Limited						−			−
Principals/teachers	Improve school meals		0			0			0	
Social workers	Provide better choices		0			0			0	
Clergy	Focus on homeless	+							0	

+ = positive, supportive attitude toward nutrition and health services; 0 = neutral or apathetic attitude toward nutrition; − = negative attitude toward nutrition. *Source:* Adapted from Kaufman M. *Nutrition in Public Health: A Handbook for Developing Programs and Services.* Gaithersburg, MD: Aspen Publishers, Inc; 1990:52.

along with data that characterize the community's health status, are needed to develop programs for a healthier living environment.

Types of Analysis

Assessment and monitoring provide measures of disease frequency and yield data to evaluate the effectiveness and efficiency of programs or interventions. *Effectiveness* means producing positive results, and *efficiency* means producing positive results at the lowest cost.

Rates can numerically express effectiveness and efficiency. They can be used to define the risk of disease in populations in specific geographic areas (such as cities, states, and countries) and in population subgroups by age, sex, ethnicity, and occupation. Rates can be defined for a specific time, such as a month or a year. As rates are monitored, change over time can be defined. Location defines a geographic unit, such as urban versus rural or institutionalized versus free living. Community characteristics can be informative, such as socioeconomic, marital, or educational status.

Rates are essential to compare or contrast groups or to establish whether a characteristic of the host is associated with a health event. Clarifying whether factors relate or do not relate and examining the extent of the relationship establishes an analytical approach to the epidemiologic process.

A rate is a single, statistical expression that defines the proportion of individuals who have experienced a specific health event. The proportion of disease occurrence is called *morbidity rate* and the proportion of deaths is called *mortality rate*. The number of individuals in the group who have a disease or have experienced a health event at a given point in time constitutes the *numerator*. The *denominator* is the population at risk of experiencing a health event. For example:

$$\text{Incidence rate} = \frac{\text{No. of new cases of a disease}}{\text{population at risk}} \text{ per time period}$$

$$\text{Prevalence rate} = \frac{\text{No. of existing cases of a disease}}{\text{total population}} \text{ at a time point}$$

Point prevalence refers to the number of cases present at a specified moment of time; period prevalence refers to the number of cases that occur during a specified period of time—for example, a year. Period prevalence consists of the point prevalence at the beginning of a specified period of time plus all new cases that occur during that period.[1]

Rates not only identify groups in the community at high risk of disease but also designate groups needing further assessment or monitoring. The high-risk group may be selected for intervention to alter risk factors that relate to the health event. Risk factor profiles of high-risk groups aid decision makers who set program priorities.[4]

To compare rates in different groups, a standardized denominator for a specified time period is needed (e.g., 100,000 in 1994). *Crude rates* are calculated by dividing the total number of events by the total population and multiplying by 1,000, 10,000, or 100,000. The crude birth rate in the United States in 1990 was 16.7 live births per 1,000 population,[28] and in 1991 it was 16.2 live births per 1,000 population.[29] The crude birth rate for 2002 ranged from 10 per 1,000 live births in Maine and Vermont to 21 per 1,000 live births in Utah.[30]

A common rate used by epidemiologists is the death rate. The crude death rate reflects deaths among the entire US population of about 300 million individuals. For the United States, the crude death rate was 861.9 deaths per 100,000 population in 1990[28] and 845.3 deaths per 100,000 population in 2002.[29]

A standardized birth or death rate is a rate that is adjusted for different age and sex distributions. This adjustment is necessary because the US composition and population profile change with time. Basic epidemiology or demography texts describe how to adjust data. This is beyond the scope of this text, but is an important aspect of community health.

If any 2 or more populations are compared for a health outcome and they differ on a characteristic that may relate to the health outcome or to a risk factor, then an adjustment must be made. This adjustment is necessary because the characteristic may confound the comparison. For example, US mortality rates increase rapidly beginning at 55 years of age. When rates are distinctly different for different ages (e.g., cancer deaths are low among children but high among older adults), one should adjust the rates for differences in the study population by calculating age-specific rates.

Age-adjusted death rates for the United States reduce the effect of age.[28] Looking at death rates from any cause—referred to as *all-cause* mortality— age-adjusted rates demonstrate a *J*-shaped curve that shows a slight elevation in infancy, low rates from 5 to 14 years, and a slow, persistent increase thereafter. Mortality from accidents, homicides, and suicides reflects age patterns influenced by societal factors.[31]

Infant mortality rate (IMR) measures death during the first year of life. IMR is calculated by dividing the number of infant deaths in a year by the number of live births for the same time. IMR is presented as a rate per 1,000 or per 100,000 live births. This rate is commonly used to compare health care among countries. The 2001 US IMR was 6.8. Table 1–3 shows IMRs for the United States in 2001 by ethnicity of the mother. The health of a country is reflected in the level of care and quality of life afforded its youngest members. In the United States, lowering the IMR among minorities is a major challenge.[5]

TABLE 1–3   Infant, Neonatal, and Postneonatal Mortality Rates by Race of Mother, 2001

Ethnic Group	IMR 2001	NMR 2001	PMR 2001
All	6.8	4.5	2.3
African American	13.3	8.9	4.4
American Indian	9.7	4.2	5.4
Asian	4.7	3.1	1.6
White	5.7	3.8	1.9

IMR = infant mortality rate, NMR = neonatal mortality rate, PMR = postneonatal mortality rate.
Source: Data from Centers for Disease Control. Available at: http://www.cdc.gov/ nchsww. Accessed May 22, 2005.

IMR equals the sum of the neonatal plus postneonatal mortality rates. *Neonatal mortality rate* is the number of deaths among infants less than 28 days old divided by the number of live births during the same year. The 2001 neonatal mortality rate in the United States was 4.5 deaths per 1,000 live births. *Postneonatal mortality rate* is the number of deaths in children between 28 days and 11 months of age divided by the number of live births. The 2001 rate was 2.3 deaths per 1,000 live births. *Maternal mortality rate* is the number of women dying from complications of pregnancy or childbirth divided by the number of live births in the same year. *Case-fatality rate* is the number of cause-specific deaths divided by the number of cases.[5]

Types of Epidemiologic Studies

Health data are collected for various reasons and use various methods. Studies using epidemiologic techniques are either controlled (experimental) or uncontrolled (observational). *Controlled* studies mean that an artificial or planned situation exists. One or more independent variables are selected and controlled or remain static. *Uncontrolled* studies are natural observations. The type of epidemiologic approach depends on the research question being asked and the time perspective (current, past, or future). Uncontrolled and controlled studies are described next, and the pros and cons of each type of study are detailed (see Figure 1–3).

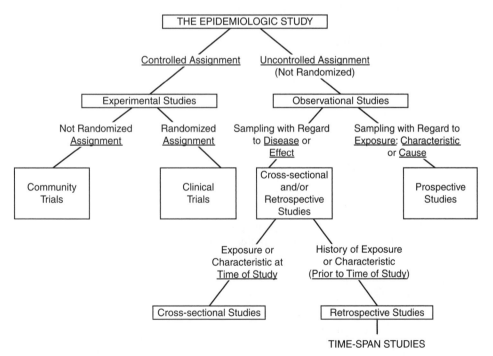

FIGURE 1–3   The anatomy of the epidemiologic study.
Source: Reprinted from Lilienfeld DE, Stolley P. *Foundations of Epidemiology.* 3rd ed. Oxford, Oxford University Press; 1994:152. Used with permission.

Uncontrolled Assignment Studies

Cross-Sectional Studies

Cross-sectional studies define the distributions of health-related characteristics in populations by taking a snapshot look at the population at 1 one point in time. Cross-sectional studies generally represent a sample from a population. Statistical inferences drawn from a sample relate to the method of sample selection. High- and low-risk groups can be identified, and hypotheses can be tested regarding the association of one variable to another.[32]

Each individual in a cross-sectional study is measured once. The same types of data are collected for all individuals in a standardized manner following protocols. Data generated create large databases for statistical analysis.

Cross-sectional studies cannot explore or test cause and effect. They can assist with formulating public health education and intervention programs. For example, one of the largest nutrition-based, cross-sectional studies in the United States is the National Health and Nutrition Examination Survey (NHANES). The first NHANES began in 1960. Direct interviews and medical examinations were included. Lipoprotein levels and prevalence rates were determined.[33,34]

Cross-sectional studies provide data to calculate prevalence rates. *Prevalence* is the number of existing health events and becomes a rate when expressed as the proportion of individuals in a population who have a certain trait.

In a cross-sectional study, associations between variables are often explored for one independent variable and one dependent variable. A *dependent variable* is the health outcome, such as blood pressure. An *independent variable* is one of several characteristics being measured, such as sodium or potassium intake. The association of independent and dependent variables can be tested with correlational data analysis.

The pros of the cross-sectional study are as follows:

- provides a quick snapshot look
- has low cost
- defines prevalence
- determines associations between variables
- generates hypotheses

The cons of the cross-sectional study are as follows:

- cannot establish cause and effect
- uses live individuals
- is insensitive to rare characteristics
- requires a sample or subsample of a population
- describes current, not past or future, events

The Behavioral Risk Factor Survey is an example of a cross-sectional study. It has been conducted since 1981 by the Centers for Disease Control and Prevention. Researchers conduct a telephone survey of adults in 47 states and the District of Columbia about their health behaviors.[35]

Telephone surveys have been used for cross-sectional data collection.[36,37] Van Horn and colleagues used telephone surveys to collect food intake data of preadolescents.

Pros of telephone surveys are as follows:

- speed of data collection
- less expensive than face-to-face interview
- less supervision
- ease of administration
- centralized procedure
- direct observation of data collection

The cons of telephone surveys are as follows:

- limited to individuals with phones
- may not reach lower socioeconomic status individuals
- decreased accuracy with self-report
- impersonal

Case-Control Studies

A retrospective approach called the case-control study compares case subjects and control subjects for the presence of antecedent variables. The flashback approach requires that case subjects and control subjects come from similar populations. Similarity of characteristics before the study begins ensures that case subjects and control subjects have the same exposure and that their health outcome is not related to one or more confounders. However, case subjects should differ from control subjects in one respect: case subjects must have the health outcome (the disease). Defining subjects requires objective criteria and their rigid application. Once case subjects and control subjects are identified, differences in antecedent exposure are investigated.

Accurate assignment or labeling as a case or control subject involves sensitivity and specificity (see Table 1–4).

Sensitivity is the percentage of individuals who have the disease and are confirmed by the test. *Specificity* is the percentage of individuals who do not have the disease and are confirmed by the test. Individuals testing positive who have the disease are called *true positives*, those testing positive who do not have the disease are *false positives*, and those testing negative who do not have the disease are *true negatives*.[1]

TABLE 1–4   Indicators of the Accuracy of a Test or Diagnostic Exam— Sensitivity and Specificity

Test or Exam	With Disease	Without Disease
Positive (disease is probably present)	*A* (true positives)	*B* (false positives)
Negative (disease is probably absent)	*C* (false negatives)	*D* (true negatives)
Totals	*A* + *C*	*B* + *D*

Source: Reprinted with permission from Lilienfeld D, Stolley, P. *Foundations of Epidemiology.* 3rd ed. Oxford: Oxford University Press; 1994:151.

The confounding effect of a variable can be avoided by selecting case and control subjects of the same age, ethnicity, and gender. This is termed *matching* and sounds easy. However, the more variables to be matched, the larger the number of subjects needed. For example, to match on age, sex, and socioeconomic class, a control subject must be similar to the case subject on all three variables (e.g., males, 24 to 30 years old, middle socioeconomic status).

Several factors must be considered when selecting case subjects. If case-control studies include patients receiving treatment, these patients may differ from control subjects on residence, income, etc. Case subjects may be limited to survivors, which demonstrates the selective-survival concept. Because only survivors are included, and not individuals with newly diagnosed cases or those with a known outcome of death, results and interpretation can be influenced.

A statistic commonly used in case-control studies is *relative risk*. It can be determined easily and is also called the odds ratio or relative odds. It is calculated as follows:

$$\frac{a \times d}{b \times c}$$

where a equals the number of case subjects who have a characteristic, d is the number of control subjects who do not have the characteristic, b is the number of control subjects with the characteristic, and c is the number of case subjects who do not have the characteristic.

A *confidence interval* is the probability (e.g., 95%) that the true value would be within a range. Confidence intervals are statistically significant if they do not include 1.0. For example, if a confidence interval for a relative risk of 2.5 is 2.1 to 3.7, it would be significant. This means that the risk is significantly greater for individuals not exposed to the variable.

Pros of the case-control study are as follows:

- Case subjects are easily available in clinical settings.
- It is relatively quick and inexpensive.
- Results support, but do not prove, causal hypotheses.
- Secondary analyses are possible, as clinical records are available and no further information from the subjects is needed.
- Sample size is small.
- Study of rare diseases is possible.

Cons of the case-control study are as follows:

- Data are from memory, which increases bias (an error that occurs in unknown ways but can produce an over- or underestimate).
- Records may be inadequate.
- Criteria for diagnoses may vary among clinicians.
- Case subjects are selected survivors.
- Case subjects may not be representative because they have come for treatment.
- Antecedent data reflect only living cases.

Cohort Studies

This type of observational study can confirm causal associations and establish secular trends between antecedent characteristics and outcomes. Cohort studies are prospective studies and can project risk estimates for future events. Results of cohort studies can be provided to decision makers who are responsible for planning and evaluating intervention, education, and treatment programs. Specifically, cohort studies confirm causation and present decision makers with specific health-related factors to modify for community wellness.[5]

A cohort study begins with a group of people who have known characteristics. The cohort is selected by virtue of an exposure or innate characteristic. Each member of the cohort is identified as free of the health event at the beginning of the study. The cohort is followed over time, maybe several years, to record health events. The number of individuals who develop the outcome are counted, creating prevalence rates that can be reported any time during the study. Any new cases reported within a select time period, such as a year, provide incidence rates.

An example of an observational cohort study is one conducted by Folsom and colleagues. This group observed the body-fat distribution and the 5-year risk of death in older women. They tested the hypothesis that both body mass index (the ratio of weight in kilograms to height in meters squared) and the ratio of waist circumference to hip circumference are positively associated with risk of death in older women.[38] A cohort of 41,837 Iowa women from 55 to 69 years old was followed for 5 years. During this time, 1,504 deaths occurred. Body mass index was associated with mortality following a *J*-shaped curve. This means that death was highest among 2 groups—the leanest and the most obese women. Waist:hip circumference ratio had a significant, positive association with mortality, which increased in increments. A 0.15-unit increase in waist:hip circumference ratio was associated with a 60% greater relative risk of death. This occurred after adjustment for age, marital status, body mass index, smoking, alcohol and estrogen use, and education. Waist:hip circumference ratio emerged as a better marker of risk of death among older women than body mass index.

Relative risk, which can be calculated in this type of study, determines the extent of risk for a health event when individuals have certain characteristics. As explained earlier, it is determined by dividing the incidence rate among individuals exposed by the incidence rate among individuals not exposed. For example, in the Framingham Heart Study, white men with high cholesterol were 2.04 times more likely to develop coronary heart disease (CHD) than white men with low cholesterol; the study results show that high serum total cholesterol is an antecedent characteristic that increases the probability of developing CHD.[5]

The potential for an association between an antecedent variable and a health outcome is increased if a larger dose produces higher rates. This concept is called "dose-response" and is applicable to the association of serum total cholesterol level and CHD incidence. Again using Framingham Heart Study data, at higher cholesterol levels, higher CHD incidence rates occur. In fact, given 4 groups, extremely high, high, moderate, and lowest, the relative risks for individuals at extremely high serum total cholesterol levels are about 3 times that for individuals at the lowest level. Accordingly, relative risk is 2 times greater for the extremely high to moderate group and 1.7 times that of the high group.

An interesting question is whether cholesterol levels of a community could be reduced to the point of preventing or lowering the incidence of CHD. The answer is yes, if a community intervention could lower all high cholesterol levels to low cholesterol levels. Further, the result could be expressed in terms of incidence rate.

For example, say IR_e is the incidence rate for the exposed group (high cholesterol), and IR_o is the incidence rate for the nonexposed group (low cholesterol). If IR_e = 154 per 1,000 and IR_o = 73 per 1,000, a reduction in the CHD rate could be realized. The risk attributed to high cholesterol equals the difference (81 per 1,000). This is called the *attributable risk*.

If an eating behavior and exercise intervention could successfully reduce every high cholesterol level to a low cholesterol level, a population's attributable risk fraction could be calculated. This is the proportion or fraction of the rate in a community that the exposed group represents. The total community rate minus the rate in the risk-free group would equal the risk contributed by individuals at risk. This is the proportion of the total rate yielding the community attributable risk proportion. For example, say the incidence rate for the total community is 73 per 1,000. For the low cholesterol group, it is 28 per 1,000. The proportion of the total population rate is calculated as 28:73 or 0.384. The interpretation is that 38% of the new cases of disease among the population would be prevented if all subjects with new cases had low cholesterol levels.[5]

Because population-attributable risk percentage specifies the reduction in health events expected if a risk factor is removed, the percentage in risk reduction can be determined for each potential factor. The cost and practicality of risk reduction can then be determined. This allows decision making based on extent of short-term risk reduction and long-term disease outcome.

Cohort studies do not prove beyond a doubt that a risk factor causes a health event. Inferences are possible and can be obtained by comparing secular trends.

Pros of the cohort study are as follows:

- increases potential for confirmation of cause and effect
- quantifies extent of effect due to risk factor
- provides baseline rates for new cases in a community
- estimates prevalence
- allows for hypothesis testing
- increases participant cooperation
- reduces information bias
- minimizes selection factors, since all members of the cohort are disease free
- follows original cohort even if individuals relocate

Cons of the cohort study are as follows:

- requires a long observation period
- increases loss to follow-up, creating selection bias
- is expensive

- enhances associations and outcomes affected or created by ecological changes
- cannot study rare diseases

Controlled Assignment Studies

The unique characteristic of an experimental study is the investigator's control over assignment of individuals to groups (random assignment). Randomization ensures comparability of individuals and groups to all known and unknown factors except the one studied. It also avoids bias and increases comparability.[1] The phrase *ceteris paribus*, meaning "all things equal," is germane. Clinical trials require randomized assignment.

An experiment evaluates what occurs after exposure to a risk factor. An intervention group receives an intervention, and a control group does not. The 2 groups are then compared. For example, a clinical trial is an experiment. A trial could test if antihypertensive drugs lower blood pressure and reduce strokes, or it could evaluate the impact of exercise or eating behavior on CHD mortality rates in a community.[5]

Experimental studies determine factors that confound a cause-and-effect association. These findings increase confidence in future studies that focus on or control known risk factors. Such an approach increases the internal validity of the study.

The basic types of experimental studies[1] are as follows:

- *Therapeutic*: An agent or procedure is given to relieve symptoms or improve survival (i.e., secondary or tertiary intervention).
- *Intervention*: Intervention occurs either before a disease has developed, after, or during a disease expression.
- *Prevention*: Intervention occurs to determine the efficacy of an agent (i.e., primary prevention).

One nonrandomized community trial involved physical fitness as an intervention. The relationship between physical fitness and risk of mortality was studied over an 8-year period among 10,224 men and 3,120 women. There were 110,482 person-years of observation. A maximal treadmill exercise test indicated level of physical fitness. The observed decline in mortality from any cause occurred for men and women due to their fitness level and lower rates of cardiovascular disease and cancer.[5]

Fitness quintiles were determined and ranged from the highest degree of fitness, quintile 5, to the lowest degree of fitness, quintile 1. An age-adjusted mortality from all causes of death declined across fitness quintiles from lowest to highest. Low physical fitness emerged as the most important risk factor attributing to death. This was true for both men and women. The least fit men had 64.0 deaths per 10,000 person-years, compared to 18.6 deaths per 10,000 person-years among the most fit men. The least fit women had 39.5 deaths per person-years, compared to only 8.5 deaths per person-years among the most fit women. These declines in death rates occurred even after controlling for age, smoking, serum cholesterol, blood pressure, blood glucose, and parental history of CHD.[39]

From 1974 to 1982, a randomized, primary prevention trial in CHD called the Multiple Risk Factor Intervention Trial involved 20 clinical centers and 12,000 men, 37 to 50 years old. The primary objective was to determine whether men at high risk of CHD death would have a significant reduction in mortality if they participated in a special intervention. A "usual care" group received basic information from private physicians, and the intervention group received intense counseling from a multidisciplinary team of physicians, nutritionists, smoking cessation specialists, and behavioral scientists. This trial provided useful but somewhat alarming data about CHD mortality. Not only did high mortality occur among participants who had high levels of cholesterol (> 200 mg%), but relatively high mortality occurred among participants with very low total cholesterol levels (< 140 mg%).[40]

Which Is Better—Observational Studies or Randomized, Controlled Trials?

Benson and Hartz[41] conducted a meta-analysis by reviewing 136 reports about 19 diverse treatments, such as calcium-channel-blocker therapy for coronary artery disease, appendectomy, and interventions for subfertility. In most cases, the estimates of the treatment effects from observational studies and randomized, controlled trials were similar. In only 2 of the 19 analyses of treatment effects did the combined magnitude of the effect in observational studies lie outside the 95% confidence interval for the combined magnitude in the randomized, controlled trials.

Benson and Hartz found little evidence that estimates of treatment effects in observational studies reported after 1984 are either consistently larger than or qualitatively different from those obtained in randomized, controlled trials.[41]

Concato et al found that for the 5 clinical topics and 99 reports evaluated in their meta-analysis, the average results of the observational studies were remarkably similar to those of the randomized, controlled trials.[42] For example, analysis of 13 randomized, controlled trials of the effectiveness of bacille Calmette-Guerin vaccine in preventing active tuberculosis yielded a relative risk of 0.49 (95% confidence interval, 0.34 to 0.70) among vaccinated patients, as compared with an odds ratio of 0.50 (95% confidence interval, 0.39 to 0.65) from 10 case-control studies. In addition, the range of the point estimates for the effects of vaccination was wider for the randomized, controlled trials (0.20 to 1.56) than for the observational studies (0.17 to 0.84).

The results of well-designed observational studies (with either a cohort or a case-control design) do not systematically overestimate the magnitude of the effects of treatment as compared with those in randomized, controlled trials on the same topic.[42]

Pocock and Elbourne[43] counter that society expects evaluation of new healthcare interventions by scientifically sound and rigorous methods. Observational studies often are cheaper, quicker, and less difficult to carry out. High-quality randomized, controlled trials, not observations, reflect personal choices and beliefs. Persuading physicians, patients, researchers, and study sponsors to collaborate on major trials with the required number of patients, treatments, outcome measures, sample sizes, and follow-up is challenging. Pocock and Elbourne believe we should build on prior approaches to serve future patients with the most reliable information possible, rather than canceling the clinical trial approach.[43]

The Link Between Eating Behavior and Chronic Disease

The growing body of epidemiologic, clinical, and laboratory data demonstrates that what a population or sample of people eats is one of the many important factors involved in the etiology of chronic diseases. During the past 40 years, scientists have been challenged with identifying dietary factors that influence specific disease and defining their pathophysiological mechanisms. Simultaneously, public health policy makers, the food industry, consumer groups, and others have been debating how much and what kind of evidence justifies giving dietary advice to the public and how best to mitigate risk factors on which there is general agreement among scientists.[44,45]

Prior reports have not been sufficiently comprehensive. They have not crossed the boundary separating the simple assessment of dietary risk factors for single chronic diseases from the complex task of determining how these risk factors influence the entire spectrum of chronic diseases—atherosclerotic cardiovascular diseases, cancer, diabetes, obesity, osteoporosis, dental caries, and chronic liver and kidney diseases.

Diet and Health[46] complemented the *Surgeon General's Report on Nutrition and Health*[47] and other efforts of government agencies and voluntary health and scientific organizations by providing an in-depth analysis of the relationship between diet and the full spectrum of major chronic diseases.

Diet and Health focused on risk reduction rather than on management of clinically manifest disease. The distinction between prevention (or risk reduction) and treatment may be blurred in conditions for which dietary modification might delay the onset of clinical diseases (e.g., the cardiovascular complications in diabetes mellitus) or slow the progression of impaired function. Risk reduction focuses on decreased morbidity as well as mortality from chronic diseases, and proponents of risk reduction believe that dietary modification should be considered to reduce the risk for both.

Ecological correlations of dietary factors and chronic diseases among human populations provide valuable data but cannot be used alone to estimate the strength of the association between diet and diseases. The effect of diet on chronic diseases has been most consistently demonstrated in comparisons of populations with substantially different dietary practices, possibly because it is more difficult to identify such associations within a population whose eating pattern is fairly homogeneous. Generally, case-control and prospective cohort studies underestimate the association within populations. In intervention studies, long exposure is usually required to manifest the effect of eating behavior on chronic disease risk. The strict criteria for selecting participants in epidemiological studies may result in more homogeneous study samples, which limit the application of results to the general population. Despite the limitations of various types of studies in humans, the committee writing *Diet and Health* concluded that repeated and consistent findings of an association between certain dietary factors and diseases are likely to be real and indicative of a cause-and-effect relationship, even though the epidemiologic data do not provide proof beyond a reasonable doubt.[46]

Experiments on dietary exposure of different animal strains can account for genetic variability and permit more intensive observation. However, extrapolation of data from animal studies to humans is limited by the ability of animal models to simulate human diseases and the comparability of absorption and metabolic phenomena among species.[48]

Six criteria can be used to evaluate the association between eating pattern and chronic diseases. There are strength of association, dose-response relationship, temporally correct association, consistency of association, specificity of association, and biologic plausibility. The strength, consistency, and amount of data and the agreement among epidemiologic, clinical, and laboratory evidence influenced the conclusions and recommendations in *Diet and Health*.[46] This report reviews the epidemiologic, clinical, and experimental data pertaining to each nutrient or dietary factor and specific chronic diseases—including cardiovascular diseases, specific cancers, diabetes, hypertension, obesity, osteoporosis, hepatobiliary disease, and dental caries—along with nutrient interactions and mechanisms of action.[46]

The evidence relating nutrients to specific chronic diseases and diet-related conditions clearly defines the role of dietary patterns in the etiology of the diseases and assessment of the potential for reducing their frequency and severity. Conclusions can be drawn directly either from the research data, where the evidence pertains to dietary patterns of foods and food groups, or from extrapolations taken from data on individual nutrients. Individuals must mature in their thinking—that is, people must change from only considering individual nutrients to considering in a stepwise manner, foods, then food groups, and then dietary patterns as they relate to the spectrum of chronic diseases:

Pathway linking food and health:
Dietary component → Food → Food group → Pattern → Disease

Proof beyond a reasonable doubt is generally accepted as a standard for making decisions and taking action. A food and health paradigm can be constructed using the strength of the evidence as one criterion for determining the course of action. Other factors include the likelihood and severity of an adverse effect, the potential benefits of avoiding the hazard, and the feasibility of reducing exposure. Current evidence supports (1) a comprehensive effort to inform the public about the likelihood of certain risks and the possible benefits of dietary modifications and (2) the use of technology and other means (e.g., production of leaner animal products) to facilitate dietary change.[46]

Synergistic and antagonistic effects of dietary interactions must be considered. Assessing potential competing risks and benefits and nutrient interactions is simplified by an inherent consistency in dietary recommendations to maintain good health.

Quantitative guidelines should be proposed when warranted by the strength of the evidence and the potential importance of recommendations to public health. Such guidelines can take into account nutrient interactions. These guidelines are less susceptible to misinterpretation when translated into food choices, and they provide specific targets that can serve as a basis for nutrition programs and policy.

Two complementary approaches[46] to reducing risk factors in the target population are as follows:

1. the public health or population-based approach, targeting the general population
2. the high-risk or individual-based approach, targeting individuals with defined risk profiles

Most chronic diseases etiologically associated with nutritional factors (e.g., atherosclerotic cardiovascular diseases, hypertension, obesity, many cancers, osteoporosis, and diabetes mellitus) also have genetic determinants, and genetic-environmental interactions play an important role in determining disease outcome. For many diseases, it is not yet possible to identify susceptible genotypes and risks to specific individuals. Major chronic disease burden, however, falls on the general population. Approximately 70% of all deaths in the US population are due to cardiovascular diseases and cancer. The greatest benefit is likely to be achieved by a public health prevention strategy to reduce dietary risk factors by means of dietary recommendations to reduce chronic disease risk in the general population.[46] By so doing, the United States may realize an increased rectangularization of the survival curve (see Figure 1–4).[48]

The public health approach to prevention recognizes that even though reduction of risk for individuals with average risk profiles might be small or negligible, people with average risk represent the great majority of the population. High-risk persons need special attention (i.e., secondary and tertiary prevention), but an effective primary prevention strategy should be aimed at the general public, and, where knowledge permits, it should be complemented with recommendations for those at high risk.

Over the past decade, clinical practice guidelines have been published to assist practitioners who detect, evaluate, and manage various diet-related diseases. The importance of medical nutrition therapy is emphasized in the report of the Joint National Committee on High Blood Pressure[49] and the expert panel reports of the National Cholesterol Education Program regarding adults,[50] children, and adolescents.[51] Prevention goals are stated in the US Department of Health and Human Services' *Healthy People 2000*[44] and *Healthy People 2010*,[45] which call for expansion of nutritional counseling by primary care providers. Practical recommendations for dietary instruction, monitoring, and follow-up are available to physicians who wish to incorporate nutritional counseling into their daily practices. The client's or patient's

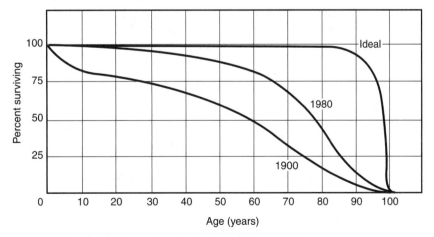

FIGURE 1–4 Increasing rectangularization of the survival curve.
Source: Reprinted from Haylick L, The cell biology of human aging. *Sci. Am.* 1980; 242:60. With permission of Scientific American, Inc.

Exhibit 1–1   Proposed Research Categories—Committee on Diet and Health,
National Research Council

- Identify foods and dietary components that alter the chronic disease risk and
  identify their mechanisms of action.
- Improve dietary assessment methods.
- Identify markers of exposure and early indicators of the disease risk.
- Quantify both adverse and beneficial effects of diet; determine optimal
  dietary ranges of macro- and micro-components.
- Conduct intervention studies to assess risk reduction potential.
- Conduct community-based programs that apply current knowledge of eating
  behavior and disease.
- Expand molecular and cellular nutrition research.

Source: From Diet and Health: Implications for Reducing Chronic Disease Risk. Reprinted
with permission from the National Academies Press, Copyright © 1989, National Academy of
Sciences.

---

failure to adhere to a recommended regimen is a major obstacle for achieving
the preventive and therapeutic nutritional goals set for the nation.[44]

Research Directions

How can nutritional epidemiology and medical nutrition therapy become
natural companions to health promotion and disease prevention? A conceptual framework for planning interdisciplinary collaborative research has
been proposed in Exhibit 1–1. Seven categories are identified. The framework encompasses different kinds of investigations: short- and long-term
experiments in vitro and in vivo, food consumption surveys, food composition analyses, uncontrolled and controlled epidemiologic studies, metabolic
studies, clinical trials in humans, and social and behavioral research.[46]

Current approaches to medical nutrition therapy, important research data
linking eating behavior with disease prevention as well as onset, and ways
community nutrition professionals can integrate and remain a vital part of
health care are all explored in the following chapters.

References

1. Lilienfeld AM, Lilienfeld DE. *Foundations of Epidemiology.* 2nd ed.
   New York: Oxford University Press Inc; 1980.
2. Last JM. *Dictionary of Epidemiology.* 2nd ed. New York: Oxford
   University Press Inc; 1988.
3. Green LW. *Community Health.* 6th ed. St. Louis, Mo: Times Mirror/CV
   Mosby Co; 1990.
4. *Principles of Epidemiology: An Introduction to Applied Epidemiology
   and Biostatistics.* 2nd ed. Atlanta, Ga: Centers for Disease Control and
   Prevention; 1992.

5. Page R, Cole G, Timmrock T. *Basic Epidemiologic Methods and Biosta-tistics.* Sudbury, Mass: Jones and Bartlett Publishers; 1993.

6. Doll R, Hill AB. Smoking and carcinoma of the lung. *Br Med J.* 1950;1:739-748.

7. Dawber TR, Kannel WB, Lyell LP. An approach to longitudinal studies in a community: the Framingham study. *Ann NY Acad Sci.* 1963;107: 539-556.

8. Berenson GS, McMahan CA, Voors AW, et al. A summing up. In: Hester AC, ed. *Cardiovascular Risk Factors in Children—The Early Natural History of Atherosclerosis and Essential Hypertension.* New York: Oxford University Press Inc; 1980:381-396.

9. Blackburn H, Luepker RV, Kline FG, et al. The Minnesota Heart Health Program: A Research and Demonstration Project in Cardiovascular Disease Prevention. In: Matarazzo JD, Weiss SM, Herd JA, et al, eds. *Behavioral Health: A Handbook of Health Enhancements and Disease Prevention.* New York: John Wiley & Sons Inc; 1984:1171-1178.

10. Farquhar JW, Fortmann SP, Maccoby N, et al. The Stanford Five City Project: An Overview. In: Matarazzo JD, Weiss SM, Herd JA, et al, eds. *Behavioral Health: A Handbook of Health Enhancements and Disease Prevention.* New York: John Wiley & Sons Inc; 1984:1154-1165.

11. Puska P, Tuomilehto J, Salonen J, et al. *The North Karelia Project: Evaluation of a Comprehensive Communication Programme for Control of Cardiovascular Disease in North Karelia, Finland, 1972–1977.* Copenhagen, Denmark: World Health Organization-EURO; 1981.

12. Caggiula AN, Christakis G, Farrand M, et al. The Multiple Risk Factor Intervention Trial (MRFIT): IV. Intervention on blood lipids. *Preventive Med.* 1981;10:443-475.

13. MacMahon B, Pugh TF. *Epidemiology: Principles and Methods.* Boston, Mass: Little, Brown, & Company; 1970.

14. *Public Health Reports.* Atlanta, Ga: Centers for Disease Control. 1923;38:2361-2368.

15. Myers GW. *History of the Massachusetts General Hospital, June 1872 to December 1900.* [unpublished manuscript]. 1929. Available in: Mary C. Egan Reference Collection, National Center for Education in Maternal and Child Health, Arlington, Va.

16. Hunt CL. *The Life of Ellen H. Richards.* Washington, DC: American Home Economics Association; 1958.

17. Egan MC. Public health nutrition: a historic perspective. *J Am Diet Assoc.* 1994;94:298-304.

18. Getting V. A modern nutrition program in a state health department. *Milbank Q.* 1947;25:3.

19. Eliot MM, Heseltine MM. Nutrition in maternal and child health programs. *Nutr Rev.* 1947;5:33-35.

20. Massachusetts Department of Public Health. Conference on standardization of qualifications and salaries of nutritional workers. [unpublished report]. 1920. Available in: Mary C. Egan Reference Collection, National Center for Education in Maternal and Child Health, Arlington, Va.

21. Association of State and Territorial Public Health Nutrition Directors. Application for a research grant. [unpublished report]. 1960. Available in: Mary C. Egan Reference Collection, National Center for Education in Maternal and Child Health, Arlington, Va.

22. Kaufman M. *Nutrition in Public Health—A Handbook for Developing Programs and Services.* Gaithersburg, Md: Aspen Publishers Inc; 1990:570.

23. Frank GC. Primary prevention in the school arena: a dietary approach. *Health Values.* 1983;7:14-21.

24. Thacker SB, Berkelman RL. Public health surveillance in the United States. *Epidemiol Rev.* 1988;10:164-190.

25. Orenstein WA, Bernier RH. Surveillance information for action. *Pediatr Clin North Am.* 1990;37:709-734.

26. Belloc NB, Breslow L. Relationship of physical health status and health practices. *Preventive Med.* 1972;1:409-421.

27. Carleton RA, Lasater TM, Assaf AR, et al. The Pawtucket Heart Health Program: community changes in cardiovascular risk factors and projected disease risk. *Am J Public Health.* 1995;85:777-785.

28. *Annual Summary of Births, Marriages, Divorces, and Deaths: United States, 1991. Monthly Vital Statistics Report.* Washington, DC: National Center for Health Statistics; September 30, 1992;40:13.

29. *Deaths: Final Data for 2002. Monthly Vital Statistics Report.* Washington, DC: National Center for Health Statistics; October 12, 2004;53:5.

30. *Trends in Characteristics of Births by State: United States, 1990, 1995, and 2000–2002. National Vital Statistics Report.* Washington, DC: National Center for Health Statistics; May 10, 2004;52:19.

31. Rosenberg HM, Curtin LR, Maurer J, et al. Choosing a standard population: some statistical considerations. In: Feinleib M, Zarate AO, eds. *Reconsidering Adjustment Procedures. Vital and Health Statistics.* Washington, DC: US Department of Health and Human Services, Public Health Service; 1984:29-67. DHHS publication 93-1466, Series 4.

32. Paffenbarger RS. Conditions of epidemiology to exercise science and cardiovascular health. *Med and Sci in Sports and Exercise.* 1988;20: 426-438.

33. Sempos CT, Cleeman JI, Carroll MD, et al. Prevalence of high blood cholesterol among US adults: an update based on guidelines from the Second Report of the National Cholesterol Education Program Adult Treatment Panel. *JAMA.* 1993;269:3009-3014.

34. Johnson CL, Rifkind BM, Sempos CT, et al. Declining serum total cholesterol levels among US adults: the National Health and Nutrition Examination Surveys. *JAMA.* 1993;269:3002-3008.

35. Frazier EL, Franks AL, Sanderson LM. Behavioral risk factor data. In: *Using Chronic Disease Data: A Handbook for Public Health Practitioners.* Atlanta, Ga: Centers for Disease Control and Prevention; 1992.

36. Van Horn L, Gerrhofer N, Moag-Stahlberg A, et al. Dietary assessment in children using electronic methods: telephones and tape recorders. *J Am Diet Assoc.* 1990;90:412-416.

37. Groves RM, Kahn RL. *Surveys by Telephone.* New York: Academic Press; 1979.

38. Folsom AR, Kaye SA, Sellers TA, et al. Body fat distribution and 5-year risk of death in older women. *JAMA.* 1993;269:483-487.

39. Blair SN, Kohl HW, Paffenbarger RS, et al. Physical fitness and all-cause mortality: a prospective study of healthy men and women. *JAMA.* 1989;262:2395-2401.

40. Jacobs D, Blackburn H, Higgins M, et al. Report of the conference on low blood cholesterol: mortality associations. *Circulation.* 1992;86: 1046-1060.

41. Benson K, Hartz A. A comparison of observational studies and randomized, controlled trials. *NEJM.* 2000;342(25):1878-1886.

42. Concato J, Shah N, Horvitz R. Randomized, controlled trials, observational studies, and the hierarchy of research designs. *NEJM.* 2000;342(25):1887-1892.

43. Pocock S, Elbourne D. Randomized trials or observational tribulations? *NEJM.* 2000. 342(25):1907-1909.

44. *Healthy People 2000: National Health Promotion and Disease Prevention Objectives.* Washington, DC: US Department of Health and Human Services; 1991. Public Health Service publication 91-50212.

45. US Department of Health and Human Services. DATA 2010—the Healthy People 2010 database. *CDC Wonder.* Atlanta, Ga: Centers for Disease Control; November 2000.

46. National Research Council. *Diet and Health: Implications for Reducing Chronic Disease Risk.* Washington, DC: National Academy Press; 1989.

47. *Surgeon General's Report on Nutrition and Health.* Washington, DC: US Department of Health and Human Services; 1988. Public Health Service publication 88-50210.

48. Haylick L. The cell biology of human aging. *Sci Am.* 1980;242:60.

49. Joint National Committee. The 1988 report of the Joint National Committee on Detection, Evaluation, and Treatment of High Blood Pressure. *Arch Intern Med.* 1988;148:1023-1038.

50. National Cholesterol Education Program. Report of the Expert Panel on Detection, Evaluation, and Treatment of High Blood Cholesterol in Adults III: final report. *Circulation.* 2002;106:3143-3421.

51. National Cholesterol Education Program. *Report of the Expert Panel on Blood Cholesterol Levels in Children and Adolescents.* Bethesda, Md: US Department of Health and Human Services, Public Health Service, National Institutes of Health, National Heart, Lung, and Blood Institute; April 1991. NIH Publication 91-2732.

NUTRITION IN THE UNITED STATES

Learning Objectives

- Enumerate the major nutrition guidelines for Americans.
- Explain the diet and health associations existing in the United States that set the stage for the *Healthy People in Healthy Communities 2010* initiative.
- Identify the role, components, and benefits of the National Nutrition Monitoring System.
- Describe the 3 levels employed by the US Department of Agriculture (USDA) to monitor food and nutrient consumption in the United States.
- Describe how the Centers for Disease Control and Prevention provide nutrition surveillance data.
- Explain how the recommended dietary allowances (RDAs) integrate with nutrition surveillance, programming, and policy development.
- Detail aspects of the Nutrition Labeling and Education Act (NLEA) regarding food labels and health claims.
- Define biotechnology and discuss its benefits and resulting new food products.
- Discuss the alternative medicine approach that uses nutraceuticals.
- Delineate the components of nutrition misinformation and disinformation.

High Definition Nutrition

Adequate intake (AI)—used when an RDA cannot be determined. Based on an observed or experimentally determined approximate nutrient intake for a subgroup of healthy people.

Antibiotic resistance—a trait in a vector DNA; only cells within which the vector DNA is incorporated are resistant to antibiotics.

Bionutrition—a vision for research that integrates the study of how genetics, molecular biology, and cell biology interact with nutrients of other environmental influences to shape more complex levels of biological organization and, ultimately, health.

Biotechnology—food engineering based on biology that benefits the quantity, value, safety, nutritional quality, desirable characteristics, and variety of foods. Examples of products are chymosin for cheese making and bovine somatotropin (BST) for milk productivity.

Clone—a group of genetically identical cells or organisms asexually coming from a common ancestor.

Dietary reference intakes (DRIs)—the new standards for nutrient recommendations to plan and to assess diets for healthy people. An umbrella term that includes estimated average requirement (EAR), recommended dietary allowances (RDA), AI, and upper level (UL).

Disinformation—unsubstantiated messages to the public about food or nutrition.

Discretionary calorie allowance—the balance of calories remaining in an individual's estimated energy allowance after allowing for the number of calories needed to meet recommended nutrient intakes eating foods low in fat or without added sugar.

Estimated average requirement (EAR)—a nutrient intake value estimated to meet the requirement of half the healthy individuals in a subgroup. Used to assess nutritional adequacy of intakes of population groups and to calculate RDAs.

Estimated energy requirement—the average dietary energy intake that will maintain energy balance in a healthy individual of a certain gender, age, weight, height, and physical activity level.

Genetic engineering—the process of changing the genetic material of a cell using restriction enzymes.

Growth retardation—defined as height-for-age below the fifth percentile of children in the National Center for Health Statistics's reference population.

Health claim—explicit and applied statement of benefit of specific composition of a food.

Moderate physical activity—3.5 to 7 kcal/min or the equivalent of 3 to 6 metabolic equivalents and results in achieving 60–73% of peak heart rate.

Nutrition assessment—selecting indicators of nutritional status and collecting those indicators among a sample or population.

Nutrition monitoring—intermittent assessment to identify change in nutritional risk of a group or community.

Nutrition screening—focused assessment generally available to a total community or group to identify at-risk individuals.

Nutrition surveillance—a sequential, community-based assessment to identify a change in the distribution or occurrence of indicators. This assessment is often used to determine a trend.

Recombinant DNA (rDNA)—DNA produced using genetic engineering techniques. Techniques involve transferring a DNA segment from 1 organism and inserting it into the DNA of another organism. The 2 organisms can be unrelated.

Recommended dietary allowances (RDA)—a goal for individuals based upon the EAR. The daily dietary intake level sufficient to meet the nutrient requirement of 97–98% of all healthy individuals in a subgroup. An EAR is required before an RDA can be proposed.

Registered dietitian (RD)—a nutrition expert in the healthcare profession. RDs provide reliable therapeutic and wellness counseling and help individuals achieve a total food intake that tastes good and ensures good health. RDs have met the requirements for credentialing by the American Dietetic Association. This involves at least a bachelor's degree, a supervised training program in an accredited/approved institution, a national registration examination, and continuing postgraduate study. A registered dietitian can be located by calling 1–800–234-RD4U.

Refuge fields—unmodified crops that are often planted adjacent to a field of pest-resistant crops.

Replication—the formation of new strands of DNA from existing DNA, permitting the reproduction of an identical new cell as the result of the division.

Sedentary behavior—little or no physical activity during leisure time.

Tolerable upper intake level (UL)—highest level of daily nutrient intake likely to pose no risks of adverse heath effects to almost all individuals in the general population. If intake increases above the UL, then the risk of adverse effects increases.

Transgenic organism—an organism that contains both parental and foreign DNA sequences within its basic genome.

Vector—a transmission agent such as a DNA vector, which is a self-replicating DNA molecule sending a piece of DNA from one host to another.

Vigorous physical activity—7 kcal/min or the equivalent of 6+ metabolic equivalents and results in achieving 74–88% peak heart rate.

Population Change

In the United States, the changing proportions of young and old persons in the population can be represented in a population pyramid. Figure 2–1 contrasts the population pyramid for 1987 with the projected pyramids for the years 2000, 2010, and 2030. Each horizontal bar in these pyramids represents a 10-year birth cohort (i.e., people born within the same 10-year period). By comparing these bars, one can determine the relative size of each birth cohort. In the first graph, the distribution of the population in 1987 had already moved from a true pyramid to one with a bulge. The bulge represents the baby boomers. This pyramid will become column-like over time.

Changes in the pyramid reflect the changes and demands on health care (e.g., the aging of babies who later need care when they are adults with chronic or long-term conditions). In the 1990s, death from acute diseases was rare. Maternal, infant, and early childhood death rates have declined considerably since the early 1900s. As a result, an increasing number of individuals survive to old age, often with clustered illness requiring long-term care.[1]

Each cohort in a population pyramid represents individuals with different healthcare needs, lifestyles, and nutrient intakes. Part II of this book addresses the lifestyles and healthcare needs of each age cohort in greater detail.

State of the Nation

While studies indicate that Americans are eating better now than they were in the late 1980s, tens of millions of Americans have poor diets and are overweight. Specific concerns currently include:

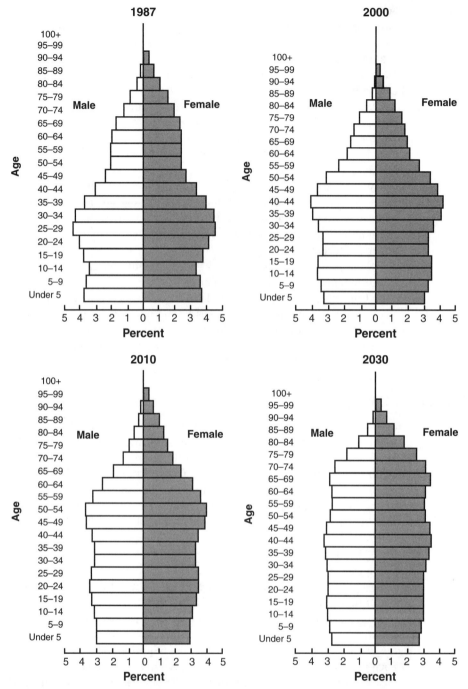

FIGURE 2–1 Age distribution of the US population: 1987, 2000, 2010, and 2030.
Source: Reprinted from US Bureau of the Census, Projections of the Population of the
US by Age, Sex, and Race: 1988-2080. *Current Population Reports*. Washington, DC:
US Department of Commerce, 1984. Series P-25, No.1018.

One in 3 nonelderly adults are now overweight. Fifty-eight million American adults ages 20 through 74 are overweight, and the number of overweight Americans increased from 25 to 65% between 1980 and 2005.

One in 5 children are at risk of being overweight. Fifteen percent of children are overweight or obese. The number of overweight children has doubled over the past 15 years, and 70% of overweight children aged 10 to 13 will be overweight and obese adults. Most of this increase has taken place in recent years; 10% of children 4 to 5 years of age were overweight in 1988 through 1994 compared with 5.8% in 1971 through 1974. Recent studies indicate that this trend is associated with low levels of physical activity rather than increased food consumption.

Obesity is linked to an increased incidence of chronic disease. Obesity is a risk factor for diseases such as coronary heart disease, certain types of cancer, stroke, and diabetes. Over $68 billion is spent each year on the direct healthcare costs related to obesity, representing more than 6% of the nation's healthcare expenditures.

Almost 90% of Americans have diets that need improvement. The Healthy Eating Index shows that 88% of Americans have diets that are poor or need improvement. Only 26% of people meet the daily dietary recommendation for dairy products, and less than 20% meet the daily recommendation for fruits. In particular, teenagers and people with low incomes tend to have lower quality diets.

Many illnesses can be prevented or mediated through regular physical activity. Regular physical activity reduces the risk of developing some of the leading causes of illness and death in the United States, including heart disease, high blood pressure, colon cancer, and diabetes. Physical activity has been demonstrated to reduce blood pressure and symptoms of anxiety and depression while maintaining healthy bones, muscles, and joints. More than 60% of adults do not engage in the recommended amount of physical activity, and approximately 25% of adults are not physically active at all.

Healthy People 2000 (HP2K), published by the US Department of Health and Human Services, established 3 overarching goals amid the complex health challenges of the 1990s.[2] They are: (1) increase the span of healthy life for Americans; (2) reduce health disparities among Americans; and (3) achieve access to preventive services for all Americans.

Basic to these goals is the premise that dietary factors are associated with 5 of the 10 leading causes of death: coronary heart disease, some types of cancer, stroke, non–insulin-dependent diabetes mellitus, and atherosclerosis. Three other major causes of death have been associated with excessive alcohol intake: cirrhosis of the liver, unintentional injuries, and suicides (see Table 2–1).[2]

Healthy People 2010 focuses on increasing the quality and years of healthy life and eliminating racial and ethnic disparities in health status. It targets healthy diet and healthy weight as critical goals. Leading health indicators in 10 areas will assess overall health of the nation via community, comparison, and improvements over time.

Twenty-eight focus areas include one for nutrition and weight and another for food safety. Strategies for combating a range of diseases, conditions, and

TABLE 2–1 The 10 Major Causes of Death in the United States: 1977, 1987, 1992, 1996, and 2002

1977	1987	1992	1996	2002
Coronary heart disease (CHD)	CHD	CHD	CHD	CHD
Cancer	Cancer	Cancer	Cancer	Cancer
Stroke	Accidents	Stroke	Stroke	Stroke
Accidents	Stroke	Chronic lung disease	Chronic lung disease	Chronic lung disease
Chronic lung disease	Chronic lung disease	Accidents	Accidents	Accidents
Pneumonia/ influenza (P/I)	P/I	P/I	P/I	Diabetes
Suicide	Suicide	Diabetes	Diabetes	P/I
Liver disease	Diabetes	HIV	HIV	Alzheimer's
Diabetes	Liver disease	Suicide	Suicide	Kidney disease
Atherosclerosis	Atherosclerosis	Homicide	Liver disease/ cirrhosis	Septicemia

Source: Data from *Healthy People 2000: National Health Promotion and Disease Prevention Objectives.* Washington, DC: US Dept of Health and Human Services; 1991. DHHS (PHS) Publication No. 91-50212, p 3; and from *Monthly Vital Statistics Report,* 43, 6S, p 5. DHHS (PHS) Publication 95-1120, 4-2415, December, 1994; Peters KD, Kochanek KD, Murphy SL. *Deaths: Final Data for 1966. National Vital Statistics Report.* Washington, DC: NCHS, CDC. 1998;47(9):1-99; *Deaths: Final Data for 2002. Monthly Vital Statistics Report.* Washington, DC: National Center for Health Statistics; October 12, 2004;53:5.

public health challenges and nutrition actions to promote health and prevent disease are identified. *Healthy People 2010* has 18 objectives that target diet and weight goals as listed in Exhibit 2–1. Focus areas linked to chronic disease are listed in Exhibit 2–2.

Inadequate and/or excessive intake of several dietary components fuel the diet and health relationships. *The Surgeon General's Report on Nutrition and Health* acknowledged that in the United States there is a disproportionate consumption of foods high in fats. This high fat intake is generally at the expense of foods high in complex carbohydrates and dietary fiber that may be more conducive to health.[3] The *Dietary Guidelines for Americans*[4] are based on the premise that staying healthy means eating a variety of foods; maintaining healthy weight; choosing a diet low in fat, saturated fat, and cholesterol; choosing a diet with plenty of vegetables, fruits, and grain products; using sugars only in moderation; using salt and sodium only in moderation; drinking in moderation if alcoholic beverages are consumed; and a focus on food safety is basic to healthy eating.[4]

New Millennium Actions for Healthy Eating

In the year 2000, 2 major actions directed the national executive branch agenda for healthy eating:

Exhibit 2-1   HP 2010 Overview

1. Cut by > 50% the proportion of children, adolescents, and adults who are overweight or obese (3 objectives).
2. Reduce growth retardation among low-income children under age 5 years (estimated at 8%) to 5%.
3. Substantially increase the proportion of people in all age categories who consume desirable levels of fruits, vegetables, grain products, saturated fats, sodium, and calcium (7 objectives).
4. Sizably reduce iron deficiency among young children, women of child-bearing age, and pregnant women (3 objectives).
5. Increase the proportion of children and adolescents whose intakes from meals and snacks at school contribute proportionally to overall dietary quality.
6. Increase to 85% (estimated at 55%) the number of work sites with 50 or more employees that offer nutrition or weight management classes or counseling.
7. Increase to 75% (estimated at 42% in 1997) the number of physician office visits that include counseling or education related to diet and nutrition for patients with cardiovascular disease, diabetes, and hyperlipidemia.
8. Achieve food security in 94% of US households (estimated at 88% of all US households in 1995).

Source: Adapted from US Department of Health and Human Services. DATA2010–the Healthy People 2010 Database. *CDC Wonder.* Centers for Disease Control. Atlanta, Ga: November 2000. www.healthypeople.org/LHI/Priorities.htm; and Tate M, Patrick S. Healthy People 2010 targets healthy diet and healthy weight as critical goals. *JADA.* March 2000;100(3):300.

1. *National Nutrition Summit.* To address the new nutritional challenges facing the country, sponsored by the Departments of Agriculture and Health and Human Services, experts explored hunger, overweight and obese Americans, and nutrition and physical activity in health promotion, and chronic disease prevention (see Exhibit 2-3).
2. *Updating the* Dietary Guidelines for Americans *(DGAs).* As the cornerstone of national nutrition policy and used to determine the content of school lunch and other federal nutrition programs, the new DGAs emphasize the need to eat whole grain foods and include:
   - *A new recommendation that both children and adults make physical activity a regular part of their routine.* The new guidelines recommend that both adults and children get at least 30 minutes of physical activity daily in order to lower risk factors for heart disease, colon cancer, and diabetes.
   - *A new guidance on how to keep food safe.* Because eating even a small portion of an unsafe food can cause illness, emphasis is placed on preparing and storing food to help protect families from foodborne illnesses. Perishable foods that require special care, i.e., eggs, meats, poultry, fish, shellfish, and milk products, are discussed.

The US Departments of Agriculture and Health and Human Services published the official report of the 2005 *Dietary Guidelines for Americans* advisory committee. This report is the basis of the actual 2005 *Dietary Guidelines for Americans*, which set policy direction, Public Law 101–445, Section 301, for

Exhibit 2–2   Healthy People 2010 Objective Focus Areas

Focus area: A specific area of health information or awareness that is tracked by the *Healthy People 2010* initiative. There are currently 28 focus areas tracked by *Healthy People 2010*. Leading health indicators are a special set of objectives selected out of the 28 focus areas. Current HP2010 focus areas:

1. Access to quality health services
2. Arthritis, osteoporosis, and chronic back conditions
3. Cancer
4. Chronic kidney disease
5. Diabetes
6. Disability and secondary conditions
7. Educational and community-based programs
8. Environmental health
9. Family planning and sexual health
10. Food safety
11. Health communication
12. Heart disease and stroke
13. HIV
14. Immunization and infectious diseases
15. Injury/violence prevention
16. Maternal, infant, and child health
17. Medical product safety: medications, biologics, and medical devices
18. Mental health and mental disorders
19. Nutrition
20. Occupational safety and health
21. Oral health
22. Physical activity and fitness
23. Public health infrastructure
24. Respiratory diseases
25. Sexually transmitted diseases
26. Substance abuse
27. Tobacco use
28. Vision and hearing

Source: Adapted from US Department of Health and Human Services. DATA2010–the Healthy People 2010 Database. *CDC Wonder.* Centers for Disease Control. Atlanta, Ga: November 2000.

the next 5 years for all government nutrition programs, including research, education, food assistance, labeling, and nutritional promotion.[4]

The *Dietary Guidelines for Americans* must be applied in menu planning programs, for example, the National School Lunch Program; in educational materials used by the Special Supplemental Nutrition Program for Women, Infants, and Children (WIC); and in setting the healthy people objectives for the nation. Using *Dietary Guidelines for Americans* helps policymakers, educators, and clinicians speak with 1 voice on nutrition and health.

The 2005 *Dietary Guidelines for Americans* advisory committee report is posted at www.health.gov/dietaryguidelines.

The committee found strong scientific support for dietary and physical activity measures that could reduce major health problems—overweight and obesity, hypertension, abnormal blood lipids, diabetes, coronary heart disease,

Exhibit 2–3 The National Nutrition Summit and the White House Conference on Food, Nutrition and Health—An Historic Perspective

Presented by Ann Gallagher and Jane White

The burgeoning problem of obesity and continuing malnourishment offer compelling evidence that the American public is not eating a healthful, well-balanced, and moderate diet. The government-sponsored National Nutrition Summit, beginning today [December, 2000] in Washington, provides a much needed opportunity for our nation to consider these problems and re-evaluate its approaches to issues of food, nutrition, and health.

For most Americans, the US food system has succeeded in providing an abundant, wholesome, and nutritious food supply. Domestic hunger, once the most significant dietary problem, has abated largely thanks to the work begun in the 1960s—the commencement of a pilot project that eventually became the Food Stamp program, the War on Poverty, and the 1969 White House Conference on Food, Nutrition and Health.

The 1969 conference was a pivotal event. The meeting, called by President Nixon and chaired by Jean Mayer, the late president of Tufts University, assembled food and nutrition experts and advocates from around the nation and world to examine what could be done to improve the nutritional status of all Americans. The result was a government-led effort to make food, nutrition, and health a national priority. It was the starting point for an agenda broader than just feeding the poor or disposing of food surpluses. Among the accomplishments since the 1969 conference: a nutrition research agenda that demonstrated the role of nutrition in good health and the dissemination of public information that paved the way to widespread "consumerism." The acclaimed Special Supplemental Nutrition Program for Women, Infants and Children, school breakfast initiatives, and the development of national dietary guidance for healthy eating also began following the 1969 event, and they continue today.

While Americans can celebrate nutrition advances over the last 31 years, there is widespread evidence of new and more complex issues related to nutrition and health. Walk through any airport or shopping mall in the country and the problem of obesity surrounds you. Today, over half of Americans are considered overweight or obese. Ironically, obesity and poor nutrition occur as Americans receive millions of messages each year that underscore the importance of diet and regular exercise. There has never been a greater demand for information to assist consumers with maintaining or improving their health, or managing disease.

At the same time, there is continued evidence of hunger in the United States. Despite our strong economy, approximately 1 in 10 households, or 30 million people, report food insecurity. There also are rising concerns that advances in food science and technology that have transformed food production and processing may have unrecognized nutritional and health risks. Outside the United States, these concerns have proven formidable barriers to new technologies, as seen in Europe where biotechnology has been sidelined. Where conventional agricultural inputs are being questioned, there is increased interest in organically grown food. The United States is not immune to these developments. It is likely that as consumer concerns are articulated, every aspect of our food production and regulatory systems could be challenged to do more to assure consumers even more wholesome, healthy diets.

The National Nutrition Summit in the year 2000 offered a new opportunity to begin a comprehensive re-evaluation of US nutrition policy. Its agenda focused largely on hunger and obesity, diet, and exercise, and it laid groundwork for

Exhibit 2–3   (Continued)

---

building consensus on food and nutrition, and defining approaches by government and industry that will have an impact in 21st century America.

Today's challenges call for a new and comprehensive approach that goes well beyond current government assistance and regulatory agendas. A new framework built upon principles that place public health at the forefront of debates affecting consumers probably can better meet America's nutrition and health needs of the coming years. That approach probably will require greater transparency to maintain public confidence, and it will be dependent upon adequate funding in order to support public and private research, regulatory functions, and public health programs to help Americans live healthier and longer lives. That is the significance of the National Nutrition Summit and its promise for the longer term.

Ann Gallagher, RD, LD, CD, President of the American Dietetic Association, 1999-2000 and Jane V. White, PhD, RD, LDN, President, 2000-2001.

Source: Gallagher A, White JV. The National Nutrition Summit and the White House Conference on Food, Nutrition and Health–An Historic Perspective. December, 2000; Washington, D.C.

---

certain types of cancer, and osteoporosis. The committee used the phrase "discretionary calories" to identify calories remaining within a person's caloric allowance after all nutrient recommendations are met. The greater the discretionary calories, the greater the chance for weight gain.

The committee focused on the potential health benefits and serious health risks of alcohol intake. Food can promote health only if it is safe to eat. Food-borne illness affects more than 76 million Americans each year, so food safety forms the basis of all dietary guidance.

Key Messages—Translating Scientific Findings Into Dietary and Physical Activity Guidance

Nine key messages will guide nutrition-related program providers, healthcare providers and educators, and those charged with the responsibility to produce the publication *Dietary Guidelines for Americans,* 2005 edition. One part identifies the scientific basis while another provides specific recommendations.

The 9 major messages and a more detailed description follow:

1. Consume a variety of foods within and among the basic food groups while staying within energy needs.
2. Control calorie intake to manage body weight.
3. Be physically active every day.
4. Choose fats wisely for good health.
5. Choose carbohydrates wisely for good health.
6. Increase daily intake of fruits and vegetables, whole grains, and nonfat or low-fat milk and milk products.
7. Choose and prepare foods with little salt.
8. If you drink alcoholic beverages, do so in moderation.
9. Keep food safe to eat.

Consume a Variety of Foods Within and Among the Basic Food Groups While Staying Within Energy Needs

Recommendations for nutrient intakes from the Institute of Medicine blend prevention and basic nutrient needs as a firm foundation for current health and for reducing chronic disease risk. Meeting recommended nutrient intakes while staying within energy needs is a basic premise of dietary guidance. Increased dietary intakes of vitamin E, calcium, magnesium, potassium, and fiber by children and adults and increased dietary intakes of vitamins A and C by adults are warranted.

Choosing a variety of foods helps, but maintaining appropriate energy balance is important. This means limiting calorie intake from added sugars, solid fats, and alcoholic beverages, which are nutrient poor.

The revised USDA food intake pattern is one method to plan diets that meet recommended nutrient intakes for different age, gender, and physical activity levels. This food pattern:

- recommends numbers of servings from the 5 food groups and from food subgroups;
- identifies good sources of nutrients relative to the calories that they provide;
- allows a choice of foods within each food group and subgroup;
- suggests ways to make substitutions across some food groups;
- lists best sources of nutrients often in short supply in US diets; and
- describes useful ways for consumers to choose popular foods to boost their intake nutrients.

Special nutrient recommendations are:

- adolescent females and women of childbearing age need extra iron and folic acid;
- persons over age 50 benefit from taking vitamin B_{12} in its crystalline form from foods fortified with this vitamin or from supplements that contain vitamin B_{12}; and
- elderly with dark skin and persons exposed to little UVB radiation may need extra vitamin D from vitamin D-fortified foods and/or supplements that contain vitamin D.

Control Calorie Intake to Manage Body Weight

Calorie intake and physical activity interact to control a person's weight. To alter the obesity epidemic, most Americans need to reduce the number of calories they consume. For weight control, calories count (not the proportions of carbohydrate, fat, and protein in the diet). Energy expended must equal energy consumed to stay at the same weight, such as a deficit by eating less, being more active physically, or combining the 2. All individuals 3 years and older have an estimated energy requirement (EER) incorporating age, weight, height, gender, and physical activity. Adults gain weight slowly over time, showing even a small calorie deficit can blunt weight gain. Fifty to 100 calories per day less would enable many adults to maintain their weight rather than continuing to gain weight each year. For children who are gaining excess fat, small decrements in energy intake can reduce the rate of weight gain, so as they age they will grow into a healthy weight. Small changes maintained over time can make a big difference in body weight.

Monitoring weight regularly helps people adjust their food intake by limiting the portion sizes or amount of physical activity to maintain their weight. Consuming large portions of raw vegetables or low-fat soups may help limit one's intake of other foods that are more energy dense. The healthiest way to reduce calorie intake is to reduce one's intake of added sugars, solid fats, and alcohol.

Be Physically Active Every Day

Lifelong moderate physical activity from childhood to adulthood for at least 30 minutes per day promotes fitness and reduces the risk of chronic health conditions such as obesity, hypertension, diabetes, and coronary artery disease. Moderate physical activity (a brisk walk at 3 to 4 miles per hour) for an hour daily increases energy expenditure by about 150 to 200 calories, depending on body size. If one does not increase calories, then this increase in physical activity could blunt weight gain.

About 60 minutes of moderate to vigorous physical activity daily prevents unhealthy weight gain. For adults who have previously lost weight, 60 to 90 minutes of moderate physical activity daily can offset weight gain. Children and adolescents need 60 minutes of moderate to vigorous physical activity daily for overall fitness and for healthy weight gain during growth.

Choose Fats Wisely for Good Health

A very low intake of saturated fat, trans fat, and cholesterol can keep low-density lipoprotein cholesterol down and reduce CHD risk. Dietary fat goals are: (1) saturated fat intake < 10% of calories; (2) trans fat intake < 1% of calories; and (3) cholesterol intake < 300 mg per day. The lower the combined intake of saturated and trans fat and dietary cholesterol intake, then the greater the cardiovascular benefit.

Animal fats are mainly found in cheese, milk, butter, ice cream, and other full-fat dairy products; fatty meat; bacon and sausage; and poultry skin and fat. Trans fats are found in foods made with partially hydrogenated vegetable oils. Dietary cholesterol is found in eggs and organ meats, especially shellfish and high-fat poultry and dairy products.

A reduced risk of both sudden death and CHD death in adults is associated with the consumption of 2 servings (approximately 8 meals) per week of fish high in n-3 fatty acids (eicosapentaenoic acid and docosahexaenoic acid). Pregnant women, lactating women, and children should avoid eating fish with a high mercury content and limit their consumption of fish with a moderate mercury content by reviewing consumer advisories to know which species of fish to limit or avoid.

Total fat intake of 20-35% of calories is recommended for all Americans age 18 years or older, 30% of energy from fat is recommended for children 2 to 3 years old, and 25% is recommended for youth 4 to 18 years old.

Choose Carbohydrates Wisely for Good Health

Carbohydrates, the sugars, starches, and fibers found in fruits, are an important part of a healthy diet and the major energy source in most diets. Sugars and starches supply energy via glucose, which is the only energy source for the red blood cell and the preferred energy source for the brain, central nervous system, placenta, and fetus and for muscle cells when they are operating anaerobically (without oxygen). Diets rich in dietary fiber help promote healthy laxation and help reduce the risk of type 2 diabetes and coronary heart disease.

When selecting foods from the fruit, vegetable, and grains groups, it is beneficial to make fiber-rich choices often. Current evidence suggests that there is no relationship between total carbohydrates intake (minus fiber) and the incidence of either type 1 or type 2 diabetes.

Increasing intake of fruits, vegetables, whole grains, and nonfat or low-fat milk or milk products is a healthy way to achieve the recommended amounts of carbohydrate. People eating small amounts of food and beverages that are high in added sugars consume fewer calories and more vitamins and minerals. Prospective studies suggest a positive association between intake of sugar-sweetened beverages and weight gain.

Sugars and starches from foods and snacks promote bacterial fermentation in the mouth, causing tooth demineralization and dental caries. Fluoridated water and fluoride-containing dental products can lower the risk of dental caries.

Increase Daily Intakes of Fruits and Vegetables, Whole Grains, and Reduced-Fat Milk and Milk Products

Fruits and Vegetables   Fruits contain glucose, fructose, sucrose, and fiber, and most fruits are relatively low in calories. In addition, fruits are important sources of at least 8 additional nutrients, including vitamin C, folate, and potassium (which may help control blood pressure). Many vegetables provide small amounts of sugars and/or starch, or are high in starch, and all provide fiber. Vegetables are important sources of 19 or more nutrients, including potassium, folate, and vitamins A and E.

Fruit and vegetable intakes are inversely associated with a decreased risk of such chronic diseases as stroke, perhaps other cardiovascular diseases, type 2 diabetes, and cancer in certain sites. Increased fruit and vegetable intake may promote and sustain weight loss.

The suggested range of intake is 2½ to 6½ cups of fruits and vegetables daily, depending on calorie needs. For persons needing 2,000 calories per day to maintain their weight, the goal is 4½ cups (or the equivalent) of various fruits and vegetables each day.

Whole Grains   Whole grains are high in starch and important sources of 14 nutrients, including fiber. Diets rich in whole grains not only reduce the risk of CHD and type 2 diabetes but can also help with weight control. Eating at least three 1-ounce equivalents per day of whole-grain foods, such as whole wheat, oatmeal, popcorn, bulgur, and brown rice, is the goal.

Nonfat and Low-Fat Milk and Milk Products   Milk and milk products provide at least 12 nutrients including calcium, magnesium, potassium, and vitamin D. Drinking 3 cups or the equivalent of milk daily can improve bone mass and may help weight maintenance.

Three cups of milk or the equivalent in milk products per day is recommended when consuming 1,600 or more calories a day. Nonfat and low-fat milk products contain very little solid fat and are very nutrient dense. Lactose-free milk or yogurt are nutrient dense as well.

Choose and Prepare Foods With Little Salt

Reducing salt (sodium chloride) intake can lower blood pressure. Bringing blood pressure to a normal range reduces one's risk of developing a stroke, heart attack, heart failure, or kidney disease. The relationship between salt intake and blood pressure is real and progressive without an apparent threshold. The higher a person's salt intake, the higher his or her blood pressure. A potassium-rich diet lowers blood pressure and blunts the effects of salt on blood pressure, and may reduce the risk of developing kidney stones or losing bone mass.

Most US adults consume too much salt frequently from processed foods. The goal is to consume < 2,300 mg of sodium per day, which can be checked for foods on the nutrition facts labels. Individuals with hypertension, blacks, and other adults benefit from lower sodium intake.

Fruits, vegetables, and most milk products are available in a variety of foods with low sodium and high potassium content.

If You Drink Alcoholic Beverages, Do So in Moderation

For middle-aged and older adults, the lowest all-cause death rate occurs at the level of 1 to 2 drinks per day. Moderate alcohol intake may be protective, especially for males older than age 45 years and women older than age 55 years. Alcohol use among young adults is associated with an increased risk of traumatic injury and death and provides little health benefit. Heavy drinking is very hazardous, contributing to automobile injuries and deaths, assault, liver disease, and other health problems. Abstention is an important option.

Moderation is defined as the consumption of up to 1 drink per day for women and 2 drinks per day for men. One drink is defined as 12 ounces of regular beer, 5 ounces of wine (12% alcohol), or 1.5 ounces of 80-proof distilled spirits.

Individuals who should not consume alcoholic beverages are those who cannot restrict their drinking to moderate levels, children, and adolescents. Some medications interact with alcohol and may be harmful. Women who may become pregnant or who are pregnant or breastfeeding should not drink. Driving or participating in activities that require attention, skill, or coordination should not be linked to drinking alcohol.

Keep Food Safe to Eat

Food-borne diseases cause approximately 76 million illnesses, 325,000 hospitalizations, and 5,000 deaths in the United States annually. Three pathogens (salmonella, listeria, and toxoplasma) are responsible for more than 75% of these deaths. Behaviors in the home that can prevent a problem with food-borne illnesses are:

- washing hands, contact surfaces, and fruits and vegetables
- separating raw, cooked, and ready-to-eat foods while shopping, preparing, or storing
- cooking foods to a safe temperature
- refrigerating perishable foods promptly
- reheating high-risk foods like deli meats and frankfurters, which may contain listeria. This is especially important for high-risk groups like infants, children, seniors, pregnant women, and those who are immuno-compromised.

New Improved Eating Patterns

Many dietary and physical activity factors influence the risk of chronic disease. The USDA recommends eating patterns that are high in fruits and vegetables, whole grains, and nonfat or low-fat milk products (consistent with recommended nutrient intakes and reducing the risk of chronic disease), and that are low in saturated fat, cholesterol, added sugars, trans fat, and sodium.

Including at least 30 minutes of moderate physical activity a day would offset excess calories, reducing the chance of weight gain.

Dealing With Health Disparities and Contributions of the Environment

Social changes and educational efforts are required to facilitate healthy eating patterns and lifestyles among racial and ethnic minorities and the economically disadvantaged. Environmental influences are often beyond the control of individuals, e.g., the large size of portions served by many food establishments, lack of information on calorie content at point of purchase, the high amount of sodium in the food supply, the trans fatty acid content of many ready-to-eat foods, the cost and availability of fruits and vegetables, and opportunities for safe and enjoyable physical activity. Positive changes could make a substantial difference in whether individuals follow the 2005 *Dietary Guidelines for Americans*.

In the 2005 DGAs, for the first time, the amount of fruits and vegetables recommended is more than *any other food group*. Proportionally, the amount is about *half the plate*. Why? The DGA advisory committee

1. identified a critical nutrient gap for potassium, fiber, magnesium, and vitamins A and C and the fruits and vegetables rich in each nutrient.
2. established a stronger role for fruits and vegetables in helping fight heart disease, high blood pressure, type 2 diabetes, stroke, and cancer.
3. established a role for fruits and vegetables in helping people lose weight or maintain a healthy weight.

US Eating Profile

US adults consume about 36% of their total calories from fat and about 13% of calories from saturated fat. At the same time that obesity is widespread, stunted growth is seen in more than 10% of young, low-income children. In 1985, US adult men consumed about 18 grams of dietary fiber, and women

19 to 50 years old consumed about 12 grams. This is only one half the amount recommended by the National Cancer Institute to reduce the risk for some types of cancer.

Approximately 9% of the total population consumes more than 2 alcoholic beverages each day. Low calcium intake is common for women and presents a special concern because the median daily intake is well below the recommended dietary allowances (RDAs).[5] For low-income women and children, a reduction in iron deficiency anemia remains a priority.

There are other broad-based nutrition concerns, but data are currently unavailable for some special groups at an increased nutritional risk. These concerns include the nutritional status of individuals in hospitals, nursing homes, and convalescent centers. The concerns extend to the physically, mentally, and developmentally disabled individuals in community settings; children with stunted growth; children in child care facilities; Native Americans on reservations; populations in correctional facilities; and the homeless. Additional data are also needed on the old (i.e., 75-84 years), oldest old (i.e., 85 years and older), and Americans living alone.

No national database exists for individuals with eating disorders such as anorexia nervosa and bulimia. Hunger is a major societal issue, but definitions of and measurements for hunger status are still evolving (see Chapter 4). Nutrition fraud has increased greatly due to increasing interest in diet and health. The costs, uses, and harms caused by fraud warrant a more careful assessment and monitoring.

With this canvas existing in the United States, *Healthy People 2010* is a guide for healthcare practice. Alliances with other health organizations, such as the Dietary Guidelines Alliance; industry partnerships, such as the ADA/ConAgra food safety campaign; and working groups with government agencies, such as the Partnership for Healthy Weight Management, enable experts to discuss the issues, find partners, and offer solutions to improve Americans' health. See the *Healthy People 2010* Web site at www.health.gov/healthypeople.[6]

All Americans must get involved, not just by personally adopting healthy behaviors but by participating in community and group action. The National Heart, Lung, and Blood Institute (NHLBI) and the Centers for Disease Control and Prevention lead the *Healthy People 2010* effort against heart disease and stroke. NHLBI has set 2 priorities—ending health disparities and using health information targeting specific needs of communities. Community-based enhanced dissemination and utilization centers exist in communities at high risk for cardiovascular disease (CVD).[7]

Healthy People 2010 objectives relevant to the chapters in this book are written at the end of each chapter, beginning with this chapter.

Food Guidance

Since the 1940s, food guidance for healthy eating has concentrated on grouping foods and recommending serving sizes and the number of servings needed for nutrient adequacy. Government guidance systems have included the Seven Food Group plan and now the Food Guide Pyramid. Each of these blueprints has met with debate during development. Advocates, nutritionists, and researchers have interacted with government agencies to improve the eating guides prior to their use.

The Food Guide Pyramid

The Food Guide Pyramid (FGP) was born, died, and born again. Political and nonpolitical groups battle to identify the most appropriate food groups—and names of the groups—to fill the pyramid.

The 2005 FGP outlines graphically what to eat each day (see Figure 2–2), from 5 major food groups, each represented as an individual section of the

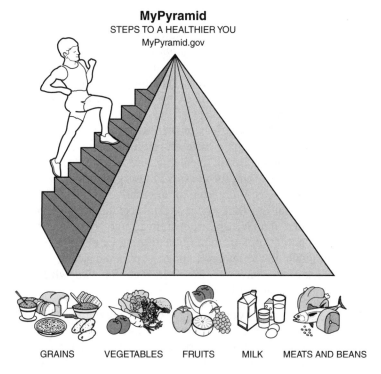

MyPyramid
STEPS TO A HEALTHIER YOU
MyPyramid.gov

GRAINS   VEGETABLES   FRUITS   MILK   MEATS AND BEANS

GRAINS Make half your grains whole	VEGETABLES Vary your veggies	FRUITS Focus on fruits	MILK Get your calcium-rich foods	MEATS AND BEANS Go lean with protein
Eat at least 3 oz. of whole-grain cereals, breads, crackers, rice, or pasta every day 1 oz. is about 1 slice of bread, about 1 cup of breakfast cereal or 1/2 cup of cooked rice, cereal, or pasta	Eat more dark-green veggies like broccoli, spinach, and other dark leafy greens Eat more orange vegetables like carrots and sweet potatoes Eat more dry beans and peas like pinto beans, kidney beans, and lentils	Eat a variety of fruit Choose fresh, frozen, canned, or dried fruit Go easy on fruit juices	Go low-fat or fat-free when you choose milk, yogurt, and other milk products If you don't or can't consume milk, choose lactose-free products or other calcium sources such as fortified foods and beverages	Choose low-fat or lean meats and poultry Bake it, broil it, or grill it Vary your protein routine—choose more fish, beans, peas, nuts, and seeds
For a 2,000-calorie diet, you need the amounts below from each food group. To find the amounts that are right for you, go to MyPyramid.gov.				
Eat 6 oz. every day	Eat 2 1/2 cups every day	Eat 2 cups every day	Eat 3 cups every day for kids aged 2 to 8 it's 2	Eat 5 1/2 oz. every day

Find your balance between food and physical activity
• Be sure to stay within your daily calorie needs.
• Be physically active for at least 30 minutes most days of the week.
• About 60 minutes a day of physical activity may be needed to prevent weight gain.
• For sustaining weight loss at least 60 to 90 minutes a day of physical activity may be required.
• Children and teenagers should be physically active for 60 minutes every day, or most days.

Know the limits on fats, sugars, and salt (sodium)
• Make most of your fat sources from fish, nuts, and vegetable oils.
• Limit solid fats like butter, stick margarine, shortening, and lard as well as foods that contain these.
• Check the Nutrition Facts label to keep saturated fats, *trans* fats, and sodium low.
• Choose food and beverages low in added sugars. Added sugars contribute calories with few, if any, nutrients.

FIGURE 2–2   MyPyramid.
Source: US Department of Agriculture, Center for Nutrition Policy and Promotion; April 2005.

pyramid, beginning with grains, then vegetables and fruits as 2 distinct groups, milk, then meat and beans.[8] The number of servings recommended from each group is based on the number of calories an individual needs. See www.mypyramid.gov.

MyPyramid assigns individuals to a calorie level based on sex, age, and activity level. Table 2-2 outlines the calorie levels for males and females by age and activity level. Calorie levels are provided for each year of childhood from 2-18 years, and for adults in 5-year increments. The *MyPyramid Food Guidance System Education Framework* is available and provides specific recommendations for making food choices that will improve the quality of an average American diet. Materials for professionals on the Web site include *Food Intake Patterns, Education Framework,* and a glossary.

Key terms in the glossary include: discretionary calorie allowance, estimated energy requirement, sedentary behavior, moderate physical activity, and vigorous physical activity. See *High Definition Nutrition* at the beginning of this chapter.

Several alternatives to the FGP have been developing. One of the most popular represents a different opinion represented by professionals in the fields of public health, medicine, and nutrition.

In June 1994, the Oldways Preservation and Exchange Trust, in Boston, Massachusetts, introduced an alternative to the FGP–the Traditional Healthy Mediterranean Diet Pyramid. The Exchange Trust joined the World Health Organization (WHO) European Regional Office, the WHO, and the Food and Agriculture Organization Collaborating Center in Nutrition at Harvard School of Public Health in developing the pyramid. This pyramid is accompanied by a list of 10 characteristics of the diet and acknowledges the need for further research and consideration[9]:

1. **Maintain your healthy weight**—Individuals gain weight if consuming more calories than they burn. Everyone should balance calories in with calories out. Each person should learn their healthy weight range and body mass index (BMI), and stay within these. Individuals should drink 8 glasses of water a day to assist all the body's systems and help maintain energy at a good level.

2. **Eat a variety of foods good for you**—Common sense about eating translates to eating foods that are good for individuals and avoiding foods that are not. Empty-calorie foods should be avoided.

3. **Eat more whole grains**—Whole grains contain fiber and many important nutrients.

4. **Eat more fruits and vegetables**—Nutrients and antioxidants in fruits and vegetables, especially if they are fresh, can protect individuals against life-limiting and crippling diseases.

5. **Reduce your saturated fats and cholesterol**—Poultry and fish have less saturated fats and cholesterol than red meat. Too much saturated fat and cholesterol are not good for the heart or blood vessels. Skim milk and reduced-fat cheese and yogurt are low in fat and cholesterol and also contain calcium.

6. **Increase your use of vegetable oils and plant oils**—Vegetable and plant oils contain monounsaturated and polyunsaturated fats, or the 'good fats,' and no cholesterol. Unrefined vegetable and plant oils contain valuable antioxidants.

TABLE 2–2 MyPyramid Food Intake Pattern Calorie Levels

MyPyramid assigns individuals to a calorie level based on their sex, age, and activity level.
The chart below identifies the calorie levels for males and females by age and activity level. Calorie levels are provided for each year of childhood, from 2-18 years, and for adults in 5-year increments.

Activity level	Males			Activity level	Females		
Age	Sedentary*	Mod. active*	Active*	Age	Sedentary*	Mod. active*	Active*
2	1,000	1,000	1,000	2	1,000	1,000	1,000
3	1,000	1,400	1,400	3	1,000	1,200	1,400
4	1,200	1,400	1,600	4	1,200	1,400	1,400
5	1,200	1,400	1,600	5	1,200	1,400	1,600
6	1,400	1,600	1,800	6	1,200	1,400	1,600
7	1,400	1,600	1,800	7	1,200	1,600	1,800
8	1,400	1,600	2,000	8	1,400	1,600	1,800
9	1,600	1,800	2,000	9	1,400	1,600	1,800
10	1,600	1,800	2,200	10	1,400	1,800	2,000
11	1,800	2,000	2,200	11	1,600	1,800	2,000
12	1,800	2,200	2,400	12	1,600	2,000	2,200
13	2,000	2,200	2,600	13	1,600	2,000	2,200
14	2,000	2,400	2,800	14	1,800	2,000	2,400
15	2,200	2,600	3,000	15	1,800	2,000	2,400
16	2,400	2,800	3,200	16	1,800	2,000	2,400
17	2,400	2,800	3,200	17	1,800	2,000	2,400
18	2,400	2,800	3,200	18	1,800	2,000	2,400

continued

TABLE 2-2 continued

Males				Females			
Activity level	Sedentary*	Mod. active*	Active*	Activity level	Sedentary*	Mod. active*	Active*
Age				Age			
19-20	2,600	2,800	3,000	19-20	2,000	2,200	2,400
21-25	2,400	2,800	3,000	21-25	2,000	2,200	2,400
26-30	2,400	2,600	3,000	26-30	1,800	2,000	2,400
31-35	2,400	2,600	3,000	31-35	1,800	2,000	2,200
36-40	2,400	2,600	2,800	36-40	1,800	2,000	2,200
41-45	2,200	2,600	2,800	41-45	1,800	2,000	2,200
46-50	2,200	2,400	2,800	46-50	1,800	2,000	2,200
51-55	2,200	2,400	2,800	51-55	1,600	1,800	2,200
56-60	2,200	2,400	2,600	56-60	1,600	1,800	2,200
61-65	2,000	2,400	2,600	61-65	1,600	1,800	2,000
66-70	2,000	2,200	2,600	66-70	1,600	1,800	2,000
71-75	2,000	2,200	2,600	71-75	1,600	1,800	2,000
76 and up	2,000	2,200	2,400	76 and up	1,600	1,800	2,000

*Calorie levels are based on the estimated energy requirements (EER) and activity levels from the Institute of Medicine Dietary Reference Intakes Macronutrients Report, 2002. Sedentary = less than 30 minutes a day of moderate physical activity in addition to daily activities; Mod. active = at least 30 minutes and up to 60 minutes a day of moderate physical activity in addition to daily activities; Active = 60 or more minutes a day of moderate physical activity in addition to daily activities.

Source: United States Department of Agriculture, Center for Nutrition Policy and Promotion; April 2005. CNPP-XX

7. **Avoid heavy use of salt and sugar**—Invisible to the eye, dissolved salt and sugar are found in foods and drinks, and when consumed in excess, are not good for overall health.

8. **For your snacks, eat fruits, peanuts, and nuts**—Moderate amounts of fresh and dried fruits, nuts, and peanuts are acceptable if not mixed with sugar, salt, preservatives, and hydrogenated fats and oils.

9. **If you drink alcoholic beverages, do so in moderation**—Moderate drinking improves health for most adults, unless they are at risk for chronic disease. Drinking with meals rather than on an empty stomach and including wines over other alcoholic beverages due to the antioxidants content is best.

10. **Be physically active every day**—Physical activity benefits overall health by its role on weight maintenance and heart health. Any kind of physical activity is better than being inactive and sedentary.

Current scientific evidence shows positive health effects from eating foods that are high in fruits, vegetables, legumes, and whole grains, while including fish, nuts, and low-fat dairy products. This eating pattern needs no total fat restriction if there are no excess calories and if the fats are predominantly vegetable oils low in saturated fats and partially hydrogenated oils. The traditional Mediterranean diet with olive oil as the principal source of fat fits this eating plan.[10] The Mediterranean diet has a specific meaning because it reflects food patterns typical of some Mediterranean regions in the early 1960s, such as Crete, parts of the rest of Greece, and southern Italy. The Mediterranean diet of the early 1960s:

- was abundant in plant foods such as fruit, vegetables, breads, cereals, potatoes, beans, nuts, and seeds;
- was minimally processed, and had seasonally fresh and locally grown foods;
- had fresh fruit as the common daily dessert and restricted sweets with concentrated sugars or honey to a few times per week;
- recommended olive oil as the principal source of fat;
- was low in saturated fat at ≤ 7-8% of energy
- included total fat that ranged from < 25% to 35% of energy and recommended:
  - dairy products, primarily cheese and yogurt daily in small amounts;
  - fish and poultry in low to moderate amounts;
  - 0-4 eggs weekly;
  - red meat in small amounts; and
  - wine in low to moderate amounts, normally with meals.

A lifestyle complementing this eating pattern includes regular physical activity and is practiced generally by adults with less obesity than rates observed in the United States (Exhibit 2–4).[10]

Eating Habits of American Families

What do Americans eat? How do they make their food selections? How can we monitor the food habits and nutrient intakes of US residents using epidemiologic techniques?

Exhibit 2–4   Issues Forming the Basics of the Mediterranean-Style Diet

A. Heart Disease
- Dietary factors important in preventing atherosclerosis:
  1. Substantial reduction of saturated fat.
  2. Substitution of saturated fats by unsaturated fats, preferably monounsaturated fats and oils.
  3. Consumption of fish.
  4. Increased consumption of vegetables, fruits, and whole grains.
- Possible mechanisms by which dietary factors decrease the risk of coronary heart disease:
  1. Improvement in the blood lipid profile (lowering LDL cholesterol and triglycerides while increasing or maintaining HDL cholesterol).
  2. Decrease oxidation of lipids.
  3. Decrease risk for atherothrombosis.
  4. Improvement in endothelial function.
  5. Improvement in insulin resistance.
  6. Decrease in ventricular irritability (lowering the risk of sudden death).
  7. Decrease in inflammation.
  8. Reduction in plasma homocysteine concentrations.

B. Diabetes
- Principal message is: "Control weight, increase physical activity, and reduce sedentary behavior."
- High-carbohydrate diets based on minimally processed cereal grains, vegetables, and fruits, and high in fiber can improve blood glucose and the lipid profile.
- The same beneficial effects can be achieved by using vegetable oils that are predominantly monounsaturated along with the foods listed above.

C. Obesity
- Obesity is primarily a disorder of energy balance.
- Obesity increases the risk of many diseases including diabetes, heart disease, hypertension, dyslipidemias, and certain cancers.
- Obesity is a common and increasing public health problem in both developed and developing countries.
- Although data are limited in population studies, no strong association has been demonstrated between dietary fat and body fatness.
- Obesity can be prevented and controlled by balancing energy intake and energy expenditure through a healthy diet and regular physical activity.
- The Mediterranean diet, though not a low-fat diet, may contribute to the prevention and treatment of obesity because of its variety and palatability, provided it is controlled in calories.

D. Cancer
There is substantial and consistent evidence that diets rich in vegetables, fruit, and whole grains reduce risk of cancer.
- Colon cancer
  1. Total fat is probably unrelated.
  2. Saturated fat may increase risk.
  3. Olive oil and marine oils may decrease risk.
  4. Antioxidants and phytosterols may decrease risk.
  5. Disagreement exists regarding the strength of the association of red meat with increased risk.

Exhibit 2–4 continued

- Breast cancer
  1. Total fat intakes in the range of 20-40% of energy are not related.
  2. Monounsaturated fats and olive oil may decrease risk.
- Prostate cancer
  Evidence exists regarding an association between intake of saturated fat and risk of prostate cancer.

E. Alcohol
- Wine is part of the traditional diet in much of the Mediterranean region, where it is the usual mealtime beverage. Light-to-moderate intake of wine and other alcoholic beverages reduces the risk of coronary heart disease and ischemic stroke by 30% or more, and it is usually associated with a reduction in all-cause mortality.
- There is less consensus on whether wine has advantages over other types of alcoholic beverages in the prevention of cardiovascular disease, as wine drinkers often have other healthy lifestyle habits that may contribute to the added protection against heart disease. Phenolics and other nonalcoholic substances in wine are well demonstrated to be powerful antioxidants and have many potentially important health effects.
- The beneficial health effects of alcohol are primarily on the risk of chronic diseases of middle-aged and elderly people.
- Consider the adverse health and societal effects of excessive or irresponsible alcohol consumption. Excessive intake of alcohol increases the risk of many cancers, especially upper aero-digestive tract cancers, and many studies indicate a slight increase in breast cancer risk even for small amounts of alcohol. Alcohol consumption is not recommended for individuals with a past history of alcohol abuse, with liver disease, or with certain other medical conditions, or for those who choose not to drink because of religious, ethical, or other reasons.

F. Antioxidants
- The Mediterranean diet contains an important amount of antioxidants: vitamins E and C, carotenoids, and various polyphenol compounds. These antioxidants are present in vegetables, fruits, nuts, whole grains, legumes, virgin olive oil, and wine.
- When absorbed, antioxidants may play an important role in the prevention of cardiovascular disease, cancer, and aging.

G. Gene/Environment Interaction
- Coronary heart disease, diabetes, cancer, hypertension, and obesity have a significant genetic predisposition.
- Higher genetic risk can be modulated by environmental factors, mainly dietary habits.
- Continuing knowledge of these genetic factors and their interaction with other foods may provide a more precise and personalized approach to preventing and treating chronic disease.

Source: Adapted from Oldways' 2000 consensus statement: dietary fat, the Mediterranean diet, and lifelong good health from the 2000 International Conference on the Mediterranean Diet; January 13-14, 2000; London, England, UK.

A national survey of 1,000 representative adults responded to a telephone interview about their families' food practices and eating habits. The study was conducted by the Food Marketing Institute and *Prevention* magazine. Respondents had primary or equally shared responsibility for food shopping for their households. A stratified, random-digit dialing was used to avoid listing bias. The number of telephone numbers randomly sampled from within a county was proportional to the county's share of telephone households in the state. Four attempts were made to complete each interview.[11]

The final sample was 27% male and 73% female; 37% were 25 to 39 years old, 20% were 40 to 49 years old, 20% were 50 to 64 years old, 9% were younger than 25, and 12% were over 64 years old. Of the respondents, 38% were high school graduates and another 29% were college graduates. Regarding income, 33% earned $25,000 or less, and 21% earned more than $50,000.

A brief summary of results[11] reveals the following:

1. Of shoppers, 45% say they have changed a food-buying decision in the last month because they read the food label.
2. Nearly 50% agree that they are concerned about fat but uncertain how to cut back on fat.
3. Of the respondents, 26% have high-fat foods (e.g., hamburger, bacon, chicken with skin, or eggs) at least 1 time a day; an additional 7% have them 15 or more times each week.
4. African Americans are much more likely than whites to consume high-fat meats; 60% have unhealthy eating patterns compared with 29% of whites.
5. Of the respondents, 60% report that a major change occurred in their eating habits during the past 10 years due to health.
6. Changes in eating patterns are more common among women over 40 years old and among more affluent consumers.
7. The most common changes are lowering fat (63%) and increasing fruit and vegetable intake (30%).
8. Overweight shoppers have particular concerns about obesity, high cholesterol, and hypertension.
9. African Americans are more motivated than whites to change food patterns due to high blood pressure rather than to heart disease.

Info Line

The 1995 Food Marketing Institute and *Prevention* magazine survey included a special oversampling of 500 African-American shoppers to contrast their views with eating habits of the total sample. The major findings were: (1) these shoppers were not different in trying to make healthful changes; (2) they experienced a higher level of confusion and frustration when making choices; (3) they were more likely to make poor food choices; and (4) they had unhealthy eating patterns more often.

For further information contact The Research Department, Food Marketing Institute, 800 Connecticut Avenue NW, Washington, DC 20008.

10. Only 20% of respondents believe their eating pattern is healthy, and only 7% consider it as healthy as possible.

11. Of the respondents, 69% are overweight (i.e., over their recommended weight using Metropolitan Life Insurance Company tables). Of 18- to 39-year-olds, 57% are overweight, and of respondents 40 years and older, 79% are overweight.

12. Over one third of those who are heavy believe they are within the proper weight range.

13. Of the respondents, 43% report regular, strenuous exercise; fewer than 1 in 10 spent time in the hospital the prior year.

How Do Consumers Think?

Analysis of focus group data regarding 5 a day fruits and vegetables shows several dominant concepts[12]:

Consumers seek moderation, not transformation. They want to eat better, not perfectly. Eating more fruits and vegetables can frequently mean "substitute for..." or "cut down on..." something else, usually red meat, high-fat foods, candy bars, potato chips, or junk food. Nutrition and health are on the consumer's agenda, but not at the top.

Price, taste, and convenience are both benefits and barriers. Good prices, taste, and convenience are benefits of buying and eating fruits and vegetables, yet men and women complain about texture, flavor, availability, and time to prepare them. Taste alone is not sufficient for increased consumption.

Women see a moral aspect of food and eating right. If one knows what is good for health, then one should strive to eat those foods.

Info Line

Dietary Guidelines for Americans 2005 is published jointly by the US Departments of Health and Human Services and Agriculture. Visit this Web site: http://www.healthierus.gov/dietaryguidelines/.

A new set of RDAs and tolerable safe upper limits of antioxidant nutrients was released by the Food and Nutrition Board of the Institute of Medicine on April 11, 2000. The recommendations include vitamins E and C and selenium, and describe the research known about nutrients' interactions in the body and their role in disease. Visit this Web site: http://www.nap.edu/books/0309069351/html/.

To substantiate claims about some common dietary supplements, the National Center for Complementary and Alternative Medicine (NCCAM) began a clinical trial on *Ginkgo biloba* in 2000. Over 3,000 men and women over 75 years old were given either 240 mg of *Ginkgo* or a placebo over the next 5 years. The purpose was to determine if *Ginkgo* can prevent the onset of dementia, including Alzheimer's disease. Studies including St John's wort, glucosamine, and chondroitin are planned. Visit this Web site: http://nccam.nih.gov.

Most consumers do not count their daily servings of fruits and vegetables, do not know how to count servings, and do not want to count. In a focus group setting, only 2 of 90 participants in 1 study counted servings because they were on a weight control program.

Favorite concepts were:

Eating 5 or more servings of fruits and vegetables a day to keep you going and not weigh you down. This concept often has the most impact of any concepts presented to consumers because it reflects their experience of preferring a light feeling with fruits and vegetables to the sluggish feeling they have when they eat high-fat or heavy meals. It may reflect the common experience of keeping up one's energy level throughout the day.

Eating 5 or more servings of fruits and vegetables is an easy way to improve my health. Although people like easy ways to prepare, serve, and carry vegetables, many are not convinced that eating 5 servings a day is easy. Health is generally viewed as a general feeling rather than avoidance of diseases.

Surveillance and Monitoring

The National Nutrition Monitoring and Related Research (NNMRR) Act (Public Law 101–445) became law on October 22, 1990, to provide timely data about food and nutrient intake and the resulting nutritional status of the public.[13]

Lack of timely nutrition data has been a persistent problem when program planners and decision makers are at the discussion and planning table. One outcome is that decisions are often made on assumptions and insufficient information. The real problems may not be addressed. Even though goals may be achieved, they may likely fall short of addressing the major problems. Nutrition data that are accurate and current are essential.

Five measurement elements spearhead the monitoring and research activities. They are as follows:

1. nutrition and health-related assessment
2. food and nutrient intake
3. knowledge, attitude, and behavior measures
4. databases about nutrients and composition of foods
5. adequacy and quality of food supply

Over 45 surveys and surveillance systems comprised the nutrition monitoring effort in the United States between 1992 and today.[14] Table 2–3 details select nutrition and health-related assessments. Food and nutrient intakes are monitored in various surveys outlined in Table 2–4. For the decade 1992 to 2002, 7 surveys documented knowledge, attitudes, and behaviors (see Table 2–5). Surveys related to nutrient databases are listed in Table 2–6. Two surveys determine adequacy and quality of the food supply: (1) the Annual Fisheries of the US, and (2) the Annual US Food and Nutrition Supply Series—Estimate of Food Available and Nutrients.[14]

Title I of the NNMRR Act established a 22-member agency board. The secretaries and undersecretaries of the US Department of Agriculture (USDA) and the US Department of Health and Human Services (DHHS) serve as chairpersons

TABLE 2-3 Nutrition and Related Health Assessments, 1992-2002

Date	Survey	Target	Department	Agency
Continuous	National Health and Nutrition Examination Survey (NHANES)	US noninstitutionalized, civilian population, aged 2 months or older; oversampling of blacks and Mexican Americans, children up to age 5 years, and individuals aged 60 years and older	DHHS	CDC/NCHS
1988-1994	NHANES III Supplemental Nutrition Survey of Older Persons	Individuals aged 50 years and older examined in NHANES III, in households with telephones	DHHS	CDC/NCHS, NIH/NIA
1991-1992	Navajo Health and Nutrition Survey	Persons aged 12 years and older residing on or near the Navajo reservation in Arizona, New Mexico, and Utah	DHHS	IHS
1992	National Home and Hospice Care Survey	A sample of home health agencies and hospices along with a subsample of patients	DHHS	CDC/NCHS
1992	NHANES I Epidemiologic Follow-up Survey	Individuals examined in NHANES I who were 25-74 years old at baseline	DHHS	CDC/NCHS
1992	NHIS on Cancer Epidemiology and Cancer Control	Individuals aged 18 years and older	DHHS	CDC/NCHS, NIH/NCI
Annual	National Health Interview Survey (NHIS)	Civilian, noninstitutionalized individuals	DHHS	CDC/NCHS
Annual	National Hospital Discharge Survey	Discharges from nonfederal, general, and short-stay specialty hospitals	DHHS	CDC/NCHS
Continuous	Vital Statistics Program	Total US population	DHHS	CDC/NCHS
Continuous	Pregnancy Nutrition Surveillance System	Low-income, high-risk, pregnant women	DHHS	CDC/NCCDPHP
Continuous	Pediatric Nutrition	Low-income, high-risk children	DHHS	CDC/NCCDPHP
Annual	National Ambulatory Medical Care Survey Surveillance System	Office visits to nonfederal, office-based physicians from birth to 17 years	DHHS	CDC/NCHS

continued

TABLE 2–3 continued

Date	Survey	Target	Department	Agency
Continuous	NHANES II Mortality Follow-up Survey	Individuals examined in NHANES II who were 35-75 years old at baseline	DHHS	CDC/NCHS
1992 Began continuous	Hispanic HANES (HHANES) Mortality Follow-up Survey	Individuals interviewed in HHANES who were 20-74 years old at baseline	DHHS	CDC/NCHS
Annual	National Hospital Ambulatory Medical Care Survey	Visits to hospital emergency and outpatient departments of nonfederal, short-stay, general, and specialty hospitals	DHHS	CDC/NCHS
Continuous	NHANES III Longitudinal Follow-up Survey	Individuals interviewed and examined in NHANES III who were aged 20 years or older at baseline	DHHS	CDC/NCHS
1993	National Mortality Follow-up Survey	Individuals aged 25 years and older	DHHS	CDC/NCHS
1994	National Survey of Family Growth	Women aged 15 to 44 years	DHHS	NCHS
Continuous	Adult Nutrition Surveillance System	Adults aged 18 years and older who were participating in local public health programs	DHHS	CDC/NCCDPHP
1995	NHIS on Health Promotion/ Disease Prevention	Individuals aged 18 years and older	DHHS	CDC/NCHS
1995	NHANES I Epidemiologic Follow-up Study	Individuals examined in NHANES I who were 55 to 74 years old at baseline	DHHS	CDC/NCHS

DHHS = US Department of Health and Human Services; CDC = Centers for Disease Control and Prevention; NCHS = National Center for Health Statistics; NIH = National Institutes of Health; NIA = National Institute on Aging; IHS = Indian Health Service; NCI = National Cancer Institute; NCCDPHP = National Center for Chronic Disease Prevention and Health Promotion.
Source: Adapted from: Kuczmarski MF, Moshfegh A, Briefel R. Update on nutrition monitoring activities in the US. *J Am Diet Assoc.* 1994;94:753-760. Used with permission of the American Dietetic Association.

TABLE 2–4 Food and Nutrient Intake, 1992-2002

Date	Survey	Target	Department	Agency
1988-1994	NHANES III and NHANES III Supplemental Nutrition Survey of Older Persons	Representative US population; elderly	DHHS	CDC/NCHS, NIH/NIA
1991-1992	Development of a National Seafood Consumption Survey Model	Individuals residing in eligible households and recreational/subsistence fishermen	DOC	NMFS/NOAA
1992	School Nutrition Dietary Assessment Study	School-aged children in grades 1 through 12	USDA	FNS
1992	School Food Authority Menu Modification Demonstration Projects	Students in elementary schools	USDA	FNS
1992	Adult Day Care Program Study	Adult day care centers and adults participating and not participating in the Child and Adult Care Food Program	USDA	FNS
Annual	Total Diet Study	Representative diets of specific age-sex groups	DHHS	FDA
Continuous	Nutritional Evaluation of Military Feeding Systems and Military Populations	Enlisted personnel of the US Army, Navy, Marine Corps, and Air Force	DOD	USARIEM
Continuous	Consumer Expenditure Survey	Civilian, noninstitutionalized population and a portion of the US institutionalized population	DOL	BLS
Continuous	Survey of Income and Program Participation	Civilian, noninstitutionalized US population	DOC	Census
1994-1996 (annual)	Continuing Survey of Food Intakes by Individuals (CSFII)	Individuals of all ages residing in eligible households nationwide; oversampling of individuals in low-income households	USDA	HNIS

continued

TABLE 2–4   continued

Date	Survey	Target	Department	Agency
Continuous	NHANES	US noninstitutionalized civilians	DHHS	CDC/NCHS
1997-1998	Household Food Consumption Survey	Civilian households and individuals residing in eligible households	USDA	HNIS
1997-1998	Low-Income Nationwide Food Consumption Survey	Low-income civilian households and individuals residing in eligible households	USDA	HNIS

DHHS = US Department of Health and Human Services; CDC = Centers for Disease Control and Prevention; NCHS = National Center for Health Statistics; NIH = National Institutes of Health; NIA = National Institute on Aging; DOC = US Department of Commerce; DOD = US Department of Defense; NMFS = National Marine Fisheries Service; NOAA = National Oceanic and Atmospheric Administration; USDA = US Department of Agriculture; FNS = Food and Nutrition Service; FDA = Food and Drug Administration; USARIEM = US Army Research Institute of Environmental Medicine; DOL = US Department of Labor; BLS = Bureau of Labor Statistics; HNIS = Human Nutrition Information Service.

Source: Adapted from: Kuczmarski MF, Moshfegh A, Briefel R. Update on nutrition monitoring activities in the US. *J Am Diet Assoc.* 1994;94:753-760. Used with permission of the American Dietetic Association.

TABLE 2–5 Knowledge, Attitude, and Behavior Measures, 1992-2002

Date	Survey	Target	Department	Agency
Biennial	Youth Risk Behavior Survey	Civilian, noninstitutionalized adolescents, aged 12 to 18 years	DHHS	CDC/NCCDPHP
1992	Infant Feeding Practices Survey	New mothers and healthy, full-term infants from birth to 1 year old	DHHS	FDA
1992	Consumer Food Handling Practices and Awareness of Microbiological Hazards Screener	Individuals aged 18 years and older in households with telephones	DHHS	FDA
1992	NHIS on Youth Risk Behavior	Civilian, noninstitutionalized adolescents, aged 12 to 21 years	DHHS	CDC/NCHS CDC/NCCDPHP
Continuous	Behavioral Risk Factor Surveillance System	Individuals aged 18 years and older residing in participating states in households with telephones	DHHS	CDC/NCCDPHP
Biennial	Health and Diet Survey	Civilian, noninstitutionalized individuals aged 18 years and older in households with telephones	DHHS	FDA
1994-1996	Diet and Health Knowledge Survey	Selected adults aged 20 years and older in households and noninstitutionalized group quarters participating in the CSFII	USDA	HNIS

DHHS = US Department of Health and Human Services; CDC = Centers for Disease Control and Prevention; NCCDPHP = National Center for Chronic Disease Prevention and Health Promotion; FDA = Food and Drug Administration; USDA = US Department of Agriculture; NCHS = National Center for Health Statistics; HNIS = Human Nutrition Information Service; CSFII = Continuing Surveys of Food Intakes by Individuals.
Source: Adapted from: Kuczmarski MF, Moshfegh A, Briefel R. Update on nutrition monitoring activities in the US. *J Am Diet Assoc.* 1994;94:753-760. Used with permission of the American Dietetic Association.

TABLE 2–6   Nutrient Databases and Composition of Foods, 1992-2002

Date	Survey	Target	Department	Agency
Annual	Total Diet Study	Representative diets of specific age-sex groups	DHHS	FDA
Biennial	Food Label and Package Survey	NA	DHHS	FDA
Continuous	Langual	NA	DHHS	FDA
Continuous	National Nutrient Data Bank	NA	USDA	HNIS
Continuous	Survey Nutrient Data Base	NA	USDA	HNIS

NA = Not applicable; DHHS = US Department of Health and Human Services; FDA = Food and Drug Administration; HNIS = Human Nutrition Information Service; USDA = US Department of Agriculture.
Source: Adapted from: Kuczmarski MF, Moshfegh A, Briefel R. Update on nutrition monitoring activities in the US. *J Am Diet Assoc.* 1994;94:753-760. Used with permission of the American Dietetic Association.

to implement and to report to the US president and to Congress. Title II established the National Nutrition Monitoring Advisory Council with 9 nonfederal members who have expertise in public health, nutrition monitoring research, or food production and distribution. This group gives scientific and technical advice and evaluates the effectiveness of the program.[14]

A 10-year comprehensive plan is mandated by PL 101-445. National, state, and local objectives are required.[14] To assist with achievement of the national objectives, the comprehensive plan outlines activities for each of the 5 measurement elements. National objectives are as follows:

- ensure a comprehensive, continuous, and coordinated program
- improve comparability and quality of data
- strengthen the research base

The state and local objectives are as follows:

- improve capacity for complementary data collection
- create more sophisticated methods of promoting comparability of data across levels
- enhance the quality of monitoring data

Surveillance and data systems can support improvement of nutrition in the United States, but will they? The National Nutrition Monitoring System intends to provide timely detection and measurement of nutritional problems, dietary practices, and nutrition-related knowledge and behaviors. Data can be collected not only for the US population in general, but also for specific high-risk groups employing nutrition screening of groups or of an entire community.[15,16] One challenge is to ensure that national and state operational objectives are met. Enthusiastic and effective management must occur at both levels, as well as sufficient funding for staff, training, and the necessary technology.

The nutrient intakes and nutritional status of the US population are periodically documented by several surveys. The Ten State Nutrition Survey—the first comprehensive US survey—focused primarily on low-income populations in California, Kentucky, Louisiana, Massachusetts, Michigan, New York, South Carolina, Texas, Washington, and West Virginia. Documentation that children and adults were experiencing hunger and malnutrition provided an essential shot in the arm for nutrition surveillance. Serial surveys now include the National Health and Nutrition Examination Surveys (NHANES) conducted by the National Center for Health Statistics (NCHS) of the Centers for Disease Control and Prevention (CDC) and the Nationwide Food Consumption Surveys (NFCS). The NFCS include the Continuing Surveys of Food Intakes by Individuals (CSFII) conducted by the Human Nutrition Information Service (HNIS) of the USDA.

Information about nutrition and health status of specific population groups, consumer knowledge and behavior, and food and diet composition is provided by other data sources. These include the Pregnancy and the Pediatric Nutrition Surveillance Systems by the CDC, the National Health Interview Surveys (NHIS) by the NCHS, the Diet and Health Knowledge Survey by the HNIS/USDA, and the Total Diet Study and Health and Diet Surveys by the Food and Drug Administration (FDA). The Pediatric Nutrition Surveillance System includes every state and assesses growth retardation, nutrient deficiency, and extreme levels of anthropometric measures. The Pediatric Nutrition Surveillance System and the Behavioral Risk Factor and Youth Risk Behavior Surveillance Systems are also conducted by the CDC. The National Institutes of Health (NIH) and the Agricultural Research Service of the USDA provide the primary research base for these nutrition-monitoring activities.

The National Nutrition Monitoring System provides data at intervals to assess progress toward national nutrition objectives.[2] However, new data collection is needed to identify the nutritional status of several groups not

Info Line

The US Department of Health and Human Services's 2004 *E-Gov Annual Report* on December 6, 2004, illustrated its implementation of the E-Government Act and initiatives through research databases for consumers and professionals as well as activities to assure homeland security and managing domestic incidents. The US food supply could be a target. The Food and Drug Administration (FDA) Emergency Operations Network Incident Management System supports the agency's counterterrorism goals and provides a Web-based connection for all FDA offices and external stakeholders to share and discuss accurate real-time information about various incidents.

US President Bush's administrative office estimates $6.1 million as the cost of a human life. One incident of food-borne pathogens could kill individuals coming into contact with it. Assuming a potential annual incident directly or indirectly related could result in 10 deaths, the benefit of early preparedness, planning, and warning would be $61 million.

Source: US Department of Health and Human Services. *2004 E-Gov Annual Report.* December 6, 2004.

routinely surveyed. New survey methods that not only increase and refine the current epidemiologic database but also identify the relationships between dietary patterns and chronic diseases are needed. As the number and type of surveys increase to establish the surveillance system, consistent methods *must* be used. Governmental agencies must remain vigilant. Standardized, valid, and reliable assessment instruments and protocols are essential across all surveys, or analysts will be forced to adjust or correct data for comparison. One persistent question is whether surveillance provides the accurate, useful data needed to profile the nutritional status of American people.

The timeliness of the data is also an issue. Researchers are attempting to make all data more readily available at both the state and local levels for program planning, evaluation, and research policy formation. Important questions are: Will the data be available when they are needed for decision making? Will the data answer our future questions, or will we always be playing catch-up because no techniques currently provide online assessment? Are new methods or adaptations of established methods needed to meet the technology and state of the nutrition science for the 21st century?

Nationwide Food Consumption

USDA surveys are used to describe food consumption behavior and to assess the nutrient composition of eating patterns.[17] Findings influence policies relating to food production and marketing, food safety, food assistance, and nutrition education. As part of the National Nutrition Monitoring System, USDA monitors food and nutrient consumption at 3 levels[17]:

1. *Food available to the US civilian population (food supply or food disappearance):* Data on production, imports and exports, military use, and beginning and year-end inventories are aggregated to describe the US food supply. Per capita data are used with tables of food composition to estimate the nutrient intake of each individual. These data have been available since 1909.
2. *Food purchased and consumed by households:* Every 10 years the cost and amount of food consumed by households over a 7-day period are surveyed. The quantities of foods reported are converted to pounds and merged with nutrient composition to estimate household nutrient content.
3. *Individual food profile:* Every 10 years, a national survey is complemented with smaller, ongoing surveys to assess foods eaten at home and away from home. The individual food profile reflects actual food ingested and provides over 25 nutrient intakes most suitable for dietary assessment purposes, for example, total energy, protein, carbohydrate, total fat, carotenes, calcium, iron, folate, and sodium. The database was expanded to provide fatty acid, antioxidant, B-vitamin, and mineral data of increasing scientific interest.[18,19]

Data from the household and individual food profiles comprise the USDA Nationwide Food Consumption Surveys. With each new but recurrent survey, various steps are taken to create a timely description of US food patterns.[17,20] These steps include the following:

A review is conducted to establish why the USDA needs the data and how the data are used by other federal agencies, food industry analysts, nutrition specialists, home economists, agricultural economists, state and local governments, and academicians. Exhibit 2–5 identifies potential uses of the data.

A review and evaluation of food consumption and related surveys conducted by the USDA, federal departments, states, and the private sector are completed.

Definitions, questions, and assumptions used previously (e.g., in Nationwide Food Consumption Surveys or the National Health and Nutrition Examination Surveys) are reviewed to improve comparability and linkages across surveys.

Methodological studies are reviewed to identify procedures appropriate for large national surveys and to demonstrate techniques for improved validity and reliability, such as whether to increase the number and quality of 24-hour dietary recalls per respondent. Because the 24-hour recall is commonly used, the trend is to collect multiple days of dietary data to accurately assess usual food intake. The rationale is:

- to estimate interindividual and intraindividual variability
- to estimate an individual's usual eating patterns, including amount and type of foods consumed

Exhibit 2–5   Potential Applications for Data From Nationwide Food Consumption Surveys

Dietary Intake Profiles
- Provide baseline data on food and nutrient intake of the population.
- Monitor the nutritional content of eating patterns.
- Project the size and nature of high-risk populations.
- Identify intervention (food assistance, fortification, or education) most appropriate for populations at risk.
- Identify socioeconomic factors associated with diets.

Economics of Food Intake
- Determine agricultural product, marketing facility, and service needs.
- Define the interplay of socioeconomic factors on the food demand and cost.
- Establish the importance of home gardens.
- Identify frequency and outcome of eating out.

Food Programs and Guidance
- Specify factors and the effect of participation in entitlement food programs on food cost and quality.
- Determine the effect of entitlement programs on food needs and requests.
- Select nutritional high-risk populations.
- Monitor the effect of eating pattern changes on health risk.
- Develop realistic food plans that address food preferences, dislikes, and restricted incomes.
- Enumerate adequate and practical amounts of foods for food entitlement programs.

Exhibit 2–5   continued

Food Safety Considerations
- Quantify intake of contaminants, additives, and natural toxic substances in foods.
- Identify extraordinary eating patterns that include additives and other specific components.
- Recommend foods that might serve as suitable substrates for additives.
- Monitor food regulations and suggest changes.
- Determine the exposure or contact with certain foods and food products that increase one's nutritional risk.

Historical Trends
- Analyze the association between food intake, nutrient profile, and disease prevalence and incidence.
- Track food intake patterns from birth to elder ages.
- Forecast food intake and nutrient profiles resulting from various economic, technical, and societal changes.

Source: From B.B. Peterkin, R.L. Rizek, K.S. Tippett, "Nationwide Food Consumption Survey", Nutrition Today, 1988:18:24. Reprinted by permission of Lippincott Williams & Wilkins.

- to evaluate prevalence of eating patterns against dietary recommendations
- to describe the distribution of nutrient intakes in different subgroups (e.g., children, ethnic groups)
- to identify intake of uncommon foods
- to encompass the variety and the consistency of different foods in an individual's eating pattern
- to control for weekday and weekend biases

To improve the quality of 24-hour recalls, an innovative survey instrument, called the Automated Multiple Pass Method (AMPM), consisting of a specialized software program, has been used to collect dietary food intake data in national surveys. The instrument is viewed as the best possible method to collect accurate information on eating patterns (see Exhibit 2–6).[21]

Research using new technology for data collection and processing is explored (e.g., evaluating the advantages of using microcomputers during household interviews or automating food coding of individual interviews).

The USDA nutrient database that is used to profile nutrient composition of foods reported in the surveys is reviewed.

Recommendations of committees within the National Research Council, the President's Task Force on Food Assistance, and the Joint Nutrition Monitoring Evaluation Committee of Congress are considered.

Emerging diet and health associations are identified.

Lifestyles altering eating patterns (e.g., increased physical activity or increased television watching) are evaluated.

The Continuing Survey of Food Intakes by Individuals (CSFII) has occurred on an annual basis since 1989.[17] CSFII monitors the dietary status of small

Exhibit 2–6   The Automated Multiple Pass Method

The Automated Multiple Pass Method (AMPM) is used in the annual national survey, "What We Eat in America." Historically, from 1994 to 1998, the survey of food intake was conducted in person by an interviewer using paper and pencil to record a respondent's replies using a 3-step method. Respondents were asked to recall, in chronological order, the foods they consumed the previous day.

In 1997, planning a transition from paper and pencil to computer-assisted interviewing instruments began, but the key strengths and weaknesses of the old method were first reviewed. Then former interviewers were queried to solicit feedback. Several new options were evaluated. It was decided that the respondents' ability to recall dietary information might improve if they were not required to report foods eaten in chronological order. A 5-step system evolved in which

1. people stated the foods they remembered eating the day before in any order,
2. interviewers probed for forgotten foods and beverages with word triggers and probes, recalling potentially forgotten foods,
3. foods were reviewed as "eating occasions," and
4. detail-oriented questions increased more detailed complete responses and summarizing invited a final recall of any missed foods.

A 1999 pilot test involved 800 randomly chosen people who were first mailed visual aids to describe quantities of foods, i.e., cups, spoons, and a ruler. Preliminary research found that the method enabled the first 100 volunteers to recall what they had eaten to within 2% of the actual calories.

A validation study involved the following:

- biochemical and physiological tests to estimate actual calories;
- 52,000 biological samples including blood, urine, saliva, and fat;
- a tiny motion detector worn around the waist to measure total daily activity to be related to calories burned;
- measuring the amount of oxygen volunteers consumed while breathing under a large, Plexiglas canopy to determine calories burned during rest;
- measuring the volunteers' heart rate to assess their fitness levels during physical exercise;
- a full body scan to assess body composition and bone density; and
- doubly labeled water with more mass than regular water, detected in body fluids by sensitive instruments to calculate how calories actually burned.

In 2002, AMPM was then used initially to collect the dietary intake component of the national survey, NHANES (National Health and Nutrition Examination Survey). After collection, the AMPM data were processed, analyzed, and then reported. The NHANES results show achievement of health-related goals reflective of the US population and influence public policy regarding food assistance and education programs.

Source: Bliss RM. Researchers produce innovation in dietary recall. *Agricultural Res*. June 2004:10-12.

---

national samples of women and young children in the general population (1,500 households) and low-income population (750 households) during interim years. Although the CSFII uses the 24-hour recall method similar to that used by the Nationwide Food Consumption Surveys (NFCS) in 1977-1978, modifications regarding fat and salt patterns, smoking, and physical activity were made. The nutrient database was expanded to include 28 food components. Results are reported annually using a moving average approach. A snapshot look at the 1987 NFCS demonstrates features of the survey design, data collection, and data management elements[17] (see Exhibit 2-7).

The NFCS is designed to obtain data from 2 probability samples: (1) the general population or basic survey, which acquires data from 6,000 households and 15,000 members, and (2) the low-income survey, comprised of 3,600 households with 10,100 members.

Exhibit 2-7 Data Elements in the Nationwide Food Consumption Survey (NFCS), 1987

HOUSEHOLD COMPONENT
Questions appear on the screen of a laptop computer. An interviewer first asks the question and then enters the participant's response directly into the computer.

Household composition and meal data for each family member
1. sex, age
2. pregnancy/lactation status
3. number of meals or snacks during the previous week
   a. at home
   b. away from home
   c. as guest or purchased
4. cost of food

Household food during the past week
1. quantity of each food
2. source (e.g., purchased, home-produced, or gift)
3. purchase unit and price
4. drinking water source

Food entitlement program participation
1. WIC (Special Supplemental Food Program for Women, Infants, and Children)
2. school lunch and breakfast
3. food stamps
4. direct distribution of cheese and butter

Household characteristics
1. race
2. ethnicity
3. income previous month
4. income previous year
5. cash assets
6. size
7. food shopping practices
8. education of male and female heads of household
9. age of male and female heads of household
10. employment of male and female heads of household
11. description of dwelling
12. kitchen equipment

Exhibit 2-7 continued

INDIVIDUAL COMPONENT

An interviewer asks each participant to recall the types and amounts of each food eaten during the 24-hour period before the interview. Information is entered onto a form. Each participant is then asked to record all foods and beverages eaten on the interview day and the next day. The resulting food records are reviewed and collected the day after the records are completed.

Three-day food records
1. time
2. eating contact (breakfast, snack, etc.)
3. situation (alone, with family, etc.)
4. description of food (descriptors in an easy-to-use instruction book are used)
5. quantity consumed (measuring utensils are provided)
6. food source (foods at home versus from restaurant, etc.)
7. preparation additions (salt, fat, etc.)
8. water intake

Other pertinent information
1. regarding food
    a. how typical
    b. healthfulness (self-evaluation)
    c. added salt at table
    d. special restrictions
    e. vegetarian
    f. supplement use
    g. calcium-rich foods
    h. alcohol intake
2. regarding respondent
    a. height and weight (self-reported)
    b. health status (self-evaluation)
    c. smoking
    d. disability, handicap
    e. diagnosed disease
    f. problem chewing food and why
    g. leisure physical activity

Note: To obtain more information on the NFCS instrumentation, contact Nutrition Monitoring Division, Human Nutrition Information Service, USDA, Federal Building, Hyattsville, MD 20782.

Source: From B.B. Peterkin, R.L. Rizek, K.S. Tippett, "Nationwide Food Consumption Survey", Nutrition Today, 1988:18:24. Reprinted by permission of Lippincott Williams & Wilkins.

Both household data and individual data are collected via household interview with trained and experienced interviewers. Each household is contacted a week before a 2-to-3-hour interview with the person most knowledgeable about meal planning and preparation. This household food manager is asked to retain store receipts, recipes, menus, or calendars that will increase the accuracy of the interview. Data collection has 3 components:

1. *Household food use component:* Using a laptop computer, the food manager is asked to recall the types and amounts of food that have

Info Line

Since 1999, the NHANES has been conducted on a continuous basis to collect examination data on 5,000 participants each year. In addition to other health endpoints, the NHANES survey measures the nutritional status of the US population and tracks changes over time by clinical observation, professional assessment, and the recording of dietary intake patterns. Its Web site is at http://www.cdc.gov/nchs/about/major/nhanes.

disappeared from home food supplies over the previous 7 days. This includes food that was prepared, eaten, discarded, left over, or fed to pets. The cost of each food is recorded.

2. *Individual intake component:* At the close of the household interview, the respondent is asked to recall the foods eaten during the previous 24 hours.
3. *Follow-up component:* The interviewer leaves 3-day food diaries for the respondent and any children in the household. Teenagers and other adults recall and record their own food intakes. Two days later, the interviewer returns to review and to collect all food records.

The data management component addresses the system by which the collected data are converted into nutrient profiles:

Household food use component: Each food is given 1 of more than 4,000 food codes linked to a food group and price. Mean prices are recorded for foods consumed, and foods are converted to pounds. A nutrient profile with 28 food components is calculated with the nutritive value of the household eating pattern compared with the RDA values. This profile indicates whether the household food was sufficient to meet RDAs for all members.

Individual food intake component. Each food is assigned a food code, and the amount consumed is converted to grams of edible portion. Individual nutrient intake for a 3-day period is determined and compared to sex- and age-specific RDAs.

The DHHS's Food and Drug Administration and the USDA's Food Safety and Inspection Service assist the Human Nutrition Information Service with a telephone survey of consumer knowledge and attitudes about certain diet/health and safety issues. The data serve as a foundation for future exploration of food intake behavior, knowledge, and attitudes using a national sample.[17]

Benefits and Disadvantages of Surveys

Combining large, decennial surveys of household food use with the smaller, continuous surveys is beneficial. Decennial surveys yield cross-sectional household and food intake data, identify differences among population segments, and elucidate factors associated with food consumption and nutritional quality of diets. Concerns include changes over time (e.g., changes in nutrient databases and food composition), potential lack of standardization due to different interviewers and training techniques, and the analytical problems of merging the data. Cost remains a concern.

Smaller surveys enable continuous monitoring of food intakes by all sex/age groups, provide data for 2 subgroups (the general public and low-income groups), are economical and flexible, and yield a format to explore issues and methodological investigations. Although small surveys are less expensive than larger surveys, concerns about them include the tendency to rely on the data for decision making because it is available sooner and the potential change or deviation in methods because the measurements are closer and observers may become lax.

The continuing survey will occur throughout most of the 6 years of NHANES III, allowing for comparisons of dietary data across surveys for validity checks and other purposes. To date, various target surveys have been conducted and others are still needed (e.g., surveys on recent immigrants, seniors, homeless persons, drug users) in the United States to establish the general health of the nation. In general, the resulting data from surveys have provided baseline profiles and temporal changes to direct policy, programs, and further surveys.[17]

The Recommended Dietary Allowances

Nutrition surveillance and monitoring can detect nutritional problems by comparing intakes against standards. In the United States, the most common standards are the recommended dietary allowances (RDAs).[17]

The RDA publication serves as a principal guide for developing nutrition programs and policies in the United States. Each edition is issued by a subcommittee of the Food and Nutrition board. With each revision, RDA may be added or changed for nutrients.[5]

Role of the RDAs

The first RDAs were published in 1941 and served as a guide for advising the federal government about nutrition problems related to national defense, especially the dietary needs of US troops during World War II. Various uses of the RDAs are listed in Table 2–7. The RDAs are based on the nutritional needs of groups rather than individuals, but they are often used to evaluate adequacy of an individual's food pattern. Until an improved standard is identified, community nutrition professionals should use RDAs for assessment of groups, employ multiple days of assessment to evaluate an individual's intake, and expand beyond dietary data (e.g., biochemical and anthropometric data) to characterize a group. The following RDA reference points (see Figure 2–3) provide a systematic way to organize scientific research data[22]:

Deficient—level of intake of a nutrient below which almost all healthy people can be expected, over time, to experience deficiency symptoms of a clinical, physical, or functional nature.

TABLE 2-7   Uses of the RDAs

Use	Model	Suggestion
Food planning and procurement	Use to develop plans for feeding groups of healthy people.	Use as an appropriate nutrient standard for a period of at least a week, but also use as one of many food-planning criteria; this should be adjusted as group varies from RDA reference individual.
	Use for food purchasing, cost control, and budgeting.	Use as an appropriate nutrient standard with knowledge of such factors as food composition, availability, acceptability, and storage changes and losses.
Food programs	Serve as a basis for the nutritional goal for feeding programs.	Use as a standard for nutritional quality of meals, along with other food-selection criteria.
	Provide the nutritional standard for the Thrifty Food Plan, the basis for allotments in the Food Stamp Program.	Use as a guideline, along with other food-selection criteria.
	Provide nutritional guidelines for food distribution programs.	Use as a standard for nutritional quality of food packages.
Evaluating dietary survey	Evaluate dietary intake of individuals.	Use as a standard for data evaluating dietary status, but not for evaluating individual nutritional status.
	Evaluate household food use.	Use as a benchmark to compare households and to identify nutrient shortfalls.
	Evaluate national food supply (food disappearance data).	Use only as a benchmark for comparison over time and to identify nutrient shortfalls.
Guides for food selection	Develop and evaluate food guides and family food plans.	Use along with other food-selection criteria.
Food and nutrition information and education	Provide guidelines for maintaining nutritious diets.	Use as a point of reference; this information becomes more useful to consumers when translated into food-selection goals.
	Use as a basis for educators to discuss individuals' nutrient needs.	Use in combination with information in the text accompanying the RDA table and with recognition that the RDAs are for reference individuals.

TABLE 2–7 continued

	Evaluate an individual's diet as a basis for recommending specific changes in food patterns and/or dietary supplements.	Use to identify nutrient shortfalls and as a tool to assess nutrient contribution of diet; do not use in prescriptive manner.
Food labeling	Provide basis for nutritional labeling of foods.	Use as a basis for labeling standards; such standards should not be used to determine nutritional intake of individuals or groups.
Food fortification	Serve as a guide for fortification for general population.	Use as a guide, but such other factors as food-consumption patterns and contribution to the total diet also must be considered.
Developing new or modified food products	Provide guidance in establishing nutritional levels for new food products.	Use in combination with information or probable products; use within the context of the total diet.
Clinical dietetics	Develop therapeutic diet manuals.	Use to assess the nutritional quality of modified diets.
	Plan modified diets.	Use as a starting point along with information on the patient's nutritional status and individual needs.
	Counsel patients who require modified diets.	Use as one basis for advice on food selection.
	Plan menus and foods served in institutions for the developmentally disabled.	Use as a starting point, but modify for individual's developmental status and body size.
Nutrient supplements and special dietary foods	Use as a basis to formulate supplements and special dietary foods.	Use as a basis in developing infant formulas and other oral supplements or foods, but also consider nutrient bioavailability and nutrient balance; RDAs cannot be used as the only guide for parenteral feeding products.

Source: Adapted with permission from: *How Should the Recommended Dietary Allowances Be Revised?* Washington, DC: National Academy of Sciences; 1994. Courtesy of the National Academy Press, Washington, DC.

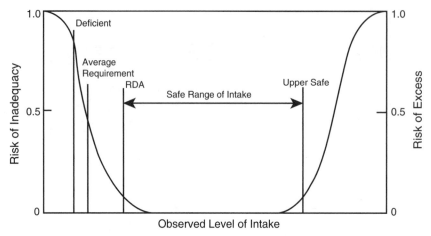

FIGURE 2–3 The concept of a safe intake range. The safe intake range is associated with a very low probability of either inadequacy or excess for an individual selected at random from the population.
Source: Adapted with permission from *Nutrient Adequacy: Assessment Using Food Consumption Surveys* by Subcommittee on Criteria for Dietary Evaluation, Coordinating Committee on Evaluation of Food Consumption Surveys, Food and Nutrition Board, National Academies Press, Copyright 1986, National Academy of Sciences.

Average requirement—mean level of intake of a nutrient or food component that appears, on the basis of experimental evidence, sufficient to maintain the desired biochemical/physiological function in a population. It is also important to know the variation in the mean requirement.

Recommended dietary allowance (RDA)—level of intake of an essential nutrient or food component considered on the basis of available scientific knowledge to be adequate to meet the known nutritional needs of practically all healthy persons. There will be a continuing need to redefine numerical recommendations. For some nutrients, other functional endpoints might be defined and included as criteria for the definition of recommended intakes.

Upper safe—level of intake of a nutrient or food component that appears to be safe for most healthy people and beyond which there is concern that some people will experience symptoms of toxicity over time.

The USDA uses the RDAs to evaluate adequacy of the US food supply, to establish standards for food assistance programs, and to determine the nutritional status of the US population. The FDA uses the RDAs to prepare product labels and to evaluate new food products.

The latest RDAs include protein, carbohydrates, and select vitamins and minerals, but some nutrients are listed using the dietary reference intake (DRI) system with an adequate intake (AI) level rather than an RDA level (see Tables 2-8 through 2-11). Recommended allowances are not given for each known nutrient because compositional data are insufficient. By eating a variety of foods that meet the RDAs, adequacy of other nutrients is likely. Otherwise, if a deficiency is observed, such as iron deficiency in women, fortification and possibly individual supplementation appear appropriate.

The RDAs are time-averaged goals, not daily objectives. When planning meals or food supplies, individuals should design eating patterns to meet all the RDAs over a 5- to 10-day interval.

TABLE 2–8   Recommended Dietary Allowances[a] Revised 1989-2001 for Achieving Good Nutrition of Healthy Individuals in the United States

Life Stage Group	Energy (kcal)	Protein (g)	CHO (g)	Vitamin A (µg RE)[b]	Iron (mg)	Zinc (mg)	Iodine (mg)
Males							
0-0.5	570	1.52	60	400	0.27	2	110
0.5-1	743	1.5	95	500	11	3	130
1-3	1,046	1.1	130	300	7	3	90
4-8	1,742	0.95	130	400	10	5	90
9-13	2,279	0.95	130	600	8	8	120
14-18	3,152	0.85	130	900	11	11	150
19-30	3,067	0.8	130	900	8	11	150
31-50	3,067	0.8	130	900	8	11	150
> 51	3,067	0.8	130	900	8	11	150
Females							
0-0.5	520	1.52	60	400	0.27	2	110
0.5-1	676	1.5	95	500	11	3	130
1-3	992	1.1	130	300	7	3	90
4-8	1,642	0.95	130	400	10	5	90
9-13	2,071	0.95	130	600	15	8	120
14-18	2,368	0.85	130	700	18	9	150
19-30	2,403	0.8	130	700	18	8	150
31-50	2,403	0.8	130	700	8	8	150
> 51	2,403	0.8	130	700	8	8	150
Pregnancy							
14-18, 1st trimester	2,368	1.1	175	750	27	13	220
2nd trimester	2,708	1.1	175	750	27	13	220
3rd trimester	2,820	1.1	175	750	27	13	220
19-50, 1st trimester	2,403	1.1	175	770	27	11	220
2nd trimester	2,743	1.1	175	770	27	11	220
3rd trimester	2,855	1.1	175	770	27	11	220
Lactating							
14-18, 1st 6 mo	2,698	1.1	210	1,200	10	14	290
2nd 6 mo,	2,768	1.1	210	1,200	10	14	290

continued

TABLE 2–8   continued

Life Stage Group	Energy (kcal)	Protein (g)	CHO (g)	Vitamin A (μg RE)[b]	Iron (mg)	Zinc (mg)	Iodine (mg)
19-50, 1st 6 mo	2,733	1.1	210	1,300	9	12	290
2nd 6 mo	2,803	1.1	210	1,300	9	12	290

a. The allowances, expressed as average daily intakes over time, are intended to provide for individual variations among most normal persons as they live in the United States under usual environmental stresses. Diets should be based on a variety of common foods in order to provide other nutrients for which human requirements have been less well defined.
b. Retinol equivalents 1 retinol equivalent =1 μg retinal or 6 μg β-carotene.

Note: This table does not include nutrients for which dietary reference intakes have recently been established (see *Dietary Reference Intakes for Calcium, Phosphorus, Magnesium, Vitamin D, and Fluoride* [1997], *Dietary Reference Intakes for Thiamin, Riboflavin, Niacin, Vitamin B$_6$, Folate, Vitamin B$_{12}$, Pantothenic Acid, Biotin, and Choline* [1998], and *Dietary Reference Intakes for Vitamin E, Vitamin C, Selenium, and Carotenoids* [2000]).
Source: Adapted from: Monsen ER. Dietary reference intakes for the antioxidant nutrients: vitamin C, vitamin E, selenium, and carotenoids. *J Am Diet Assoc.* 2000;100:637-640.

TABLE 2–9   Dietary Reference Intakes: Recommended Intakes for Individuals

Life Stage Group	Calcium (mg/d)	Phosphorus (mg/d)	Magnesium (mg/d)	Vitamin D (mg/d)	Fluoride (mg/d)
Infants					
0-6 m	210*	100*	30*	5*	0.01*
7-12 m	270*	275*	75*	5*	0.5*
Children					
1-3 y	500*	460	80	5*	0.7*
4-8 y	800*	500	130	5*	1*
Males					
9-13 y	1,300*	1,250	240	5*	2*
14-18 y	1,300*	1,250	410	5*	3*
19-30 y	1,000*	700	400	5*	4*
31-50 y	1,000*	700	420	5*	4*
51-70 y	1,200*	700	420	10*	4*
> 70 y	1,200*	700	420	15*	4*
Females					
9-13 y	1,300*	1,250	240	5*	2*
14-18 y	1,300*	1,250	360	5*	3*
19-30 y	1,000*	700	310	5*	3*
31-50 y	1,000*	700	320	5*	3*
51-70 y	1,200*	700	320	10*	3*
> 70 y	1,200*	700	320	15*	3*

continued

TABLE 2–9 continued

Life Stage Group	Calcium (mg/d)	Phosphorus (mg/d)	Magnesium (mg/d)	Vitamin D (mg/d)	Fluoride (mg/d)
Pregnancy					
≤ 18 y	1,300*	**1,250**	**400**	5*	3*
19-30 y	1,000*	**700**	**350**	5*	3*
31-50 y	1,000*	**700**	**360**	5*	3*
Lactation					
≤ 18 y	1,300*	**1,250**	**360**	5*	3*
19-30 y	1,000*	**700**	**310**	5*	3*
31-50 y	1,000*	**700**	**320**	5*	3*

Note: This table presents recommended dietary allowances (RDAs) in **bold type** and adequate intakes (AIs) in ordinary type followed by an asterisk (*).
Source: National Academy of Sciences, Institute of Medicine (IOM). Dietary reference intakes for thiamin, riboflavin, niacin, vitamin B_6, folate, vitamin B_{12}, pantothenic acid, biotin, and choline. Washington, DC: National Academy Press; 2001. Available at: http://www.nap.edu.

Table 2–10   Dietary Reference Intakes: Recommended Intakes for Individuals for Water Soluble Vitamins and Folate

Life Stage Group	Thiamin (mg/d)	Riboflavin (mg/d)	Niacin (mg/d)	Vitamin B_6 (mg/d)	Folate (mg/d)	Vitamin B_{12} (μg/d)	Vitamin C (mg/d)
Infants							
0-6 m	0.2*	0.3*	2*	0.1*	65*	0.4*	40*
7-12 m	0.3*	0.4*	4*	0.3*	80*	0.5*	50*
Children							
1-3 y	**0.5**	**0.5**	**6**	**0.5**	**150**	0.9*	15*
4-8 y	**0.6**	**0.6**	**8**	**0.6**	**200**	1.2*	25*
Males							
9-13 y	**0.9**	**0.9**	**12**	**1.0**	**300**	**1.8**	45*
14-18 y	**1.2**	**1.3**	**16**	**1.3**	**400**	**2.4**	75*
19-30 y	**1.2**	**1.3**	**16**	**1.3**	**400**	**2.4**	90*
31-50 y	**1.2**	**1.3**	**16**	**1.3**	**400**	**2.4**	90*
51-70 y	**1.2**	**1.3**	**16**	**1.7**	**400**	**2.4**	90*
> 70 y	**1.2**	**1.3**	**16**	**1.7**	**400**	**2.4**	90*
Females							
9-13 y	**0.9**	**0.9**	**12**	**1.0**	**300**	**1.8**	45*
14-18 y	**1.0**	**1.0**	**14**	**1.2**	**400**	**2.4**	65*
19-30 y	**1.0**	**1.1**	**14**	**1.3**	**400**	**2.4**	75*

continued

Table 2–10   continued

Life Stage Group	Thiamin (mg/d)	Riboflavin (mg/d)	Niacin (mg/d)	Vitamin B_6 (mg/d)	Folate (mg/d)	Vitamin B_{12} (μg/d)	Vitamin C (mg/d)
31-50 y	**1.1**	**1.1**	**14**	**1.3**	**400**	**2.4**	75*
51-70 y	**1.1**	**1.1**	**14**	**1.5**	**400**	**2.4**	75*
> 70 y	**1.1**	**1.1**	**14**	**1.5**	**400**	**2.4**	75*
Pregnancy							
≤ 18 y	**1.4**	**1.4**	**18**	**1.9**	**600**	**2.6**	80*
19-30 y	**1.4**	**1.4**	**18**	**1.9**	**600**	**2.6**	85*
31-50 y	**1.4**	**1.4**	**18**	**1.9**	**600**	**2.6**	85*
Lactation							
≤ 18 y	**1.4**	**1.6**	**17**	**2.0**	**500**	**2.8**	115*
19-30 y	**1.4**	**1.6**	**17**	**2.0**	**500**	**2.8**	120*
31-50 y	**1.4**	**1.6**	**17**	**2.0**	**500**	**2.8**	120*

Note: This table presents recommended dietary allowances (RDAs) in **bold type** and adequate intakes (AIs) in ordinary type followed by an asterisk (*).
Source: National Academy of Sciences, Institute of Medicine (IOM). Dietary reference intakes for thiamin, riboflavin, niacin, vitamin B_6, folate, vitamin B_{12}, pantothenic acid, biotin, and choline. Washington, DC: National Academy Press; 2001. Available at: http://www.nap.edu.

TABLE 2–11   Dietary Reference Intakes: Recommended Intakes for Individuals for Pantothenic Acid, Biotin, Choline, Vitamin E, and Selenium

Life Stage Group	Pantothenic Acid (mg/d)	Biotin (μg/d)	Choline (mg/d)	Vitamin E (mg/d)	Selenium (μg/d)
0-6 m	1.7*	5*	125*	4*	15*
7-12 m	1.8*	6*	130*	6*	20*
Children					
1-3 y	2*	8*	200*	**6**	**20**
4-8 y	3*	12*	250*	**7**	**30**
Males					
9-13 y	4*	20*	375*	**11**	**40**
14-18 y	5*	25*	550*	**15**	**55**
19-30 y	5*	30*	550*	**15**	**55**
31-50 y	5*	30*	550*	**15**	**55**
51-70 y	5*	30*	550*	**15**	**55**
> 70 y	5*	30*	550*	**15**	**55**
Females					
9-13 y	4*	20*	375*	**11**	**40**
14-18 y	5*	25*	400*	**15**	**55**

TABLE 2–11   continued

Life Stage Group	Pantothenic Acid (mg/d)	Biotin (μg/d)	Choline (mg/d)	Vitamin E (mg/d)	Selenium (μg/d)
19-30 y	5*	30*	425*	**15**	**55**
31-50 y	5*	30*	425*	**15**	**55**
51-70 y	5*	30*	425*	**15**	**55**
> 70 y	5*	30*	425*	**15**	**55**
Pregnancy					
≤ 18 y	6*	30*	450*	**15**	**60**
19-30 y	6*	30*	450*	**15**	**60**
31-50 y	6*	30*	450*	**15**	**60**
Lactation					
≤18 y	7*	35*	550*	**19**	**70**
19-30 y	7*	35*	550*	**19**	**70**
31-50 y	7*	35*	550*	**19**	**70**

Note: This table presents recommended dietary allowances (RDAs) in **bold type** and adequate intakes (AIs) in ordinary type followed by an asterisk (*).
Source: National Academy of Sciences, Institute of Medicine (IOM). Dietary reference intakes for thiamin, riboflavin, niacin, vitamin B_6, folate, vitamin B_{12}, pantothenic acid, biotin, and choline. Washington, DC: National Academy Press; 2001 Available at: http://www.nap.edu.

Dietary Reference Intakes

Dietary reference intakes provide quantitative estimates or estimated average requirements of nutrient intakes and replace and expand the past 50 years of periodic updates and revisions of the recommended dietary allowances (RDAs).[23] DRIs include current concepts about the role of nutrients and food components in long-term health. For example,

Energy, carbohydrate, fiber, fat, fatty acids, cholesterol, protein, and amino acids: The data tape was released on September 5, 2002. Adults should get 45-65% of their energy intake from carbohydrates, 20-35% from fat, and 10-35% from protein. Acceptable ranges for children are similar, except that infants and younger children need 25-40% of energy from fat. Added sugars should comprise no more than 25% of total energy; protein intake should be 0.8 grams per kilogram of body weight for adults and 0.88 g/kg/day for women during pregnancy. Recommendations include linoleic acid (n-6 FA) at 17 g/day for men and 12 g/day for women, and alpha-linolenic acid (n-3 FA) at 1.6 g/day for men and 1.1 g/day for women. Protein during the last 2 trimesters of pregnancy increases 21 g/day over prepregnancy requirements.
- Recommended level of protein intake is 0.8 grams per kilogram of body weight for adults.
- No maximum level is set for saturated fat, cholesterol, or trans fatty acids, as increased risk exists at levels above 0.

- For cardiovascular health, regardless of weight, adults and children should achieve one hour of moderately intense physical activity each day.
- Added sugars should comprise no more than 25% of total calories consumed. Major sources include soft drinks, fruit drinks, pastries, candy, and other sweets.
- Recommended total fiber intake for adults no older than 50 years is 38 grams for men and 25 grams for women. For men and women older than 50, it is 30 grams and 21 grams per day, respectively, due to decreased food intake.

Folate, other B vitamins, and choline: The DRI report including folate, thiamin, riboflavin, niacin, vitamin B_6, vitamin B_{12}, pantothenic acid, biotin, and choline is available at http://books.nap.edu/catalog/6015.html.

Antioxidants: The *Dietary Antioxidants and Related Compounds* report established DRIs for vitamins C and E, selenium, beta carotene, and other carotenoids. *Proposed Definition and Plan for Review of Dietary Antioxidants and Related Compounds* can be found at http://books.nap.edu/catalog/6252.html.

Micronutrients: The Micronutrient Panel is reviewing the estimated average requirements, tolerable upper intake levels, and bioavailability for iron, zinc, copper, iodine, chromium, boron, manganese, molybdenum, nickel, silicon, and vitamins A and K.

Uses and interpretation: The Subcommittee on Uses and Interpretation of the DRIs has 2 reports. The first report discusses assessing diets using the DRIs. The second report focuses on using the DRIs to plan diets.

Upper reference levels: *DRIs: A Risk Assessment for Establishing Upper Intake Levels for Nutrients* describes the model for risk assessment of nutrients and food components that were used to develop upper levels (ULs). See Table 2-12 and visit http://www.iom.edu/fnb.

DRIs for Macronutrients

A study of dietary reference intakes for macronutrients including protein, amino acids, dietary fat and individual fatty acids, phospholipids, cholesterol, complex carbohydrates, simple sugars, dietary fiber, energy intake, alcohol intake, and energy expenditure began with NHANES III. New data on dietary intake, supplement use, and their relation to markers of health as measured in the NHANES and the Continuing Survey of Food Intake by Individuals is included.

Antioxidants' Role in Chronic Disease Prevention Uncertain as Huge Doses Considered Risky

Insufficient evidence exists to support claims that taking megadoses of dietary antioxidants, such as selenium and vitamins C and E, or carotenoids, including beta-carotene, can prevent chronic diseases.[24] Extremely large doses may lead to health problems rather than confer benefits. The dietary reference intakes report calls for increases in daily intakes of vitamins C and E to exploit their role in maintaining good health, and recommends an even

TABLE 2–12 Dietary Reference Intakes: Tolerable Upper Intake Levels (ULs) for Certain Nutrients and Food Components

Life Stage Group	Calcium g/day	Phosphorus g/day	Magnesium mg/day	Vitamin D µg/day	Fluoride mg/day	Niacin mg/day	Vitamin B$_6$ mg/day	Folate µg/day	Choline g/day
0-6 m	ND	ND	ND	25	0.7	ND	ND	ND	ND
7-12 m	ND	ND	ND	25	0.9	ND	ND	ND	ND
1-3 y	2.5	3	65	50	1.3	10	30	300	1.0
4-8 y	2.5	3	110	50	2.2	15	40	400	1.0
9-13 y	2.5	4	350	50	10	20	60	600	2.0
14-18 y	2.5	4	350	50	10	30	80	800	3.0
19-70 y	2.5	4	350	50	10	35	100	1,000	3.5
> 70 y	2.5	3	350	50	10	35	100	1,000	3.5
Pregnancy									
≤ 18 years	2.5	3.5	350	50	10	30	80	800	3.0
19-50 y	2.5	3.5	350	50	10	35	100	1,000	3.5
Lactation									
≤ 18 y	2.5	4	350	50	10	30	80	800	3.0
19-50 y	2.5	4	350	50	10	35	100	1,000	3.5

Source: Adapted with permission from *Dietary Reference Intakes: Guiding Principles for Nutrition Labeling and Fortification,* 2003. National Academies Press.

larger amount of vitamin C for smokers. It does set a limit on daily consumption of selenium and vitamins C and E to reduce the risk of adverse side effects from overuse. American and Canadian adults ingest sufficient quantities of these 3 nutrients from food alone.

Dietary antioxidants are nutrients that help protect cells from a normal but damaging physiological process known as oxidative stress. They are natural components of many fruits and vegetables. They have been added to some foods and are available as dietary supplements. Antioxidants may have a role in reducing the risk of cancer, cardiovascular disease, eye disease, and Alzheimer's and Parkinson's diseases. A direct connection between intake and prevention remains.

Insufficient evidence exists to conclude that these nutrients, even in very high doses, will reduce the risk of diseases such as cancer; cardiovascular disease; cataracts; age-related macular degeneration, a common form of blindness in elderly people; diabetes mellitus; and neurodegenerative diseases. Tolerable upper intake levels (TUIL) for vitamins C and E and selenium are not a recommended amount but the maximum intake posing no risk of adverse health effects in almost all people in the general population. Recommendations:

> *Vitamin C*—achieve maximum saturation in the body, i.e., women 75 milligrams per day, and men 90 milligrams daily. Smokers suffer from damaged cells and depleted vitamin C, requiring an additional 35 milligrams per day. Food sources are citrus fruit, potatoes, strawberries, broccoli, and leafy green vegetables. Upper intake level from both food and supplements is 2,000 milligrams per day for adults. Higher intakes may cause diarrhea.

Much research focuses on vitamin C. Currently the RDA for adults is 60 mg/day. Tissues near saturation levels are 200 mg/day and 1,000 mg/day for full saturation. Criteria for determining recommended intakes of vitamin C include but are not limited to dietary availability, steady-state concentrations, bioavailability, urinary excretion, and adverse effects. An EAR of 100 mg/day and a UL of 1 gm/day can limit adverse conditions.[25]

Humans differ from plants and animals because of their inability to synthesize ascorbic acid from glucose. No functional markers exist for assessing optimal status. Dietary intake, plasma and tissue levels, gastrointestinal absorption, and urinary levels affect vitamin C status. The most common measure is fasting plasma ascorbic acid concentration. Stable functional markers, however, are needed to distinguish the different categories of vitamin status. Functional markers (molecular, biochemical, or physiological) can be used in conjunction with current methods for assessing intake and status. Two potential biochemical markers are free carnitine and a deoxypyridinoline: pyridinoline collagen index. Functional assessment, e.g., a vitamin's antioxidant defense ability and free radical and lipid peroxidation levels may be practical alternatives.[26]

Factors that affect plasma ascorbate acid levels include dose, age, body weight, physical activity, stress, and prior depletion-repletion. Sixty-eight men, 30–59 years old, completed depletion-repletion cycles and reported behavioral and psychosocial factors daily. The men did not smoke, drink alcohol, or take aspirin during the study, and breakfast and dinner bag lunches, snacks, and weekend meals were provided. After a 1-month period of stabilization on

60 mg/d of vitamin C, the men consumed 9 mg/d (depletion) for 1 month, then 117 mg/d (repletion) for 1 month; the cycle was repeated. Total body weight was a slightly stronger predictor of loss of lean body mass. During the first repletion period, dose per kg of body weight was strongly associated with extent of repletion; younger men and those weighing less had greater repletion. Heavier men had lower plasma ascorbate levels. Recommendations are that repletion levels of 117 mg/d may be inadequate to replace body stores and reach a maximum plasma level; and repeated depletions may occur among the poor, chronically ill, and elderly; a public health policy is needed.[27]

Vitamin E—both women and men should consume 15 milligrams—or 22 international units (IU)—of alpha-tocopherol from food each day. Alpha-tocopherol is the only type of vitamin E that human blood can maintain and transfer to cells. Food sources are nuts, seeds, liver, and leafy green vegetables. Upper level, based only on intake from vitamin supplements, is 1,000 milligrams of alpha-tocopherol per day for adults. This equals 1,500 IU of d-alpha-tocopherol, sometimes labeled as natural source vitamin E, or 1,100 IU of dl-alpha-tocopherol, a synthetic version of vitamin E. Consuming more than this amount increases one's risk of hemorrhagic damage because the nutrient can act as an anticoagulant.

Selenium—ingest the amount associated with the highest activity of enzymes, which minimize oxidants in the body, or 55 micrograms daily for women and men. Food sources are seafood, liver, meat, and grains. Upper intake level is 400 micrograms per day based on nutrients from all sources. Higher intakes can cause selenosis, a toxic reaction causing hair loss and nail sloughing.

Beta-carotene and other carotenoids—antioxidants, with inconsistent and contradictory effects in humans. No recommend daily intake level or an upper intake level is given for carotenoids. Beta-carotene supplementation should occur only for the prevention and control of vitamin A deficiency.

General Rule

Healthy people should not routinely exceed upper intake levels. Well-controlled clinical trials are essential not only to investigate role of dietary antioxidants and carotenoids in the prevention of chronic diseases, but also to explore the nutrient needs of children, the elderly, and individuals with compromised health. The ways selenium, vitamins C and E, and beta-carotene interact with each other and with other food components is also an important factor.[24]

Nutrient Information on Food Labels

The best guide for individuals to evaluate how well their eating pattern meets the RDAs is found on the food label. In addition, the most visible and accessible format for nutrition education for the public is the food label. The regulatory authority for food labeling rests with the FDA, the USDA, and the Federal Trade Commission (FTC). The USDA regulates poultry according to the Poultry Products Inspection Act and regulates meat under the Federal Meat Inspection Act. Under the Food, Drug and Cosmetic (FD&C) Act, FDA regulates the labeling of all other foods. Manufacturers must obtain prior approval by the USDA for any label.[28] The FTC challenges product claims when products cross state boundaries.

The FDA can challenge mislabeled products, and it maintains persistent monitoring. A committee sponsored by both the FDA and the USDA met in 1989 and published recommendations in 1992 about how food labels could be improved to help consumers with healthy eating. One recommendation was that the FDA and the USDA adopt mandatory and uniform nutrition labeling requirements. A second recommendation was that Congress endorse the authority of the FDA and the USDA to mandate nutritional labeling.

President George Bush signed the Nutrition Labeling and Education Act (NLEA) on November 8, 1990.[29,30] On January 6, 1993, the FDA issued the final rule implementing the NLEA.[29,30] Provisions became effective May 8, 1993.[31]

The NLEA is considered the most powerful piece of legislation about food and labeling since the 1938 FD&C Act.[32-34] It is a landmark effort because it requires standard food labels and nutrition information on practically all foods produced and sold in the United States. The NLEA mandated the following:

- nutrition labeling for conventional foods
- FDA regulation of claims about health (e.g., low fat to prevent cancer and heart disease, low sodium to prevent hypertension, and calcium to prevent osteoporosis)

The nutrition label is required to include information on total calories, calories from fat, total fat, saturated fat, cholesterol, sodium, total carbohydrates, dietary fiber, sugars, protein, vitamin A, vitamin C, calcium, and iron.[31] Manufacturers may volunteer information on calories from saturated fat and on amounts of polyunsaturated and monounsaturated fat, soluble and insoluble fiber, sugar alcohol, other carbohydrate, potassium, additional vitamins, and minerals with established reference daily intakes (RDIs), and the content of vitamin A as beta-carotene. The nutrition label information must characterize the packaged product accurately prior to consumer preparation.

The final FDA rule establishes a standard format for nutrition information on food labels.[31-34] This information includes the quantitative amount per serving for each nutrient except vitamins and minerals, the amount of each nutrient as a percentage of the daily value for a 2,000-calorie diet, a footnote with reference values for selected nutrients based on 2,000-calorie and 2,500-calorie diets, and caloric conversion information.

Some foods are exempt from mandatory nutrition labeling requirements. These include foods offered for sale by small businesses; foods sold in restaurants or other establishments in which food is served for immediate human consumption; foods similar to restaurant foods (e.g., ready-to-eat but not for immediate consumption), but primarily prepared on site and not offered for sale outside the premise; foods that contain insignificant amounts of all nutrients subject to this rule (e.g., coffee and tea); dietary supplements, except those in conventional food form; infant formula; medical foods; custom-processed fish or game meats; foods shipped in bulk form; and donated foods.[31] Manufacturers that make a nutrient content claim or health claim on an exempted food forfeit the exemption.

Some food products are not required to include food label information due to special labeling provisions. These include foods in small packages with less than 12 square inches available for labeling (an address or telephone number is required for consumers to obtain nutrition information); packages with 40 square inches or less (these may list the required information in tabular or linear fashion if the package shape cannot accommodate the other information in the specified format); food for children less than 2 years of age (these products must not declare information concerning calories from fat, fatty acids, and cholesterol); foods for children less than 4 years of age (these must not include daily value information); raw fruits, vegetables, and fish (these should follow voluntary nutrition labeling guidelines); packaged single-ingredient fish or game meat (these may provide information on an as-prepared basis); foods sold from bulk containers and game meat products (these may provide information on labeling); shell eggs (these may provide the required nutrition information inside the egg carton); multi-unit packages (only the outer package of unit containers must provide nutrition information); and gift packs of food (manufacturers may provide information on labeling according to the special requirements).[31]

Government authorities in the United States and Canada recommend using the current DRI values to update nutrition information on food and dietary supplement labels so that consumers can compare products more easily and make informed food choices based on the latest science. The recommended changes would help consumers use food and dietary supplement labels to choose healthier diets.

In the United States, current label information is based on the 1968 RDAs; however, 10 guiding principles are considered for incorporating current scientific information into nutrition labeling, and 6 principles are being used to guide discretionary fortification, or voluntary addition of nutrients to food by manufacturers. Technical issues will be addressed by government scientists and policymakers.[35] See Table 2–13.

Consumers tend to shop for and purchase foods without applying formal learning. Consumers are influenced by factors present at the point and time of purchase. Two marketing tools, nutrition labels and targeted marketing strategies, affect a consumer's food purchase and are powerful change agents. Shoppers like nutrition labels on foods but only 34% of consumers read them most of the time. Shoppers report that label information is difficult to understand, but when given instructions, they use labels more frequently. If labels are only in English, some ethnic groups may not be able to use the information. Shelf stickers, brochures, posters, menu labels, table tents, and prominent, colorful signage affect choices.[36]

Lang et al evaluated the awareness and use of a supermarket-shelf labeling program designed to encourage shoppers to make food choices that promote heart health in 18 supermarkets serving minority communities in Detroit, Michigan (Figure 2–4). Three hundred sixty-one adults, 66% female, 67% African American, and mean age of 51.6 years + 18.5 s.d., were given an exit survey to determine awareness and use of the program.[37]

Overall awareness of the program was 28.8% with awareness among minorities significantly higher compared with whites, 35.3% vs 20.8%; p = 0.02. Gender, age, and education level were not predictive of program awareness. Individuals who had been screened for cardiovascular disease risk factors the previous year had greater awareness than those not screened, 32.6% vs 13.6%, p = 0.06. The program was used by 56% of individuals aware of the program. There was no significant difference by gender, age, or ethnicity.[37]

TABLE 2–13   Guiding Principles for Nutrition Labeling and Discretionary Fortification

Issue	Number	Principle

Labeling

1. Nutrition information in the nutrition facts box expressed as a percentage of daily value (% DV).

2. The daily value (DV) based on a population-weighted reference value.

3. A population-weighted estimated average requirement (EAR) as the basis for DVs for those nutrients for which EARs have been identified.

4. If no EAR for a nutrient, then a population-weighted adequate intake (AI) used as the basis for DVs.

5. The acceptable macronutrient distribution ranges (AMDRs) as the basis for the macronutrients protein, total carbohydrates, and total fat.

6. Two thousand calories used, when needed, as the basis for expressing energy intake when developing DVs.

7. The DVs for saturated fatty acids, *trans* fatty acids, and cholesterol set low for an achievable health-promoting diet.

8. General population identified as all individuals 4 years of age and older, with 4 distinctive life stages when nutrient needs are physiologically different from the main population, i.e., infancy, toddlers ages 1 to 3 years old, pregnancy, and lactation.

9. The supplement facts box should use the same DVs as the nutrition facts box.

10. Absolute amounts should be included in the nutrition facts and supplement facts boxes for all nutrients.

Discretionary fortification

1. Justification for fortification of foods based on documented public health needs.

2. Intake data should be used with the UL to provide evidence to explain how current exposure to the nutrient would be altered by fortification.

3. Consideration given to fortification with nutrients up to the amount for products to meet the criteria as good or excellent sources of the nutrient.

4. Potential changes to long-standing discretionary fortification practices carefully reviewed because they may be central to the maintenance of nutrient adequacy in the population.

5. Continuous review of the severity of the adverse affect on which the UL is based.

6. The intended use of the targeted food as the standard against which the nutrient content is assessed.

Source: Adapted from Dietary reference intakes: guiding principles for nutrition labeling and fortification. Released 2003. USDA. Washington, D.C.

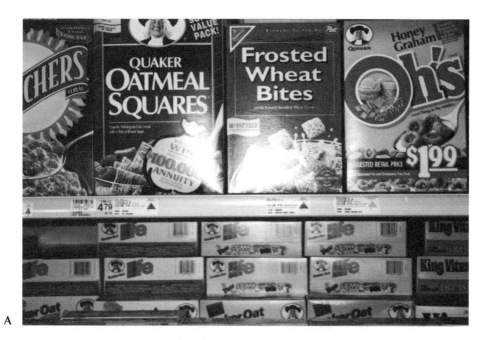

A

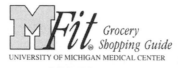

BEST
CHOICE

COLUMBO
LIGHT NONFAT YOGURT
ALL FLAVORS

1

BEST
CHOICE

DANNON
BLENDED FAT FREE YOGURT
B **ALL FLAVORS**

1

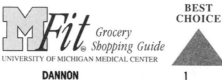

ACCEPTABLE
CHOICE

COLUMBO   5
SHOPPE STYLE GOURMET
C **CAPPUCCINO COFFEE BEAN**

ACCEPTABLE
CHOICE

21000- **BREYERS**   5
27021 **REDUCED FAT ICE CREAM**
D **PRALINE ALMOND CRUNCH**

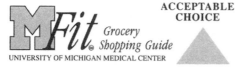

FIGURE 2–4 A photo of the Michigan *M-Fit Supermarket Program* (A) demonstrates placement of a label beneath cereal products. The label gives consumers information and guidance by designating if the product is an acceptable choice or a best choice. See yogurt and
ice cream, and cappuccino products (B, C, D).
Source: University of Michigan Medical Center.

Awareness of the shelf-labeling program was highest among African Americans and those recently screened for cardiovascular disease risk. Shelf labels may increase the selection of foods that promote heart health in predominately low-income, minority populations.[37]

Reference Daily Intakes and Daily Reference Values

The final FDA rule establishes the reference values for the food label. The Dietary Supplement Act of 1992 requires FDA to retain current US recommended daily allowance values for vitamins and minerals (i.e., values that had been developed chiefly by selecting the highest RDA value from among the various sex/age groups listed in RDA tables published in 1968).[31] The Dietary Supplement Act of 1992 establishes label reference values for 19 vitamins and minerals. The description for those values changes from US recommended daily allowance to reference daily intake (RDI). The Dietary Supplement Act of 1992 did not establish reference values for infants, children less than 4 years of age, pregnant women, or lactating women.

The FDA regulation expands the label reference values to include 8 other nutrients, including fat, cholesterol, and fiber. These values are called daily reference values (DRVs) and are established for nutrients of public health importance. They serve as a point of reference for adults and children 4 years of age and older.[31] An energy intake of 2,000 calories per day is used as the basis for reference values. The resulting nutrients with DRVs are: fat (65 g), saturated fat (20 g), cholesterol (300 mg), total carbohydrate (300 g), fiber (25 g), sodium (2,400 mg), potassium (3,500 mg), and protein (50 g). To reduce confusion, all reference values on food labels are called daily values, or DVs.

Serving Sizes

A serving size regulation that does the following was established:

- defines serving size based on the amount of food usually consumed per eating occasion.
- establishes reference amounts usually consumed for 139 specific food product categories and establishes a petition process of modifying the list.
- provides rules for using the reference amounts to determine serving sizes for specific food products.
- requires both common household and metric measures on the label (e.g., 1 cup [240 mL] for milk, 1 slice [28 g] for sliced bread).
- permits optional declaration of serving size in US measures (ounces or fluid ounces) in addition to the household and metric measures (e.g., 1 cup [240 mL/8 fl oz]).
- allows a second column on the nutrition label to express the nutrition content per 100 g or 100 mL or per 1 oz for all products; per unit for products in discrete units (e.g., sliced products such as bread, muffins, cookies, ice cream bars, etc.); and per cup popped for popcorn.
- defines a single-serving container as any package that contains less than 200% of the reference amount for the food product category. The reference amount for soft drinks is 8 fl oz. A 12-fl-oz can of soft drink is a single-serving container. Its nutrient content must be based on the entire contents of the can. If products contain more than 150% but less

than 200% of the reference amount when the reference amount is 100 g or 100 mL or larger, the manufacturer may determine whether to declare 1 or 2 servings. If 245 g is the reference amount for soups, a 15-oz can of soup may be labeled as 2 servings.

- defines a unit of product in discrete segments (e.g., sliced bread or a single muffin). If multiserving containers are sold, a single serving is allowed on the label if the unit weighs more than 50% but less than 200% of the reference amount. For bread, the reference amount is 50 g and the serving size of sliced bread is 1 slice if a slice weighs more than 25 g.
- allows claims such as "low sodium" if the product qualifies based on the reference amount for the product category. When serving size differs from the reference amount but the product qualifies for the claim, the claim must be followed by the criteria (for example, "very low sodium, 35 mg or less per 240 mL or 8 fl oz").[31]

Definition of Descriptor Terms

FDA defines the terms *free, low, light* or *lite, reduced, less,* and *high*, along with selected synonyms. The terms *good source, very low* (for sodium only), *lean, extra lean, fewer, more,* and *added* (or *fortified* or *enriched*) are also identified. The terms *healthy* and *fresh* are defined, but *natural* is not.

Free equates to an amount that is nutritionally insignificant. The following can be labeled as zero: sodium, less than 5 mg; calories, less than 5 calories; sugars, less than 0.5 g; saturated fat, less than 0.5 g; and trans fatty acids not exceeding 1% of total fat; and cholesterol, less than 2 mg. Foods that do not undergo a special process to reduce the nutrient are basically free and must be labeled as such (e.g., "leaf lettuce, a sodium-free food").

A *cholesterol-free* claim is only allowed on foods containing 2 g or less of saturated fat per reference serving. Foods having more than 13 g total fat per reference serving must list the total fat content per serving immediately adjacent to the cholesterol claim.

Criteria for the term *low* are based on reference serving sizes. The values for different components include: sodium, less than 140 mg; calories, less than 40 calories; fat, less than 3 g; saturated fat, less than 1 g and not more than 15% of calories from saturated fat; and cholesterol, less than 20 mg. If the food is naturally low in a nutrient, the label must explain that all similar foods are low (e.g., "frozen bagel, a low-fat food," or "very low sodium" describes a food with a sodium value less than or equal to 35 mg of sodium).

High and *good source* are based on a percentage of the daily value of the specific nutrients in a reference serving. *High* means 20% or more of the daily amount, whereas *good source* is between 10% and 19% of the daily amount.

For *light, reduced,* and *added,* the reference food must be similar to the product bearing the claim (e.g., a *lite* potato chip must be similar to regular potato chips). The terms *added, fortified,* and *enriched* are used interchangeably. All related claims must be accompanied by information on the identity of the reference food and the percentage or fraction by which the nutrient has been modified. The amount of the nutrient in the labeled product compared to the amount in the reference food must appear on the information panel.

The terms *reduced, less,* or *fewer* refer to a food with at least 25% less of the nutrient than the reference food; *more* or *added* defines a food with 10%

or more of the daily value per reference serving. *Light* or *lite* means a food has at least 50% less calories from fat if the reference food has 50% or more of its calories from fat. Reference foods with 50% of calories from fat require the *light* foods be reduced in fat by at least 50% or in calories by at least one third.

A food labeled *light in sodium* must have at least a 50% reduction in sodium content compared to an appropriate reference food. The words *light in sodium* must be printed in the same size, style, color, and prominence as the remaining label. *Light* may also be used to describe an organoleptic quality if specific (e.g., "light in color").

Descriptions of percentage and amount for nutrients may be given on a food label, if such statements are truthful and not misleading (e.g., "6 g fat per serving, but not a low-fat food").

Lean describes fish or game meat if the food contains less than 10 g fat, less than 4 g saturated fat, and less than 96 mg cholesterol per reference serving and per 100 g. *Extra lean* defines a product with less than 5 g fat, less than 2 g saturated fat, and less than 95 mg cholesterol per reference serving and per 100 g.

Meal and main-dish product definitions are similar to single-nutrient definitions of *free*. *Free* is based on the specific nutrient value per 100 g. *High* and *good source* are not applicable to meal-type products. These terms refer to a single food in the meal that meets the definition. The term *low calorie* means 120 calories per 100 g. To use the word *light*, the product must show which component the meal meets (e.g., "light, a low-fat meal," or "light in sodium").

The term *fresh* implies that a food is unprocessed, in its raw state, and never frozen or thermally processed. Fresh bread and fresh milk are not affected by this regulation.

The terms *lightly salted*, *no added sugar*, and *% fat free* are allowed on food labels if specific definitions are used. Implied claims are restricted. The term *healthy* can be printed on foods with less than 480 mg sodium or less than 60 mg cholesterol per serving.

Definition of *Healthy* Finalized

The FDA and the USDA published final rules defining the term *healthy* and its derivatives, *healthful* or *healthier*, as a nutrient content claim in food labeling effective May 8, 1994, with total compliance by January 1, 1996. The rule that applies to meat and poultry product labels became official November 10, 1995. The term *healthy* may be used as an implied nutrient content claim on individual, FDA-regulated foods if the food complies with the following:

- contains 3 g fat or less per reference amount
- contains 1 g or less of saturated fatty acids per reference amount, which accounts for no more than 15% of calories
- contains at least 10% of the RDI or DRV of one of the following micronutrients per reference amount and per serving: vitamin A, vitamin C, protein, calcium, iron, and fiber (except for raw fruits and vegetables)
- contains 360 mg or less of sodium per reference amount and per serving after January 1, 1998

Restaurant menus are not within the scope of the regulations. If claims are made, restaurant foods must meet these definitions, but the claims can be based on nutrient database calculations.

Consumers also need assistance when eating out, but menus do not contain nutrient information. The US Congress exempted restaurants from nutrient labeling in the Nutrition Labeling and Education Act in 1990.[38] Congress continues to debate legislation that would require nutritional labels in restaurants with 20 or more outlets.[39] A growing tendency is to provide nutrition information in public schools and universities to establish eating habits to last a lifetime.

The Obesity Working Group of the US Food and Drug Administration recommends that nutrient information be posted at the point of selection to promote wise food choices.[40] Studies have shown a positive relationship between nutrient label reading on food packages and dietary practices in the general population.[41,42] A study on the relationships among food label knowledge, attitudes, and behaviors of college students exposed to some form of nutrition label reading information about packaged food found that these students had favorable attitudes toward the labels and an increased use of labels in making food choices.[43]

Standardized Foods

A product with a nutrient content claim must have performance characteristics similar to those of the standardized food. The product must contain the ingredients used in the standardized food and any other safe and suitable ingredients. Water and approved fat substitutes can replace fat and calories.[31]

Declaration of Ingredients

The ingredient list on a food label lists all ingredients in order by weight, with the most predominant ingredient listed first. All certified color additives and protein hydrozylates must be identified by their common name (e.g., "FD&C blue No. 1," or "hydrolyzed soy protein"). Commonly used flavor enhancers may be added as a parenthetical term (e.g., "contains glutamate"). All ingredients in foods that are identified by a standard of identity must be listed. A sulfating agent having a functional effect or present in at least 10 parts per million must be identified.[31]

Preservative coatings on fresh fruits and vegetables can be listed by a generic name. Caseinate must be identified as a milk derivative if it is an ingredient and the food label states that the product is nondairy.

The standard of identity of canned tuna requires the words, "includes soybeans" in the name, if soybeans are a vegetable extract in the broth.[31] The delimiter "and/or" can be used for sweeteners in soft drinks (e.g., "sugar and/or high-fructose corn syrup").

Juice Beverages

The ingredient statement on beverages containing fruit or vegetable juice must include the percentage of total juice. Criteria for naming juice beverages include the following:

- A beverage with less than 100% juice is a *juice beverage* or *juice drink*, not a *juice.*

- A multijuice beverage can list the names of the juices present, but if minimal in amount, the label must describe and give a 5% range (e.g., "strawberry-flavored juice blend" or "juice blend, 2-7% strawberry juice").

A 100% juice beverage must state *from concentrate* if it is made from concentrated juice. Modified juice beverages must describe their modification and accurately calculate the percentage of total juice present.[31]

New Organic Standards

New labeling rules may assist consumers by setting standards for organic foods that farmers must follow. The rules may define organic, define a mandatory planning process that requires the use of materials from a restrictive list, and establish a procedure to verify farming prices. State, country, and private agencies will enforce the rules. The rules match industry standards and exclude irradiated and genetically engineered products. Industry sales reached $6 billion in 1999 and a projected growth of 20-25% a year is anticipated.[44]

A consumer survey conducted for the National Center for Public Policy Research, a nonpartisan, nonprofit education foundation, concluded that the rules for labeling organic food products "will seriously mislead consumers into thinking the products are safer, better in quality or more nutritious." The national consumer poll found 7 out of 10 or 69% of consumers would think the products are better for the environment and 4 out of 10 or 43% would believe they would be more nutritious. See the National Center for Public Policy Research Web site at http://www.nationalcenter.org.

Trans Fatty Acids on Nutrition Facts Labels

The Food and Drug Administration has proposed that manufacturers list grams of trans fatty acids when listing the number of grams of saturated fat in products. If a serving of a food has 4 grams of saturated fat and 2 grams of trans fatty acids, the number 6 will appear in the listing for saturated fat. A footnote saying how many grams are actually trans fat will appear at the bottom of the label.[45]

A label will not be allowed to have the words "low saturated fat" if the food is low in saturated fat but not low in trans fats. The FDA estimates that 1 out of 7-8 packaged foods will be affected, most notably margarines, crackers, cookies, pastries, and deep-fried products, along with candy bars, boxed cakes, and TV dinners. A serving of pound cake could easily have 4 grams of trans fatty acids, while doughnuts, microwave popcorn, french fries, crackers, and chocolate candies could have 2 to 3 grams. Industry is responding by producing stick margarines that were once high in trans fatty acids now trans fat free.

Trans fats don't raise LDL cholesterol quite as much as saturated fats. The intake of both should be less than 10% of total calories. Saturated fat makes up an average of 12-14% of the calories in the American diet; trans fatty acids contribute only about 2-3% of total calories.[45]

FDA Final Rule on Structure-Function Claims

An FDA final rule that enacts new labeling regulations for structure claims for dietary supplements was effective on February 7, 2000. The new regulations become part of the Code of Federal Regulations 21 CFR 101.93 (f) and (g). See Appendix 2–A.

Products marketed for the first time 30 or more days after publication of the final rule and any new claims made for the first time for an existing product on or after that date must comply. Small businesses with products and claims existing prior to January 6, 1999, had until July 6, 2001 to comply.[46]

The new regulations outline the rationale for structure/function and mechanism claims. The final rule represents substantial improvements over the proposed rule published on April 29, 1998. From a business perspective, there are both strengths and weaknesses warranting further evaluation by legal counsel.[46]

Supplement Considerations

Considerations of supplements include their efficacy, safety, dosage, side effects, interactions with medications and foods, and how dietary supplements affect medical conditions. Guides are available to assist the Community Nutrition Professional (CNP) to:

- evaluate the science behind supplements
- determine how certain dietary supplements may fit into current wellness and treatment strategies
- understand potential adverse effects, drug-nutrient interactions, and indications for commonly used dietary supplements
- communicate effectively with patients and clients regarding dietary supplements and answer questions about their use
- understand the ethical, legal, and regulatory challenges related to dietary supplements
- access essential resources for reliable information regarding botanicals and nutrient products
- educate other healthcare professionals, including physicians and nurses

In 1998, total sales of dietary supplements were estimated to be $13.9 billion in the United States, and sales were expected to increase from 10 to 14% by 2001.

Nearly one half of Americans reported taking a daily vitamin or mineral supplement.[47] Americans remain ambivalent about herbal supplements. Only 12% reported using herbal supplements on a daily basis while 80% said they rarely or never use them.[47]

In 2000, the FDA merged 2 offices within the Center for Food Safety and Applied Nutrition (CFSAN). The CFSAN's Office of Food Labeling and Office of Special Nutritionals were combined not only to form a single unit but also to maximize the resources. The new office is Office of Nutritional Products, Labeling and Dietary Supplements (ONPLDS).

The United States market for herbal supplements approaches $4 billion a year. The fastest growth has been recorded for St John's wort, an herbal antidepressant whose sales increased in 1 year by 2,800%. Doctors question if rigorous trials exist to show that herbal treatments are efficacious. Systematic reviews of trials of herbal medicines appears on the *British Medical Journal's*

Web site: www.bmj.com. Single studies do not convince skeptics, but an increasing body of evidence from systematic reviews and meta-analyses of randomized clinical trials can influence attitude and practice. Research suggests that some herbal medicines are efficacious.

The increased demand for St John's wort was initiated by press reports of a meta-analysis of 32 randomized trials of almost 2,000 patients with mild or moderate depression. The research suggested that extracts of hypericum were significantly more effective than placebo, odds ratio (O.R.) 2.67; 95% confidence interval (C.I.) of 1.78 to 4.01 and as effective as conventional antidepressants, O.R. 1.10; 93 to 1.31 in alleviating the symptoms of mild to moderate depression.[48]

A review of 9 placebo-controlled, double-blind randomized trials of *Ginkgo biloba* for dementia, involving 1,497 patients, showed that *Ginkgo* was more effective than placebo in delaying the clinical course of dementia. Concerns about herbal supplements exist, such as:

- understanding how herbal supplements actually work;
- which component is pharmacologically active;
- whether benefits outweigh risks; and

Info Line

DANGERS RELATED TO SUPPLEMENTS

DHEA

DHEA (dehydroepiandrosterone) turns into hormones such as estrogen and testosterone in the body, and the risk of hormone-related cancers like endometrial, breast, and prostate cancers may increase with supplementation. Other ill effects of taking this hormone may include acne, body hair growth, aggressive behavior, and liver enlargement. Over 2,600 reports of adverse events which consumers link with using DHEA have been received by the FDA.[35]

Further information regarding assessment of public health risks associated with the use of ephedrine alkaloid-containing dietary supplements is available at www.accessdata.fda.gov/scripts/oc/ohrms/index.cfm.

Interactions with Prescription Drugs

Functional foods may interact with prescription medications. The American Society of Anesthesiologists issued a warning to consumers not to take herbal preparations (and herbal-containing functional foods) for 2 weeks prior to receiving anesthesia because of possible cardiovascular instability, prolongation of anesthesia, and bleeding. Medications for heart disease, seizures, cancer, and birth control may be compromised if taken simultaneously with St John's wort as extracts contain at least 10 different constituents that may contribute to the pharmacological effects.

Sources: American Institute for Cancer Research Newsletter 66, Winter 2000; California Nutrition Council Newsletter, Fall 1999, p 10; FDA Public Health Advisory February 10, 2000; Quin-Ying Y, Berquist C, Gerden B. Safety of St. John's wort. *Lancet.* 2000;355:575-577.

- whether a possibility of herb-drug interactions and serious adverse effects exists. For example, when combined with warfarin, ginseng's antiplatelet activity might cause overanticoagulation.

Interactions between herbal remedies and synthetic drugs are possible. The following and other healthcare issues are destined to play a role in the debate about the safety of phytomedicines.[48]

- Can herbal medicines save money?
- Are doctors, pharmacists, and other healthcare professionals sufficiently knowledgeable to advise their patients responsibly?
- Should detailed questions about use of herbal drugs form an essential part of taking a medical history?
- Can the perceived benefits and adverse effects of self-prescribed herbal treatments be monitored?

Selected dietary supplements are associated with serious safety problems that were originally cited in a 1993 FDA document, *Unsubstantiated Claims and Documented Health Hazards in the Dietary Supplement Marketplace*.[49] Please visit the FDA Web site at http://vm.cfsan.fda.gov/~dms/ds-ill2.html. FDA does not endorse or recommend products or services visible on the Web site. The NIH's Office of Dietary Supplements (ODS) electronic mailing list can be accessed at http://dietary-supplements.info.nih.gov.

No federal guidance or mandate exists for the collection, documentation, or evaluation of consumer health complaints associated with the use of dietary supplements. The Life Sciences Research Office convened an independent panel to review data associated with the use of dietary supplements and evaluate their application when signaling potential product problems. Postmarketing surveillance programs and an effective system to monitor and respond to health complaints associated with the use of dietary supplements use will be developed.[50]

General Reqiurements for Health Claims on Food Labels

The Nutrition Labeling and Education Act mandates nutrition labels for conventional foods and requires FDA to regulate any claims printed on labels.[29,30,51,52] Several key words on labels have specific, defined meanings. If a health claim is made, then the food must have a certain composition. Table 2–14 identifies key label issues and consumer messages surrounding dietary supplements.

The term *health claim* is defined for food labels to encompass both explicit and implied claims. Food labeling can include health claims, but the claims must be supported by valid and substantial scientific evidence. The claims must also be those FDA has specifically identified by regulation. The final rules exist for health claims relating nutrients and conditions: calcium and osteoporosis, dietary saturated fat and cholesterol and risk of coronary heart disease, dietary fat and cancer, sodium and hypertension, fiber-containing foods and cancer, fiber-containing foods and coronary heart disease, and folic acid and neural tube defects. Health claims that are not authorized include those concerning zinc and immune function in the elderly and omega-3 fatty acids and coronary heart disease.[51,52]

TABLE 2-14 Comparison of Nutrition Labels Claims and Messages for Food Products and Dietary Supplements

	Food Products	Dietary Supplements
Title	Nutrition Facts	Supplement Facts
Serving size information	Serving size based on reference amounts. Wording for heading specified (e.g., "Amount per serving").	Manufacturer determines serving size. Manufacturer determines wording for heading (e.g., "Each tablet contains").
Nutrient list	14 mandatory nutrients must be included in main list or in footnote. 24 nonmandatory nutrients may be listed optionally, unless added to product or a claim is made about them. Only mandatory or the aforementioned 24 nonmandatory nutrients may be listed. Order of nutrients is specified.	14 mandatory nutrients listed only when present. Same provisions for nonmandatory nutrients. Different order of nutrients specified. Can list sources of nutrients (e.g., vitamin C as ascorbic acid).
Ingredients	Cannot be included in nutrition facts box.	Included in supplement facts box. List part of plant when botanicals (e.g., root, leaves). List below nutrients, separated by heavy line.
Footnotes	"Percent DV based on a 2,000-calorie diet." "Not a significant source of . . ." used for mandatory nutrients at insignificant levels.	"Percent DV based on a 2,000-calorie diet." "+ DV not established" flags other dietary ingredients and subcomponents of nutrients.
Design and layout	Strict rules that pertain to Type size Leading (space between lines) Rules Bolding Box	Same basic format. Some requirements more relaxed. Can use smaller type to accommodate pill-size bottles.

Permissible and Prohibited Claims

Types of Prohibited Statements	Examples of Prohibited Disease Claims	Examples of Permissible Structure/Function Claims
Effect on a specific disease or class of diseases	Protects against the development of cancer. Reduces pain and stiffness associated with arthritis.	Helps promote urinary tract health. Helps maintain cardiovascular function. Promotes relaxation.
Drug or substitute for a drug	Antibiotic/antiseptic. Laxative. Diuretic. Antidepressant. Herbal Prozac.	Energize. Rejuvenate. Promotes regularity.
Effect on signs or symptoms of a disease	Lowers cholesterol. Reduces joint pain.	Maintains healthy cholesterol levels. Reduces stress and frustration.
Role in body's response to disease	Supports body's antiviral capabilities. Supports body's ability to resist infection.	Supports immune system.
Treats, prevents, or mitigates adverse effects of a medical therapy or procedure	Helps avoid diarrhea associated with antibiotic use. Reduces nausea associated with chemotherapy.	Helps maintain healthy intestinal flora.

Key Messages About the Supplement Facts Label

Feature of Label	Key Messages
Product name	If the term *dietary supplement* or *supplement* is in the product name, the product is not a conventional food.
	Dietary supplements are intended to be used as an adjunct to, not replacement for, a balanced diet.
Ingredients	The supplements facts box and ingredients or other ingredients information tells what is in a product.
Claims	Dietary supplement labels can carry statements of nutritional support (often referred to as structure/function of claims) without obtaining premarketing authorization of FDA.

continued

TABLE 2-14   continued

Key Messages About the Supplement Facts Label

Feature of Label	Key Messages
	Structure/function claims can address how nutrients and/or dietary ingredients support or promote healthy functioning of the body.
	Supplement labels that contain a structure/function claim must also carry a disclaimer prominently displayed and in boldface type that states: **"This statement has not been evaluated by the Food and Drug Administration. This product is not intended to diagnose, treat, cure, or prevent any disease"**
	Supplement companies must maintain substantiation files to support structure/function claim; however, substantiation files are not generally reviewed by FDA and vary in content.
	Health and nutrient content claims on dietary supplement and food product labels are subject to provisions set forth in the Nutrition Labeling and Education Act of 1990 and the FDA Modernization Act of 1997 and must be authorized by FDA prior to the product's being sold in the marketplace.
Percent daily value	This column provides information on how the nutrient content of the product compares to the recommended intakes.
Serving size and daily dosage	Manufacturers determine the serving size and are free to make a label statement about how many servings to consume in a day.
	Many nutrients and other dietary ingredients found in supplements can be toxic if taken in excessive amounts. Consumers should be cautioned about taking supplements with more than 100% of the daily value.
Footnotes	"Daily values based on a 2,000-calorie reference diet." Individual needs may be higher or lower, depending on necessary energy intake. "+ Daily value not established" Comparative information for some nutrients and dietary ingredients is not included because recommended intakes have not been determined.

Source: Storlie J. DSHEA revisited: understanding and using the supplement facts label. *Scan's Pulse.* Winter 1999;18(1):5-9.

A general health claim rule exists. It defines *disqualifying nutrient levels* and refers to specified levels of total fat, saturated fat, cholesterol, and sodium. A food will be disqualified from making any health claim if it contains 1 or more of these nutrients in amounts above widely accepted guidelines for reducing the risk. A higher value is allowed for main dish and meal products.[51,52]

A food bearing a health claim must be a good source of either vitamin A, vitamin C, iron, calcium, protein, or fiber before addition of other nutrients. Claims on infant and toddler foods are prohibited unless under a special permit. The final rule identifies the FDA process to review food label petitions and the information required for the review.[51,52] Rationale for and examples of model health claims are presented in the following sections.

Fiber-Containing Grain Products, Fruits, Vegetables, and Cancer

Food labeling health claims relating low-fat, high-fiber foods and cancer are allowed. Research data show an association between fiber-containing grain products, fruits, and vegetables and below-normal rates of some cancers. The exact role of total dietary fiber and fiber components is not fully understood.

To have a health claim for fiber-containing grains, fruits, vegetables, and a reduced risk of cancer, a food must qualify as a low-fat food and contain, without fortification, a good source of dietary fiber. The claim cannot give any credit for cancer risk reduction to low-fat and fiber-rich foods, and it cannot specify types of dietary fiber that may relate to cancer risk.[31]

> *Model Health Claim:* "Low-fat diets rich in fiber-containing grain products, fruits, and vegetables may reduce the risk of some types of cancer, a disease associated with many factors."[31]

Fruits, Vegetables, and Grain Products That Contain Fiber, Particularly Soluble Fiber, and Risk of Coronary Heart Disease

Sufficient scientific evidence and scientific agreement exist that show that an eating pattern low in saturated fat and cholesterol and rich in fruits, vegetables, and grain products with certain dietary fibers may enhance coronary heart disease (CHD) risk reduction. Numerous scientific and professional organizations recommend that Americans consume foods low in saturated fat and cholesterol and rich in fruits, vegetables, and grain products. These foods are rich sources of soluble fiber, which is associated with lowering blood cholesterol. This claim clearly exemplifies applied nutritional epidemiology. That is, epidemiologic data provided the foundation linking food with nutrition and health; the science of nutrition identified the specific protective foods to promote health; and nutrition education of the public about food selection at the point of purchase has become the channel to communicate the message. Nutrition and epidemiology thereby became essential partners in the identification of the problem and the promotion and prevention of disease.

To bear a health claim relating fiber-rich fruits, vegetables, and grain products to CHD, a food must contain, without fortification, at least 0.6 g of soluble fiber in the common serving. The claim cannot give a numeric value to the potential risk reduction.[31]

> *Model Health Claim:* "Diets low in saturated fat and cholesterol and rich in fruits, vegetables, and grain products that contain some types of dietary fiber may reduce the risk of heart disease, a disease associated with many factors."[31]

Calcium and Osteoporosis

Sufficient scientific evidence exists to demonstrate an association between inadequate calcium intake and osteoporosis. Risk factors include the following:

- increased age
- being a female of the white or Asian race
- menopausal women experiencing loss of the hormone estrogen
- an inadequate amount of calcium throughout life
- lack of regular exercise
- an unhealthy eating pattern

For individuals at greatest risk of osteoporosis, an adequate calcium intake can increase bone mass during the teens and early adult life. Bone loss begins at about age 35; however, women and men with higher bone mass before age 35 delay their bone loss and pending bone fractures.[31]

To list a calcium–osteoporosis-related health claim, a food or supplement must contain at least 20% (at least 200 mg) of the calcium RDI. The food or supplement should not contain excess amounts of other nutrients (e.g., fat or sodium) that are contrary to overall good health. The form of the calcium in the food must be bioavailable and dissolve well. In addition, the amount of phosphorus cannot exceed the amount of calcium. Labels of products having more than 40% of the RDI or 400 mg must indicate that a total dietary calcium intake greater than 200% of the RDI for calcium (2,000 mg) does not give additional benefit to bone health. This claim is another excellent example of applied nutritional epidemiology.

> *Model Health Claim Appropriate for Most Conventional Foods:*
> "Regular exercise and a healthy diet with enough calcium help teens and young adult white and Asian women maintain good bone health and may reduce their high risk of osteoporosis later in life."[31]

Dietary Fat and Cancer

Scientific data show a significant association between dietary fat and some cancers. Eating behaviors, heredity, and exposure to environmental factors are the major risk factors for cancer. Scientific data support a link between high fat intake and some cancers, but not specific fatty acids and cancer. Individuals at risk for cancer cannot be clearly identified; however, the public in general is at risk due to the high average fat intake. A lower fat intake is preventative and advised.[31]

To have a health claim of this type, a food must be a low-fat food. This health claim is the third excellent example of applied nutritional epidemiology.

> *Model Health Claim:* "Development of cancer depends on many factors. A diet low in total fat may reduce the risk of some cancers."[31]

Dietary Saturated Fat and Cholesterol and Risk of CHD

The data linking (1) an eating pattern high in saturated fat and cholesterol with an increased risk of heart disease, and (2) an eating pattern low in saturated fat and cholesterol linked with decreasing CHD risk are strong, convincing, and consistent. Excessive intakes of saturated fat and cholesterol are the major determinants of total cholesterol, low-density-lipoprotein cholesterol (LDL cholesterol), and an increased risk of CHD.

Foods that are low in saturated fat, low in cholesterol, and low in fat can have a health claim. Fish and game meats must be extra lean. The health claim must state that eating patterns low in saturated fat and cholesterol "may" or "might" reduce the risk of heart disease and that CHD has many causal factors.[31]

The effects of dietary changes in saturated fat and cholesterol on the total and LDL cholesterol levels of blood vary among individuals. However, most individuals will benefit from diets low in saturated fat and cholesterol. Acceptable recommendations for all Americans are to follow eating patterns with less than 30% of calories from total fat, less than 10% from saturated fat, and less than 300 mg of cholesterol per day. Each individual recommendation and the aggregate of all the recommendations exemplify applied nutritional epidemiology.

> *Model Health Claim:* "While many factors affect heart disease, diets low in saturated fat and cholesterol may reduce the risk of this disease."[31]

Fruits and Vegetables and Cancer

Foods that are low in fat and are a good source of dietary fiber, vitamin A as beta-carotene, or vitamin C can lower an individual's cancer risk. Health claims linking antioxidant vitamins themselves to reduced cancer risk are not authorized. FDA has concluded that, based on the totality of scientific evidence, there is significant scientific agreement that eating patterns low in fat and high in fruits and vegetables reduce the risk of cancer.[31]

The health claim must say that low fat and high fruit and vegetable intakes "may" or "might" reduce the risk of "some cancers" or "some types of cancer." No specific level of cancer risk reduction can be stated. Each food with a claim must be or contain a fruit or vegetable, be a low-fat food and a natural good source of vitamin A, vitamin C, or dietary fiber. This link between fruits, vegetables, and cancer prevention again demonstrates applied nutritional epidemiology.

> *Model Health Claim:* "Low-fat eating patterns rich in fruits and vegetables and low in fat but high in dietary fiber, vitamin A, or vitamin C may reduce the risk of some types of cancer, a disease associated with many factors. Broccoli is high in vitamins A and C, and is a good source of dietary fiber."[31]

Sodium and Hypertension

High blood pressure is correlated to a family history of hypertension, aging, obesity, excess alcohol intake, and an eating pattern high in sodium. Sodium chloride, commonly known as table salt, is 40% sodium. Sodium occurs naturally in many foods, but an excess intake is unnecessary and potentially harmful. Individuals need only 500 mg of sodium each day. A total intake of 2,400 mg of sodium per day exceeds basic needs, even though a typical intake is between 3,000 and 6,000 mg.

Foods with a claim must state that a low-sodium eating pattern "may" or "might" reduce high blood pressure risk and that high blood pressure is multi-factorial. A specific statement about the magnitude of risk reduction expected with a low-sodium eating pattern is not allowed. Foods eligible for the sodium claim must be low in sodium and have acceptable levels of fat, saturated fat, and cholesterol.[31] Applying the nutritional science to the selection of foods to reduce high blood pressure is yet another example of how nutrition can be applied in the community to improve the health of the nation.

> *Model Health Claim:* "Diets low in sodium may reduce the risk of high blood pressure, a disease associated with many factors."[31]

Dietary Sugar Alcohol and Dental Caries

Between-meal eating of foods high in sugar and starches may promote tooth decay. Sugarless candies made with certain sugar alcohols do not. Typical foods are sugarless candy and gum. Foods must meet the criteria for sugar free. The sugar alcohol must be xylitol, sorbitol, mannitol, maltitol, isomalt, lactitol, hydrogenated starch hydrolysates, hydrogenated glucose syrups, erythritol, or a combination of these. When the food contains a fermentable carbohydrate, such as sugar or flour, the food must not lower plaque pH in the mouth below 5.7 while it is being eaten or up to 30 minutes afterward. Claims must use "sugar alcohol," "sugar alcohols," or the name(s) of the sugar alcohol present and "dental caries" or "tooth decay" in discussing the nutrient-disease link. Claims must state that the sugar alcohol present "does not promote," "may reduce the risk of," "is useful in not promoting," or "is expressly for not promoting" dental caries.

> *Model Health Claim:* Full claim: "Frequent between-meal consumption of foods high in sugars and starches promotes tooth decay. The sugar alcohols in this food do not promote tooth decay." Shortened claim (on small packages only): "Does not promote tooth decay."

Folic Acid and Neural Tube Defects

For most women who have problems due to inadequate folate intake, these problems develop before they are aware they are pregnant. Adequate folate protects unborn babies from spina bifida, in which the backbone does not fully form around the nerves of the spinal cord. The spinal cord is exposed and may be damaged when the child is born. This can result in paralysis. Foods that are fortified with 140 mg of folic acid per 100 g of bread and grain product can make a health claim.

> *Model Health Claim:* "Daily consumption of folate by women of child-bearing age may reduce the risk of neural tube defects in their offspring."[31]

Soy Protein and Heart Disease

The Food and Drug Administration allows health claims on labels stating that foods containing soy protein may reduce the risk of heart disease when included in a diet low in both saturated fat and cholesterol. Aggregate research strongly suggests that soy protein lowers both total cholesterol and LDLs ("bad," low-density-lipoprotein cholesterol).

To have the claim, a food must contain at least 6.25 g of soy protein per serving, i.e., one fourth the 25 g/d recommended to lower cholesterol. To lower LDLs by 5-7%, 4 servings a day are suggested, unless the food is made from whole soybeans, which are naturally high in heart-healthy unsaturated fats.

Soy protein and isoflavones are the plant chemicals giving additional heart benefits, protecting against cancer, strengthening bones, and relieving menopausal symptoms. Most soy beverages, tofu, tempeh, and soy-based meat and dairy alternatives contain the isoflavones.

For heart health, the goal is 25 g/d of soy protein and 30 mg/d of isoflavones (the FDA allows soy health claims on labels).

> *Model Health Claim:* "Daily intakes of 25 grams of soy protein may reduce the risk of heart disease when eaten as part of a low saturated fat and cholesterol eating plan."

Plant Stanols and CHD

The US FDA on September 5, 2000, issued a rare interim final rule on plant stanol/sterol esters that will allow labeling on Benecol foods stating that they have been proven to lower cholesterol and may lower the risk of heart disease when part of a diet low in saturated fat and cholesterol. This is only the 12th food health claim ever issued by the FDA. The FDA took this action on the basis of the public health significance of the cholesterol-lowering benefit of Benecol.

> *Model Health Claim:* "3.4 grams of plant stanol esters consumed daily, added to a diet low in saturated fat and cholesterol, may reduce the risk of heart disease. Benecol spread contains 1.7 grams of stanol esters per serving."

Soluble Fiber from Certain Foods and Risk of Coronary Heart Disease

> *Model Health Claim:* "Soluble fiber from foods such as [name of soluble fiber source, and, if desired, name of food product], as part of a diet low in saturated fat and cholesterol, may reduce the risk of heart disease. A serving of [name of food product] supplies __ grams of the [necessary daily dietary intake for the benefit] soluble fiber from [name of soluble fiber source] necessary per day to have this effect."

Claims Authorized Based on Authoritative Statements by Federal Scientific Bodies

- Whole grain foods and risk of heart disease and certain cancers
  Food must contain 51% or more whole grain ingredients by weight.

> *Model Health Claim:* "Diets rich in whole grain foods and other plant foods and low in total fat, saturated fat, and cholesterol may reduce the risk of heart disease and some cancers."

- Sodium, potassium, and the risk of high blood pressure and stroke

> *Model Health Claim:* "Diets containing foods that are a good source of potassium and that are low in sodium may reduce the risk of high blood pressure and stroke."

- Monounsaturated fat from olive oil and reduced risk of CHD

> *Model Health Claim:* "Limited and not conclusive scientific evidence suggests that eating about 2 tablespoons (23 grams) of olive oil daily may reduce the risk of coronary heart disease due to the monounsaturated fat in olive oil. To achieve this possible benefit, olive oil is to replace a similar amount of saturated fat and not increase the total number of calories you eat in a day. One serving of this product [Name of food] contains [x] grams of olive oil."

Info Line

> Pam cooking spray, introduced in 1959, was novel, allowing consumers to spray a fine mist of vegetable oil on pans prior to cooking or baking, thus reducing the amount of fat needed. Fill-it-yourself oil canisters are now available. Canisters allow greasing of baking pans with any preferred oil, spraying oil evenly, and misting pasta. Several brands use a pump in the cap to pressurize the contents and a spray valve that releases a very fine mist. The original EcoPump, in a clear plastic bottle, is about $15; the Misto, in stainless steel, is about $20, or in brushed aluminum is about $15; Kitchen Mister, is about $7.
>
> *Source:* Move over Pam … for refillable oil misters. *Environmental Nutrition.* Dec. 1999; 22:(12).

Designing Foods

High-protein and low-carbohydrate foods were mainstreamed in the United States to meet consumer demands. Most snack foods are made from high-starch ingredients such as corn flour, and they contain only 3-5 % protein, fats, and sweeteners.

To increase the protein in such foods as breakfast cereals, corn puffs, cheese curls, and energy bars by 35%, whey proteins left over from cheese making are added without reducing the crunchiness of the end product. The right temperature and moisture content needed to blend corn flour with whey protein isolate has been determined.[53]

On the other hand, 2 frequent processes to lower carbohydrates are:

- replace wheat flour with soy flour, nuts, or wheat protein containing fiber to add weight and texture; and
- replace sugar with sugar alcohols—maltitol, lactitol, and sorbitol, containing half the carbohydrate of sugar. Because sugar alcohols have less effect on blood insulin and blood sugar, food producers often advise consumers to subtract all sugar alcohols to get effective carbs or net effective carbs. The problem is that the carbohydrate number on the nutrition facts panel is correct. *Low carbohydrate* is not an approved term and has no legal definition.[54]

Foods Outside the Home

Americans average about half of their food dollars on meals and snacks in restaurants, hotels, hospitals, and schools. In 2001, food away from home exceeded $400 billion as consumers chose larger portions and newer foods. How eating away from home affects nutrition and health isn't clear. On the average, adults have experienced a threefold increase in the percentage of total energy intake from food away from home and chosen one fourth of their meals as food away from home. Restaurant dining has a positive impact on body fatness. Using food frequency questionnaires with energy and macronutrient intakes, a cross-sectional study of 73 older adults reported a positive association between eating away from home frequency and body fatness, controlling for education, smoking, alcohol intake, and physical activity. Total energy, fat, and saturated fat intakes increased as eating away from home increased. Most respondents were white and from a middle to upper-middle economic level.[55]

Consumers who eat healthy may be more selective of restaurant type.[56] Healthy restaurants could be distinguished by their menus and whether they provide nutrient analysis. A study of New Jersey consumers showed they were aware of the link between diet and health and believe that heart disease and other chronic diseases are related to diet.[57] Knowledge, however, may not impact consumers' decisions when choosing foods outside the home.

Research Needs

Food and nutrition are integrative disciplines that invite other specialties to join their research and program agenda. Together these disciplines develop new avenues of thought when presented with human nutrition problems facing both individuals and groups. The problems may surface from surveillance or monitoring or from development or adaptation of products for human use. A recurrent challenge is to keep the research agenda for food and nutrition invigorated by innovations in the biological sciences.[58] Major research themes of the Institute of Medicine (see Chapter 3) were identified as nutrients in human development, genes, food, and chronic disease, determinants of food intake, enhancing the food supply, and food and nutrition policies. The committee recognizes that food and nutrition policies involve social, economic, and biological issues.[58-61]

Efforts are being made to evaluate the efficacy of nutrition research. Uniform and up-to-date reporting methods of research costs include the Human Nutrition Research and Information Management System. This is an online retrieval system to identify and categorize federally funded human nutrition research projects in all government agencies.[62]

Analysis of the cost-effectiveness of the research shows whether investments in nutrition are worthwhile. Research investments and their benefits, especially for basic research, are difficult to measure.[63] Nutrition research can provide the best available knowledge to address national problems and goals and to help the United States maintain a leadership position in technologies that affect industrial and economic performance.[64]

The Relationship Between Nutrition and Disease

In today's food-selection environment, the roles of several dietary factors in the etiology and prevention of chronic diseases—including cancer, osteoporosis, and stroke—have been elucidated. We have a fairly clear understanding of the childhood dietary patterns that will best provide adequate intake of calories and nutrients essential for growth and development, yet prevent the early onset of chronic diseases. The effects of maternal nutrition on the health of the developing fetus remain pivotal for young mothers in their teen years as well as for women over 20 years of age. Nutrient and energy requirements of older adults need to be extended to include the effects of nutrition on age-related impairment of organ system functions (e.g., cardiovascular, gastrointestinal/oral cavity, immune, musculoskeletal, and nervous systems). In addition, comprehensive dietary recommendations for older adults should reflect common comorbidity patterns.[58]

The relationship of total body fat and body fat distribution to health outcomes (i.e., a health-related definition of obesity) needs further study. Research efforts could be directed toward the epidemiology of weight gain and successful weight loss, the health effects of weight loss and regain (weight cycling), and the healthy nutritional practices that best promote weight loss.

Conversely, the etiology, epidemiology, prevention, and treatment of eating disorders such as anorexia nervosa and bulimia need exploration. Nutrition-to-drug interaction research and delineation of the definition and measurement of hunger are needed.

Determining valid and reliable biochemical markers of dietary intake remains a challenge, yet credible markers will improve the ability of community nutrition professionals to monitor the effectiveness of dietary intervention.

Research efforts are needed to translate nutrient requirements and dietary recommendations into healthful dietary patterns. The 2005 USDA

Exhibit 2–8   Research in USDA–the 2005 Strategic Action Plan in Human Nutrition

The 2005 research plan in human nutrition within the USDA is a strategic action plan divided into the 7 major and relevant components.

Component 1: Nutrition Requirements
Performance goal–human nutrition requirements: Determine requirements for nutrients and other food components of children, pregnant and lactating women, adults, and elderly of diverse racial and ethnic backgrounds.

The challenge regarding nutrient requirements is to identify essential nutrients, determine their effects on reproduction, development, function, and longevity, and to provide information useful for developing standards. The standards can optimize human health, well-being, and genetic potential throughout the life cycle.

Component 2: Diet, Genetics, Lifestyle, and the Prevention of Obesity and Disease
Performance goal–human nutrition requirements: Determine requirements for nutrients and other food components of children, pregnant and lactating women, adults, and elderly of diverse racial and ethnic backgrounds.

The interaction among nutrient intakes, genotypes, and living environments that affect individual health and biological function are the focus. Inadequate intakes and metabolism of many nutrients are associated with an increased risk of both chronic and infectious disease. Effects are modifiable. Age and life stage, overall health and nutritional status, intakes of other nutrients and food components, and exposure to environmental agents influence the effect. In addition, lifestyle and medical factors such as physical activity, smoking, alcohol and medications, reproductive history, and genetic factors including sex, race, and genetic polymorphisms all have a role in the disease process.

Component 3: Nutrition Monitoring
Performance goal–food composition and consumption: Develop techniques for determining food composition, maintain national food composition databases, monitor the food and nutrient consumption of the US population, and develop and transfer effective nutrition intervention strategies.

USDA has been conducting nationwide surveys on the food consumption of Americans since the 1930s. The goal is to continue to monitor the diets of Americans to assess food and nutrient intakes as required by the National Nutrition Monitoring and Related Research Act of 1990 (PL 101-445). The USDA/ARS nationwide food consumption surveys provide the data needed to monitor and assess food consumption and related behavior of the US population, and for food and nutrition-related programs and policy decisions.

Ongoing methodology research and development is a priority. This supports effective and efficient large-scale survey operations. For example, exploring whether technology can enhance the accuracy of 24-hour dietary recalls and the development of computerized systems to collect and process dietary data is important. Continuous research and development are required to assure that nutrition monitoring data are provided to all customers in a timely, comprehensive, and accurate manner.

Component 4: Composition of Foods
Performance goal–food composition and consumption: Develop techniques for determining food composition, maintain national food composition databases,

Exhibit 2–8   continued

monitor the food and nutrient consumption of the US population, and develop and transfer effective nutrition intervention strategies.

Food composition data form the basis of nutrition research, nutrition monitoring, medical treatment, and development of national nutritional policy. These data must be accurate and current for the US food supply. Due to the wide variety of foods, a continuous introduction of new foods, scientific discoveries regarding biologically active food components, and the need to expand analytical methodology, maintaining a quality database is essential. The USDA/ARS reference National Nutrient Databank includes diverse agricultural commodities and processed, multicomponent, ethnic, and restaurant foods. Values for nutrients and other components must be available to support diverse needs. Characterization of the food supply requires analytical methods suitable for large-scale analyses. These methods must be simultaneously sophisticated (to extract, identify, and quantify the components of interest) and robust (automated, rapid, and user-friendly).

Component 5: Health Promoting Intervention Strategies for Targeted Populations
Performance goal–food composition and consumption: Develop techniques for determining food composition, maintain national food composition databases, monitor the food and nutrient consumption of the US population, and develop and transfer effective nutrition intervention strategies.

Coronary heart disease, cancer, diabetes, and obesity are caused in different ways by unhealthful dietary and physical activity behaviors. Preventing these diseases means changes in eating patterns like adding more fruit and vegetables and physical activities. Research will focus on the design, implementation, and evaluation of intervention programs to improve ineffective strategies. Basic behavioral research is needed to understand current dietary and physical activity behaviors and to determine dietary and lifestyle interventions that motivate a positive, long-term behavioral change.

Component 6: Health Promoting Properties of Plant and Animal Foods
Performance goal–nutritious plant and animal products: Develop more nutritious plant and animal products for human consumption.

Many foods contain components other than traditional nutrients that may affect fetal/child development and aging. This occurs from altering body function. Foods have the potential to improve general health and prevent certain chronic diseases. These phytonutrients/phytochemicals may come from plants, others may come from animal foods like meat, milk, or eggs, and alternative treatment and supplementation of usual foods as vitamins, minerals.

Component 7: Bioavailability of Nutrients and Food Components (e.g., Phytonutrients and Phytochemicals)
Performance goal–nutritious plant and animal products: Develop more nutritious plant and animal products for human consumption.

Bioavailability, the fraction of an ingested nutrient or food component that is absorbed and utilized or stored within the body, is influenced by the nutrient or food component in the food. Bioavailability and knowledge of the nutrient or component in the food is the focus to determine human requirements for the nutrient and the component.

Source: US Department of Agriculture. *2005 Strategic Action Plan in Human Nutrition.* Washington, DC: US Dept of Agriculture; 2005.

strategic action plan is outlined in Exhibit 2–8. How to achieve appropriate food choices and sustained behavioral changes for various subpopulations needs further exploration. Creating, evaluating, and communicating information about food by using labels that are more informative can be a part of social research efforts to evaluate behavior change. The goal of creating healthy foods rather than changing eating habits has fostered the development of biotechnology.[58,59,65]

Biotechnology

Traditional biotechnology involves plant and animal breeding and mutation, collection, selection, and natural products. New biotechnology produces genetic modification at the molecular level opening the doors for a new field of bionutrition. The American Medical Association and the American Dietetic Association both support biotechnology for food uses,[66,67] while others oppose it.[68] Surveys of consumer awareness and acceptance of biotechnology demonstrate the greatest consumer trust in independent health organizations, such as the American Medical Association, and least trust in grocery stores, activist groups, and chefs.[69,70]

Biotech Foods

In April 2000, the National Academy of Sciences identified foods from biotechnology (bt) crops as safe, with oversight needed. A Gallup poll reported 14% of Americans with limited awareness and 80% believing grocery store foods are safe to eat. About one third of Americans believe foods made with bt present a health hazard to consumers, leaving one half to disagree and one fifth unsure. These proportions have not changed since the first Gallup poll on this topic in the fall of 1999. See www.gallup.com, April 11, 2000.

In molecular biotechnology or genetic engineering, genes are isolated and chemically characterized and the protein produced by the gene and its function are known. Using replication and with this knowledge, vegetables can be cloned using a vector that transmits the DNA to produce the new and identical cells. A modern case study involved a tomato gene and the Flavr Savr tomato.[71-77]

Molecular biotechnology allows genes to be moved from one unrelated organism to another to produce a *transgenic organism*. The gene for chymosin, the milk coagulant used in cheese production, has been isolated in pure form from calves and introduced into *Escherichia coli* K-12. This enhances fermentation and isolation of pure chymosin. An impure renin from the stomachs of slaughtered calves does not have to be used. The chymosin is identical in form and function to the chymosin from calves.[65] Another transgenic product, bovine somatotropin (BST), has increased efficiency of milk production of cows by 10-20%. Several organizations provide position papers, pamphlets, and information sheets on biotechnology (see Table 2–15).

Other food products are being developed as a result of advances in biotechnology. Microbial *Bacillus thuringiensis* toxin (BT) is a biological insect control agent[78] that produces a protein that is toxic to insects but not to mammals.[79] Crops treated with BT are planted in refuse fields adjacent to pest-resistant crops.Transgenic potato contains the BT gene and eliminates the use of synthetic chemical pesticides.[74,80]

TABLE 2–15   Abbreviated List of Resources About Food Biotechnology

Organization Name	Address	Resources
American Council on Science and Health, Inc	1995 Broadway, 2nd Floor New York, NY 10023-5860 (212) 362-7044	• Public perception of food safety, *Priorities for Long Life & Good Health*, Summer 1991 • Leaner meat: a product of biotechnology, *Priorities for Long Life & Good Health*, Summer 1992 • Biotechnology—the new designer genes, *Priorities for Long Life & Good Health*, Spring 1993
American Culinary Federation, Inc	10 San Bartola Road St Augustine, FL 32085-3466 (904) 824-4468	• Biotechnology: beyond the hysteria, *The National Culinary Review*, November 1992
The American Dietetic Association	216 W Jackson Blvd Suite 800 Chicago, IL 60606-6995 (312) 899-0040	• Position of the American Dietetic Association: biotechnology and the future of food, *J Am Diet Assoc*, February 1993
Council on Scientific Affairs, The American Medical Association	515 N State St Chicago, IL 60610 (312) 422-2922	• Biotechnology and the American agricultural industry, *JAMA*, March 20, 1991
Food and Drug Administration	5600 Fishers Lane Rockville, MD 20857 (301) 443-3170	• Genetically engineered foods: fears & facts—an interview with FDA's Jim Maryanski, FDA *Consumer*, January-February 1993 • Question and answer sheet, FDA's statement of policy: foods derived from new plant varieties
International Food Information Council	1100 Connecticut Ave NW Suite 430 Washington, DC 20036 (202) 296-6540	• Consumers support use of food biotech, *Food Insight*, September-October 1992
Institute of Food Technologists	221 N LaSalle St Chicago, IL 60601 (312) 782-8424	• *Journal of the Institute of Food Technologists*
Produce Marketing Association	1500 Casho Mill Road PO Box 6036 Newark, DE 19714-6036 (302) 738-7100	• Position paper on biotechnology, October 1992
Science magazine	1333 H St NW Washington, DC 20005 (202) 326-6500	• The safety of foods developed by biotechnology, *Science*, June 26, 1992;48:36

Source: List compiled from *School Food Service J.* 1994;48(8):36.

Some transgenic plants have improved nutritional and healthful qualities. Potatoes with a higher starch content produce french fries and potato chips that absorb less fat.[81] Vegetable oils in transgenic plants have less saturated fats and can eliminate hydrogenation.[82] Transgenic corn or soybeans contain a balance of essential amino acids producing a higher quality animal feed. In time, researchers may be able to remove allergens from foods.[83] Vaccines using transgenic bananas for oral immunization of children in developing countries may become available, costing less than 2 cents per "vaccine" fruit.[84] BST has been approved for use with dairy cows, but the process has met opposition.

The Industrial Research Institute, a nonprofit organization representing 260 major food companies, reports that the United States is putting more money than ever into research and development in food technology. Aggregate research and development investment by industry increased from $97.1 billion in 1994 to $100 billion annually. About 70% will be spent on development activities such as engineering, prototypes, and testing; 22% involves applied research for products, processes, and services; and 7% for discovery-type research. Dramatic increases are noted for life science, generally biotech research. Federal spending in fiscal 2000 for research and development activities was $83.3 billion with approximately 50% going to defense-related research. See Appendices 2–B and 2–C for an update regarding consumer and expert views about biotechnology.

Benefits of Recombinant DNA (rDNA) Technology

Increased antibiotic resistance and biological resistance to specific pests and diseases include those caused by viruses. Biotechnically changed or bt corn with the *Bacillus thuringiensis* gene to withstand the corn borer pest resulted in increased yields and reduced pesticide use; e.g., 26% of farmers in the Midwest who planted the modified corn in 1998 decreased insecticide use and about 50% did not use any insecticides.[85] No evidence demonstrates that transferring genes between unrelated species will convert a harmless organism into a hazardous one. A beneficial trait may be expressed in the organism for which the targeted gene is transferred.

More than 15 years of laboratory research and field trials with rDNA-engineered plants indicate that the risks are not any greater than or different from the risks posed by traditionally grown plants.

> The agency is not aware of any information showing that foods derived by these new methods differ from other foods in any meaningful or uniform way, or that, as a class, foods developed by the new techniques present any different or greater safety concern than foods developed by traditional plant breeding.[86]

Food producers have a responsibility to ensure that their foods are safe and in compliance with applicable legal requirements. This means that they do not contain substantially increased levels of previously known toxic substances, new hazardous substances, or different levels of nutrients present in traditional counterparts; and they state whether known or potentially new allergens have been transferred to the modified product.

Info Line

MONARCH BUTTERFLY AND CORN BORER

Monarch butterflies belong to the same order of insects (*Lepidoptera*) as the corn borer. Bt corn pollen has the potential to harm monarch larvae if they eat it. This is not a surprise. The key questions are: Are monarch butterflies exposed to bt corn pollen and, if so, to what degree? Would their larvae eat plants with bt pollen instead of plants without it? What amount of pollen could be harmful to the larvae? Does milkweed, the primary source of monarch food, grow close enough to corn fields to be exposed to bt corn pollen? Up to what distance is pollen drift possible? Research in both the private and public sectors may answer these questions.

LABELING OF GENETICALLY MODIFIED FOODS

Labels imply warning. Labeling rDNA-engineered foods may not be economical because thousands of common foods containing small amounts of bt ingredients, such as soybean and corn products, would have to be labeled. Costs would be passed to producers and consumers, especially farmers, who would absorb costs for equipment to separate bt crops from non-bt ones.

Allergens are the centerpiece of health worries since allergies result from proteins, and bioengineering research already has demonstrated that genes from often-allergenic foods, like nuts, can produce allergies when transferred to new plants. Pioneer Hi-Bred stopped production of a new soybean variety with a Brazil nut gene in 1995 because people allergic to Brazil nuts became allergic to the soybeans. The Brazil nut gene would have made the soybean more nutritious as animal feed.

Industry and consumer polls show a slow but steady rise in the number of Americans who support mandatory labeling. In a 1999 *Time* magazine poll, 58% of US respondents reported they would avoid bt foods if they were labeled as such.

Fears about health risks from bt foods are not generally based on hard science, but are motivated by industry flight from biotech crops. Frito-Lay may stop the use of genetically modified corn in its corn chips but will still use biotech corn syrup in its soft drinks.

Position of the American Dietetic Association: Biotechnology and the Future of Food

Position Statement

> It is the position of the American Dietetic Association that biotechnology techniques have the potential to be useful in enhancing the quality, nutritional value, and variety of food available for human consumption and in increasing the efficiency of food production, food processing, food distribution, and waste management.[87]

ADA states that potential public health hazards posed by introduction of a food product produced by bt include an increase in toxins that naturally occur in the parent line, entrance of either a new and potentially allergenic protein from the original genetic material or of unnaturally occurring hormones, and possible pathogenic strains of bacteria.[88]

FDA states that bt foods present no inherent risk and, therefore, are regulated as food. Because of the federal Food, Drug, and Cosmetic Act, FDA uses characteristics of the food as the basis for regulation and decision making. FDA provides a decision tree, or series of testing procedures, so food processors can anticipate safety concerns and consult FDA during product development. Assessment involves toxicant characteristic of the host and donor species; the potential for food allergen transfer; the concentration and bioavailability of nutrients; and the safety and nutritional value of any new proteins, carbohydrates, or fats.[88] Toxicology and product safety data are required in the application for approval of the food product or bt ingredient.

Golden Rice

Golden rice could help prevent blindness in 500,000 children in developing countries each year. The product is enhanced through biotechnology to contain high levels of beta-carotene, which the body converts to vitamin A. About 230 million children are at risk of vitamin A deficiency, which can lead to irreversible blindness. Product availability and deployment are expected to be in 2007.[89]

Ketchup!

You may not think of pizza, spaghetti sauce, and salsa as health foods, but if these products were enhanced through biotechnology, they could contain 3 times the amount of lycopene and beta-carotene than in conventional tomatoes. The tomato may help prevent heart disease and reduce the risk of developing some cancers. The higher levels of these carotenoids may also help combat the incidence of blindness associated with vitamin A deficiency.[89]

Nutraceuticals

An alternative medicine movement has begun in the United States. This has in part occurred as more foods and specific nutrients are linked to disease prevention and promotion (e.g., linking high-fat foods with heart disease and cancer) via epidemiologic studies. As individuals take an increasing responsibility for their health, health-preventing behaviors include the use of alternative approaches.

The term *nutraceuticals* is being used in today's health care arena. The term was coined by the Foundation for Innovation in Medicine (FFIM) in 1989.[90] *Nutra* comes from the Latin word for nourish, and *pharmaceutical* is derived from the Greek term meaning a medicinal drug.*

Nutraceuticals range from isolated nutrients, to dietary supplements, to real food, and even diet plans (see Table 2–16). Genetically engineered designer foods, herbal products, and processed foods such as cereals, soups, and beverages are also included.[91]

In Japan, nutraceuticals are known as functional foods or foods derived from naturally occurring substances that are consumed as part of a daily diet or that regulate or affect certain body processes. The Japanese have instituted

*Unpublished position papers are available from FFIM, 411 North Avenue East, Cranford, NJ 07016.

TABLE 2–16 Nutraceutical Foods to Prevent Illness

Food	Action
Carrots, sweet potatoes, orange squash	Contain beta-carotene to prevent cancer.
Chili peppers	Contain capsaicin to treat infections by killing bacteria and increasing acidity of urine.
Cranberry juice	Prevents urinary tract infections by killing bacteria and increasing acidity of urine.
Cruciferous vegetables (broccoli, brussels sprouts, cabbage) and fish oil	Contain vitamin A to fight cancer, omega-3 fatty acid to prevent heart disease by lowering blood triglyceride levels.
Garlic	Lowers cholesterol and reduces blood clotting.
Green tea	Contains tannins and suppresses tumors in mice.
Licorice root	Contains prostaglandin inhibitors to inhibit cancer, ulcers, and tooth decay.
Soybeans	Contain genistein to stop tumor growth.

Source: Adapted from Dunkin A. Eat nine cloves of garlic, and call me in the morning. *Business Week.* February 25, 1993. By special permission from McGraw-Hill, Inc.

new rules for food for specified health use. The first approvals were to occur in 1993, although tension between the food and pharmaceutical industries influenced these approvals. The new rules deal with products that fall between traditional drugs and foods. It is predicted that this market will rocket to more than $500 billion by the year 2010.[90]

The definition of nutraceuticals in the United States has created a real dilemma for regulatory agencies. Many of the nutraceutical products make a health claim. The FDA regulates products based on claims, not on their manufacture. Biopharmaceuticals are judged by their safety and effectiveness for the intended use claimed by their manufacturer. The same is true for foods created by biotechnology. Health claims for foods have therefore become one of the main regulatory issues of the day.[92] The federal Food, Drug and Cosmetic Act defines drugs as substances used in the diagnosis, cure, treatment, or prevention of disease in man and animals. Drugs are also considered any article other than food that is intended to affect the structure or function of the body. Foods are subject to the drug laws if therapeutic claims are made.

A nutraceutical may be considered a food additive. If so, it must be shown to be safe by the "generally recognized as safe" regulation. Nutraceuticals may also be considered a medical product with intended use only under medical supervision.

Medical Foods

FDA requires that *medical foods* be used for oral or tube feeding and make a therapeutic claim. They must be labeled if intended for dietary management

Info Line

On September 26, 2000, Kraft Foods announced a nationwide recall of taco shells containing StarLink, a genetically modified (gm) corn approved for animals but not for humans. The recall reflects the practical difficulties involved in labeling of gm foods. Questions include the reliability of testing, the extent to which conventional grains and foods realistically can be kept separate from those that are gm, and the definition of gm food.

These issues are confronting the European Union, Australia, Japan, and other countries that require labeling or are transitioning to it, with different countries or even different supermarkets in the same country adopting different standards.

In the United States, about two thirds of processed food contains ingredients made from gm corn, soybeans, potatoes, or other crops. Congress is sponsoring bills requiring labeling and safety testing of these foods.

A coalition opposed to bt foods learned that taco shells sold under the Taco Bell brand contained small amounts of a gm corn known as "StarLink." The corn has a gene for pest resistance but has only been approved for use as animal feed, not for human consumption, since the protein has characteristics of an allergen. Labeling gm products on store shelves would establish a higher level of responsibility from industry.[93]

of a specific condition (Section 5[b] of the Orphan Drug Act [21 USC 360 ee(b)]).[94] Medical foods do not require premarket approval. They are distinguished from conventional foods that make health claims. Medical foods are not foods simply recommended by a healthcare provider to reduce disease risk or medical conditions.

Medical foods are not all foods fed to patients, rather they are specially formulated and processed foods. This contrasts with naturally occurring foodstuffs used in their natural state. Medical foods were considered drugs prior to 1972, when the FDA reclassified them as foods. They are used today for the dietary management of lung, kidney, heart, and liver diseases. Information about medical foods is important for community nutrition professionals, as more individuals are being cared for at home during rehabilitation. These individuals must draw from community services to meet their needs. Home care is a growing, progressive field, and community nutrition services in health departments and health maintenance organizations are beginning to expand home health services.

Many questions remain. Bran can lower serum cholesterol in blood. Is bran a drug? Is psyllium, a biopolymer that reduces blood cholesterol and glucose levels, a drug?

Amino acids used for total parenteral nutrition are used therapeutically in hospitals and fall into the health claims controversy. The same problem exists for L-dopa in Parkinson's disease, and beta-carotene for cancer prevention.

A 1992 legislative action, the Hatch-Richardson Bill, defined a *dietary supplement* as different from a food additive or a drug. It permits health claims without government approval if there are adequate data to support the claim.[95]

Misinformation/Disinformation

A constant consumer challenge is to decipher the volumes of nutrition information beaming from magazines, television, billboards, and product advertisements. Often the media take bits and pieces of nutrition data from epidemiologic studies and extrapolate it to mass application, creating mass confusion. Or manufacturers adapt a nutrition finding, such as the benefit of a vitamin by creating a new product or "magic bullet." The truth about the benefit of the vitamin may be stretched or taken out of context. Ironically, the public may not view the fields of nutrition, epidemiology, and nutritional epidemiology as credible due to the confusion, and the public may view business and industry as the knowledgeable group responding to help the consumer.

Disinformation is a term that describes statements, testimonials, and messages given to the public but unsubstantiated by scientific research or credible sources.[96] Seven situations or statements, that should be questioned are listed in Table 2–17 and explained further as follows[97]:

1. Beware of a dramatic or unusual statement that is not supported by a recognized organization, such as advice cited by a single individual speaking on his/her own behalf or a single individual speaking alone about his/her specific research that does not fit into mainstream research. The advocate may claim to be ahead of the times. Be concerned about a small, unknown or little-known advocacy group that could be representing facts or statements with no consensus agreement from a reputable organization. For example, "Milk is bad for all children" is not a valid claim.
2. Beware of a story that covers very diverse subjects and then leads to an overall conclusion that represents a very narrow interpretation of the information.
3. Beware when the spokesperson is a star figure whose expertise is not in the subject area that he or she is discussing. Testimonial and anecdotal nutrition statements by Hollywood stars, such as protest statements regarding Alar on apples, should make you suspicious.
4. Beware of promises or implications that there will be dramatic benefits from the use of a product or regimen. Be wary of statements implying that individuals can eat anything they want when using a particular

TABLE 2–17   Seven Situations of Concern

1. Dramatic or unusual statements not supported by a recognized organization.
2. Diverse story covers with narrow interpretation.
3. Spokesperson is star figure.
4. Promises or implies that dramatic benefits will occur.
5. Nutritional advice does not meet *Dietary Guidelines for Americans*.
6. Nutrition recommendations from politically based environmental groups.
7. Nutrition recommendations disregard differences for life stages.

Source: FDA Backgrounder: Top Health Frauds. Washington, DC: Food and Drug Administration; 1990:1-2.

substance or regimen, promising dramatic weight loss or renewed vigor, or claiming that use of a familiar food can alter a behavior. Review situations that carefully encourage the purchase of special products, involve an expensive regimen, or claim that products contain a unique nutritional ingredient unavailable in the normal food supply (for example: 'Wheatgrass cleanses the body of toxins,' 'Sugar causes hyperactivity in children,' or 'These particular fish oils and oat bran lower risk of heart disease and cancer').

5. Beware of nutrition advice that does not meet the *Dietary Guidelines for Americans*. Question recommendations that advocate eating very small or very large amounts of specific foods or that recommend exclusion of all foods from one or more food groups.

6. Beware of nutrition recommendations that come from politically based environmental groups rather than from a health or medicine perspective. For example, the Physicians' Committee for Responsible Medicine decries all children's consumption of cow's milk without offering reasonable nutrient alternatives. This is an animal rights group, representing less than 1% of all physicians in this country.

7. Beware of nutrition recommendations that leave no room for differences in life stages, such as for pregnant or lactating women, seniors, adolescents, and children. For example, question an unsupervised vegan diet for young children or pregnant women without referral to a medical or trained healthcare specialist for guidance.

The public can believe the nutrition messages[97] outlined next and summarized in Table 2–18:

- Messages that comment on reputable confirmed research or represent the consensus opinion of a recognized professional organization or government agency, including the DHHS, FDA, and USDA. Volunteer health organizations, such as the American Cancer Society, the American Diabetes Association, and the American Heart Association, are credible sources of nutrition information. Reputable consumer organizations include the Better Business Bureau, the Consumers Union, and the National Council Against Health Fraud. Credible scientific and professional organizations include the American Dietetic Association and any state dietetic association, the Society for Nutrition Education, the American Medical Association, and the American Academy of Pediatrics.

TABLE 2–18   Nutritional Stories One Can Believe

Stories that:

- comment on reptuable confirmed research
- suggest a range of food choices
- describe a reputable diet for real conditions
- differentiate between needs for children versus adults
- explain when new research is preliminary

Source: FDA Backgrounder: Top Health Frauds. Washington, DC: Food and Drug Administration; 1990:1-2.

- Messages that suggest a range of food choices based on the food grouping system represented by the USDA food guide pyramid.
- Messages that describe a special diet that severely restricts food groups in the USDA food group pyramid, if they are backed by a recognized professional organization that provides specific, practical food recommendations for adequate nutrients normally provided by the missing food groups.
- Messages that identify children's nutrient needs and eating habits as different from adults.
- Messages about new, preliminary research using 50 to 100 or more participants and a rigorous research design.

Fraud and Quackery

Obstacles to optimal health habits and positive eating behaviors include nutrition misinformation, fraud, and quackery.[97] An epidemic of quick cures, magic foods, perfect diets, and easy remedies overshadows simple truths about healthy eating. Certain situations appear to fuel nutrition quackery, such as[98]:

- *'Magic bullets':* These include just about anything that can be sold and generally labeled as a dietary supplement.
- *Nutrition publications:* These are numerous and are protected by the First Amendment of the US Constitution.
- *The title 'nutritionist':* This can be used to describe one who assumes he or she is an expert because he or she likes to eat, one who likes to cook, or one who completes a college degree.
- *Premature presentation of research:* The practice of presenting research findings is very common when only preliminary work is completed and not replicated or validated. Although findings may contradict a science base, they may seem just as important to novice consumers as a volume of sound research.

One of the greatest areas of nutrition quackery relates to sports nutrition. A competitive edge is sought by athletes and health-conscious individuals who may believe that the potential for success is greater with ergogenics.[98] As many as 50% of team members may use ergogenics.[99]

The array of ergogenic items includes more than 700 brands, products, or ingredients.[99] The buyer is receptive and unaware of the potential danger of the products. Deceptive tactics include the following[98]:

- selecting only pieces of published research to prove a point
- displaying unauthorized endorsement or support of professional organizations
- falsely stating that research has been conducted or is continuing
- providing inaccurate documentation of research
- substituting testimonials as research
- patenting products without evaluating them
- using mass media to publicize and to promote products

Another area where fraud and quackery are common is the weight-loss industry. Fraudulent products and programs are unscrupulous and persuasive[100] (see Exhibit 2–9). Many registered dietitians (RDs) work in weight-loss programs and decipher the fraudulent practices and products for their clients. Community nutrition professionals must be astute in recognizing the demands of competitive athletes for a winning edge and health-conscious adults for vitality, and the role played by pseudonutrition products.[98,101,102] Continuing education provides professionals who are not athletes with some of the necessary background to organize workshops or group presentations for parents, coaches, and athletes. It is necessary to counter quick results and

Exhibit 2–9   Weight Loss Fraud and Quackery—Guidelines for Identification

Message
- Claims or implies a large, fast weight loss—often promised as easy, effortless, guaranteed, or permanent.
- Implies weight can be lost without restricting calories or exercising, and discounts the benefits of exercise.
- Uses typical quackery terms such as miraculous, breakthrough, exclusive, secret, unique, ancient, accidental discovery, doctor developed.
- Claims to get rid of cellulite.
- Relies heavily on undocumented case histories, before-and-after photos, and testimonials by satisfied customers.
- Misuses medical or technical terms, refers to studies without giving complete references, claims government approval.
- Professes to be a treatment for a wide range of ailments and nutritional deficiencies as well as for weight loss.

Program
- Promotes a medically unsupervised diet of less than 1,000 calories per day.
- Diagnoses nutrient deficiencies with computer-scored questionnaire and prescribes vitamins and supplements. Recommends them in excess of 100% of recommended dietary allowance.
- Requires special foods purchased from the company rather than conventional foods.
- Promotes aids and devices such as body wraps, sauna belts, electronic muscle stimulators, passive motion tables, ear stapling, aromatherapy, appetite patches, and acupuncture.
- Promotes a nutritional plan without relying on at least 1 author or counselor with nutrition credentials.
- Fails to state risks or recommend a medical exam.

Ingredients
- Uses unproven, bogus, or potentially dangerous ingredients such as dinitrophenol, spirulina, amino acid supplements, glucomate, human chorionic gonadotrophin (HCG) hormone, diuretics, slimming teas, echinacea root, bee pollen, fennel, chickweed, and starch blockers.
- Claims ingredients will block digestion or surround calories, starches, carbohydrates, or fat, and remove them from the body.

Mystique
- Encourages reliance on a guru figure who has the ultimate answers.
- Grants mystical properties to certain foods or ingredients.

Exhibit 2–9   continued

- Bases plan on faddish ideas, such as food allergies, forbidden foods, or magic combinations of foods.
- Declares that the established medical community is against this discovery and refuses to accept its miraculous benefits.

Method of Availability
- Is sold by self-proclaimed health advisors or nutritionists—often door to door, in health food stores, or a chiropractor's office.
- Distributes through hard-sell mail order advertisements or through ads that list only a toll-free number without an address, indicating possible Postal Service action against the company.
- Demands large advance payments or long-term contracts.
- Uses high-pressure sales tactics, one-time-only deals, or recruitment for a pyramid sales organization. Displays prominent money-back guarantee.
- Available at popular locations such as fitness centers, beauty salons, spas, health food stores, drug stores, and grocery stores.

Source: Adapted from Berg FM. Prevention of obesity gets top billing. *Healthy Weight Journal.* 1995;9(5):2.

Info Line

The National Council Against Health Fraud, Inc
Post Office Box 1276
Loma Linda, CA 92354–1276
The following Web sites separate fact from fiction:
www.quackwatch.org, www.urbanlegends.about.com/index.htm, and www.netsquirrel.com/combatkit

'magic bullet' products, which are attractive but may present risks. Informed presentations and media messages with alternatives that are science-based may correct faulty nutrition knowledge and improve approaches to athletic training and performance. This arena is growing, and methods are needed to label products with accurate claims about their composition and benefit much in the same way the NLEA functions.

Healthy People 2010 Actions

Community nutrition professionals must be actively involved in developing and implementing programs to help consumers and their clients become nutrition smart. The knowledge base of the public influences its ability to make healthy food choices (see Exhibit 2–10). Kaufman formulated model nutrition objectives for reducing risk factors for disease and for increasing public and professional awareness[103] (Exhibit 2–11). Acronyms commonly used in community nutrition are listed in Appendix 2–D.

Exhibit 2-10 DATA 2010: *The Healthy People 2010* Database—November 2000 Edition Focus Area: 11-Health Communication

Objective	Baseline Year	Baseline	Target 2010
Households With Internet access	1998	26%	80%
Race and ethnicity			
American Indian or Alaskan native	1998	NA	80%
Asian or Pacific Islander	1998	NA	80%
Asian	1998	NA	80%
Native Hawaiian and other Pacific Islander	1998	NA	80%
Black or African American	1998	NA	80%
White	1998	NA	80%
Hispanic or Latino	1998	13%	80%
Not Hispanic or Latino	1998	NA	80%
American Indian or Alaska native, not Hispanic/Latino	1998	19%	80%
Asian or Pacific Islander, not Hispanic/Latino	1998	36%	80%
Black or African American, not Hispanic/Latino	1998	11%	80%
White, not Hispanic/Latino	1998	30%	80%
Gender (head of household)			
Female	1998	NA	80%
Male	1998	NA	80%
Education level (head of household)			
Less than high school	1998	NA	80%
High school graduate	1998	14%	80%
At least some college	1998	NA	80%
Family income level			
Poor	1998	NA	80%
Near poor	1998	NA	80%
Middle/high income	1998	NA	80%
Geographical location			
Urban (metropolitan statistical area)	1998	28%	80%
Rural (nonmetropolitan statistical area)	1998	22%	80%

Source: Adapted from US Department of Health and Human Services. DATA 2010—the Healthy People 2010 Database. *CDC Wonder.* Atlanta, Ga: Centers for Disease Control; November 2000.

Exhibit 2-11   Model Nutrition Objectives for Reduced Risk Factors

By 20__, the following contaminants will not be present in the state food supply above toxic/hazardous levels as defined by state or federal agencies:

- Agricultural: pesticides, fertilizers, growth regulators
- Drugs: antibiotics, steroids/hormones, growth regulators
- Environmental: organics, inorganics/heavy metals
- Food additives: preservatives, colors, flavors, sweeteners, stabilizers
- Industrial: organics, inorganics/heavy metals, radioactives
- Microbial: bacteria, molds, fungi, viruses, protozoa, and related toxins
- Naturally occurring toxins: carcinogens, mutagens, neurotoxins

Source: Adapted from Model State Nutrition Objectives, The Association of State and Territorial Public Health Nutrition Directors, 1988.

References

1. Hooyman NR, Kiyak HS. *Social Gerontology.* 3rd ed. Needham Heights, Mass: Simon & Schuster, Inc; 1993.
2. *Healthy People 2000: National Health Promotion and Disease Prevention Objectives.* Washington, DC: US Dept of Health and Human Services; 1991. Public Health Service publication 91-50212.
3. *The Surgeon General's Report on Nutrition and Health.* Washington, DC: US Dept of Health and Human Services; 1988. Public Health Service publication 88-50210.
4. *Dietary Guidelines for Americans.* Washington, DC: US Dept of Agriculture and US Dept of Health and Human Services; 2005.
5. National Research Council. *Recommended Dietary Allowances.* 10th ed. Washington, DC: National Academy Press; 1989.
6. Tate MJ, Patrick S. Healthy People 2010 targets healthy diet and healthy weight as critical goals. *J Am Diet Asso.* 2000;100(3):300.
7. National Heart, Lung, and Blood Institute. *NIH Heart Memo.* Bethesda, Md: Office of the Director; Spring 2003:36.
8. *The Food Guide Pyramid.* Washington, DC: US Dept of Agriculture, Human Nutrition Information Service; April 2005. Available at: http://www.mypyramid.com.
9. Oldways Preservation and Exchange Trust. *The Traditional Healthy Mediterranean Diet Pyramid.* Boston, Mass: Oldways Preservation and Exchange Trust; 1993.
10. Oldways' 2000 consensus statement: dietary fat, the Mediterranean diet, and lifelong good health. 2000 International Conference on the Mediterranean Diet; January 13-14, 2000. London, England, UK. Available at: http://www.oldwayspt.org.
11. Food Marketing Institute and *Prevention* Magazine. *Shopping for Health, 1994; Eating in America: Perception and Reality.* Washington, DC: Food Marketing Institute and *Prevention* Magazine; 1994.
12. Balch G, Loughrey K, Weinberg L, Lurie D, Eisner E. Probing consumer benefits and barriers for the national 5 A Day Campaign: focus group findings. *JNE.* 1997;29:178-183.
13. Public Law No. 101-455.
14. Kuczmarski MF, Moshfegh A, Briefel R. Update on nutrition monitoring activities in the US. *J Am Diet Assoc.* 1994;94:753-760.

15. *Nutrition Monitoring in the United States: A Progress Report from the Joint Nutrition Monitoring Evaluation Committee.* Washington, DC: US Dept of Health and Human Services and US Dept of Agriculture; 1986:356.

16. US Department of Health and Human Services and US Department of Agriculture. *Joint Implementation Plan for a Comprehensive National Nutrition Monitoring System.* Report to Congress; August 1981:59.

17. Peterkin BB, Rizek RL, Tippett KS. Nationwide Food Consumption Survey, 1987. *Nutr Today.* 1988;18:24.

18. *Nationwide Food Consumption Survey, Continuing Survey of Food Intakes by Individuals: Women 19-50 Years and Children 1-5 Years, 1 Day, 1985.* Washington, DC: US Dept of Agriculture, Human Nutrition Information Service; 1985:102.

19. *Nationwide Food Consumption Survey, Continuing Survey of Food Intakes by Individuals: Women 19-50 Years and Children 1-5 Years, 4 Days, 1985.* Washington, DC: US Dept of Agriculture, Human Nutrition Information Service; 1987:182.

20. *Research on Survey Methodology: Proceedings of a Symposium Held at the 71st Annual Meeting of the Federation of American Societies for Experimental Biology, April 1987.* Washington, DC: US Dept of Agriculture, Human Nutrition Information Service; 1987:77. Administrative report 382.

21. Bliss RM. Researchers produce innovation in dietary recall. *Agricultural Res.* June 2004;10-12.

22. Food and Nutrition Board, Institute of Medicine. *How Should the Recommended Dietary Allowances Be Revised?* Washington, DC: National Academy Press; 1994.

23. Food and Nutrition Board, Institute of Medicine, The National Academies; Food and nutrition board update; Fall 1999; Washington, DC.

24. Institute of Medicine, Food and Nutrition Board. *Dietary Reference Intakes for Vitamin C, Vitamin E, Selenium, and Carotenoids.* Washington, DC: National Academy Press; 2000.

25. Ausman LM, Mayer J. Criteria and recommendations of vitamin C intake. *Nutr Rev.* 1999;57(7):222-229.

26. Benzie IFF. Vitamin C: prospective functional markers for defining optimal nutritional status. *Proc Nutr Soc.* 1999;58:469-476.

27. Block G, Mangels AR, Patterson BH, Levander OA, Norkus EP, Taylor PR. Body weight and prior depletion affect plasma ascorbate levels attained on identical vitamin C intake: a controlled-diet study. *J Am Coll Nutr.* 1999;18(6):628-637.

28. McNamara SH. New food labeling legislation enacted. *Regulatory Affairs.* 1990;2:483-487.

29. 21 *CFR* Part I, *Federal Register.* January 6, 1993;58 Book II:2302-2964.

30. Tillotson JE. United States Nutrition Labeling and Education Act of 1990. *Nutr Rev.* 1991;49:273-276.

31. The FDA's final regulations on health claims for foods [editorial]. *Nutr Rev.* 1993;51:90-93.

32. Shank FR. The Nutrition Labeling and Education Act of 1990. *Food and Drug Law J.* 1992;47:247-252.

33. Final rule: mandatory status of nutrition labeling and nutrient content revision, formal for nutrition label. *Federal Register.* January 6, 1993;58:2079.

34. Kessler DA. Restoring the FDA's preeminence in the regulation of food. *Food Drug Cosmetic J.* 1991;46:391-394.

35. National Academy of Sciences, Institute of Medicine. *Dietary Reference Intakes: Guiding Principles for Nutrition Labeling and Fortification.*

Washington, DC: National Academy of Sciences, Institute of Medicine; 2003. Available at: http://www.IOM.edu/.

36. Traux B. Influencing Consumer Food Choices. *DBC Dimensions*; 1999:7.

37. Lang J, Mercer N, Tran D, Mosca L. Use of supermarket shelf-labeling program to educate a predominately minority community about foods that promote heart health. *J Am Diet Assoc.* 2000;100:804-809.

38. Nutrition Labeling and Education Act of 1990, Publ L. No. 101-535, 104 Stat 2353.

39. Martin A. Nutrition labels for restaurant meals urged: but firms doubt it will curb obesity. *Chicago Tribune.* November 21, 2003.

40. US Food and Drug Administration. Counting Calories: Report of the Working Group on Obesity. 2004. Available at: http://www.cfsan.fda.gov/~dms/owg-rpt.html. Accessed on March 30, 2004.

41. Kreuter LK, Scharff DP, Lukwago SM. Do nutrition label readers eat healthier diets? Behavioral correlates of adults' use of food label. *Am J Prev Med.* 1997;13:277-283.

42. Szykman LR, Bloom PN, Levy AS. A proposed model of the use of package claims and nutrition labels. *Public Policy Marketing.* 1997;16(2): 228-241.

43. Marietta AB, Welshimer KJ, Anderson SL. Knowledge, attitudes, and behaviors of college students regarding the 1990 Nutrition Labeling Education Act food labels. *J Am Diet Assoc.* 1999;99:445-449.

44. Associated Press. New organic standards finally ready. *USA Today* Health, January 21, 2000. Available at: http://www.usatoday.com. Accessed March 2000.

45. Tufts University. *Health and nutrition letter: trans fatty acids expected to appear on nutrition facts labels.* February 2000; 17(12):3. Medford, Mass.

46. Center for Food Safety and Applied Nutrition. US Food and Drug Administration. FDA final rule on structure-function claims; Washington DC: US Food and Drug Administration; February 2000.

47. American Dietetic Association. Nutrition and you: trends 2000 survey. Chicago: American Dietetic Association. National Center of Nutrition and Dietetics; 2000.

48. Ernest E. Herbal medicines: where is the evidence? *BMJ.* 2000;321: 395-396.

49. Devine N. Dangerous combinations: understanding the risks of mixing herbal products and drugs. *Nurse Week.* 2000;13(8):26.

50. News breaks: panel reports adverse event monitoring program for dietary supplements. *Nutr Today.* 2004;39(5):192-193.

51. Final rule: general requirements for health claims for foods. *Federal Register.* January 6, 1993;58:247.

52. Mandatory nutrition labeling—FDA's final rule [special report]. *Nutr Rev.* 1993;51:101-105.

53. Onwulata C. More protein in snacks. *Agricultural Res.* June 2004;23.

54. How do food manufacturers remove the carbs? Tufts University *Health & Nutrition Letter.* October 2003;21(8)4.

55. McCrory MA, Fuss PJ, Hays NP, Vinken AG, Greenberg AS, Roberts SB. Overeating in America: association between restaurant food consumption and body fatness in healthy adult men and women ages 19 to 80. *Obes Res.* 1999;7:564-571.

56. Lin B, Frazao E, Guthrie J. Contribution of away from home foods to American diet quality. *Fam Econ Nutr Rev.* 1999;12:85-89.

57. Bhyuyan S, Stewart H, Govindasamy R. Satisfaction evaluation of food-away-from-home choices by consumers. Presented at: annual conference of the Food Distribution Research Society; Summer 2002; Miami, Fla.

58. Dwyer J. Nutrition research for the year 2000 and beyond. *Contemporary Nutr.* 1993;18:1-2.

59. National Institutes of Health. *Ad Hoc Bionutrition Group, NIH Bionutrition Initiative Nutrition Notes: Draft Guidance Document April 29, 1993.* Bethesda, Md: American Institute of Nutrition; 1993;29:7-9.

60. Taylor H, Voivodas G. *The Bristol-Myers Report: Medicine in the Next Century.* New York: Louis Harris and Assoc; 1986.

61. Shafter MO, Story M, Houghton B. *Report: Survey of the Association of Graduate Faculty Programs in Public Health Nutrition* [unpublished manuscript]. Minneapolis, Minn; 1993.

62. National Institutes of Health. *Fourteenth Annual Report of the NIH Program in Biomedical and Behavioral Nutrition Research and Training, Fiscal Year 1990.* Bethesda, Md: National Institutes of Health; 1990. NIH publication 91-2092.

63. Office of Technology Assessment, US Congress. *Research Funding as an Investment: Can We Measure the Returns?* Washington, DC: US Government Printing Office; 1986.

64. Committee on Science, Engineering and Public Policy of the Academies and the Institute of Medicine. *Science, Technology and the Federal Government: National Goals for a New Era.* Washington, DC: National Academy of Sciences; 1993.

65. Hardy RWF. Biotechnology and food. *Contemporary Nutr.* 1994;19:2.

66. Council on Scientific Affairs, American Medical Association. Biotechnology and the American agricultural industry. *JAMA.* 1991;265:1429-1436.

67. Brewer MS, Kendall P. Position of the American Dietetic Association—Agricultural and food biotechnology. Chicago. *J Am Diet Asso.* 2006; 106:285-293.

68. Vines G. Guess what's coming to dinner. *New Sci.* 1992;136:13-14.

69. Hoban TJ, Woodrum E, Czaia R. Public opposition to genetic engineering. *Rural Sociol.* 1992;57:476-493.

70. Hoban TJ. *Consumer Awareness and Acceptance of Bovine Somatotropin (BST).* Raleigh, NC: NC State University; 1994:15.

71. National Research Council. *Field Testing Genetically Modified Organisms.* Washington, DC: National Academy Press; 1989:170.

72. Kramer MG, Sheehy RE, Hiatt WR. Progress toward the genetic engineering of tomato fruit softening. *Trends Biotechnol.* 1989;7:191-194.

73. Kramer MG. *NABC 2.* Ithaca, NY: Boyce Thompson Institute; 1990: 127-130.

74. Hiatt WR. Tomato transgene structure and silencing—nature biotechnology. In: Setlow JK, ed. *Genetic Engineering.* New York: Plenum Pub Corp; 1989:49-63.

75. National Cancer Institute. *Frequently Consumed Vegetables.* Washington, DC: National Cancer Institute; 1993.

76. Redenbaugh K, Berner T, Emlay D, et al. Regulatory issues for commercialization of tomatoes with an antisense polygalacturonase gene. *In Vitro Cell Dev Biol.* 1993;29:17-26.

77. Redenbaugh K, Hiatt W. Field trials and risk evaluation of tomatoes genetically engineered for enhanced firmness and shelflife. *Acta Hort.* 1993;336:133-146.

78. Marrone PG, Sandmeier R. *NABC 3.* Ithaca, NY: Boyce Thompson Institute; 1991:228-237.

79. Goldburg RJ, Tjaden G. Are BTK plants really safe to eat? *Bio/Technol.* 1990;8:1011-1015.

80. Perlak FJ, Fischhoff DA. Transgenic Indica Rice Breeding Line. IR58. *Advanced Engineered Pesticides.* New York: M. Dekker; 1993:199-211.

81. Stark DM, Timmerman KP, Barry GF, et al. Regulation of the amount of starch in plant tissues by ADP glucose pyrophosphorylase. *Science.* 1992;258:287-292.

82. Ohlrogge JB. Design of new plant products—engineering of fatty acid metabolism. *Plant Physiol.* 1994;104:821-826.

83. Flora F, ed. *Naturally Occurring Substances in Traditional and Biotechnologically Derived Foods.* Washington, DC: US Dept of Agriculture, CRS; 1992:29.

84. Arntzen CJ. Edible vaccines. *Public Health Rep. J US Public Health Service.* Boston, Mass. 1997;112:191-197.

85. National Corn Growers Association. President Roger Pine. March 3, 1999, testimony before the House of Agriculture Subcommittee on Risk Management, Research and Specialty Crops.

86. Food and Drug Administration. Statement of policy: foods derived from new plant varieties. *Federal Register.* May 29, 1992;57:22984-23005.

87. Brewer M, Kendall P. Position of the American Dietetic Association: Biotechnology and the future of food. *JADA.* December 1995;95:12.

88. Zeneca Ag Products, May 16, 2000. Available at: http://www.ZenacaAg.com; World Health Organization.

89. Romer S, et al. Elevation of the provitamin A content of transgenic tomato plants. *Nature Biotechnol.* 2000;18:666-669.

90. De Felice SL. The nutraceutical revolution. Global implications. *Regulatory Affairs.* 1993;5:169-172.

91. Dunkin A. Eat nine cloves of garlic, and call me in the morning. *Data Business Week.* February 15, 1993.

92. Chew NJ. Nutraceuticals: using food to treat disease. *BioPharm.* July-August 1993:18-19.

93. Dabkowski R. Concerns regarding genetically modified foods [consumer submission to FDA]. April 4, 2001. Available at: fdadockets@oc.fda.gov.

94. Pub. Law. No. 101-535, 104 Stat 2353 (1990), preprinted in *Regulatory Affairs.* 1990;2:488-504.

95. LaBell F. Experts ask policy change on health claims. *Food Processing.* April 1993:52-57.

96. California Dietetic Association. *Help or Harm.* San Diego, Calif: California Dietetic Association; 1992:2.

97. Position of the American Dietetic Association: identifying food and nutrition misinformation. *J Am Diet Assoc.* 1988;88:1589-1591.

98. Short SH. Health-quackery: our role as professionals. *J Am Diet Assoc.* 1994;94:607-611.

99. Philen RM, Ortiz DI, Auerbach SB, et al. Survey of advertising for nutritional supplements in health and bodybuilding magazines. *JAMA.* 1991;268:1008-1011.

100. Berg FM. *Obesity and Health.* Hettinger, ND: Healthy Living Institute; 1990.

101. Stare FJ. Combating misinformation—a continuing challenge for nutrition professionals. *Nutr Today.* 1992;27:43-46.

102. Marquart LF, Sobal J. Vitamin/mineral supplement use among athletes [abstract]. *J Am Diet Assoc.* 1992;92(suppl):A56.

103. Kaufman M. *Nutrition in Public Health—A Handbook for Developing Programs and Services.* Gaithersburg, Md: Aspen Publishers, Inc; 1990:570.

CHAPTER THREE

THE COMMUNITY NUTRITION PROFESSIONAL

Learning Objectives

- Define community nutrition and community nutrition research and how they fit within the scope of research, from basic research to community application.
- List the vocabulary common to professionals in community nutrition research.
- Describe various communication skills needed to relate effectively with the media and the viewing audience.
- Enumerate the educational needs and skills of individuals functioning as community nutrition educators or researchers.
- Identify the factors that motivate community nutrition research.
- Identify the characteristics of defendable nutrition research methods.
- Outline a nutrition research agenda for community nutrition professionals.

High Definition Nutrition

Community development—planned and organized effort to assist individuals to acquire the attitudes, skills, and concepts required for their democratic participation in formulating effective solutions that will affect their health.

Distance learning—any formal instruction process in which the educator and the student are in different locations.

Empowerment—process of change that provides the opportunity, authority, resources, support, or encouragement to take action or solve problems.

Entrepreneurialship—a tenor that reflects a creative spirit, a dedication to persist, and a problem-solving nature.

Leadership—the art of bringing together people with diverse talents, interests, ideas, and backgrounds to voluntarily participate in a shared approach toward common or compatible goals.

Nutrition counseling—an extension of nutrition teaching to assist individuals to change old and to maintain new eating behaviors.

Nutrition education—the process of imparting knowledge for improved nutritional status of the public.

Nutrition information—information about food and nutrition and their relationship to good health and to disease.

Nutrition teaching—providing information through nutrition instruction to individuals or groups.

Nutrition education research—a 5-stage process often using a number of methodologies to increase a knowledge content base.

Technology—the types of equipment and methods used to complete tasks at various levels of performance.

Avenues of Opportunity in Community Nutrition

Community nutrition activities form an umbrella needed to implement many objectives stated in *Healthy People 2010.*[1] Although the nutrition field in general and community nutrition specifically are considered primarily service professions, community nutrition professionals perform multiple services, including high-quality research.

Community nutrition professionals (CNPs) are challenged to use scientific methods to study, interpret, promote, and apply findings to remediate public health problems. To do so, community nutrition professionals need requisite skills (e.g., research skills, the ability to critique and to determine the usefulness of research, a broad knowledge base, and an entrepreneurial tenor). Requisite skills involve a focused education about public health problems, training and technical skill development, and first-hand experience with people and organizations that function at the community level.

Knowledge is essential and must include not only a general base, but a level of expertise in a chosen area (e.g., the needs of pregnant women, older individuals, or migrant individuals). A creative spirit and a dedication to persist and to solve problems are both essential.

There are many relevant issues for community nutrition as a practice and as a research effort. Toward 2010, meeting multiethnic needs is a major issue in community nutrition. Using computer technology efficiently, choosing defendable research methods, and using valid and reliable instrumentation are also major issues. Further, community nutrition professionals must understand nutritional needs across the life cycle when planning, implementing, evaluating, and reporting programs and research efforts. To venture down the community nutrition research path, individuals should pause to appreciate the scenery and the human road signs along the way. Each contact enriches the community nutritionist's art of creating ways to improve the world through nutrition.[2]

The flow of research as defined by the National Heart, Lung, and Blood Institute (NHLBI) identifies how the research community moves from basic research to application (see Figure 3–1).[3] In basic, applied, or clinical research, the individual—a plant or an animal—is generally the unit of intervention and

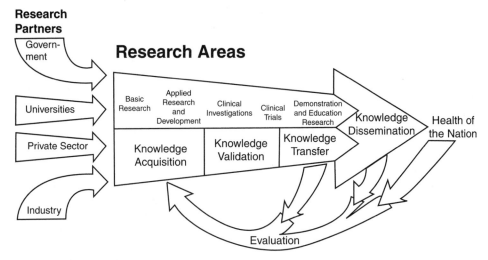

FIGURE 3–1   The flow of research from basic research to application.
Source: Adapted from Stone E. Obtaining an NIH grant: basic building blocks. *Cardiovasc Nurs.* 1989;25(2):7-11. Used with permission of the American Heart Association.

analysis. If a sufficient number of units have been observed and tests have been conducted, researchers can document the failures and successes. If success is linked to either a therapy or an approach to remediate disease morbidity or mortality, then research efforts may move from individual units of experimentation to a broader human application. This may include demonstration and education research to integrate a successful treatment into a public health domain.

Community nutrition research is usually identified at the level of demonstration and education research in the NHLBI model, because community implies groups of individuals linked by a commonality. On the other hand, community nutrition research often evolves as either a product of knowledge transfer, application, and inquiry, or of evaluation research (see Figure 3–2). Baseline data are often collected on a group participating in a nutrition program or intervention. The endpoint data may be a repetition of the same data elements to see if a change has occurred because of the intervention. Using this repeat or test-retest approach as a model, evaluation defines a format for nutrition research: develop a nutrition intervention, select a target population or high-risk group, collect baseline data, apply the intervention, and then repeat the baseline assessment.

Another way to look at community nutrition is either as a bidirectional flow from assessment to program, or as a sophisticated, community-oriented program akin to a research effort. There is a strong belief that eating behavior still remains insignificant and is not a powerful intervention to bring about health change. Pharmacological approaches continue to have a leading edge and certainly require more of the healthcare dollar than dietary intervention. Current technological advances and surgical procedures appear more effective than dietary intervention as a modality for health change, but it doesn't need to stay that way.

It is important to establish the point at which a nutrition program begins. Nutrition intervention that precedes the onset or the diagnosis of a disease is called *primary prevention*. Programs that are implemented after a diagnosis

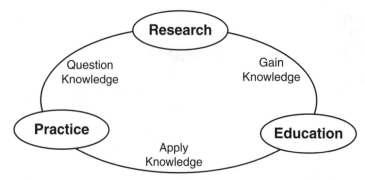

FIGURE 3–2 A conceptual framework linking community nutrition research, education, and practice via different levels of knowledge transfer.
Source: Adapted from Stone, E. Obtaining an NIH Grant: Basic Building Blocks, *Cardiovascular Nursing,* vol. 25, no. 2, pp. 7–11, with permission of the American Heart Association, © 1989.

as a result of services given to a target group are called *secondary prevention* or *secondary intervention*. Nutrition programs provided to an individual or group after disease symptoms appear and the disease expresses itself with increasing morbidity and pending mortality are known as *tertiary care*. Tertiary care or intervention is an attempt to offset early mortality.

Moving to the Future Model: Developing Community-Based Nutrition Services

The health care environment is shifting from direct individual services to community services. To institute the change, CNPs need the knowledge, skills, and attitudes necessary to develop community-based nutrition programs. A resource, *Moving to the Future: Developing Community-Based Nutrition Services Handbook, Workbook and Training Manual*, helps the community planning process, and provides 5 steps to develop community-based nutrition programs: (1) community assessment; (2) priorities, goals, and objectives; (3) the nutrition plan; (4) implementation; and (5) monitoring and evaluation.[4]

To bring community nutrition into the classroom for training CNPs, one must present an enormous amount of material in an active and meaningful way.[4] Three important community nutrition messages exist: a sense of community, an appreciation of the importance of good nutrition in community health, and a recognition of the nutrition professional's integral role in community health. Four features seem to aid accomplishment of the messages. These include the community definition chart, the resource checklist, the opinion survey, and the nutrition plan.[5]

Dietetic internships that provide workshop experiences for students can increase their awareness of community issues, provide tools to use in the community setting, and increase the interns' likelihood of participating in community nutrition activities.[4]

Examples are:

- A 2-part workshop in which the first 3-hour workshop involves collection of data for a simulated community followed by the second workshop with a computer lab to access health information and learning how to build coalitions with stakeholders to implement a nutrition intervention.[4]

- The Virginia Department of Health internship, which allows nutritionists to complete the program and continue to work in their local health department. Relocation is not required, and learning experiences increase the level of care provided by the nutritionists to health department clients. In addition, an 8-hour workshop can include a detailed explanation on assessing nutrition data in the community through a simulated community activity and a case study.[4]

To assess self-identified needs for training in leadership and community development, all of the 61 members of the Caribbean Association of Nutritionists and Dietitians (CANDi) residing in the Caribbean were mailed a questionnaire. Community development was defined as a planned and organized effort to assist individuals to acquire the attitudes, skills, and concepts required for their democratic participation in formulating effective solutions that will affect their health. Leadership was defined as the art of bringing together people with diverse talents, interests, ideas, and backgrounds to voluntarily participate in a shared approach toward common or compatible goals.[6]

Four major skills and a few examples of subactivities needed for CNPs were identified as: (1) planning—evaluating outcomes, assessing needs, and identifying resources; (2) management—presenting proposals, problem solving, and team building; (3) communication—networking, writing letters and reports, negotiating, and listening; and (4) teaching—varying leadership styles, motivating others, leading groups, and counseling. A rank order of the specific communication skills identified as priorities for a CNP from the CANDi survey is as follows[6]: writing for the public, networking, lobbying, writing letters/memos, public speaking, negotiating, advocating, providing feedback, and listening.

What Motivates Community Nutrition Research?

Three major motivational forces for community nutrition research are:

1. The public health problems that exist in our society. (These are often termed the *morbidity* and *mortality* within a population and quantified with *rates*, such as the number of new cases of hypertension in a given year. See Chapter 1.)
2. The scientific and professional consensus regarding relevant needs, severity of a disease, and resulting health goals. (*Healthy People 2010* is a major document identifying a research agenda for community nutrition in the United States.[1,7])
3. Advocacy as demonstrated by research involving women's health issues, which has lagged behind research on men until recently.

In addition, resource dollars motivate community nutrition research. Generally, funding agencies, called *sponsors*, must be addressed when planning nutrition research projects or evaluating the state of health of a community. Sponsors may select certain topics or health problems as priorities and earmark only these for research dollars. Federal or state funding is often received in the form of block grants. Community nutrition research is often based on soft moneys that may be available only for a period of 1, 2, or 3 years and may focus on only certain health concerns. Because the major governmental or sponsorship concerns will shift, the community nutrition research focus must be flexible.

Healthy People 2010 is the current national directive to increase a healthy life span, reduce disparities among groups within the population, and increase access to service. The directive lists 289 specific objectives within 22 priority areas, including nutrition. The objectives are quantifiable and specific and give the rationale for a community nutrition research agenda.[1] These objectives create the ideal research opportunity for community nutrition professionals.

Research is the foundation of the dietetics profession and provides the scientific principles that form the basis of practice.[8] Research and scientific evidence help make decisions about which programs and services to offer and about needed resource and financial commitments.[9,10] The American Dietetic Association (ADA) encourages the use of research to prepare evidence-based practice guides and to integrate findings into daily practice.[11]

The Dietetic Practice Based Research Network (DPBRN) has as its goal to conduct, support, promote, and advocate for research in practice settings.[12] See http://www.eatright.org/.

A practitioner-driven DPBRN can guide: (1) decisions and services provided through programs to make a positive difference in the lives of older adults; (2) research to improve practice by creating evidence-based best practices; and (3) standardized data collection to document program and consumer outcomes, services, need for funding, and to influence policy.

Current ADA research priorities relate to older adults—prevention and treatment of obesity and chronic disease, effective nutrition and lifestyle change intervention, effective nutrition indicators and outcome measures, delivery of and payment for dietetic services, access to a safe and secure food supply, and customer satisfaction.

In addition, *Healthy Youth 2000*, a directive of the American Medical Association, focuses on priorities for youth 10 to 24 years of age. These priorities include many that are related to nutrition, such as the need to address obesity, inadequate calcium intake, iron deficiency anemia, and inability to choose foods using food labels.[13]

An astute community nutrition professional serving a target group can create a research agenda by focusing on and advocating for 1 or 2 priorities related to nutrition of this target group. For example, the professional may choose to reduce obesity to less than 20% of the youth; to have at least 50% of children receiving adequate calcium intakes; to decrease iron deficiency anemia to less than 3%; or to increase the use of food labels in making nutritious choices among 85% of the youth.

Requirements for Conducting Community Nutrition Research

Community nutrition professionals need skills, knowledge of research techniques, advanced knowledge, and an entrepreneurial tenor to conduct quality research.

Knowledge of Research Techniques

To conduct community nutrition research, individuals need technical training to acquire field or hands-on experience. A common vocabulary aids communication.[2] Important terms are divided into 3 general domains: design, implementation, and analysis.[14,15] All 3 domains overlap, but what is important is that students and CNPs understand and apply them correctly.

Design

- *Population*—the target group that receives the program, is involved in the research, or is in greatest need for nutritional intervention.
- *Sample*—denotes a subset within a population.
- *Sampling frame*—the collection area and description of the population from which the sample is chosen.
- *Randomization*—the process by which individuals in a group have an equal chance of being selected.
- *Matching*—a statistical procedure to control for potential confounders and to ensure that individuals are alike on important characteristics before they are assigned to treatment or control conditions.

Implementation

- *Methods*—procedures, techniques, and instruments.
- *Protocols*—procedures for assessing, implementing, or evaluating the program or research.
- *Quality control*—a reflection of how carefully data collection, interventions, or methods are conducted. Examples include protocols for each technique, training of interviewers or observers in a standardized fashion, duplicate measures, and data editing prior to computer entry.
- *Time lines (Gantt charts)*—a formal delineation of activities across time. One can track progress and clearly show the order of specific events. For example, a time line states *when* researchers do something, *what* they are doing, and in *what order* they are doing it.
- *Coalitions*—combinations of organizations and individuals with a common goal. Coalitions might involve groups such as the American Cancer Society, a district dietetic association, the Cooperative Extension Service, or a nursing agency addressing a colon cancer screening and education program.
- *Sponsors*—those who fund a program or research study.

Analysis

- *Statistics*—analysis of data. Descriptive statistics, such as measures of central tendency (mean, mode, and median) are quite different than inferential statistics, such as reporting how well 2 or more variables relate (correlation) or if one variable predicts another.
- *Confounder*—a characteristic that appears to have an influential role in the nature of an outcome. Potential confounders must be controlled in the sampling or analysis.
- *Evaluation/accountability*—a process for comparing a measure against a standard or objective. If a *Healthy Youth 2000* objective was chosen, the evaluation research could analyze how close the baseline and endpoint measures were to the objective (e.g., less than 20% of youths overweight); or analysts could evaluate effectiveness (e.g., whether a change from 30% overweight to 25% overweight was achieved with the program); or

analysts could evaluate *efficiency* (if a change from 30% to 25% was achieved spending $1,200 per child).

- *Paradigm*—defines a design, how different components link (O = observation, X = intervention), and if a random (R) or quasi-experimental design is being used (e.g., R . . . O . . . X . . . O).
- *Framework*—the organization of health education or health promotion work. Models such as PRECEDE and PROCEED are examples of defining modifiable (fat intake) and nonmodifiable (gender) variables for intervention in the community's environment.[10]

Qualifications

Experience helps professionals to develop their skills. Community nutrition professionals find that each year of experience strengthens their basic skills, alerts them to improved techniques, and allows them to streamline their efforts in the community to enlarge their population or study sample.

Since 1920, various professional groups have met to review the functions and qualifications of community nutrition professionals.[16] The University of Tennessee was the first graduate training program in nutrition to receive Title V Maternal and Child Health Services funding for public health nutrition training grants. This funding was followed by awards to the University of California Berkeley, Case Western Reserve University, the University of Michigan, the University of North Carolina, and Harvard University. The training awards were expanded with Title VII of the Public Health Act in the mid-1970s.[17]

During the past 75 years, qualifications of community nutrition professionals have been carefully documented and demonstrate a commitment to high educational standards in an evolving field that responds to the nutritional needs of individuals and the community. Chronologically, educational qualifications are briefly outlined as follows[17]:

- 1937—minimum qualifications for home economists and nutritionists were identified for health and welfare agencies.
- 1950—objectives for preparation of public health nutritionists were enumerated.
- 1962—educational qualifications of nutritionists in healthcare agencies were listed.
- 1989—a description of personnel in public health nutrition for the 1980s was outlined.
- 1990—strategies for successful graduate programs in public health nutrition were identified.

Competencies

Today, standard entry-level skills for minimal knowledge and understanding of community nutrition can be acquired through a didactic program in dietetics or a dietetic internship.[18] At the completion of these programs, entry-level competencies should include the following:

- knowledge of and ability to apply the scientific research method across all age and ethnic groups for primary, secondary, and tertiary prevention

- a basic understanding of how to work with and communicate with groups to recruit and retain research and program participants
- an understanding of how to target and pinpoint high-risk individuals for assessment and intervention
- the ability to develop, program, and delegate responsibilities to a variety of trained individuals during research, implementation, and analysis stages

These competencies are needed to implement the community nutrition program that may be the center of the research endeavor. Specific educational needs of an individual who plans to conduct research in the community require a minimum of an MPH or MS degree with courses in research methods, statistics, sampling, interpretation, and communication. A doctoral program with an emphasis in research would refine these skills. A DrPH or a PhD program that includes coursework in research methods, statistics, sampling, communication, accounting, and ethics is important in today's world (see Appendix 3–A), because community nutrition professionals are managers. Their positions require skills in managing staff as well as managing delivery programs, implementing research objectives, and conducting research studies.

Knowledge of multinutrient databases and the ability to establish complex data management systems to articulate and integrate collected data are important. Familiarity with the personal computer versions of statistical packages for data management and with simple, user-friendly, educational software packages is essential.

Several terms are commonly used by educators of practitioners in public health/community nutrition and nutrition research. Students and CNPs would benefit from learning and applying these terms in written and verbal communications[19] (see Appendix 3–B).

Future Training

A current concern of nutrition professionals is the continual training of students to meet the changing community nutrition environment. One avenue for training public health/community nutritionists is the practice environment. Representatives of the Food and Nutrition Service, the National Association of WIC Directors, and the Association of State and Territorial Public Health Nutrition Directors convened in June 1992 to study the issue of recruitment and retention of qualified nutritionists in public health/community nutrition programs. The working group solicited the assistance and support of the American Dietetic Association (ADA) in developing effective recruitment strategies.

A meeting was held with ADA and other interested national agencies on May 11, 1993, to identify specific actions to be taken. Eleven actions were proposed, of which 2 were specific to programs sponsored by public health/community nutrition programs:

1. *Increase the number of programs in public health/community nutrition programs.* The Food and Nutrition Service is committed to the development of more training sites for WIC (Special Supplemental Food Program for Women, Infants, and Children). The sponsoring of a practice program by a public health/community nutrition program can serve as a training program for WIC nutritionists to improve their skills and, at the same time, to acquire professional credentials. Further, the sponsoring of a

program by a WIC agency can serve as an effective recruitment/reten-tion tool for state and local programs. Over a dozen programs are spon-sored by either a state or local health department. Interest continues as these programs are developed within state WIC agencies.

2. *Develop a prototype self-study for use by health departments.* The Food and Nutrition Service has developed a national self-study prototype for development of programs, which can be adaptable for use by state and local WIC directors. The prototype can be expanded and applied to other child nutrition programs.

Info Line

FOUR UNIVERSITIES OFFER MATERNAL AND CHILD NUTRITION TRAINEESHIPS

Four universities offer education and training opportunities in mater-nal and child nutrition to registered dietitians (RDs) seeking a master's degree in public health nutrition. The programs vary in their empha-sis and length of study, but all provide support in the form of tuition assistance, fees, and a monthly stipend. Their funding source is the Maternal and Child Health Bureau, Health Resources and Services Administration, US Department of Health and Human Services.

The 4 universities and mailing addresses are:

University of Minnesota
Division of Epidemiology
School of Public Health
Suite 300, WBOB
1300 S 2nd Street
Minneapolis, MN 55454-1015

University of North Carolina
Department of Nutrition
CB No 7400
McGavron-Greenberg Hall
Chapel Hill, NC 27599-7400

University of Tennessee
Department of Nutrition
1215 W Cumberland Avenue
229JHB
Knoxville, TN 37996-1900

University of California
Los Angeles School of Public Health
Community Health Sciences
650 Charles E. Young Drive
Los Angeles, CA 90095-1772

Several private higher education institutions with a public health orientation offer nutrition and dietetics degrees linked to public health. St Louis University has as its primary goal to prepare nutrition specialists to work in many types of public health and voluntary agencies, medical care, and educational settings.

Several professional positions are available for the CNP. See Table 3–1. A clear role for the CNP who is a registered dietitian is managing the care of community residents with specific health conditions, such as celiac disease, cancer, or renal failure.

An independent consensus panel of healthcare practitioners and researchers recommended 6 key strategies for managing celiac disease, the first of which is to consult a skilled dietetics professional. Convened by the National Institutes of Health of the US Department of Health and Human Services, the panel assessed all available scientific evidence on celiac disease under contract with the Agency for Healthcare Quality and Research.[20]

Based on its assessment of an extensive collection of medical literature and expert presentations, the panel identified 6 elements essential to treating celiac disease once it is diagnosed:

C: Consultation with a skilled registered dietitian (RD)
E: Education about the disease
L: Lifelong adherence to a gluten-free diet
I: Identification and treatment of nutritional deficiencies
A: Access to an advocacy group
C: Continuous long-term follow-up

Previously believed to be rare, celiac disease is present in 0.5-1% of the US population, 10 times higher than former estimates. For more information, see http://consensus.nih.gov/cons/118/118cdc_intro.htm.

Professionalism

A *professional* has certain distinct characteristics. The professional is generally employed full time in an occupation, possesses strong motivation for making a particular career choice, and possesses a specialized body of knowledge and skills acquired in a set academic course. A professional has a service orientation, interprets client needs without moral judgment, and allows peers to judge his or her knowledge and performance. Participating in a professional association, following a code of ethics, and demonstrating both leadership and status in an area of expertise further distinguish a professional from a nonprofessional.[21-24]

To measure differences between professional attitudes of dietetics students and practitioners, Spears et al[25] developed a 5-item questionnaire with a Likert response scale. The professional statements that loaded at a 0.36 or greater level using factor analysis were considered significant. The researchers identified 12 scales and noted differences in the way students versus experienced members responded. For example, the score for social service orientation, which assessed responsibility and commitment to help others, was higher for younger respondents than for experienced practitioners.[25] Table 3–2 provides an index for individuals to evaluate the extent of their professionalism.

TABLE 3–1   Major Community Nutrition Employment Positions

Position Title	Summary	Primary Responsibilities
Cooperative extension educator	The cooperative extension educator provides leadership and overall coordination in improving county residents' lives through an educational process that provides practical information and guidance in response to local, state, and national issues. Primary responsibilities include planning, developing, and implementing nutrition and health-related extension programs; developing and implementing a network of volunteer leadership; collaborating with community groups and agencies to further program goals; and maintaining professional competency and skills required for professional practice.	Program planning and development Volunteer leadership development Interagency collaboration Community development Business/supervisory functions Professional development
Corrections dietitian	The corrections dietitian plans, organizes, and directs food and nutrition services for inmates in a correctional facility. Primary responsibilities include planning regular and therapeutic diets for inmates; supervising the preparation and service of therapeutic diets; assessing the nutritional status of inmates, and providing nutrition counseling as needed; organizing and conducting training programs for food service personnel; assisting in the administration of the food service department; and maintaining professional competency and skills required for professional practice.	Therapeutic diets Nutrition care Food service administration Professional development

Public health nutritionist	The public health nutritionist plans, develops, implements, and evaluates nutrition services within the community. Primary responsibilities include assessing community nutrition needs; developing and implementing community events and programs; providing nutrition services and medical nutrition therapy to individuals and groups; collaborating with state and community agencies; planning and delivering in-service training and education activities for public health personnel; and maintaining professional competency and skills required for professional practice.	Program planning and evaluation Patient care services Training and education Business and public relations Professional development
Home care nutritionists (usually registered dietitians)	The home care nutritionist plans, develops, implements, and monitors medical nutrition therapy for a broad range of clients who live in a noninstitutional residence or independently in their homes or with family members. Primary responsibilities include assessing individual clients, receiving diet orders from physicians or nurse practitioners; creating a care plan for individual clients, arranging appointments and delivering onsite assessment, education, and monitoring; recording in medical progress notes; and reporting outcome of appointments to appropriate health care providers.	Medical nutrition therapy planning, implementation, and evaluation Communicating with healthcare professionals Traveling to client homes Recording activities

Source: Adapted from: The American Dietetic Association. *Job Descriptions: Models for the Dietetics Profession.* Chicago, Il: American Dietetic Association; 2003.

TABLE 3–2 Professional Self-Assessment Form

	Belief Level of Agreement[a]				
	Strongly Disagree				Strongly Agree
I believe the profession of dietetics is important.	1	2	3	4	5
I believe continuing education for dietitians is important.	1	2	3	4	5
I believe dietitians have a responsibility to help others.	1	2	3	4	5
I believe that it is important for dietitians to be active in the political process.	1	2	3	4	5
I believe that it is important for dietitians to be active in professional organizations.	1	2	3	4	5
I believe that a career in dietetics provides intellectual growth and job challenges.	1	2	3	4	5
I believe dietetics is important to society.	1	2	3	4	5
I believe dietitians should have professional autonomy.	1	2	3	4	5
I believe dietitians have an obligation to uphold the profession's code of ethics.	1	2	3	4	5
I believe dietitians make a substantial contribution to the provision of quality health care.	1	2	3	4	5

[a]Agreement codes are 1 = strongly disagree; 2 = disagree; 3 = not sure; 4 = agree; 5 = strongly agree.
Source: Adapted from: Spears MC, Simonis PL, Vaden AG. Professional attitudes of dietetics students and practitioners. *J Am Diet Assoc.* 1992;92:1522-1526. Used with permission of the American Dietetic Association.

Community nutrition professionals can continue their education in a specific direction or they can enlarge their knowledge base by joining professional organizations such as the Society of Nutrition Education, the American Public Health Association, or a council in the American Heart Association. Professionals may also join one or more dietetic practice groups (DPGs) of the American Dietetic Association (see Appendix 3–C). The focus of the DPGs ranges from Public Health Nutritionists, a large US network composed primarily of practicing community nutritionists; to the Hunger and Malnutrition DPG, which enrolls nutrition professionals from across the United States; to the Nutrition Research DPG, whose members range from university professors conducting research to clinical RDs involved in randomized trials. These professionals may or may not work directly with social problems. They may contribute ideas, volunteer time in their own communities, or incorporate messages into their writings or newsletters for other groups to aid campaigns.

A description of personnel in public health nutrition reflects a corps of dedicated, trained professionals.[26] In 2000, community nutrition professionals continued to serve the public; however, the nature of their service was more research based. Community nutrition professionals must strengthen their research skills and remain vigilant about improving their basic tasks to plan, assess, define, target, develop, train, implement, monitor, evaluate, and report community nutrition activities.

Important Issues Relevant to Community Nutrition Research

Six important issues related to community nutrition research must be addressed:

1. Participants must be informed prior to consent. They need to understand the risks and benefits of participating in research or demonstration studies. Written, signed, and witnessed documents are essential.

2. Studies should focus on multiethnic groups, children, women, and older adults during the next decade. For example, in San Francisco, a study of the hypertension morbidity among the Vietnamese community has enriched the efforts of nutrition professionals and produced important information regarding the influence of beliefs and structure on medical and health decisions of this population, including youth and adult (using ethnic-sensitive program titles, e.g., "Suc Khoe la Vang!" or "Health is Gold!").[27]

3. It is important to conduct surveys of various groups across the age spectrum to understand the needs of individuals in different stages of the life cycle. Instruments that identify and characterize eating behaviors of children and seniors should be developed.[28]

4. Methods and instruments should be developed and evaluated so they can be used to assess multicultural population patterns, eating behaviors, physical activities, and decision-making patterns. Methods and instruments must be clearly defined and defendable. Four characteristics of defendable methods are as follows[14]:
   * *Reliable*—relates to how well a method can be repeated in a similar setting and give the same answer.
   * *Valid*—relates to whether an instrument measures what one is trying to measure.
   * *Comparable*—means being able to contrast results for 2 or more different studies.
   * *Transportable*—means that an approach tested or applied in one setting can be transferred and applied to another setting. Transportability reduces the need to reinvent the wheel.

   An example of a defendable method is the fat-cholesterol avoidance scale, a quick, handy tool with a relative validity to assess the extent of fat avoidance in a study sample. Researchers validated the instrument in both adult and pediatric populations. They reported differences between Mexican American and Anglo samples in 2 different states.[29,30]

   Frequency tools are evolving and allow researchers to assess multiple days of intake including a representative group of 50-80 foods to characterize an overall pattern.[31,32] Frequencies are valuable when categorizing individuals into broad groups (e.g., low-fat versus high-fat consumers). One-to-one interview techniques or individual self-reports involve shorter time periods. Three-day or 7-day food records are essential for identifying specific nutrient intake instead of food group intakes.[28]

5. Because community nutrition research is fluid, researchers must learn to ask questions and integrate new questioning techniques for mass data collection (e.g., telephone surveys).[33] Interactive video, use of computer networks, and e-mail for "survey monkey" and the Internet for simucasts are viable options for data collection, transfer, and communication.

6. Community nutrition professionals must quantify their value in any nutrition research study. One way is to establish a value or cost for each task and the value of professional time to complete each task. Individual costs can be aggregated to establish total project cost. Community nutrition managers must document staff responsibilities for program implementation, data collection, and analysis. Knowledge of the cost or value of a task can assist with salary negotiations. Establishing competitive salaries also helps to maintain high-quality staff. Salary differential should be real for experienced compared with new researchers. Women in research positions and with varying degrees of experience should evaluate and seek salary equity compared to male peers in similar positions and with similar education and experience.

Research Agenda

Nutrition research in the United States can address national problems and identify national goals. Nutrition research strengthens technology, which affects the US industrial and economic agenda.[34]

Food science and nutrition are integrative disciplines that incorporate other specialties into their research and program agendas. New avenues of thought develop when researchers confront human nutrition problems that face both individuals and groups. A recurrent challenge is to keep the research agenda for food science and nutrition invigorated. One recommendation is to infuse the field with innovations from the biological sciences by developing a field of bionutrition.[35] Bionutrition is integrative and concerns the interaction of genetics, molecular biology, and cell biology with dietary components, and environmental influences and the outcome in terms of more complex levels of biological organization and human health.[36]

The Committee on Opportunities in the Nutrition and Food Sciences, the Food and Nutrition Board, and the National Academy of Sciences have published a landmark report that identifies nutrition research opportunities for health promotion and disease prevention.[37] Major research themes for the new millennium include: nutrients in stages of human development spanning from conception to death (specific areas are cell differentiation, growth, aging, physiological functions, and wellness); genetic mapping; food and degenerative disease; determinants of eating patterns in multicultures; development of new health-promoting, high-quality, economic, and wholesome foods that are environmentally safe; and effective food and nutrition policies for improved access to and acceptance of food programs and surveillance of nutritional status across the life cycle.[35]

Others have identified social, economic, and biological issues.[38,39] These include prevention and treatment of obesity, effective lifestyle change interventions, delivery of and payment for dietetic services and consumer satisfaction. In addition, the Human Nutrition Research and Information Management System is an online retrieval system that identifies and categorizes federally funded human nutrition research projects in all government agencies.[40]

Research must be considered worthwhile and show cost-effectiveness. This is often difficult for nutrition research, where examples of both cost-benefit and cost-effectiveness are lacking and needed.[41-43]

There are numerous opportunities for research on issues related to dietetic manpower.[44,45]

Specific opportunities can be identified for community nutrition. Several terms are useful to understand the research opportunities and approaches[45]:

- *Distance learning* describes formal instruction in which a majority of teaching and learning occurs while the educator and the student are at a distance from one another. One distance education course that was piloted with 9 students studying nutrition included a print study guide, written assignments, and an e-mail component. The e-mail component allowed for discussion. The method of delivery of the course did not appear to affect students' impressions of the content. Students also rated the e-mail interaction positively. Students especially seemed to like having the chance to have their questions answered in a timely manner. [46]
- *Nutrition counseling* is an extension of nutrition teaching that is intended to help an individual adjust to change required to achieve and to maintain new eating behaviors. It can be an individualized process by which a client is helped to acquire the ability to manage nutritional care, and it requires a relationship between a professionally trained, competent nutritionist/dietitian and an individual. It may also involve a group of individuals who seek help in following a special diet, gaining knowledge or self-understanding, improving decision-making skills, or changing behavior.
- *Nutrition education* is the process of imparting knowledge to the public aimed at the general improvement of nutritional status through elimination of unsatisfactory dietary practices, promotion of adequate food habits and better food hygiene, and more efficient use of food resources. Nine issues are relevant to professionals working in research, teaching, or nutrition education for the public.[47] If these issues (listed below) are not addressed adequately, nutrition improvement programs for developing and developed countries may be rendered ineffective with severe consequences for both individuals and society as a whole.
  1. all the public needs to be reached
  2. "total diet" versus "single nutrients" concept
  3. rational, food-based dietary guidance
  4. informing and motivating
  5. building trust and self-reliance
  6. stimulating collaboration among sectors
  7. using the mass media
  8. acknowledging strengths and limits of nutrition education
  9. developing human resources for nutrition education
- *Nutrition information* is a generic term that refers to routine information that meets an individual's or group's need for knowledge about food and nutrition, and their relationship to good health and disease. Its purpose is generally to improve the ability of an individual or group to self-manage any dietary change.
- *Nutrition teaching* involves providing instruction and information that seeks to promote specific changes in eating behaviors and improved self-management of dietary treatment.
- *Nutrition education research* is a process that can be described in 5 stages: (1) hypothesis development; (2) methods development and

message focus; (3) intervention-effectiveness test; (4) efficacy in the real world; and (5) dissemination of the intervention. A number of methodologies can be used for achieving a better understanding of a knowledge content base.

- The level of *technology* is defined by the types and patterns of activity, equipment, material, and knowledge or experience used to perform tasks.

Seven major arenas of change in the United States and the relevance for CNPs involved in nutrition education and research are briefly discussed next. Potential researchable questions are listed for each arena of change.

Societal Change

The Institute of Medicine identifies 2 factors that will affect the future demand for nutrition services: (1) consumer desire for nutrition information and direction; and (2) the potential willingness of the consumer to pay for the service.[48] In both 1988 and 1992, the strategic plan for the American Dietetic Association identified the following influential societal trends[49,50]:

- cost containment
- lifestyle and demographic changes
- awareness of the relationship of diet to health
- governmental influence on health care
- changing technology
- environmental issues
- nutrition information channels

One of the most important demographic trends is the aging of the US population and the extended longevity of the aging cohort. One result is an increased use of medical services by individuals over 65 years of age. From 1982 to 1983, healthcare expenses equaled 4.4% of the total expenditures of all consumer units. This contrasts with 9.9% of the total expenditures for consumer units with heads of household over 65 years of age.[51] Further, an increase in the number of 85-year-old individuals living independently will challenge home health services.

Potential manpower-related research questions for community nutrition research are as follows:

- What community nutrition services will be essential due to the increasing number of consumer units over 65 years of age?
- What educational opportunities or hands-on experiences are currently available to train community nutrition professionals to work with individuals over 65 years of age?
- Are community nutrition professionals currently providing nutrition services to individuals in their homes? If so, what are the services? If not, what services are needed?

Changes in Lifestyle

Two changes that are important for community nutrition professionals are: (1) the restructuring of careers (i.e., no more 25-year careers in 1 position or setting[51]); and (2) the mobility of the work force on a daily basis, resulting in an increasing demand for quick, convenient foods that bear nutrition information (e.g., point-of-choice nutrition information).[52]

Researchable questions include the following:

- What new career paths are of interest to and within the reach of established community nutrition professionals?
- How well do community nutrition professionals practice healthy eating behaviors on a daily basis?
- What types of information do community nutrition professionals use to make their own food choices?

Technological Change

Increased skill in the use of nutritional databases, communication and retrieval systems, and robotics is needed. Timely strategies for training professionals in communication skills are needed.[53] This includes expanded use of computer-assisted instruction, videotapes, distance education, telephone menus for messages and hot lines, television programming (both live and cable access), and immediate information regarding nutritional content of foods at the point of choice.[54-60]

Researchable questions include the following:

- Are community nutrition professionals aware of and using contemporary computerized nutritional analysis systems?
- What costs are involved in using up-to-date technology in nutrition information transmission?
- What skills are needed for community nutrition professionals to use robotics, computer-assisted instruction, videos, and live television?
- What is the effectiveness of these methods in changing eating behaviors of groups and communities?

Changes in Business and Industry

Technological changes generally challenge community nutrition professionals to become actively involved in business and industry, which are likewise experiencing their own changes. The demands for community education are due in large part to the Nutrition Labeling Education Act, the appeal of radio and television for entertaining education, and innovative marketing and advertising approaches of the food and nutrition supplement industries. Community nutrition professionals with a broad knowledge base can become skilled management consultants and open new fields of employment and new outreach techniques, such as self-employment, working at home, and telephone conferencing.[61]

Researchable questions include the following:

- What employment opportunities exist for community nutrition professionals who have an entrepreneurial approach to their career and who wish to develop a business-oriented career track?
- What marketing and communication skills are part of the training of community nutrition professionals?

Changes in Health Care

Several new target groups have been identified for community nutrition programs, including individuals who have tested positive for HIV (human immunodeficiency virus), pregnant teens, adolescents with alcohol problems, and children and adults with eating disorders and vacillating weight-management skills.[62] Segmented health care delivery and shifts from hospital to clinic-, outpatient-, and work site-based health care all influence the community nutrition approach.[61] Specialization of healthcare professionals and the need for certification (e.g., certified health education specialists and state licensure for community nutrition professionals) create new continuing education demands.[63]

Researchable questions include the following:

- What are the differences in effectiveness and cost of delivering community nutrition services in various health and employment settings?
- Are community nutrition professionals ready and willing to practice their profession in a variety of settings from physicians' offices to community-based clinics, and from school-based clinics to work sites?

Changes in Dietetic Education

The fairly small pool of doctoral-trained academicians in community nutrition may face retirement within the next decade.[64] Early retirement due to university downsizing negatively influences the educational arena. Refining undergraduate programs and merging similar programs (e.g., health education, community nursing, epidemiology, public health nutrition, etc.) may redefine the education of community nutrition professionals.

Researchable questions include the following:

- What is the magnitude of the time line for retirement of current university professors in community nutrition?
- Are specific strategies in place to strengthen a new pool of community nutrition professionals?
- Why are men not entering the community nutrition profession as rapidly as women?
- What are the similarities between programs in nutrition, nursing, sociology, health education, and epidemiology? Are there untapped areas of overlap that could be strengthened to allow interdisciplinary and multicultural training?

Changes in Student Profile

The community nutrition professional is often female and white.[65,66] Men have not entered the field as quickly as women. Many universities are opening their doors to adult reentry students who are changing their careers or finishing ones they began before they started families.[67] Communities are becoming more culturally diverse, and skilled professionals from all cultural groups are needed to improve communication and acceptance of nutrition programs by the diverse US population.[68]

Researchable questions include the following:

- Are university training programs preparing a multiethnic cadre of professionals to mirror the US population?

- Do training programs acknowledge and address the differing needs of male, adult reentry, and minority students?

Professional Skill Development

A community nutrition practitioner needs certain skills to function effectively, including creativity, communication skills, and developing a professional presence. Covey has defined 7 habits of highly effective people.[63] Professionals in a community nutrition practice or research setting can practice these habits to strengthen their skills and performance. The habits are as follows[69]:

1. *Be proactive.* The habit of being proactive, or the habit of personal vision, means taking responsibility for one's attitudes and actions.
2. *Begin with the end in mind.* The habit of personal leadership means to begin each day with a clear understanding of the desired direction and destination.
3. *Put first things first.* The habit of personal management involves organizing and managing time and events according to the personal priorities identified in habit 2.
4. *Think win-win.* Win-win is the habit of interpersonal leadership. In families and businesses, effectiveness is largely achieved through the cooperative efforts of 2 or more people. Win-win is the attitude of seeking mutual benefit. Win-win thinking begins with a commitment to explore all options until a mutually satisfactory solution is reached, or to make no deal at all. It begins with an abundance mentality, a belief that by synergistically increasing the pie, there are pieces enough for everybody.
5. *Seek first to understand, then to be understood.* The habit of communication is one of the master skills in life, the key to building win-win relationships, and the essence of professionalism.
6. *Synergize.* Synergizing is the habit of creative cooperation or teamwork. For those who have a win-win abundance mentality and exercise empathy, differences in any relationship can produce synergy, where the whole is greater than the sum of its parts.
7. *Sharpen the saw.* The habit of self-renewal is the foundation for the first 6 habits of successful people. The habit of sharpening the saw regularly means having a balanced, systematic program for self-renewal in the physical, mental, emotional-social, and spiritual components of life.

Creativity

A creative edge is needed to enhance both individual and organizational innovation and bring them to their fullest potential.[70] New ways of solving problems, handling situations and relationships, and managing change must be considered. To overcome barriers to creativity, restricted mindsets must be guided to use linear and intuitive techniques. These techniques promote new approaches and new questions.

Every idea should be communicated and encouraged. Linear methods redirect how information is organized (e.g., information is examined from a new angle). A linear model begins at 1 point and moves in small steps toward a goal. A linear approach called matrix analysis uses a 2- or 3-dimensional matrix to explore new ideas. It is constructed like a crossword puzzle or spreadsheet. One axis is labeled "market needs" and the other is labeled "available technology." Intersections between market needs and available technology establish or mark a new goal or position.

Intuitive techniques draw upon stored data to synthesize solutions. Often imagery is used as a window to intuitive, creative thought. Brainstorming is an intuitive technique in which one states the problem and then participants give random ideas to solve the problem. Meditation is not only an intuitive technique but also a focused state of related attention. A mind in a quiet state can give quick, new responses to questions that otherwise seem puzzling.

Creativity within an organization should ideally evolve in the context set by the organization's vision. Strategies that will propel an individual or an organization toward its goals can then be identified. Effective change addresses all groups and processes and occurs under the guidance of a committed leadership.[70]

Individuals can propose creative processes and a creative climate by opening their minds and making contributions. If an organization is to have a creative edge, 4 activities must occur[70]:

1. promoting the organization's status in a market or with a service
2. confronting the frontiers of marketing technology and health care
3. participating in change
4. exploring and developing of each employee's creativity

When individuals are creative, they tend to possess one or more of the following distinct characteristics[70]:

- *Spontaneous*: The individual is fresh, curious, willing to take risks; has sense of humor.
- *Persistent*: One is energetic, courageous, assertive, independent, determined.
- *Inventive*: The person looks at problems in new ways, likes challenge, is sometimes skeptical, is comfortable with ambiguity.
- *Rewarding*: One is willing to share credit, values personal satisfaction and peer recognition over money.
- *Inner openness*: The individual is intuitive, easily switches from logic to fantasy, is open to emotions, can think/act/create/innovate in different modes.
- *Transcendent*: Someone who sees situations realistically, fantasizes how he/she wants things to be, is confident he/she can effect change, chooses growth over fear.
- *Evaluative*: The person is discerning, discriminating, judgmental at appropriate times.
- *Democratic*: One values and respects people, seeks stimulation from a variety of people, is responsible, promotes the highest benefits of all concerned.

Creativity can be blocked due to a variety of reasons. The more common ones are emotional patterns including guilt and anger over previous experiences, personal or cultural perceptions that evoke narrow-mindedness, and social blocks such as fear of rejection or the unwillingness to collaborate. Creativity can also be blocked by an individual's or group's preference for how to solve problems, skills or training, stress, or lack of imagination.[70]

Within an organization, creativity is spurred by external forces. These include the economy, which is both global and information based; competition;

technical evolution; changes in social mores and demographics; and a growing awareness of the relationships between lifestyle and health.[70] However, a basic tenet of a successful individual or organization is the need to possess a sense of purpose and vision. Purpose is related to values; vision shows the path for achieving the purpose. Statements of purpose and vision set the standard for evaluating day-to-day and year-to-year success and give direction to actions. The American Dietetic Association periodically articulates and updates its mission and vision[71] (see Exhibit 3-1).

Highly effective community nutrition professionals realize that their creativity can be demonstrated and enhanced by communicating with the public and that skills are needed to communicate in several media.

Empowerment Versus Power

Empowerment is a process of change that provides the opportunity, authority, resources, support, or encouragement to take action or solve problems. Based on the belief that power can be expanded and transferred from one person to another, it has the potential to:

- influence the behavior of others
- change the course of events in someone's life
- overcome resistance
- awaken people to do what they normally wouldn't do

Personal power varies by how individuals gain, develop, choose, and use it. Negative power happens when someone is forced to respond using fear, manipulation, guilt, criticism, or control tactics. This act does not empower but removes power from people and weakens them.[72]

Positive power promotes behavioral change by sharing or transferring authority, knowledge, or skills. This occurs through teaching, coaching, listening, or other enabling activities. When empowered, people want to learn, experiment, and maintain healthy behaviors.

Exhibit 3-1   The American Dietetic Association Mission, Vision, and Areas of Interest

Mission:	Leading the future of dietetics.
Vision:	ADA members are the most valued source of food and nutrition services.
Areas of interest:	ADA's commitment to helping people enjoy healthy lives brings the association into the forefront of 5 critical health areas facing all Americans: • Obesity and overweight • Aging • Complementary care and dietary supplements • Safe and nutritious food supply • Human genome and genetics

Source: Adapted from the American Dietetic Association Web site: www.eatright.org. Accessed June 20, 2005.

Power Types

CNPs, by virtue of position, embody power to make decisions and teach clients. Their power is considered to be expert power. Expert power comes through advanced education, work experience, and specialized skills.[72] Several types of power exist, including:

> *Reward power*—This type of power is displayed when one gives incentives to clients, compliments, praise, or flatter them to encourage and to reinforce certain behaviors. Reward power can promote behavioral compliance, but its effects diminish after the reward or punishment is discontinued. CNPs possess varying degrees of reward power.
> *Referent power*—This means how well you are liked by others (ingratiation). People are more likely to listen, cooperate, and trust people they like. Referent power, created through rapport or friendly communication, is a strong motivational tool to influence and promote change.
> *Coercive power*—This type of power is ineffective in motivating behavioral change and may create resistance.
> *Expert and legitimate power*—These power types provide credibility when counselors clearly explain to clients why behavioral change is needed.

Understanding and using referent, expert, and legitimate power combined with actions that exert an influence (e.g., flattery, rationalization, self-esteem building) can effectively persuade people to adopt and commit to new behaviors.

Two barriers to counseling for behavior change are giving too much information and presenting it too quickly. This overwhelms most clients and creates a barrier to learning. Providing too little information can lead to misunderstanding and nonadherence. Skill is required to identify and balance a client's learning needs with his health needs and deliver it frequently but within a brief time frame.

Tailored messaging can meet the unique, critical learning needs of clients. Brief, clear messages motivate and empower clients to own their health and adopt healthy, yet self-caring and directed behaviors. Table 3–3 lists personal power enhancers and deflaters.[72]

Speaking Effectively

Community nutritionists are frequently called upon to give formal presentations to public and professional groups as a recruitment technique. Developing verbal and nonverbal skills increases their effectiveness and improves their chance of becoming popular speakers. Community awareness, nutrition education, and coalition building rely on the communication skills of professionals[66] (see Table 3–4).

Preliminary steps are essential for preparing an effective presentation. If you are asked to speak, learn about the organization and audience. Analyze the situation by asking about the purpose of the talk and who and what else is on the program. Find out where the talk will be given and check out the physical environment of the room. Is it classroom or theater style? Ask if there will be a head table, a podium, a microphone, and visual projection equipment.

TABLE 3–3 A Contrast of Counseling Techniques

Technique	Enhance	Power
		Deflate
Be empathetic	Compassionate	Judging and blaming attitude
Be respectful	Polite, courteous, and aware of client's time	Late for appointments; inappropriate language
Be upbeat	Enthusiastic to motivate client in a direct and positive way to make lifestyle changes	Having a bored, deadpan, or sour expression on your face when counseling (this suggests you're not interested in the client)
Communicate openly and honestly	Direct giving honest, objective information and feedback when requested	Keeping important information from clients
Establish rapport	Talk informally	Not friendly or approachable
Identify client's needs	Seek client wants and health needs	Placing personal assumptions above client's needs or wants
Listen actively	Practice motivational listening skills	Interrupting clients when they speak slowly; using negative body language
Monitor client's expressions	Monitor client's expectations while you counsel to ensure the expectations are being met	Forgetting to check with the client if the session is meeting his or her needs or if the client has any questions or concerns
	Periodically evaluate if client believes his or her needs are being met	
Network with peers	Work with other healthcare professionals who can complement your skills	Timid and limiting client referrals to other professionals
Share decision-making power	Encourage choice of options	Limiting clients' choices in their healthcare plans
Share goal setting	Query client's choice of options for learning goals and assist client in setting his or her own behavioral goals	Determine clients' behavioral goals for them (when you do this it suggests your clients aren't capable of making their own decisions)

continued

TABLE 3–3   continued

Technique	Enhance	Power Deflate
Upskill	Demonstrate expert power	Lack recent education on current health topics of interest to clients
Use persuasion and influencing tactics	Explain in a logical fashion the reason for new lifestyle behaviors	Practice negative power to enforce change; don't force, nag, preach, or talk condescendingly to clients
Use the right tools	Allow clients to identify how they learn Practice various teaching methods in your counseling	Lecture format during counseling
Watch speed	Insert questions and answers throughout counseling session to allow for questions	Brief, quick sessions cramming in much information

Source: Adapted from: Gehling E. Are you using your power? *Diabetes Care.* 2004;25(5):14-16.

TABLE 3–4   Verbal and Nonverbal Skills

Skill	Point
Rate and volume voice	Vary the volume of your voice and rate of speech, using a slightly louder voice when opening, closing, and when emphasizing important points. Making slash marks in the text will remind you to pause or change volume.
Articulation	Pronounce words precisely, but not artificially. Use formal or informal language depending upon the situation. Do not sacrifice simplicity and clarity for formality.
Vary sentence length	Use short statements to emphasize key points. Avoid reading to the audience. This will eliminate monotony.
Be concise	The more concise you are, with memorable statements, the more impact you will have. Don't try to fill a 1-hour time slot if what you have to say takes only 45 minutes.
Eye contact	Establish eye contact; move your eyes around the room, but don't let them roam. It is helpful to focus your attention on a few interested and responsive people in various areas of the room.
Body language	Maintain an open and natural style, using gestures and enthusiasm to give meaning to your words. Avoid handling paper clips, rubber bands, or other items when you are speaking. Avoid placing your hands in your pockets, clenching them in front or back of you, or keeping them glued to your sides. Try to keep your hands at waist level in a natural position. If there is a podium, do not clutch it or hide behind it. Remember that your message is important—the audience came to hear you!
Maintain interest	Use funny stories or jokes when appropriate, if it feels natural. Ask the audience questions to garner interest. Inject personal anecdotes to make your point come alive.

Source: Data from Ambassador Roundtable, American Dietetic Association annual meeting; October 1993; Anaheim, Calif.

Analyze the audience, including its size, age, education, and gender. Decide what the audience has in common. Does the audience know the topic? Use a speaker's checklist (Table 3–5) to assist in planning and evaluating the talk.

When sitting down to write a speech, think about how to write a persuasive talk but keep it entertaining and informative. Plan the speech with the following 3 components.

1. *Introduction.* Get your audience's attention. Give them a clue that what you have to say will be good. The primary objective in the introduction is to capture your audience's attention and establish rapport. Keep it simple. The statement of purpose should be short. Let your audience know what they can expect to get from the meeting. Include a few objectives and goals, a statement of the problem or situation, and your solution.
2. *Body.* In the body of the talk, support themes or points with evidence that is clear and easy to follow.
3. *Conclusion.* The conclusion becomes the message an audience leaves with and remembers. Summarize the key objectives or messages. For example, "If there's one thing I'd like to leave with you today, it is the feeling of confidence and skill in being an effective speaker."

TABLE 3–5   Speaker's Checklist

Do You . . .	Action
___	Check room, equipment, podium, and lighting, prior to speech?
___	Focus on communications objectives?
___	Keep control of: ___ self?
	___ environment?
	___ materials?
___	Project a strong, positive image?
___	Maintain direct eye contact with audience?
___	Use gestures effectively for emphasis and to convey feeling?
___	Eliminate distracting body language (swaying, clutching podium, etc.)?
___	Remain calm and relaxed?
___	Exhibit enthusiasm?
___	Project voice adequately?
___	Smile and use humor?
___	Vary tone, pitch, volume, and pace?
___	Avoid undue dependence on notes (script, outline)?
___	Enunciate clearly?
___	Maintain sincerity, credibility?
___	Avoid nervous habits (clearing throat, shuffling papers)?
___	Maintain clarity in providing technical information?
___	Use personal examples, anecdotes?
___	Use visual aids appropriately and effectively?
___	Anticipate questions?
___	Listen carefully to questions?

Keep visual aids simple by limiting each slide or overhead to 7 lines per page. Make visuals easy to read and understand. Use large lettering and styles that have eye appeal.

Allow the audience to ask questions at the close of the talk. Repeat each question in your own words, and then give evidence to support your point. End on a positive note and never demean a question or the person asking the question.

Developing and Nurturing Media Relations

Community nutritionists must learn techniques to build and maintain positive and productive media relationships. The media is a channel for communicating, educating, and recruiting for nutrition programs and research. Key elements of a positive media relationship include building a media resource inventory, becoming a reliable media source, understanding time pressures, and keeping track of the media (see Exhibit 3–2).

Build a media resource inventory. Check with your local chamber of commerce, United Way, or government public information office to see if a

Exhibit 3-2   Keys to Becoming a Reliable Media Source

---

1. Keep current. Be dynamic, consumer-oriented, informed, and reliable.
2. Stay tuned in to media happenings. Know what allies and adversaries say.
3. Provide your business card. Ensure that you are in reporters' resource files.
4. Send an occasional pitch letter. Provide articles or leads that will be of interest to a reporter.
5. Offer background information, recipes, graphics, audiovisual materials, or other contacts (health professionals, consumers) to make a story more exciting.
6. Do the interview if at all possible. Too many obstacles and too many *nos* are sure to exclude you from a reporter's resource file.
7. Be honest. Take the interview only if you can handle it; refer the request to another media resource if you cannot handle it.

Source: Data from Ambassador Roundtable, American Dietetic Association annual meeting; October 1993; Anaheim, Calif.

---

compiled list of local media exists. If not, abstract information from the yellow pages or media directories in libraries. For newspapers, the managing editor's office can supply names of specialized reporters. Check newspapers for lifestyle, health and fitness, food, medical, science, and consumer writers. Writers' names may appear on articles as bylines. Food sections often appear midweek (e.g., Tuesday, Wednesday, or Thursday), and community calendars usually run weekly.

For radio programming opportunities, include public service announcements, community calendar announcements, public affairs shows, daily news reports, call-in shows (question-answer format), and specialty shows (health/fitness). For television, the challenge is to identify the gamut of air opportunities and not only learn how to access them but to achieve a positive media presence and high marks for meeting the public's needs (see Figure 3-3).

Understanding the Media World

On June 2, 2003, the Federal Communications Commission (FCC) ended the long-standing federal checks and balances on corporate media power. Companies supporting the measure include the powerful Rupert Murdoch's News Corp/Fox, General Electric/NBC, Viacom/CBS, Disney/ABC, Tribune Corp, and Clear Channel. After the FCC rules were changed, more mergers and buyouts for radio and TV stations, major newspapers, and even TV networks occured. A single conglomerate could control most of a community's major media outlets, including cable systems and broadband Internet service providers. As a result, there will be fewer owners nationally of all major media outlets of communication.[73]

At the same time, more of the public is willing to stand up and express their unhappiness with the way media conglomerates are using the public airwaves. The media conglomerates seek more control and an end to media ownership limits. Existing FCC rules weaken the ability of mainstream journalism to serve as a critical public safeguard.

Info Line

The early methods used to describe the audience that listened to radio were crude. Usually the announcer's closing remarks would be something like, "to keep this fine program coming your way, send a postcard to our sponsor and let him know how much you enjoyed the program." Once the postcards were received and sorted, they were weighed. The weight reflected the popularity and audience size.

A.C. Nielsen Sr sought a more reliable method and purchased a patent for a radio meter developed for the Lever Brothers Company. Between 1938 and 1945, the meter was modified and tested, and it finally entered the market as the *Nielsen Rating*. Today a small electronic computer called a "People Meter" is installed in a cross-sectional sample of 4,000 households.

Each Nielsen audiometer links by telephone to a central computer, which polls the sample responses nightly. Ratings are calculated and transmitted to the subscribers early the following morning. Reports using slightly different methods are also produced for tracking the television-viewing audience for 210 major metropolitan areas.

Subscribers include broadcasters, advertisers and their agencies, program producers, and talents. The goal of the service is to determine fair and equitable prices for the broadcasts and commercials, based upon the size and demographics of the sample tracked by the audiometer. The Nielsen method is used not only in the United States but in many other countries where television is an important advertising medium.

Massive consolidation in cable TV and with online communications, e.g., the merger of Comcast and AOL Time Warner, may be legally permitted to own almost all of the nation's cable TV systems. Critical safeguards may be eliminated, which will enable cable and telephone giants to dominate high-speed Internet access.

As for radio, Clear Channel Communications (the company now owns more than 1,200 radio stations) is creating conformity and commercialism. In contrast, back in 1996, only 115 stations were owned by the 2 largest radio chains. A less known trend is the model of local news from a central source thousands of miles away from the market.

Congress will be involved in the legislation and will not be silent about the most significant changes in media diversity rules since the Reagan era and in the agency's history. The outcome could have the most profound effects on how Americans receive their news and information. Less stringent rules would cause a far greater concentration of media power in the hands of fewer and fewer huge companies—even more concentration than already exists. This will minimize competition and diversity of viewpoints.

To discover the best way to use local television to promote health, phone or write the television station's public service director. Request a local programming schedule and personnel guide. Watch the station to identify the style and topics discussed. Focus on opportunities such as community calendar announcements, public service announcements, daily news reports (consumer, medical, or health), weekly public affairs shows, and entertainment talk programs.

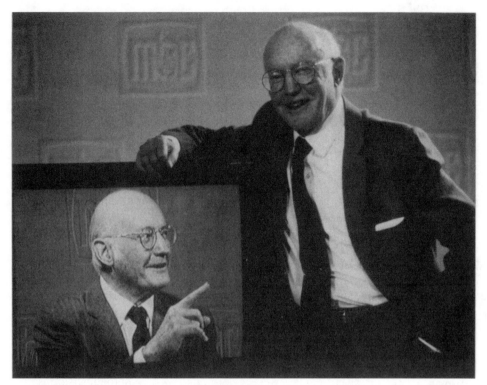

FIGURE 3–3   The Nielsens. A.C. Nielsen Jr and his father developed the popular Nielsen Ratings for television, which reflect the importance of meeting the public's interest. RDs on television are not evaluated by the Nielsen Ratings, but they are sensitive to the power of this media.
Source: Courtesy of A.C. Nielsen Jr, Northbrook, Ill.

Understand time pressures because the media, both print and electronic, work on a minute-to-minute basis. Being sensitive to their time crunch strengthens your chance to serve as a resource.

Being a resource means responding to a reporter's questions on the spot (your education and experience should enable you to respond to many nutrition issues without major research) or referring the reporter to the appropriate expert.

To track the media, use data sheets and document who you work with and the final outcome of your contact. As you widen your circle of media contacts, you become more adept at responding to inquiries and you become more visible to the community as a valuable resource. CNPs are sophisticated career men and women who frequently volunteer to create effective messages for the public's nutritional and health benefit, as shown in Figure 3–4.

Working Effectively With Print

To work effectively with the media, story angles that sell are a must! Five tips for success are outlined in Exhibit 3–3. Creative topics for print media are topics that hold a reader's interest or explore a hot issue. Food trends, food myths, and food and health never grow old. Every January, print media address

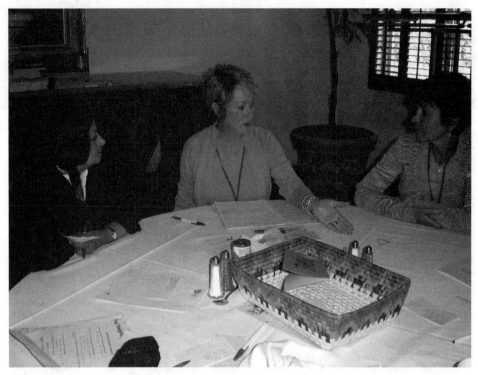

FIGURE 3–4   American Dietetic Association president from 2006-2007, Connie Diekman, MS, RD, FADA, from St. Louis, Mo, was a former media spokesperson for the ADA. She is shown here (center) working closely with 2 other former ADA spokespersons, Wahida Karmally, DrPH, RD (left), of New York, and Leslie Bonci, MS, RD (right), of Pittsburgh, Pa. They are preparing media messages to educate consumers about the availability of 29 lean cuts of beef that are high in protein, low in fat, and nutrient dense

Exhibit 3–3   Five Tips for Success With Print Interviews

1. Understand that interviews will be edited, so an interviewee may say a lot but only be quoted a little. It's important to be relaxed and friendly but stay with the agenda. If answers are concise, there is less chance of being misquoted.
2. Provide solid, well-researched information. Reporters are usually unfamiliar with the subject and rely on the nutritionist's expertise. Explain technical terms in lay language. Answer irrelevant questions, but learn to bridge to a more relevant topic.
3. If pressed due to a reporter's deadline, ask reporter to call back so interviewee can collect thoughts, write a brief outline, and then honor the interview.
4. A negative impression is difficult to change. Think of the reporter as a live microphone. Only say what you wouldn't mind having quoted.
5. Make yourself available for follow-up and fact checking. Ask for a copy of the published article, and send a thank-you note after publication.

Source: Data from Ambassador Roundtable, American Dietetic Association annual meeting; October 1993; Anaheim, Calif.

weight loss and how to rebound from the holiday overload. Sports nutrition and fitness occupy most summer issues, and the fall turns to packing healthy school lunches, after-school snacks, and dormitory food. Winter thrives on holiday and food pleasures. Community nutritionists can provide local angles to any story and help the reader to identify with real-life events.

When working with print media, especially newspaper, create a health calendar and pitch story ideas accordingly. For example, November is Diabetes Month and April is Cancer Month. Link preventive care or medical nutrition therapy with eating behavior. Your choice of topics depends on which area you feel most well versed.

Working Effectively With Television

The purpose of television interviews is to inform, provide a service, promote, or entertain.[66] To work successfully with television, nutritionists should differentiate between the types of interviews they may experience and decide which ones will most effectively present their message to the community. The most common types of interviews for television are news shows, talk shows, consumer-interest segments, and public service announcements.

News shows can include hard news, such as 2-to-4-minute segments on timely issues, or 15-second interviews to represent specific viewpoints. Talk shows are generally entertainment-oriented. Visuals are frequently used and can help "sell" a viewpoint. Consumer-interest segments are 1-to-7-minute spots that are presented as regular news features for a brief discussion of a current topic.

Public service announcements are 10 to 60 seconds in length and pre-taped as educational segments. These announcements are informative and are not commercials.

Prior to the television interview, it is important to profile the audience by watching similar shows. Specifically identify who is listening and what their interests are. Consider visuals to support the message. The media professional thinks about the audience while the amateur thinks about the topic!

Clarify on paper your key messages before beginning. Define your single overriding communication objectives. Focus on these objectives and don't wait for the right question to be asked. Bridge the questions to fit your objective. When the interview begins, address the interviewer by his or her first name. Reiterate each message 2-3 times during the interview. Help to build the story. Don't leave it up to the interviewer to make the points understood, because that allows the interviewer to direct the story (see Exhibit 3–4).

Working Effectively With Radio

Five formats are used for programming in the radio broadcast media. The community nutritionist needs to match his or her message and style to the radio medium.[71]

When giving nutrition information on the radio, the community nutritionist is allowed more time for verbal illustration of points. Audience retention is better than with television. Radio stations have an ongoing need for guests with timely, interesting, and controversial topics, and nutrition remains one of those hot topics. The radio host is usually prepared for the interview

Exhibit 3–4   General Guidelines for Television Interviews

- *Behavior*: Be punctual. At the end of the show, keep still until you hear the all clear signal from the director. Maintain correct posture and gestures for television interviews.
- *Chairs*: As the guest, lean forward in your chair to show involvement and interest. Sit at a 45-degree angle to the interviewer. This will cause you to lean slightly to one side, resting your elbow on the armrest and freeing your hands for gesturing. Don't swivel.
- *Hands*: Use gestures constructively. They look natural and illustrate your speech.
- *Legs*: Cross your legs at the ankles. If you do cross your legs at the knees, be sure to avoid bouncing your foot up and down.
- *Eyes*: The audience will unconsciously be studying your eyes in search of confidence, credibility, and enthusiasm. Have regular eye contact with the interviewer. This makes you appear interested and attentive. When 2 people are being interviewed, look at the guest who is speaking, but bring your eyes directly back to the interviewer afterward.
- *Speech*: Before the show, the audio person may ask for a sound check. At this time, say the alphabet or count to 10 at normal speaking volume. Speak clearly and distinctly. Mumbling sounds worse on television than it does in real life. Speak with a normal volume, but don't be afraid to be excited or animated. Remember that you're answering the questions; therefore, you hold the advantage over the interviewer and audience since the answers given will dictate what type of message is being communicated.

Source: Data from Ambassador Roundtable, American Dietetic Association annual meeting; October 1993; Anaheim, Calif.

---

with some knowledge of the topic; however, the host's knowledge base may not always be accurate, or the host may have a strong opinion. Being prepared and specific is the best preparation. Learn to provide facts and examples without being defensive. Five radio formats are as follows:

1. *News shows.* Scripts that are 30-60 seconds long are common. Hard news outlines research, an occurrence, or a discovery. The purpose is to inform the listener about current information in a timely manner. It is best to address the issues from the public's point of view and to keep it simple. The first 85 words are the ones most likely to be included in a taped interview. People tend to remember the first thing that is said in an interview, not the last.

2. *Talk shows.* Time slots of 10, 30, or 60 minutes are frequently used to discuss topics of broad interest to inform and entertain listeners. The show may be live or taped. The host is usually well informed and/or opinionated and includes himself or herself in the discussion. Use the host's first name, and don't be afraid to ask the host a question.

   Use hooking, bridging, and flagging techniques to help direct the conversation and to allow important points to be covered. If there are other guests, know the credentials, place of employment, areas of interest and expertise, and published works of these individuals. Avoid being scheduled head to head on a controversial topic.

3. *Call-in shows.* This format provides the longest time slot of 30-120 minutes since there are many interruptions and breaks. The time of day the show airs determines the audience. Programming is almost always live, and guests are generally scheduled a few weeks in advance.

Keep the discussion on target, but be flexible enough to handle varied questions from the callers. Consumer information is typically dealt with in an entertaining manner. Plan to speak in personal terms and use the caller's first name. Prepare an outline and rehearse by practicing in front of a mirror. Smile frequently to make you more relaxed and to project a more personable voice.

4. *Public affairs programs.* This programming format may be 10, 30, or 60 minutes in length and usually airs on Sundays or off-hours. The purpose of this format is to inform, educate, or provide a service. Generally the shows are taped.

5. *Editorial or rebuttal segments.* A single issue is covered in this 30-to-60-second spot. Facts are presented in a concise, direct manner, and the segment is often pretaped.

Evaluation of media's influence on the credibility of nutrition science and nutrition scientists exists.[74] According to a 1997 Roper Center survey, American distrust of news that sensationalizes, manipulates biases, and uses testimonials is real.[75] The increasing consumer confusion about diet and health undermines the scientific base and general eating guidelines.[76] When 78% of household food gatekeepers believe it very likely or somewhat likely that experts will flip-flop their views about healthy foods,[77] mistrust is more dominant than trust.[74]

Nutrition has become fodder for entertainment. Educating the reader about the process has emerged and Wellman et al[74] identified actions for quality reporting (Table 3-6) and 3 important issues, such as:

- *Publicizing single studies*—to give the public what they want to know, e.g., the latest insight, before they draw their conclusions and make dietary choices. Fostering a logical discovery is the preferred atmosphere.

TABLE 3–6 Actions for Quality Nutrition Reporting

- *Training for scientists*—garner resources for professional groups to train their members in writing and media skills.

- *Collaboration with the media*—establish scientist-journalist exchanges, increase access of journalists to nutrition research, and develop training programs for science writers.

- *Process information for dissemination*—preview new research by peer scientists, publicize scientific consensus statements and position papers.

- *Create consumer filters for science news*—create a Web site registry for responsible nutrition information and define type of research, e.g., observational versus randomized clinical trials.

Source: Wellman et al. An American Society for Nutritional Sciences controversy session Report. *Am J Clin Nutr.* 1999;70:802-805.

- *Negative effect of publicizing single studies*—individual studies are usually only one link in a process for scientific disclosure, are nonconclusive, and may be in conflict with the current state of knowledge.
- *Role of individual nutrition scientists reporting single studies*—promotes a celebrity status and a "magic bullet" cure rather than promoting a laudable investigator building sound evidence for beneficial health practice.

Guidelines exist for communicating emerging science on nutrition, food safety, and health.[78] CNPs and nutrition scientists have a professional responsibility to select a reputable journal, put their findings in perspective, identify whether findings affect public health recommendations or individual behavior and focused health, and minimize controversy by cooling the flames of debate with simple statements of factual information.

Tips to Communicate Information From the Lab to the Table

In a world of media activities, these recommendations are useful when CNPs explain to the public how to evaluate media messages.[79]

1. Serve as a go-between rather than an expert. CNPs who give clear and concise information help clients make their own decisions.
2. Present science as a gray area wherein every PhD has an equal and opposite PhD showing, for example, that a functional food is either beneficial or not, maybe even harmful.
3. Explain how to evaluate the science by instructing clients to identify the truth and the fluff about functional food or other nutritional stories, e.g.:
   - What does the study really report?
   - Was the study conducted in a quality, scientific manner?
   - Is the study applicable or superficial to community nutrition problems?
   - What quantity must be eaten for an effect?
   - Can the substance be incorporated easily into an eating pattern?
   - Who are the researchers?
   - Who funded the research?
   - Present critical thinking and reasoning as essential rather than changing after every published study.
   - Keep food as the focus for eating well and healthfully. CNPs can strive to lead clients to positive food action, not elimination and restriction.

At the *Healthy People 2010* conference, a panel examined how public health practitioners can make health news by making their stories relevant to people's lives. George Strait, a former reporter with ABC News, stated,

> If you put out good information, and you do it in the right way, it really does connect with people. The media play a major role in our society as brokers, mediators, and translators of health information. Furthermore, surveys show that people trust the information they get from the media.

Sally Squires, health and medical reporter for the *Washington Post*, explained, "The media is a partner in public health." Her tips for working with the media were:

- Health news must grab the reader's attention. A story must have impact, importance, and interest. Figure out your story's potential impact before you pitch it to a reporter.
- Keep in mind that your news competes with other news, and that available space and air time are shrinking. Condense your information.
- Consider enhancing a public health program by forming partnerships with the media. The media will be more inclined to cover it.
- Be creative in using the media. For instance, don't forget about Internet news services.
- Offer a variety of spokespersons to deliver your message.
- Put a face on your story. Real people add interest to a story and make it more appealing.

John Ford, president of Discovery Health Media Inc, stated health news is ". . . one of the most important reporting genres. . . . Its complexity makes it one of the most difficult reporting jobs."

He believed that public health practitioners should expect to see more media convergence or the use of different media by a single news organization, a television network giving a brief report or the story on the evening news, and then providing more information on its Web site.

Communication guidelines were developed by an advisory group convened by the Harvard School of Public Health and the International Food Information Council Foundation.[80] Specific recommendations for scientists, journal editors, journalists, industry, and consumer groups are a subset of general guidelines, which follows:

General Guidelines (Questions) for All Stakeholders in the Communication Process

1. Will your communication enhance public understanding of diet and health?
2. Have you put the study findings into context?
3. Have the study or findings been peer reviewed?
4. Have you disclosed the important facts about the study?
5. Have you disclosed all key information about the study's funding?

Communication Guidelines (Questions) for Scientists

1. Have you provided essential background information about the study in your written findings, or to journalists or others requesting it, in a language that can be understood?
2. Have you clarified dietary risks and benefits?
3. Have you met the needs of the media?

Communication Guidelines (Questions) for Journal Editors

1. Does your embargo policy enhance public communication?
2. Do you encourage responsible media reporting on study findings?
3. Have you considered the effects of the study findings on consumers?
4. Does your submission policy permit scientists to clarify results of abstract presentations with the media?

Communication Guidelines (Questions) for Journalists

1. Is your story accurate and balanced?
2. Have you applied a healthy skepticism in your reporting?
3. Does your story provide practical consumer advice?
4. Is your reporting grounded in basic understanding of scientific principles?

Guidelines (Questions) for Industry, Consumer, and Other Interest Groups

1. Have you provided accurate information and feedback to the media?
2. Do you adhere to ethical standards in providing diet and health information?

Food for Thought III—Reporting of Diet, Nutrition, and Food Safety

The Center for Media and Public Affairs (CMPA) examined the coverage in 39 local and national news outlets from May through July 1999 and compared the results to findings from the same 3-month period in 1997 and 1995.[76] The snapshots provide a reliable measure of both the changes and the constants in the information the media made available to consumers. An innovation in the 1999 study was an examination of the food and nutrition news posted on 5 major media Web sites: http://abcnews.com, http://www.cbsnews.com, http://www.msnbc.com, http://www.cnn.com, and http://www.washingtonpost.com.

These Web sites were not remarkably different from their counterparts, offering information that had already appeared in conventional forms, and they seemed to retain information based on established health advice, not fad news.

Major Findings

- In 1999, food news was up 53% over 1997 and 32% over 1995. Notably, the *Atlanta Journal-Constitution* gave heavy coverage to contaminated soft drink products in Europe while in 1997, CNN dropped "On the Menu," and food news at CNN declined by 70%.
- In 1999, disease prevention, disease risk reduction, and discussions about the benefits of certain foods were aligned center stage with news coverage. The biggest beneficiaries were soybeans and garlic.
- The number of claims of health benefits from food or diet outpaced claims of harm associated with foods, 57% versus 43%.
- The threat of food-borne illness was the most frequently discussed health risk.
- News accounts focusing on specific nutrients or components were 26% more frequent in 1999 than in 1997 and twice that of 1995.
- Both an increase in the number of new research reports and the number of scientific experts cited as sources were observed.
- Consumer and environmental groups were referenced more in 1999 than in 1997, but ranked fourth as a major source.
- In 1995 and 1997, genetically modified foods was not a media issue, but in 1999 it involved 6% of all discussions.
- Context regarding amounts, frequency, and target groups was mentioned as frequently in 1997 or 1999.

TABLE 3–7 Ten Most Frequent Nutrition Topics in News at 4 Different Years, *Food for Thought Survey*, International Food Information Council, Washington, DC

1995		1997		1999		2001	
Topic	%	Topic	%	Topic	%	Topic	%
Fat intake	18	Food-borne illness	10	Disease prevention	13	Biotechnology	12
Disease prevention	10	Fat intake	10	Food-borne illness	7	Disease prevention	9
Food-borne illness	6	Disease prevention	8	Biotechnology	6	Food-borne illness	8
Vitamin/mineral intake	6	Disease causation	5	Fat intake	6	Vitamin/mineral intake	5
Disease causation	5	Food trends	5	Functional foods	6	Allergic reactions	5
Caloric intake	4	Vitamin/mineral intake	4	Disease causation	6	Fat intake	4
Antioxidants	3	Caloric intake	4	Vitamin/mineral intake	4	Functional foods	4
Cholesterol intake	2	Food labels	3	Fiber intake	3	Disease causation	3
Sugar intake	1	Antioxidants	3	Antioxidants	3	Food labels	3
Fiber intake	1	Weight loss	3	Caloric intake	3	Antioxidants	2
All others	44	All others	45	All others	44	All others	44
Total	100	Total	100	Total	100	Total	100

Source: From S. Rowe, "Are Consumers, 'getting the message?' ", Nutrition Today, 2002:38(5):170–173. Reprinted by permission of Lippincott Williams & Wilkins.

- Reporting the method of exposure, i.e., what was ingested, and the basic research design, e.g., epidemiological or clinical, were mentioned about the same all 3 years.[81]

Another major area of concern regarding nutrition information in the media is the context in which it is presented. Contextual information is basic not only to public understanding of science, but also to the application of the information for improved health.[82]

International Food Information Council's (IFIC) 4 *Food for Thought* surveys alert CNPs that most nutrition and food stories tell consumers what to eat or not to eat but rarely detail how much, how often, or name the primary target group. When a food was linked to a specific harm or benefit, 7% of the stories listed how much of the food to eat and 4% stated how often a food should be eaten to yield an effect.[81]

For contextual information to be adequate, it should include but not be limited to:

- dosage/amount/frequency of food/nutrient consumption
- information about the study population
- expression of risk (absolute versus relative)
- risk/benefit trade-offs
- cumulative effects
- how the study compares with the current science research and body of knowledge

Table 3–7 contrasts the most frequent topics in the media from 1995 to 2001 as noted in 4 *Food for Thought* surveys.

Exhibit 3–5   *Healthy People 2010* Health Status Objectives Targeting Professionals

01–08a	Racial and ethnic representation in health professions	1996-97	2010
	American Indian or Alaska native	0.6%	1.0%
	Asian or Pacific Islander	16.2%	4.0%
	Black	6.7%	13.0%
	Hispanic	4.0%	12.0%
		1997	2010
23–01	Public health employee access to the Internet	UK	UK
02	Public access to information and surveillance data	UK	UK
05	Data for leading health indicators	UK	UK
09	Training in essential public health services	UK	UK
10	Continuing education and training by public health agencies	UK	UK

UK = unknown
Source: Adapted from: US Department of Health and Human Services. DATA2010–the *Healthy People 2010* Database. *CDC Wonder.* Atlanta, Ga: Centers for Disease Control; November 2000.

Healthy People 2010 Actions

Community nutrition professionals are the focus of several *Healthy People 2010* objectives and the driving force to achieve them (see Exhibit 3–5). Objectives are defined for working with the media, maintaining continuing education at the professional level, and increasing multiethnic representation among healthcare professionals.

References

1. US Department of Health and Human Services. DATA 2010—the *Healthy People 2010* database. *CDC Wonder*. Atlanta, Ga: Centers for Disease Control; November 2000.
2. Frank GC. On the road to research: avenues of opportunity in community nutrition. Presented at American Dietetic Association Annual Meeting; October 1991; Dallas, Tex.
3. National Heart, Lung, and Blood Institute. *National Institutes of Health Conceptual Model for Research*. Bethesda, Md: NHLBI; 1991.
4. Silverstein S, Costello L, Pazzaglia, G. Moving to the future: developing community based nutrition services. A model to meet community competencies. *Dep-Line*. 2000;21(2):10-15.
5. Costello C. Incorporating community competencies in a generalist emphasis hospital-based internship. *Dep-Line*. 2000;21:11.
6. Corby L. Assessment of community development and leadership skills required by Caribbean nutritionists and dietitians: research and international collaboration in action. *JNE*. 1997;29:250-257.
7. US Department of Health and Human Services. *Promoting Health/ Preventing Disease: Objectives for the Nation*. Washington, DC: US Government Printing Office; 1980.
8. Weddle D. Improving practice through research: gerontological nutritionists can make a difference. *Gerontological Nutritionist*. Summer 2004:4.
9. Manore MM, Myers EF. Research and the dietetics profession: making a bigger impact. *J Am Diet Assoc*. 2003;103(1):108-112.
10. Trostler N, Meyers EF. Blending practice and research: practice-based research networks an opportunity for dietetics professionals. *J Am Diet Assoc*. 2003;103(5):626-632.
11. Castellanos VH, Myers EF, Shanklin CW. The ADA's research priorities contribute to a bright future for dietetics professionals. *J Am Diet Assoc*. 2004;104(4):678-681.
12. ADA. *What Is a Dietetic Practice Based Research Network?* 2004. Available at: http://www.eatright.org/eps/rde/xchg/ada/hs.xsl/career_1708_ENU_HTML.htm Accessed April 14, 2004.
13. American Medical Association. *Healthy Youth 2000*. Chicago, Ill: American Medical Association; December 1990.
14. Miller DC. *Handbook of Research Design and Social Measurement*. 5th ed. Los Angeles, Calif: Sage Publications; 1991.
15. Green LW, Kreuter MW, Deed SG, et al. *Health Education Planning: A Diagnosis Approach*. Palo Alto, Calif: Mayfield; 1980.
16. Massachusetts Department of Public Health. Conference on standardization of qualifications and salaries of nutritional workers. Unpublished report. 1920. Available in Mary C Egan Reference Collection, National Center for Education in Maternal and Child Health, Arlington, Va.
17. Egan MC. Public health nutrition: a historic perspective. *J Am Diet Assoc*. 1994;94:298-304.

18. *Directory of Dietetic Programs.* Chicago, Ill: American Dietetic Association; 1994.
19. University of Tennessee. *Guide for Field Experiences in Community and Public Health Nutrition.* Knoxville, Tenn: University of Tennessee Press; 1978.
20. *ADA Times.* American Dietetic Association. 2004;2(1):7.
21. Vollmer HM, Mills DL. *Professionalization.* Englewood Cliffs, NJ: Prentice-Hall; 1966.
22. Wilensky HL. The professionalization of everyone? *Am J Sociol.* 1964;70:137-158.
23. Laramae SH. Entry-level practice: challenges, obligations, and opportunities. *J Am Diet Assoc.* 1989;89:1247-1249.
24. Hill L. Women's changing work roles: implications for the progress of the dietetic profession. *J Am Diet Assoc.* 1991;91:25-27.
25. Spears M, Simonis PL, Vaden AG. Professional attitudes of dietetics students and practitioners. *J Am Diet Assoc.* 1992;92:1522-1526.
26. Dodds JM, Kaufman M, eds. *Personnel in Public Health Nutrition for the 1990's.* Washington, DC: The Public Health Foundation; 1991.
27. McPhee SJ, Hung S. Suc Khoe La Vang. *Health Is Gold!* Health program for the Vietnamese. San Francisco, Calif: Department of Health Services and the University of California, San Francisco; 1990-1993.
28. Frank GC. Taking a bite out of eating behavior: food records and food recalls of children. *J School Health.* 1991;61:198-200.
29. Knapp JA, Hazuda HP, Haffner SM, et al. A saturated fat/cholesterol avoidance scale: sex and ethnic differences in a biethnic population. *J Am Diet Assoc.* 1988;88:172-177.
30. Frank GC, Zive M, Nelson J, et al. Fat and cholesterol avoidance among Mexican American and Anglo preschool children and parents. *J Am Diet Assoc.* 1991;91:954-961.
31. Frank GC, Nicklas TA, Webber LS, et al. A food frequency questionnaire for adolescents: defining eating patterns. *J Am Diet Assoc.* 1992;92: 313-318.
32. Willett W, Sampson LS, Stampfer MJ, et al. Reproducibility and validity of a semi-quantitative food frequency questionnaire. *Am J Epidemiol.* 1985;122:51-65.
33. Van Horn L, Gernhofer N, Moag-Stahlberg A, et al. Dietary assessment in children using electronic methods: telephones and tape recorders. *J Am Diet Assoc.* 1990;90:412-416.
34. Committee on Science, Engineering and Public Policy of the Academies and the Institute of Medicine. *Science, Technology and the Federal Government: National Goals for a New Era.* Washington, DC: National Academy of Sciences; 1993.
35. Dwyer J. Nutrition research for the year 2000 and beyond. *Contemporary Nutr.* 1994;18(6):1-2.
36. Ad Hoc Bionutrition Group. *NIH Bionutrition Initiative Nutrition Notes.* Bethesda, Md: American Institute of Nutrition; 1993. National Institutes of Health, Draft Guidance Document. April 29, 1993;29:7-9.
37. Committee on Opportunities in the Nutrition and Food Sciences. *Opportunities in the Nutrition and Food Sciences: Research Challenges and the Next Generation of Investigators.* Washington, DC: National Academy Press; 1993.
38. Taylor H, Voivodas G. *The Bristol-Myers Report: Medicine in the Next Century.* New York: Louis Harris and Associates, Inc; 1986.

39. Shafer MO, Story M, Houghton B. Survey of the association of graduate faculty programs in public health nutrition. Unpublished report. Minneapolis, Minn; 1993.

40. National Institutes of Health. *Fourteenth Annual Report of the NIH Program in Biomedical and Behavioral Nutrition Research and Training, Fiscal Year 1990.* Bethesda, Md: National Institutes of Health; 1990. NIH publication 91-2092.

41. Office of Technology Assessment, US Congress. *Research Funding as an Investment: Can We Measure the Returns?* Washington, DC: US Government Printing Office; 1986.

42. Raiten DJ, Berman SM. *Can the Impact of Basic Biomedical Research Be Measured? A Case Study Approach.* Bethesda, Md: Life Sciences Research Office, Federation of Associated Societies for Experimental Biology; 1993.

43. National Institutes of Health. *Cost Savings Resulting from NIH Research Support.* Bethesda, Md: National Institutes of Health; 1990. *NIH* publication 90-3109.

44. Cassell J. Professional supply and demand of dietetic practitioners. In: *The Research Agenda for Dietetics: Conference Proceedings ADA, May 14-15, 1992.* Chicago, Ill: American Dietetic Association; 1993: 104-117.

45. American Dietetic Association. *The Research Agenda for Dietetics: Conference Proceedings.* Chicago, Ill: American Dietetic Association; 1993.

46. McDonnell E, Achterberg C. Development and delivery of a nutrition education course with an electronic mail component. *JNE.* 1997; 29:210-214.

47. Lupien J, Clay W, Albert J. Challenges for nutrition education in developing countries: the FAO response. *Food and Agriculture Organization.* 1999;24(3).

48. Institute of Medicine. *Allied Health Services: Avoiding Crises.* Washington, DC: National Academy Press; 1989.

49. *Dietetics in the 21st Century: A Strategic Plan for the American Dietetic Association.* Chicago, Ill: American Dietetic Association; 1988.

50. *Achieving Competitive Advantage: The American Dietetic Association 1992 Strategic Thinking Initiative.* Chicago, Ill: American Dietetic Association; 1992.

51. Kutscher RE. Overview and implications of the projections to 2000. In: *Projections 2000.* Washington, DC: US Dept of Labor; 1988:1-7. Bureau of Labor Statistics bulletin 2302.

52. Mayer JA, Dubbert PM, Elder JP. Promoting nutrition at the point of choice: a review. *Health Ed Q.* 1989;16:31-43.

53. Gillespie A, Shafer L. Position of the American Dietetic Association: nutrition education for the public. *J Am Diet Assoc.* 1990;90:107-110.

54. Disbrow D. The cost-benefit of nutrition services. In: *The Research Agenda for Dietetics: Conference Proceedings ADA, May 14-15, 1992.* Chicago, Ill: American Dietetic Association; 1993:118-126.

55. Dennison KF, Dennison D, Ward JY. Computerized nutrition program: effect on nutrient intake of senior citizens. *J Am Diet Assoc.* 1991;91:1431-1433.

56. Luker KA, Caress AL. The development and evaluation of computer assisted learning for patients on continuous ambulatory peritoneal dialysis. *Computer Nurs.* 1991;9:15-21.

57. Bethea CD, Stallings SF, Wolman PG, et al. Comparison of conventional and videotaped diabetic exchange lists instruction. *J Am Diet Assoc.* 1989;89:405-406.
58. NCND launches consumer hotline. *ADA Courier.* 1992;31:1.
59. Levine J, Gussow JD. Better than we think? A reassessment of "Feeling Good." *J Nutr Ed.* 1991;23:296-302.
60. Shannon B, Mullis RM, Pirie PL, et al. Promoting better nutrition in the grocery store using a game format: the shop smart game project. *J Nutr Ed.* 1990;22:183-188.
61. Personick VA. Industry output and employment through the end of the century. In: *Projections 2000.* Washington, DC: US Dept of Labor; 1988:28-43. Bureau of Labor Statistics bulletin 2302.
62. Sargent J, Pfleeger J. The job outlook for college graduates to the year 2000. *Occupational Outlook Quarterly.* 1990;34(2):2-8.
63. National Commission for Health Education Credentialing. *Certification Examination for Certified Health Education Specialists.* New York, 1989.
64. Bryk JA, Kornblum TH. Report on the 1990 membership data base of the American Dietetic Association. *J Am Diet Assoc.* 1991;91:1136-1141.
65. Kaufman M, Heimendinger J, Foerster S, et al. Survey of nutritionists in state and local public health agencies. *J Am Diet Assoc.* 1986;86: 1566-1570.
66. *Minorities and Women in the Health Fields.* Washington, DC: US Dept of Health and Human Services, Public Health Service; 1990.
67. Sawyer TR. Re-entry and second career. In: *Abstracts of the American Dietetic Association 71st Annual Meeting.* Chicago, Ill: American Dietetic Association; 1988:21.
68. Gitchell R, Fitz PA. Recruiting minority students into dietetics: an outreach and education project. *J Am Diet Assoc.* 1985;85:1293-1295.
69. Covey S. *The Seven Habits of Highly Effective People.* New York: Simon & Schuster, Inc; 1989.
70. Miller WC. The creative edge. In: *Executive Book Summaries.* Bristol, Vt: Sandview Executive Book Summaries; 1988;10(1, part 3):1-8.
71. American Dietetic Association. ADA ambassador roundtables. Presented at ADA annual meeting; October 1993; Anaheim, Calif.
72. Gehling E. Are you using your power? *Diabetes Care.* 2004;25(5):14-16.
73. Chester J, Haxen D. Showdown at the FCC. May 3, 2003. Available at: http://alernet.org/story/15796.
74. Wellman N, Scarbrough E, Ziegler R, Lyle B. Do we facilitate the scientific process and the development of dietary guidance when findings from single studies are publicized? An American Society for Nutritional Sciences controversy session report. *Am J Clin Nutr.* 1999;70:802-805.
75. Institute for Social Inquiry/Roper Center, University of Connecticut. Attitudes about the news, media. Washington, DC: Freedom Forum Media Studies Center and Newseum; 1997.
76. International Food Information Council and Center for Media and Public Affairs. *Food for Thought II: Reporting of Diet, Nutrition and Food Safety.* Washington, DC: International Food Information Council and Center for Media and Public Affairs; 1998.
77. Food Marketing Institute and *Prevention* Magazine. Shopping for health 1997: balancing convenience, nutrition and taste. Washington, DC: Food Marketing Institute and *Prevention* Magazine; 1997.
78. Improving public understanding: guidelines for communicating emerging science on nutrition, food safety and health. *J Natl Cancer Inst.* 1998;9(3):194-199.

79. Feder D. What do I tell my clients? The American Dietetic Association Annual Meeting; October 18, 1999; Atlanta, Ga.

80. Fineberg H, Rowe S. Improving public understanding: guidelines for communicating emerging science on nutrition, food safety, and health. *J Nat Cancer Inst.* 1998;90(3):194-199.

81. International Food Information Council. *Food for Thought IV: Reporting of Diet, Nutrition and Food Safety.* Washington, DC: International Food Information Council and Center for Media and Public Affairs; 2002.

82. Rowe S. Are consumers "getting the message"? *Nutr Today.* 2002;38(5): 170-173.

WORKING WITH SPECIAL GROUPS IN A COMPLEX ENVIRONMENT

Learning Objectives

- Define the ways community nutrition professionals can acquire cultural competence.
- Identify how to develop and to evaluate nutrition education materials for multiethnic groups.
- Describe the wasting syndrome common among individuals with HIV and how secondary infections affect morbidity and mortality of HIV-positive individuals.
- Discuss the historic development of the US policy to identify and alleviate hunger.
- Describe the composition of a vegetarian eating pattern, and explain the health benefits of such a pattern.

High Definition Nutrition

Acculturation–repeated exposure to influences from a different culture. The process is related to age, education, frequency of interaction, and income and occurs on a continuum.

Cachectin factor–the ability to promote catabolism in fat cells; cytokines exhibiting this property include interleukin-1 and interferons alfa, beta, and gamma; also called the cytokine tumor necrosis factor.

Cultural broker–an individual who arbitrates/mediates on behalf of individuals from different cultures.

Cultural competence–the ability to increase one's understanding and appreciation of cultural differences and commonalities by developing knowledge and interpersonal skills.

Cultural sensitivity–recognition that cultural differences and similarities exist.

Cultural universal—structures and functions common to every culture (e.g., a family unit, marriage, parental roles, education, health care, and occupations).

Cultural values—standards that characterize groups.

Culturally appropriate—an entity that is sensitive to cultural differences and commonalities and often uses cultural symbols to communicate a message.

Culture—unique values, customs, language, and history. It can transcend time or change with time.

Enculturation—the process of learning the beliefs, attitudes, and behaviors of a group.

Ethnic—the commonality of a group expressed by its nationality, language, or race.

Ethnocentric—perception or belief that one's own values, beliefs, and practices are superior to those of another culture.

Food deprivation—an inability of individuals to obtain sufficient food to meet their nutrient needs.

Food poverty—an incapacity of households to access food (as opposed to a national scarcity of food).

Food security—level of assurance in which any individual could obtain a culturally acceptable and nutritionally adequate eating pattern from non-emergency food sources at any time.

Homeless person—an individual unable to secure permanent and stable housing without special assistance.

Household—the basic socioeconomic unit that decides how and when investments, including the acquisition of food, are made for its members.

Hunger—involuntary, inadequate food intake, reducing physical activity and reducing mental ability.

Lactovegetarian—an individual who eats a diet of fruits, vegetables, grains, dairy foods, and eggs.

Malnutrition—the consequence of changes in any of the processes involved in nutrition or in those factors affecting it (i.e., over- or undernutrition). Undernutrition, associated with deficiencies of one or more nutrients, is caused by one or more primary causes, such as inadequate ingestion, absorption, or utilization, or increased excretion and requirement.

Multicultural—composed of 2 or more unique cultures.

Nationality—the homeland of an individual or group.

Nutrition—the sum total of the processes involved in the ingestion and use of nutrients that are involved in the growth, repair, and maintenance of the body's components and their functions. These processes include ingestion, digestion, absorption, metabolism, and functional use of nutrients. Accessibility of a balanced diet is influenced by an array of physical, sociocultural, economic, behavioral, genetic, and medical factors.

Race—a genetically linked population.

Religion—a structure involving worship and beliefs about a higher power.

Society—people unified by a common culture and geography.

Subculture—the knowledge, beliefs, and values common to a segment of a society (e.g., socioeconomic or age groups).

Vegan—an individual who does not eat meat, fish, fowl, eggs, or dairy products.

Community Nutrition Professionals and Diversity

The United States is a land of beautiful diversity—diversity of peoples, religions, educations, and work experiences, to name a few[1] (see Table 4–1). The richness of this mosaic creates challenges for community nutrition professionals who attempt to meet the various nutritional needs of diverse individuals and groups.

The needs of a multiethnic society differ from the needs of subgroups with risk factors for and complications of devastating disease such as acquired immune deficiency syndrome (AIDS). The potential nutritional cures or remedies for the complications and the wasting syndrome experienced by individuals who test positive for the human immunodeficiency virus (HIV) challenge community nutrition professionals to present accurate information and interpretation of these remedies.

In another arena, community nutrition professionals who work with multiethnic groups need cultural competence to assess eating behavior and nutritional status as part of nutritional epidemiology, and also to provide effective nutrition education as a primary, secondary, or tertiary intervention. A nutrition professional may formulate a program to alleviate hunger one day, and the next day either instruct pregnant vegetarian mothers how to plan nutritionally adequate meals for themselves and their families or visit a convalescing stroke patient at home to monitor low-sodium eating. These clients and their families may come from any one of several ethnic groups.

These real-life situations demand new skills, increased knowledge, and sincere efforts by community nutrition professionals (CNPs) to practice their profession. Working in a culturally diverse environment is not new, but it remains a daily challenge.

TABLE 4–1   The Broad Scope of Diversity Surrounding the Individual

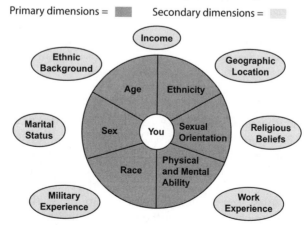

Source: Jones and Bartlett Publishers, 2007.

Working in a Multicultural Environment

The US population today is one of multiethnic groups living in geographic areas that do not resemble their homelands. Working successfully in a multicultural environment demands an understanding of the culture of each group, and the cultural universe as well as the values unique to each ethnic group.

California, for example, is the first US mainland state with a majority of minorities.[2] To address the challenge, strategies for California and companion states facing multiethnic majorities include intra-assessment. This assessment identifies factors influencing health and illness specific to population groups other than middle-income whites, the usual standard. Gaps in health status may then be reduced, and US health statistics may then be improved. Central to the endeavor is understanding the various cultures.

Culture has been defined as the accumulation of a group's beliefs, assumptions, customs, and values that direct the lifestyle of the group's members.[3-9] Beliefs stem from the knowledge, opinions, and faith individuals or groups have and often precipitate customs or common practices. Values are beliefs deemed important by an individual or group, whereas assumptions are statements that are taken for granted. Values expressed by one culture may not be honored in another culture.[3]

Cultural sensitivity is awareness of one's own cultural beliefs and the ability to understand and to acknowledge the values and customs of another culture. Cultural sensitivity during nutrition education sessions or programs may simply mean that nutrition professionals do not express their personal bias about individuals from ethnic groups different from their own.[10]

One early cultural group immigrating to the United States consisted of white, Anglo-Saxon Protestants (WASPs), who remain distinct by their eye, skin, and hair colors.[11] Current immigrants to the United States range from Southeast Asians to South and Central Americans. Each group embodies its own customs, languages, beliefs, and appearances.[6,7] Each new group has been challenged during enculturation to the US, with its melting pot of cultures originally from Northern Europe.

Cultural competence is the acquisition of knowledge and requisite skills to identify and appreciate differences and commonalities of various groups.[12] Knowledge alone does not produce cultural competence. Understanding the codes and mores of a group and its numerous subgroups equips nutritionists with powerful communication and evaluation skills. As professionals recruit

Info Line

E. Randall-David's *Strategies for Working With Culturally Diverse Communities and Clients* (Washington, DC: Office of Maternal and Child Health, US DHHS; 1989) is designed to assist healthcare providers by increasing their understanding of the cultural aspects of health and illness so they can work effectively with clients and families from culturally diverse communities. The book is available from the Association for the Care of Children's Health, 7910 Woodmont Avenue, Suite 300, Bethesda, MD 20814; 301-654-6549.

Exhibit 4-1   Community Nutritionist Self-Evaluation About
Diversity Awareness

Do I . . .

- Know about the rules and customs of different cultures?
- Know and admit that I hold stereotypes about other groups?
- Feel equally comfortable with people of all backgrounds?
- Actively associate with those who are different from me?
- Find it satisfying to work on a multicultural team?
- Find change stimulating and exciting?
- Like to learn about other cultures?
- Show patience and understanding with individuals who speak limited English?
- Find that more gets done when I spend time building relationships?
- Feel that both newcomers and society need to make an effort to change?

Source: Adapted from: Gardenswartz L, Rowe A. What's your diversity quotient? *Working World.* August 31, 1992, with permission of Rhodes Publications, Inc.

---

participants into studies and programs, develop assessment tools, interpret data, and employ staff to complete projects, cultural competence is essential. A self-evaluation instrument is given in Exhibit 4-1.[13]

To respect and accept a cultural group's beliefs and behaviors, the CNP may have to study individuals and their broader community-based structure. Incorporating community leaders into decision-making positions, forming coalitions, and employing residents from within the community are actions a community nutritionist can take to acquire cultural sensitivity and respect.[11]

To minimize an ethnocentric attitude, although one's cultural pride is important, CNPs need to be culturally competent.

Four stages identify the process of acquiring cultural competence. These are (1) *cultural awareness* of one's own values by self-assessment; (2) *cultural knowledge* of the target group using books, lectures, film, and personal contact; (3) *cultural skill* in communication, interpretation, and definition of the target group's beliefs and customs; and (4) an increased frequency of *cultural encounters* that expand understanding and ease communication while enhancing respect.[3] A checklist for gathering information about culturally diverse communities to aid organizations that wish to work with diverse groups is presented in Exhibit 4-2. A quick guide to assist community nutrition and other health professionals who counsel multicultural groups was developed by the US Department of Agriculture (Exhibit 4-3). The guide addresses activities to prepare for counseling, enhance communication, and promote positive change.[14] See Appendix 4-A for a list of questions for clients to evaluate their eating environment.

A framework for counseling different ethnic groups is called LEARN (listen, explain, acknowledge, recommend, and negotiate). Using this framework, nutrition educators can improve their communication skills.[15] The components include listening to the client's statement of his or her problems, explaining what was heard, acknowledging similarities and differences, projecting a common understanding, recommending changes, and negotiating an action plan.

Exhibit 4–2   Checklist for Information Gathering

Check the items as you complete the important steps to your own satisfaction.

- Have you gathered information on and increased your understanding of the following?
  ___ The demographics of the target community
  ___ The major historical issues of the community
  ___ The community's economic and political concerns
  ___ The major cultural beliefs, values, and practices of the target community
  ___ The health problem as it can be addressed within the cultural context(s) of this community
  ___ Other questions you have chosen to explore

- Have you also consulted the following sources?
  Library resources, such as the following:
  ___ Census data, government documents, reports, and statistics
  ___ Public health literature
  ___ Behavioral and social science literature
  ___ Local newspapers

  Experts, such as the following:
  ___ Academicians with knowledge or experience working with specific ethnic or cultural groups
  ___ Health professionals who work in similar communities or with similar problems
  ___ Other professionals working in diverse communities or in the target community
  ___ Individuals from the target community

- Have you prepared your staff to work in the community through the following activities?
  ___ Summary of research findings in a report for your staff
  ___ Discussion of this information with staff's input
  ___ Exploration of staff's cultural attitudes and beliefs and how these might influence staff members' behavior in the community
  ___ Assessment of your and your staff's past experiences in working with diverse communities to determine who has the necessary skills
  ___ Training and/or ongoing support for staff to help them resolve personal and professional issues as they arise in the community

Source: Adapted from: Health promotion section, *Multi-Ethnic Health Promotion Task Force Reports.* Sacramento, Calif: California Department of Health and Human Services; 1991.

Preparing Information for and Counseling Multiethnic Groups

All information intended to reach people of a particular culture must pass through cultural filters before it is received and acted upon. If information is culturally appropriate, it will be more readily received. As information goes through these filters, it is colored by social norms, values, traditions, and

Exhibit 4–3   Quick Guide for Cross-Cultural Counseling

Preparing for Counseling

- Understand your own cultural values and biases.
- Acquire basic knowledge of cultural values, health beliefs, and nutrition practices for client groups you routinely serve.
- Be respectful of, interested in, and understanding of other cultures without being judgmental.

Enhancing Communication

- Determine the level of fluency in English and arrange for an interpreter, if needed.
- Ask how the client prefers to be addressed.
- Allow the client to choose seating for comfortable personal space and eye contact.
- Avoid body language that may be offensive or misunderstood.
- Speak directly to the client, whether an interpreter is present or not.
- Choose a speech rate and style that promotes understanding and demonstrates respect for the client.
- Avoid slang, technical jargon, and complex sentences.
- Use open-ended questions or questions phrased in several ways to obtain information.
- Determine the client's reading ability before using written materials in the process.

Promoting Positive Change

- Build on cultural practices, reinforcing those that are positive, and promoting change only in those that are harmful.
- Check for client understanding and acceptance of recommendations.
- Remember that not all seeds of knowledge fall into a fertile environment to produce change. Of those that do, some will take years to germinate. Be patient and provide counseling in a culturally appropriate environment to promote positive health behavior.

Source: Adapted from: *Cross-Cultural Counseling: A Guide for Nutrition and Health Counselors.* Washington, DC: US Dept of Agriculture; 1986.

---

history. This filtering process is essential for information directed toward any ethnic group living in the United States. When working on prevention and treatment programs among various ethnic groups, community nutritionists may interact with cultural brokers and must understand cultural filters that influence the comprehension and, ultimately, the behavior of the group. Professionals who are sensitive to the values and traditions of the multiethnic groups are more likely to overcome barriers that may exist to prevention, intervention, or treatment.[16]

Two good resources are Randall-David's *Stategies for Working with Culturally Diverse Communities and Clients*, Office of Maternal and Child Health, US Department of Health and Human Services; and Sue and Sue's *Counseling the Culturally Different: Theory and Practice.*[9,17]

Hispanics/Latinos

The Hispanic/Latino population in the United States includes nationalities such as Mexican Americans, Puerto Ricans, and Cuban Americans; immigrants from El Salvador, Nicaragua, and the Dominican Republic; and immigrants from other Central and South American countries. The people in each Hispanic/Latino subgroup have different needs and experiences that have shaped their attitudes toward health, family, and nutrition. Lack of awareness and sensitivity to this fact can build formidable barriers in reaching Hispanic/Latino audiences.[16]

According to US Census Bureau statistics, Hispanics/Latinos in the continental United States number nearly 20 million, and Puerto Rico has 3 million inhabitants. Approximately 62% are Mexican Americans; 13% are mainland Puerto Ricans; 5% are Cuban Americans; 12% are of predominantly Central and South American origins; and 8% are of other Hispanic origins. Undocumented laborers and illegal immigrants are not included.[16]

Hispanics/Latinos constitute the second largest minority in the United States, after African Americans. They represent 8% of the total US population and are expected to remain the largest minority group. The Hispanic/Latino population is increasing 3 times faster than the non-Hispanic US population and may account for one quarter of the nation's growth during the next 20 years. They are the fastest-growing and the youngest minority, with a median age of 25. About 40% are under 21.[16]

Hispanics/Latinos are difficult to reach primarily because of language and cultural barriers. Program planners or CNPs can learn Spanish and become sensitive to the myriad of ethnic nuances that can make or break interpersonal relationships. Subgroups may differ by education, income level, health status, and degree of assimilation to mainstream American culture. Professionals can also employ, train, and guide local community paraprofessionals whose fluency and acceptance by the subgroup may be greater than that of the professional.

A potential reason the Hispanic/Latino population may neglect health care is that money is often scarce. About 26% of all Hispanic families in the United States live below the poverty line and comprise a growing subculture. Many do not have the basic insurance to cover treatment. In addition, as a rule, Hispanics/Latinos are very proud and very private when it comes to family problems. It is difficult for a family to help a member who has problems, such as with alcohol, and still more difficult to recommend external help. For Hispanic/Latino families, revealing secrets and looking for answers outside the strong family unit is adverse to their culture.[16]

Hispanic/Latino families work as a team with their focus on the good of the whole or the good of others. Interdependence, rather that independence, is encouraged. This value influences receptivity to community nutrition programs and printed materials. Community nutrition programs may be more attractive if advertisements appeal to individual members' commitment for the common good of the family. A publication might start out with the appeal that "It will benefit your husband . . . children . . . sister, if you learn more about healthy eating."

The Hispanic/Latino family bond, or *carino*, evokes a deep sense of unqualified caring and protection. All family members are equal, unconditionally accepted, and valued simply because they are, not because of what they have done or not done. Machismo among Hispanics/Latinos is accepted, and men are expected to be dominant, protective, and authoritarian. Hispanic/Latino women are expected to conform to the female ideal of purity, discipline, and self-sacrifice in body, mind, and spirit.

General recommendations for working with Hispanic/Latino populations are[16]:

- Target prevention and intervention efforts to the entire family and their religious leaders.
- Help Hispanic/Latino fathers recognize how important their role is to their children. Encourage mothers to learn strategies for including their spouses in family interactions.
- Educate mothers and daughters to reduce the shame associated with asking for help.
- Emphasize the family as a unit in printed materials. Tailor separate versions for males and females.
- Emphasize participation in healthy eating and exercise programs to adjust to the American culture without abandoning their own.
- Reach Hispanic/Latino audiences through Spanish-speaking, community-level organizations and leaders.
- Educate community nutritionists and assistants about traditional gender roles to aid their efforts. Nontraditional religions are very powerful, especially in Puerto Rican and Cuban-American communities. Two popular nontraditional religions draw heavily from the traditions of the Catholic church and mix the belief in saints with psychic powers and the spirit world. *Espiritismo* is popular among Puerto Ricans, and *santeria* is likely to be found in Cuban-American communities. The believers regularly follow spiritual leaders called *espiritistas* and *santeros/santeras*, respectively, who are supposedly born with or develop psychic powers and knowledge of spells, charms, and incantations.[16]

Nutrition education and prevention program planners must explore the demographic characteristics and religions of their target group. This translates into several tasks:

- Obtain approval of the local *espiritistas* or *santeros/santeras*, because they may tell their followers that the prevention program is not good and thereby destroy a community effort.
- Do not attempt to hold joint meetings, seminars, or fund-raisers with different religious groups.
- Ensure that learning about the different religions is a part of the planning process, because insulting religious beliefs due to ignorance may be fatal for a community-based program.

African Americans

The term *soul food*, coined in the 1960s, refers to traditional African-American Southern cuisine, which is a symbol of ethnic solidarity, identity, and heritage. The soul food tradition is interwoven with the slave experience, foods and food preparation styles from Africa, changes due to US slavery, and Southern foods, creating new foodways.[18]

Eleven states comprise the South and its 74 million people and include Alabama, Arkansas, Florida, Georgia, Louisiana, Mississippi, North Carolina, South Carolina, Tennessee, Texas, and Virginia. Kentucky is frequently considered a Southern state. The majority of the South is white, with African Americans, Hispanics, Native Americans, and Asian Americans comprising the minority groups.

The Southern states produce 60% of US farm income from poultry and poultry products and 15% of pork production. Rice, cotton, tobacco, sugarcane, and soybeans are common.

Soul foodways have their origins in Europe and Africa. Slaves working on the Southern plantations brought with them new ingredients, including okra, sesame (or benne) seed, and black-eyed peas, peanuts, and other legumes. They also brought cookery methods, such as frying and boiling. Indigenous Southern foods, such as corn, pumpkin, and oysters, were added to those of Europe and Africa.

Nutrition counseling for individuals eating African-American/soul foods requires knowledge of and sensitivity to a spiritual actuating principle of nutriment in solid form.[19] This belief stemmed from a slave culture that identified an escape and means of nourishing the tired and weary.[20-23] The types of foods that embody soul food reflect West African fare, limited resources in the United States, seasoning to improve taste, and extended boiling to tenderize tough and coarse foods.[24] Table 4–2 contrasts traditional versus contemporary food choices among different ethnic groups.

The basics of soul food are inconsistent with 3 of the 2005 *Dietary Guidelines for Americans*[25]:

- Guideline 4: Eat more fruits and vegetables, whole grains and nonfat or low-fat milk and milk products.
- Guideline 5: Choose fats wisely.
- Guideline 7: Choose and prepare foods with little salt.

Young African Americans have high-fat eating patterns, and African Americans in general consume about 36% of total calories from fat and exceed 300 mg of cholesterol each day.[26] On the other hand, African Americans enjoy many nutrient-rich, cruciferous vegetables and fruits high in vitamins A and C. Intakes of high-fiber cereal and grain products are not common.[27] Use of cured and salted meats and the addition of salt during cooking and eating are common, resulting in a high sodium intake.[28] Counseling for African Americans should address the following points to improve healthy eating and reduce health risk[19]:

- Lower total fat, animal or saturated fat, and cholesterol intake.
- Try new cooking procedures and new tastes; attend cooking demonstrations.
- Taste food before seasoning with salt; order unsalted fast foods.

Native Americans

It is estimated that 20,000 to 50,000 years ago, a land bridge across the Bering Strait provided the means for about 400 Indian and Alaskan nations to enter North America. Many moved to the territory we now call the United States.

TABLE 4–2 Traditional Versus Contemporary Food Choices of Multiethnic Groups

Ethnic Group	Traditional	Contemporary
Hispanic	**Breakfast** • Corn tortillas, eggs with chorizo (sausage), salsa • Mexican sweet bread and fruit • Hot chocolate or coffee with milk **Lunch** • Corn tortillas; rice and beans; beef, chicken, or pork stewed with chilis and tomatoes • Soft drinks or coffee with milk **Dinner** • Enchiladas, rice, and beans • Cactus with pork and onion, beans, and corn tortillas • Soft drinks or coffee with milk	**Breakfast** • Traditional foods or Americanized choices such as bacon, eggs, and toast, or cold cereal with milk • Milk, fruit juice, or coffee with milk **Lunch** • Traditional foods at home or fast food including pizza, hamburgers, burritos, and sandwiches • School lunch for most children • Milk, fruit juice, or soft drinks **Dinner** • Traditional food choices such as rice, beans, a meat dish, and tortillas • Typical Americanized food choices such as spaghetti or barbecued chicken, corn, salad, and bread • Fruit juice, soft drinks, or coffee with milk
African American	**Breakfast** • Eggs, country ham with red-eye gravy, biscuits, and fried potatoes or grits • Coffee or milk **Dinner (the traditional luncheon meal)** • Fried chicken or catfish, boiled cabbage and potatoes • Beef-vegetable stew with cornbread • Fruit cobbler • Buttermilk and fruit-flavored drinks	**Breakfast** • Much lighter than traditional • May include toast; eggs and bacon; cream of wheat, oatmeal, or grits **Lunch** • Typical fast-food choices: hamburgers, hot dogs, sandwiches, pizza • School lunches for most children • Milk, fruit juice, or coffee

continued

TABLE 4-2 continued

Ethnic Group	Traditional	Contemporary
	Supper (the traditional dinnertime meal) • Boiled legumes or greens with ham hocks, coleslaw, and cornbread • Buttermilk or fruit-flavored drinks	**Dinner** • Baked chicken with bread stuffing, green beans, green salad, bread and butter • Macaroni and cheese • Cobblers • Coffee, tea, fruit-flavored drinks, or milk
Filipino	**Breakfast** • Broiled fish, leafy vegetables with fish sauce, rice • Dried salty fish, rice, and fruit • Coffee with milk and sugar **Lunch** • Bamboo shoots with shrimp and coconut milk, eggplant sauce, rice, and fruit • Stir-fried rice with leftover meat and vegetables • Coffee with milk and sugar **Dinner** • Dried, salted fish, sauteed okra, rice, and fruit • Beef or chicken and vegetable stew with rice • Soy milk, coffee with milk and sugar, or tea	**Breakfast** • Rice with egg or meat dish • Toast or cold cereal with milk • Coffee with milk **Lunch** • Meat dish with vegetables and rice • School lunch for most children • Milk and fruit juice **Dinner** • Sauteed meat, long green beans, and rice • Typical westernized meals: roast beef with vegetables and bread, barbecued meats, corn, salad, and bread • Soft drinks, fruit drinks, or coffee with milk
Chinese	**Breakfast** • Rice porridge seasoned with small amounts of meat or fish • Bowl of noodles with vegetables and meat	**Breakfast** • Similar to traditional choices but may include westernized selections of cold cereal with milk, or eggs with toast

Lunch • Rice or fried noodles, Chinese greens, and a seasoned meat dish with clear soup • Tea **Dinner (a larger version of lunch)** • Rice, tofu with sausage, several vegetable dishes, and clear soup • Tea or soup (In northern China, soup is usually the beverage at meals; in southern China the beverage is usually tea.)	**Lunch** • Traditional choices including rice with leftovers • Sandwiches and other take-out foods • School lunch for most children • Tea, fruit juice, or milk **Dinner** • Most similar to traditional pattern including rice, meat or fish dishes, sauteed vegetables with soy sauce or oyster sauce, and clear soup • Tea, fruit juice, or milk
Vietnamese **Breakfast** • Soup with rice noodles, sliced meat, bean sprouts, and mustard greens • Boiled egg with meat and pickled vegetables on French bread **Lunch** • Rice, fish with lemon grass, string beans, clear soup with vegetables, and fruit **Dinner** • Rice, sauteed pork, leeks, clear soup, and fruit • Coffee with sweetened condensed milk, tea, or fruit drinks (drunk after meal)	**Breakfast** • French bread with fried eggs • Toast with butter and sugar sprinkled on top • Instant noodles **Lunch** • Rice with seasoned beef, sauteed vegetables, and clear soup • School lunch for most children **Dinner** • Similar to the traditional dinner with rice, a meat or fish dish, stir-fried vegetables, clear soup, fruit for dessert • Coffee with sweetened condensed milk, tea, or soft drinks

Source: Data from Dairy Council of California. 17 pgs. *A Celebration of Culture: A Food Guide for Educators.* Sacramento, CA; 1994.

Their languages were only verbal, not written, so the record of early food habits is scarce. What is known is that several centers of Indian culture flourished (for example, the Cherokees, Chickasaws, Choctaws, Creeks, and Seminoles in the southeast; the Iroquois in the northeast or New York State; and the Pueblo community near the Rio Grande and the Little Colorado River in the southwest).[29]

The socioeconomic status of Native Americans declined dramatically with forced migration in the 19th century. This was most notable when tribal nations moved to areas with limited agricultural resources. Indian food habits reflect the land and its climate and vegetation. Much of the daily endeavor of traditional American Indians focused on hunting, gathering, and preparing food.

Staples common to most American Indians were beans, corn, and squash. Traditional foods included blueberries, cranberries, grapes, beans, corn, pumpkins, lobster, moose, pigeon, rabbit, squirrel, and turkey on the East Coast; peanuts, potatoes, sweet potatoes, and tomatoes in the South; salmon and fruit on the Pacific Cost; chili peppers, melons, and squash in the Southwest; and buffalo and wild rice on the plains. Only a few US cities serve most residents of the Native-American population today. These include in descending order of population: Los Angeles, San Francisco, Tulsa, Minneapolis and St. Paul (combined), Oklahoma City, Chicago, and Phoenix. The remaining American Indians live in rural areas and on reservations.[28] For further information, contact the Indian Health Service (IHS), US Department of Health and Human Services, Washington, DC.

American Indians hold food in high spiritual regard and link physical health, balance, and harmony with food. Corn has a special healing significance; agave leaves assist with wound healing, chilis remediate arthritis and warts, and mint tea eases gastrointestinal ailments. Certain tribes practice dietary restrictions to correct health problems. For example, cabbage, eggs, fish, onions, organ meat and other meats, and milk may be restricted in general; cod, halibut, and certain types of salmon are restricted for a short period after childbirth.

Traditional foods are not as visible in the eating patterns of American Indians today. If the food gatekeeper (i.e., the individual who plans, purchases, and cooks the meals) inherited traditions, then these are reflected in foods; however, native greens, wild game meats, cornmeal mush, hominy, and wild sumac berry pudding are rare today.[30-33] Meal patterns may be repetitive, with fried foods for breakfast and lunch and boiled meat for dinner. Today, fast foods are purchased and consumed with more frequency by each new generation.[30]

Over the past few decades, the total energy, protein, and fiber intakes, as well as calcium, iron, phosphorus, vitamins A and C, and riboflavin intakes of American Indians have declined among certain tribes.[31] With lifestyle changes, health changes have also been identified. Infant mortality and maternal mortality rates for American Indians are 2.5 and 4 times the US average, respectively. Obesity, diabetes, heart disease, and alcoholism are the major health problems. There have been dramatic increases for diabetes, heart disease, and hypertension among American Indians.[29]

Healthcare providers who counsel American Indians must recognize traditional beliefs and practices. For example, all individuals speak for themselves, as no other can speak for them; "yes" and "no" are considered complete responses, and explanations are not thought to be warranted (see Appendix 4–B). In-depth interviews are not consistent with the belief in personal autonomy in the American Indian culture, and direct eye contact is not common.[29]

Asians

Asian immigrants to the United States include people from China, Japan, Korea, and Southeast Asian countries, such as Thailand, Taiwan, Laos, Burma, Cambodia, Vietnam, Philippines, and Malaysia. The major Chinese immigration began in the 1850s with the gold rush to California. Koreans immigrated beginning in the mid-1950s, and refugees from Vietnam and Cambodia arrived in the United States beginning in the 1970s.[29]

Chinese

Chinese enjoy a broad range of foods; however, dairy products are not common, and polished white rice is the staple. Wheat is used for crepes and wrappers of many foods, noodles, and wontons. Meat, fish, and poultry are common but generally served in small portions reflecting food habits originating in generations of famine in China. Soybeans are considered the "poor man's cow," because they are transformed into many milk-type products, soy milk, bean curd/tofu, black beans, soy sauce, and hoisin and oyster sauces. Hot soup and tea are common accompaniments. Wines, beers, and distilled alcohols are made from starches, such as bamboo-leaf green, hua diao, and red rice wine. Raw fruits, often unripe, are served for dessert. Stir-frying and deep-fat frying of bite-size portions is common.[29] See Figure 4–1.

Meal patterns for Chinese generally reflect 3 meals and several snacks. A *yin* (cold) and *yang* (hot) balance is complemented with a *fan* and *ts'ai* balance. *Fan* refers to foods made of grains and served in individual dishes; *ts'ai* is the meat/vegetable combination served on a platter for all to pass and take a serving. It is proper to raise the rice bowl to the mouth when using chopsticks, and the *ts'ai* is served in small portions on the rice with the sauce flowing to the bottom.[34]

Food among the Chinese symbolizes harmony of the body with the *yin/yang* and the *fan/ts'ai* foods. Tiredness and early winter postpartum months signal use of hot foods; dry lips, irritability, and summer months evoke consumption of cold foods. Disease is considered either a hot disease (e.g., measles and sore throats) that is treated with cold foods, or a cold disease (e.g., anemia) that is treated with hot foods.[34]

Dietary Guidelines and the Food Guide Pagoda   *The Dietary Guidelines for Chinese Residents* were founded on principles of nutritional science, food culture, and the current agricultural condition.[35] Prepared by experts, the guidelines for the general population are:

1. Eat a variety of foods, with cereals as the staple.
2. Consume plenty of vegetables, fruits, and tubers.
3. Consume milk, beans, or dairy or bean products every day.

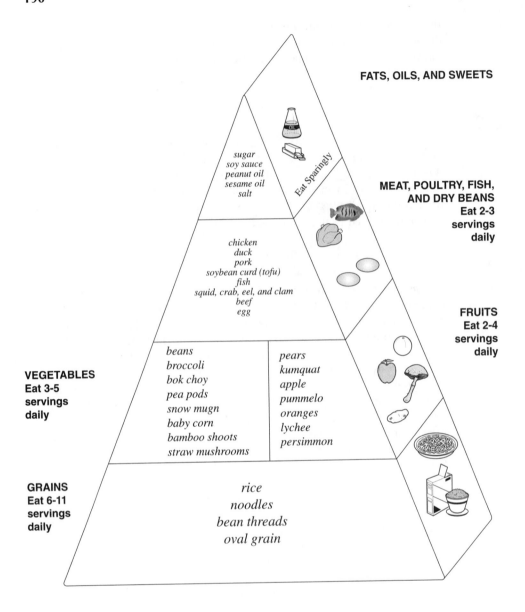

FIGURE 4–1   Food guide pyramid for popular Chinese foods.
Source: Author interpretation of a traditional Chinese food pyramid.
*Note: Dairy products are not a part of the traditional Chinese diet.

4. Consume appropriate amounts of fish, poultry, eggs, and lean meat. Reduce fatty meat and animal fat in the diet.
5. Balance food intake with physical activity to maintain a healthy body weight.
6. Choose a light diet that is also low in salt.
7. If you drink alcoholic beverages, do so in limited amounts.
8. Avoid unsanitary and spoiled foods.

Info Line

> A publication entitled *The Recommendations for Particular Groups of People* contains guidelines for all groups across the life cycle and presents daily food recommendations in the form of a pagoda.[35] Additional information includes:
>
> - daily requirements
> - varied menus by exchanging food items within each level of the pagoda
> - wise distribution of the daily food intake among the 3 meals
> - use of local foods
> - making a lifetime commitment to the recommended principles

Japanese

Japanese immigration to the United States began after 1890. Basic beliefs and practices include a strong sense of family and community commitment, suppression of emotions, visibility of politeness and respect, and care of elders.[29,36] Japanese food preparation is unique, but it includes the traditional *yin* and *yang* concepts. Identification of all ingredients in meals and visual pleasure are most important. Basic foods are soybeans, rice, and tea. Sushi is an English word that means rice together with toppings. Teriyaki sauce is comprised of soy sauce and a sweet rice wine called mirin. Seaweed and algae are common and used as either seasoning or made into a wrapping.[29]

Meals have a distinct composition with a traditional pattern of 3 meals plus a snack called an *oyatsu*; breakfast consists of a salty sour plum, rice soup and pickled vegetables; lunch often includes rice and leftovers from the night before; dinner consists of rice, soup, a main dish of fish or shellfish, and pickled vegetables (*tsukemono*). Sweets, rice crackers, and fruit comprise the snacks; sweet bean jelly and dumplings are common.[29] Japanese believe that certain foods have harmful or beneficial effects. For example, they believe that cherries and milk cause illness; they use hot tea and pickled plums therapeutically to alleviate constipation.

Even though traditional Japanese foods are low in fat and cholesterol, increased incidence of several chronic diseases have signified the impact of Western food fare on coronary heart disease (CHD) and cancer mortality rates. Japanese experienced a progressive increase in CHD mortality and colon cancer as they migrated to Hawaii and then to the United States, primarily the San Francisco area. High sodium intakes, low red meat and iron intakes, and insufficient calcium intakes are common among older persons. Lactose intolerance is frequent.[37]

Southeast Asians

Large numbers of individuals from the Philippines, Vietnam, Cambodia, and Laos have immigrated to the United States. Many "boat people" arrived in the United States, fleeing from political conflicts and wars in their countries. They arrived with no material or financial resources. Vietnamese live primarily in urban areas in extended families; Cambodian and Laotian refugees are often dependent on US government services until they obtain employment. All groups have a high regard for family, respect elders, and rely on families for support.[38]

Traditional food habits include rice, soybeans, and tea as staples, and rich desserts (e.g., cream-filled French pastries or custard flan). Filipino food preparation is based on 3 principles: (1) do not cook any food alone; (2) use garlic in olive oil or lard to fry foods; and (3) prepare foods with a sour-cool taste. The French introduced many ingredients and foods into the Southeast Asian food pattern that have remained: strong coffee, asparagus, French bread, meat pâtés, and pastries. A Chinese influence is noted in the use of chopsticks, stir-frying, individually served foods, long-grain rice, and *yin-yang* concepts. A fermented fish paste or sauce is substituted for salt throughout Southeast Asia. Coconut is a common food in the Pacific Islands. Soy milk, tofu, uncooked vegetables, fish, shellfish, pork, and fresh herbs and spices including basil, ginger, mint, and lemon are common in Vietnamese foods.

Filipinos enjoy 3 meals and 2 snack breaks with fritters, sweets, or an egg roll. Vietnamese likewise eat 3 meals with an optional snack. A traditional Vietnamese breakfast is a soup with noodles, and perhaps an egg or pickled vegetables on French bread. Lunch and dinner are composed of a soup, rice, fish/meat, and a vegetable. Coffee with sugar and condensed milk is common. Holidays in the Philippines involve midnight suppers, holiday fiestas, parties, and celebrations, with food central to the event.[29]

Folklore regarding foods is common in the Philippines; Vietnamese believe that eating organ meats benefits that organ. Lifestyle changes have occurred as the immigrants have become westernized. Health screening identifies diabetes mellitus, gout, and hypochromic microcytic anemia among Filipinos. Low-birth-weight infants and poor maternal weight gain are noted among Vietnamese.[39]

When counseling individuals from these ethnic groups, it is important to understand that they do not use direct eye contact unless to express anger or sexuality. Relatives are important to the success of rehabilitation, treatment, or dietary behavior change. Social harmony is important, yet grouping all Southeast Asians into 1 room or 1 interview area may be unproductive and offend the individuals.

Major Immigrant Populations

Jews

There are approximately 6 million Jews residing in the United States, with most coming to the United States for an improved lifestyle and to escape war and persecution. Having emigrated from all over the world, distinct food traditions exist. Two broad groups of Jews are Ashkenazic Jews, from central and eastern European countries such as Russia, Germany, Poland, and Romania, and from South Africa. The second group is composed of Sephardic Jews originally from Spain and Portugal. Most large Jewish populations reside in New York, Los Angeles, Chicago, Atlanta, and Boston.

Three subgroups of religious practice within Judaism are orthodox, conservative, and reform. Orthodox Jews usually observe the Jewish dietary laws, whereas conservatives may not; reform Jews are the least likely to follow them. Jewish dietary laws called *kashrut* and holiday traditions cross all subgroups. Jewish foods such as bagels with cream cheese, rye bread, corned beef, and pastrami are popular Ashkenazic foods for Americans of many ethnic backgrounds. The Jewish dietary laws prescribe foods for the soul and are viewed as divine commandments, possibly avoiding gluttony, protecting unity of beliefs at marriage, and promoting a spiritual and hygienic quality.[40]

The word *kosher* means fit, proper, or in accordance with the religious law and criteria.[41] The word *trefe* refers to foods that are ritually unfit.[42] The most widely accepted kosher symbol is Ⓤ, designating approval by the Union of Orthodox Jewish Congregations of America, and it designates supervision of a *mashigiach*, someone who oversees the *kashrut* procedures. The letter *K* is also used to denote kosher foods but rabbinical supervision is not required, thus the symbol is not valid.

The basic rules of *kashrut,* or keeping kosher, are the Jewish dietary principles set forth in the Torah, the Jewish book of written laws, which encompass the 5 books of Moses. Several misconceptions exist about keeping kosher, such as[43]:

Myth: All Jews abide by the Jewish dietary law. In fact, this varies.
Myth: Only a few Jews really practice all the rules of keeping kosher. Some individuals may not restrict their foods, others may avoid pork and shellfish products, and others may never eat meals any place other than their home. Someone brought up in a strictly kosher home may choose not to keep a traditional kosher kitchen, instead that person may eat pork and shellfish but not mix milk with meat either in preparation or at a single meal.
Myth: The laws of *kashrut* are an ancient health measure. The truth is that pork products are not consumed because dietary laws only allow Jews to eat animals that both chew their cud and have cloven hooves, such as cows, sheep, and lambs.

Holiday and Ritual Food Customs and Celebrations   The Jewish religion has a long history of table- and family-centered holiday celebrations with foods symbolic to that occasion, such as bar mitzvahs and weddings. For example:

- *Sabbath* is the most important day of the week. It begins at sundown on Friday and ends on Saturday at sundown. For those who strictly observe the sabbath, there is a total abstinence from any labor, including cooking or reheating food. Food is often left on a warm burner during the Sabbath and is eaten at Saturday's noon meal after attending synagogue. Jewish housewives in Europe developed a stew called *cholent* that was prepared on Friday and left on a low heat on the stove. Traditionally, Friday evening's meal is a special one where the Sabbath bread, *hallah*, is served, often with roasted chicken as the entrée. Ashkenazis Jews eat a chicken soup with matzoh *knaidlach*, potato or noodle *kugel*, often called *lokshen kugel*.
- *Rosh Hashanah*, a high holy day each fall, marks the beginning of the Jewish new year and includes a sweet on the holiday table. Honey, raisins, carrots, and apples represent optimism and a sweet future.

- *Yom Kippur* is observed 8 days following Rosh Hashanah. It is the day of atonement, asking God's forgiveness for sins. A festive meal of bland foods is usually served on the eve of the holiday to prevent excessive thirst while fasting. Fasting begins at sundown on the eve of the holiday and ends at sundown the next day. At sunset of Yom Kippur, families and friends gather to break the fast with a brunch, serving a dairy-based meal. For Ashkenazic Jews, this meal typically contains bagels, noodle kugel, eggs, smoked salmon and other smoked fish, herring, fruits, and light cakes.
- *Sukkot* marks the gathering of the harvest and the commencement of autumn. Often a little booth or hut (called a sukka) is built in the back-yard with a roof made of thatched straw and containing hanging fruits.
- *Hanukkah*, the festival of lights, is celebrated in early to late December when potato latkes, potato kugel, and a wide variety of sweets are served.
- *Passover*, or Pesach, is a very significant holiday in the Jewish religion, lasting 8 days and marking the exodus from Egypt and the release of the Jews from bondage. During Passover, no leavened products are eaten, which is why matzoh, the unleavened bread, is served to symbolize the bread eaten by Jews who fled Egypt. The first 2 nights of Passover are the most significant and are observed with a festive meal, or *seder* (meaning order), and the story of the exodus from Egypt. Many foods are consumed: for example, Ashkenazic Jews include gefilte fish, matzoh balls with chicken soup, chopped liver, matzoh stuffing, poultry, and *tzimmes*.

Limited epidemiologic data identify Jews with diabetes. Jewish law or the kashrut accepts that medical conditions such as diabetes may warrant excep-tion to the observance of dietary law. For example, individuals with insulin-dependent diabetes mellitus are not expected to fast on Yom Kippur. A rabbi or other religious counselor should be consulted if individuals have questions about food restrictions for their health condition.[43]

East Indian Ethnic and Regional Food Practices

India and Pakistan are part of the Asian subcontinent. They become separate countries in 1947. Bangladesh, which was part of Pakistan, became indepen-dent in 1971. The 3 countries share some similarities in food practices.[44]

The terms *Asian Indian* and *Pakistani*, designated by the US Census Bureau in 1980, represent varied religions and differences in eating prac-tices. Indian immigrants come from a country that is 83% Hindu, 11% Muslim, 2% Christian, 2% Sikh, 0.7% Buddhist, 0.5% Jain, and about 0.4% other, including Parsi and Jewish (1981 Indian census), reflecting about 850 languages and dialects. The official language of India is Hindi, but English is widely taught and spoken. Pakistani immigrants come from a number of cultural groups, each with its own language or dialect, but Urdu is the offi-cial language and English is widely spoken. Most Pakistanis are Muslims, and a small percentage are Christian, Parsi, or Hindu.[44,45]

These ethnic groups are among the fastest growing in the United States, i.e., Indians compose 11% of the US Asian/Pacific Islander population and are the fourth largest component after the Chinese, Filipino, and Japanese. The Pakistani community is small but increasing. Both groups are relatively young, literate communities consisting of academicians, technical professionals, individuals who own or work in commercial establishments such as retail stores, restaurants, movie houses, and insurance and travel agencies, students pursuing higher education, and their dependents (spouses, children, parents, and siblings).[46]

East Indian immigrants to the United States between 1820 and 1920 were mainly agrarian Sikhs. As immigration and naturalization laws were liberalized through the mid-1950s for students pursuing higher studies, many chose to stay while others returned to their homeland. The Immigration Act of 1965 enabled the Indian and Pakistani populations to grow dramatically. The 1990 census reports 815,447 Indians and 81,000 Pakistanis. The year 2000 US Census lists 1,678,765 for the total Asian Indian population. Thirty-five percent of Indians live in the Northeast, followed by 24% in the South, 23% in the West, and 18% in the Midwest. A similar distribution pattern is noted for the Pakistani community, with most having settled in the Chicago, Houston, Los Angeles, and Washington, DC, areas.[44,46]

The holy Vedic scriptures (believed by Hindus to be ageless) categorize commonly used foods and emphasize the connection between foods, moods, fitness, and longevity (*Bhagavad Gita.* 17th chapter; verses 2–22). Foods are divided into 3 major categories, depending on the kind of mind-altering, mood-provoking, and physiologic influences they are believed to exert. *Sattvic* foods, like milk and milk products (except cheese made from rennet), rice, wheat, *ghee,* most legumes, and some other vegetables, are believed to contribute to the making of a person who is serene, enlightened, healthy, and long lived. Calling a person "sattvic" is a high tribute. *Rajasic* foods, like some meats, eggs, and foods that are very bitter, sour, salty, rich, and spicy, are believed to contribute to aggression, acquisitiveness, passion, and a desire for power. Warriors were encouraged to eat these foods. *Tamasic* foods, like garlic and pickled, preserved, stale, or rotten foods and alcohol and drugs used for pleasure and in excess, are believed to contribute to lust, malice, confusion, slothfulness, and dullness.[44]

Health-related Hindu customs include yoga, a word that means "to rein in," "harness," or "tune the body," which consists of structured physical exercise and body positions best suited as a morning workout; mental exercises and meditation, reputed to reenergize from daily stresses; and controlled leisure activities (the tenet of simple living–high thinking is held in high esteem).

The classical system of Indian medicine called *Ayurveda* (the Code of Life and Longevity) is used widely during illness and is based on the belief that humors in the body and in foods can interact to preserve a homeostatic harmony or cause imbalance.[44] Ayurvedic remedies, listed next, are prescribed for various ailments, including colds, coughs, constipation, and stomach pains.

- *Kapha* foods include white sugar, millet, and buttermilk, and are thought to be heavy, dense, and mucus-producing, and are to be avoided by those with respiratory ailments.
- *Vata* or *vayu,* translated as the "wind" or gas-producing foods, like some legumes, are thought to be unpredictable and are to be avoided during states of distention.
- Hot or *ushna* foods include black gram or mung bean, cowpea, ripe eggplant, and papaya, and are believed to promote digestion.

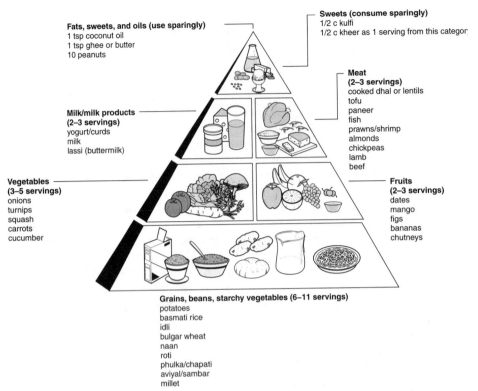

Sweets (consume sparingly)
1/2 c kulfi
1/2 c kheer as 1 serving from this categor;

Fats, sweets, and oils (use sparingly)
1 tsp coconut oil
1 tsp ghee or butter
10 peanuts

Meat
(2–3 servings)
cooked dhal or lentils
tofu
paneer
fish
prawns/shrimp
almonds
chickpeas
lamb
beef

Milk/milk products
(2–3 servings)
yogurt/curds
milk
lassi (buttermilk)

Vegetables
(3–5 servings)
onions
turnips
squash
carrots
cucumber

Fruits
(2–3 servings)
dates
mango
figs
bananas
chutneys

Grains, beans, starchy vegetables (6–11 servings)
potatoes
basmati rice
idli
bulgar wheat
naan
roti
phulka/chapati
aviyal/sambar
millet

FIGURE 4–2 Indian and Pakistani food guide pyramid. The pyramid is helpful when counseling individual clients or groups with diabetes, hypertension, or obesity. *Source:* Author interpretation of a typical Indian/Pakistani food pyramid.

- Cool or *seeta* foods are thought to impart strength and nourishment and include cereals, rice, wheat, mung beans, kidney beans, most fruits and vegetables, milk from most animals except goats, butter, and *ghee.*

Traditional beliefs firmly advocate moderation even when eating the proper foods.[44] See Figure 4–2. Obesity is disfavored and laws of food consumption dictate that solid food should fill half the stomach, liquid one fourth, and the remainder left empty for smooth digestion.[44]

In the United States, diabetes prevalence data for Indians and Pakistanis are scarce, but estimates are that the risk of diabetes is greater than 50% for all minority groups.[44] One study of 153 Indian immigrants found a high genetic predisposition to diabetes in 15% of families, possibly due to increased caloric intake and inadequate exercise patterns. A different study of 62 Indian vegetarians showed a tendency for glucose intolerance. Indian vegetarians in the United States may be at high risk for type 2 diabetes mellitus. A common underlying thread appears to be the interplay of genetics with dietary and lifestyle changes.[44]

Potential Medicinal Effects of Asian Indian Spices and Herbs Several Asian Indian spices and herbs, listed below, are thought to have a physiologic effect in the body.[47]

Tips for Healthy Meal Planning

- Eat meals and snacks at regular times every day.
- Eat about the same amount of food every day.

- Try not to skip meals.
- If you want to lose weight, cut down on your portion sizes.

Fats and oils	Sweets
• Eat less fat and saturated fat. Saturated fat is found in foods like ghee, coconut, coconut milk, and meats. Limit coconut based dishes; use coconut as a garnish. • Limit fried condiments like pappads, chips, or pickles. • Add less fat to starch dishes.	• Choose sweets less often. When you do eat sweets, make them a part of your healthy diet, not extras. • Add less or no sugar while cooking. • Limit fried sweets like jamun, milk sweets, sweets with fruit and nuts like halwas, and the use of honey and jaggery. **Alcohol** • If you choose to drink alcohol, limit the amount and have it with a meal. Check with your health care professional about a safe amount for you.
Milk	**Meat and others**
• Choose fat-free or low-fat milk, yogurt, cheese, and buttermilk. • Yogurt has natural sugar and may have added sugar. • When making desserts with milk or yogurt, use sugar substitutes as directed, or less sugar. • Reduced milk desserts like khoa, rasmalai, peda, or kheer contain sugar. Limit these dishes, their portion sizes, and fats used in preparation. • Use low-fat milk to make paneer.	• Select lean cuts and trim visible fat. Use skinless poultry and fish more often. • Steam or broil rather than deep-fat fry: limit oil when stir-frying. • Use spices rather than fats to season dishes. • Add less malai or creams to cooked dishes. • Use dhals and legume dishes like rajma often. Limit fried legume dishes like vada or fried channa dhal. • Count the meat added to mixed dishes, for example, in mutton biriyani.
Vegetables	**Fruits**
• Use nonstarchy vegetables more often. Choose leafy green and deep yellow vegetables like broccoli, spinach, and carrots. • Increase vegetable portion sizes and use less sauce, fat, and salt. • Use limited oil for seasoning. • Limit the use of preserved vegetables. Be aware of the oil and salt content of pickled vegetables. • Use brinjal, okra, karela, or moong bean sprouts to make stir-fried curries, using less oil and salt for seasoning. • Eat deep-fried vegetables such as bhajjis less often.	• Eat fruit instead of drinking juices. Eat only one serving of fruit at a time. • Choose fruit rather than traditional sweets like khulti, kheer, or rasmalai. Eat fewer dried fruits like dates. • Limit sugared fruits such as aam pappad, honeyed jackfruit, banana chips, and sugared dried ginger.

Grains, beans, starchy vegetables
- Choose whole grains such as whole-wheat flour (for rotis), bran cereals, and brown rice (basmati or plain). Use steamed rice instead of fried pulao or biriyani.
- Use dhals and legumes like rajma, loor dhal, and moong dhal. They are good sources of fiber.
- Choose phulka or idli instead of high-fat starches like paratha or dosa.
- Pita bread can be used like phulaka. Count the fat in high-fat starches like dosa, paratha, and puri as part of your meal plan. Use less fat when preparing dhansak, dhokla, matki usal, and poha.
- Limit fried snacks like chivda or ghatia; instead, use fresh vegetables or dry roasted chickpeas.

Special Considerations for Indian and Pakistani Clients

- Try not to skip meals, If you observe fasts, eat nutritious meals before and after the fast. Consult your physician before fasting, especially if you take medicines to control diabetes. If you do fast, drink less coffee and tea before the fast.

- if you are vegetarian, try to include foods rich in vitamin B12 (like fat-free or low-fat milk). Unless well planned, a vegetarian diet can be high in fat, salt, and sugar and low in fiber.

- Encourage your family to drink water instead of juice with meals.

FIGURE 4–2 continued

- *Fenugreek*—mixture of ground nuts, spices, brown sugar, and ghee (clarified butter). It is often made into a ladoo (round ball) or a brownie. It tastes sweet and provides needed energy along with other health benefits.
- *Asafoetida (heeng)*—may contain sulfur compounds in its volatile oil, which may protect against fat-induced hyperlipidemia. It may contain coumarin constituents with anticoagulant activity.
- *Capsicum, clove, ginger, and onion*—these herbs commonly used in Indian cooking have anticoagulant/antiplatelet potential.

- *Coriander*—a rich source of vitamin C, calcium, magnesium, potassium, and iron. In animals, coriander has shown hypoglycemic activity.
- *Cumin*—may have hypoglycemic effects.
- *Garlic*—has been shown to improve blood glucose control. Active ingredients allicin (diallyl disulfide oxide) and allyl propyl disulphide are hypoglycemic. Researchers have noted that garlic use may be associated with increased serum insulin and improved liver glycogen storage.

Translating Nutrition Materials

Literal translation of nutrition materials does not work. For example, the Spanish-speaking population in the United States includes at least 7 Hispanic/Latino subgroups. It is ideal to adapt/test to a neutral, simple, and grammatically correct language that can be understood by the subgroups of the region.

Once a publication has been adapted to the comprehensive language, it should be tested with focus groups to ensure that the text does not contain inappropriate language or insulting expressions. To provide effective nutrition education to different ethnic groups, consider assessing their current food purchasing and preparation procedures. Use of a rapid assessment tool (see Appendix 4–A) can form the basis for understanding how the group is currently making food choices and how westernized its members have become.

Nutrition and HIV Infection

A new challenge facing nutrition professionals is the need to understand and work effectively with the growing population of people with HIV infection. These high-need men and women reside in many US towns and cities. Many need nutritional counseling to maintain their health and well-being.[48]

> The enormous burden of grief and loss that AIDS will impose on our society has yet to be felt fully, and the work in care, prevention, and research must be not merely sustained but accelerated just to keep pace. . . . The human immunodeficiency virus (HIV) has profoundly changed life on our planet. America has not done well in acknowledging this fact or in mobilizing its vast resources to address it appropriately. Many are suffering profoundly because of that failure, and America is poorer because of this neglect.[48]

The clinical course of HIV infection in adults varies greatly from one individual to the next. Usually, there is a sudden onset of a mononucleosis-like syndrome. The onset is about 1-2 weeks in length and relates to the seroconversion process. Referred to as a *primary* HIV infection, the condition occurs between 2 and 4 weeks after exposure and may include various neurologic, dermatologic, and other pathophysiologic problems.[49] The next period is asymptomatic and may include a persistent, generalized lymphadenopathy. This stage is often followed by the early manifestations of HIV infection, which include fatigue, seborrhea, eczema, fevers, diarrhea, muscle pain, night sweats, weight loss, oral candidiasis, herpes zoster, and other opportunistic infections. None of these conditions are life threatening. The cluster of these signs and symptoms is referred to as AIDS-related complex (ARC) and is the antecedent of AIDS.

TABLE 4–3 Classification System for HIV Infection and Expanded AIDS Surveillance Case Definition for Adolescents and Adults*

CD4+ Cell Categories	Clinical Categories		
	A Asymptomatic or PGL**	B Symptomatic, Not A or C Conditions	C AIDS-Indicator Conditions
1. ≥ 500/mm³	A1	B1	C1
2. 200-499/mm³	A2	B2	C2
3. < 200/mm³	A2	B3	C3

*Persons in Category C are reportable to every health department. Individuals in Categories C1/C2/C3/ A3/B3 are reportable as AIDS cases in the United States and its territories.
**PGL = persistent generalized lymphadenopathy. Category A includes acute (primary) HIV infection.
Source: Reprinted from *HIV Classifications.* Atlanta, Ga: Centers for Disease Control and Prevention; 1992.

The Centers for Disease Control and Prevention (CDC) has developed a classification system for HIV infection and AIDS surveillance among adolescents and adults[50] (see Table 4–3). The adult and adolescent case definitions for AIDS for surveillance purposes is found in Appendix 4–C. The cumulative number of cases by age and other demographic data are outlined in Appendix 4–D.

Considerations for HIV-Infected Pediatric Patients

In 1997, HIV infection was the 11th leading cause of death in the United States among children 1 to 4 years of age.[51] HIV infection remains a leading cause of death among persons 25 to 44 years old, particularly among blacks and Hispanics. More than 16,000 perinatally HIV-infected children have been born since the beginning of the epidemic in the United States.[52] Perinatal transmission of HIV accounts for 90% of pediatric AIDS cases and almost all new HIV infections in children.[53] Worldwide, a total of 1.1 million children are estimated to be living with HIV infection, almost 90% living in sub-Saharan Africa and the developing countries of Asia.[54] Considerable advances have been made in the understanding of the pathogenesis, diagnosis, treatment, monitoring, and prevention of HIV in the United States. The 1994 Pediatric AIDS Clinical Trials Group (PACTG) protocol 076 demonstrated that zidovudine (ZDV) therapy administered to selected HIV-infected pregnant women and their newborn infants reduced the rate of perinatal HIV transmission from 25 to 8% and was the first major prevention breakthrough in the HIV epidemic.[55,56]

Malnutrition, growth failure and weight loss are still significant and common problems for children with HIV infection.[57,58] As reported by the Centers for Disease Control (CDC), weight loss and muscle wasting remain significant clinical problems even in the era of potent antiretroviral therapy.[59] It is well documented that nutritional status is predictive of survival and functional status during the course of HIV infection.[60-62] Moreover, the nutritional implications of HIV infection for children are often more devastating than for adults because children have the added nutritional demands of growth and development. Common problems for HIV-infected children include poor weight gain, failure to thrive, slowed linear growth, growth stunting, malnutrition, and wasting.[63] Compromised nutrition increases the risk of infection and prolongs the recovery from acute illness.

Early identification of nutritional problems is vital to successful prevention and treatment. Screening for nutritional status by a dietitian is a strategic part of an early intervention effort to prevent the loss of crucial body tissue, especially since crucial body tissue, such as lean body mass, is where the metabolism of nutrients and medications occur. In addition to nutrition education for symptom management due to opportunistic infections, many HIV-infected children also require care for comorbidities such as renal disease, hyperlipidemia, pancreatic dysfunction, liver disease, encephalopathy, and others. Nutrition interventions are specific for HIV-infected children and should be individualized. With a skilled and comprehensive medical team that includes a dietitian, such interventions can maintain optimal nutritional status.

HIV infection in infants and children may result in children who are asymptomatic or critically ill. Most children experience lymphadenopathy, hepatosplenomegaly, oral candidiasis, low birth weight, failure to thrive, weight loss, diarrhea, chronic eczematoid dermatitis, or fever.[64] Serious bacterial infections with *Streptococcus* pneumonia, *Hemophilus* influenza, salmonella, and other organisms are common manifestations of AIDS.

Many HIV-infected children are more susceptible to various opportunistic and pathogenic microorganisms because they never developed appropriate immunity prior to infection. A majority are partially affected by a common encephalopathy that causes developmental delay or reduced motor and intellectual function.[64] Lymphocytic interstitial pneumonitis is rare in adults, but common in children; the reverse is true of Kaposi's sarcoma and HIV-associated lymphomas.[50]

Some infants are born with passively acquired antibodies from their HIV-infected mothers.[65] Conventional tests cannot detect the difference between passively acquired antibodies and those that have been endogenously produced. A diagnosis for HIV infection in very young children should include direct identification of live virus, HIV-specific nucleic acids, or HIV-specific antigens.[65]

Nutritional Risk of HIV-positive Children

Heller et al developed a simple and effective instrument to evaluate and monitor the nutritional risk of children infected with the human immunodeficiency virus. Consultants who included 5 physicians, 5 nutritionists, and 5 social workers with expertise in caring for HIV-infected children plus a medical record review provided 19 sociodemographic, 10 anthropometric, 4 biochemical, 6 dietary intake, and 19 medical variables of potential inclusion.[66]

To evaluate the instrument, anthropometric data were obtained on 39 HIV-infected children. The caregiver was asked to complete a 3-day diet record. The most recent CD4+ T-cell numbers and serum HIV p24 antigen and plasma HIV-RNA levels were included.

The severity or degree of potential nutritional risk based on anthropometric, biochemical, dietary intake, and medical data was established using 0-4 where 0 indicated low risk and values were summed across categories.

Info Line

HIV DISTANCE LEARNING TECHNOLOGY AIDS SERVICE

Given adequate support, AIDS prevention programs effective in research settings can be adapted to developing countries. Popular leaders in one community can educate other communities about avoiding the disease. Researchers from the Medical College of Wisconsin have tested whether distance learning techniques using computers and CD-based interactive programs could reach and teach people from remote locations. A popular opinion leader model was used for dissemination to adapt across cultures and use the power of a community for protection from AIDS. A group of leading nongovernmental organizations (NGOs) worked in AIDS prevention in 78 countries. Countries in Africa and those of the former Soviet Union in Eastern Europe, and Central Asia, Latin America, and Caribbean countries were divided into either an experimental group or a control group.

- The control group attended an orientation meeting and the members were given a computer, Internet service, and access to a study Web site to network with other NGOs, and they received information about grant writing, program evaluation, needs assessment, and organizational management.
- The experimental group received the same supports plus a self-paced 3-4 week curriculum on CD to train staff on how to implement the program. Each was paired with a behavioral science consultant to adapt and tailor the model.

In-depth follow-up telephone interviews 15 months later showed that 43% of organizations with distance training had developed new programs versus only 17% of the control group. Fifty-five percent of the experimental group incorporated the intervention into existing programs whereas 27% of control organizations did such.

Sources: Medical College of Wisconsin. *Medical News.* September 23, 2004: 1-3; Jeffrey. Distance communication: transfer of HIV prevention interventions to service providers. *Science.* September 24, 2004;305(5692):1953-1955.

Reliability of internal consistency and validity were determined. Pearson product moment correlations were calculated for 6 selected dependent variables: weight-for-height, weight-growth velocity, lean body mass, serum albumin level, CD4+ T-cell numbers, and quantitative plasma HIV-RNA levels.

Thirty-eight variables were analyzed for their reliability. Those found to be reliable indicators of nutritional risk were height-for-age, weight-for-age, clinical class, somatic protein stores, mid-arm circumference, weight-for-height, serum albumin, immunologic status, body mass index, energy intake, and opportunistic infection. The 8 weakest predictors not used in the final instrument were zinc level, splenomegaly, protein intake, time spent eating, sweets intake, consumption of multivitamin, HIV-RNA level, and consumption of nutrition supplements.[66]

Info Line

BREAST MILK TREATMENT

HIV is heat sensitive and is inactivated by pasteurization at temperatures between 56 and 62°C.[67] Breast milk banks in developed countries use expensive, thermostatically controlled pasteurizing equipment that is not available in resource-poor settings. A low-cost, low-tech method, the Pretoria pasteurization method, makes use of passive heat transfer from water that has been heated to a boiling point, to milk that is contained in a glass jar standing in the water. The woman expresses her milk into a clean glass jar, which is then placed into a 1-L aluminium cooking pot. Water is boiled by any method and when it is boiling vigorously, the hot water is poured into the cooking pot in which the jar of milk is standing. The jar and milk are left to stand in the hot water until the water is a comfortable temperature, approximately 25 minutes. The final temperature reached by the milk and the duration for which it remains at that temperature are dependent on the volume of boiling water and the sizes and materials of the milk and water containers. Using water at boiling point has the advantage that it can be achieved every time without the need for a thermometer or thermostat. Several sets of apparatus were investigated and the glass jar and aluminum pot were found to provide the best results. The desired temperature range is between 56 and 62°C, as this will maintain a large proportion of the secretory IgA within the milk.[68] The method was tested and found to be reliable under a wide range of conditions.[69]

The Pretoria pasteurization method has been shown to reliably inactivate HIV in the milk of HIV-infected women.[70] The experience from these studies suggests that both exclusive formula feeding (EFF) and exclusive breast feeding (EBF) are acceptable and feasible options to HIV-positive women to reduce mother-to-child transmission (MTCT) of HIV. The decision-making process and the ability to achieve these depend on the personal motivation of the HIV-infected women, the support of partners and close family, and the practical support of healthcare staff.[70]

Nutrition Concepts and HIV

Data derived from experimental studies regarding the role of nutrition in HIV infection and AIDS is limited but increasing. The involuntary weight loss or wasting indicative of severe protein–energy malnutrition observed in many patients with HIV infection demands nutritional care.[71] Nutrition and specific nutrients play an intimate and inextricable role in immunocompetence.[72] For many diseases, the nutritional status of the individual will have an impact on morbidity and mortality, irrespective of the disease process.[73,74]

Several questions remain unanswered regarding the relationship between nutrition and HIV disease, including:

- What is the impact of nutritional status or specific nutrients on the progression of the HIV infection?
- What is the impact of the HIV and subsequent infections and/or neoplasms on general or specific nutritional needs?

- What are the potential iatrogenic effects of current treatments on nutritional status?

Community nutrition health workers must recognize the importance of a conceptual framework based on an understanding of fundamental concepts of nutrition and nutritional assessment in order to address these issues and to develop effective secondary and tertiary prevention programs.

To interpret studies relating nutrition to any disease, including HIV infection, it is necessary to use appropriate nutritional assessment methodologies to identify the stage of a nutritional deficiency.[75] A deficiency may progress from manifestations such as weight loss or lethargy, to specific biochemical and anatomic lesions and eventual death. In HIV, clinical assessments should progress from general, nonspecific, sensitive indicators of overall nutrient intake and nutritional status to specific, sensitive biochemical measures. Further, the method should document if the result reflects immediate food intake or long-term eating status. Interpretation of the biochemical assessment must address dietary intake, dietary supplements, and drug use (both recreational and therapeutic).

Some research studies focus only on very ill AIDS patients, while other studies include patients who are HIV positive and asymptomatic or patients who have AIDS. The physiology, immunocompetence, and nutritional status of patients who are HIV positive and asymptomatic vary greatly from those with terminal stages of AIDS. Generalizations should not be made about changes observed in AIDS patients or the application of treatment to all HIV-positive patients.

In addition, most published studies have examined adult males with AIDS; about one third of the studies are from peer-reviewed, refereed scientific journals. Studies are rarely prospective and tend to have inadequate sample sizes and inappropriate control groups. Many reported studies are preliminary abstracts or letters to the editor, reflect small samples, and are observational rather than investigative.

Wasting is a major cause of morbidity and mortality in people with AIDS.[76-78] To understand the wasting process, it is important to understand the mismatch between energy intake and total energy expenditure, as well as the processes that accelerate negative nitrogen balance or protein wasting. In both the absence of disease and in AIDS, starvation leads to death when body weight is 66% of ideal.[77,79-82] Studies suggest that it is the degree of wasting rather than its specific cause that leads to death. Thus,

Info Line

The word AIDS is popular but not the preferred description. HIV infection defines the problem and leadership must focus on the full course of HIV infection rather than concentrating on the later stages like ARC and AIDS. A lack of focus on the entire spectrum of HIV infection has left our nation unable to deal adequately with the epidemic.

Source: Report of the Presidential Commission on Human Immunodeficient Virus Epidemic; 1988.

theoretically, therapies that maintain body cell mass could prolong life. Many studies document that even after AIDS-related illnesses begin, wasting is not inevitable. This finding suggests that wasting is not a component of immunodeficiency.[76,83-86] AIDS differs from simple starvation in that the metabolic disturbances prevent nitrogen sparing and allow adipose tissue conservation.[76,81,82,87] Body cell mass may be lost, but there may be minimal body fat loss.[76,77]

The host response to infection appears to cause the changes in metabolism. It is now generally accepted that cytokines mediate the host immune response and metabolic changes.[88-93] Each metabolic disturbance must be considered in the context of total energy balance.[94-98] Animals that eat more to compensate for metabolic disturbances maintain weight, whereas animals that do not lose weight.[99]

Numerous studies suggest that synergistic interactions between cytokines may be necessary for the wasting syndrome to develop.[100] Plasma triglyceride concentrations are very high in patients with AIDS and slightly elevated in HIV-positive individuals compared with controls,[83,101] and they may persist for a long time without substantial wasting.[83]

In one study, increased levels of cachectin factor (tumor necrosis factor) were reported for patients with AIDS.[102] It has been proposed that tumor necrosis factor is responsible for the cachexia of AIDS.[102-104] Numerous follow-up studies have uncovered no significant differences in tumor necrosis factor levels between patients with AIDS and appropriate controls.[85,101,105-107]

Patients with AIDS have persistently high serum levels of interferon alfa.[106] In AIDS, triglyceride levels correlate positively with circulating levels of interferon alfa.[101,106,108] There is an even stronger correlation between levels of interferon alfa and both the decrease in triglyceride clearance and the increase in hepatic synthesis of fatty acids while fasting.[101]

AIDS and Energy Balance

To maintain weight, total energy expenditure must equal food energy (caloric) intake. Total energy expenditure equals resting energy expenditure plus dietary thermogenesis plus energy expenditure in activity. If energy intake exceeds total energy expenditure, the excess calories are stored as either body cell mass or fat. On the other hand, if total energy expenditure exceeds the energy absorbed, an energy deficit results. This promotes the breakdown of protein or fat for use as energy. Energy deficiency can be due to a decrease in consumed or absorbed energy, an increase in total energy expenditure, or both. In AIDS, a malfunction may occur for each component of the energy-balance equation. To understand the wasting process in AIDS, both the metabolic disturbances due to HIV infection itself and those due to secondary infections must be analyzed.

In 1 study, the average weight of randomly selected patients with HIV infection or full-blown AIDS was stable in the absence of active secondary infections.[83] Patients with AIDS and active secondary infections had an average weight loss of 5% within 28 days.[86] Data suggest that accelerated protein breakdown and negative nitrogen balance occur in patients with AIDS who also have active secondary infections. Levels of interferon alfa are chronically elevated in AIDS. Tumor necrosis factor, interleukin-1, and related cytokines are thought to be activated during secondary infection. The synergy between these cytokines may mediate the accelerated weight loss.[85,86]

In industrialized countries, most patients with AIDS do not experience continuous wasting.[83-86] They experience stable weight interspersed with rapid wasting, which generally occurs during active secondary infections. In developing countries, such as those in Africa, treatment is usually not available for disease caused by indigenous pathogens or opportunistic infections. Wasting then becomes relentless, and AIDS is known as the "slim disease."[109]

Decreased physical activity may conserve body cell mass by countering the metabolic disturbance. Physical activity helps to maintain muscle mass. Inactivity and the stressful symptoms of an infection cause both a decrease in muscle mass and an inability to rebuild the muscle after a period of wasting.[110] HIV infection creates a series of metabolic disturbances, i.e., increased resting energy expenditure and decreased rate of protein synthesis. Secondary infection in the presence of cancer leads to anorexia. A limited food intake and an elevated resting energy expenditure create rapid weight loss and negative nitrogen balance. Debilitation and weight loss set the individual back after each weight loss episode. The result is progressive debilitation, along with increased morbidity and mortality.[101] Figure 4–3 outlines the flow of these processes.

In light of the unconventional diets and questionable information reaching HIV-positive individuals, the American and Canadian Dietetic Associations have taken a position, stating that nutrition intervention and education are essential components of complete care for individuals infected with HIV[111] (see Exhibit 4–4).

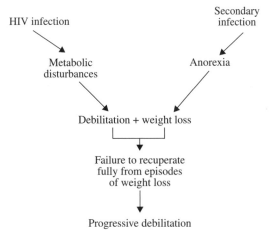

FIGURE 4–3 Debilitation and wasting in AIDS. Pathways of progressive debilitation and wasting are shown. In addition, primary HIV infection may lead to relative anorexia, and secondary infection may cause other metabolic disturbances. Malabsorption may also decrease the intake of nutrients.
Source: Reprinted from Grunfeld C, Feingold RR. Metabolic disturbances and wasting in the acquired immunodeficiency syndrome. *Semin Med.* 1992;327(5):334; Massachusetts Medical Society, with permission of the *N Engl J Med.*

Exhibit 4–4   Components of Nutrition Education of HIV-Infected Persons

- Healthful eating principles: what nutrients are important and why, use of vitamin/mineral supplements, frequency of eating
- Healthful eating plan: what to eat and recommended amounts
- Food-safety issues: food storage, food preparation, dining away from home
- Managing nutrition-related symptoms: how to deal with poor appetite, early satiety, nausea/vomiting, diarrhea, food intolerances, mouth sores, swallowing difficulties, and fever
- Alternative feeding methods: use of nutritional supplements, tube feeding, or parenteral nutrition support
- Guidelines for evaluating nutrition information and products: special diet plans, individual vitamin/mineral supplements, or other suggested nutrition practices

Source: Adapted from: James JS. *AIDS Treatment News-Issues.* 1989;1-75, with permission of the American Dietetic Association.

Info Line

A useful tool to measure the severity of an illness is the skinfold caliper, an instrument that measures skinfold thickness gathered from various parts of the body. Tricep skinfold is a useful measurement for the CNP. Combining it with midarm circumference and using a simple mathematical equation, the approximate muscle stores or lean body mass can be determined. Changes in body composition such as when assessing nutritional status change among children and adults with human immunodeficiency virus (HIV) are important.

The skinfold calipers provide a simple, noninvasive technique using only the caliper itself and a tape measure. The low-level technology operates without batteries and is relatively inexpensive and extremely mobile, posing no health risk to the patient or the CNP.[112]

A free training video is available from the Centers for Disease Control and Prevention, National Health and Nutrition Examination Survey III: Anthropometric. The video outlines procedures and provides demonstrations and explanations of various anthropometric measurements, including skinfold calipers. A web-based anthropometry course developed by Cade Fields-Gardner is free and available at www.nutritionclassroom.com.

Source: Heller L, Fox S, Hell KJ, Church JA. Tricep skinfold calipers for assessing nutritional risk. *J Am Diet Assoc.* 2000;100(3):329.

HUNGER

In November 1989, 23 experts met at the Rockefeller Foundation Conference Center in Bellagio, Italy, to address the problem of world hunger. They produced the Bellagio Declaration,[113] which identified methods to reduce world hunger by 50% by the year 2000.[113] That did not happen. Recent projections are that over 100% of the world population could be fed on a basic vegetarian

TABLE 4–4   The Estimated Number of Individuals Supported by the 1992 Global Food Supply

Food Pattern (2,350 kcal/day)	Billions of Individuals	Percentage of World Population
Basic:	6.3	115
Purely vegetarian cereals, fruits, roots, vegetables		
Improved:	4.2	77
15% of kcal from animal products		
Complete:	3.2	59
25% of kcal from animal products		

Source: Adapted from: Uvin P. The state of world hunger. *Nutr Rev.* 1994;52(5):151-161.

diet of 2,350 kcal/day, but improving the quality of the diet with animal food products would reduce the number of individuals receiving available foodstuffs worldwide[114] (see Table 4–4).

No single document defines the way to end hunger in the United States and also appeals to multiple contingencies. The 1990 Brown University World Hunger Conference suggested that US organizations concerned with domestic hunger create a domestic Bellagio declaration. The result was the Medford Declaration to End Hunger in the United States, written during a meeting at Tufts University in Medford, Massachusetts.[115]

Hunger in the United States is serious, but remediable. In the 1970s, the United States mobilized bipartisan support to address hunger.[116] Programs reduced the problem, but hunger returned and remains a widespread phenomenon. The Medford Declaration described the economic costs and simple unacceptability of domestic hunger and how this problem could be ended. Estimates are that 5 million US children from birth to 12 years of age are hungry, and 6 million are at risk. Approximately 25 million adults experience hunger. Using medium-range estimates and 3 methods, projected hunger estimates among Americans are as follows[116,117]:

- epidemiologic model: 28.1 million Americans
- state hunger surveys: 31.6 million Americans
- Breglio survey: 32.4 million Americans

The hunger problem is magnified by the fact that the United States is still considered one of the most desirable countries in which to live. Hunger data from task force reports, polls, hunger estimates for older adults, harvest estimates, and child hunger surveys shows that over 20 million US residents have been identified in each assessment. Exhibit 4–5 shows the prevalence of food hunger in households with children.

The US National Committee to the International Union for Nutritional Sciences (IUNS) of the Food and Nutrition Board (FNB) reviews documents such as the Food and Agriculture Organization's (FAO) *Plan of Action on Food Security Solutions to Hunger.* A central theme is partnerships among private and public institutions to advance research. Other projects of the FNB include evaluation of USDA's methodology for estimating eligibility and participation

Exhibit 4–5   Prevalence of Food Security, Food Insecurity, and Hunger

According to the USDA's Economic Research Service, the prevalence of food insecurity rose from 10.7% in 2001 to 11.1% in 2002, and the prevalence of food insecurity with hunger rose from 3.3 to 3.5%. The number of food-insecure households increased from 11.5 million in 2001 to 12.1 million in 2002, an increase of 4.7%, and the number of households that were food insecure with hunger rose from 3.5 million to 3.8 million, an increase of 8.2%. During this period, the total number of households in the United States grew by 0.7%.

Households with children by year	Total households (thousands)	With hunger among children (thousands)	Percentage
1998	38,036	331	0.09
1999	37,884	219	0.06
2000	38,113	255	0.07
2001	38,330	211	0.06
2002	38,647	265	0.07

Source: USDA's Economic Research Service, Household Food Security in the United States, 2002. Available at: www.ers.usda.gov/publications/fanrr26/fanrr26-10.

for the Women, Infants, and Children (WIC) Program. The scientific basis of the dietary risk assessment methods used to determine participant eligibility will be reviewed. Their review will assess methods to determine individuals at risk for dietary inadequacy, using the concepts of failure to meet dietary guidelines, highly restrictive diets, markers of dietary patterns that increase the risk of nutritional inadequacy, and methods to assess inadequate diets, including food consumption behavior patterns.

US Hunger Policies

Policies regarding hunger were first developed in the United States during the Great Depression of the 1930s.[118] Warehouses of surplus food were destroyed, while the poor were jobless, standing in breadlines, and unable to buy food. The Federal Emergency Relief Administration distributed surplus farm products as food relief and assisted farmers as well as the poor.[119] Policies regarding farm prices and production in 1933, food distribution in 1935, and a school lunch program using donated surplus commodities in 1936 all established hunger-based policies in the United States. A food stamp concept was tested between 1939 and 1943, and in 1946 the National School Lunch Act converted food aid to cash subsidies. Overall, the decade of the 1930s witnessed the use of surplus agricultural products as the basis of food distribution rather than feeding the poor.[118,120]

The United States prospered from 1950 to 1960, and hunger was thought to be impossible until 1961. In that year, President John F. Kennedy initiated a pilot food stamp program in poverty areas. The program became nationally available in 1964 and was followed in 1966 with the School Breakfast Program.

Info Line

PLANNING FOOD DRIVES—SUGGESTIONS FOR SUCCESS

- Ask for donations of gift certificates for grocery stores and or discount stores located near low-income areas.
- Deliver certificates to the agency working with families in need. This approach not only maintains confidentiality and allows families and individuals to shop for their own food, but it also reduces problems with food safety and storage at food banks and pantries.
- In addition to food items, purchase basics for personal hygiene, e.g., soap, wash cloths, tooth brushes, etc. Wrap and label for "boy child," "adult woman," etc., and take to shelters.
- Communicate with organizations that serve the public, e.g., the Salvation Army or the Red Cross, and discuss their program goals and needs.
- Consider cash donations preferred by many organizations.
- Establish semiannual food drives and events at Valentine's Day, National Nutrition Month, at Passover and Easter, or for Mother's or Father's Day.
- Focus on one kind of food so all people serviced by the organization receive the same donation. Include easy-to-follow recipes and all ingredients. Minimize donating homemade or leftover food due to food safety issues. Foods often needed are: infant formula and baby food, pasta, rice, whole grain cereals, canned vegetables like kale, spinach, carrots, and sweet potatoes; canned fruits; dried fruits; instant potatoes; canned beans like black, garbanzo, navy, lima, and baked beans; canned protein foods like tuna, salmon, chicken, beef, or peanut butter; and canned or dried dairy products.

Source: Bass H. Planning food drives—suggestions for success. *Ped Nutr Prac Group Post.* 2003;10(3):3,8.

Hunger was not identified as a major issue until 1968, when "Hunger USA," a report by the Citizens' Board of Inquiry Into Hunger and Malnutrition in the United States, and a television documentary, *Hunger in America*, evoked national attention.[121] The Senate Select Committee on Nutrition and Human Needs introduced legislation to expand food assistance.[122] In 1969, President Richard M. Nixon convened the first White House Conference on Food, Nutrition, and Health to establish a national forum and policy direction.[123]

During the 1970s, the purchasing power of families and individuals at the poverty level increased via cash subsidies and vouchers to address and reduce food poverty. The Special Supplemental Food Program for Women, Infants, and Children and nutrition programs for the elderly evolved. Federal food assistance increased from $1.2 billion to $8.3 billion between 1969 and 1977.[122] A second *Hunger in America* report not only acknowledged the continued presence of hunger, but clarified how difficult hunger was to capture and to mediate.[118,124]

During the 1980s, the states and the private sector became more accountable for welfare programs. A new poor group was identified, consisting of children, unskilled and unemployed youths, and families with limited financial security and limited incomes.[118] Reports documented an increasing demand for food assistance across most states and various high-risk groups.[125] The Food

Research and Action Center in Washington, DC, compiled 250 reports of hunger studies from 1970 to 1991.[125]

By defining hunger in economic terms, the Physician Task Force on Hunger in America identified 12 million children and 8 million adults in 1985 whose income fell below the poverty line or whose food stamp benefits were inadequate.[118,126] Over 40 million US citizens received food assistance to the tune of $21 billion in the 1989 USDA budget alone.[127-130]

Most policy makers are skeptical of data on hunger; they view malnutrition, the extreme of hunger, as a rare occurrence and find it difficult to link malnutrition with hunger. Many believe hunger data are soft, anecdotal, and unconfirmed. There are a number of real methodological concerns about data on hunger[131]:

- Many surveys underrepresent the homeless, migrants, and ethnic minorities at risk for hunger and malnutrition.
- Advocates who lack social survey skills, rather than trained researchers, conduct many of the surveys and construct the methods. Generalizability of the data is limited due to inadequate reliability and validity. The issue of generalizability is paramount to any survey.
- The link between hunger and a defined disease outcome is hard to document (e.g., the onset of hypertension after inadequate balance of nutrients for several years leading to weight gain, then obesity, then elevated blood pressure, hence hypertension). There is no easily defined chain reaction showing that hunger leads to abnormal biochemical measures, which lead to poor health status, which leads to disease.[118]
- Ways to successfully bring individuals and families out of the vicious poverty and hunger cycle have not been documented.
- Measuring the extent of hunger is very difficult. The result of acute hunger is not as far-reaching as chronic hunger, which promotes undernutrition and disease. It is difficult to judge who is the most hungry or who has the greatest need. Special concerns relate to persons who are homeless.[132]

Homelessness affects from 250,000 to 2.2 million people in the United States.[133] Socioeconomic and health factors increase the homeless person's nutritional risk. Relevant demographic characteristics of persons who are

Info Line

Methodological concerns regarding collection of data about hunger include:

- underrepresentation of homeless, migrants, and ethnic minorities
- managing errors in data from advocates lacking survey skills and who conduct surveys
- generalizability is paramount but may be lacking
- articulating the hunger-to-disease link
- documenting the breakdown that occurs with the hunger/poverty cycle
- characterizing the magnitude or extent of hunger

Source: Bickel G, Nord M, Price C, Hamilton W, Cook J. *Guide to Measuring Household Food Security.* Alexandria, Va: US Dept of Agriculture, Food and Nutrition Service; 2000.

homeless include family status, age, education, duration of homelessness, income sources, household size, race, sex, social network, and veteran status.[134]

Research on homeless and housed poor children find that eating patterns of homeless children tend to be unbalanced, with a heavy reliance on fast food, and plagued by periods of food deprivation. Obesity and iron deficiency in children 6 months to 2 years old are common.[134]

Health problems of homeless adults include, among others: dental problems, cardiovascular disease, anemia, hypertension, and alcoholism.[135] Dietary records of 55 urban homeless persons indicated high intakes of fat, cholesterol, and sodium.[136] Anthropometric measures indicated low levels of lean body mass and increased levels of body fat. Nutritional deficiencies commonly found in the homeless include protein-calorie malnutrition and deficiencies of B vitamins, vitamin C, zinc, calcium, thiamin, folic acid, and iron.[132]

Measuring clinical or biochemical indices of malnutrition in cross-sectional surveys is expensive. The result has been a cadre of surrogate indicators such as food insecurity, low income, or unemployment.[118] Use of multiple indicators is proposed as a means of increasing the reliability of the measures.[137]

Nestle and Guttmacher[138] reviewed hunger studies authorized by 11 states between 1984 and 1988.[139-149] These studies employed various methods to estimate hunger and food insecurity in the samples, and they commonly used subjective data from questionnaires or interviews.[139-149] Hunger and food insecurity were frequently reported, as was the need for increased food assistance amid inadequate federal, state, and private resources.[139-149] High-risk subgroups were women, children, and older adults.[139,141-143,145,146,148,149] Many were members of minority groups.[139-141,143,149] Causal factors ranged from poverty and the high costs of housing to inadequate welfare and food assistance benefits.[138] Nestle and Guttmacher's findings show that:

- Food insufficiency is a chronic US problem.
- Food insufficiency does not reflect food shortages.
- People with lack of access to resources are at greatest risk of hunger.
- The federal poverty level is an inappropriate index of hunger.
- The US social welfare system does not insulate individuals and families from repetitive economic insults.
- Voluntary activities and private charity cannot cure the hunger problem.
- Hunger, poverty, unemployment, and the costs of housing and basic needs are interrelated.

These studies identified strategies to resolve the hunger problem, and many of the studies' recommendations overlap. They include increasing the federal contribution to state food and welfare assistance programs and enhancing client access to welfare benefits,[139-146,148,149] increasing employment opportunities,[139,142-144,148] higher wages,[149] on-the-job training, accessibility of low-cost housing,[139,143,149] and income redistribution.[149]

Food assistance is currently needed by a large portion of the low-income, minority, single-head-of-household, and older adult US population. Current entitlement programs do not appear sufficient. Table 4–5 outlines the 2003 poverty income guidelines used for WIC, the Commodity Supplemental Food Program, and the Seniors Program.[150]

CNPs can use information about these programs, e.g., benefits, eligibility, education given, and participation, as demographic or eating behavior data

**TABLE 4–5   Poverty Income Guidelines Showing Maximum Income for Eligibility
to Receive Commodity Supplemental Food Program, Women, Infants, and Children
Assistance, and Seniors Program**

No. in Household	Pregnant/Postpartum Women/Children (185% PIG)			Seniors Program (130% PIG)		
	Annual $	Month $	Week $	Annual $	Month $	Week $
1	16,613	1,384	319	11,674	973	225
2	22,422	1,869	431	15,756	1,313	303
3	28,231	2,353	543	19,838	1,653	382
4	34,405	2,837	655	23,920	1,993	460
5	39,849	3,321	767	28,002	2,333	539
6	45,658	3,805	879	32,084	2,674	617
7	51,467	4,289	990	36,166	3,014	696
8	57,276	4,773	1101	40,248	3,354	774
For each additional family member add	5,809	484	112	4,082	340	79

PIG = Poverty income guidelines
Source: United States Department of Agriculture Poverty Income Guidelines/Rates effective
February 7, 2003.

for program planning and implementation. The data can serve as baseline
data or sequential variables to monitor individuals and groups.

Today, the attack on hunger in the United States reflects policies of the
1930s and integrates hunger with employment status, poverty, and wages.[151-153]
In the 21st century, the hunger problem continues, and its resolution has eluded
the US political scene. Empowering low-income groups by training them for
jobs and expanding the job market may be a proactive approach toward reducing hunger, as well as a step in the right direction toward reducing health risks
and health care costs.

Hunger is directly related to poverty and affects more people than the more
extreme condition, homelessness. Hunger reflects the cumulative effects of an
economic downturn, concerns about the war on terrorism after September 11,
2001, and uncertainties about both the future and the job market. Millions of
people in the United States struggle to meet basic human needs, living just
above, at, or below the poverty line when hunger becomes a daily phenomenon. When financial resources are very low, families tend to secure shelter and
spend resources for transportation to work. This leaves less money for food.
With insufficient nutrition, individuals have less energy, increased illness, and
fewer opportunities to work.

Reasons that people turn to a food pantry or soup kitchen are either temporary, e.g., severe medical crisis, loss of job, or a chronic condition, e.g., unemployment, mental illness, or a low-paying job. Coping behaviors often result in
consuming smaller food quantities, then substituting cheaper and less nutritious
foods, and then skipping meals. Parents often skip meals so children have
food.[154]

In 2003, food pantries reported that more working poor and families come for food. Community hunger coalitions provide referral lists of organizations offering either emergency groceries (donated items, USDA Government Surplus Commodities, etc.) or prepared meals, and information about supplemental food resources and government programs like WIC, the Commodity Supplemental Food Program (CSFP), food stamps, and cooperative buying programs.

Agencies and sites providing USDA government surplus commodities must ensure that the individual and family participants are eligible. Supplemental food resources include the following:

- *The Food Stamp Program*—provides funding for food to eligible low-income households with a gross income < 130% of the federal poverty level and a net income equal to or below the poverty level.
- *Expedited Food Stamps*—a government program for individuals in food crisis situations who need food immediately and are eligible for the Food Stamp Program.
- *Summer Food Service Program for Children*—eligible children are served at school sites during summer months when regular school lunch and breakfast programs are closed.
- *Food Co-Ops*—provide low-income families foods in brown bags or family share bags.
- *Food Finders*—volunteers deliver prepared or semiprepared salvaged food from restaurants and other donor sources to agencies.
- *Senior Citizens*—Congregate Title IIIC meals at centers and Meals on Wheels for homebound seniors.
- *WIC*—a supplemental food program meeting the nutritional needs of low-income, pregnant, and postpartum women, as well as infants and young children up to the age of 5.

Food Assistance Programs

US food assistance programs are designed to improve the nutrition and health status of target recipients/beneficiaries by improving their access to food. Another aim of these programs is to support agriculture and ultimately to reduce food insecurity in many US households.[155] In Los Angeles County, the Division of Chronic Disease Prevention and Health Promotion assessed 1,868 low-income participants defined as those households at or below 300% of the federal poverty threshold. Data were based on results from the 1999-2000 Los Angeles County Health Supplemental Survey. Fair or poor health was more often perceived by households with greater food insecurity (see Figure 4–4).[156]

Dimensions of Food Assistance Programs

Three dimensions are identified to explore the impact of food assistance programs on nutrition status, health status, and quality of life for low-income populations: economic, sociopolitical, and nutrition dimensions.

The Economic Dimension   This generally addresses the effects of actions and programs on recipients, society, and delivery costs.[155] Short-term outcomes tend to focus on changes in food intake and immediate indicators of nutritional

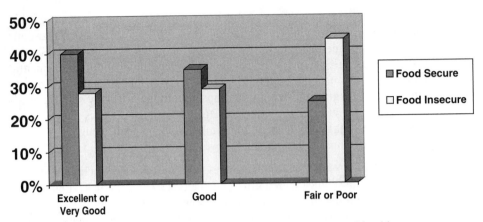

FIGURE 4–4   Food security in Los Angeles County by self-perceived health status among 1,868 low-income participants. Low-income participants = households at or below 300% of federal poverty threshold.
Source: County of Los Angeles, Department of Health Services, Division of Chronic Disease Prevention and Health Promotion, Nutrition Program. 1999-2000 Los Angeles County Health Supplemental Survey. January 2001.

status (e.g., weight gain in pregnancy, growth in children, and hemoglobin level). Knowledge change denotes short-term outcome. Unless participants are followed in a longitudinal manner, actual impact is difficult to assess.

Medicaid cost savings for newborns was an outcome measure for the cost-benefit evaluation of the WIC program.[157] Noticeable improvements were seen in birth outcomes, with healthier babies and less medical care. Medical care costs were less when women participated in WIC, and program costs were less than medical care costs for these high-risk women. The cost benefit precipitates strong national support for the WIC program.[155,157]

Intermediate outcomes of food assistance programs include behaviors, attitudes, and preferences. Eating patterns, food handling procedures, child-care alternatives, and medical services all affect nutrition and health status.[155]

Long-term outcomes are reflected in an adequate food and nutrient intake, positive mental and physical development of infants and youths, increased productivity of adults and seniors, and job security of adults.[155]

The Sociopolitical Dimension   The sociopolitical dimension challenges food and nutrition policy makers to reduce individual and household food insecurity by distributing resources to meet immediate as well as chronic needs. In addition, 2 values must be considered: (1) access to food is a basic right; and (2) individuals have the right to free choice.[155] The concepts of hunger and food insecurity include 4 components[158]:

1. sufficiency
2. suitability and nutritional adequacy
3. anxiety, lack of choice, or feeling of deprivation
4. acceptability of receiving food

Effective intervention programs must enhance the household's capacity to achieve household goals. Food assistance programs may influence consumer behavior but still allow independent food choice (e.g., food stamps).

Or, on the other hand, programs may target specific nutrient deficiencies and package foods accordingly (e.g., WIC coupons).

Cashing out of food stamps has been tested in Washington State; San Diego, California; and several counties in Alabama. It substitutes a cash transfer for food stamps. A credit card format has also been tested. Recipients are given a plastic card and personal identification number to use at the checkout counter. A debit is made to the recipient's food account, which is similar to a bank account. These alternatives promote choice and lower administrative costs more than cash payments would. Concern remains, however, about the nutrient quality of products actually purchased and the proportion of the purchase spent on nonfood purchases.[159]

The Nutrition Dimension   The nutrition dimension addresses dietary factors that influence morbidity and premature mortality among poorly nourished individuals. Malnourished children are more vulnerable to lead and environmental toxins, infectious diseases, school absenteeism, and a muted intellectual achievement. Malnutrition can promote reduced productivity and impaired socialization of young and middle-aged adults. Frail older adults may experience a reduced mobility, impaired digestion and absorption, and an increased risk of malnutrition.[155]

There is no question that hunger exists in the United States. Its presence should motivate the nation to tackle a problem within its borders. From a global perspective, a complex, holistic approach to hunger has been proposed for the world by the International Conference on Nutrition.

In the United States, food security and nutritional well-being arising from food consumed by households is determined by at least 5 interrelated factors:

1. availability of food through market and other channels
2. ability of households to acquire whatever food the market and other sources have to offer, which is a function of household income levels and flow and the resource base for subsistence farming
3. desire to buy specific foods available in the market or to grow them for home consumption, which is related to food habits, intrahousehold income control, and nutritional knowledge
4. mode of food preparation and to whom the food is fed, which is influenced by income control, time constraints, food habits, and nutritional knowledge
5. health status of individuals, which is governed by the nutritional status of the individual, nutritional knowledge, health and sanitary conditions at the household and community levels, and caretaking, among others[160]

Info Line

The Dannon Institute provides awards for excellence in community nutrition to highlight innovative programs improving the community through nutrition.

Source: Community Nutritionary. Spring 2000;3(1):3.

Vegetarianism

Vegetarians frequently experience lower mortality rates from chronic degenerative diseases than nonvegetarians.[161-162] Diet and other lifestyle patterns of vegetarians are health promoting (e.g., maintaining desirable weight, having regular physical activity, not smoking, not drinking alcohol, and not using illicit drugs). The National Restaurant Association Gallup survey showed that about 20% of US customers seek a restaurant that offers vegetarian items. A study revealed that only 3-7% of students at the University of Missouri at Columbia are vegetarians, but as many as 25% of students consistently order vegetarian meals. The National Restaurant Association and the National Association of College and University Foodservice reported that approximately 20% of college students in 1999 were vegetarians.[163]

The vegetarian diet is generally composed of fruits, vegetables, legumes, grains, seeds, and nuts. Eggs, dairy products, or both may be included. Vegetarian diets can vary considerably, depending on the extent to which animal products are avoided.[164]

Total serum cholesterol and low-density lipoprotein cholesterol levels are usually lower among vegetarians. The levels of high-density lipoprotein cholesterol and triglyceride reflect the type of vegetarian diet.[165,166] Low-fat, low-cholesterol, vegetarian diets may decrease apoproteins A, B, and E. Platelet composition and platelet function are altered, and plasma viscosity may decrease. Reversal of severe coronary artery disease has been shown without the use of lipid-lowering drugs. A vegetarian diet with less than 10% of its energy from fat, smoking cessation, stress management, and moderate exercise have shown a combined effect on reducing artery stenosis.[165]

The Gurmat (Sikh) faith allows meat, but many sikhs are primarily vegetarian and consume lentils, legumes, wheat or corn, and buttermilk. At a langar or community meal, Sikhs eat a vegetarian meal so they do not offend anyone. Parsis follow a mainly nonvegetarian diet and eat eggs, fish, shrimp, chicken, or goat. Eggs are symbols of fertility and are placed on trays together with raw rice, coconut, fresh flowers, and oil lamps at weddings, birthdays, and other special occasions. Fish is an auspicious food. Common Asian Indian foods for vegetarians are[44]:

Badaam: Almonds.
Bhaji: Generic term for cooked vegetables. Other names for vegetable
    dishes include curry, bharta, sabzi, and sag.

Info Line

Vegetarianism is commonly practiced in India, and it stems from religious beliefs of nonviolence toward animals and contributing to self-improvement and well-being. The lactovegetarian diet is the most common, then lactoovovegetarian, and vegan diets are also popular. Nonvegetarians eat vegetarian meals on auspicious or religious occasions except when fish or meat is allowed. Beef consumption is forbidden as the cow is considered a cosmic symbol, a universal mother, and the producer of dairy products that are all predominant in the vegetarian diet.[44]

Chenna: Chickpeas or garbanzo beans, either whole or hulled and split (when it is known as channa dhal).

Chutney: A sweet or salty dip or relish made to be eaten as a dip with a variety of dishes.

Dahi: Also known as curds, a homemade yogurt.

Haram: Food that observers of the Islamic faith regard as forbidden or tainted.

Karela: A widely used bitter vegetable, believed to have medicinal value.

Roti: A generic term for bread, a staple for most people in northern India and Pakistan.

Tandoor: A clay, charcoal-heated oven for baking and broiling.

Vagaar: Different.

Vegetarians experience hypertension and non-insulin-dependent diabetes mellitus less often than nonvegetarians.[167] A study of 55 Chinese Buddhist vegetarians and 59 nonvegetarian Chinese medical students shows major benefits of the Buddhist vegetarian diet, which contained 58-63% of energy from carbohydrate and 25-30% fat. Benefits in lower blood cholesterol were noted, as were a lower ratio of apolipoprotein A-I to B, and reductions in glucose and uric acid. No positive effect was noted for blood risk factors.[168]

One group of vegetarians of particular interest are the Seventh-Day Adventist vegetarians. They have lower rates of mortality from colon cancer than the general population.[169] Their eating pattern promotes high amounts of fiber, less fat and saturated fat, reduced cholesterol and caffeine, and large amounts of fruits and vegetables.

Lactovegetarians consume abundant amounts of calcium. The vegan eating pattern may produce physiologic changes that retard colon cancer.[170] Less meat and animal protein has been associated with decreased colon cancer. A vegetarian eating pattern may lower lung cancer rates, decrease risk for breast cancer, and lower body weight.[171-173]

Because vegetarians have a relatively high intake of complex carbohydrates and fiber, their carbohydrate metabolism may be improved, yielding lower basal blood glucose levels.[174]

A Health-Promoting Eating Pattern

Plant proteins can provide sufficient amounts of the essential and nonessential amino acids if protein sources are varied and an individual eats sufficient calories. Guidelines to assist vegetarians with meal planning are outlined in Exhibit 4–6. Whole grains, legumes, vegetables, seeds, and nuts are excellent sources of essential and nonessential amino acids. Soy protein is equivalent to proteins of animal origin.[175]

Most vegetarian diets meet or exceed the recommended dietary allowances for protein.[176] A lower protein intake may improve calcium retention in vegetarians and enhance kidney function in individuals with prior kidney damage. Lower protein intake often leads to lower fat intake.[164]

Plant carbohydrates are rich sources of dietary fiber, which may prevent and/or treat certain diseases such as diverticulosis and colon cancer. In a vegetarian eating pattern, adequate iron intake reflects the amount of dietary iron consumed and absorbed. Inhibitors and enhancers affect nonheme iron absorption.

Exhibit 4-6   Guidelines to Assist Vegetarians With Meal Planning

Emphasize a variety of foods to meet energy needs. Recommend the following:

- Limit low-nutrient-dense foods, such as sweets and fatty foods.
- Choose whole or unrefined grain products and use fortified or enriched cereal products.
- Use a variety of fruits and vegetables.
- Eat a good food source of vitamin C.
- Use low-fat or nonfat milk or dairy products.
- Limit egg intake to 3 to 4 yolks per week.
- Have a reliable source of vitamin B_{12} (fortified commercial breakfast cereals, fortified soy beverages, or a cyanocobalamin supplement).
- Take vitamin D supplement if exposure to sunlight is limited.
- Give vegetarian and nonvegetarian infants who are solely breastfed past 4 to 6 months of age a supplement of iron and vitamin D if exposure to sunlight is limited.

Source: Adapted from: Position of the ADA: vegetarian diets. *J Am Diet Assoc.* 1993;11:1317-1319, with permission of the American Dietetic Association.

Vegetarians are not at an increased risk of iron deficiency if they consume abundant amounts of ascorbic acid, which enhances nonheme iron absorption. Vegetarians in developing countries consume food staples low in iron. They have fewer sources of ascorbic acid and drink more tea containing tannin. This counters iron absorption and promotes iron deficiency.

Vitamin B_{12} is found in all animal products including milk and milk products. Bacteria produce vitamin B_{12} in the human gut. The site of vitamin B_{12} production is beyond the ileum, where B_{12} is absorbed in the intestine.[164,177] Lack of intrinsic factor in the stomach is the most common cause of vitamin B_{12} deficiency. Atrophic gastritis and the resulting bacterial overgrowth in the upper gut may also contribute to vitamin B_{12} deficiency, especially in older adults.

Plants do not contain vitamin B_{12}. In developing countries, vegans ingest vitamin B_{12} from foods contaminated with organisms that produce the vitamin (e.g., unwashed fruits or vegetables). In Western societies, sanitation is better and the vitamin B_{12} deficiency among vegans may be greater.

Cyanocobalamin, the active form of vitamin B_{12}, is available from vitamin supplements or fortified foods such as commercial breakfast cereals, soy beverages, and some brands of nutritional yeast.[164]

Calcium deficiency among vegetarians is rare.[176] Calcium from low-oxalate vegetable greens, such as kale, has been shown to be absorbed as well as or better than calcium from cow's milk.[178] Zinc is necessary for proper growth and development. Vegetarians in Western countries generally consume adequate amounts of grains, nuts, and legumes and have adequate zinc intake.[164,179]

Infants, children, and adolescents who follow or are fed a vegetarian eating pattern need a reliable source of both vitamin B_{12} and vitamin D.[180,181] Louwman et al found that children raised on foods without meat and dairy foods are more likely to be B_{12} deficient and may score lower on intelligence tests. This may affect how well a child evaluates abstractly and finds logical solutions to problems, so ensuring that a reliable source of vitamin B_{12} is available is important.[182]

If exposure to sunlight is limited, vitamin D supplementation may be required. Vegan diets tend to be high in complex carbohydrate and fiber, creating a feeling of fullness. Daily food intake should be abundant to meet energy needs in infancy and during weaning. Premature infants or infants who are solely breastfed past 4 to 6 months of age need a vitamin D supplement if exposure to sunlight is limited. In addition, infants should be given iron from 4 to 6 months of age.[183] Vegetarians need iron and folic acid supplements during pregnancy. In addition, a regular source of vitamin B_{12} is recommended during pregnancy and lactation.[183,184]

Recent research findings demonstrating the benefits of a vegetarian eating pattern are outlined in Appendix 4–E. It is the position of the American Dietetic Association and Dietitians of Canada that appropriately planned vegetarian diets are healthful and nutritionally adequate. About 2.5% of adults in the United States and 4% of adults in Canada follow vegetarian diets. Many restaurants and college food services offer vegetarian meals routinely.[185]

Healthy People 2010 Actions

Many of the *Healthy People 2010* objectives are directed toward improving access to health care, nutrition education, and health education for minorities and other high-risk groups (Exhibit 4–7). These specific objectives are integrated

Exhibit 4–7 Healthy People 2010 Objectives to Promote Health Among a Multicultural US Population

Objective		1996-97	2010
07-11	Culturally appropriate and linguistically competent community health promotion programs in the following:		
07-11b	arthritis, osteoporosis, and chronic back conditions	UK	UK
07-11c	cancer	30%	50%
07-11d	chronic kidney disease	UK	UK
07-11e	diabetes	UK	UK
07-11f	disability	UK	UK
07-11g	community-based education	33%	50%
07-11j	food safety	UK	UK
07-11m	CHD and stroke	28%	50%
07-11n	HIV	45%	50%
07-11s	nutrition and overweight	44%	50%
07-11u	oral health	25%	50%
07-11v	physical activity and fitness	21%	50%
07-11z	substance abuse, including alcohol	26%	50%

UK = unknown

Source: Adapted from: US Department of Health and Human Services. DATA2010–the *Healthy People 2010* database. *CDC Wonder.* Atlanta, Ga: Centers for Disease Control; November 2000.

within the chapters of this book that deal with the specific disease or disorder (e.g., cancer, cardiovascular disease, and hypertension). Community nutrition professionals have important roles in all aspects of health care delivery, medical nutrition therapy, and general nutrition education of minorities, high-risk groups, and healthy subgroups such as vegetarians.

References

1. Loden M, Rosener JB. *Workforce America!* Homewood, IL. Business One Irwin; 1990.
2. California Department of Health Services. *Health Promotion Section, Multiethnic Health Promotion Task Force Reports.* Sacramento, Calif: California Department of Health Services; 1991.
3. Bronner Y. Cultural sensitivity and nutrition counseling. *Top Clin Nutr.* 1994;9(2):13-19.
4. Wright PA, Hatamiya F, Kane-Williams E. Cultural competence: applications to designing materials to prevent alcohol, tobacco, and other drug problems. Presented at: the Third Annual National Conference on Social Marketing. Public Health: A New Strategy in Health Promotion; May 1993; Clearwater Beach, Fla.
5. US Department of Commerce. *Statistical Abstracts of the United States.* 112th ed. Washington, DC: US Government Printing Office; 1992.
6. Orlandi MA, Weston R, Epstein LG. *Cultural Competence for Evaluators: A Guide for Alcohol and Other Drug Abuse Prevention Practitioners Working With Ethnic/Racial Communities.* Rockville, Md: US Dept of Health and Human Services, Public Health Service, Alcohol, Drug Abuse, and Mental Health Administration, Office of Substance Abuse Prevention; 1992.
7. Bryant CA, Courtney A, Markesbery BA, et al. *The Cultural Feast: An Introduction to Food and Society.* St. Paul, Minn: West Publishing Co; 1985.
8. Kittler-Goyan P, Sucher KP. *Food and Culture.* New York: Van Nostrand Reinhold; 1989.
9. Randall-David E. *Strategies for Working With Culturally Diverse Communities and Clients.* Washington, DC: Association for the Care of Children's Health; 1989.
10. US Department of Agriculture. *Cross Cultural Counseling. A Guide for Nutrition and Health Counselors.* Washington, DC: US Government Printing Office; 1986.
11. Riordan J, Auerbach KA. *Breastfeeding and Human Lactation.* Sudbury, Mass: Jones and Bartlett Publishers, Inc; 1993.
12. Campinha-Bacote J. *The Process of Cultural Competence. A Culturally Competent Model of Care.* Wyoming, Ohio: Transcultural CARE Associates; 1991.
13. Gardenswartz L, Rowe A. What's your diversity quotient? *Working World.* August 31, 1992.
14. US Department of Agriculture. *Cross-Cultural Counseling: A Guide for Nutrition and Health Counselors.* Washington, DC: US Department of Agriculture; 1986.
15. Berlin EA, Fowkes WC Jr. A teaching framework for cross-cultural health care: Application in family practice. *West J Med.* 1983;139:934.
16. *The Fact Is, Reaching Hispanic/Latino Audiences Requires Cultural Sensitivity.* Rockville, Md: National Clearinghouse for Alcohol and Drug Information; September 1990. Publication 20852.

17. Sue DW, Sue D. *Counseling the Culturally Difficult: Theory and Practice.* 2nd ed. New York: John Wiley & Sons, Inc; 1990.

18. Burke CB, Raia SP. *Ethnic and Regional Food Practices, a Series: Soul and Traditional Southern Food Practices, Customs, and Holidays.* The American Dietetic Association; 1995.

19. Bronner Y, Burke C, Joubert B. African-American soul foodways and nutrition counseling. *Top Clin Nutr.* 1994;9(2):20-27.

20. Watkins EL, Johnson AE, ed. *Removing Cultural and Ethnic Barriers to Health Care. Proceedings of a National Conference. Chapel Hill, NC.* Washington, DC: US Dept of Health, Education, and Welfare, Bureau of Community Health Services, Office of Maternal and Child Health; 1985.

21. Orlandi MA, Weston R, Epstein LG. *Cultural Competence of Evaluators: A Guide for Alcohol and Other Drug Abuse Prevention Practitioners Working With Ethnic/Racial Communities.* Rockville, Md: US Dept of Health and Human Services, Public Health Service, Alcohol, Drug Abuse, and Mental Health Administration, Office of Substance Abuse Prevention; 1992.

22. Gittler JB. *Understanding Minority Groups.* New York: John Wiley & Sons, Inc; 1964.

23. Bryant CA, Courtney A, Markesbery BA, et al. *The Cultural Feast: An Introduction to Food, Society, and Change.* St. Paul, Minn: West Publishing Co; 1985.

24. Bennett L. *Before the Mayflower: A History of the Negro in America, 1619-1964.* Baltimore, Md: Penguin; 1966.

25. *Dietary Guidelines for Americans.* Washington, DC: US Dept of Agriculture and US Dept of Health and Human Services; 2005.

26. Block G, Rosenberger WF, Patterson BH. Calories, fat, and cholesterol: intake patterns in the US population by race, sex, and age. *Am J Public Health.* 1988;78:1150-1155.

27. Lanza E, Jones DY, Block G, et al. Dietary fiber intake in the US population. *Am J Clin Nutr.* 1987;46:790-797.

28. Kerr GR, Amante P, Decker M, et al. Ethnic patterns of salt purchase in Houston, Texas. *Am J Epidemiol.* 1982;115:906-916.

29. Kittler PG, Sucher K. *Food and Culture in America.* New York: Van Nostrand Reinhold; 1989.

30. Bass MA, Wakefield LM. Nutrient intake and food patterns of Indians on Standing Rock Reservation. *J Am Diet Assoc.* 1974;64:36-41.

31. Wolfe WS, Sanjur D. Contemporary diet and body weight of Navajo women receiving food assistance: an ethnographic and nutrition investigation. *J Am Diet Assoc.* 1988;88:822-827.

32. Jackson MY. Nutrition in American Indian health: past, present, and future. *J Am Diet Assoc.* 1986;86:1561-1565.

33. Storey M, Bass MA, Wakefield LM. Food preferences of Cherokee teenagers in Cherokee, North Carolina. *Ecology Food Nutr.* 1986;19:51-59.

34. Chau PP, Lee HS, Tseng R, et al. *Dietary Habits, Health Beliefs, and Health-Related Food Practices Among Chinese Elderly: A Pilot Study* [master's project]. San Jose, Calif: San Jose State University; 1987.

35. Chinese Nutrition Society. Dietary Guidelines and the Food Guide Pagoda. *J Am Diet Assoc.* 2000;100(8):886-887.

36. Leonard AR, Jang VL, Foester S, et al. *Dietary Practices, Ethnicity and Hypertension: Preliminary Results of the 1979 California Hypertensive Survey.* Sacramento, Calif: California Department of Health Services; 1981.

37. Reischauer EO. *Japan: The Story of a Nation.* New York: Alfred A Knopf, Inc; 1974.

38. Tong A. Food habits of Vietnamese immigrants. *Family Economic Review.* 1979;2:28-30.
39. Davis JM, Goldenring J, McChesney M, et al. Pregnancy outcome of Indochinese refugees, Santa Clara County, California. *Am J Public Health.* 1982;72:742-743.
40. Higgins C, Warshaw H. *Ethnic and Regional Food Practices. Jewish Food Practices, Customs, and Holidays.* Chicago, Ill: ADA and American Diabetes Association, Inc; 1989.
41. Donin H. The dietary laws: a diet for the soul. In: *To Be a Jew: A Guide to Jewish Observance in Contemporary Life.* New York: Basic Books, Inc; 1972.
42. Siegel R, Strassfeld M, Strassfeld S. Kashrut: food, eating and winemaking. In: *The Jewish Catalog.* Philadelphia: The Jewish Publication Society of America; 1973.
43. Higgins C, Warshaw H. *Ethnic and Regional Food Practices, Jewish Food Practices, Customs, and Holidays.* Chicago, Ill: American Dietetic Association and American Diabetes Association; 1989.
44. Balagopal P, Ganganna P, Karmally W, Kulkarni K, Raj S, Ramasubramanian N. *Ethnic and Regional Food Practices: Indian and Pakistani Food Practices, Customs and Holidays.* Chicago, Ill: ADA and American Diabetes Association, Inc; 2000.
45. Allen J, Turner E. *We Are the People: An Atlas of America's Ethnic Diversity.* New York: Macmillan Publishing Co; 1988.
46. Kumanyika S. Diet and chronic disease issues for minority populations. *J Nutr Educ.* 1990;22:89-95.
47. Patel G. Food practices of Asian Indians. *Diabetes Care Education.* 2004;5:5,8.
48. Osborne JE, Rogers DE. *AIDS Frontline Healthcare Conference Summary.* Washington, DC: Health, Education Resources Foundation; 1989.
49. Life Sciences Research Office. *Nutrition and HIV Infection: A Review and Evaluation.* Bethesda, Md: Federation for Experimental Biology American Societies; November 1990.
50. Centers for Disease Control and Prevention. *HIV Classifications.* Altanta, Ga: CDC; 1992.
51. Lindegren ML, Steinberg S, Byers J. Epidemiology of HIV/AIDS in children. *Pediatr Clin North Am.* February 2000;47:1
52. Davis SF, Byers RJ, Lindegren ML, et al: Prevalence and incidence of vertically acquired HIV infection in the United States. *JAMA.* 1995; 274:952-955.
53. Centers for Disease Control and Prevention *HIV/AIDS Surveillance Report.* 1999;11(1):1-24.
54. UNAIDS/WHO: Joint United Nations Programme on HIV/AIDS (UNAIDS), World Health Organization. *Report on the Global HIV/AIDS Epidemic.* Geneva, Switzerland: WHO;June 1998.
55. Connor EM, Sperling RS, Gelber R. Reduction of maternal-infant transmission of human immunodeficiency virus type 1 with zidovudine treatment. *N Engl J Med.* 1994;331:1173-1180.
56. ADA. *Medical Nutrition Therapy Across the Continuum of Care—Pediatric HIV Nutrition Management.* Chicago, Ill: ADA;1998.
57. Miller TL. Nutrition assessment and its clinical application in children infected with the human immunodeficiency virus. *Pediatr.* 1996; 129(5):633-636.
58. Peters VB, Rosh JR, Mugridithian L, et al. Growth failure as the first expression of malnutrition in children with human immunodefiecieny virus infection. *Mt Sinai J Med.* 1998;65:1-4.

59. Centers for Disease Control and Prevention. *HIV/AIDS Surveillance Report.* 1997;9(2):18.

60. Kotler DP, Tierney AR, Francisco A, Wang J, Pierson RN. The magnitude of body cell mass depletion determines the timing of death from wasting in AIDS. *Am J Clin Nutr.* 1989;50:444-447.

61. Palenick J, Graham N. Weight loss prior to clinical AIDS as a predictor of survival. *JAIDS.* 1995;10:366-373.

62. Suttman U, Ockenga J. Incidence and prognostic value of malnutrition and wasting in human immunodeficiency virus-infected outpatients. *JAIDS.* 1995;8:239-246.

63. Heller LS. Nutrition support for children with HIV/AIDS. *AIDS Reader.* 2000;10(2):109-114.

64. Falloon J, Eddy J, Roper M, et al. AIDS in the pediatric population. In: DeVita VT, Hellman S, Rosenberg SA, eds. *AIDS: Etiology, Diagnosis, Treatment, and Prevention.* 2nd ed. New York: JB Lippincott Co;1988:339-351.

65. Goedert JJ, Blattner WA. The epidemiology and natural history of human immunodeficiency virus. In: DeVita VT, Hellman S, Rosenberg SA, eds. *AIDS: Etiology, Diagnosis, Treatment, and Prevention.* 2nd ed. New York: JB Lippincott Co; 1988:33-60.

66. Heller L, Fox S, Hell K, Church J. Development of an instrument to assess nutritional risk factors for children infected with human immunodeficiency virus. *J Am Diet Assoc.* 2000;100:323-329.

67. Orloff SL, Wallingford JC, McDougal JS. Inactivation of human immunodeficiency virus type 1 in human milk: effects of intrinsic factors in human milk and of pasteurization. *J Hum Lact.* 1993;9:13-19.

68. Wills ME, Han VEM, Harris DA, et al. Short-time, low-temperature pasteurization of human milk. *Early Hum Dev.* 1982;7:71-80.

69. Jeffery BS, Mercer KG. Pretoria pasteurization: a potential method for reduction of postnatal mother-to-child transmission of the human immunodeficiency virus. *J Trop Pediatr.* 2000;47:219-233.

70. Rollins N, Meda N, Becquet R, et al. Preventing postnatal transmission of HIV-1 through breast-feeding: modifying infant feeding practices. *J Acquir Immune Defic Syndr.* 2004;35(2):188-194.

71. Kotler DP, Wang J, Pierson RN. Body composition in patients with the acquired immunodeficiency syndrome. *Am J Clin Nutr.* 1985;42: 1255-1265.

72. Chandra RK. Nutrition, immunity, and infection: present knowledge and future directions. *Lancet.* 1983;1:688-691.

73. Krause MV, Mahan LK. *Food, Nutrition, and Diet Therapy.* 7th ed. Philadelphia, Pa: WB Saunders; 1984.

74. Herbert V, Fong W, Gulle V, et al. Low holotrans-cobalamin II is the earliest serum market for subnormal vitamin B_{12} (cobalamin) absorption in patients with AIDS. *Am J Hematol.* 1990;34:132-139.

75. Brin M. Drugs and environmental chemicals in relation to vitamin needs. In: Hathcock JN, Coon J, eds. *Nutrition and Drug Interrelations.* New York: Academic Press; 1978.

76. Kotler DP, Wang J, Pierson RN. Body composition studies in patients with the acquired immunodeficiency syndrome. *Am J Clin Nutr.* 1985;42:1255-1265.

77. Grunfeld C, Feingold RR. Metabolic disturbances and wasting in the acquired immunodeficiency syndrome. *Semin Med Beth Israel Hosp (Boston, Mass).* 1992;327:329-337.

78. Chlebowski RT, Grosvenor MB, Bernhard NH, et al. Nutritional status, gastrointestinal dysfunction, and survival in patients with AIDS. *Am J Gastroenterol.* 1989;84:1288-1293.

79. Brozek J, Wells S, Keys A. Medical aspects of semistarvation in Leningrad siege (1941-1942). *Am Rev Soviet Med.* 1946;4:70-86.

80. Fliederbaum J. Clinical aspects of hunger disease in adults. In: Winick M, ed. *Hunger Disease: Studies by the Jewish Physicians in the Warsaw Ghetto.* Osnos M, trans. New York: John Wiley & Sons, Inc; 1979:11-43.

81. Keys A, Brozek J, Henschel A, et al. *The Biology of Human Starvation.* Minneapolis, Minn: University of Minnesota Press; 1950.

82. Cahill GF Jr. Starvation in man. *N Engl J Med.* 1970;282:668-675.

83. Grunfeld C, Kotler DP, Hamadeh R, et al. Hypertriglyceridemia in the acquired immunodeficiency syndrome. *Am J Med.* 1989;86:27-31.

84. Kotler DP, Tierney AR, Brenner SK, et al. Preservation of short-term energy balance in clinically stable patients with AIDS. *Am J Clin Nutr.* 1990;51:7-13.

85. Hommes MJ, Romijn JA, Godfried MH, et al. Increased resting energy expenditure in human immunodeficiency virus-infected men. *Metabolism.* 1990;39:1186-1190.

86. Grunfeld C, Pang M, Shimizu L, et al. Resting energy expenditure, caloric intake, and short-term weight change in human immunodeficiency virus infection and the acquired immunodeficiency syndrome. *Am J Clin Nutr.* 1992;55:455-460.

87. Brennan MF. Uncomplicated starvation versus cancer cachexia. *Cancer Res.* 1977;37:2359-2364.

88. Grunfeld C, Feingold RR. The metabolic effects of tumor necrosis factor and other cytokines. *Biotherapy.* 1991;3:143-158.

89. Rosenberg ZF, Fauci AS. Immunopathogenic mechanisms in HIV infections. *Ann NY Acad Sci.* 1988;546:164-174.

90. Patton JS, Shepard HM, Wilking H, et al. Interferons and tumor necrosis factors have similar catabolic effects on 3T3-L1 cells. *Proc Natl Acad Sci USA.* 1986;83:8313-8317.

91. Beutler BA, Cerami A. Recombinant interleukin I suppresses lipoprotein lipase activity in 3T3-L1 cells. *J Immunol.* 1985;135:3969-3971.

92. Keay S, Grossberg SE. Interferon inhibits the conversion of 3T3-L1 mouse fibroblasts into adipocytes. *Proc Natl Acad Sci USA.* 1980; 77:4099-4103.

93. Beutler B, Cerami A. Cachectic: more than a tumor necrosis factor. *N Engl J Med.* 1987;316:379-385.

94. Patton JS, Peters PM, McCabe J, et al. Development of partial tolerance to the gastrointestinal effects of high doses of recombinant tumor necrosis factor-alpha in rodents. *J Clin Invest.* 1987;80:1587-1596.

95. Tracey KJ, Wei H, Manogue KR, et al. Cachectin/tumor necrosis factor induces cachexia, anemia, and inflammation. *J Exp Med.* 1988; 167:1211-1227.

96. Socher SH, Friedman A, Martinez D. Recombinant human tumor necrosis factor induces acute reductions in food intake and body weight in mice. *J Exp Med.* 1988;167:1957-1962.

97. Stovroff MC, Fraker DL, Swedenborg JA, et al. Cachectin/tumor necrosis factor: a possible mediator of cancer anorexia in the rat. *Cancer Res.* 1988;48:4567-4572.

98. Mullen BJ, Harris RBS, Patton JS, et al. Recombinant tumor necrosis factor-alpha chronically administered in rats: lack of cachetic effect. *Proc Soc Exp Biol Med.* 1990;193:318-325.

99. Mulligan HD, Tisdale MJ. Lipogenesis in tumor and host tissues in mice bearing colonic adenocarcinomas. *Br J Cancer.* 1991;63:719-722.

100. Bartholeyns J, Freudenberg M, Galanos C. Growing tumors induce hypersensitivity to endotoxin and tumor necrosis factor. *Infect Immun.* 1987;55:2230-2233.

101. Grunfeld C, Pang M, Doerrler W, et al. Lipids, lipoproteins, triglyceride clearance and cytokines in human immunodeficiency virus infection and the acquired immunodeficiency syndrome. *J Clin Endocrinol Metab.* 1992;74:1045-1052.

102. Sarin PS, Gallo RC, Scheer DI, et al. Effects of a novel compound (AL721) on HTLV-III infectivity in vitro. *N Engl J Med.* 1983;309:445-448.

103. Bennett J. NIH-sponsored clinical trials begin for antiviral drug AL721. *Am J Nurs.* 1988;88:432.

104. Mildvan D, Armstrong D, Antoniskis D, et al. An open label dose-ranging trial of AL721 in PGL and ARC (abstract). In: *Proceedings of the Fifth International Conference on AIDS.* Montreal, Canada; June 4-9, 1989:403.

105. Snipes W, Person S, Keith A, et al. Butylated hydroxytoluene inactivate lipid-coated viruses. *Science.* 1975;188:64-66.

106. James JS. *AIDS Treatment News-Issues.* 1989: Issues 1-75 (April 1986-March 1989) and 76-125 (April 1989-April 1991).

107. Shlian DM, Goldstone J. Toxicity of butylated hydroxytoluene. *N Engl J Med.* 1986;314:648-649.

108. Langsjoen PH, Vadhanavikit S, Folkers K. Response of patients in classes III and IV of cardiomyopathy to therapy in a blind and crossover trial with coenzyme Q-10. *Proc Natl Acad Sci USA.* 1985;82:4204-4244.

109. Folkers KS, Shizukuishi K, Takemura K, et al. Increase in levels of IgG in serum of patients with coenzyme Q-10. *Res Commun Chem Pathol Pharmacol.* 1982;38:335-338.

110. Berger SM. *Dr Berger's Immune Power Diet.* New York: Penguin Books; 1985.

111. American Dietetic Association and Dietitians of Canada. *Position: Nutrition Intervention in the Care of Persons With Human Immuno-deficiency Virus Infection.* Approved February 17, 1989, in effect until December 31, 2008. Chicago, Ill: American Dietetic Association and Dietitians of Canada; 2005.

112. Thompson B, Demark-Wahnefried W, Taylor G, McClelland JW, Stables G, Havas S. Tricep skinfold calipers for assessing nutritional risk. *J Am Diet Assoc.* 100;3:329.

113. *Bellagio Declaration.* Bellagio, Italy: Rockefeller Foundation Conference Center; 1992.

114. Uvin P. The state of world hunger. *Nutr Rev.* 1994;52:151-161.

115. The Medford declaration to end hunger in the United States [editorial]. *Nutr Rev.* 1992;50:240-242.

116. Goodwin MY. Can the poor afford to eat? In: Wright HS, Sims LS, eds. *Community Nutrition: People, Policies and Programs.* Sudbury, Mass: Jones and Bartlett; 1981.

117. Center on Hunger, Poverty and Nutrition Policy. *Summary of US Hunger Estimates.* Medford, Mass: Tufts University School of Nutrition; 1994.

118. Nestle M, Guttmacher S. Hunger in the United States: rationale, methods, and policy implications of state hunger surveys. *Nutr Rev.* 1992;24:18s-22s.

119. Poppendieck J. *Breadlines Knee-Deep in Wheat: Food Assistance in the Great Depression.* New Brunswick, NJ: Rutgers University Press; 1986.

120. Kerr NA. The evolution of USDA surplus disposal programs. *Natl Food Rev.* 1988;11(3):25-30.

121. Citizens Board of Inquiry into Hunger and Malnutrition in the United States. *Hunger USA*. Boston, Mass: Beacon Press; 1968.

122. US Senate Select Committee on Nutrition and Human Needs. *Final Report*. Washington, DC: US Government Printing Office; December 1977.

123. White House Conference on Food, Nutrition, and Health. *Final Report: December 24, 1969*. Washington, DC: US Government Printing Office; 1970.

124. Kotz N. *Hunger in America: The Federal Response*. New York: Field Foundation; 1979.

125. Food Research and Action Center. *Hunger Survey Index*. Washington, DC: Food Research and Action Center; 1993.

126. Physician Task Force on Hunger in America. *Hunger in America: The Growing Epidemic*. Middletown, Conn: Wesleyan University Press; 1988.

127. *President's Task Force on Food Assistance Report*. Washington, DC: The White House; January 18, 1984.

128. Matsumoto M. Recent trends in domestic food programs. *Natl Food Rev*. 1989;12(4):34-36.

129. *Hunger Counties: Methodological Review of a Report by the Physician Task Force on Hunger*. Washington, DC: US General Accounting Office; March 1986. GAO/PEMD-86-7BR.

130. US House of Representatives, Select Committee on Hunger. *Food Security in the United States*. Washington, DC: US Government Printing Office; 1990.

131. Nestle M. National nutrition monitoring policy: the continuing need for legislative intervention. *J Nutr Ed*. 1990;22:141-144.

132. Strasser JA, Damrosh S, Gaines J. Nutrition and the homeless person. *J Community Health Nurs*. 1991;8:65-73.

133. Wiecha JL, Dwyer JT, Dunn-Strohecker M. Nutrition and health services needs among the homeless. *Public Health Rep*. 1991;106:364-374.

134. Acker PJ, Fierman AH, Dreyer BP. An assessment of parameters of health care and nutrition in homeless children. *Am J Dis Child*. 1987;141:388.

135. Breakey WR, Fischer PJ, Kramer M, et al. Health and mental health problems of homeless men and women in Baltimore. *JAMA*. 1989; 262:1352-1357.

136. Luder E, Boey E, Buchalter B, et al. Assessment of nutritional status of urban homeless adults. *Public Health Rep*. 1989;104:451-457.

137. Anderson SA, ed. Core indicators of nutritional state for difficult-to-sample populations. *J Nutr*. 1990;120(suppl):1559-1600.

138. Nestle M, Guttmacher S. Hunger in the United States: rationale, methods, and policy implications of state hunger surveys. *Nutr Rev*. 1992;24:18s-22s.

139. *Hunger in Florida: A Report to the Legislature*. Tallahassee, Fla: Department of Health and Rehabilitative Services and the Florida Task Force on Hunger; April 1, 1986.

140. *Results of the Iowa Food and Hunger Survey*. Des Moines, Iowa: Iowa Department of Human Services and the Governor's Advisory Committee on Commodity Food and Shelter Programs; March 1984.

141. State of Maryland, Governor's Task Force on Food and Nutrition. *Interim Report, November 1984; Final Report, Executive Summary, November 1985*. Annapolis, Md.

142. Michigan Department of Public Health. *A Right to Food: Food Assistance— The Need and Response*. Proceedings and recommendations of the Food and Nutrition Advisory Commission Hearings; Lansing, Mich; May 1984.

143. New Jersey Commission on Hunger. *Hunger: Report and Recommendations.* Trenton, NJ: New Jersey Commission on Hunger; 1986.

144. Ohio Senate Hunger Task Force. *Final Report, 1984.* Columbus, Ohio.

145. The Interim Study Committee on Hunger and Nutrition in South Carolina. *Accounting for Hunger: Hunger and Nutrition in South Carolina.* Columbia, SC; September 1986.

146. Senate Interim Committee on Hunger and Malnutrition. *Faces of Hunger in the Shadow of Plenty: 1984 Report and Recommendations.* Austin, Texas: Senate of Texas; November 30, 1984.

147. Utahns Against Hunger and Utah Department of Health. *Utah Nutrition Monitoring Project: Study of Low Income Households, Utah 1985.* Salt Lake City: Utah Governor's Office; May 1986.

148. Governor's Task Force on Hunger. *Hunger in Vermont.* Montpelier, Vt: Governor's Office; June 1986.

149. Governor's Task Force on Hunger. *Hunger in Washington State.* Olympia, Wash: Governor's Office; October 1988.

150. United States Department of Agriculture. *Poverty Income Guidelines Rates Effective February 07, 2003.* Washington, DC: US Dept of Agriculture; 2004.

151. Ellwood DE. *Poor Support: Poverty in the American Family.* New York: Basic Books; 1988.

152. Domestic Policy Council Low Income Opportunity Working Group. *Up From Dependency: A New National Public Assistance Strategy.* Washington, DC: The White House; December 1986.

153. Matsumoto M. Recent trends in domestic food programs. *Natl Food Rev.* 1990;13(2):31-33.

154. *Basiotis 1992. Family Policy Center.* New York: Hunter College. 1992.

155. Splett PL. *Food Assistance Programs: Economic, Sociopolitical, and Nutrition Dimensions.* Chicago, Ill: ADA Research agenda conference proceedings; 1993:127-142.

156. County of Los Angeles, Department of Health Services, Division of Chronic Disease Prevention and Health Promotion. *Nutrition Program.* Los Angeles; January 2001.

157. Mathematica Policy Research, Inc. *The Savings in Medicaid Costs for Newborns and Their Mothers From Prenatal Participation in the WIC Program.* Volume I. Washington, DC: US Dept of Agriculture, Food and Nutrition Service; 1990.

158. Radimer KL, Olson CM, Green JC, et al. Understanding hunger and developing indicators to assess it in women and children. *J Nutr Ed.* 1992;24(suppl):36S-44S.

159. Blanciforti L. Food stamp program effects in Puerto Rico. *Natl Food Rev.* 1983;23:27-29.

160. Food and Agriculture Organization of the United Nations. *The State of Food and Agriculture 1992.* Rome, Italy: Food and Agriculture Organization of the United Nations; 1992.

161. Burr ML, Butland BK. Heart disease in British vegetarians. *Am J Clin Nutr.* 1988;48:830-832.

162. Fraser GE. Determinants of ischemic heart disease in Seventh-Day Adventists: a review. *Am J Clin Nutr.* 1988;48:833-836.

163. Stein K. Keeping up with a current trend in food service. *J Am Diet Assoc.* 2004;104:1343-1344.

164. American Dietetic Association. Position of the ADA: vegetarian diets. *J Am Diet Assoc.* 1993;11:1317-1319.

165. Ornish D, Brown S, Scherwitz L, et al. Can lifestyle changes reverse coronary heart disease? *Lancet.* 1990;336:129-133.

166. Kestin M, Rouse I, Correll R, et al. Cardiovascular disease risk factors in free-living men: comparison of two prudent diets, one based on lactoovovegetarianism and the other allowing lean meat. *Am J Clin Nutr.* 1989;50:280-287.

167. Beilin LJ, Rouse IL, Armstrong BK, et al. Vegetarian diet and blood pressure levels: incidental or causal association? *Am J Clin Nutr.* 1988;48:806-810.

168. Pan W-H, Chin C-J, Sheu C-T, Lee M-H. Hemostatic factors and blood lipids in young Buddhist vegetarians and omnivores. *Am J Clin Nutr.* 1993;58:354-359.

169. Philips R, Snowdon D. Association of meat and coffee use with cancers of the large bowel, breast, and prostate among Seventh-Day Adventists: preliminary results. *Cancer Res.* 1983;45(suppl):2403-2408.

170. Turjiman N, Goodman GT, Jaeger B, et al. Diet, nutrition intake and metabolism in populations at high and low risk for colon cancer: metabolism of bile acids. *Am J Clin Nutr.* 1984;4:937.

171. Colditz G, Stampfer M, Willett W. Diet and lung cancer: a review of the epidemiological evidence in humans. *Arch Intern Med.* 1987;147:157.

172. Chen J, Campbell TC, Li J, et al. *Diet, Life-Style and Mortality in China. A Study of the Characteristics of 65 Counties.* New York: Cornell University Press; 1990.

173. Began JC, Brown PT. Nutritional status of "new" vegetarians. *J Am Diet Assoc.* 1980;76:151-155.

174. Nieman DC, Underwood BC, Sherman KM, et al. Dietary status of Seventh-Day Adventist vegetarian and non-vegetarian elderly women. *J Am Diet Assoc.* 1989;89:1763-1769.

175. Young VR. Soy protein in relation to human protein and amino acid nutrition. *J Am Diet Assoc.* 1991;91:828-835.

176. Food and Nutrition Board. *Recommended Dietary Allowances.* 10th ed. Washington, DC: National Academy Press; 1989.

177. Herbert V. Vitamin B-12: plant sources, requirements, assay—First International Congress on Vegetarian Nutrition. *Am J Clin Nutr.* 1988;48:452.

178. Heaney R, Weaver C. Calcium absorption from kale. *Am J Clin Nutr.* 1990;51:656.

179. Hambige K, Casey C, Krebs N. Zinc. In: Mertz W, ed. *Trace Elements in Human and Animal Nutrition*, II. 5th ed. Orlando, Fla: Academic Press; 1986.

180. Sabate J, Lindsted K, Harris R, et al. Attained height of lactoovovegetarian children and adolescents. *Eur J Clin Nutr.* 1991;45:51-58.

181. O'Connell J, Dibley M, Sierra J, et al. Growth of vegetarian children: the farm study. *Pediatrics.* 1989;84:475-480.

182. Louwman M. Signs of impaired cognitive function in adolescents with marginal cobalamin status. *Am J Clin Nutr.* 2000;72:762-769.

183. Food and Nutrition Board, Institute of Medicine. *Nutrition During Lactation.* Washington, DC: National Academy Press; 1991.

184. Food and Nutrition Board, Institute of Medicine. *Nutrition During Pregnancy.* Washington, DC: National Academy Press; 1991.

185. Mangels AR, Messina V, Vesanto M. *ADA Position Paper: Vegetarian Diets.* Adopted October 18, 1987, effective until December 31, 2007. Chicago, Ill: American Dietetic Association and Dietitians of Canada; 1987.

NUTRITION POLICY, HEALTHCARE REFORM, AND POPULATION-BASED CHANGE

Learning Objectives

- Describe why nutrition care and nutrition services fit within a basic health/medical benefit package.
- Define the major components of a nutrition policy.
- Identify the committees of the US House of Representatives and the US Senate that consider food, nutrition, and health issues.
- Define and give examples of US entitlement programs.
- Explain how to identify state and national legislators.
- Define managed health care and the new healthcare vocabulary.
- Identify community-based programs and professional skills, e.g., grant writing, that strengthen local resources and return nutrition back to individuals and their community.

High Definition Nutrition

Capitation—a risk-adjusted fixed monthly or annual payment to a community health network to cover all services provided. The priority and focus are on wellness. This is the opposite of the fee-for-service payment system, which requires payment for each service provided.

Clinical pathway—a course of treatment for a specific diagnosis that considers all elements of care, regardless of the effect on patient outcomes.

Critical pathway—a treatment regimen established by a consensus of clinicians. The pathway includes only essential components shown to affect patient outcomes.

Entitlement programs—programs funded directly by Congress for which persons qualify because of certain income or other eligibility requirements. Food stamps and most other food assistance programs are entitlement programs.

Global budgeting–an across-the-board limit on the total public and private
health care spending by the federal government. Limits would likely be
imposed on states and regions of states.

Health alliance–a group effort by employers and the unemployed to purchase
the highest quality of health service for the most economical price from
community health networks.

Health maintenance organization (HMO)–a health plan based on relationships between participants and primary care physicians, offering individuals defined benefits monthly or annually with a fee, copayment, or
deductible.

Managed care–a system where the care of individuals is carefully planned
and monitored. Primary care physicians are assigned, and referrals require
preauthorization.

Managed competition–a system by which community health networks compete
with one another and provide care based on quality and satisfaction of
service by enrollees.

Nutrition policy–"a concerted set of actions, often initiated by government,
to safeguard the health of the whole population through the provision of
safe and healthy food" (World Health Organization, 1989).

Outcome-based monitoring–a statistical approach to measurement, analysis,
and reporting of patient recovery rates using categories of illness and
injury.

Physician hospital organization (PHO)–a cooperative relationship between
hospitals and physicians to form integrated organizations to contract
jointly with an employer, managed care plan, insurer, or governmental
entity for health services.

Policy making–a dynamic, evolutionary response of individuals or groups to
situations and circumstances to improve the public environment, which
remains tempered by budget realities.

Preferred provider organization (PPO)–an organizational structure that develops and coordinates contracts among providers and enrollees who
purchase service.

Primary care–the first contact made with the health care system resulting in
routine medical or preventive care in a physician's office or an ambulatory-
care setting.

Tertiary care–specialized, long-term health services, such as burn treatment,
organ transplants, and other highly advanced technical procedures, occurring in a specialty care health facility.

Universal access–health care and insurance available to every American.

Vertical integration–a process to organize all services needed by a specific
group with the intent to provide a full continuum of care.

Healthcare Reform

Healthcare and welfare reform are exciting and far-reaching initiatives
influencing community nutrition today. Then-US President William Clinton's
initial proposal for potential global budgeting and health care was presented
to the nation on Wednesday, September 22, 1993. It included the following
pathbreaking nutrition components:

- The proposal specifically said local health plans may cover health education and training, and it mentioned nutrition counseling as an example of what that might be.
- Home health coverage for infusion therapy, which is the administration of drugs or nutrients through a tube or intravenously for those unable to swallow or digest, would be covered for the first time.
- The president requested increased funding for the National Institutes of Health (NIH) for research into disease prevention and how nutrition plays a major role.

In 1993, then-President Clinton presented the administration's Health Security Act to Congress. The American Dietetic Association (ADA) recommended that the basic healthcare package include medical nutrition therapy. This would establish nutrition as part of therapy and cover costs of treatment for some of the most devastating and long-term medical conditions and diseases.[1]

Medical conditions such as cancer, acquired immune deficiency syndrome (AIDS), kidney disease, heart disease, high-risk pregnancy, and diabetes can be positively affected by including nutrition therapy in their course of treatment. Medical nutrition therapy, which relies on the science of nutrition, is practiced by highly trained registered dietitians (RDs) who work on a medical team with physicians and other health professionals. It was rare for an insurance policy to cover nutrition therapy in 1995. Patients who could not pay for the services of a dietitian out of their own pockets much more frequently ended up hospitalized and in surgery than patients who could pay for RD services.

Data collected casually by nutrition professionals show that for every dollar spent on nutrition therapy, between $3.25 and $600 in later medical costs is saved, depending upon the severity of the condition. Multiplied by the estimated 17 million patients in the medical system who could benefit from nutrition therapy, the potential benefit for the economy and the cost of health care is enormous.

Several organizations share the same views on including nutrition in health care reform.[2,3] The Coalition for Nutrition Services in Health Care Reform has endorsed a position statement as outlined in Exhibit 5–1. Member organizations of this coalition include the following: American Dietetic Association, Association of State and Territorial Health Officials, American Public Health Association, Center for Science in the Public Interest, American Society for Clinical Nutrition, The Oley Foundation, American Society for Parenteral and Enteral Nutrition, National Association of WIC Directors, Association of the Faculties of Graduate Programs in Public Health Nutrition, and the Society for Nutrition Education.[3]

Dietetics practitioners take creative steps to increase private health plan coverage and reimbursement of nutrition services. The ADA facilitates this progress by linking and coaching ADA leaders via teleconferences. More providers cover medical nutrition therapy (MNT) with verification of referral by a medical doctor.

Questions and Answers About Nutrition and Healthcare Reform

The debate about nutrition and healthcare reform has raised many questions. The ADA has responded to several general questions posed about nutrition's role in health care.[1]

Exhibit 5-1   Position Statement of the Coalition for Nutrition Services in Healthcare Reform

Preventive, therapeutic, and rehabilitative nutrition services compose an essential, though often underappreciated component of health care. Appropriate nutrition is important to all stages of the life cycle–from prenatal care and infancy to long-term care of the elderly; from developing healthy eating practices and cholesterol screening to high-tech interventions requiring specialized nutrition support services.

It is the position of the Coalition for Nutrition Services in Health Care Reform that:

- Quality health and nutrition services must be available, accessible, and affordable to all Americans.
- Quality nutrition services are essential to meeting the preventive, therapeutic, and rehabilitative health care needs of all segments of the population.
- Any basic benefits plan must include the following nutrition services: screening, assessment, counseling, and treatment for individuals receiving primary care, acute care, outpatient services, home care, and long-term care.
- Quality nutrition services must be reimbursable and provided by qualified professionals.
- Nutrition intervention and education programs that promote health and prevent disease are fundamental to health care reform and must be funded.
- Nutrition services should be coordinated with supplemental food programs and other food assistance programs and be delivered in a variety of settings that are both traditional and innovative.

> "If you are among the two out of three Americans who do not smoke or drink excessively, your choice of diet can influence your long-term health prospects more than any other action you might take." *Surgeon General's Report on Nutrition and Health*. Washington, DC: US Dept of Health and Human Services, 1988. Public Health Service Publication 88-50210.

Nutrition programs that promote health and prevent disease must foster personal and community responsibility for healthy behaviors and lifestyles and be delivered in primary care, public health, and community settings. To maximize the benefit, these nutrition programs must meet the needs of the vulnerable and frequently underserved segments of our population, assure access to a nutritious diet, be culturally appropriate, and be included in preventive care, maternal and child health care, and in healthcare services for older Americans.

Nutrition services that prevent or ameliorate malnutrition can avert chronic illness or the need for expensive hospital care. For persons suffering from serious illness, specialized nutrition support services such as enteral (tube) and parenteral (intravenous) feeding can save lives as well as promote healing and reduce the length of hospitalization.

A quality health care system must be available, accessible, and affordable; contain mechanisms for monitoring and evaluating the public's health; assure that providers of nutrition care programs and services are qualified and have advanced training or education in nutrition; use clinical and applied research to improve healthcare practice; and maintain a comprehensive federal, state, and local public health infrastructure to protect the community's health.

Source: Adapted from Position Statement on Coalition for Nutrition Services in Health Care Reform, 1993.

Q: How can people pay for new services, like nutrition assessment and therapies, when they can't even afford the services that insurance and the government currently cover?

A: Nutrition services can reduce spending for health care by reducing the need for hospitalization among those with acute and chronic illnesses that have a nutrition component. The issue really is: How can we afford *not* to cover nutrition services?[4]

Q: Won't managed care plans simply provide nutrition services since they are cost effective?

A: Nutrition services must be available to all patients whose health places them at risk of malnutrition. The lack of reimbursement for nutrition services in our current system has meant that providers learn to practice without these vital services, even when they know that they would be very beneficial to their patients. Managed-care plans currently cover more nutrition services than fee-for-service plans, but these services are not universally available. Fee-for-service plans may extend to nutrition services that make medical treatment more effective and less costly.

Q: Every provider wants to be covered. Why should the plan cover RDs and not others?

A: Nutrition assessment and therapies reduce hospital stays, the need for drug therapies, and dialysis; enhance effectiveness of treatments such as chemotherapy; and help people recover from disease faster. Coverage of nutrition services in general results in better outcomes and more efficient use of all provider services.

Q: Registered dietitians aren't well known in the community. Are they really part of the medical treatment team?

A: Yes. RDs provide services to clients who are referred by physicians for nutrition services. Many RDs have a private practice, giving group education and 1-to-1 counseling. RDs collaborate with nurses and other professionals to include a nutrition component in each patient's plan of care. For example, practice guidelines for the care of diabetic and end-stage renal disease patients explicitly call for nutritional assessments, monitoring, and education for routine, effective primary care.

Q: Why can't physicians provide nutrition therapy?

A: Physicians receive extensive training in health and medicine, but their training does not provide the in-depth knowledge of nutrition science and human health. For example, physicians are not trained to provide physical therapy and need physical therapists to provide the physical therapy they prescribe. Dietitians are among the community nutrition professionals who have the vital, in-depth scientific knowledge for medical nutrition therapy.

Q: How are RDs trained, and what are their qualifications?

A: Registered dietitians (RDs) are highly trained in the science of nutrition and its application to human health. RDs, at a minimum, have a bachelor's degree in nutrition science, have passed a national registration exam, and serve an internship with a minimum of 900 hours. Over 40% of RDs exceed these minimum qualifications and have completed master's or doctoral degrees.

Q: How do RDs affect patient outcomes?

A: Nutrition therapies are designed to establish a balance of nutrient intake that may offset any malabsorption or varied nutritional needs due to the illness. Once appropriate nutrient levels are achieved, the healing process works more effectively. The body can expend its energy on healing rather than dealing with malnutrition (e.g., malnourished HIV-positive individuals who have impaired immune systems are far more susceptible to secondary infections).

Q: Aren't nutrition services just fancy terms for weight-loss clinics and products?
A: No. Nutrition assessment and therapies are part of the medical treatment protocols for many diseases and conditions that have nutritional components. Weight-loss programs can be important to the public health in general, but they do not include the breadth of nutrition services that should compose the medical insurance system.

Q: Shouldn't people do this on their own? How is eating a legitimate part of the healthcare system?
A: For people who have conditions or diseases with a nutritional component, eating right is not enough. People who have diabetes, are pregnant, or have renal disease must pay very careful attention to their intake of sugar, protein, fats, calories, and electrolytes. For many, no matter how well they balance their diet, consultation with an expert in the science of nutrition is essential to determine the nutrition therapy most appropriate to their disease.

Q: Why should Congress specify this level of benefit coverage? What organization/agency should define specific benefits?
A: Congress should specify a comprehensive benefit package that includes a broad range of primary care, preventive, acute, therapeutic, and rehabilitative services including nutrition services. The establishment of a board that could provide detailed study and rules regarding specific benefit issues may be necessary. Given the historic neglect shown to nutrition services, nutrition professionals would prefer to see Congress specify nutrition services among those that would be covered.

Important events have occurred in the new millennium, including[5]:

- The US House Ways and Means Health Subcommittee approved the Medicare Refinement and Benefit Improvement Act, which establishes medical nutrition therapy as a Medicare benefit and registered dietitians as Medicare providers. It provides for a nationwide, permanent benefit that would enable Medicare patients to seek MNT in an outpatient setting upon physician referral for diabetes and renal disease, but cardiovascular disease coverage was not included.
- MNT is included in the final Medicare package Part B. A permanent, nationwide benefit that covers cardiovascular, renal, diabetes, and other disease forms the strong foundation needed to ensure that all seniors receive coverage.
- On January 1, 2001, MNT was included and approved in the final Medicare package and the 3 current procedural terminology codes (CPT) for MNT were released by the Health Care Financing Administration (HCFA) and the American Medical Association as 97802: initial individual assessment for 15 minutes; 97803: reassessment and individual

intervention for 15 minutes; and 97804: group (2 or more individuals) assessment for 30 minutes.[6]

Other provisions in past US President Clinton's original Health Security Act that have been positive for MNT include:

- Medical nutrition therapy covered if medically appropriate.
- Clinical preventive services including nutrition counseling.
- Nutrition counseling identified as an example of health education and training that health plans cover.
- Home infusion therapy covered for the administration of drugs or nutrients through a tube or intravenously for those unable to swallow or digest.
- The Special Supplemental Food Program for Women, Infants, and Children (WIC) would be fully funded.
- Public health nutrition was identified with grant funding as a core public health function.
- School health education programs that include nutritional health developed.
- All health services research initiatives focusing on promoting health and preventing diseases such as breast cancer, heart disease, and stroke contain a nutrition component.

Managed Health Care—The New Paradigm

Delivering health care in an organized and integrated system is called managed health care. Its goals are as follows[7]: to improve the clinical quality of medical services, to improve the social and client service component of health care, and to reduce costs of delivering quality health care.

Managed care is an organized approach to buying and receiving the correct service for a specific health need. Physician hospital organizations (PHOs), health maintenance organizations (HMOs), and preferred provider organizations (PPOs) are types of managed care. The new paradigm is presented simply as $Q/C = V$, where Q = quality service, C = cost, and V = value.

In managed care, clients are assigned to 1 primary physician who refers clients as he or she deems necessary. In this way the single physician manages the care via critical pathways and clinical pathways, and the client pays a fixed monthly payment called capitation. Organizations charge the same price for a doctor's visit (e.g., capitation of $40.00). Clients can evaluate different managed-care programs by comparing the type of service provided when the cost is the same. This would be considered the quality of care. Higher quality care when the cost is the same results in higher value. Healthcare reform in the United States includes this new paradigm and uses an outcome-based system to monitor patient service.

Nutrition care may become a standard component of the preventive approach. It may not only tilt the balance in favor of higher quality service but be a component of health service for which individuals have universal access. As employers form a health alliance, managed competition can occur. Ideally, health care would be universal for individuals with and without insurance coverage, and not specific or concentrated for only employed or economically advantaged individuals, called vertical integration.

Info Line

> The US debate for expanding healthcare coverage with an apparent political resistance includes using a federal worker's health plan, expanding Medicaid, and financing increased cost with a value-added tax on select US goods and services.
>
> *Source:* Project Hope. "Health Affairs." The People-to-People Health Information, Inc. www.healthaffairs.org/press/marapr0301.htm. March 5, 2003. Bethesda, Md.

Public Policy

Policy is a framework to make decisions and guide actions that aid the public good.[8,9] Public policies exert significant impact on societal behavior; they are developed when science, economics, social, and political situations evoke government response and direction to meet a need or solve a problem.[8]

Local government is expected to provide a leadership role to ensure that the needs of local communities are being met. The challenge is for public health professionals to establish the importance of food system and nutrition issues on the local government agenda. Yeatman[10] identified a range of opportunities for health professionals in Australia to engage local governments in improving the local food system and to influence the nutrition of residents. Health professionals in the United States can initiate collaborative opportunities with various organizations in their communities to:

- clarify the roles and responsibilities of different levels of government
- identify how legislative changes and program initiatives affect local government and identify opportunities to collaborate on food and nutrition issues
- advocate for legislative and program changes to strengthen local public health capacity
- investigate traditional and future links between local government to components of the food system and identify opportunities for collaboration on food and nutrition issues in the future
- strategically plan comprehensive, but simply presented, local food system data
- apply food system discussions and case studies to aid local health management when planning programs
- identify opportunities to interact with local government

In the United States, the legislative branch, or Congress, has the responsibility of creating policy by passing laws (Appendix 5–A). The executive branch, directed by the president, executes all legislation. The judicial branch, or court system, interprets the laws and settles legal disputes. These 3 branches formulate, implement, and interpret US laws, respectively (see Table 5–1).

Congress passes laws that initiate, modify, authorize, and appropriate funds for all programs and services administered by the federal government.

TABLE 5–1 Federal Structures to Initiate, Implement, and Influence Nutrition Policy

Policy Element	Congressional Committees (Legislative Branch) — House	Senate	Administrative Regulatory Agencies (Executive Branch)	External Structures
Providing adequate food at reasonable costs	Agriculture	Agriculture, Nutrition and Forestry	USDA	American Farm Bureau Federation, National Farmers Union, Farm Credit Council, National Grange, NCA, Responsible Industry for a Sound Environment, Sierra Club
Ensuring quality, safety, and wholesomeness of food supply	Agriculture, Energy and Commerce, Science, Space and Technology	Agriculture, Nutrition and Forestry, Labor and Human Resources	USDA: Food Safety and Inspection Service, Animal and Plant Health Inspection Service; DHHS: FDA; EPA: Office of Pesticides and Toxic Substances	Public Voice for Food and Health Policy, CSPI, National Food Processors Association, Grocery Manufacturers of America, Food Marketing Institute, Americans for Safe Food
Ensuring food access and availability	Agriculture, Education and Labor	Agriculture, Nutrition and Forestry, Labor and Human Resources	USDA: Food and Nutrition Service; DHHS: Administration on Aging	Food Action Resource Center, Children's Defense Fund, Community Nutrition Institute, Center for Budget and Policy Priorities, Bread for the World, American School Food Service Administration, National Association of WIC Directors, etc.
Provide research-based information and education programs	Education and Labor, Agriculture, Energy and Commerce	Agriculture, Nutrition and Forestry, Labor and Human Resources	USDA: Cooperative Extension Service, Food and Nutrition Service, Human Nutrition Information Service, FNIC, FSIS; DHHS: FDA; NIH: National Heart, Lung, and Blood Institute, National Cancer Institute	Society for Nutrition Education, American Dietetic Association, National Association of Extension Home Economists, National Exchange for Food Labeling Education

continued

TABLE 5–1 continued

Policy Element	Congressional Committees (Legislative Branch)		Administrative Regulatory Agencies (Executive Branch)	External Structures
	House	**Senate**		
Supporting an optimal science/ research base for food and nutrition	Agriculture Science, Space and Technology Energy and Commerce	Agriculture, Nutrition and Forestry Government Affairs Labor and Human Resources	USDA: Agriculture Research Service, Cooperative State Research Service, Human Nutrition Information Service DHHS: NIH, National Center for Health Statistics, FDA	FASEB, American Institute of Nutrition/ASCN, National Association of State Universities and Land Grant Colleges, NAS, Food and Nutrition Board
Improving access to nutrition services and integrating them with medical services	Energy and Commerce Ways and Means	Labor and Human Resources Finance	DHHS: Health Care Financing Administration, Public Health Services, NIH	American Dietetic Association, American Public Health Association, American Medical Association, American Nurses Association

Notes: Authorizing committees for the 103rd Congress are identified. All nonentitlement programs are reviewed by the House and Senate Appropriations Committees.
ASCN = American Society of Clinical Nutrition
CSPI = Center for Science in the Public Interest
DHHS = US Department of Health and Human Services
EPA = Environmental Protection Agency
FASEB = Federation of American Societies for Experimental Biology
FDA = Food and Drug Administration
FNIC = Food and Nutrition Information Center
NAS = National Academy of Sciences
NCA = National Cattlemen's Association
NIH = National Institutes of Health
USDA = US Department of Agriculture
Source: Adapted from: Sims LS, Smith JS. 1993 public policy in nutrition: a framework for action. *Nutr Today.* March/April 1993:10–20, with permission of Williams & Wilkins.

See Appendix 5-A, How a Bill Becomes a Law—Typical Path to Passage of Legislation. Between 10,000 and 15,000 bills are introduced annually. Committees or subcommittees review, conduct hearings, amend, and "kill" or recommend a bill for full congressional action.[8]

Food, nutrition, and health issues are considered by the US Senate in the Agriculture, Nutrition and Forestry Committee and the Labor and Human Resources Committee. In the US House of Representatives, the Agriculture Committee, the Education and Labor Committee, and the Energy and Commerce Committee are primarily responsible for nutrition issues.[8]

Since members of Congress seek information on the benefits of nutrition education, services, and MNT, community nutrition professionals (CNPs) should pose questions to candidates for political offices,[11] such as:

1. Would you support increasing the National Institutes of Health funding for medical research into diseases linked to nutrition? Would you support giving states the funding they need for community nutrition education programs?
2. Would you support government initiatives for community nutrition education about obesity, improved eating patterns, and increased physical activity in our schools and communities?
3. Would you support programs that reduce the incidence of heart attacks and improve the quality of life for survivors?
4. Do you support Congress granting the Food and Drug Administration (FDA) the same oversight over tobacco that it has for over-the-counter medicines, or even orange juice?
5. Would you help save lives by supporting clean indoor air policies, increased tobacco taxes, and prevention programs that keep kids from starting to smoke and eating unhealthy snacks?

Federal programs are either entitlement or nonentitlement programs. Nonentitlement programs compete for funds through the congressional appropriation process and establish eligibility requirements for recipients. WIC and the National School Lunch Program (NSLP) are examples. Entitlement programs guarantee eligible individuals the program benefits. Each year the federal budget may reduce or increase allotments for either type of program. Nutrition policy issues and the level of importance placed on certain programs influence the funded amount. Individuals and organizations can testify at congressional hearings and make recommendations to modify specific programs.[12]

In the United States, nutrition policy issues are represented at the federal level primarily by the US Department of Agriculture (USDA) and the US Department of Health and Human Services (DHHS). USDA ensures the availability of a sufficient, wholesome, and nutritious supply of food and provides information to allow individuals to select a healthful diet (see Exhibit 5-2). DHHS directs its efforts toward food and health and how dietary excesses and imbalances increase an individual's or group's risk for chronic diseases.

Regulatory agencies of the executive branch place restrictions and guidelines on general laws they implement. Regulations may include eligibility criteria, the target audience, amount and type of benefits, and qualifications for service providers. The final rules are as powerful as the original law.[14]

Exhibit 5–2   National Nutrition Summit 2000

The U.S. Department of Health and Human Services (DHHS) and the U.S. Department of Agriculture (USDA) sponsored the National Nutrition Summit in Washington, D.C., on May 30 and 31, 2000. The Summit provided an opportunity to highlight accomplishments in the areas of food, nutrition, and health since the landmark 1969 White House Conference on Food, Nutrition, and Health; to identify continuing challenges and emerging opportunities for the nation in these areas; and to focus on nutrition and lifestyle issues across the lifespan, particularly those related to the nation's epidemic of overweight and obesity. Several overarching themes emerged from the National Nutrition Summit, including the need for research and action:

- Publicize that food security is the foundation of a healthy lifestyle by raising awareness of the links among poverty, hunger, and health.
- Encourage and support healthy dietary and physical activity behaviors across all levels of society to improve health status. Conduct research to understand which factors bar behavioral change and identify changes that can be made to facilitate change.
- Prevent overweight and obesity among U.S. citizens through creation of a supportive environment for promoting healthy lifestyles and encouraging people to practice appropriate nutrition and activity behaviors.
- Conduct applied and behavioral research to identify cost-effective and exemplary health promotion practices and programs
- Educate public about various nutrition and physical activity requirements for different populations (e.g., infants, children, reproductive-aged women, elderly) to facilitate the appropriate implementation of prevention and intervention strategies.
- Deliver more expertly effective communication of nutrition and health messages intended to raise awareness that hunger continues to exist and raise recognition that poor dietary practices, overweight, and lack of physical activity contribute to poor health.

Source: Adapted from the National Nutrition Summit, National Institute of Health, US Department of Health and Human Services. National Nutrition Summit 2000 background and overarching themes. Available at: http://www.nns.nih.gov/default.htm. Accessed August 23, 2007

Regulatory Activities

The *Federal Register* publishes the proposed rules and notices. The final rules that guide the operation of federal programs appear in the Code of Federal Regulations (CFR). This document is revised and published annually. Technical reports or position papers focus on specific subject matter. For example, *Dietary Guidelines for Americans* reflects the federal government's dietary guidance policy.[13]

Problems surfaced after the decision of the US Court of Appeals for the District of Columbia that granted dietary supplement manufacturers First Amendment rights to make health claims as long as the claim was accompanied by a disclaimer of preliminary evidence.[14] In 1999, the FDA proposed, though it was not enacted, to limit the lenient application of the disclaimer to dietary supplements, not foods. Rules are expected to protect consumers from claims based on unsound science.

USDA's Food Safety and Inspection Service requires that foods labeled as "healthy" on individual meat and poultry products must contain no more than 360 milligrams (mg) of sodium, and meal-type products no more than 480 mg of sodium.[14]

The FDA conducts science forums to review the safety and timely approach for risk management of FDA-regulated products. Forums included FDA scientists, industry academia, government agencies, consumer groups, and the public.[14] See http://vm.cfsan.fda.gov/~frf/forum00/finprog.htm.

The USDA found that allowing consumers to use food stamps to purchase vitamin and mineral supplements would cause 2 concerns[14]:

1. Allowing the purchase of supplements could possibly lead food stamp recipients to abandon foods.
2. It could reduce the sales of agricultural products.

The impact on food purchases is estimated to be $0 to $0.94 per household per month; the impact of agricultural sales is estimated at $5 million (0.008% of current sales) to $19 million (0.03% of current sales).[15]

Vitamin and mineral intakes from food are a concern because 25% of people receive less than two thirds of the old recommended daily allowance (RDA) for calcium, vitamin E, and zinc, and 50% of the adult population consumes less than two thirds of the RDA for folic acid; women of childbearing age receive only 50%.

Food stamp recipients are free to buy supplements with their non-food stamp income, but supplement use is lower among food stamp recipients than among other low-income families. Only 31% of food stamp recipients use supplements, compared to 42% of low-income persons in general, whereas 50% of higher income individuals use vitamin or mineral supplements.

A public policy issue question is, "should USDA prohibit food stamp users from purchasing vitamin, mineral, or other supplements?" Given that dietary supplements are regulated as foods and the USDA policy permits food stamp participants a full range of free choice in the food category, making an exception for dietary supplements is a concern. Low-income people with the greatest need for nutritional supplementation could be kept from purchasing them.[14-15]

Info Line

The Organization for Economic Cooperation and Development (OECD) discusses current international issues: pesticides, residues, regulations on hormones, acceptability of irradiated food products, acceptability of cheese from unpasteurized milk, genetically modified organism (GMO) crops and food products, sanitary controls, and food labeling requirements and restrictions. Food safety and quality issues have an increasing impact on world trade. New technologies in the production and processing of foodstuffs merge with global economic developments, giving food safety a broader base.

Source: Organization for Economic Cooperation and Development. *Food Safety and Quality: Trade Considerations.* Washington, DC: Organization for Economic Cooperation and Development; 1999.

Formulating Nutrition Policy

Two major considerations when formulating nutrition policy are providing wholesome food at an affordable cost and recognizing the potential health outcomes resulting from nutrition policy.[16] Nutrition influences health, and it involves individual choice and the social environment. Nutrition is susceptible to modification through social policy changes.[17] No single comprehensive nutrition policy exists in the United States.[18] Instead, a mosaic of separate but related health, social, and food-related programs exist. Each program establishes its own objectives and expected outcomes. The cost-effectiveness of each program is evaluated independently from the others and at various stages of delivery (e.g., after 1 year versus 2 years of participation). The effect of program participation on nutritional or health status may not be reported if adequate and well-defined assessments are not designed and implemented. If Congress mandates evaluation within the legislation, evaluation occurs.

Figure 5–1 illustrates the process and factors innate to nutrition policy. Input involves issues (e.g., agricultural issues including distribution and marketing) that affect the quantity and quality of available food. Process represents events and situations that affect use of the food supply. Food consumption and selections affect the food production. Output refers to range outcomes (e.g., individual health or sustainable food environments).[8,19]

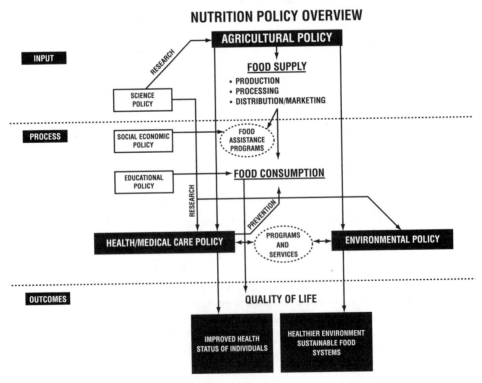

FIGURE 5–1   The components of nutrition policy.
Source: Reprinted from McNutt K. Integrating nutrition and environmental objectives. *Nutr Today.* 1990;25(6):40-41, with permission of Williams & Wilkins.

Agricultural policy initiates a nutrition policy process because it influences the quantity and quality of the food supply and the costs of foods presented in the grocery store to the consumer. Health, medical, and environmental policies influence consumer food intake patterns. Health promotion and disease prevention include nutrition as an essential component of any chronic disease prevention policy.[14, 20]

Science policy influences funding priorities for research and new food product development.[14] Almost $400 million was spent annually for nutrition research and training in 1988; about 78% was used by DHHS, 18% by USDA, and 2% by the Human Nutrition Research and Information Management (HNRIM) system.

Socioeconomic policy affects food costs and food assistance programs when it establishes eligibility criteria. Educational policy affects nutrition education programs and the capability of consumers, youths, and adults to make educated food choices.[14, 21]

Some federal food assistance programs are designed to help economically disadvantaged individuals and families, while other programs are available to any individual. The general types of food assistance programs are family nutrition, child nutrition, supplemental food, and food distribution. Over $22 million was funded for the Food Stamp program, which served about 25 million individuals in 1992 and 27 million individuals in 2006, which costs $33 million.[8]

Five major child nutrition programs exist:

1. National School Lunch Program (NSLP), which is the largest and the oldest
2. School Breakfast Program (SBP)
3. Child and Adult Care Food Program
4. Special Milk Program
5. Summer Food Service Program

WIC provides coupons for a monthly supply of nutritious foods for low-income women and children, nutrition education, health screening, and referral. WIC is generally regarded as one of the most effective of the nutrition programs (see Chapter 7). Several food distribution programs link surplus commodities obtained through farm price supports with people in need (e.g., the Temporary Emergency Food Assistance Program [TEFAP] and the Nutrition Program for the Elderly).[14]

Policy Elements in Nutrition

There are a limited number of policy options that are considered under the rubric of nutrition. Exhibit 5–3 lists the more common elements of a nutrition policy. Various institutions and groups must be actively involved in the policy formation process because they affect the orientation of the final policy.[8,14,18]

Policy Element 1: Provide an Adequate Food Supply at Reasonable Cost

Food production issues are under the jurisdiction of the Agriculture Committee in the House of Representatives and the Agriculture, Nutrition and Forestry

Exhibit 5–3   The Elements of a Nutrition Policy

- Provide an adequate food supply at reasonable cost to consumers.
- Ensure the quality, safety, and wholesomeness of the food supply.
- Ensure food access and availability to those lacking resources or the ability to obtain sufficient foods.
- Provide research-based information and educational programs to encourage the public to make informed food choices.
- Support an adequate science/research base in food and nutrition.
- Improve access to and integration of nutrition services into preventive health care and medical services.

Source: Adapted from: Sims LS, Smith JS. 1993 public policy in nutrition: a framework for action. *Nutr Today.* March/April 1993; 38(2):10-20, with permission of Williams & Wilkins.

Committee in the Senate. Implementation rests with USDA in the executive branch. Various farm, environmental, and consumer groups influence this element.

Policy Element 2: Ensure the Quality, Safety, and Wholesomeness of the Food Supply

The Agriculture Committee and the Energy and Commerce Committee in the House, and the Agriculture, Nutrition and Forestry Committee and Labor and Human Resources Committee in the Senate are responsible for food safety and quality. The Science Committee and Space and Technology Committee in the House oversee food enrichment and fortification issues. The USDA oversees meat and poultry products. The FDA in the DHHS and the Office of Pesticides and Toxic Substances in the Environmental Protection Agency (EPA) collaborate on issues of food safety and quality. Public Voice for Food and Health Policy and trade associations like the National Food Processors Association, Grocery Manufacturers of America, and the Food Marketing Institute all influence this element.

Policy Element 3: Ensure Food Access and Availability to Those Lacking Economic Resources or the Ability to Obtain Sufficient Food

The Education and Labor Committee and Agriculture Committee in the House, and the Committee on Agriculture, Nutrition and Forestry in the Senate oversee issues of domestic hunger and food assistance programs. The Food and Nutrition Service of the USDA implements almost all programs. Elderly Feeding Programs are under the Senate Committee on Labor and Human Resources and are administered by the Agency on Aging in the DHHS. Advocacy groups such as the Food Action Research Center, the Children's Defense Fund, and the Community Nutrition Institute, and associations such as the American School Food Service Association direct their actions toward access and availability.[22]

Policy Element 4: Provide Research-Based Information and Educational Programs to Encourage the Public to Make Informed Food Choices

The congressional committee that is assigned to oversee an educational program depends on the agency conducting the program. Educational programs are administered by the Cooperative Extension Service, and dietary guidance programs are directed by the Human Nutrition Information Service. Both programs are administered by the USDA. Educational initiatives of the DHHS are under the Education and Labor Committee in the House, and the Labor and Human Resources Committee in the Senate.

These 2 committees oversee labeling programs (e.g., the Nutrition Labeling and Education Act, which is administered by the FDA). Meat and poultry labeling initiatives are in committees that oversee USDA programs. Advocacy groups include professional associations such as the Society for Nutrition Education and the American Dietetic Association. The American Association of Family and Consumer Sciences and the National Association of Extension Home Economists have also been strong advocates for nutrition education and training programs. The National Exchange for Food Labeling Education convenes trade associations and professional and voluntary health associations to promote nutrition education for the public.

Policy Element 5: Support an Adequate Science/Research Base in Food and Nutrition

Research and nutrition monitoring programs are under the direction of the Agriculture Committee, the Science, Space and Technology Committee, and the Energy and Commerce Committee in the House of Representatives. Governmental Affairs; Agriculture, Nutrition and Forestry; and Labor and Human Resources oversee these activities in the Senate. The nutrition research/monitoring activities of the Agricultural Research Service, the Cooperative State Research Service, and the Human Nutrition Information Service are under the executive branch.

In the DHHS, these responsibilities are mainly assigned to the National Institutes of Health (NIH) and the National Center for Health Statistics (NCHS). The Centers for Disease Control and Prevention (CDC) oversee NCHS activities. Trade associations and professional groups such as the National Association of State Universities and Land Grant Colleges closely monitor the areas targeted for research, since their staff and faculty may apply for government research initiatives and funding.

Policy Element 6: Improve Access to and Integration of Nutrition Services Into Preventive Health Care and Medical Services

Healthcare delivery and healthcare reform have been top priorities for legislators since 1994. This focus illustrates the formation of a new healthcare paradigm directed toward prevention. The Education and Labor Committee in the House and the Labor and Human Resources Committee in the Senate oversee this area. The Health Care Financing Administration in the DHHS and the Public Health Service (PHS) are posed to respond to healthcare issues.

Info Line

> The USDA and the DHHS was sued by the Physicians' Committee for Responsible Medicine (PCRM), a national advocacy group, in December 1999 for undue influence in designing its food pyramid dietary guidelines. The suit was thrown out of court within weeks, but the action demonstrates the level of interest and control occurring in the US food arena.

Info Line

> TELEMEDICINE UPDATE
>
> Long-term trends may change the way health care is delivered, including heightened patient awareness of treatment alternatives and the growing impact of the Internet on disease treatment.
>   *Source:* Trend Watch E-Bulletin. Available at: healthtrends@ healthtrends.net.
>   Remote access to major medical centers, telehomecare, and medical e-commerce will expand opportunities for community nutrition practitioners. The American Telemedicine Association (http://www.atmeda.org) reports how telemedicine can improve patient outcomes and reduce health care costs. Services provided by the registered dietitian and the CNP may blend well with patient needs.[22]

In response to the new paradigm, the American Dietetic Association has mounted an effort to include medical nutritional services in the basic benefit package of any pending healthcare reform legislation. The American Medical Association, the American Public Health Association, the American Nurses Association, and the American Dental Association likewise represent their constituents in the healthcare debate.

Home Care Community Nutrition Professionals

Home care is diverse. Gilchrist and Williams define culture as "the assumed beliefs and norms of a group, its shared sense of reality."[23] To understand this definition, home care must include a variety of cultures like the culture of home care therapists versus the culture of families of children with special healthcare needs. Although very different, these 2 cultures must integrate to succeed.

Until 1977, the primary service provided in the home was nursing.[24] Home nutrition support was a new area of work for dietitians and primarily involved parenteral and enteral support.[20] See Table 5–2.

The prevalence of infants and children requiring medical or therapeutic assistance is increasing. This need has expanded with the advent of improved technology, success of neonatal care, multiple births, and more aggressive screening practices to identify children with special needs.[21] Currently, about 1 of 6 youth 17 years old or younger have had a developmental disability[25] and 10-15% of the school-age youth have chronic illnesses.[26] The demand for

TABLE 5–2   Considerations for a Community Nutrition Professional in a Home Care Environment

Advantages	Concerns	Impact
Set own schedule	Lack of schedule may appear chaotic	Be flexible, tolerant of last-minute cancellations and no-shows; able to accept an inconsistent paycheck; understand no reimbursement for telephone calls, gas, continuing education, or state-required meetings; and necessity to work evenings and weekends.
Work from home	Home-based office, cost, variety of skills (clinical, management, secretarial, marketing).	Organize and separate family/home from work responsibilities; create an organized traveling office.
Work with multiple disciplines	Increased number of therapists, physicians, and coordinators making communication challenging, in the evening, and continuous.	Appreciate multiple disciplines. Become self-learner, motivated, eager to attend a variety of seminars in and out of primary field of practice. Knowledgeable and respectful of families' culture. Provide education despite language.
Multiple diagnoses are challenging for nutritional assessments	Overwhelmed feeling with information demand or limited resources.	Identify quality resources, skilled peers, a mentor, and/or a confidant to discuss confusing cases.
Independence	Independence can be lonely, creating an out-of-touch feeling.	Increase attendance at conferences, local council meetings to network and to meet peer professionals, increase activity in district dietetic association.
Mobility	Driving costs and personal safety.	Embellish strong directional skills, knowledge of area geography, and maintain a functional car. Become selective with clients if personal safety is at risk.
Growth	Identify time for collaboration and continuing education.	Be patient and able to present positive ideas.
Relaxed dress	Select casually appropriate dress that doesn't intimidate.	Create a relaxed atmosphere and clothing not drawing attention to the therapist.

Source: Adapted from: Pantalos DC. Home health care: a new worksite for dietitians monitoring nutrition support. *J Am Diet Assoc.* 1993;93:1146-1151; and Cole LW. Building block for life. *Culture of Home Healthcare.* Spring 2003;26:(3)1-7.

services has influenced hospitals and pediatric offices and strengthened the home health industry. Home health care for children is one of the fastest growing areas in health care.[21]

Home Diagnostics

Today's health care is self-care with self-monitoring of blood glucose and blood cholesterol level innovations. There are problems, however, when patients care for themselves, including inappropriate use of the test and incorrect interpretation of the findings. Usually, this occurs because patients have no conversation with a physician to make sense of the findings.[27]

Elements of Change

Primary, secondary, and tertiary prevention are interventions to change health risk, morbidity, and mortality, respectively. Community nutrition can be positioned in the healthcare delivery system to improve the health and well-being of US citizens by providing primary, secondary, and tertiary prevention programs.

Healthcare agencies and organizations are constantly functioning in a changing environment to meet the challenge of a changing healthcare delivery system. In order to adapt, it is necessary that they initiate several internal activities[28]:

- *Build a sense of urgency:* People tend not to change without discomfort or anxiety. Discomfort with the way something is done creates a sense of urgency that can empower people to accept a new approach to a problem.
- *Create a clear tomorrow:* Create a sense of urgency by showing people what benefits could be possible if a newly defined approach to health care is instituted (e.g., primary prevention efforts directed toward food gatekeepers).
- *Show the way:* Present a clear vision, and then encourage individuals to learn and to practice activities that support the vision. Develop an energizing, inspiring vision that invites individuals in the organization to act. Identify why employees and clients should support the vision. Take the time to lead by giving examples at every opportunity.
- *Create tomorrow:* Select a strategic planning model to achieve goals.
    Lead from strength.
    Do what's familiar.
    Stay a little bit ahead.
- *Remember that vision makes the difference:* Vision is the difference between short-term moves to improve the bottom line and long-term change. Vision translates strategies on paper into a way of life. Vision empowers people and paints a picture of direction. Recommendations include the following:
    Focus the vision on strategic advantages.
    Think about how an organization adds value to others.
    Make the vision clear, so it can be used to make decisions.
- *Support the vision:* Employees should be able to ask, "Does my action support the vision?" and the vision statement should answer the question.
- *Set the pace with actions:* Demonstrate the vision in action to empower managers and employees. Ensure that managers know that the vision represents what the organization leaders think, feel, and understand. Emphasize the need to change. Use urgency to motivate. Generate specific, concrete actions that support the vision. Emphasize short-term actions to demonstrate immediate change.
- *Expect change or forget it:* Establish quantifiable goals that are short term and realistic. Review goals continuously to empower and to reinforce individuals. Small successes can build large achievements.

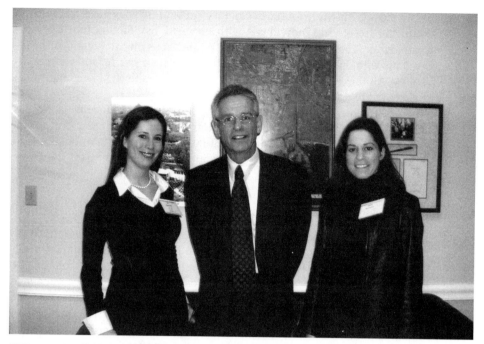

FIGURE 5–2 California State University Long Beach Master of Science graduate students, Siri Perlman, BS, RD and Amanda Mathews, BS, RD, attended the California Dietetic Association Legislative Day in Sacramento, Calif. They met with California Senator Alan Lowenthal to update him on community nutrition interests, concerns, and their interests in nutrition legislation.

Political action should be practical, but consistent with these caveats[29] (see Figure 5–2):

- Learn the art of compromise.
- Focus on high-priority issues.
- Recognize the role of professionals as experts.
- Coalitions are important, but so are personal contacts.
- The split between the nutrition community's antihunger and pronutrition groups is a problem, because resources are limited, and priorities are often set by putting one's issue above another's.
- Often federal legislation has local implications.
- Grassroots efforts are most useful when there is legislation that can be fully supported in getting general support for specific provisions on bills and there is high interest by members (see Figure 5–2).
- Authorizations alone are not enough because they require appropriations.

Nonlegislative Programs and Approaches

Healthcare delivery takes many different forms, and government policy can mold the process. In community nutrition, nutrition education and general awareness of the availability of nutritious foods may be the goal. Primary prevention efforts may be focused on a specific high-risk target group such as physically inactive youth. Secondary prevention may take the form of recruiting free-living individuals with elevated risk factors into a special treatment or study. Tertiary prevention might focus on interventions for individuals with diabetes or hypertension to lower their risk for further complications. All these different forms bring health care into the home and to the kitchen and dining room tables.

For example, an urban farmer's market can bring produce from various agricultural regions to inner-city children and adults, primary prevention efforts for adolescents via planning and intervention may involve grants to community-based organizations, and an international strategy to coordinate prevention and control activities may extend worldwide.

Community Awareness—The Reading Terminal Farmers' Market Trust

The Reading Terminal Farmers' Market Trust is a charitable organization founded in 1991 to promote better nutrition in low-income communities in Philadelphia. The trust is a core member of a large collaborative program, the Regional Infrastructure for Sustaining Agriculture. M. Sutnick, in a 1994 personal communication, said that the mission of the trust is to promote the benefits of fresh foods, cultivate links between regional farmers and urban markets, and establish a nutritious food distribution system for low-income residents. Several situations motivated the trust to establish programs:

- In Philadelphia, 25% of Reading Terminal Market coupons issued to WIC clients are not redeemed because of the inability of recipients to reach designated markets.
- Local residents are not able to provide input about urban renewal and community programs in their own areas.
- Job training opportunities are limited unless new programs begin in low-income areas.
  The trust sponsors several programs:
- The Reading Terminal Community Farmers' Market Program, which brings fresh, nutritious foods to low-income communities in Philadelphia. Ten neighborhood markets with high-quality fruits and vegetables at low cost are each open a half day a week (see Figure 5–3).
- A food learning network, which teaches low-income school children about healthy foods by having them visit the Reading Terminal Market in downtown Philadelphia; tasting fresh fruits, vegetables, and whole-grain breads; and learning how and where the foods are grown (see Figure 5–4).
- The Regional Infrastructure for Sustaining Agriculture, a 3-year project that was funded by the Kellogg Foundation to promote adoption of sustainable agriculture in southeast Pennsylvania. Producer-only farmers' markets and a contract program to link low-income consumers with area farmers for fresh foods are components of the project.

Primary Prevention of Global Proportions—the INTERHEALTH Nutrition Initiative

The World Health Organization's Division of Noncommunicable Diseases (WHO-NCD) initiated a global program for health in 1986 to prevent and control the common risk factors for chronic diseases throughout the world.[30] The noncommunicable diseases include cardiovascular diseases, cancer,

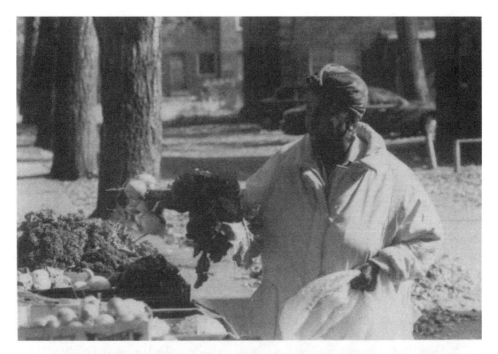

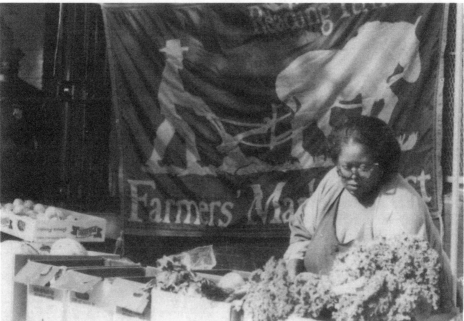

FIGURE 5–3   The Reading Terminal Community Farmers' Market Program, Philadelphia, Pennsylvania, unites regional agriculture with local access to fresh produce.
Source: Courtesy of Mona Sutnick, The Reading Terminal Farmers' Market Trust, Philadelphia, Pennsylvania.

diabetes, and osteoporosis. Strategies acceptable by participating countries emphasize total community involvement, health promotion activities, behavioral interventions, and prevention and control activities implemented through existing primary healthcare systems and community structures.[31,32]

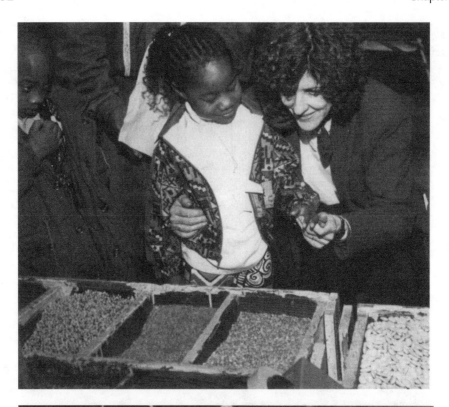

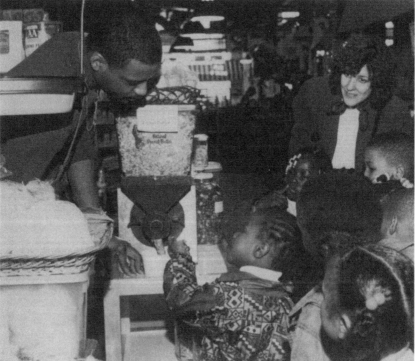

FIGURE 5–4   Low-income children are taught about agriculture in Pennsylvania by on-site visits to the Reading Terminal Market.
Source: Courtesy of Mona Sutnick, The Reading Terminal Farmers' Market Trust, Philadelphia, Pennsylvania.

The INTERHEALTH Nutrition Initiative seeks to coordinate prevention and control activities simultaneously for multiple diseases.[31] This approach supports comprehensive population-based screening, developing standardized protocols, and teaching healthy lifestyle behaviors to reduce noncommunicable disease risk factors at the population level. Countries implementing activities to various degrees include Tanzania, Mauritius, Chile, Cuba, United States, Cyprus, Finland, Malta, Lithuania, Russia, Thailand, Sri Lanka, China, Australia, and Japan.

The multi-country activities range from baseline screening to monitoring change in population disease rates and risk factor levels, and from public health policy and nutrition policy development to population-based nutrition interventions focused on chronic diseases.[31] This multi-country approach to common health problems is a global acknowledgment of the ability to prevent and to control noncommunicable disease risk factors. Nutrition intervention is recognized as a viable approach to reduce risk. Future activities with a global perspective may strengthen dietary change activities within each country.[33] The goal is to standardize the dietary assessment method so food and nutrient intake can be monitored as dietary modification programs are implemented.[33]

Global Activities

Italy

From the early 1980s until 1992, Italy formulated a health programming policy and defined assistance levels for citizens. Implementation was given to independent regional authorities and health agencies. Accreditation standards for public and private facilities and professional self-regulation have been initiated by scientific companies and associations. In 1994, a legal framework defined a dietitian, and uniform training was established. The Associazione Nazionale Dietisti (ANDID) lobbied the Ministry of Health and achieved legal recognition for the profession in 1995, establishing a 3-year university curriculum for dietitians. Defining dietitians' services and fee scale in the regional tariff tables is a future goal. Future activities include developing a self-regulatory system for assessing quality in the work practices of dietitians, a code of ethics for the profession, competencies for various categories of service, and a fee scale for private professionals.[34]

South Africa

The XIX International Vitamin A Consultative Group meeting and the International Nutritional Anaemia Consultative Group symposium have addressed national problems. The belief in South Africa is that global efforts to combat vitamin A and iron deficiencies should be multifaceted. Supplementation should not take place in isolation, but should be one of multiple micronutrient supplementation and fortification efforts. These approaches should address multiple micronutrient deficiencies and counter actions that affect the bioavailability of the micronutrients. Integrating efforts with national immunization, dietary diversity, promotion of breastfeeding, and parasite control is envisioned. [35]

Switzerland

Since 1984, Swiss dietitians must complete 3 years of training to receive a professional certificate that is countersigned and registered by the Swiss Red

Exhibit 5–4   Model Nutrition Objective for Improved Health Status

---

By 20___, the prevalence of nutrition-related growth and developmental anomalies and/or risk factor(s), namely [*risk factor**] among [*target group*] will be reduced from _____ to _____.

By 20___, the incidence/prevalence/morbidity/mortality associated with nutrition-related chronic disease (abnormal exercise stress test, angina, coronary bypass surgery, cancers, hypertension, strokes, diabetes, osteoporosis, dental problems, malnutrition) will be reduced from _____ to _____ among (*target group*).

* Low birth weight, delayed growth, underweight, iron deficiency, fetal alcohol syndrome, inappropriate infant feeding practices, inadequate pregnancy weight gain, dental caries, eating disorders, inborn errors of metabolism (specific conditions), and children with special needs conditions (specify).

Source: Adapted from: *Model State Nutrition Objective.* Washington, DC: The Association of State and Territorial Public Health Nutrition Directors; 1988.

Exhibit 5–5   Model Nutrition Objectives for Improved Services/Protection

---

By 20__, the State Health Agency (in cooperation with other officials, professionals, voluntary agencies, organizations, and industry) will establish dietary guidance recommendations for the general public and [*target population*] and promote the availability, accessibility, and consumption of a nutritionally adequate and prudent diet in [*restaurants, food markets, schools, media, work sites, and institutions*].

By 20__, _____ percent of restaurants and _____ percent of secondary school districts will provide/include nutrition education as part of required comprehensive school health education; and _____ percent of school food service programs will comply with established state or federal recommendations for implementation of the dietary guidelines.

By 20__, _____ percent of restaurants, _____ percent of work site cafeterias, and _____ percent of food markets exceeding _____ size will participate in point-of-purchase nutrition education and promotion programs.

By 20__, the state will be protected by an operational system of inspection, surveillance, reporting, investigation, intervention, enforcement, follow-up, and training for protection against hazardous chemical or biological contamination of food.

By 20__, the state will have a [*mass media, training, professional seminar*] program to educate the public on the issues of normal nutrition, diet and disease, food safety, and nutrition fraud.

By 20__, __ percent of [*well-child care; prenatal visits; screenings for coronary heart disease or cancer risk factors; medical management of diabetes, hypertension, elevated cholesterol; preventive care of the elderly*] contacts should include some element of nutrition screening, assessment, counseling, or education provided by the health professionals in [*publicly funded programs, private medical care, health fairs, etc.*].

Source: Adapted from: *Model State Nutrition Objectives.* Washington, DC: The Association of State and Territorial Public Health Nutrition Directors; 1988.

Exhibit 5–6   Model Nutrition Objectives for Improved Surveillance and Evaluation

---

By 20__, the State Health Agency will have a nutrition monitoring system that will assess and report on any or all of the following:
- nutritional status of various population groups
- food intake patterns
- quantity, quality, and distribution of the food supply including the adequacy of public and private food assistance
- availability and quality of nutrition services and staff
- nutrition education needs

By 20__, the State Health Agency will establish and implement a quality assurance mechanism for monitoring, evaluating, and auditing current activities to measure progress; identify factors that interfere with program effectiveness; and determine the need for continuation or modification of operations and compliance with nutrition standards.

By 20__, the State Health Agency will have a systematic, comprehensive nutrition program plan.

By 20__, the State Health Agency will establish standards for the following:
- nutritional status of the population
- dietary intake of the population
- public and professional nutrition education
- delivery of nutrition services (e.g., nutrition screening, assessment, referral, intervention, and follow-up)
- nutrition personnel qualifications and performance

By 20__, mechanisms will be established to finance and/or recover costs for public health nutrition program/services utilizing [*federal funds, state and local funds, fee-for-service, third-party reimbursements, grants, contracts, donations, in-kind contributions*].

Source: Adapted from: *Model State Nutrition Objective*. Washington, DC: The Association of State and Territorial Public Health Nutrition Directors; 1988.

Cross and acknowledged by the government. In 1999, the title of "registered dietitian" was government protected. A foreign certificate is accepted if the applicant's skills meet the requirements for obtaining a Swiss degree in dietetics and if the applicant meets the following conditions:

- is a cross-border commuter or Swiss resident
- holds a valid certificate by a sanctioned body
- has the ability to write and speak either German, French, or Italian
- has work experience.[36]

Healthy People 2010 Actions

Community nutrition professionals are closely linked to nutrition policy, healthcare reform, and population-based change in the United States. Improving the overall health status of the US public is the intended outcome of these 3 broad movements. Specific nutrition objectives can be established by community nutrition professionals to support the effort. Exhibits 5–4 through 5–6 provide a framework for developing nutrition objectives to improve health status and services.

References

1. American Dietetic Association. *Health Care Reform Statement.* Chicago, Ill: American Dietetic Association; 1994.
2. *Surgeon General's Report on Nutrition and Health.* Washington, DC: US Dept of Health and Human Services; 1988. Public Health Service publication 88-50210.
3. Coalition for Nutrition Services in Health Care Reform. *Position statement.* Washington, DC: Coalition for Nutrition Services in Health Care Reform; 1993.
4. California Dietetic Association. *Cost of services.* Playa del Rey, Calif: California Dietetic Association; 1994.
5. White J. *Statement on Medical Nutrition Therapy Legislation.* Chicago, Ill: October 2000.
6. Chima LS, Pollock HA. Nutrition services in managed care. *JAM Dietetic Asso.* 2002;102:1471-1478.
7. Smith JS. *Managed Health Care.* Boston: Arthur D. Little Inc; 1993.
8. Sims LS. Public policy in nutrition: a framework for action. *Nutr Today.* 1993;28(2):10-20.
9. Chapman N. Consensus and coalitions—key to nutrition policy development. *Nutr Today.* 1987;22(5):22-29.
10. Yeatman H. The food system and local government in Australia: the current situation and opportunities for the future. *J Nutr Ed.* 1997; 29:258-266.
11. American Heart Association. *Take Heart 2004.* 2004. Available at http://www.americanheart.org.
12. Matz M. School food service and nutrition. *Am Sch Food Serv J.* 1994;48(7):82-83.
13. US Department of Agriculture and US Department of Health and Human Services. *Dietary Guidelines for Americans.* Washington, DC: US Dept of Agriculture and US Dept of Health and Human Services; 2005.
14. The American Dietetic Association. *On the Pulse.* Chicago, Ill: American Dietetic Association; December 1999.
15. Sheldon J, Pelletier D. Nutrient intakes among dietary supplement users and nonusers in the food stamp population. *FAM ECON and Nut. Rev.* 2003;15(2):3-14.
16. World Health Organization. *Developing a Nutrition Policy Statement.* Helsing, Switzerland: WHO; 1989.
17. Spasoff RA. The role of nutrition in healthy public policy. *Rapport.* 1989;4:6-7.
18. Sims LS. Nutrition policy through the Reagan era: feast or famine? Presented at: Pew/Cornell Lecture Series on Food and Nutrition Policy; 1988; Ithaca, NY.
19. McNutt K. Integrating nutrition and environmental objectives. *Nutr Today.* 1990;25(6):40-41.
20. Pantalos DC. Home health care: a new worksite for dietitians monitoring nutrition support. *J Am Diet Assoc.* 1993;93:1146-1151.
21. Agosta J, Melda K. Supporting families who provide care at home for children with disabilities. *Except Child.* 1995;62:271-281.
22. Johnson R. American Dietetic Association child nutrition reauthorization. Testimony given before the Senate Agriculture, Nutrition and Forestry Committee; 1994.
23. Gilchrist VJ, Williams RL. Key informant interviews. In: Crabtree BF, Miller WL, eds. *Doing Qualitative Research.* Thousand Oaks, Calif: Sage; 1999:71-88.

24. Meisenheimer CG. *Quality Assurance for Home Health Care*. Rockville, Md: Aspen Publishers; 1989.
25. Boyle CA, Decoufle P, Yeargin-Allsopp M. Prevalence and health impact of developmental disabilities in US children. *Pediatrics*. 1994;93:399-403.
26. Mattsson A. Long-term physical illness in childhood: a challenge to psychosocial adaptation. *Pediatrics*. 1972;50:801-811.
27. Tufts University. Your guide to living healthier longer: putting home tests to the test. *Health Nutr Let*. October 2003;21(8):9-12.
28. Belasco JA. Teaching the elephant to dance. In: *Executive Book Summaries*. Bristol, Vt: Soundview Publishers; 1990:1-8.
29. Nutrition Legislation. News breaks. *Nutr Today*. 2004;39(5):192-194.
30. Litrak J, Ruiz L, Restrepo HE, et al. The growing burden of noncommunicable diseases: a challenge for the countries of the Americas. *Bull Pan Am Health Organ*. 1987;21:156-169.
31. Posner BM, Quatromoni PA, Franz M. Nutrition policies and interventions for chronic disease risk reduction in international settings: the INTERHEALTH nutrition initiative. *Nutr Rev*. 1994;52:179-187.
32. Epstein FH, Holland WW. Prevention of chronic diseases in the community—one-disease versus multiple-disease strategies. *Int J Epidemiol*. 1983;12:135-137.
33. Posner BM, Franz M, Quatromoni P, and the INTERHEALTH Steering Committee. Nutrition and the global risk for chronic disease: the INTERHEALTH nutrition initiative. *Nutr Rev*. 1994;52:201-207.
34. Cecchetto G. Quality assessment of dietetics practice. In: *Dietetics Around the World*. Chicago: ICDA. October 1999;6(2):4.
35. Kassier S. Programs explore micronutrient interventions. In: *Dietetics Around the World*. Chicago: ICDA. October 1999;6(2):4
36. Oliveira S. Professional certification in Switzerland. In *Dietetics Around the World*. Chicago: ICDA. October 1999;6(1):5.

PART 2

PRIMARY PREVENTIONS OF DISEASE

FOOD-BORNE ILLNESS

Learning Objectives

- Contrast infectious disease with noninfectious disease.
- Define the progressive sequence that occurs in a food-borne illness.
- Enumerate the basic food service sanitation procedures, including the steps in the hazard analysis and critical control points (HACCP) system.
- List the major bacteria causing food-borne illnesses.
- Define the role of pesticides in food production.
- List the components of an emergency survival kit.

High Definition Nutrition

Bioterrorism—food-borne pathogens, chemical toxicities, or systems used intentionally to harm people.

Endemic—a persistent but low to average disease expression.

Epidemic outbreak—occurrence exceeds the expectation.

Food hazard—a source of danger that is contained within an edible food. Microbial food poisoning or allergic reactions create an immediate effect.

Food risk—an indicator of the probability and severity of harm to human health after exposure to a food hazard. Scientists determine food risk when they identify a hazard; determine the relationship between the dose, amount, or potential for the hazard; and determine the dose or exposure.

Food safety—an estimate of acceptable risk from consuming foods containing potential hazard. A substance in food is considered safe if the risks are estimated as acceptable.

Hyperendemic—persistently high occurrence.

Infectivity—the proportion or ratio of exposed persons who become infected to those who do not become infected.

Irradiation—a pencil-thin high energy e-beam, which, upon striking food, damages or destroys DNA.

Pandemic—an epidemic that occurs in several countries or continents.

Pathogenicity—the proportion or ratio of infected persons who develop clinical disease in relation to those exposed.

Sporadic—an irregular occurrence.

Virulence—the proportion of persons with clinical disease who experience morbidity and/or mortality.

Infectious and Noninfectious Diseases

Community nutrition professionals are generally employed in jobs that address chronic disease rather than infectious disease. The new millennium is witnessing an increasing number of food-borne illnesses, disasters, and deaths from both types of disease. Identifying the cause of a food-borne illness and employing procedures to eliminate the cause have given community nutrition professionals opportunities to apply their skills to food production, provide in-service education for employees and the public, and inspect food facilities. Preparing for and managing disasters such as earthquakes and floods means adequate food supplies must be kept safe and sanitary. This chapter addresses the infectious disease process, food-borne illness, pesticides, sanitation procedures, and preparing for community emergencies and homeland security.

In infectious disease, health outcomes are influenced by exposure to a causal factor. Some individuals are infectious, yet have no subclinical disease. They are called *carriers*, because they are incubating a disease or infection. The reservoir for an agent is the habitat in which the agent exists. Reservoirs may be humans, animals, or the environment. The reservoir could be the transmission source by which an agent moves to a host. *Clostridium botulinum* exists in the soil, but the medium for infection is often improperly canned food containing the *C. botulinum* spores. Humans and animals are common reservoirs for infectious disease. An infection transfer model begins with disease transmission that occurs when the agent leaves a reservoir or host through a portal of exit and is transferred to another host via a portal of entry. This process is called the *chain of infection*.[1,2]

In contrast, in the noninfectious disease process, or chronic disease progression, coinhabitants in 1 environment (e.g., a family living in 1 house) may follow similar unhealthy eating and exercise patterns. These individuals are unaware of their risk and are simply blind targets. Does this situation create an invisible chain of disease progression? Does the parent or guardian become the *initiator* of a habit and the environment a *promoter*, with the child an unknowing or passive *recipient*?

Asymptomatic individuals remain at risk. They lack knowledge of their own risk. These individuals are undiagnosed and therefore unable to receive or to attempt intervention to forestall the disease progression. The environment is a major agent for disease progression. Its magnitude of influence can range from minimal (if genetics has a large influence), to maximum (if genetics has little influence). In chronic disease development the environment becomes the home, neighborhood, norms, and policies that influence the knowledge, attitudes, and practices of individuals and communities.

Portal of Exit and Entry

Portal of exit is the path or route an agent takes to leave its source host. Generally the exit corresponds to the site by which the agent creates exposure to others.

When an agent leaves its natural reservoir, it can enter a susceptible host directly, indirectly, mechanically, or biologically. *Direct transmission* is an immediate transfer to a susceptible host usually by direct contact. *Indirect transmission* requires an intermediary. *Mechanical transmission* describes the process by which an agent does not grow or alter its form but is physically placed in the vector. *Biologic transmission* refers to the transfer of an agent to a host followed by an agent modifying its form.[2]

Indirect vehicles (e.g., food, fomites such as plates, forks, and cups) can transmit agents. A dented can of food is an inviting receptacle for *C. botulinum*, which produces the fatal botulism toxin.

Agents enter susceptible hosts through a *portal of entry*. For example, a fecal-oral transmission involves an intestinal agent that lives in and is excreted by a host's gastrointestinal tract. Later the agent enters the intestinal tract of a new host through another vehicle (e.g., food, water, or an eating utensil).[2]

A susceptible *host* becomes the final stage for infection transfer. Genetic factors, immunity, and nutritional status influence the individual's susceptibility. *Herd immunity* describes the condition of a group when its characteristics slow or limit the dissemination of the disease. Disease can occur at different levels of intensity.[2] Epidemics occur under several conditions, as follows:

- An adequate number of agents and hosts exist simultaneously.
- An agent moves with ease within a group of susceptible hosts.
- Virulence of an agent has increased.
- An agent has entered a new, receptive environment.
- New transfer methods have occurred.
- Host susceptibility or entry has changed.

Bacteria and Food-Borne Illness

Bacteria cause 90% of the cases of food-borne illness, and symptoms are variable (see Appendix 6–A). Foods containing either a poison or toxin produced by bacteria, chemicals, or viruses can produce a food-borne illness.[2-5]

Bacteria are often transferred by infected food handlers, but unsanitary equipment or storage procedures can create the problem. Bacteria and toxins contaminate foods through a chain of factors. The sequence is:

$$\text{food} \rightarrow \text{bacteria} \rightarrow \text{employee} \rightarrow \text{moisture} \rightarrow \text{temperature} \rightarrow \text{time}$$

The Centers for Disease Control and Prevention (CDC) estimates that about 76 million cases of illness and as many as 9,000 deaths are related to food-borne disease annually in the United States.[3] In California, 324 outbreaks with almost 10,000 illnesses were reported from 1983 to 1992. From 1993 to 1997, 2,751 outbreaks were reported, causing a reported 86,058 persons to become ill. The agent and transmission mode are illustrated in Figure 6–1.

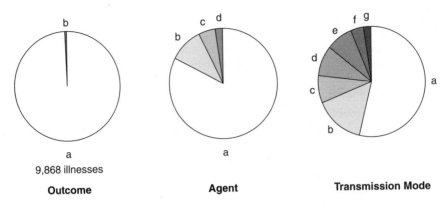

Key:
Outcome: a = illness 99.6%; b = deaths 0.4%
Agent: a = bacterial pathogen 83%; b = chemical agent 10%; c = virus 5%; d = parasite 2%
Transmission mode: a = improper storage or handling temperature 54%
                            b = poor personal hygiene 15%
                            c = other mishandling 8%
                            d = unsafe source 9%
                            e = contaminated equipment = 8%
                            f = inadequate cooling 4%
                            g = other, unknown 2%

FIGURE 6–1   A profile of food-borne illness outbreaks, California, 1983-1992 (324 reported outbreaks, with 9,868 cases of illness).
Source: Bruhn C. *Safety and Quality of Foods in California* [white paper]. Sacramento: California Nutrition Council Symposium—Future directions for nutrition policy in California. December 13, 1994.

Factors

Food

Different bacteria have different food needs. Bacteria that cause illness prefer nonacidic foods, such as milk, eggs, meat, poultry, and fish because bacteria thrive best in them. Since most vegetables are slightly acidic, bacteria within them multiply slowly. Fruits, made acidic by adding vinegar or lemon juice, are not good media for bacterial growth. Surprisingly, baked potatoes, refried beans, and cooked rice can be potentially hazardous when kept barely warm during a long serving period.

Bacteria

Many bacteria are beneficial to humans because they assist with the production of cheese, yogurt, buttermilk, and sauerkraut. The majority of bacteria are neither beneficial nor harmful to humans. There are harmful bacteria, however, including *Salmonella, Campylobacter, Clostridium perfringens, Staphylococcus aureus, Escherichia coli,* and *Clostridium botulinum.*

Handling Procedures

Food service workers control the amount of time and the temperature of food during preparation. If proper handling procedures are not followed, then food held for 2 hours even at ideal temperatures may initiate a food-borne illness. In-service education of employees and quality controls are essential. Hair nets, caps, chef hats, or painters' caps must be worn in all food preparation and service areas. Clothes, uniforms, and aprons must be clean and free from odors. Employees should brush off their shoulders and clothing after combing or brushing their hair when in restrooms. Hands and fingernails must be kept clean, and dangling jewelry and nail polish should not be allowed.

Smoke-free environments are essential near food storage, preparation, and service. "No smoking" signs must be posted in all food preparation, storage, service, and cleanup areas. Hands must be washed after eating, smoking, blowing one's nose, sneezing, or coughing. Signs about washing hands after using the toilet facilities must be posted in all restrooms.

Food handlers must be free from infections and communicable diseases. All cuts on hands must be covered with a bandage and plastic glove and reported to supervisors.

Inspections of food service facilities are usually conducted by trained staff in the local environmental health agency. Inspection criteria are generally detailed in the state's uniform retail food facilities law.

Nearly 10% of Americans admitted to a hospital acquire an infection while a patient. Most hospital infections are sporadic and transmitted from one patient to another by doctors, nurses, and other healthcare workers. Hospital infections can be virulent and contribute to the deaths of nearly 90,000 patients in the United States each year, adding about $4.5 billion to medical costs. The solution—washing hands, a bar of medicated soap, or a disinfectant alcohol rub. These precautions can reduce rates of infection by one third. Wearing latex gloves isn't necessarily a good substitute, since taking them off improperly can lead to recontamination. Hospital staff generally follow hand-washing guidelines less than 40% of the time and nurses may be better than doctors at washing their hands.[6]

Many states require that newly built hospitals have at least 2 sinks per room: 1 for the patient, another for the medical staff. This eliminates the chance a person feels they were intruding by using the patient's sink to wash their hands and can reduce the pathogenicity of an infection. Researchers at the Mayo Clinic College of Medicine in Rochester, Minn, recommend that the healthcare workers carry alcohol hand rubs in their pockets to make disinfecting easier. Lately, some hygiene experts have suggested that patients ask doctors and nurses whether they've washed their hands before an examination. The public should feel comfortable saying, "if it's important for healthcare staff to wash their hands often, even if you're busy, please wash your hands for my safety before you examine me."[6]

Moisture

Water or liquid is necessary for bacterial growth. Therefore, milk, water, sauces, soups, gravies, and juice are viable sources.

Temperature

Temperatures from 45 to 140°F promote bacterial growth with fastest growth between 72 and 98°F. Some bacteria thrive at 113°F or higher and can initiate

Exhibit 6-1   Refrigerator Checklist to Evaluate Proper Storage

- Is the refrigerator temperature 40°F or below? Yes___ No___
  If your answer is no, then record the temperature of the refrigerator and
  report it to your supervisor.
- Are the foods placed in the proper section? Yes___ No___
  If no, explain.
- Are foods stored in the correct type of containers? Yes___ No___
  If no, explain.
- Are the foods that give off odors separated from those that absorb odors?
  Yes___ No___
  If no, explain.
- Is the refrigerator overcrowded? Yes___ No___
- Are foods in the refrigerator labeled and dated? Yes___ No___
  If no, explain.
- Are similar foods stored in the same general area? Yes___ No___
  If no, explain.
- Are older foods brought to the front so that they will be used first?
  Yes___ No___
  If no, explain.

spoilage in canned foods stored in hot areas. Other bacteria that thrive in
cool places can spoil foods stored for extended periods in the refrigerator.
A refrigerator checklist can be used to evaluate proper storage procedures
(see Exhibit 6-1). Freezing food slows multiplication of bacteria but does not
destroy them. During thawing, bacteria start to multiply at about 45°F. Two
safety zones that kill and retard the growth of bacteria are 165°F and higher
or 40°F and below, respectively.

Hazardous foods must be rapidly cooled to an internal temperature of
40°F or below and checked with a food thermometer. Large quantities of hazardous foods should be placed in shallow pans, stirred frequently, and cooled
rapidly. When transporting hazardous foods, refrigerating them ahead of time
to 35°F and holding them at 40°F or below are essential.

The golden rule to minimize a food hazard is: keep hot food hot (140°F
or hotter) and cold food cold (40°F or colder).

Time

At favorable temperatures, bacteria double about every 20 minutes. Contaminated foods begin with thousands of bacteria.

Food Service Sanitation Procedures

Certain procedures are recommended for maintaining sanitary food service
conditions to eliminate acute and to avoid hyperendemic food-borne illnesses.[7]

Protection From Food Safety Hazards

Food must be protected from potential contamination when stored, prepared, displayed, served, or transported. Dust, insects, rodents, unclean equipment and utensils, unnecessary handling, coughs and sneezes, flooding, drainage, and overhead leakage or overhead drippage from condensation are all potential sources of contamination and increased food risk.

Refrigerator Storage Practices

Refrigerators need visible internal thermometers to monitor temperature regularly. A temperature of 40°F or lower is safe. The preferred refrigerator storage procedures for specific foods are listed in Table 6–1. Food containers should be:

- covered to protect the food from contamination
- arranged for ease of cleaning and air circulation
- stored 6 inches or more above the floor in walk-in refrigerators

TABLE 6–1   Guidelines for Refrigerating Specific Foods

Food	Procedure
Butter	Wrap butter to prevent absorption of odors and to protect it from exposure to light and air, which hastens rancidity. Remove soiled shipping container.
Cheese	Wrap cheese lightly to prevent drying out. Do not freeze, because freezing breaks the grain and causes cheese to crumble (or shred cheese and then freeze it).
Dairy products and eggs	Refrigerate milk, cheese, butter, and eggs immediately. Store dairy products and eggs away from strong-flavored foods. Cross-stack egg crates for air circulation.
Fresh fruits and vegetables	Refrigerate fresh fruits and vegetables immediately to preserve color, flavor, texture, and nutritive value. Leave paper wrappings on fruits to prevent spoilage and moisture loss. Store fruits and vegetables so cold air can circulate. Examine produce for freshness before storing. Use very ripe items immediately.
Meats, fish, and poultry	Refrigerate fresh meats, fish, and poultry immediately. For most items, remove outer paper wrapping and cover lightly.
Cooked foods	Use clean, covered containers that promote quick cooling. Quick cool (within 2 hours) hot foods to refrigeration temperature to avoid food poisoning. Keep precooked foods refrigerated until serving (e.g., cream- or custard-filled pastries, puddings, salads, sandwiches, cold meats). Use foods within 2 to 3 days, preferably within 24 hours. Discard cooked foods if they have been removed from refrigeration and reheated for serving more than 2 times.

Does the date mean "too late"? Table eggs are labeled with a sell-by date. Testing of the quality and use of eggs was conducted after 10 weeks of storage, which exceeds the 30-day industry standard for keeping eggs on the store shelf. Results showed that properly refrigerated eggs are safe to eat for 4 to 5 weeks beyond the pack date.[8]

A family of bacteria called *Enterobacteriaceae* includes *Salmonella, Escherichia, Enterobacter, Klebsiella,* and *Yersinia,* which can contaminate eggshells. With improper handling or processing, bacteria can remain on the shells.

Most eggs are sterile at creation, but can be contaminated as they exit the hen's body or sit on a surface. Cleaning protects the consumer from the bacteria. Eggs are washed with water between 90 and 120°F, rinsed with water and chlorine, and placed in refrigeration. No *Enterobacteriaceae* bacteria contamination occur the fifth week after processing.[8]

Eggshell and membranes under the shell provide a barrier that limits the ability of organisms to enter the egg. With 7,000 to 17,000 tiny pores, moisture and carbon dioxide move out and air moves in. A natural protective coating called "cuticle" preserves freshness and prevents microbial contamination. This coating is damaged or removed by processing, however, so a thin layer of oil is applied.

Using eggs within 10 weeks of storage showed no marked decrease in quality. Cooking foods with eggs at a high temperature actually destroyed harmful microbes.[8]

Review The Food Safety (Animal and Plant Products), and ARS National Program (No. 108) at www.nps.ars.usda.gov.

Freezer Storage Practices

Frozen foods should be frozen at 0°F or below. A thermometer should be kept in freezers, and foods should be arranged to allow air to circulate. Proper packaging can prevent freezer burn and protect foods. Potentially hazardous foods must be thawed in refrigerators below 40°F, under clean running water of 70°F or below, or in a microwave and must then be cooked immediately.

Dry Storage Practices

Dry storerooms should be monitored to protect the food from insects, rodents, high temperatures, and high humidity. A range of 55 to 70°F discourages bacterial action and food deterioration.

Hot Storage Practices

Potentially hazardous foods must have an internal temperature of 140°F or above during service or transportation.

Food Preparation and Service Procedures

Food should be touched rarely by human hands. Disposable plastic gloves are essential. Clean and sanitary utensils and preparation surfaces are essential to prevent cross-contamination from other foods. Raw fruits or vegetables should be thoroughly washed with clean, running water before being cooked or served. Poultry, poultry stuffing, stuffed meats, and stuffing containing meat must be cooked to 165°F or higher. Pork and any food containing pork must be cooked to at least 165°F. Rare roast beef must be cooked to an internal temperature of at least 130°F. Food served to a customer but not eaten should be discarded.

Food Transportation Practices

To prevent contamination during transportation (e.g., transfer to a school or congregate feeding site), food and food utensils must be covered, completely wrapped, or packaged. Hot foods must be 165°F or higher before they are placed in transport carts or containers, and cold foods must be at a temperature of 35°F. Written records of food temperatures before transport, upon arrival, and prior to service should be kept for a year.

A Review of Food Code 2005

To monitor and prevent food-borne diseases and ensure that consumers are provided the safest possible foods, the biennial food code revisions since 1999 have contained important components.[9]

- A food employee may drink from a closed beverage container if the container doesn't cross-contaminate their hands, other food, clean equipment, and cooking utensils.
- In certain settings, hand sanitizers and automatic hand-washing facilities may be used. Signage must be visible in lavatories to alert employees to wash their hands.
- A food employee may not wear fingernail polish or artificial fingernails when working with exposed food unless they wear intact gloves.
- Touching ready-to-eat food is prohibited. Only deli tissue, spatulas, tongs, single-use gloves or dispensing equipment can be used.
- In-use utensils and food contact surfaces must be cleaned and sanitized. Utensils used in preparation may be stored in water kept at or above 140°F.
- Food must be cooked so certain temperatures are achieved in all parts of the item, such as 145°F for pork and 158°F for hamburger.
- Raw or undercooked beef may be served if the surface is seared on both sides to a temperature of 145°F or above and a cooked color change is evident on all external surfaces.
- Fruits and vegetables may be washed using approved chemicals.
- Equipment and utensils used with potentially hazardous food may be cleaned less than every 4 hours, if they are kept below 41°F.

Food Code 2005 has 7 annexes:

- Annex 1: requirements for compliance and enforcement.
- Annex 2: references.
- Annex 3: the public health reasons/administrative guidelines.
- Annex 4: management of food safety practices—achieving active managerial control of food borne illness risk factors.
- Annex 5: conducting risk-based inspections.

Info Line

> The National Restaurant Association states that Americans eat 54 billion meals each year at 1 of 870,000 restaurants in the United States. Twenty-one percent of all meals are now carried away or delivered from a restaurant.
>
> Of the 70% of people who eat a carry-out meal at least once a week and the 90% who bring home leftovers, more than half didn't know the proper temperature for reheating a meal: 165°F. At least 75% admitted they would like a helpful reminder from restaurants about properly storing and reheating food.
>
> In June 2003, every leftovers and take-out container from a Francesca restaurant included a sticker with food safety information based on key messages from the ADA/ConAgra Foods Home Food Safety . . . It's in Your Hands consumer education initiative.
>
> The carry-out labels also include space for patrons to record the date they purchased the food and feature the Home Food Safety Web site address, www.homefoodsafety.org. The site offers consumers additional information on proper cooking and storage of food.
>
> Source: *ADA Times,* March-April 2004.

- Annex 6: food-processing criteria.
- Annex 7: model forms, guides, and other aids.

The complete Food Code 2005 is available at http://www.cfsan.fda.gov. Hard copies can be ordered at 703/605-6000, or the National Technical Information Service, 5285 Port Royal Road, Springfield, VA 22161. The order number is PB 2005-102200, and the cost is $60.

One 2005 dietary guideline regards keeping food safe. Safe equates to no or minimal risk of food-borne illness.

High-Risk Groups for Food-Borne Illness

Several groups are considered at high risk if they eat contaminated seafood. This includes individuals with liver disease, diabetes mellitus, immune disorders, and gastrointestinal disorders (see Exhibit 6–2). Children, pregnant women, older adults, individuals receiving chemotherapy or radiation treatment, and individuals suffering from a debilitating disease (e.g., diabetes) or who have a human immunodeficiency virus infection are at high risk for severe illness if they acquire a food-borne illness.[10,11]

Extra precautions for high-risk groups are:

- Do not eat or drink unpasteurized juices, raw sprouts, raw (unpasteurized) milk, and products made from unpasteurized milk.
- Do not eat raw or undercooked meat, poultry, eggs, fish, and shellfish (clams, oysters, scallops, and mussels).

Exhibit 6-2   FDA Warning and High-Risk Groups

The FDA warns that patients with diabetes are at serious risk of *Vibrio* infection from eating raw shellfish. While this infection is not a threat to most healthy patients, certain susceptible patients can be exposed to the infection by eating raw or undercooked molluscan shellfish (oysters, mussels, clams, and whole scallops). The population groups that are particularly vulnerable to severe illness or even death if they ingest contaminated seafood are those with liver disease, diabetes mellitus, immune disorders, and gastrointestinal disorders.

The high-risk season for raw shellfish consumption begins in April, when warmer water encourages the growth of the bacteria *Vibrio vulnificus*. The symptoms of the infection include fever, chills, nausea, vomiting, and abdominal pain. The bacteria are killed when shellfish are thoroughly cooked.

More information is available in a series of 4 brochures entitled, *Get Hooked on Seafood Safety*. For a free copy, write to: FDA, Seafood Brochures, HFI-40, 5600 Fishers Lane, Rockville, MD 20857. Indicate which brochure you want: diabetes mellitus, gastrointestinal disorders, immune disorders, or liver disease.

Source: American Diabetes Association. *Professional Section Newsletter.* Summer 1993.

A convenience sample of 40 assisted-living facilities provided samples from 4 contact surfaces (food preparation table or counter, steam-jacketed kettle or mixing bowl, and 2 cutting boards) and from 1 refrigerator or freezer handle. All samples were analyzed for aerobic plate count, *Enterobacteriaceae*, and *Staphylococcus aureus*. Using standard colony-forming units, aerobic plate counts were highest for cutting boards. Thirty-three facilities meet the standard for all 5 samples.[12]

Cross-contamination is possible even after cutting boards are sanitized in the dish machine. This is especially true if employees are noncompliant with hand washing. Almost one fourth of the cutting boards sampled had an *S. aureus* count indicating either inadequate sanitation or recontamination.

Implications for community nutrition professionals are that when supervising or consulting in assisted-living facilities[12]:

- standard operating procedures related to cleaning and sanitation should address cross-contamination
- cross-contamination may occur after cutting boards and equipment have been sanitized
- proper hand washing is important to reduce contamination
- hand washing between handling dirty and clean dishes must be emphasized

Control Procedures

In a report from the Centers for Disease Control and Prevention (CDC), 97% of most food illnesses are preventable if individuals would use improved food-handling practices.[3] A copy of the form developed by the CDC to investigate food-borne outbreaks is given in Exhibit 6-3.

Exhibit 6–3   Form for Investigating Outbreak of Food-Borne Illness

1. Where did the outbreak occur?	**2. Date of outbreak:** (Date of onset 1st case)
State _____	MO/DA/YR
City or town _____	Country _____

3. Indicate actual (a) or estimated (e) numbers:	4. History of exposed persons:	5. Incubation period (hours):
Persons exposed _____	No. histories obtained ____	Shortest ____ Longest ____
Persons ill _____	No. persons with symptoms ___	Approx. for majority ____
Hospitalized _____	Nausea _____	6. Duration of illness (hours) ____
Fatal cases _____	Diarrhea _____	Shortest ____ Longest ____
		Approx. for majority ____

7. Food-specific attack rates.

Food items served	Number of persons who *ate* specified food _____				Number who did *not* eat specified food _____			
	Ill	Not	Total	Percent ill	Ill	Not	Total	Percent ill

8. Vehicle responsible (food item incriminated by epidemiological evidence): _____

9. Manner in which incriminated food was marketed : (Mark all applicable)

			10. Place of preparation of contaminated item:	11. Place where eaten:
(a) Food industry	(c) Not wrapped........ Y N		Restaurant 1	Restaurant 1
Raw......... Y N	Ordinary wrapping.... Y N		Delicate 2	Delicatessen 2
Processed Y N	Canned.................... Y N		Cafeteria 3	Cafeteria 3
Home produced	Canned-vacuum sealed Y N		Private home 4	Private home 4
Raw......... Y N	Other (specify).......... Y N		Caterer 5	Picnic 5
Processed Y N			Institution:	Institution:
(b) Vending machine Y N	(d) Room temperature Y N		School 6	School 6
	Refrigerator.............. Y N		Church 7	Church 7
	Frozen...................... Y N		Camp 8	Camp 8
	Heated...................... Y N		Other, specify 9	Other, specify 9

If a commercial product, indicate brand name and lot number _____

Source: Reprinted with permission of the Centers for Disease Control and Prevention. US Department of Health and Human Services. Public Health Service. Atlanta, Ga.

The most common food-borne pathogens remain the same, decade after decade, creating an endemic rather than an epidemic or pandemic outbreak. The ways they can be controlled rarely change. The problems are the lack of basic knowledge by consumers and food handlers, and the lack of personal commitment to acceptable, safe procedures. For all foods, individuals should check the dates on the packages and not violate the keep refrigerated, sell-by, and use-by dates. Some specific guides for reducing exposure to or proliferation of common bacteria that cause food-borne illness follow.

Campylobacter jejuni

Campylobacter jejuni is commonly found in raw foods of animal origin.[13] Everyone should wash hands and utensils that contact raw meats prior to using the utensils with cooked foods. Use warm, soapy water. Cook ground meats (e.g., beef, pork, veal, and lamb) to an internal temperature of 160°F, and cook ground poultry to 165°F. Reheat leftovers to 160°F. Don't drink unpasteurized milk or other unpasteurized dairy products, don't drink untreated water, and don't eat raw or undercooked foods from animals. Do not allow dogs and pets in restaurants or other food preparation environments.

Clostridium perfringens

Clostridium perfringens contributed to major food-borne outbreaks recorded from 1978 to 1987.[3] CNPs should instruct food service employees to divide leftover roasts, turkey, stuffing, soups, stews, and casseroles into 2-inch-deep portions before cooling or freezing. They should reheat to 160°F and wash all soil off vegetables.

Escherichia coli

Escherichia coli has appeared as a major public health problem for North America.[3] The CNP must instruct food service staff to cook all ground meats to a uniform internal temperature of at least 160°F, ground poultry to 165°F, and non-ground meat cuts to 145°F. They should reheat foods to 160°F. They must avoid serving unprocessed fruit and vegetable juices and unpasteurized milk and milk products.

Salmonella

Salmonella was one of the most common microorganisms to cause food-borne illness during the past 30 years.[3] (Note: *Salmonella* always causes the largest percentage of cases.) Instruct employees to thaw poultry and meat in the refrigerator or microwave and cook them immediately after thawing. Food service workers should avoid cross-contamination of raw and cooked foods, utensils, and work surfaces. No one should ever eat unpasteurized, raw, or undercooked animal products. Cooks should cook ground meats to an internal temperature of 160°F, ground poultry to 165°F, and non-ground meat to 145°F. Keep cold foods at 40°F. Reheat leftovers to 160°F. Buy eggs from refrigerated cases.

Warning Associated With Raw Sprouts

The FDA has strongly advised consumers of the risks associated with eating raw sprouts, e.g., alfalfa, clover, and radish—for all persons, not just children, the elderly, and the immune-compromised—and told individuals not to eat raw sprouts due to their health risks.

In the past decade in the United States, raw sprouts have been implicated in over 1,300 cases of food-borne illness, involving *Salmonella* and *E. coli* 0157:H7. The growing time, temperature, water activity, pH, and nutrients are ideal for the rapid growth of bacteria.

The FDA issued and implemented 2 guidance documents:

1. *Steps to reduce microbial hazards.* These steps are common to sprout production, e.g., seed disinfection with solutions such as calcium hypochlorite.

Info Line

FDA ISSUES IMPORT ALERT ON CANTALOUPES
FROM MEXICO

On October 28, 2002, the FDA issued a nationwide import alert on
cantaloupes from Mexico because of unsanitary conditions that had
resulted in 4 salmonellosis outbreaks in the previous 3 years in the
United States. These outbreaks were responsible for many illnesses,
including 2 deaths and at least 18 hospitalizations. The import alert
recommended that officials detain, without physical examination,
cantaloupe from Mexico offered for entry at all US ports.

Investigations of *Salmonella* outbreaks between 2000 and 2002
showed unsanitary conditions in the growing and packing of cantaloupe in Mexico. In addition, FDA sampling of imported produce
found some samples of cantaloupe from most growing regions in
Mexico tested positive for *Salmonella*. The samples were collected
during both the fall/winter and spring/summer seasons. This import
alert expands prior import alerts that targeted specific shippers and
growers whose products were linked to outbreaks or tested positive
for *Salmonella*.

The FDA announced that it will continue to work with the
Mexican government on a food safety program for production, packing, and shipping of fresh cantaloupes. The Mexican government has
proposed a certification program based on good agricultural practices and current good manufacturing practices (CGMP) that would
allow FDA to identify farms that have adopted and implemented a
food safety program.

Salmonella is an organism that can cause serious and sometimes
fatal infections in young children, elderly people, and others with
weakened immune systems. Healthy persons infected with *Salmonella*
often experience fever, diarrhea (which may be bloody), nausea,
vomiting, and abdominal pain. In rare circumstances, infection with
Salmonella can result in the organism getting into the bloodstream
and producing more severe illnesses such as arterial infections,
endocarditis (an infection of the lining of the heart), and arthritis.

Source: Center for Food Safety and Applied Nutrition. *Enforcement Stories 2003.*
Washington, DC: FDA; 2003.

---

2. *Testing irrigation water.* The FDA monitors sprout safety and the
   adoption of prevention practices and enforces actions against
   producers without preventive controls.[14]

Cheese Preservative Kills Superbugs

Breukink et al studied a peptide called nisin, which is added to cheese to kill
botulism. It is both nontoxic to human beings and highly effective in killing

Info Line

GROCERY CHAIN RECALLS GROUND BEEF AFTER *E. COLI* OUTBREAK

In December of 2000 ground beef suspected of *E. coli* contamination was pulled off the shelves at Cub grocery stores in Minnesota, Wisconsin, Chicago, Illinois, and Indiana. American Foods Group Inc recalled 1.1 million pounds of ground beef sent to stores in 15 states in early November.

The Minnesota Department of Health investigated 22 cases of *E. coli* poisoning with links to ground beef in which 8 people were hospitalized, including a 2-year-old girl who suffered from life-threatening complications of the infection.

---

gram-positive bacteria.[15] In a unique process, it blocks the development of the lipophilic cell membrane and seeks out Lipid II, punching a hole in the cell wall, killing the bacteria cell in less than 1 minute. The US Food and Drug Administration lists nisin as a generally recognized safe food additive, and it is safe for human beings even in larger doses. [16]

New Food-Borne Pathogens

We are experiencing an era of new food-borne pathogens (see Table 6–2). Much of this is the result of environmental and societal changes, especially lifestyle. For example, the organic and natural food industry had over $4 billion in sales in the 1990s even though these products cost 20 to 25% more than conventional items.[5,17] The demand for natural foods, minimally processed foods, novel or innovative food processes, and changes in agricultural practices and distribution are some of the factors behind this new order of food-borne pathogens.

TABLE 6–2   Food-Borne Pathogens for the 21st Century

Pathogen Status	Type
Previously unrecognized	*Salmonella enteritidis* *Vibrio vulnificus* Norwalk virus *Escherichia coli* 0157:H7
Not previously recognized as agents of food-borne disease	*Yersinia enterocolitica* *Listeria monocytogenes* *Campylobacter jejuni*
Recognized as an agent of food-borne disease, now able to grow in unique situations	*Clostridium botulinum* Conventional botulism Infant botulism

Source: Adapted from: Matthews ME, Theis M. Relationship between the environment, the food supply and the practice of dietetics: research agenda conference. *J Am Diet Assoc.* 1993; 93(9):1045-1049.

Listeria monocytogenes (L. monoc) is a bacterium that can cause a serious infection in humans called listeriosis, producing an estimated 2,500 serious illnesses and 500 deaths annually.

When this affects pregnant women, it can result in miscarriage, fetal death, and severe illness or death of a newborn infant. Older adults and those with weakened immune systems are at risk for severe illness or death. In May 2000, then-President Clinton directed the Secretary of Health and Human Services and the Secretary of Agriculture, who co-chair the President's Council on Food Safety, to identify aggressive steps to reduce significantly the risk of illness and death from *L. monoc* in ready-to-eat foods.

The intent was a 50% reduction in the number of *Listeria*-related illnesses by 2005, which was 5 years ahead of the previously established *Healthy People 2010* target. Risk assessment will predict the potential relative risk of listeriosis among perinatal, elderly, and intermediate-age people from eating ready-to-eat foods within 20 categories or principal sources of *L. monoc*. Potential vehicles of listeriosis are fresh soft cheeses, smoked seafood, frankfurters (hot dogs), and some foods from deli counters. Factors affecting consumer exposure are:

- amount or frequency of consumption of a food
- frequency and levels of *L. monoc* in ready-to-eat food
- potential to support growth of *L. monoc* in food during refrigerated storage
- refrigerated storage temperature
- duration of refrigerated storage before consumption

To ensure food safety and because *Listeria monoc* grows at refrigerator temperatures, the FDA and Food Safety and Inspection Service (FSIS) advise all consumers to reduce the risk of illness by using perishable items that are precooked or ready to eat as soon as possible; cleaning their refrigerators regularly; and using a refrigerator thermometer to ensure a temperature of 40°F or below.

Info Line

USDA Meat and Poultry Hotline—Monday-Friday, 10 AM-4 PM (Eastern time), (800) 535-4555

Centers for Disease Control and Prevention Food-borne Illness Line 24-hour recorded information: (404) 332-4597. In Washington, DC: (202) 720-3333

National Live Stock and Meat Board—Consumer Information Department, 444 North Michigan Ave, Chicago, IL 60611. Monday-Friday, 9:30 AM to 5:30 PM (Eastern time), (312) 467-5520

County Extension Home Economists—Look in phone book under county government, cooperative extension service, or a state university.

Food and Drug Administration, Rockville, Md, (888) SAFE-FOOD, www.foodsafety.gov.

Preparing for Community Emergencies

A community emergency is an unforeseen combination of circumstances that calls for immediate action, such as an earthquake, flood, hurricane, or tornado. Such a definition can encompass a wide array of circumstances, even in the area of food and nutrition. The first rule is for households to always keep a supply of familiar, easy-to-prepare, nonperishable basic foods on hand, replacing each item as it is eaten.

Water is an absolute necessity for life, and in times of emergency it may be the scarcest resource. A 72-hour supply (3 gallons per family member) is needed for food preparation and personal cleansing. In an emergency, immediately shut off the water and use the uncontaminated supply in the toilet tank and water heater. Use discarded water to flush commodes. If one suspects that the water supply is contaminated, purify by boiling, or by using 16 drops of household bleach per gallon or 24 drops of iodine per gallon, until water appears clear. Purification tablets may also be used and can be purchased at local sporting goods stores.[18]

Authorities recommend that at least a 3-day supply of food for each family member be available in the event of an emergency. Ideally, these foods should be stored separately, apart from the cupboard basics. A nutrition survival plan should include the following[18]:

- the top 10 staples (see Exhibit 6–4)
- infant food needs
- pet food (for the family friend)
- barbecue and briquettes (outdoors only)
- comfort foods, such as instant coffee, cocoa, nuts, raisins, instant pudding

Minimum quantities should be planned per family member for a 3-day period:

- milk: four 12-oz cans low-fat, evaporated milk
- fruits and vegetables: five 15-oz cans, assorted

Exhibit 6–4   The Top 10 Long-Lasting, Nutritious, and Inexpensive Staples for Emergency Use

---

- pasta, rice, and canned or instant potatoes
- all-purpose biscuit mix
- canned fruits, vegetables, and juices
- peanut butter
- canned meats, chicken, and fish
- powdered and canned milk
- canned stew or other main dishes
- canned or dried beans (all types)
- quick-cooking or enriched dry cereals
- canned or dried soups

Source: California Dietetic Association. *Nutrition Survival Plan: A Food Guide for Emergencies, Big and Small.* Playa del Rey, Calif: CA Dietetic Asso; 1990.

- protein: three 6-oz cans of meat, or three 1-cup servings of beans
- cereals, pastas, and crackers: 9 cups or 72 crackers

Storage and maintenance tips include:

- Store foods in a dry, cool area, below 70°F.
- Containers should be water resistant and dated.
- Store in basement or garage.
- Rotate foods into normal eating patterns every 3-6 months to maintain freshness.

In case of an emergency, items in Table 6–3 provide a 3-day supply in the form of a supply checklist. A smaller version of this kit should be stored in the trunk of your car. All items should be kept in sturdy, easy-to-carry containers such as backpacks, duffel bags, or sealable plastic containers (like trash containers or storage bins). Keep important family documents in an easy-to-access waterproof and fireproof container. Put copies of vital records in a safe deposit container. Consider photographing or videotaping all valuables and keeping those records in the safe deposit box as well. Personal identification may be required for emergency food, shelter, and medical care.

Hazard Analysis and Critical Control Points in Food Service

HACCP, pronounced "haysap," is an acronym for hazard analysis and critical control points. This is a term for a food safety system for food service directors to prevent contamination of the food served to clients.[19]

HACCP was created in 1965 by Pillsbury Company. Pillsbury was selected by the National Aeronautics and Space Administration to provide food for US astronauts during extended space missions. The food had to be virtually 100% free of contamination. Pillsbury devised a prevention-oriented system of quality control by starting at the very beginning of food preparation. This HACCP system is applied in all steps of the preparation process. It starts with the selection of vendors and ends when the meal is eaten.

Community nutrition professionals (CNPs) are generally not involved in the inspection or remediation process, but it might be wise to rethink the situation. A merger between CNPs, who plan and oversee food production, and environmental specialists, who inspect and monitor food production facilities, seems practical.

The *HA* in HACCP, *hazard analysis*, is the identification of any potentially hazardous ingredient or food preparation method. The *CCP* in HACCP, *critical control point*, is any food preparation step where loss of control could result in an unacceptable health risk (see Exhibit 6–5).

Food Service Standards and Regulations

Regulations and standards for food service sanitation and safety are enforced at the local, state, and federal levels. Local environmental health departments manage these tasks to reduce infectivity in hospitals, schools, nursing homes, correctional facilities, and any type of food production or preparation and service facility. Standards require that appropriate safeguards against contamination exist. HACCP principles can be integrated into existing regulations and standards using *HACCP Principles for Food Production*.[20]

TABLE 6–3 Three-Day Emergency Supply Checklist

One gallon of water per person per day (stored water supplies should be replaced every 3 months).	A battery-powered radio.	An ax.	Feminine hygiene supplies.
Food that won't spoil (stored food supplies should be replaced every 6 months).	A flashlight.	A shovel.	Toilet paper.
One change of clothing, sturdy shoes, a rain poncho, and one blanket or sleeping bag per person.	A whistle.	A broom.	Paper towels.
A first aid kit that includes your family's prescription medications (check dates).	Extra batteries, all sizes.	A tool kit (including a screwdriver, pliers, a hammer, and an adjustable wrench for turning off the gas main).	A nonelectric can opener.
An extra pair of glasses.	Heavy gloves.	A coil of ½-inch rope.	Plastic utensils, paper plates, cups.
A credit card, cash, and coins (ATM machines will not work during power outage).	Light sticks.	Large plastic trash bags.	A cooking stove, aluminum foil, and at least one small pan.
An extra set of car keys.	A knife or razor blades.	Tarps.	Pet supplies: leashes, food, water.
A city map.	An ABC-type fire extinguisher approved for use on regular and electric fires.	Soap, detergent, and shampoo.	Special items for infant, elderly, or disabled family members.
Paper, pens, and stamps.	A water-purification kit or household bleach.	Toothpaste/toothbrushes.	

Source: "Three-Day Emergency Supply Checklist" from www.redcross.org. Courtesy of the American National Red Cross. All rights reserved in all countries.

Exhibit 6-5   Steps in the HACCP System

---

1. Assess hazards.
2. Determine critical points.
3. Establish limits.
4. Develop monitoring plan.
5. Devise corrective action.
6. Organize recordkeeping.
7. Verify reliability of system.

Source: HACCP: making the system work. *Food Engineering.* August 1988;7:70-80.

Food service employees are trained in food safety precautions to maintain acceptable standards and can be taught HACCP principles during ongoing in-service sessions. *Applied Food-Service Sanitation,* a resource for directors, covers HACCP guidelines and employee sanitation training.[7]

Food manufacturers can analyze their products for microbes before they are distributed to the general public.[21] Major microbes in food, where they are found, and how to control them are as follows: *Salmonella* found in poultry, meat, and eggs is controlled by cooking thoroughly; *S. aureus* found in high-protein foods and foods kept at room temperature for prolonged periods can be controlled by keeping hot foods hot and cold foods cold; *C. perfringens* found in beef, poultry, and leftover foods is controlled by cooking thoroughly, chilling rapidly, and reheating leftovers thoroughly; *C. jejuni* found in meat, poultry, and fish must be cooked thoroughly to control; and *C. botulinum* found in home-canned foods and tightly wrapped cooked potatoes, meatloaf, meat pies, and stews can be controlled by using commercially canned foods, chilling rapidly, and reheating leftovers thoroughly. The importance of preparing a safe product for clients is clear because there is no opportunity for second chances in a food service setting. Food-borne illness can have devastating consequences.

Developing a HACCP System

Not all products require extensive methods for quality control. Individually packaged prepared food products, such as crackers, muffins, chips, and cookies, have a low potential for food-borne illness.

The important first step is to identify and to evaluate any food products or preparation procedures that have potential for causing food-borne illness. For example, the potential hazards in serving canned peaches would be far less than the potential hazards for preparing ground beef for tacos. Ground beef has a high potential for bacterial contamination and goes through several critical steps in its preparation—storing, thawing, cooking, and holding. Canned peaches are free from bacterial contamination and do not require many handling steps by the food service workers.

Ground beef for tacos is used as an example to illustrate the steps of the HACCP system:

Step 1: Assess hazards associated with growing and harvesting raw materials and ingredients, processing, manufacturing, distributing, marketing, preparing, and consuming the food. Each food item served by the food service organization would undergo this assessment. The hazard associated with ground beef is the potential for bacterial contamination.

Step 2: Determine critical control points required to control the identified hazards. The critical control points for ground beef preparation are those steps when hazardous microorganisms need to be controlled or destroyed. Vendor selection is important to ensure that the raw product is processed and handled according to US Department of Agriculture protocol. Storing, defrosting, cooking, holding, and possibly chilling and reheating are all critical steps for control of bacterial contamination.

Step 3: Establish the critical limits that must be met at each identified critical control point. Each critical control point in food preparation must have specific limits, such as time and temperature. For example, ground beef should be kept frozen in a freezer no higher than 0°F. The meat should be defrosted in such a way as to keep its temperature below 45°F, and it should be held at a temperature of greater than 140°F. Raw ground beef should be kept separate from cooked or prepared foods at all times.

Step 4: Develop procedures to monitor critical control points. A monitoring schedule must be established. The temperature of the freezer in which the ground beef is stored is probably already monitored in an organization. Continuous monitoring of critical control points is important because of the possibility for food contamination if these limits are not met (e.g., freezer temperature greater than 0°F).

Step 5: Devise corrective action to be taken when there is a deviation identified by monitoring a critical control point. The limit for the critical control point of cooking ground beef is that the beef must be cooked to 165°F. If the supervisor sees an area of beef that is not fully cooked and still pink, then this likely occurred because the cook failed to stir the ground beef thoroughly while cooking. A corrective action would be to stir the ground beef immediately to attain even heating. Long-term correction of this problem would be to add this step of frequent stirring to the list of critical limits.

Step 6: Organize effective recordkeeping systems to document the HACCP plan. This step is important because the food service director may keep and use these records for continuous improvement of the organization. These records may also be made available to regulatory agencies to show compliance to specific standards.

Step 7: Verify that the HACCP system is working correctly. This step is carried out by retracing the flow of ground beef during its path to reach the consumers. Reports of food poisoning should be reviewed and recorded. Controls and procedures can be reviewed periodically. Adjustments can be made to improve the food preparation process.

Food safety, along with sensory quality and client acceptance, has always been a top priority among food service operations. Over the years, food service systems in the United States have done a good job preventing food contamination. However, an immaculate and sanitary kitchen will not suffice for preventing food contamination. HACCP is an approach to ensure that food safety is integrated into the whole food path from purchase to service.

Four Priority Areas for Reducing Food-Borne Disease

Doyle outlined 4 priority areas for reducing food-borne disease.[22] These are:

1. *Emphasize risk analysis, management, and communications.* Since many foods carry an inherent risk because of the occurrence of microbial pathogens, foods could be regulated on the basis of risk. Information systems can identify foods most often associated with illnesses, identify minimum infectious dose of harmful microorganisms, determine the survival and growth characteristics of food pathogens, and determine which pathogens may or may not be tolerable in certain foods.
2. *Develop innovative approaches to produce pathogen-free foods from animals.* Innovative yet practical approaches to reduce external contamination of foods during slaughter and processing are needed to reduce the conveyance of pathogens by animals.
3. *Conduct research to support the implementation of effective HACCP programs.* Current areas needing further research are procedures to detect and to isolate pathogens in the facilities where food is processed.

Info Line

The routine measures that can be used to control further food-borne outbreaks are as follows:

1. Collect appropriate specimens for laboratory analysis, and then destroy remaining foods to prevent their consumption.
2. Prevent a recurrent event by:
   a. educating food handlers in proper food preparation and storage techniques; stress the importance of time-temperature associations
   b. acquiring necessary equipment for properly cooking, cooling, serving, and storing foods
   c. eliminating sources of contaminated food when applicable
3. Implement basic principles in prevention of the pathogen, such as for *C. perfringens*:
   a. Cook all foods to minimum internal temperature of 165°F.
   b. Serve immediately or hold at > 140°F.
   c. Discard any leftovers, or immediately chill and hold food at < 40°F in shallow pans.
   d. Reheat all leftovers and hold at proper temperatures.

The rationale for working up an outbreak is as follows:

1. to identify factors associated with the outbreak occurrence and to institute the necessary measures to prevent future recurrences
2. to document that a premeditated and deliberate act of poisoning was not involved
3. to demonstrate that public health officials can react promptly to a problem and identify causative factors using epidemiologic methods

Source: Reproduced with permission of Paige R, Cole G, Timmrock T. *Basic Epidemiologic Methods and Biostatistics.* Boston, Mass: Jones and Bartlett Publishers; 1993.

Procedures currently take 1-4 days to isolate pathogens. Tests that require minutes or hours would allow processors to respond with quick, corrective action when pathogens are detected. Steps can be applied at critical points to destroy pathogens. Innovative, practical methods are needed in food-processing plants.

4. *Develop innovative approaches to educate consumers and food preparers about proper food-handling practices.* Improper handling of foods by consumers at home and by employees in commercial food preparation has increased the incidence of salmonellosis. New approaches are needed to educate consumers and food preparers about proper food preparation and storage techniques and to clarify the risks of food-borne illness from eating raw or undercooked foods of animal origin.

Pesticides in Foods

To combat damage to crops by insects, pesticides were introduced. Americans are as concerned about exposing their families to pesticides as they are about food-borne illnesses. Foods are not the only source of pesticides in the environment. Pets, home gardens, parks, and specialty gardens can all embody pesticides and residues. However, home and private application of pesticides is not monitored by the FDA to the degree that growers are regulated. Reports from recent federal and state monitoring indicate no detectable residues in 90% or more of food test samples. When residues are detected, however, they are only a fraction of the FDA tolerance level.[23]

The FDA's total diet study is performed annually and gives a very accurate comparison of pesticide exposure estimates using health criteria.[24] The procedure involves purchasing foods at retail outlets and in table-ready form. Analysis reveals that infants and children are exposed to pesticide residues at less than 1% of the allowable level based on long-term animal toxicology studies.

Important information that frames the discussion about pesticides includes the fact that different quantities of different pesticides produce a toxic effect on humans. A child's exposure to pesticides is greater than an adult's, because children tend to eat a narrower range of foods, consume more processed foods, and ingest more food per kilogram of body weight. The exposure of children to pesticides varies by geographic region.[23]

The Environmental Working Group's 1994 report, *Washed, Peeled, Contaminated: Pesticide Residues in Ready-to-Eat Fruits and Vegetables*,[25] has voiced selective concern for pesticide exposure to children. The report recommends an increase in the availability and promotion of certified organic foods.[26] Reviewers of the report make the following points[25]:

- Dose makes the poison. It is the amount of pesticide residue—not merely its presence or absence—that determines harm.
- The report did not include a risk assessment to calculate estimates of infant and child exposures to pesticides.
- The wording of the report implies that washing and peeling do not eliminate residues, which is incorrect.
- It is important to differentiate between *reduction* and *elimination* of pesticide residues.

Info Line

The Food and Drug Administration publishes an annual pesticide program report, Residue Monitoring, in the *J AOAC Int.*

A well-publicized scare involved daminozide (trade name Alar) in 1989. Daminozide is a plant growth regulator that has been used on apples and other fruits. The Natural Resources Defense Council released a report, *Intolerable Risk: Pesticides in Our Children's Food.* After the hysteria from the report and an apple boycott, factual information emerged. This included acknowledging that no human cancers had ever been linked to Alar and that no well-designed clinical trials had ever been conducted on Alar to warrant a ban on its use. Later, in a well controlled study with mice, a dose more than 250,000 times the highest amount thought consumable by children was used. No tumors were noted in the mice.[27]

Pesticides

Pesticides have 2 major functions: to regulate plant growth and to prevent crop damage caused by insects, weeds, and plant disease. Herbicides are the most common pesticides and are used to control weeds. Insecticides and fungicides control insects and plant disease. As a result of the concern over pesticides in foods and the cost of pesticides, new ways have been developed to produce crops and to replace the exclusive use of pesticides. One approach is the use of compounds that are highly specific to certain pests and that require only a small dosage. A new agricultural approach called integrated pest management (IPM) seeks alternatives that produce the least impact on the environment.[23]

IPM techniques have been used by the state of Washington apple growers to control mites, moths, and apple scab. To control mites, miticides are replaced with predator mites. The codling moth is controlled by the use of pheromone, a natural sex-attractant odor that traps moths by disrupting mating patterns. To control apple scab, a fungal disease that attacks leaves and fruit, farmers use a moisture timetable and spray at the peak of potential attack.[28]

Irradiated Foods

A new germ-killing technology has evolved from research at the University of Missouri and Iowa State University. Food processors can irradiate their products with an electron beam accelerator. Titan Corporation unveiled e-beam technology, or SureBeam, in Sioux City, Iowa, where chicken and ground beef producers will use the SureBeam to irradiate frozen meat for test marketing. Suppliers of soft drinks, produce, fruit juices, baked goods, and even pet foods are interested in using the technology due to public concern about food poisoning.[29] With an estimated 76 million cases of food-borne illness annually in the United States, e-beams can eliminate *Salmonella, E. coli, Campylobacter, Listeria,* and other disease-producing germs. The electron beam accelerator has a cathode creating a stream of electrons while a simultaneous high voltage is applied to accelerate the electrons. In effect, a pencil-thin, high-energy e-beam strikes the food. The DNA of bacteria dies or becomes unable to reproduce as the beam damages or destroys it instantaneously. After the process, consumers must handle and prepare the irradiated foods; food safety remains in the hands of the preparer. In January 2000, the USDA published regulations governing irradiation of pork chops, hamburger, steaks, and other raw meat.

Consumer Acceptance of Irradiated Foods

Consumer demand for irradiated foods increased twofold in the year 2000 above usual demand. One company expanded its distribution of irradiated meat patties from Minnesota to 4 other states in 2000 and expected further expansion. Irradiation is approved for disinfecting poultry, spices, fruit, and vegetables. The real challenge is convincing the public that the food is safe. Irradiation may destroy substantial amounts of vitamins and may cause chemical reactions in foods that create cancer-causing substances. The latter condition scares the public and will remain an area of research. Another issue is that processors cannot turn to irradiation instead of improving sanitation to keep contaminants off meat.

Carol Tucker Foreman, a distinguished fellow with the Consumer Federation of America, a coalition of consumer groups, believes the scientific evidence. She supports use of irradiated foods first to hospitals and nursing homes, and then to people with weakened immune systems, such as AIDS patients. The USDA is requiring that irradiated products carry a statement of treatment and be labeled with the international symbol for irradiation, called a radura. [29] The issue will solicit a debate well into the new millennium.

Info Line

HISTORY OF FOOD IRRADIATION

Food irradiation is not new to the United States. The first patents for the process were granted to the United States and the United Kingdom in 1905. A French scientist in the 1920s recognized that irradiation extended the life of easily perishable foods. US Army scientists studied irradiation effects on fruits, dairy products, vegetables, and meat during World War II. These studies tested irradiation effects on microorganism and nutrient content and on potential toxicity.

The Food and Drug Administration approved irradiation for poultry, pork, fruits, vegetables, grains, and spices. The benefits include increasing the shelf life of sweet onions to 3 months, for example, or for mushrooms to 3 weeks without browning or cap separation.[30]

Food Safety Comes to the Media

A joint national campaign promoting food safety was initiated by the American Dietetic Association and ConAgra in 1999. CNPs can interpret and convert food science and hygiene tenets into 4 key messages:

1. *Wash hands often.* Nearly 50% of people wash their hands during meal preparation; however, significantly more women than men wash their hands throughout the cooking process. Frequent hand washing could eliminate nearly half of all cases of food-borne illness.
2. *Keep raw meats and ready-to-eat foods separate.* About 75% of people use 2 separate plates: 1 for raw meats, poultry, or seafood, and 1 for cooked foods when grilling, but 40% of men shake off the plate and reuse it for cooked meats. When juices from raw meats touch cooked or ready-to-eat foods, cross-contamination occurs.
3. *Cook to proper temperatures.* Eight out of 10 people don't believe that a thermometer helps meats taste better. Cooking to proper temperatures is a major way to ensure food safety, not alter taste.
4. *Refrigerate promptly below 40°F.* Three quarters of people know that foods should be refrigerated in hot weather (> 90°F). More men than women, however, believe that it's OK to leave food out longer than 1 hour. Storing foods promptly at under 40°F slows the growth of bacteria and prevents food-borne illness.

FDA's Strategic Priorities

The FDA has the following 4 strategic priorities to reinforce *prevention* as their primary response to the nation's health and safety[31]:

1. *Assuring a safe food supply*: to assure the safety of 80% of the US food supply and annually monitor more than 4 million food import entries into the United States. That includes 50% of all seafood and > 20% of the fresh fruits and vegetables consumed by Americans. The FDA is working with partners to significantly reduce food-borne illnesses and deaths. Prevention strategies based on strong scientific research and risk assessment are implemented through a nationwide inspection program in partnership with the states.
2. *Assuring medical product safety*: to ensure that drugs, vaccines, and medical devices are safe. The FDA conducts more than 15,000 inspections each year to assure proper manufacturing and distribution by monitoring performance and use.
3. *Managing emerging hazards*: to assess and effectively reduce risks associated with unexpected threats to Americans, e.g., bioterrorism, AIDS, and bovine spongiform encephalopathy (BSE), or mad cow disease.
4. *Bringing new technologies to market*: to ensure that the products of new technologies are available to consumers, e.g., medicines, biologics, and medical devices.

Bioterrorism

The devastating events of September 11, 2001, have caused Americans to take many defensive measures to prepare for another possible attack. Concerns include food-borne pathogens, chemical toxicities, or systems that have evolved to control the unintentional harm to food. The induction of the HACCP monitoring system in many food service operations is an example of a science-based process implemented to regulate and enforce food safety concerns. While it remains important to ensure food is safe for consumption and to protect food and water from contamination against food-borne illnesses, we also have the responsibility to protect food and water supplies from intentional contamination. Past terrorist actions have prompted federal, state, and local agencies and organizations to develop preventive and awareness plans to protect against intentional tampering with our country's most vulnerable resource.[32]

The World Health Organization has passed a resolution to respond to natural occurrence, accidental release, or deliberate use of biological and chemical agents or radionuclear material that affect health. Four main areas are: international preparedness; global alert and response; national preparedness; and preparedness for selected disease and intoxication to serve as a guide to strengthen existing international networks of experts on various aspects of chemical and biological agents.[33]

The Department of Homeland Security (DHS) is responsible for protecting the United States against further terrorist attacks by analyzing threats and coordinating response during emergencies. Twenty-two federal agencies collaborate to confront any threats to the country, educate other organizations and citizens, and prepare for future emergencies. DHS enhances public services, such as natural disaster assistance and citizenship services and dedicates offices to these important missions.[34] The US Congress passed the Public Health Security and Bioterrorism Preparedness and Response Act of 2002 (Bioterrorism Act of 2002). The Bioterrorism Act of 2002 requires institutions to notify the DHHS or the USDA of the possession of specific pathogens or toxic agents and provides for expanded regulatory monitoring of these agents and procedures for limiting access to them.[35]

Food and water are essential to life; the food and water supplies are vulnerable biological and chemical targets. Agriculture, food processors, and food service operations such as those found in hospitals and schools may become direct targets or may be threatened in any part of the food chain. The Food and Drug Administration has designed 4 guidance documents designed to minimize the risk of malicious tampering with the food and water supplies. With responsibility for more than 80% of the nation's food supply, the FDA has initiated the following new activities[36]: (1) formulate partnerships with the food industry to reduce threats, (2) increase the surveillance of the domestic food industry, (3) increase monitoring of imported foods, and (4) enhance collaboration with other government agencies.

The National Food Service Management Institute (NFSMI), supported by the USDA's Food and Nutrition Service, has developed a comprehensive guide for school food service operations. Many schools and hospitals serve as sites for emergency shelters during times of crisis and are also vulnerable potential targets for terrorist attacks. The Emergency Readiness Plan: A Guide for the School Foodservice Operations serves as a comprehensive guide for school food service departments to ensure the health and safety of customers and employees.

The 6-step plan also has forms to assist school food service organizations with organizing and developing their facility's emergency management plan.[37]

Most hospitals and long-term care facilities are required to also prepare and implement emergency management plans. The Joint Commission on Accreditation of Healthcare Organizations (JCAHO) has developed a bioterrorism plan for healthcare facilities to modify their existing emergency management plan. The new plan encourages healthcare organizations to integrate departmental emergency plans into a single, integrated system of response. The plan will require organizations to conduct annual emergency drills to ensure that the plan is functional for various types of emergencies and to correct any problem identified during the drill. JCAHO will also require facilities to educate their employees about potential hazards and establish reporting procedures to officials and the community.[38]

Animal Hazards

Foot-and-Mouth Disease Questions and Answers

Q: What is foot-and-mouth disease?
A: Foot-and-mouth disease (FMD) is an incurable, highly contagious, and economically devastating disease that affects cattle, pigs, sheep, goats, deer, and other cloven-hooved ruminants. The disease spreads widely and rapidly. Nearly every exposed animal becomes infected. If the disease grew to be widespread in any country, the economic impact could be severe. The disease is rarely fatal. It can result in decline in milk production from dairy cattle and goats, decline in meat production, possible sterility of animals, chronic lameness, and chronic mastitis. The most serious effects would result from the need to destroy animals—infected as well as healthy—in order to eradicate the disease. In March, Great Britain reported that more than 170,000 sheep, cows, and pigs had been slaughtered since an outbreak that began in February 2001.
Q: Is FMD a danger to people?
A: No. The disease does not affect food safety or people.
Q: How many cases have been reported in the United States?
A: None since 1929, in which there was an outbreak that was quickly contained and eradicated. In March 2001, USDA said: "As part of a routine foreign animal disease investigation, the US Department of Agriculture can confirm that no cases of foot-and-mouth disease exist in the United States."[39]
Q: What is the government doing to protect the United States from foot-and-mouth disease?
A: USDA regularly monitors for any disease among US cattle herds and takes steps to prevent FMD from spreading to the United States whenever there is an outbreak in other countries. In February 2001, USDA restricted the importation of live swine and ruminants and any fresh swine or ruminant meat (chilled or frozen) or products from Great Britain or Northern Ireland, retroactive to imports since mid-January.[39]
Q: What should travelers do if they are planning to visit a farm or are in contact with livestock while abroad?
A: Baggage of all returning travelers who indicate they have been on a farm or in contact with livestock will be inspected. Soiled footwear should be disinfected with detergent and bleach. If travelers are around livestock in the United Kingdom and have livestock at home in the United States, they

should avoid contact with their animals for 5 days after returning. Soiled clothing must be washed and disinfected prior to returning to the United States.

Bovine Spongiform Encephalopathy

Table 6–4 provides detailed questions and answers regarding the USDA management of bovine spongiform encephalopathy.

Hepatitis C

Approximately 1.8% of the US population and over 170 million people worldwide have been infected with hepatitis C. In California, 500,000 may be infected with hepatitis, and many do not know they are sick. Chronic disease is estimated nationally at 2.7 million people.

TABLE 6–4 Bovine Spongiform Encephalopathy Questions and Answers

Question	Answer
What is mad cow disease?	Formally known as bovine spongiform encepahlopathy, or BSE, it is a transmissible, degenerative, and fatal disease affecting the central nervous system of adult cattle. BSE was first diagnosed in 1986.
How does the United States handle a BSE diagnosis?	The US Department of Agriculture announced on December 23, 2003, a presumptive diagnosis of BSE in an adult Holstein cow from Washington State. Beef products from Washington, Oregon, California, Nevada, Alaska, Hawaii, Montana, Idaho, and Guam were recalled from estabishments that may have received these products.
Does BSE affect humans?	BSE is believed to be linked to a brain-wasting illness in humans known as variant Creutzfeldt-Jakob disease (vCJD).
How many cases of vCJD have been reported?	The Centers for Disease Control and Prevention documents 153 vCJD cases reported worldwide as of December 1, 2003. Of these, 143 cases occurred in the United Kingdom.
Is vCJD presently in the United States?	According to the CDC, there have been no reported cases of vCJD in the United States, except one case who was a young woman and likely contracted it while living in the United Kingdom.
What should I do if I purchase beef in one of the states affected by a recall?	Contact the store where you purchased the beef.
What is the risk for contracting vCJD?	Risk is very low after eating BSE-contaminated beef in the United States, even following the December 2003 announcement.
Why is the risk so low?	According to the USDA, the agent that causes mad cow disease is found only in cattle's central nervous system tissue, such as the brain and spinal column. It is not found in muscle tissue—the source of roasts, steaks, and other beef cuts.

continued

TABLE 6–4 Bovine Spongiform Encephalopathy Questions and Answers   continued

Question	Answer
If I'm still concerned about what types of beef to eat, what should I do?	If you remain concerned, choose cuts of muscle meats; make your own ground beef from muscle cuts, or buy ground muscle cuts in the market.
Can BSE infection be transmitted through milk?	Research studies show no evidence of transmission of BSE infection through milk or milk products.
What safeguards are in place to protect consumers in the United States from BSE?	Since 1997, the FDA has restricted the importation of live animals and products including meat and meat-and-bone meal not only from countries where BSE is known to exist, but also from countries thought to be at high risk for BSE, even if the disease hasn't been identified in those countries. FDA prohibits the use of most mammalian protein in the manufacture of animal feeds given to ruminants because this kind of feeding practice is believed to have initiated and amplified the outbreak of BSE in the United Kingdom.
Does the United States import beef from countries where BSE is present in animals?	No. USDA's Animal and Plant Health Inspection Service restricts the import of live ruminants, like cows and sheep, and food products from these animals from BSE countries since 1989, and from all European countries since 1997. No meat products used in human, animal, and pet foods from the 31 countries identified as having BSE or at risk for having BSE are allowed into the United States. Milk and milk products continue to be imported into the United States from these countries.
Where can I call for the latest information?	Consumers with food safety questions can phone the USDA's toll-free English and Spanish Meat and Poultry Hotline at 888/MPHotline; 10 A.M. to 4 P.M. (Eastern time), Monday through Friday. Recorded food safety messages are available 24 hours a day; or visit http://www.fsis.usda.gov/Food_Safety_Education/USDA_Meat_&_Poultry_Hotline/index.asp.
Where can I find more information on BSE?	From the following Web sites: American Dietetic Assoctiation: www.eatright.org. Click on the Food and Nutrition Information tab in the left of the ADA home page. ADA's position statement on food and water safety: www.eatright.org/ US Department of Agriculture: www.usda.gov and www.aphis.usda.gov/lpa/issues/bse/bse.html Food and Drug Administration: www.fda.gov Centers for Disease Control and Prevention: www.cdc.gov/ncidod/diseases/diseases/index.htm National Cattlemen's Beef Association: www.bseinfo.org Pan American Health Organization: www.paho.org World Health Organization: www.who.int/esr/disease/bse/en American Culinary Federation: www.acfchefs.org/media/

Sources: Compiled from information provided by the USDA, FDA, CDC, Beef Association, PAHO, WHO, and ACF.

TABLE 6–5 Travel Precautions—Dietary Alerts

	What?	How?	Signs and Symptoms	What Considerations?
HIV/AIDS	HIV is a virus that attacks the immune system. HIV may lead to AIDS. Currently, there is no cure for HIV or AIDS. AIDS kills 3 million people in the world each year.	HIV is passed by exchanging body fluids (blood, semen, vaginal fluids) during sex (anal, oral, or vaginal) or while sharing needles with another person. HIV can also be passed from mother to baby.	The only way to know if you have HIV or AIDS is to take a test. Some people with HIV are tired all the time, lose weight, or have a fever. Some people with HIV have *no* symptoms.	Condoms help protect against HIV during sex. Do not share needles to inject drugs or other substances with another person. HIV testing and counseling are available at many places.
Tuberculosis (TB)	TB is caused by a bacterium that gets into the lungs. This disease kills 2 million people in the world each year.	When someone with TB coughs or sneezes, the bacteria can be spread to other people.	People infected with TB may develop a cough that doesn't go away, fever, weight loss, feeling weak, or night sweats.	You can get a TB skin test or chest X-ray at your doctor's office or at a clinic.
Malaria	Malaria is a disease caused by a parasite. Malaria is not common in the United States, but you can get it if you travel, especially to warm, tropical areas such as South America, Africa, or Asia.	Malaria is passed to people when they are bitten by infected mosquitoes.	Malaria causes fever, sweating, chills, body aches, and headache. Some cases of malaria need to be cared for in a hospital.	Malaria can be prevented by taking pills before traveling, using bug spray, and wearing protective clothing such as long-sleeved shirts and long pants.
Diarrheal diseases	Diarrheal diseases are those that cause loose, watery feces, stomach cramps, and similar stomach problems.	There are many causes for diarrhea, such as viruses, bacteria, parasites, medicines, and travel. Many times, people get diarrhea from food they eat.	Loose, watery feces, stomach pain, and cramps. A person who has diarrhea for more than a week should see a doctor or go to a clinic right away.	Diarrhea can cause serious problems for babies and people over age 65. Take steps to protect yourself while traveling, such as only drinking boiled or bottled water.
Influenza	Influenza (the flu) is caused by a virus. The flu can lead to serious problems in some people, especially young children and people over age 65. Healthy people can get over the flu easily by resting and drinking lots of fluids for a few days.	If a person has the flu, it is very easy for him/her to pass it to another person through coughing, sneezing, or touching. Washing your hands often can help protect you from getting the flu.	Chills, high fever, weakness, a dry cough, body aches, and headache.	A flu shot is available each fall to protect people against the flu. See your doctor about medicines that can help you get over the flu more quickly.

Source: Long Beach Chapter United Nations Association, 2001-2002 Global Health Initiative.

Hepatitis C is a virus that causes inflammation of the liver. Some people may develop cirrhosis and other problems associated with this disease. Hepatitis C can be transmitted in a multitude of ways: blood transfusions prior to 1992, intravenous and contaminated needle use, infected mother to unborn child, and perhaps intranasal cocaine. Other risk factors may include body piercings, tattoos, and potential sources of blood where the virus is present and enters the blood stream. This is not an airborne or food-borne disease; however, it affects liver functions and metabolism, stressing the body's nutritional status.

Most people with hepatitis C do not have symptoms and are leading normal lives. They were probably infected many years ago. This does not infer that the disease is not damaging to the liver. Medical care and evaluation are essential.[40]

International Travel Precautions

Global travel means daily alerts to major health issues such as malaria, tuberculosis (TB), HIV/AIDS, diarrheal diseases, and influenza. Immunizations and precautions are essential for continued health. See Table 6–5.

Exhibit 6–6   Healthy People 2010 Objectives Targeting Food-Borne Outbreaks

Objective Number		Baseline 1997	Target 2010
10-01a	Food-borne infections—*Campylobacter* per 100,000, persons of all ages	24.6	12.3
	American Indians or Alaska native	UK	12.3
	Asian or Pacific Islander	UK	12.3
	Black	UK	12.3
	White	UK	12.3
	Hispanic	UK	12.3
	Female	21.7	12.3
	Male	27.5	12.3
10-01b	Food-borne infections—*Escherichia coli* 0157:H7 per 100,000, persons of all ages	2.1	1.0
10-01c	Food-borne infections—*Listeria monocytogenes* per 100,000, persons of all ages	0.5	0.25
10-01d	Food-borne infections—*Salmonella* species per 100,000, persons of all ages	13.7	6.8
10-02a	Outbreaks of food-borne infections—*Escherichia coli* 0157:H7 (number of cases; all ages)	22	11
10-02b	Outbreaks of food-borne infections—*Salmonella* serotype *Enteritidis* (number of cases; all ages)	44	22
10-04	Food allergy deaths—anaphylaxis (persons of all ages)	UK	UK
10-05	Consumer food safety practices (adults of all ages)	72%	79%

UK = unknown.

Source: Adapted from: US Department of Health and Human Services. DATA2010–the *Healthy People 2010* database. *CDC Wonder.* Atlanta, Ga: Centers for Disease Control; November 2000.

Exhibit 6–7   Model Nutrition Objectives for Reduced Risk Factors

By 20__, the following contaminants will not be present in the state food supply
above toxic/hazardous levels as defined by state or federal agencies.
- Agricultural: pesticides, fertilizers, growth regulators
- Drugs: antibiotics, steroids/hormones, growth regulators
- Environmental: organics, inorganics/heavy metals
- Food additives: preservatives, colors, flavors, sweeteners, stabilizers
- Industrial: organics, inorganics/heavy metals, radioactives
- Microbial: bacteria, molds, fungi, viruses, protozoa, and related toxins
- Naturally occurring toxins: carcinogens, mutagens, neurotoxins

Source: Reprinted with permission from *Healthy People 2000: National Health Promotion
and Disease Prevention Objectives.* Washington, DC: US Dept of Health and Human Services;
1991. DHHS (PHS) publication 91-50212.

Exhibit 6–8   Model Nutrition Objectives for Increased Public and Professional
Awareness

By 20__, there will be an ongoing interdisciplinary information program for
public health and food industry professionals on food safety, labeling,
health claims, nutrition fraud, and the reporting of food-borne illness.

Source: Kaufman M. *Nutrition in Public Health—A Handbook for Developing Programs and
Services.* Gaithersburg, Md: Aspen Publishers, Inc; 1990:570.

Healthy People 2010 Actions

Specific *Healthy People 2010* objectives target food-borne outbreaks and actions that can be taken in the home as well as in institutional food service
settings (see Exhibit 6–6). Model nutrition objectives for community nutrition professionals are given in Exhibits 6–7 and 6–8.[41]

References

1. Centers for Disease Control and Prevention. *Principles of Epidemiology:
An Introduction to Applied Epidemiology and Biostatistics.* Atlanta, Ga:
Centers for Disease Control and Prevention; 1992.
2. Page R, Cole G, Timmrock T. *Basic Epidemiologic Methods and
Biostatistics.* Boston, Mass: Jones and Bartlett Publishers; 1993.
Olsen SJ, MacKinon LC, Goulding JS, Bean NH, and Slutsker L.
Surveillance for Foodborne disease outbreaks. U.S., 1993-97.
3. Centers for Disease Control and Prevention. CDC surveillance summaries
food-borne disease outbreaks, 5-year summary: 1983-1987. *MMWR.*
2000;49(SS01);1-51.

4. Matthews ME, Theis M. Relationship between the environment, the food supply and the practice of dietetics: research agenda conference. *J Am Diet Assoc.* 1993;93(9):1045-1049.

5. Expert Panel on Food Safety and Nutrition. Government regulation of food safety: interaction of scientific and societal forces. *Food Technol.* 1992;46(1):73-80.

6. Gorman C. *Wash Those Hands!* Rochester, Minn: Mayo Clinic College of Medicine; 2003.

7. National Restaurant Association; The Education Foundation. *Applied Foodservice Sanitation.* 4th ed. New York: John Wiley & Sons, Inc; 1992.

8. Durham S. Does the date mean "too late"? *Agricultural Res.* June 2004:17.

9. Puckett R. A review of food code 1999. *DBC Dimension.* Fall 1999:3.

10. American Diabetes Association and the Diabetes Care and Education Practice Group of the American Dietetic Association. *Maximizing the Role of Nutrition in Diabetes Management.* Alexandria, Va: American Diabetes Association; 1994.

11. Fields GC, Ayoob KT. Position of the American Dietetic Association and Dietitians of Canada: nutrition intervention in the care of persons with human immunodeficiency virus infection. *J Am Dietetic Assoc.* 2000;100(6):708-717. American Diabetes Association. *Professional Section Newsletter.* June 1993.

12. Sneed J, Strohbehn C, Mendonca A, Gilmore S. Microbiological evaluation of foodservice contact surfaces in Iowa assisted-living facilities. *J Am Diet Assoc.* 2002;104:1722-1724.

13. Ryser ET, Marth EH. "New" food-borne pathogens of public health significance. *J Am Diet Assoc.* 1989;89:948-956.

14. McDonald, J. Warning to consumers of risks associated with raw sprouts. *California Nutrition Council Newsletter.* Fall 1999.

15. Breukink E, Widemann I, van Kraaij C, Kulpers OP, Sahl H-G, de Kruijft B. Use of cell wall precursor lipid II by a pore-forming peptide antibiotic. *Science.* 1999;286:2361-2364.

16. Ferber D. Food Preservative or Potential Antibiotic? Nisin Z Could Be Both. Dec 16, 1999. WebMD Medical News. Available at: http://aolsvc.health.webmd.aol.com/content/article/20/1728_53477.htm. Accessed December 6, 2006.

17. "Green consumers" boost organic sales over $1 billion. *Magic Mill Newsletter Food, Health Environ Issues.* 1992;2(1):1.

18. California Dietetic Association. *Nutrition Survival Plan: A Food Guide for Emergencies, Big and Small.* Playa del Rey, Calif: California Dietetic Association; 1990.

19. Stier RF. Food Safety: as strong as your weakest link. Available at: http://www.foodengineeringmag.com. Accessed October 2006.

20. National Advisory Committee for Microbiological Criteria for Foods. *HACCP Principles for Food Production.* Washington, DC: US Dept of Agriculture, Food Safety and Inspection Service; 1989.

21. *Bacteria That Cause Foodborne Illness.* Washington, DC: US Dept of Agriculture, Food Safety and Inspection Service; December 1990. FSIS-40.

22. Dolye MP. Reducing food-borne disease—what are the priorities. *Nutr Rev.* 1993;51:346-347.

23. Committee on Pesticides in the Diets of Infants and Children. *Pesticides in the Diets of Infants and Children.* Washington, DC: National Academy Press; 1993.

24. Yess NJ. FDA monitoring program: residues in foods. 1990. *J Assoc Anal Chem.* 1991;74:121a-141a.
25. Winter CK. *Washed, Peeled, Contaminated: Pesticide Residues in Ready-to-Eat Fruits and Vegetables: A Critical Review* [position paper]. Davis: University of California, Davis; 1994.
26. Expert Panel on Food Safety and Nutrition. Organically grown foods. *Food Technol.* 1990;44(12):123-130.
27. Smith K. *Alar Three Years Later: Science Unmasks a Hypothetical Health Scare.* New York: American Council on Science and Health; 1992.
28. Washington Apple Commission. *Apple Production Information.* Wenatchee, Wash: Washington Apple Commission; 1992.
29. Duffy S. Eliminating bacteria from foods. AP News. *NY Times.* December 28, 1999.
30. Food and Drug Administration. FDA gives green light to red meat irradiation. *Commodity Alert.* Washington, DC. Fall 1998:1-2.
31. FDA. *The Nation's Premier Consumer Protection and Health Agency.* Washington, DC: DHHS 01-1316.
32. Position of the American Dietetic Association: dietetics professionals can implement practices to conserve natural resources and protect the environment. *J Am Diet Assoc.* 2001;101:1221.
33. World Health Organization, Fifty-fifth World Assembly. *Deliberate Use of Biological and Chemical Agents to Cause Harm.* April 16, 2002. Available at: http://www.who.int/gb/ebwha/pdf_files/whas5/ea5520.pdf. Accessed April 21, 2003.
34. US Department of Homeland Security. DHS Organization: Building a Secure Homeland. Available at: http://www.dhs.gov/dhspublic/ theme_home1.jsp. Accessed April 21, 2002.
35. Public Health Security and Bioterrorism Preparedness Act of 2002, June 12, 2002. Pub No. 107-188: 107th Congress. Available at: http://www.fda.gov/oc/bioterrorism/PL107-188.html. Accessed April 21, 2002.
36. US Food and Drug Administration. *Plans for Developing Bioterrorism-Related Food Regulations.* 2003. Available at: http://www.fda.gov/ oc/bioterrorism/titlelll.html#recordkeeping. Accessed April 25, 2003.
37. National Food Service Management Institute. *Emergency Readiness Plan: Guide and Forms for the School Foodservice Operation.* Oxford, Miss: University of Mississippi; 2003.
38. Joint Commission on Accreditation of Healthcare Organizations. Facts About the Emergency Management Standards. October 2002. Available at: http://www.jcaho.org/accredited+organizations/hospitals/standards/ ems+facts.htm. Accessed April 25, 2003.
39. USDA. APHIS Strategic Plan 2003-2008. Washington, DC. February 2006. Available at: http://www.aphis.usda.gov/oa/fmd/index.html, http://www.usda.gov/ocfo/usdasp/pdf/sp0-05.pdf.
40. University of California Irvine Liver Disease Program. *Back to Life–Southern California: Hepatitis C Support and Education Project.* Irvine: University of Calfornia; 2004.
41. Kaufman M. *Nutrition in Public Health–A Handbook for Developing Programs and Services.* Gaithersburg, Md: Aspen Publishers, Inc; 1990:570.

CHAPTER SEVEN

HEALTHY EATING IN EARLY LIFE— INFANTS AND PRESCHOOLERS

Learning Objectives

- Describe the development of a healthy eating pattern for children.
- List the factors influencing normal growth and development of young children.
- Identify the nutrition programs available for all infants and preschoolers and low-income children in particular.
- Enumerate the major nutrition issues in early life.
- Identify the roles and responsibilities of caregivers including community nutrition professionals in providing a safe and healthy eating and playing environment for infants and preschoolers.

High Definition Nutrition

Atherogenic—description of an eating pattern that promotes heart disease.

Day care center—a facility licensed by a sponsor to keep more than 12 infants or children and be responsible for their safety, well-being, and food.

Day care home—a personal residence licensed by a sponsor to keep 12 or fewer infants or children and be responsible for their safety, well-being, and food.

Food neophobia—a reluctance or refusal to try unfamiliar foods.

Kid culture—commonalities among day care centers and home facilities regarding foods served to children (e.g., spaghetti, fish sticks, hot dogs, potato chips, and cookies) that may be extremely popular but nutrient poor.

Salutogenic—health-promoting quality of food or eating pattern.

Introduction

The nutritional health of a child depends on the foods ingested and how the body uses them. Excess weight predisposes children to high blood cholesterol and sets them on a track for chronic disease.[1] At the other extreme, underweight and malnourished children present a different mosaic of nutritional problems, many of which begin during infancy and the preschool years.

The most common problems among Massachusetts Head Start children were excess weight (13%), short stature (13%), and iron deficiency anemia (12%). About 20% of physically or developmentally disabled children had short stature compared with 15% of the Asian children. Acute undernutrition was not prevalent. Excess weight among Hispanic, African-American, and white children was 17%, 13%, and 11%, respectively.[2]

Migrant children are a special group of children suspected of receiving inadequate nutrition prior to school entrance. These children experience poor housing with limited cooking facilities. They are victims of a lack of prenatal care, because their mothers have inadequate money for nutritious foods. Migrant children exist at a poverty level that has negative effects on their health and school potential.[3]

Infants and preschoolers are fun to watch, to teach, and to love. Their vitality, exuberance, and innocence capture the eye of parents, relatives, and caregivers. The nutritional needs of young children are as important as their emotional and social needs. Children who do not grow according to a standard growth chart or who remain either listless or overactive at school may not be receiving their nutrient needs on a daily basis. These nutrient needs may have escaped the living environment of the child when still a fetus.

Adult concerns for preschoolers' health should begin at conception or even before. The foundation for healthy infants and preschoolers remains an adult task. For each cohort born in the United States annually, attention must be paid not only to how well but also to how poorly the nutrient needs of young children are met.

A free school breakfast program evaluation showed that eating breakfast improved the children's daily nutrient intake, and significant improvements in their performance in school with reductions in school absenteeism occurred. In addition, the children had fewer hunger pangs and increased psychological functioning.[4,5]

Current scientific research links cognitive development of infants and children to nutrition. The Center on Hunger, Poverty and Nutrition Policy at Tufts University School of Nutrition summarized the research findings[6]:

- Undernutrition, along with environmental factors associated with poverty, can permanently retard physical growth, brain development, and cognitive functioning.
- The longer a child's nutritional, emotional, and education needs go unmet, the greater the likelihood of cognitive impairments.
- Iron deficiency anemia, affecting nearly 25% of low-income children in the United States, is associated with impaired cognitive development.
- Low-income children who attend school hungry perform significantly below their nonhungry, low-income peers on standardized tests.
- There exists a strong association between family income and the growth and cognitive development of children.

- Improved nutrition and environmental conditions can modify the effects of early undernutrition.
- Iron repletion therapy can reduce some of the effects of anemia on learning, attention, and memory.
- Supplemental feeding programs can help to offset threats to children's capacity to learn and perform in school that result from inadequate nutrient intake.
- Once undernutrition occurs, its long-term effects may be reduced or eliminated by a combination of adequate food intake and environmental support—both at home and at school.

US infant mortality rates (IMRs) have declined by almost two thirds since 1970. However, IMRs for African-American and Native American infants remain at 14 and 9 per 1,000 live births, respectively, compared to 7 per 1,000 live births for the total population (see Figure 7–1, and see Chapter 9 for prenatal nutrition). The Special Supplemental Program for Women, Infants, and Children (WIC) reaches high-risk pregnant mothers, infants, and children to change the direction of their health.

	1983	1998	2002
All mothers	11	7	7
White	9	6	6
Black or African American	19	14	14
American Indian or Alaska Native	15	9	9
Asian or Pacific Islander	8	6	5
Hispanic or Latino	10	6	6

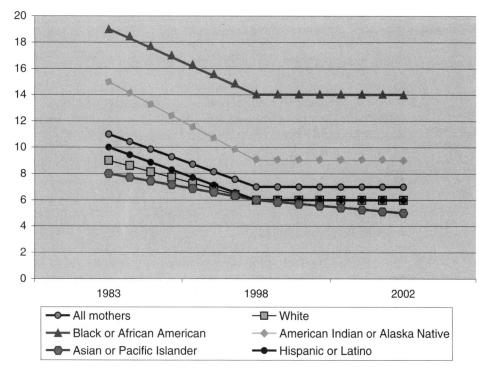

FIGURE 7–1 Infant mortality rates (IMR) by ethnicity of mother, US, 1983-2002. *Source:* CDC; 2005.

TABLE 7–1   Recommendations for Dietary Supplements for the Full-Term Infant

Vitamin D	400 IU daily for at-risk infants. At-risk infants include those whose sun exposure is:
	< 30 minutes per week, when clad in diaper only
	< 2 hours per week, when dressed, but head bare
Vitamin K	To be given at birth
Vitamin B_{12}	0.3-0.5 mcg/day if the strict vegetarian mother is not receiving vitamin B_{12} supplements
Fluoride	0.25 mg daily, after 6 months of age if water is not adequately fluoridated (< 0.3 ppm)
Iron	Choose high-iron weaning foods beginning at approximately 6 months of age

Source: PHNPG. Breastfeeding success: you can make the difference. *Digest.* Fall 1999.

WIC has been shown to dramatically reduce infant mortality by 25-66% among Medicaid beneficiaries who are WIC participants, compared to non-WIC Medicaid beneficiaries. The incidence of low-birth-weight babies can be lowered by 3.3%, and preterm births can be reduced by 3.5% (see Chapter 9). Nutrient requirements for full-term infants are outlined in Table 7–1.

The First Food for Newborns

Milk remains the first choice, and breast milk remains the best choice to feed a newborn. The reasons are as follows[7]:

- Breastfeeding protects from disease and infections. There is less illness and hospitalization of breast-fed babies than bottle-fed babies. Breast milk contains many immunological factors that protect babies.
- Breast milk is less allergenic. Breast milk rarely causes allergic reactions in babies, whereas cow's milk formula may create these problems.
- Breastfeeding improves learning. Breastfeeding has a positive effect on learning, memory, and other brain functions of young children.
- Breastfeeding reduces cancer risk. Cancer of the breast, ovaries, and cervix are less common among women who have breastfed an infant.
- Breastfeeding improves the mother's shape. Breastfeeding allows a woman to lose weight after pregnancy and reduces uterine bleeding. Milk production requires an additional 300 to 600 calories daily, which is partially obtained from the fat stores accumulated during pregnancy.
- Breastfeeding reduces overfeeding. A mother becomes more sensitive to her baby's satiety cues and does not simply empty a bottle.
- Breastfeeding promotes bonding. Having skin contact, smelling the mother, and hearing the mother's heartbeat all contribute to the baby's bond to its mother. The mother feels special because she is providing her baby's food.
- Breastfeeding provides optimal nutrient content. The protein, fat, mineral, vitamin, and calorie content of breast milk is superior to any other form of milk. It is made by humans for humans, and its nutrient content changes as the baby's needs change.

- Breastfeeding is convenient. When a baby is hungry, the milk is always there. Milk is at the right temperature and is clean, with no bottles to heat and no formula to prepare.
- Breastfeeding is economical. It is less expensive to breastfeed than to formula feed. Breast pumps are not a requirement.
- Breast milk is digestible. It is made by humans for humans, is easy to digest, and it creates less constipation and diarrhea.
- Breastfeeding is natural. It is the natural extension of a pregnancy; 95% of all women can be successful with encouragement, support, and basic information.
- Breastfeeding is safe. It is bacteriologically safe and always fresh.
- Breastfeeding promotes infant bone formation. The breast-fed infant has good jaw and tooth development.

To ensure success for both mother and infant, a guide is provided in Table 7–2 to evaluate whether a mother and infant will be successful with breastfeeding.

Even with the benefits of breastfeeding known, cow's milk is commonly used for infants early in life. The role of cow's milk or cow's milk-based

TABLE 7–2   Critical Assessment of the Breastfeeding Dyad

Information Type	Detail
General	Age of the infant, birth weight, and current weight if known.
	Underlying health problems of either mother or infant.
	Medications of mother or infant, including contraceptives.
Infant intake (if weights are not known)	Can you tell if your baby is swallowing?
	Describe what it is that you see or hear that you consider to be swallows.
	How many wet diapers has the baby had in the last 24 hours?
	Can you easily tell that the baby has urinated?
	How many bowel movements has the baby had in the last 24 hours?
	What do they look—color and amount?
	Describe your baby's behavior
	How often is your baby waking up to request a feeding?
	How does your baby act when the feeding is over?
	Do you need to wake your baby for feeds?
Maternal breast comfort	Are you having pain with the feedings? If yes, is it getting better or worse?
	How do your nipples feel?
	How do your breasts feel?
	How do you feel?
	Do you have any illness symptoms?
Maternal concerns	Questions or concerns the mother has about breastfeeding.
	Situations that worry the mother about how she or the baby is doing.

Source: Adapted from PHNPG. Breastfeeding success: you can make the difference. *Digest.* Fall 1999.

Info Line

Professional organizations that provide information about breastfeeding include:
- American Academy of Pediatrics (www.aap.org)
- American Dietetic Association (www.eatright.org)
- International Board of Lactation Consultant Examiners (www.iblce.org)
- International Lactation Consultant Association (www.ilca.org)
- La Leche League International (www.lalecheleague.org)

Advocacy groups and sites with general breastfeeding information include:

- Baby Friendly Hospital Initiative (www.dshs.state.tx.us/wichd/bf.shtm)
- Baby Milk Action (www.gn.apc.org/babymilk)
- *Healthy People 2010* (http://web.health.gov/healthypeople)
- National Alliance for Breastfeeding Advocacy (http://naba-breastfeeding.org)
- National Center for Education in Maternal and Child Health (www.NCEMCH.org)
- United States Food and Drug Administration (www.fda.gov/fdac/features/895_brstfeed.html)
- World Alliance for Breastfeeding Action (www.waba.org.myr)
- World Health Organization (www.who.int)

Source: Darby P. Breastfeeding resources on the World Wide Web. PHNPG. *Digest.* Fall 1999.

---

formula in food allergy remains unclear, but it is generally thought that increased intestinal permeability early in life contributes significantly to the development of food allergies. Cow's milk protein is the most common food allergy in childhood, affecting 0.4-7.5% of infants.[7] Milk, both bottle and breast, is implicated in 20% of colicky infants who persistently cry and are sleepless and irritable during the first 3-4 months of life.[8] Breast milk is contraindicated when women are HIV positive, drug abusers, or required to take multiple or powerful drugs.

A recurring question is whether breast-fed infants have a slower growth rate after the second or third month compared with bottle-fed infants. In the DARLING Study (Davis Area Research on Lactation, Infant Nutrition and Growth), researchers observed 46 breast-fed and 41 formula-fed infants, 2,500 to 5,000 g at birth, who were given no solid food before 4 months. At 3-month intervals of observation, formula-fed infants drank a significantly higher total energy and protein intake. No difference was noted in weight, length, lean body mass, or fat mass during the first 3 months of life, but the breast-fed infants had a slower weight gain from 3 to 9 months. From 3 to 12 months, the breast-fed infants consistently showed a positive correlation between total energy ingested and lean body mass gain. Fat mass deposition was more apparent for the formula-fed infants. A higher incidence of illness from 6 to 9 months occurred for infants having higher protein intakes.[9]

General recommendations for infants and young children less than 2 years old are that fat not be restricted.[10] Breast milk and commercial infant formula contain 50% of energy as fat. Risks associated with low-fat diets appear to outweigh the theoretical risk associated with a high-fat intake. Lower-fat milk is a good source of protein, calcium, and vitamin D for older children.

Breastfeeding

The first Surgeon General's workshop on breastfeeding and human lactation occurred in 1984 when breastfeeding initiation rates peaked at 59.7% and then declined but rose to 58.7% in 1995.[11] US rates do not reach the *Healthy People in Healthy Communities 2010* goal of 75% initiating and 50% breast-feeding at six months.[12]

US healthcare professionals recommend breastfeeding exclusively for the first 6 months of life, and then feeding some complementary foods in addition to breast milk for the first year.[13]

Achieving 2 *Healthy People 2010* objectives for breastfeeding could improve the overall health of infants and reduce US medical costs. The value is due to decreased morbidity and mortality, protection against infections, and decreased acute and chronic diseases along with psychological and physical advantages for the mothers.[14] Two *Healthy People 2010* goals have been achieved in 6 states and involve breastfeeding duration—50% of infants breast-feeding at 6 months of age and 25% breastfeeding at 12 months of age. More work is needed as the national average is 33.2-36% of all infants are breast-feeding at 6 months of age. Increased breastfeeding has occurred for Hispanic women and non-WIC participants; however, only 17-20% of all US infants are breast fed for 12 months. The United states is behind as internationally 79% of infants are still breastfeeding at 12 months of age.[15] See Figure 7–2.

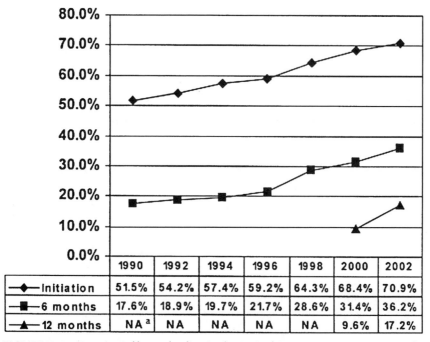

	1990	1992	1994	1996	1998	2000	2002
—♦—Initiation	51.5%	54.2%	57.4%	59.2%	64.3%	68.4%	70.9%
—■—6 months	17.6%	18.9%	19.7%	21.7%	28.6%	31.4%	36.2%
—▲—12 months	NA[a]	NA	NA	NA	NA	9.6%	17.2%

FIGURE 7–2 Duration of breastfeeding in the United States over a 12-year period. *Source:* Reproduced with permission of the American Dietetic Association (ADA). *Position Paper on Promoting and Supporting Breastfeeding.* Adopted by the ADA House of Delegates on March 16, 1997, and reaffirmed June 6, 2003.

Health professionals report lack of training and clinical experience in the promotion and support of breastfeeding, leading to feelings of discomfort and resulting in mismanagement of lactation issues.[16-18] Only 22% of women have persisted in breastfeeding until 6 months.[11] Nutrition professionals have positive attitudes about breastfeeding,[19] but in the hospital setting may be the least likely source of information, support, or assistance for the woman and her breastfeeding infant.[20] The breastfeeding position paper of the American Dietetic Association (ADA) recommends client- and profession-centered programs.[15] Client-centered issues include prenatal education, continuous assistance with lactation, and support of cultural mores so barriers to lactation are minimized. Professionals can develop standards for training students and staff to strengthen their understanding of lactation management and involvement in research.[21]

Info Line

HERBS AND LACTATION

Natural does not equal safety. Most drugs originate from herbs, but unlike drugs, herbs are regulated as dietary supplements. The FDA does not review and approve ingredients for supplements or the supplements themselves before marketing, causing concern about purity, concentration, and standardization.

The herbal industry has sales between $2 billion and $3 billion annually, warranting safety concerns. When companies isolate 1 ingredient in a plant and then concentrate it far beyond what it was meant to contain in nature, CNPs should be concerned. Herb quality, potency, and efficacy depend on date of harvest, drying process, and storage.

For women considering herbs while breastfeeding, CNPs should alert them to benefits versus risks. General guidelines include:

- Choose standardized products with standardized ingredients.
- Avoid diuretics and herbs that inhibit milk production.
- Avoid herbs that are contraindicated for infants or small children.
- Monitor the infant's changes in mood, sleeping habits, and/or the number of wet diapers after initiating herb use.
- Avoid herbal antihistamines, for example, *Ephedra* or ma huang.
- Avoid herbs containing steroid-like ingredients such as licorice, ginseng, sage, black walnut, and yarrow.
- If the infant has a fever, avoid mint teas. The salicylic acid found in peppermint, wintergreen, and spearmint, if in the breast milk, may lead to Reye's syndrome.
- Check for possible drug interactions.
- Consult a knowledgeable physician or a qualified herbalist before using any herb.

Source: PHNPG. The use of herbs during lactation. *Digest.* Fall 1999.

SHAPING FOOD PATTERNS IN YOUNG CHILDREN

Eating behaviors and food choices are formed early in life. Primary prevention efforts to reduce the onset of chronic disease might be improved if the factors shaping food patterns early in life were understood. Parents influence food-related behaviors, but several factors interact to shape food choices. These factors include but are not limited to nutrition attitudes and knowledge of parents and child-care providers, economic and social status of the family, birth order of the child, and number of siblings. Peers, media and advertising, access to the healthcare system, and the source of food (ranging from the home, to day care, to fast-food restaurants) all shape children's food choices.

A conceptual model to identify the determinants of eating behavior and the outcome of actual nutrient intakes is given in Table 7–3. This model suggests that actual nutrient intake is the end result of a progressive sequence of actions. The actions begin with a stimulus, which may be physiological or environmental. The stimulus creates a response—the child's eating behavior. The behavior causes food to be ingested, which is the first stage of response. The second stage of response is the resulting nutrient intake.

This model relates to the theory of reasoned action, which has been successful in predicting intent to perform health behaviors including eating in a fast-food restaurant.[22] *Reasoned action* postulates that one's behavior is predictable and based on the individual's intention to perform that behavior. *Intention* is a function of attitude about the behavior and the perception that one has about the way significant others would feel if one performs the behavior.

Four elements are inherent to the definition of the behavior: specified action, target for the action, context in which the behavior occurs, and time frame for the action. For example, fat avoidance is the specified action; it is reflected in the target for action as total fat intake or the percentage of energy from fat. The context for the behavior might be the home-prepared meals or eating out. The time frame for action might be the one half hour around mealtime.

Factors that have been evaluated for their influence on the eating pattern of young children are texture, taste, familiarity of food, preferences of the child compared with those of parents and other significant adults, and interaction patterns of parents and children around food. The child's willingness to eat is affected by the sensory appeal of the food, immediate hunger and nutritional status, the child's prior experience with food (both good and bad), and the child's personal beliefs and feelings about food.

TABLE 7–3   Conceptual Model to Identify Determinants of Eating Behavior of Children

Stimulus (Determinants)	→	Response (Behaviors*)	→	Result (Nutrients)
Parents		Fat avoidance or excess		Fat
School		Salt use or limit		Saturated fatty acids
Siblings		Snacks eaten or limited		Sodium
Environment		Meals eaten or missed		Energy
Physiology		Sugar use or amount		Carbohydrate

* An abbreviated list of possible behaviors for demonstration purposes.

Concern of parents about their child's refusal to try unfamiliar foods has stimulated research on neophobia but studies have involved older children.[23] Falciglia et al enrolled all fourth- and fifth-grade children in the Princeton School District of Cincinnati, Ohio, in a study to test whether food neophobia in children would be reflective of a similar neophobia in parents, if food neophobia would affect the child's nutritional status when compared with normative data, and if food neophobia in children would be supported by both parents and child behaviors. Results were that neophobic children did not appear to have neophobic parents, but neophobic children's diets were high in saturated fat, low in vegetable servings, and low in variety compared with children of the same age. Parental food practices neither supported food neophobia nor promoted the use of a variety of foods.[23]

Preference for a sweet taste is expressed early in life but appears modifiable.[24] Beauchamp et al demonstrated that to maintain a newborn's level of preference for sugar water, sweetened water must be repeatedly offered to the infant.[25] With no exposure during the newborn period, the relative acceptance of the sweetened water decreases.

Dislike of bitter tastes appears early in life, and an infant's reaction to salty tastes tends to be indifference.[24] The preference for a salt taste begins at about 4 months of age, as different foods are entered into the newborn's eating repertoire. Young children and infants prefer a salty taste; in fact, studies have shown that preschoolers favor higher levels of salt compared to adults.[26]

For preschool children, sweetness and familiarity enhance choice; familiarity is less important to older children.[27] Preference rankings of preschool children are highly correlated with consumption,[28] yet their preferences are strongly influenced by their peers. Fear of new foods decreases with exposure to the food. Food preferences of young children are influenced by parents and child-care staff, but not unequivocally.[28]

Burt and Hertzler observed that the mother and father can equally influence a child's food preferences, if weight is given to the father's preferences, specifically at mealtime.[29] Birch reported that adults from the same ethnic group as the child, but not related to the child, influence the child's food preferences as much as the parents.[30] When parents are involved in nutrition education, the eating patterns of their children are more nutritious than when the parents are not included.[31]

Evaluations of mother-child choices generally show a stronger influence of what the mother chooses rather than what the father chooses. As a child advances through the preschool years, the parental and child food choices become more similar and stronger than when the child was younger, for example, at age 2. Food choices of younger children also mirror those of the child's siblings.[32]

EATING BEHAVIOR OF CHILDREN

Interactions

Eating interactions form a continuum influenced by parental attitudes, values, interests, and beliefs and the child's cognitive, physical, and emotional maturity. Parent-child interactions determine children's acceptance of healthy and not-so-healthy foods and attitudes toward eating. Parents are often anxious and may pressure children to eat. In response, children often assume control of the eating environment. Battles may intensify, and a child's nutrient intake may suffer. Disordered eating including excessive weight, obesity, and failure to thrive may occur.

Parent-child eating interaction is complex and reciprocal. Each response to an action can cause future behaviors, both healthy and unhealthy. Eating behavior becomes both the cause and the effect of other behaviors. Because of the dependence of children on parents and caregivers for food, this section will address the role of adult-child interactions on food intake and nutrient intake. Community nutrition professionals may learn new ways to approach old problems.

Parent-child interactions can be initiated by the child and influence the child, as seen by the cries of a hungry infant stimulating the parent or guardian to respond with food. Eating behaviors increase, stay the same, or decrease, depending on the consequence that follows initial eating. In fact, the consequences can reinforce or punish.[33] Determining what is reinforcing rather than punishing depends on the outcome or preceding event.

Reinforcers can be either positive or negative. Positive reinforcement—such as a smile, food, or money—can create a positive environment. Negative reinforcement, such as silence, often removes or ends a behavior. All reinforcers increase the behavior that follows. However, positive reinforcement adds pleasure, and a negative reinforcement removes something. Shouting is a punisher that adds reinforcement to a child who eats something that she or he should not eat.

Peterson suggests considering interaction in terms of A (antecedent events), B (behavior), and C (consequences).[34] For example, a father takes his 4-year-old son to a baseball game. The boy asks for candy and cries when the father refuses to buy it. The child cries and kicks the seat in front of him, and the father ends up buying the candy. In buying the candy, the father reinforced the kicking and the crying, but the father received negative reinforcement because the kicking stopped after he gave candy. By giving candy, he stopped something annoying to him. Both father and son were reinforced for their behaviors (i.e., the son was positively reinforced for kicking; the father was negatively reinforced, because the kicking stopped when he gave in). The tendency would be for each person to repeat their behavior. Table 7–4 classifies the behaviors and consequences of similar situations—a negative reinforcement for a parent and a positive reinforcement for a child.[35]

Parents and caregivers often become trapped and unable to see their own ineffectiveness in directing their children's eating behavior. Mealtimes can create difficult, volatile eating interactions. Affection, praise, and touch often create secondary reinforcement when they are paired with a positive eating event. Money can become a reinforcer, and food is often used as a reinforcer for various other behaviors such as physical activity.[35]

Assessing the antecedent behaviors of eating is pivotal for community nutrition professionals to understand why children eat certain foods or persist with certain behaviors. Assessment is essential if effective behavioral change is needed for primary prevention and health promotion. Adults can review the foods that are reinforcers, help children learn appropriate behaviors, and then use the foods with other reinforcers—such as affection and praise—until the

TABLE 7–4   Flow of Parent and Child Food Interaction

Negative Reinforcement for Parent and Positive Reinforcement for Child

A (Mother)	B (Child)	C (Mother)
1. Pours milk into glass	2. Starts crying	3. "Drink your milk."
	4. Cries	5. Removes milk and gives child soda
	6. Stops crying and drinks soda	

Circular Interaction to Reinforce a Child's Control of Eating Environment and Solution

A (Mother)	B (Child)	C (Mother)
Interaction in which child controls eating		
1. Presents applesauce to toddler in high chair	2. Cries and whines, points to the refrigerator	3. "What do you want?"
	4. Cries, points to cupboard	5. "Do you want a cracker?
	6. Cries, points to cupboard and refrigerator	7. "What do you want? Here is some cereal."
	8. Cries, points to refrigerator	9. "No, you can't have ice cream."
	10. Screams	11. "OK, here is some ice cream."
	12. Stops crying	
Solution—Interaction in which parent controls eating		
1. Presents applesauce to toddler in high chair	2. Cries, points to cupboard	3. Leaves room (can see child but child can't see her)
	4. Slowly stops crying, starts eating applesauce	5. Returns and says "My, what a big boy!"
	6. Child laughs and keeps on eating	

Source: Adapted from Pipes PLC. Management of mealtime behavior. In: *Nutrition in Infancy and Childhood.* 4th ed. Boston, Mass: Times Mirror; 405, 1989.

child understands how the 2 behaviors reinforce one another. Then the food can be removed as the reward but the secondary reinforcer retained. A circular interaction that reinforces a child's control of eating and a possible solution is given in Table 7–4.[35]

Selections

Young children learn to differentiate food from nonfood substances and place items into edible and inedible categories. Very young children show a high to moderate level of acceptance of all categories of food and nonfood items, but the acceptance of dangerous, disgusting, or unacceptable substances (e.g., ketchup on mashed potatoes) decreases with age.[36]

Energy regulation appears keener for children than adults. When given a high-calorie instead of a low-calorie snack before lunch, 95% of the children and 60% of adults ate less lunch.[37] Food contingencies, for example, "eat this and you can do this," can discourage rather than encourage food consumption among preschoolers, and variety increases intake.[38,39]

When asked to group foods, children group foods based on commonalities, such as sweet foods or foods served at breakfast, but not based on nutritional value.[40] Categories tend to match the cognitive level of children (e.g., food recognition is based on sensory perceptions or differentiating animal versus plant sources).[41]

For decades, the basic food groups have been a common grouping to teach children about food selection. However, not all children know and use the food groups correctly. In one study, all children identified a sweets group; one half put foods in a fruit, vegetable, or beverage group; one fourth identified a dairy group; and one fifth identified a breads and cereals category.[40] The US Department of Agriculture (USDA) 2005 Food Guide Pyramid is the current visual aid for grouping foods and the focus of games, mobiles, and refrigerator magnets.[42]

Other Factors

The extent to which nutrition knowledge is used in family and child-care menu planning may relate to a child's self-esteem, problem-solving skills, and family organization.[43] Older children, by virtue of their age, appear to influence the mother's food selection more than younger siblings, irrespective of the mother's nutrition knowledge.[44] Day care providers who report limited nutrition knowledge still value the role they play in influencing eating patterns of children.[45] Further, family role modeling and reinforcement may set the stage for strong interactive environmental conditioning.[46] Differences have been observed between thin parents and their thin children, compared with heavy parents and their children. Birch[47] observed more interaction and positive reinforcement for thin children and their mothers compared to their heavier counterparts.[46]

Food rewards can influence food preferences of children.[48] Nonfood rewards such as stickers, sports equipment, amusement tickets, and sports cards are preferred incentives in behavior modification. Reinforcement procedures of cueing have been used to redirect snack choices, but once the cues are removed, prior habits return.[49] Satter views the parent or caregiver as the individual who is responsible for what is offered to the child. The child is responsible for the amount of food eaten.[50,51]

Role of Media

The role of mass media has increased proportionately to the amount of time children are in contact with the media. Young children are mesmerized by television before they can speak, and the preschooler cannot differentiate between commercials and actual programs. There appears to be an inverse association between income and the amount of time children spend watching television. The specific television segments that influence children are advertisements. On the average, children watch 3 hours of advertisements per week and 19,000 to 22,000 commercials over a year. Advertisements categorize foods by first establishing their enjoyability and pleasure in terms of sweetness and richness. Children's repeated exposure to messages that do not build positive images about crisp, fresh vegetables or the bone-building capacity of milk and dairy products has motivated national healthy eating campaigns directed toward children, such as the 5 A Day campaign.[52-56]

Since preschool children may spend over 26 hours a week watching television, physical activity may be displaced by sedentary activities. Six- to 16-year-olds still average 25 hours of television watching per week.[57] Understanding and trusting commercials has been explored among children; it appears that older children recognize commercials as sales pitches and not educational, and they even tend to distrust the information.[53]

An overriding concern of health professionals and educators has been the long-term impact of television commercials and messages on the health of all children, including preschoolers. When television can influence what a family purchases and which snacks are provided to children and confuses the role of food with other outcomes—smoking, sexual appeal, and popularity—then the real message about healthy eating has been lost. The more television children watch, the greater the tendency for weight gain. This can be considered from 2 perspectives. First, fewer calories are expended when sitting, and one is more likely to eat while watching television. Second, seeing thin, active children eat gooey chocolate and high-fat foods on television is interpreted as an acceptable habit that does not cause excess body weight.

Children in the United States spend an average of at least 2 hours more each day watching television or playing video games compared to other activities. Sedentary behavior provides a setting for increased snacking and exposure to food on commercials. Television viewing may decrease resting metabolic rate, although the data are limited.[57]

ATHEROGENIC VERSUS SALUTOGENIC EATING PATTERNS

Data from the Nationwide Food Consumption Survey in the 1990s indicated that children 1 to 19 years old averaged 35-36% of their total calories from fat. Saturated fat was 14% of their intake, polyunsaturated fat was 6%, and monounsaturated fat was 13-14%; dietary cholesterol levels were 193-296 mg. This eating pattern predisposed children to a health-risk behavior resulting in

Info Line

The 2005 *Dietary Guidelines for Americans* (DGAs) emphasize overall modifications in eating patterns for individuals older than 2 years to reduce the risk of diet-related chronic diseases.

Source: The United States Department of Agriculture and United States Department of Health and Human Services. *Dietary Guidelines for Americans.* Washington, DC: US Dept of Agriculture and US Dept of Health and Human Services; 2005.

excess weight and high blood cholesterol levels. At least 25% of American children exceed the acceptable 170 mg% serum cholesterol level. However, recent data show adolescents are consuming less total fat, saturated fat, and cholesterol.[58]

Fat-avoiding behaviors have been observed in a cross-sectional sample of Mexican-American preschoolers and their parents.[59] Significantly higher fat-avoiding scores were noted for 143 Anglo-American preschoolers than 198 Mexican-American preschoolers (maximum score = 7.0, sum score = 4.85 compared to 4.35, $p < 0.0001$).[60]

The eating patterns of young children 2 to 5 years of age reflect intraindividual and interindividual variability. To evaluate the influence of food choices on actual health risk, nutrient intake can be compared with a standard. A conceptual guide that characterizes the salutogenic (health-promoting) quality of food versus the atherogenic (heart disease-promoting) quality of an eating pattern is outlined in Table 7–5.

Standards used as cutoff points reflect consensus recommendations of such organizations as the American Heart Association, the American Cancer Society, and the National Cholesterol Education Program. Achieving the standards means achieving a healthy eating pattern. If young children can be taught to make wise food choices and if their parents and other adults plan and prepare healthy meals and snacks, then a primary prevention effort can unfold. If the salutogenic approach (i.e., health promotion) is consistent, then

TABLE 7–5   Conceptual Model for Describing Eating Patterns of Children and Their Relation to Health Risk Versus Health Promotion

Component	− Health Risk +		
	Salutogenic*	*Standard*	*Atherogenic**
Total fat	25-29% kcal	30%	> 30%
Saturated fat	8-9% kcal	10%	> 10%
Polyunsaturated fat	8-9% kcal	10%	< 8%
Monounsaturated fat	12-14% kcal	10-12%	< 10%
Carbohydrate	55-60% kcal	53-55%	< 53%
Starch	30-40% kcal	28-30%	< 28%
Cholesterol	100-150 mg/kcal	140-150 mg/kcal	> 150 mg/kcal
Sodium (1-3 y)	< 975 mg	325-975 mg	> 975 mg
(4-6 y)	< 1,350 mg	450-1,350 mg	> 1,350 mg
Potassium (1-3 y)	> 1,650 mg	550-1,650 mg	< 1,650 mg
(4-6 y)	> 2,325 mg	775-2,325 mg	< 2,325 mg
Fiber	> 10 g	10-20 g	< 5 g
CSI[†]	< 37	35-37	> 37
FAS[‡]	> 3.5	3.5	< 3.5

*Both accepted (American Heart Association and National Cholesterol Education Panel) and author-hypothesized values

†Cholesterol saturated fat index

‡Fat/cholesterol avoidance scale

over time the eating pattern will promote positive health of the child. If the usual eating pattern is atherogenic rather than salutogenic, then the risk factors for chronic disease may appear early in the life of a child.

FACTORS IN CHILDHOOD THAT PREDISPOSE TO ADULT DISEASE

Obesity

Obesity among preschool children has increased among all ethnic groups disproportionately and is linked to excessive energy intake and not expending the excess calories, among several other factors.[61] A 20-year longitudinal study reported that 41% of children defined as fat at 1 year of age maintained their fat into early childhood, preadolescence, and adulthood 21 years later.[62] Heights, weights, and triceps skinfold measures for boys and girls from 6 months to 5 years old are collected in the Health and Nutrition Examination Survey and the Hispanic Health and Nutrition Examination Survey. In the fall of 2000, new growth and head circumference charts were available for boys and girls up to 6 months as shown in Appendix 7–A.

Obese infants at 6 months of age are at an increased risk of being obese adults, and tracking of obesity is more pronounced for children at or above the 95th percentile for age-specific measures. A higher percentage of Hispanic children are obese compared to their white and African-American peers. Obesity increases the risk of hypertension, high serum cholesterol, adult-onset diabetes mellitus, and certain cancers. Hispanic subgroups in the United States demonstrate a 2-4 times higher risk for developing non-insulin-dependent diabetes mellitus primarily linked to body weight. High sodium intake and excess body weight promote high blood pressure.[63-67]

The correlation between a child's body fat and his or her responsiveness to caloric-dense cues was observed for 77 preschoolers, 2 to 4 years old. Children at higher levels of body fat were not able to regulate energy intake as well as children at lower levels. More parental control over intake lessened the child's ability to self-regulate ($r = -0.67$; $p < 0.0001$).[68]

Researchers in North Dakota examined the association between beverage consumption (fruit juice, fruit drinks, milk, soda, and diet soda) and changes in weight and body mass index among preschool children.

The study sample included 1,345 children age 2 to 5 years participating in the WIC clinics on 2 visits 6 to 12 months apart. The study did not show an association between beverage consumption and changes in weight or body mass index in this population of low-income preschool children in North Dakota.[69]

High Blood Pressure and Hyperlipidemia

Blood pressure and serum total cholesterol are indicators of a child's health status. Direct relationships are reported between incidence of coronary heart disease (CHD) and both the average level of adult serum total cholesterol ($r = 0.80$) and the amount of saturated fat in the diet ($r = 0.84$).[70] Serum total cholesterol and blood pressure have been shown to track or remain in a set position for some children relative to their peers.[71] Determining a child's dietary intakes, serum total cholesterol, and blood pressure levels (Appendix 7–B) establishes a baseline to forecast and to track associations and future risk.

The Pediatric Nutrition Surveillance System provides the opportunity to explore the tracking question. Using serum total cholesterol data of a multi-ethnic group of 1,169 preschoolers from low-income families in Arizona, an initial level was compared with a follow-up level about 13 months later.[72] The correlation of the 2 measures was $r = 0.54$ and did not vary by ethnicity, sex, relative weight, or changes in weight. Association increased when the age was higher at the initial measure. The correlation of $r = 0.64$ for 4-year-olds and their follow-up measure was identical to that observed by the Bogalusa Heart Study.

Of the children, 34%, or 5 times the number expected, had an initial and follow-up cholesterol level equal to or greater than 200 mg/dL. This contrasts with 25% who had their subsequent measure at less than 170 mg/dL. Although intravariability exists, multiple measures portray the cholesterol and subsequent risk beginning in childhood.[72]

Eating pattern models that integrate both the nutrient intakes and the behaviors of preschoolers are needed to explore the combined role of eating patterns on the chronic disease process early in life. How well these eating patterns and blood levels persist or whether new practices that become habits can be taught remain areas of interest and research.

NUTRITION GUIDELINES FOR PRESCHOOL CHILDREN

General nutrition guidelines for children have evolved over the years. For proper growth and development, all young children need an array of nutrients on a daily basis. The recommended dietary allowances (RDAs) and daily reference intakes (DRIs) are the standards used to evaluate the sufficiency of a child's total daily food intake.[73] RDAs are set for energy, protein, 10 vitamins, and 7 minerals. Minimum requirements are set for sodium, chloride, and potassium (see Chapter 2 for a listing of the RDAs for infants and young children).

The USDA bases the meal planning guide for child care, day care, summer foods programs, and home meals on the assumption that children should consume one third of the RDAs for lunch and about one fourth of the RDAs for breakfast.[74]

To reduce heart disease, the current recommendation is to lower fat and saturated fat consumption. Current dietary recommendations call for energy reduction and a concomitant replacement of dietary fat with complex carbohydrate.[75,76] The 2005 *Dietary Guidelines for Americans*[76] apply to healthy individuals 2 years and older and address the progression of chronic diseases (e.g., CHD and hypertension). General goals include choosing fats wisely and choosing and preparing foods with little salt. Specific goals address the following:

- total fat 30% or less
- saturated fat < 10%
- fewer animal sources of fat
- less salt and sodium in cooking, at the table, and when planning meals.

NUTRITION GUIDELINES FOR TODDLERS AND INFANTS

Specific statements are made in the National Cholesterol Education Panel (NCEP) III report regarding healthy food choices early in life.[75] Toddlers 2 and 3 years of age are in a transition period during which they gradually adopt the eating patterns of the rest of the family. The RDAs for zinc, iron, and calcium are high for young children, and preschoolers generally do not meet the RDAs for iron and zinc. Foods that provide these nutrients are lean meat for iron and zinc and low-fat dairy products for calcium. Fortified or enriched bread and cereal products, beans, and peas supply iron.[76-78]

The NCEP excludes newborns to 2 years of age from dietary fat recommendations. These infants require energy-rich foods and a higher percentage of calories from fat than older children. The American Academy of Pediatrics, the American Heart Association, the National Institutes of Health Consensus Development Conference on Lowering Blood Cholesterol, and the NCEP all recommend that fat and cholesterol should not be restricted during infancy.[75]

Breast milk is recommended as the main source of nutrients from birth to 6 months of age, with infant formula substituted when breastfeeding is not possible. Breast milk and infant formula have a caloric density of about 0.7 kcal/mL and 50% of energy from fat to sustain growth and meet the small volume held by the stomach. After 4 to 6 months of age, pureed and mashed table foods, which provide fewer calories from fat than breast milk or formula, can be added gradually to replace some milk or formula. Fatty acid content of breast milk fat is partially influenced by a woman's eating pattern and by her body fat stores. In fact, a low saturated fat or total fat eating pattern has limited effect on a woman's breast milk.[10,74]

The NCEP does not recommend feeding skim milk to infants because it provides a very high solute load per calorie from mineral salts and protein. This requires extra water for excretion in the urine and may lead to serious dehydration of the infant. The NCEP's recommended eating pattern for toddlers does not require major changes from what young children currently eat. Preschool children have lower energy and nutrient needs per kilogram of body weight compared to toddlers, but protein and other nutrient needs are higher. Reduction in saturated fatty acids and total fat from the dairy and meat groups is recommended. A wide variety of foods from all food groups; regular, scheduled mealtimes; and low-fat snacks at midmorning, midafternoon, and bedtime are advised since toddlers have a limited capacity for food at one sitting.

These recommendations form the basis of primary prevention efforts early in life[79] and include the following:

- studies that report, for example, an average decrease among adults of 1-10% in plasma cholesterol from a higher intake of fiber-rich fruits, vegetables, grains, and legumes
- the integration of nutrition education into preschool education for children and parents to encourage healthy behaviors (e.g., the Fun Kit with puppets, music cassettes, and stickers)[80]
- documentation that positive mealtime behavior of child-care providers (e.g., eating alongside children and giving positive comments about food) is associated with structured activities such as cooking and baking, tasting new foods, artwork, and storytelling

Info Line

> Although food labels for infants less than 2 years old look like labels on adult foods, there are differences:
>
> - Food labels for infants do not list calories from fat, saturated fat, or cholesterol, but they do show total fat content.
> - Serving sizes for infant foods are based on average amounts usually eaten at one time.
> - Daily values are listed only for protein, vitamins, and minerals; they do not include fat, cholesterol, sodium, potassium, carbohydrate, or fiber.
>
> *Source:* Adapted from National Center for Nutrition and Dietetics. *Nutrition Fact Sheet. Food Labels for Infants Under Two Years.* 1994:1.

ROLE OF CAREGIVERS

In 1992, 24,361 child care centers (CCC) and 161,533 day care homes were participating in the USDA Child and Adult Care Food Program. This program involved approximately 1.9 million children who ate at least 1 meal on the premises.[81]

Much of the protection and health promotion of children rests with caregivers. Today's parenting lifestyle often includes assigning responsibility of infants or preschoolers to caregivers for the majority of the waking hours. Caregivers are responsible for encouraging healthful behavior patterns including exercise, sleep, and play and for practicing healthful food preparation, sanitation, and safety procedures. The latter are necessary to reduce the potential of food-borne illness (see Chapter 6).

Most communicable illnesses are transferred from one child to another in group settings via coughing; sneezing; and improperly sanitized eating utensils, toys, and toilets. Simple hand-washing procedures and proper toileting and handling of colds and diarrhea can reduce the spread of illness.[82]

Meeting the nutrient need of infants and children in group care settings requires attention to the following:

- *A variety of foods:* Presenting different foods promotes awareness and generates interest.
- *Interesting shapes, colors, and temperatures:* Children enjoy crisp, finger-size foods that are easy to chew and handle. Cool and warm foods are preferred to hot and very cold foods, since a child's mouth is sensitive to temperatures. Foods that can cause choking include tough or stringy meat, grapes, nuts, small pieces of hard raw vegetables and fruits, miniature hot dogs, popcorn, and small pieces of fried foods. Single foods rather than mixed foods or casseroles are preferred. Individually wrapped servings teach self-service and dexterity.
- *Appropriate servings:* Preschoolers can meet the RDAs for their age group by eating small servings rather than adult servings (1 tablespoon per year of age).

- *Ethnic variety and awareness:* Table manners and common foods of preschoolers vary by ethnic group. For example, Japanese often wash their faces and hands with a wet towel at the table before the meal and use a low table for eating; Asians often drink soup directly from the bowl; Europeans may cut fruit and some sandwiches with a knife and fork. Children may be used to certain foods with their meals. For example, tortillas are common with Mexican Americans, sliced bread with Anglo-Americans, and biscuits or cornbread with African Americans. Activities that develop an awareness of the richness of many cultures include the following:

  1. activities that build on the shared experiences of all people, not on the emphasis of difference
  2. programs that reach outside the immediate child-care environment
  3. projects that use racial, cultural, and socioeconomic backgrounds of the children in care
  4. planned curricula with incidental teaching opportunities giving a multicultural perspective

- *Frequent feedings:* Preschoolers' small stomachs, small appetites, and short attention spans demand an eating approach that provides nutrient-dense foods in small and frequent feeding times. Snacks of fruit, dairy products, or cereal should be served 2 hours from meals.
- *Family-style meal service:* Providing bulk quantities of each food allows teaching staff to serve small portions of single foods first and then to promote second helpings. This encourages capacity building among the children, for example, acquiring the capacity to eat a variety of foods rather than focusing on any one favorite food.
- *Avoidance of certain foods:* Foods to avoid include foods that are hard to control, chew, or swallow such as whole nuts and grapes, raw carrots, and hard candies. Remove obvious hazards such as fruit pits and fish bones (except canned salmon, which has bones that can be mashed into the meat). Quarter breads and sandwiches.
- *Elimination of conflict around food:* Conflicts about food and preoccupation with eating can lead to negative attitudes and behaviors about food. Realistic and positive expectations by parents and food service staff about food are essential if eating is to be a primary prevention training ground for children and if children are to establish positive eating behaviors early in life.

Skinner et al compared relationships between family socioeconomic status (SES) and dietary patterns of children 24 to 36 months of age focusing on caffeine intake.[83,84] One hundred twenty-four children from families of middle and upper SES and 49 children from families of lower SES form the sample. All children were white and resided in an urban, southeastern US city. Random home interviews occurred when children were 24 to 36 months old. Three-day data sets including a weekend day reflected one 24-hour recall and 2 days of food records.

No consistent differences were noted in any nutrient intake between groups. Mean intakes for both SES groups met 100% of the most recent RDA or AI level except for iron (88-97% RDA), zinc (60-75% RDA), and vitamin E (55-80% RDA). Average daily intake of caffeine consumed in both groups was less than the amount in a can of cola; many children consumed no caffeine. Forty-three percent of children in the upper SES group had no caffeine in their diets compared with 29% in the lower SES group, but 15% in the upper SES group had 20+ mg of caffeine or more per day. Cola beverages, tea, and chocolate were the primary contributors to dietary caffeine. Boys' intake of caffeine was higher than that of girls at 24 and 32 months, $p = 0.04$ and $p = 0.05$, respectively.[83,84]

Recommendations regarding CN professionals are:

- Dietitians should evaluate with parents and other caregivers whether beverages with caffeine are appropriate for young children. Intakes of 100% fruit juice and milk have been reported as inversely related to consumption of carbonated beverages.[83] Carbonated beverages substitute for nutritious beverages and since many provide caffeine, when consumed in high amounts regularly, undesirable effects may result.[83-85]
- Parents' knowledge of the caffeine content of foods and the stimulating effect should be evaluated. On a body weight basis, 20 mg of caffeine in a 14-kg child would be equal to 80 mg caffeine, or the amount in about 20 oz of cola, in a 56-kg adult. Cola beverages have 3.9 mg caffeine per ounce, tea 5.9 mg per ounce, and chocolate bars 7.3 mg per ounce.
- CNPs should promote a daily intake of nutritious beverages and nutrient-dense foods for young children and then address reduction of dietary caffeine.

NUTRITION STANDARDS FOR CHILD-CARE PROGRAMS

Caring for Our Children—National Health and Safety Performance Standards: Guidelines for Out-of-Home Child Care Programs is a joint publication of the American Academy of Pediatrics and American Public Health Association. It provides a consensus of direction regarding how to provide quality care for children in child-care programs. A written plan for the food and nutrition services is a key standard; a comprehensive plan written under the direction of a nutrition specialist is preferred. Three guiding principles set the tone of the nutrition section of the standards[86]:

1. Food should help to meet the child's daily nutritional needs and reflect individual and cultural differences. Foods should provide an opportunity for learning, and activities should complement and supplement those of the home and the community. The facility can assist the child and family to understand the association between nutrition and health and various ways to meet the nutritional needs.
2. A nutrition specialist or food service expert is a vital member of the facility's planning team to ensure the implementation of an efficient and cost-effective food service.
3. To prevent food-borne illness, proper equipment and food handling are essential.

The American Dietetic Association (ADA) has published a position paper entitled, *Benchmarks for Nutrition Program Standards in Child Care Settings.*[87] The standards cited by ADA reflect those of the following groups:

- US Department of Health and Human Services (DHHS) as established for the Head Start Program
- USDA for the Child and Adult Care Food Program

- American Public Health Association for home child care
- American Academy of Pediatrics for home child care
- Society for Nutrition Education and Behavior for child-care facilities

General recommendations include the following:

- *Meal plans:* One third of the RDAs should be met if the child is present 4 to 7 hours per day; one half to two thirds of the RDAs should be met for a child present 8 or more hours per day. Meals and snacks with a variety of nutritious foods should make up the foods offered. Attention should be given to cultural food patterns, appetizing colors and textures, and appropriate portions.
- *Preparation and food service:* Salt, fat, and sugar should be kept to a minimum. Fruits, vegetables, and whole-grain foods should be promoted. Preparation that promotes nutrient retention is essential.
- *Nutrition consultation and guidance:* Registered dietitians (RDs) knowledgeable of the child-care environment and the nutrient needs of infants and preschoolers should be employed to review and guide a quality program.
- *Nutrition education and training:* Education for children, parents, and caregivers should be routine. Parents can serve as instructors and facilitators.
- *Physical and emotional environment:* A positive, enjoyable interaction among children and adults is preferred.
- *Compliance with local and state regulations:* All tasks to ensure wholesomeness of foods and the sanitation and safety of the facility should be followed.

HEALTHY MENU PLANNING IN CHILD AND FAMILY DAY CARE CENTERS

Briley et al examined meal and snack consumption before and after children attended child care. Six nonprofit CCCs cared for 51 children aged 3 to 6 years. Most children had inadequate vegetables, bread, cereal, pasta, and rice intakes. Average percentage of energy from fat was 33% ±4%; total days' intake showing deficiencies were energy, iron, sodium, and zinc. Given this profile, menus at CCCs become important, as CCC menus in 10 states were not consistently nutritionally adequate. The variety of foods is often limited, servings of cruciferous fruits and vegetables are rare, and fat content is high.[88]

To evaluate the menu planning process, Briley et al used a mailed survey to 300 CCCs located across 6 US states in different geographic regions. One hundred fifty-three menu planners were described and included the following: 98% were female, 46% were older than 45 years of age, 80% were full-time employees, 72% were at current site more than 5 years, and 36% were program directors. The study reported 40% of the menu planners served as cook at the center, 66% received training in food service, 58% received training on the job, 41% completed college-based training, and 33% used home study courses.[88]

Factors that influence menu planning in CCCs with children from different ethnic groups have been reported as the food program requirements, staff perceptions of children's food preferences, the background of the food program, and the fee for the child-care service. Evaluators concluded that[89]:

- Menu improvement is needed
- Training for center or home care staff should be sensitive to ethnic composition of the center's client base
- Staff's nutrition knowledge has an indirect influence on menu quality
- Program requirements and monitoring activities need revision.

The California Department of Education, Child Nutrition and Food Distribution Division has developed a healthy meal pattern planning guide, called The New SHAPE Meal Pattern[90] for CCCs that feed children from 1 to 12 years of age (see Table 7-6).

For infants, meal planning centers around breast milk or formula for the first 4 to 6 months of age. Solid foods are introduced between 4 and 6 months. Portions listed are the minimum amount needed to ensure achievement of the RDAs. The meal planning guide uses whole milk for children from 1 to 2 years of age and emphasizes 2% low-fat milk for children 2 years and older. A raw fruit or vegetable must be offered at least once a day, and foods rich in vitamin A and vitamin C must be served daily. One half of all bread/bread alternates served must be from 25 to 33% whole grain or list whole grain as the first ingredient. Emphasis must be placed on lean and lower sodium choices. At least one eighth cup of beans must replace one half ounce of meat or meat alternate each week.

While several changes would have to be made to incorporate these guidelines into child-care food programs outside of California, an overriding goal is to lower the fat intake of young children. This message motivates menu planning in many programs throughout the United States due to the recommendations of the National Cholesterol Education Panel (NCEP).[75]

The extent of limiting fat in preschool menus depends on the age of the child and the primary prevention population approach to be used. Some skeptics have asked if 30-35% of energy from fat can provide adequate calories for 2- to 6-year-old preschoolers. To lower fat and still meet the recommendations for all nutrients including fat, meals and snacks must provide variety and adequate amounts of fruits, vegetables, grains, breads, cereals, and legumes each day. Low-fat dairy products and moderate portions of lean meats and poultry must be served.[91] While targeting a lower fat content means lowering the fat in food, menu planners must address the smaller appetites of preschoolers and control the salt and sugar content of the foods planned. A transition phase may be warranted to lower the fat, salt, and sugar content while maintaining taste and visual appeal.[92]

Zimmerman et al used computer modeling to determine menu planning components to reduce fat but retain two thirds of the RDAs for young children.[93] The following techniques were applied: medium-fat meats (MMt) replaced high-fat ones; lean meats (LMt) replaced higher-fat ones; lean meats were used with 3 high-fat meats a week (LMt-mod); skim milk replaced whole milk and 2% milk; fat-modified products (FMP) were used; low-fat preparation techniques (PrP) were used; and extraneous sources of fat (EF) were removed.

TABLE 7–6   The SHAPE Meal Pattern for California Child Care Food Programs

Meal and Meal Components	Age	
	1 to 3 years	*3 to 6 years*
Breakfast		
Milk, fluid	$\frac{1}{2}$ C	$\frac{1}{2}$ C
Bread/bread alternates (whole grain or enriched)	$\frac{1}{4}$ C	$\frac{1}{2}$ C
Vegtable, fruit, or full-strength juice	2 servings total*	4 servings total*
• Bread	$\frac{1}{2}$ slice	$\frac{1}{2}$ slice
• Cornbread, rolls, muffins, biscuits	$\frac{1}{2}$ serving	$\frac{1}{2}$ serving
• Cold dry cereal (volume or weight, whichever is less)	$\frac{1}{4}$ C	$\frac{1}{2}$ oz
• Cooked cereal, pasta, noodle products, or cereal grains	$\frac{1}{4}$ C	$\frac{1}{4}$ C
Lunch/Supper		
Milk, fluid	$\frac{1}{2}$ C	$\frac{1}{2}$ C
Vegetable and/or fruit (2 or more kinds)	$\frac{1}{4}$ C total	$\frac{3}{4}$ C total
Bread/bread alternates (whote grain or enriched)	2 servings total*	2 servings total*
• Bread	$\frac{1}{2}$ slice	$\frac{1}{2}$ slice
• Cornbread, rolls, muffins, biscuits	$\frac{1}{2}$ serving	$\frac{1}{2}$ serving
• Cold dry cereal (volume or weight whichever is less)	$\frac{1}{4}$ C	$\frac{1}{2}$ oz
• Cooked cereal, pasta, noodle products, or cereal grains	$\frac{1}{4}$ C	$\frac{1}{4}$ C
Meat/meat alternates[†,‡]		
• Lean meat, fish, or poultry (edible portion as served)	1 oz	$1\frac{1}{2}$ oz
• Cheese, cottage cheese	1 oz	$1\frac{1}{2}$ oz
• Egg	1 egg	1 egg
• Cooked dry beans or peas[†]	$\frac{1}{4}$ C	$\frac{1}{2}$ oz
• Peanut butter, soy nut butter, or other nut or seed butters	2T	3T
• Peanuts, soy nuts, tree nuts, seeds	$\frac{1}{2}$ oz[‡]	$\frac{1}{2}$ oz[‡]
• An equivalent quantity of any combination of the above meat/meat alternates		
AM or PM Supplement (Snack)—Select 2 of these 4 components:		
Milk, fluids[§]	$\frac{1}{2}$ C	$\frac{1}{2}$ C
Vegetable, fruit, or full-strength juice[§]	$\frac{1}{2}$ C	$\frac{1}{2}$ C
Bread/bread alternates (whole grain or enriched)	2 servings total*	2 servings total*
• Bread	$\frac{1}{2}$ slice	$\frac{1}{2}$ slice
• Cornbread, rolls, muffins, biscuits	$\frac{1}{2}$ serving	$\frac{1}{2}$ serving
• Cold dry cereal (volume or weight, whichever is less)	$\frac{1}{4}$ C	$\frac{1}{2}$ oz
• Cooked cereal, pasta, noodle products, or cereal grains	$\frac{1}{4}$ C	$\frac{1}{4}$ C

Meat/Meat Alternates[†‡]

• Lean meat, fish, or poultry (edible portion as served)	$^1/_2$ oz	$^1/_2$ oz
• Cheese or cottage cheese	$^1/_2$ oz	$^1/_3$ oz
• Egg	$^1/_2$ egg	$^1/_2$ egg
• Cooked dry beans or peas[†]	$^1/_3$ oz	$^1/_2$ oz
• Peanut butter, soy nut butter, or other nut or seed butters	1 t	1 t
• Peanuts, soy nuts, tree nuts, seeds, or yogurt	$^1/_2$ oz[‡]	$^1/_2$ oz[‡]
• An equivalent amount of any combination of the above meat/meat alternates	$^1/_4$ C	$^1/_4$ C

[*] Any combination of bread/bread alternates may be served, as long as the required number of serving is met.

[†] In the same meal service, dried beans or dried peas may be used as a meat alternate or as a vegetable; however, such use does not satisfy the requirement for both components.

[‡] No more than 50% of the requirement shall be met with nuts or seeds. Nuts or seeds shall be combined with another meat/meat alternate to fulfill the requirement. For the purpose of determining combinations, 1 oz of nuts or seeds is equal to 1 oz of cooked lean meat, poultry, or fish.

[§] Juice may not be served when milk is served as the only other component.

Note: General selection guides:

Milk:
• Use breast milk or iron-fortified formula for children under 1 year of age.
• Use whole milk for children 1 to 2 years of age.
• Emphasize use of 2% low-fat milk for children 2 years and older.

Fruits/Vegetables:
• Must offer raw fruits or vegetable at least once a day.
• Serve vitamin A and vitamin C rich foods daily.

Bread/Bread Alternates:
• One half of all bread/bread alternates served must be a minimum of 25% whole grain (with recommended levels of 33% or more whole grain) or list whole grain as first ingredient.

Meat/Meat Alternate:
• Emphasize lean and lower-sodium choices.
• At least $^1/_8$ cup beans per week must be served as replacement for $^1/_2$ ounce meat/meat alternate.

Source: Adapted from California Department of Education; Nutrition Services Division. *Improving Children's Health Through a Comprehensive Nutrition Approach.* Sacramento, Calif: California Dept of Education; 2001. Available at: http//www.cde.ca.gov/re/di/or/division.asp?id=nsd.

For children 2 and 3 years old, single strategies of LMt, LMt-mod, skim, FMP, EF, and a combined strategy of MMt + PrP achieved the goal of less than 30% (±1%) of calories from fat, and reduced energy intake by 54 to 107 kcal. Only strategies Skim and MMt + PrP also met the criteria of providing at least

67% of the RDAs for 1- to 3-year olds. Zinc and vitamin D were low. Menus were made isocaloric or the same by adding carbohydrates. Then strategies LMt, FMP, and LMt-mod also achieved both goals. All techniques led to a decrease in saturated fatty acids and monounsaturated fatty acids. Only the isocaloric strategy Skim approached the recommended ratio of saturated to monounsaturated to polyunsaturated fatty acids.

For children 4 and 5 years old, strategies LMt, LMt-mod, Skim, FMP, EF, and MMt + PrP achieved the goal of less than 30% (±1%) of calories from fat, met at least 67% of the RDAs, and reduced energy intake by 58 to 131 kcal. When strategies LMt and Skim were made isocaloric, saturated fatty acids and monounsaturated fatty acids fell to levels at or below 10% (±1%) of total calories.

Several strategies can be used to lower total fat in the menu for preschoolers. Planners must recognize and alter saturated and monounsaturated fatty acid sources. Menus must be isocaloric if variety is to be achieved, but they must be nutrient rich to ensure micronutrient adequacy.[93]

ROLE AND STATUS OF CHILD-CARE EMPLOYEES

A major responsibility of staff in CCCs and family child care homes is to protect young children from any hazards in the eating environment and to provide enjoyable and nutritious foods. Specific information needed by all employees includes the following[87]:

- basic concepts of nutrition, including nutrition issues in the child-care setting
- interpretation and application of nutrition information and resources
- likes and dislikes, cultural beliefs and practices, and the food acceptability of preschoolers
- procurement and production techniques with attention to specifications, labels, storage, cost, nutrient retention, and standardized production

One avenue to disseminate the information is continuing education activities that enrich the skills of employees. Management can provide these activities with hands-on learning experiences, discussions, simulations, and problem-solving exercises. Often, connecting the daily activities of the center or home to a state or national initiative (e.g., 5 A Day) increases staff commitment and gives direction. Integrating parents into program planning with staff and providing incentives for staff participation in continuing education strengthen the chances that employees will buy into the activities.

What is a typical child-care facility? A statewide survey of CCCs was conducted in California.[94] A mass mailing of 707 questionnaires was sent to agencies that sponsored a Child Care Food Program (CCFP). These respondents were called *sponsors*. A 20% random sample (23) of the 114 agencies that only sponsor day care homes was identified. Day care homes are actual residences in which an individual takes care of children as a daytime job. This random sample of agencies received the sponsor questionnaire and a questionnaire for day care home providers.

Completed questionnaires were returned by 445 CCFP sponsors for a 63% response rate. Of these, 40% represented urban areas; 16% represented rural areas; 25% served both rural and urban areas; and 13% served the suburban areas of California. Of the respondents, 34% served metropolitan areas with more than 250,000 people; 15% served towns with less than 25,000 people. The title of the respondents included director, coordinator, administrator, nutrition coordinator, and program director. Of the respondents, 47% had served in their current position between 1 and 5 years; 39% were 41 to 50 years of age, and 30% were 31 to 40 years of age; 39% had either a BA or BS degree, and 28% held a master's degrees. Only 4% of the respondents were registered dietitians.

Agencies provided various incentives for their director or supervisor to gain professional training. Paid time for training was provided for 59% of the directors/supervisors, whereas only 3% had received a single salary increase and 1% a single promotion after additional training. Of the respondents, 9% had both pay increases and promotion when they participated in continuing education and training, but 26% reported receiving no incentive (neither paid time for training, salary increase, or promotion) for continuing education. Of the sponsors, 54% managed some developmentally disabled children. Due to the multiethnic population in California, 59% of nutrition staff members were bilingual. Of the sponsors, 19% employed a nutrition education specialist.

Average daily participation at CCCs varied (i.e., 63% had fewer than 200 children, 15% kept 200 to 799 children, and 7% cared for more than 800 children). The number of centers sponsored by a single sponsor across the state ranged from 1 to over 20; 68% sponsored 1 to 5 centers, 17% sponsored 6 to 10 centers, 4% sponsored 11 to 20, and 6% sponsored more than 20 day care centers. Agencies reported sponsoring up to 1,500 individual home child-care providers.

Sponsors were asked how well prepared they felt on topics related to their job. Over 40% of the sponsors felt very well prepared on the topics of food sanitation, interpersonal skills, organization management, healthy menu planning, personnel management, and arranging pleasant mealtimes. They reported feeling not at all prepared for special feeding concerns (53%), infant feeding (31%), recycling waste (28%), cultural foods (23%), and disaster planning (19%).

Of the sponsors, 18% had a regular quarterly or annual training schedule for their staff members that commonly used demonstrations, handouts, and videotapes. On-the-job training was continuous. Demonstrations, handouts, group discussions, and on-the-job training were common for home care providers. Menu and food service system characteristics included 54% of sponsors preparing meals on-site, 13% subcontracting, and 13% using bulk preparation at a central kitchen. Of the sponsors, 37% followed a menu planning system consistently. Breakfast and lunch were commonly served at centers and homes. About one half of centers and homes served dinner. Snacks were also popular at both types of facilities.[94]

TECHNIQUES TO ASSESS FOOD LIKES OF PRESCHOOLERS

A common procedure in child-care facilities is to regulate a child's food intake to reduce food waste and to control overeating. A 29-day study assessed self-selected feeding of 20 preschool children who were 3 years old and 20 who were 4 years old. Preschoolers could select and eat as much as they

Info Line

> A kid culture or child-care culture may exist in day care centers and home facilities. Common menu items served include spaghetti, fish sticks, hot dogs, potato chips, and cookies, which may be extremely popular but are nutrient poor.[95]

wanted. Using a 2×2 factorial design, a significant interaction of class and feeding method was noted. Four-year-olds increased their intake more than three-year-olds; but no significant difference was noted in plate waste, whether self-selection or portion control was used. A significant difference was noted in plate waste by age; younger children wasted more than older children.[96] Based on this study, child-care providers should review their menu planning and portion-control procedures.

It has been the norm to use adult food preferences when planning meals and snacks for children.[97] Several techniques that have been useful to day care center staff to include children in decisions about foods are as follows:

- *A facial hedonic scale:* This has shown consistency by having children rate preferences for a sample of food by circling the face that reflects how they feel about a food.
- *A ranking scale:* With this method, preschoolers are presented with a group of foods, asked to taste them, and then asked to identify the ones they like the best. The preferred item can be removed and the procedure repeated to establish a list of preferred foods.
- *Plate waste method:* This technique is used when a standard portion is served to a child. The amount remaining is subtracted from the standard portion to determine how much was eaten.
- *Informal tasting with sample bites:* By using this method, children can sample foods at a classroom learning center in science or health and associate what they eat with their health.

SUMMER FOOD SERVICE PROGRAM

The summer can often create a time of deficit food intake for children. Organizations may sponsor a Summer Food Service Program (SFSP), but sponsorship is limited to the following[98]:

- public and private nonprofit school food authorities, residential summer camps, and colleges and universities that participate in the summer programs for youth
- private, nonprofit organizations that meet specific criteria defined in SFSP regulations
- local, county, municipal, state, or federal government units

Both private, nonprofit organizations, and governmental units must have direct operational control over each site under their sponsorship. This means that they will be responsible for managing site staff, including such areas as hiring, conditions of employment, and termination; and exercising management control over SFSP operations at sites during the period of program participation.[98]

Potential sponsors must demonstrate that they have the necessary financial and administrative capability to meet SFSP objectives and to comply with program regulations. They must also accept final financial and administrative responsibility for all sites under their auspices. Approved sponsors must operate the program according to the federal and state regulations. Management responsibilities cannot be delegated below the sponsor level. The quality of the meal service, the conduct of site personnel, and the adequacy of record keeping reflect the sponsor's performance, which is subject to audit by the administering agency, by the USDA Office of the Inspector General, and by the General Accounting Office.

Sponsors may operate the SFSP at one or more sites (i.e., the physical locations where program meals are served to children). Regular sites and sites primarily for homeless children may be approved to serve up to 2 meals daily, either lunch and breakfast or lunch and a snack. Sites serving primarily migrant children and camps may be approved to serve up to 4 meals per day—breakfast, snack, lunch, and supper.[98] Sponsors must demonstrate that their proposed open sites are located in areas in which poor economic conditions exist. Two methods to demonstrate this are use of school data and use of census tract data. Sponsors of sites where meals are served only to an enrolled group of children must document eligibility based on statements of the household size and income, food stamp numbers, or Aid to Families with Dependent Children (AFDC) case numbers of children enrolled at each site. Sponsors must demonstrate that at least 50% of the enrolled children have been individually determined to be eligible for free or reduced-price school meals.

Sponsors may either prepare their own meals, obtain meals from a school food service authority, or obtain meals from a food service management company. Meals must meet meal pattern requirements as outlined in Appendix 7–C. Sponsors must comply with the following rules[98,99]:

- Serve the same meal to all children.
- Ensure that children eat all meals on-site. Site personnel must be sure to supervise all children on the site while they are eating meals. Only meals that children eat on-site are eligible for reimbursement.
- Serve meals during the times of meal service posted and approved by the administering agency.
- Ensure that all children at the site receive 1 meal before any child is served a second meal.
- Ensure that there is a 3-hour interval between meals. When nonresidential camp sites and sites serving primarily migrant children serve lunch and supper with no afternoon snack between the 2 meals, a 4-hour interval must occur between lunch and supper.
- Except at feeding sites for homeless children, ensure that the meal service period is no more than 2 hours for lunch and supper and no more than 1 hour for all other meals, including snacks.
- Adhere to local health and sanitation regulations.
- Arrange for delivery and adequate storage of meals if not prepared at the site.

Several job positions are essential to conduct an effective and efficient summer food service program. These include the director, the bookkeeper, site monitors, and the site supervisor. The responsibilities of these positions are listed in Appendix 7–D.

SPECIAL NUTRITION-RELATED CONCERNS

Several of the special nutrition concerns during gestation, infancy, and childhood are discussed briefly next.

Fetal Alcohol Syndrome

Data from the last decade show that several kinds of birth defects and mental retardation may result from ingestion of alcohol by pregnant women. This condition is known as fetal alcohol syndrome. Fetal alcohol syndrome is considered the third leading cause of birth defects and mental retardation among newborns. These harmful effects on fetal development occur in the first few weeks or months of prenatal development, which is when much of the nervous system is being formed. The level of alcohol in the fetus's blood might be 10 times greater than the blood alcohol content of the mother. A few drinks during pregnancy can endanger normal fetal development.[100]

Neural Tube Defects

In 1960, researchers discovered that folic acid deficiency causes birth defects in animals. A deficiency of folic acid during pregnancy paired with a family history of birth defects appear to increase the risk of neural tube defects (NTDs) in humans. Studies have shown that women with no previous history of giving birth to children with NTDs can reduce their risk by 60-75% by taking a supplement of 0.4 mg to 0.8 mg of folic acid each day.[101]

Often, defect of the neural tube occurs in an embryo before a woman is aware that she is pregnant. Incidence in the United States is 1 to 2 infants per 1,000 live births. Annually, about 2,500 babies are born with NTDs. Many other pregnancies result in miscarriage or stillbirth. About 70% of NTDs could be prevented if every woman in the United States had 400 micrograms of folic acid every day. The March of Dimes, the National Council on Folic Acid, and the American Dietetic Association are united in recommending that women of childbearing age take 400 micrograms of synthetic folic acid daily, from fortified foods and/or supplements, in addition to consuming food folate from a varied diet.[102]

The average daily intake of folic acid for women is 0.2 mg. The FDA fortifies foods to ensure an adequate intake among childbearing women (i.e., 140 micrograms per 100 grams or 3.5 ounces of bread, rolls, buns, corn grits, cornmeal, rice, noodles, and farina). Good sources of folic acid include leafy green vegetables, citrus fruits, beans, and fortified breakfast cereals.

An FDA regulation became fully implemented in January 1998, requiring the addition of 140 mcg of folic acid to each 100 grams of currently enriched grain products, including most flours, corn meals, pasta, rice, baked goods made with the fortified flours, and breakfast cereals up to 400 mcg per serving. This is the first new fortification since 1943, and it is the first time foods have been fortified to prevent birth defects. Manufacturers of foods with high folic acid levels can advertise and place claims on the labels that this vitamin can prevent NTDs. This is the eighth health claim that FDA allowed for foods. The expected outcome is an increase in the folic acid intake of childbearing women by 100 mcg a day.[103]

There are 2 types of NTDs: anencephaly, which means that a baby does not develop a brain, and spina bifida, which is a defect of the spinal column. An infant with anencephaly dies soon after birth. In an infant with spina bifida, the bones of the spinal column may surround the spinal cord but do not fuse correctly within the first month after conception. As a result, the cord or spinal fluid bulge in the lower back. Paralysis and incontinence occur. The severity of the condition ranges from a mild, often undiagnosed form to spina bifida aperta, which creates a sac called a meningocele on the infant's back. Symptoms range from hydrocephalus, to foot and knee deformities that require braces, to obesity due to limited ability to move.[101]

About 100 mcg of additional folic acid a day can reduce the risk of an NTD by 22%, and 200 mcg could reduce the risk by 41%. About 2,500 women each year deliver infants with spina bifida or anencephaly, and of these, about 1,500 women terminate the pregnancies before birth. Conversely, if the total folic acid intake is > 1,000 mcg a day, the hematologic symptoms of pernicious anemia may not be apparent, especially for individuals who don't absorb vitamin B_{12}.[103]

Pernicious anemia of adults and seniors is prevented by folic acid, but the neurological damage can progress silently. The condition is significant for seniors since gastric acidity and absorption decline with age. Including a serum B_{12} test for seniors may evolve.

A Gallup poll reported in the August 8, 1997, *MMWR* that between 1995 and 1997:

- There was a 5% increase among nonpregnant women taking a vitamin supplement with folic acid.
- 19% of nonpregnant women < 25 years old were taking a supplement.
- < 20% of women having 39% of all pregnancies met the guidelines for folic acid supplementation.
- 65% of the women knew about folic acid, but only 22% knew the recommended intake.[102]

Also, women pregnant in 1995 only increased supplementation by 3%

Phenylketonuria

Phenylketonuria (PKU) is a metabolic disorder characterized by a deficiency of phenylalanine hydroxylase. Hyperphenylalaninemia occurs when phenylalanine is not metabolized to tyrosine. A screening test, the Guthrie bacterial inhibition assay, is performed on blood from the heel of newborns within 28 days of life. Undiagnosed PKU infants without diet alteration (i.e., a low-phenylalanine diet, primarily Lofenalac formula) are severely mentally retarded and function with an IQ of about 40. Diagnosed and treated infants have a normal range of functioning and intelligence.[104]

Iron Deficiency Anemia

A significant decline in the prevalence of iron deficiency anemia has been observed among healthy children from 1969 to 1986, with credit given to improved prenatal and infant care among recipients of WIC (see Chapter 9). Iron deficiency (less than 3.5 mg%) remains the most common nutrient deficiency among US children 6 months to 3 years of age.[105]

According to the 1996 Continuing Survey of Food Intake by Individuals (CSFII), about 95% of formula-fed infants up to 12 months of age meet the RDA for iron and 77% meet their need for zinc. Breast milk is a relatively poor source of iron and zinc, but the bioavailability and absorption are higher in breast milk than in infant formulas. Full-term infants exclusively breast fed are rarely at risk for iron or zinc deficiency during the first 4 to 6 months, but intake of both dietary iron and zinc emerge at 6 months of age when the liver's stores typically become depleted. Breast milk content drops steadily over 7 to 9 months of lactation. The RDA for iron increases at 6 months of age, while the RDA for zinc remains constant throughout the first year of life. Infants aged 9 to 18 months are at the highest risk of any age group for iron deficiency due to their rapid growth and inadequate intakes. All these factors influence iron and zinc status.[105]

Serial screening of infants and young children at high risk for iron deficiency anemia is recommended. For example, screen the following high-risk children for iron deficiency anemia between 9 and 12 months, 6 months later, and annually from ages 2 to 5 years: children from low-income families, children eligible for WIC, migrant children, and recently arrived refugee children. At ages 9 to 12 months and 6 months later, screen infants with the following risk factors for iron deficiency anemia: preterm or low-birth-weight, not breast fed, received non–iron-fortified infant formula for more than 2 months, introduced to cow's milk before 12 months, and breast-fed infants with insufficient iron from supplementary foods. Annually assess children aged 2 to 5 years and screen children with the following risks for anemia: low-iron diet, limited access to food because of poverty or neglect, and special healthcare needs.[105]

Researchers placed preschool children ages 3 to 5 on either a 500-mg low-calcium diet or a high-calcium diet with about 1,000 mg. There was no difference in iron absorption. Children who increased their calcium intakes of milk, cheese, and yogurt foods increased their calcium absorption, which may benefit bone growth and development. This benefit may occur without negatively affecting iron absorption and not increasing the risk of iron deficiency anemia.[106] The NAS daily calcium recommendations for children ages 1 to 3 is 500 mg/day; ages 4 to 8, 800 mg/day; and ages 9 to 18, 1,300 mg/day.

Lead Poisoning

Lead exposure has now become the most common environmental disease of childhood. A strong relationship between blood lead level, hematocrit, and age has been noted. The higher the blood lead level, the greater the probability of iron-deficiency anemia; a toxic level is from 10 to 25 μg/dL. Lead affects nutrition by displacing essential divalent cat-ions (e.g., iron, zinc, and calcium) in several metabolic functions; thereby, lead toxicity is associated with deficiencies of iron, zinc, and calcium. Since the body absorbs lead more efficiently during times of growth, children and infants are susceptible to toxicity.[107]

Even at low levels, lead can affect the central nervous system, hearing, blood pressure, and physical growth. Initial signs of lead poisoning include diarrhea, irritability, and lethargy. The long-term effects of exposure include lower IQ scores, poorer speech and language performance, impaired attention, and an increased risk of attention deficit disorder and hyperactivity.

In one study, 55% of African-American children living in poverty had blood lead levels greater than 10 μg/dL. The blood lead levels of 579 children, aged 1 to 5, who lived near a lead smelter ranged from 11 to 164 μg/dL. The younger children with higher blood lead levels had a higher probability of anemia.[107]

Hyperactivity

Many dietary links to hyperactivity are presented as testimonials, parental reports, and case studies. Feingold's alarming statement in 1975 regarding food additives made many parents fearful of food additives, but clinical trials have not supported the allegations.[108] Only preschool children who had extremely high levels of food dyes or who were allergic to food dyes were observed to have adverse effects from diet.[109]

Sugar and aspartame have been reported to produce behavioral problems including hyperactivity among young children. A double-blind, controlled trial involving 25 normal 3- to-5-year-olds and 23 sugar sensitive 6- to 10-year olds was conducted by Wolraich and colleagues.[110] Three consecutive 3-week modified diets were followed by the children and their families: (1) a diet with about 5,600 mg of sucrose per kg and no artificial sweeteners; (2) a diet low in sucrose with 38 g aspartame/kg; and (3) a diet low in sucrose but containing 12 mg saccharin as a placebo sweetener. None of the test foods had additives, artificial food coloring, or preservatives.

School-age children were given about 4,500 mg of sucrose/kg, 32 mg of aspartame per kg, and 9.9 mg saccharin per kg. The results showed that for 39 different behavioral and cognitive variables measured during the 3 diets, only preschool parents reported significantly better cognition during the sucrose diet versus the aspartame and saccharin diets and that a decreased pegboard performance occurred when the sucrose diet was followed. No significant differences were noted for the school-age children, and no adverse reaction occurred when children followed the sucrose or aspartame diets.[110] Overall, sugar, saccharin, and aspartame do not appear to affect behavior and cognitive functioning of young children.

Obesigenic Eating Environment

Obesigenic eating environments often reflect larger portion sizes of inexpensive, palatable, energy-dense foods.[111-114] Portion sizes have become mammoth, especially for foods that are consumed outside the home.[115] Restaurant portions may approach the recommended daily number of servings from several food groups in a single entrée.[116] US families spend 1 of every 3 food dollars on foods and beverages consumed away from the home, creating an almost constant exposure to large portions.[116]

Restrictive child-feeding strategies are associated with overeating and overweight in young children.[117-119] In addition, the risk of overweight has been linked to both neglectful family environments during childhood and limited maternal knowledge of children's intake of sweets.[120-122]

Researchers asked the question, "Do large portion sizes affect children's eating behavior?" Their objectives were to determine the effects of repeated exposure to a large portion of an entrée on preschool-aged children's awareness of portion size, self-selected portion size, and food intake; and to evaluate associations of children's responsiveness to portion size with weight status and overeating.[122]

Thirty children at 2 different lunches were presented with either an age-appropriate portion or a large portion of an entrée. At a different time, children's self-served portions, their weight, height, and tendency to overeat were assessed. The researchers observed that when doubling an age-appropriate portion of an entrée, the child's entrée and total energy intake were increased at lunch by 25% and 15%, respectively. This was due to increases in the average size of the children's bites of the entrée without compensatory reduction in the intake of other foods served at the meal. The children were unaware of changes in portion size but generally their response to the portion size was overeating. The children consumed 25% less of the entrée when allowed to serve themselves than when served a large portion.[122]

Large entrée portions may constitute an obesigenic environmental influence for preschool-aged children by producing excessive intake at meals. Children who can't or don't recognize satiety may consume large portions. Allowing children to select their own portion size may be the best plan.

RECAP OF COMMUNITY NUTRITION SERVICES— A PUBLIC HEALTH PERSPECTIVE

Since the 1920s, the United States has supported public health programs for infants and children. Title V of the Social Security Act of 1935 confirmed a state and federal collaboration to address the needs of this cohort. During the last 20 to 30 years, the US Congress has responded with appropriations for programs including the WIC; the Food Stamp Program; Maternal and Child Health Services Block Grant Programs; the Preventive Health Services Block Grant Programs; the Medicaid Early Periodic Screening, Diagnosis and Treatment Program; and programs in the Indian Health Service. WIC has been a highly funded program, primarily because evaluation has been conducted and positive results are visible.[123] For example:

- WIC lowers the rate of anemia among participating children ages 6 months to 5 years. The data show an average decrease in the anemia rate of more than 16% for each year from 1980 to 1992.
- WIC significantly improves children's diets, particularly when it comes to vitamins and nutrients including iron, vitamin C, thiamin, protein, niacin, and vitamin B_6.

- Four- and 5-year-olds who participate in WIC in early childhood have better vocabularies and digit memory scores than comparable children who do not participate in WIC.
- WIC participants have higher rates of immunization against childhood diseases.

Approximately 15,000 community nutrition professionals, commonly referred to as public health nutritionists, function at the local, state, and federal levels to assess the needs of infants and children, to develop and direct programs, and to evaluate the impact of WIC and other programs.[124]

Head Start

Head Start is a comprehensive early childhood program established in 1965 to ameliorate the effects of poverty on preschool children and their families. Initially the program was an 8-week summer program that gradually expanded its scope of activities, length of operation year, and funding base. Over 1,400 grantees in the United States, Puerto Rico, the US Virgin Islands, and the Pacific Trust territories provide services to more than 750,000 children and their families annually through a $4.3 billion federal government US DHHS appropriation. Since 1965, Head Start has served more than 14 million at-risk children. Legislation in 1994 funded infant/toddler projects. About 200 grantees operate an Early Head Start program.[125]

Head Start is a family-focused, comprehensive child development program providing education, health, nutrition, social services, and parent involvement to birth through 5-year-old at-risk children and their families. Center-based and home-based program options are available. At least 10% of enrolled children have been professionally diagnosed as having a disability.

Children are screened and assessed for cognitive development activities in the classroom; screened for dental and medical problems and provided appropriate follow-up services where needed; fed at least one third of their daily nutritional requirements when attending classes through the US Department of Agriculture's Child and Adult Care Feeding Program; and observed by mental health professionals to ensure that emotional and psychological needs are being met. Individual education plans are developed and implemented for disabled children in addition to regular program services.

As members of the policy council, parents are decision makers for the program and provide input into classroom activities by participating in center committees. They are invaluable volunteers in the classroom and other component areas. Parents are informed of community resources available to them through the social services component and are offered both formal and informal training on a variety of topics, such as preventive health practices, parenting skills, child abuse awareness and avoidance, and sound nutrition planning for the family.[125]

Method Alert

Sobo and Rock transcribed audiotaped caretaker-assisted, 24-hour dietary recalls to quantify measures of caretaker-child interaction. The Olestra Post-marketing Surveillance Study in San Diego involved 34 children 7 to 11 years old. Measures of participation for caretaker-child pairs were compared, and within-group differences were examined. Caretakers contributed first by adding food details, and second, by prompting children. Children were remarkably knowledgeable of food details, and they rejected many items reported by caretakers. Gender was not a factor, but male caretakers reduced the extent of details voiced by children. The investigators reported that questions should be directed toward children, even when caretakers are present and professionals should limit caretaker participation, even excusing them at the end of the interview so children respond freely.[126]

HEALTHY PEOPLE 2010 ACTIONS

Currently in the United States, public programs combine with the newer wave of community-based primary prevention activities of schools, universities, professional organizations, hospitals, clinics, and private industry to provide services and interventions for young children. The collaborative and complementary efforts of these groups are needed to address immediate health and nutrition needs, as well as long-term goals for a healthier population of children in the United States.

Eating behaviors and nutrient intakes early in life set the stage for lifelong habits. *Healthy People 2010* objectives include ensuring healthy body weight from birth to the preschool age (see Exhibit 7–1). Breastfeeding, iron deficiency anemia, and diarrhea are nutrition-related topics.[79] The meal and snack pattern and its blend with appropriate physical activity set the agenda for preschool and day care facilities. Community nutrition professionals have a visible role and responsibility to work with children, parents, teachers, administrators, and caregivers who work with preschool and day care facilities to achieve these *Healthy People 2010* objectives.

Exhibit 7–1   DATA 2010: The *Healthy People 2010* Database—November 2000
Edition, Focus Area: 16—Maternal Infant and Child Health

Objective No.	Objective	Baseline Year	Baseline %	Target 2010 %
16-01a	Fetal and infant deaths—fetal deaths at 20 or more weeks of gestation (rate per 1,000 live births plus fetal deaths)	1997	6.8	4.1
16-01b	Fetal and infant deaths—during perinatal period (28 weeks of gestation to 7 days after birth) (rate per 1,000 live births plus fetal deaths)	1997	7.3	4.5
16-01c	Fetal and infant deaths—all infant deaths (within 1 year) (rate per 1,000 live births)	1998	7.2	4.5

16-01d	Fetal and infant deaths—neonatal deaths (within first 28 days of life) (rate per 1,000 live births)	1998	4.8	2.9
16-01e	Fetal and infant deaths—postneonatal deaths (between 28 days and 1 year) (rate per 1,000 live births)	1998	2.4	1.2
16-01h	Fetal and infant deaths—sudden infant death syndrome (SIDS) (rate per 1,000 live births, infants aged under 1 year)	1998	0.72	0.25
16-02a	Child deaths (rate per 100,000 children aged 1 to 4 years)	1998	34.6	18.6
16-04	Maternal deaths (rate per 100,000 live births)	1998	7.1	3.3
16-06a	Prenatal care—beginning in first trimester	1998	83	90
16-06b	Prenatal care—early and adequate	1998	74	90
16-08	Very-low-birth-weight infants born at level III hospitals (age under 1 year)	1996-1997	73	90
16-10a	Low birth weight and very low birth weight—low-birth-weight (LBW) infants aged under 1 year	1998	7.6	5.0
16-10b	Low birth weight and very low birth weight—very-low-birth-weight (VLBW) infants aged under 1 year	1998	1.4	0.9
16-12	Weight gain during pregnancy	UK	UK	UK
16-15	Spina bifida and other neural tube defects (new cases per 10,000 live births)	1996	6	3
16-16a	Optimum folic acid levels—females who began pregnancy with at least 400 µg of folic acid each day (females aged 15 to 44 years)	1991-1994	21	80
16-16b	Optimum folic acid levels—females who began pregnancy with median RBC folate level (number in ng/mL, females aged 15 to 44 years)	1991-94	160	220
16-19a	Breastfeeding—in early postpartum period	1998	64	75
16-19b	Breastfeeding—at 6 months	1998	29	50
16-19c	Breastfeeding—at 1 year	1998	16	25

UK = unknown

Source: Adapted from: US Department of Health and Human Services. DATA 2010—The *Healthy People 2010* Database. *CDC Wonder.* Atlanta, Ga: Centers for Disease Control; November 2000.

REFERENCES

1. Berenson G. Causation of cardiovascular risk factors. In: *Children—Perspectives on Cardiovascular Risk in Early Life*. New York: Raven Press; 1986:408.
2. Wiecha JL, Grandon CA, Fisher-Miller P, et al. *Nutrition Counts: Massachusetts Nutrition Surveillance System, FY90 Annual Report*. Boston, Mass: Department of Public Health; 1991. ERIC Document Reproduction Service No. ED 338; 423.
3. Good ME. *A Needs Assessment: The Health Status of Migrant Children as They Enter Kindergarten*. San Jose, Calif: San Jose State University; 1990. ERIC Document Reproduction Service No. ED 338; 460.
4. Kleinman RE, Hall S, Green H, et al. Diet, breakfast, and academic performance in children. *Ann Nutr Metab*. 2002;46(suppl 1):S24-S30.
5. Friedman BJ, Hurd-Crixell SL. Nutrient intake of children eating school breakfast. *J Am Diet Assoc*. 1999;99:219-221.
6. Center on Hunger, Poverty and Nutrition Policy. *The Link Between Nutrition and Cognitive Development in Children*. Medford, Mass: Tufts University School of Nutrition; 1994:16.
7. American Academy of Pediatrics, Committee on Nutrition. The use of whole cow's milk in infancy. *Pediatrics*. 1992;89:1105-1109.
8. Clyne PS, Kulczycki A. Human breast milk contains bovine IgG: relationship to infant colic? *Pediatrics*. 1991;87:439-444.
9. Heinig MJ, Nommsen LA, Peerson JM, et al. Energy and protein intakes of breast-fed and formula-fed infants during the first year of life and their association with growth velocity: the Darling study. *Am J Clin Nutr*. 1993;58:152-161.
10. American Academy of Pediatrics. Breastfeeding and the use of human milk. *Pediatrics*. 1997;100:1035-1039.
11. Ryan AS. The resurgence of breastfeeding in the United States. *Pediatrics*. 1997;99(4):e12.
12. US Department of Health and Human Services. Maternal, infant, and child health. *Healthy People 2010: Understanding and Improving Health*. 2nd ed. Washington, DC: US Government Printing Office, November 2000;61-1-16-2.
13. Black RE, Morris SS, Bryce J. Child survival I: where and why 10 million children die every year? *Lancet*. 2003;361:2226-2234.
14. Wolf JH. Low breastfeeding rates and public health in the United States. *Am J Public Health*. 2003;93:2000-2010.
15. The American Dietetic Association. Position of the American Dietetic Association: breaking the barriers to breastfeeding. *J Am Diet Assoc*. 2001;101:1213-1220.
16. Bagwell JE, Kendrick OW, Stitt KR, Leeper JD. Knowledge and attitudes toward breast-feeding: differences among dietitians, nurses and physicians working with WIC clients. *J Am Diet Assoc*. 1993;93:901-804.
17. Freed GL, Clark SJ, Sorenson J, Lohr JA, Cefalo R, Curtis P. National assessment of physicians' breasfeeding knowledge, attitudes, training and experience. *JAMA*. 1995;472-476.
18. Michelman DF, Faden RR, Gielen AC, Buxton KS. Pediatricians and breastfeeding promotion: attitudes, beliefs, and practices. *Am J Health Prom*. 1990;4:181-186.
19. Barnett E, Sienkiewicz M, Roholt S. Beliefs about breastfeeding: a statewide survey of health professionals. *Birth*. 1995;22:15-20.
20. Helm A, Windham CT, Wyse B. Dietitians in breastfeeding management: an untapped resource in the hospital. *J Hum Lactation*. 1997;13(3):221-226.

21. PHNPG. Breastfeeding success: you can make the difference. *Digest.* Fall 1999.
22. Ajzen I, Fishbein M. *Understanding Attitudes and Predicting Social Behavior.* Englewood Cliffs, NJ: Prentice Hall; 1980:250.
23. Falciglia G. Neophobia and lack of variety of food in children's diets—child nutrition and health campaign. Presentation at: ADA Annual Meeting; 1998; Kansas City, Kan.
24. Lawless H. Sensory development in children: research in taste and olfaction. *J Am Diet Assoc.* 1985;85:577.
25. Beauchamp GK, Cowart BJ. Congenital and experimental factors in the development of human flavor preferences. *Appetite.* 1985;6:357.
26. Cowart BJ, Beauchamp GK. The importance of sensory context in young children's acceptance of salty tastes. *Child Dev.* 1986;57:1034.
27. Birch LL. Dimensions of preschool children's food preferences. *J Nutr Ed.* 1979;11:77.
28. Birch LL. Preschool children's food preferences and consumption patterns. *J Nutr Ed.* 1979;11:189-192.
29. Burt JV, Hertzler AA. Parental influence on the child's food preference. *J Nutr Ed.* 1978;10:127.
30. Birch LL. The relationship between children's food preferences and those of their parents. *J Nutr Ed.* 1980;12:14.
31. Kirks BA, Hughes C. Long-term behavioral effects of parent involvement in nutrition education. *J Nutr Ed.* 1986;18:203.
32. Pliner P, Pelchant ML. Similarities in food preferences between children and their siblings and parents. *Appetite.* 1986;7:333.
33. Cooper JO, Heron TE, Heward WL. *Applied Behavior Analysis.* Columbus, Ohio: Charles E. Merrill Publishing Co; 1987.
34. Peterson LW. Operant approach to observation and recording. *Nurs Outlook.* 1967;15:28.
35. Pipes PC. *Nutrition in Infancy and Childhood.* 4th ed. Boston, Mass: Times Mirror/Mosby College Publishing; 1989:405.
36. Rozin P, Hammer L, Osler H, Horowitz T, Marmora Y. The child's conception of food: differentiation of categories of rejected substances in the 16 months to 5 year age range. *Appetite.* 1986;7:141.
37. Birch LL, Deysher M. Conditional and unconditioned caloric compensation: evidence for self-regulation of food intake in young children. *Learning and Motivation.* 1985;16:341.
38. Birch LL, Marlin DW, Rotter J. Eating as the 'means' activity in a contingency: effects on young children's food preferences. *Child Dev.* 1984;55:431.
39. Rolls BJ. Experimental analysis of the effects of variety in a meal on human feeding. *Am J Clin Nutr.* 1985;42:932.
40. Michela JL, Contento IR. Spontaneous classification of foods by elementary school-aged children. *Health Ed Q.* 1984;11:57.
41. Bybee RW, Sund RB. *Piaget for Educators.* 2nd ed. Columbus, Ohio: Charles E. Merrill Publishing Co; 1982.
42. *The Food Guide Pyramid.* Washington, DC: US Dept of Agriculture, Human Nutrition Information Service; April 2005. Available at www.mypyramid.com.
43. Swanson-Rudd J. Nutrition orientations of working mothers in the North Central region. *J Nutr Ed.* 1982;14:132.
44. Phillips DE, Bass MA, Yetley E. Use of food and nutrition knowledge by mothers of preschool children. *J Nutr Ed.* 1978;10:73.
45. Gillis DEG, Sabry JH. Daycare teachers: nutrition knowledge, opinions, and use of food. *J Nutr Ed.* 1980;12:200.

46. Hertzler AA. Obesity—impact on the family. *J Am Diet Assoc.* 1981;79:525.
47. Birch LL. Mother-child interaction patterns and the degree of fatness in children. *J Nutr Ed.* 1981;12:17.
48. Birch LL, Zimmerman SI, Hind H. The influence of social-affective context on the formation of children's food preferences. *J Nutr Ed.* 1981;13:115.
49. Stark LJ, Collins FL, Osnes PG, Stokes TF. Using reinforcement and cueing to increase healthy snack food choices in preschoolers. *J Appl Behav Anal.* 1986;19:367.
50. Satter EM. The feeding relationship. *J Am Diet Assoc.* 1986;86:352.
51. Satter E. *Child of Mine.* Palo Alto, Calif: Bull Publishing Co; 1991.
52. Somers AR. Violence, television, and the health of American youth. *N Engl J Med.* 1976;294:811.
53. Blatt J, Spencer L, Ward S. A cognitive developmental study of children's reactions to television advertising. In: Rubinstein EA, Comstock GA, Murray JP, eds. *Television and Social Behavior.* Washington, DC: US Government Printing Office; 1972. *Television in Day to Day Life: Patterns of Use*; vol 4.
54. Reid LN, Bearden WO, Teel JE. Family income, TV viewing, and children's cereal ratings. *Journalism Q.* 1980;57:327.
55. Choate R. Statement presented before the House Subcommittee on Communications of the Committee on Interstate and Foreign Commerce, US House of Representatives. Washington, DC: US Government Printing Office; 1975.
56. California Department of Health Services. *The California Nutrition Network for Healthy, Active Families and the California 5 a Day for Better Health! Campaign.* Sacramento, Calif: California Department of Health Services; 2005. Available at: http://www.dhs.ca.gov/ps/cdic/cpns/ca5aday/.
57. Calamaro CJ, Faith MS. Preventing childhood overweight: television viewing. *Nutr Today.* 2004;39(5):194-195.
58. NHLBI study shows reduced fat intake to lower cholesterol is safe and beneficial for children [news release]. Washington, DC: National Cholesterol Education Program; February 5, 2001.
59. Knapp JA, Hazuda HP, Haffner SM, et al. A saturated fat/cholesterol avoidance scale: sex and ethnic differences in a biethnic population. *J Am Diet Assoc.* 1988;88:172-177.
60. Frank GC, Zive M, Nelson J, et al. Fat and cholesterol avoidance among Mexican American and Anglo preschool children and parents. *J Am Diet Assoc.* 1991;91:954-961.
61. Armstrong J, Dorosty AR, Reilly JJ, Emmett PM. Coexistence of social inequalities in undernutrition and obesity in preschool children: population-based cross sectional study. *Arch Dis Child.* 2003;88(8):671-675.
62. Rolland-Cachera MF, Deheeger M, Avons P, et al. Tracking adiposity patterns from 1 month to adulthood. *Ann Hum Biol.* 1987;14:219-222.
63. Charney E, Goodman HC, McBride M, et al. Childhood antecedents of adult obesity: do chubby infants become obese adults? *N Engl J Med.* 1976;295:6-9.
64. Gutin B, Basch C, Shea S, et al. Blood pressure, fitness, and fatness in 5- and 6-year-old children. *JAMA.* 1990;264:1123-1127.
65. US Department of Health and Human Services. *Surgeon General's Call to Action to Prevent and Decrease Overweight and Obesity.* Washington, DC; 2001. Available at: http://www.surgeongeneral.gov/topics/obesity.

66. Centers for Disease Control and Prevention. Prevalence of overweight for Hispanics—United States, 1982-1984. *JAMA*. 1990;263:631.
67. Heinbach JT. Sodium, hypertension and the American public: second tracking survey. *Public Health Rep*. 1985;100:371.
68. Johnson SL, Birch LL. Parents and children's adiposity and eating styles. *Pediatrics*. 1994;94:1-9.
69. Newby PK, Peterson KE, Berkey CS, Leppert J, Willett WC, Colditz GA. Beverage consumption is not associated with changes in weight and body mass index among low-income preschool children in North Dakota. *J Am Diet Assoc*. 2004;104:1086-1094.
70. Keys A. Coronary heart disease in seven countries. *Circulation*. 1970;41:1-211.
71. Webber LS, Cresanta JL, Voors AW, et al. Tracking of cardiovascular disease risk factor variables in school-age children. *J Chronic Dis*. 1983;36:647-660.
72. Freedman DS, Byers T, Sell K, et al. Tracking of serum cholesterol levels in multiracial sample of preschool children. *Pediatrics*. 1992;90:80-85.
73. National Academy of Sciences, Food and Nutrition Board, National Research Council. *Dietary Reference Intakes (DRI) and Recommended Dietary Allowances (RDA)*. Available at: http://www.nal/usda.gov/fnic/etext/000105.htm. Accessed June 26, 2004.
74. US Department of Agriculture. *Food Buying Guide for Child Nutrition Programs*. Washington, DC: US Government Printing Office; 1981. Program aid 1331.
75. National Heart, Lung and Blood Institute. National Cholesterol Education Program. Implications of recent clinical trials for the National Cholesterol Education Program adult treatment panel III guidelines. *Circulation*. 2004;110:227-239.
76. *Dietary Guidelines for Americans*. Washington, DC: US Dept of Agriculture and US Dept of Health and Human Services; 2005.
77. Gleason P, Suitor C. *Changes in Children's Diets: 1989-1991 to 1994-1996*. Alexandria, Va: Office of Analysis, Nutrition and Evaluation. Food and Nutrition Services. United States Dept of Agriculture; January 2001. Report No. CN-01-CD1.
78. National Cholesterol Education Program. *Report of the Expert Panel on Population Strategies for Blood Cholesterol Reduction*. Bethesda, Md: US Dept of Health and Human Services, Public Health Services, National Institutes of Health, National Heart, Lung, and Blood Institute; November 1990. NIH pub no 90-3046.
79. *Healthy People in Healthy Communities 2010: National Health Promotion and Disease Prevention Objectives*. Washington, DC: US Dept of Health and Human Services. DHHS (PHS).
80. Portland Unified School District. *"Fun Kit" Preschool Curriculum*. Portland, Ore: Portland School Food Service Department; 1992.
81. US Department of Agriculture. *Facts About the Child and Adult Care Food Program*. Alexandria, Va: Food and Nutrition Services. FNS Public Information 703-305-2286. Available at http://www.fns.usda.gov/cnd/Care/CACFP/. Accessed June 29, 2005.
82. Duyff RL, Giarratano SC, Zurich MF. *Nutrition, Health and Safety for Preschool Children*. New York: Glencoe-McGraw-Hill; 1994:238,210-211.
83. Skinner J, Carruth B, Moran J, Houck K, Coletta F. Fruit juice intake is not related to children's growth. *Pediatrics*. 1999;103:58-64.
84. Skinner J, Carruth B, Houck K, et al. Longitudinal study of nutrient and food intakes of infants aged 2 to 24 months. *J Am Diet Assoc*. 1997;97:496-504.

85. Arbeit M, Nicklas T, Frank G, Webber L, Miner M, Berenson G. Caffeine intakes of children from a biracial population: the Bogalusa Heart Study. *J Am Diet Assoc.* 1988;88:466-471.

86. American Public Health Association and American Academy of Pediatrics. *Caring for Our Children—National Health and Safety Performance Standards.* 2nd ed. Ann Arbor, Mich; 2004.

87. American Dietetic Association. *Benchmarks for Nutrition Programs in Child Care Settings* [position paper]. Chicago, Ill: ADA; July 23, 2002.

88. Briley ME, Coyle E, Roberts-Gray C, Sparkman A. Nutrition knowledge and attitudes and menu planning skills of family day-home providers. *J Am Diet Assoc.* 1989;89:694-695.

89. Briley ME, Roberts-Gray C, Simpson D. Identification of factors that influence the menu at child care centers: a grounded theory approach. *J Am Diet Assoc.* 1994;94:276-281.

90. California Department of Education, Nutrition Services Division. *Executive Summary: Improving Children's Health Through a Comprehensive Nutrition Approach—An Evaluation of Nutrition Education in SHAPE California.* Sacramento, Calif; 2001. Available at: http://www.cde.ca.gov/re/di/or/division.asp?id=nsd

91. American Dietetic Association. Position of the American Dietetic Association: Dietary guidance for healthy children ages 2-11 years. *J Am Diet Assoc.* 2004;104:660-677.

92. Obarzanek E, Kimm YS, Barton BA, et al. Long-term safety and efficacy of a cholesterol-lowering diet in children with elevated low-density lipoprotein cholesterol: seven-year results of the dietary intervention study in children (DISC). *Pediatrics.* 2001;107:256-264.

93. Zimmerman SA, Kris-Etherton P, Sigman MJ. Nutrient adequacy and effectiveness of dietary fat reduction techniques for preschool children. *American Dietetic Association Annual Meeting Abstracts Supplement.* 1992;92(9):A-112.

94. Frank GC, Adsen MA. *Final Termination Report of the Statewide Survey of Child Care Food Program Sponsors.* Long Beach: California State University Long Beach, Child Nutrition Program Management Center; 1993:1-144.

95. Hobbie C, Baker S, Bayerl C. Parental understanding of basic infant nutrition: misinformed feeding choices. *J Pediatr Health Care.* 2000;14:26-31.

96. Branen L, Fletcher J. Effects of restrictive and self-selected feeding on preschool children's food intake and waste at snacktime. *J Nutr Ed.* 1994;26:273-277.

97. Bourcier E, Bowen DJ, Hendrika M, Moinpour C. Evaluation of strategies used by family food preparers to influence healthy eating. *Appetite.* 2003;41:265-272.

98. US Department of Agriculture, Food and Nutrition Service. *Summer Food Service Program for Children. Sponsor's Handbook.* Washington, DC: US Dept of Agriculture; 1991. FNS-206.

99. Briley ME, Jastrow S, Vickers J, Roberts-Gray C. Dietary intake at child-care centers and away: are parents and care providers working as partners or at cross-purposes? *J Am Diet Assoc.* August 1999; 99(8):950-954.

100. US Department of Health and Human Services. *US Surgeon General Advisory on Alcohol Use in Pregnancy.* Washington, DC; February 21, 2005. Available at: www.surgeongeneral.gov.

101. Williams RD. FDA proposes folic acid fortification. *FDA Consumer.* 1994;11-14.

102. March of Dimes. *Folic Acid* [abstract]. White Plains, NY: Pregnancy and Newborn Health Education Center; June 27, 2005. Available at: www.marchofdimes.com.

103. Daly S, Mills JL, Molloy AM, et al. Minimum effective dose of folic acid for food fortification to prevent neural-tube defects. *Lancet.* December 6, 1997;350(9092):1666-1669.

104. Mahan LK, Escott-Stump S. *Krause's Food Nutrition and Diet Therapy.* 11th ed. Philadelphia, Pa: WB Saunders Company; 2000:197,399.

105. Centers for Disease Control and Prevention. Iron deficiency—United States, 1999-2000. *MMWR.* October 11, 2002;51(40):897-899.

106. Ames S, Gorham BM, Abrams SA. Effects of high compared with low calcium intake on calcium absorption and incorporation of iron by red blood cells in small children. *Am J Clin Nutr.* 1999;70:44-48.

107. US Environmental Protection Agency. *Protect Your Child from Lead Poisoning—Lead in Paint, Dust, and Soil.* Washington, DC; 2004. Available at: http://www.epa.gov/.

108. Feingold BF. Hyperkinesis and learning disabilities linked to artificial food flavors and colors. *Am J Nurs.* 1975;75:797-803.

109. Weiss B, Williams JH, Margen S, et al. Behavioral responses to artificial food colors. *Science.* 1980;207:1487-1489.

110. Wolraich ML, Lindgren SD, Stumbo PJ, et al. Effects of diets high in sucrose or aspartame on the behavior and cognitive performance of children. *N Engl J Med.* 1994;330:301-307.

111. Hill JO. Genetic and environmental contributions to obesity. *Am J Clin Nutr.* 1998;68:991-992.

112. Poston WS, Foreyt JP. Obesity is an environmental issue. *Atherosclerosis.* 1999;146:201,209.

113. Hill JO, Goldberg JP, Russell RP, Peters JC. Introduction. Summit on promoting healthy eating and active living: developing a framework for progress. *Nutr Rev.* 2000;59:S4-S6.

114. French S, Story M, Jeffrey R. Environmental influences on eating and physical activity. *Annu Rev Public Health.* 2001;22:309-335.

115. Young L, Nestle M. Portion sizes in dietary assessment: issues and policy implications. *Nutr Rev.* 1995;53:149-158.

116. Tufts University. Portion distortion. *Tufts University Health and Nutrition Letter*; February 2001. Available at http://healthletter.tufts.edu/. Accessed March 15, 2001.

117. Fisher JO, Birch LL. Restricting access to foods and children's eating appetite. *Appetite.* 1999;32:405-419.

118. Birch LL, Fisher JO. Mother's child feeding practices influence daughters eating and weight. *Am J Clin Nutr.* 2000;71,1054-1061.

119. Fisher JO, Birch LL. Eating in the absence of hunger and overweight in girls from 5 to 7. *Am J Clin Nutr.* 2002;76:226-231.

120. Lissau I, Sorensen TI. Parental neglect during childhood and increased risk of obesity in young adulthood. *Lancet.* 1994;343:324-327.

121. Lissau I, Breum L, Sorenson T. Maternal attitude to sweet eating habits and risk of overweight in offspring: a ten-year prospective population study. *Int J Obes.* 1993;17:125-129.

122. Fisher J, Rolls BJ, Birch LL. Children's bite size and intake of an entrée are greater with large portions than with age-appropriate or self-selected portions. *Am J Clin Nutr.* 2003;77:1164-1170.

123. US Department of Agriculture. *Loving Support Makes Breastfeeding Work.* Available at: http://www.fns.usda.gov/wic/Breastfeeding/lovingsupport.htm. Accessed December 16, 2004.

124. International Board of Lactation Consultant Examiners. *Certification Information*. Available at: http://www.iblce.org. Accessed June 30, 2005.

125. United States Department of Health and Human Services. *HeadStart*. Washington, DC: US Dept of Health and Human Services; 2005. Available at: http://www.dhhs.gov/children/index.shtml.

126. Sobo EJ, Rock CL. You ate all that!?!: caretaker-child interaction during children's assisted dietary recall interviews. *Med Anthropol Q*. 2001; 15(2):222-244.

NUTRITION FOR SCHOOL-AGE CHILDREN

Learning Objectives

- Identify a healthy eating pattern for children.
- Name the major child nutrition responsibilities of schools, families, and health care professionals.
- Define *comprehensive school health education* and identify how child nutrition fits within the definition.
- Describe preventive efforts directed toward youth, such as Guidelines for Adolescent Preventive Services (GAPS), *Healthy Youth 2010* efforts, and specific community-based initiatives.
- Name the *Healthy People 2010* objectives that are specific for child nutrition.

High Definition Nutrition

Comprehensive school health education—a primary prevention strategy for teaching life skills for disease prevention and health promotion to children and parents, involving a planned, sequential pre-K through 12th-grade curriculum that addresses the physical, mental, emotional, and social dimensions of children.

Guidelines for Adolescent Preventive Services—an initiative to address current adolescent morbidity and mortality in the United States. It is a part of the Healthier Youth 2000 Project of the American Medical Association and directed to primary and secondary prevention.

Iron deficiency—the most common nutrient deficiency among US adolescents. It is defined as a hemoglobin level less than 3.5 mg/dL.

National School Lunch Program—the program for school-age children established by Public Law 79-396 for the purpose of protecting the health and well-being of all US children with nutritious foods.

> *School Breakfast Program*—the program for school-age children established by the Child Nutrition Act of 1966, Public Law 89-642, as a pilot program but extended to all schools in 1975 for the purpose of providing a nutritious breakfast to all US children.

Nutrition and School-Age Children

An overriding concern about school-age children (ages 6 to 18) is the general lack of acceptance of 2 concepts: (1) eating behavior influences health; and (2) eating behavior in childhood initiates adolescent and adult eating patterns. Parents and other adults who are responsible for the foods served to children must understand and acknowledge the benefits of nutrition for children's long-term health (e.g., prevention of cancer, heart disease, obesity, and osteoporosis). Further, they must integrate facts and recommendations into their meal planning and any formal or informal nutrition education they provide.[1]

Healthy children have better athletic performance, mental prowess, and physical attractiveness than unhealthy children. They have good skin and hair quality and body leanness complemented with a small amount of body fat. Good nutrition contributes to positive feelings and an energetic nature.

Children associate with desirable role models (e.g., athletes and entertainers) and the eating patterns they project. Teachers influence eating patterns via the knowledge they impart and the personal habits they practice, especially among elementary students. Peers emerge as an adolescent's major role model, and peers who practice unhealthy eating habits may serve as negative role models. Overemphasis of lean bodies with no fat may lead students to distorted body perceptions, lack of interpersonal trust, and bizarre weight control methods.

On the other hand, hunger still exists. This is especially true for low-income families where children face additional pressures in school due to their high-risk status. The eating patterns and nutritional well-being of school children are influenced by the multiple environments of their daily living (see Figure 8–1). This means that the home and family, school with teachers and food services, all forms of media, the healthcare setting, fast food establishments, and peer groups all influence what a child chooses to eat. The effect can be positive or negative on the overall health of the children[2] and their future health as adults.[3,4]

The nutritional well-being of a child depends on the foods ingested and how the body uses them. During the school-age years, growth and development will be a continuous process. Recommended daily nutrient intakes may or may not be achieved with the child's meal and snack choices. The child's eating pattern—both in and outside of school—contributes to overall intake.

Growth and Development

Growth and development are monitored by 2 common nutritional indicators, height and weight. Many US students today exist at one of the extremes: they are either too heavy or too light for age or height. Children who exceed their recommended weights either are considered *at risk for overweight* or *overweight*.

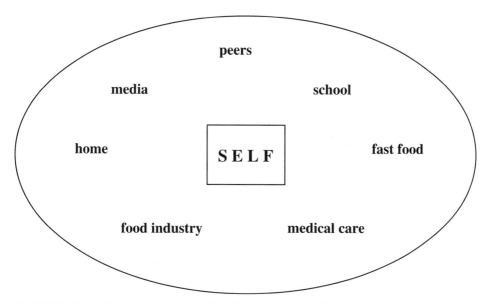

FIGURE 8–1 Multiple environments of youth that influences daily living.

Overweight is defined as body mass index (BMI) greater than the 95th percentile for age and sex, and *at risk for overweight* for a BMI greater than the 85th percentile for age and sex.[5] In the fall of 2000, new growth and BMI charts were available; see Appendix 8–A.

Excess weight predisposes children to high blood cholesterol and sets them on a track for chronic disease, and in the year 2000, recognition of the early onset of type 2 diabetes was evident.[6,7] At the other extreme, underweight and malnourished children present a different mosaic of nutritional problems, many of which begin during infancy and the preschool years.[1]

HHANES found that Mexican-American children were shorter than non-Hispanic whites but had larger anthropometric measurements and greater weight-for-height than average American children. Hispanic children in all age groups were heavier than non-Hispanic children, and their excess weight represented increased fatness in the trunk. Of these Hispanic children, 23% had an abnormal weight for their age: 19% were overweight and 4% were underweight. Of these Hispanic children, 10% had abnormal hemoglobin and/or hematocrit levels, and this increased to 23% when borderline cases were counted.[1]

Access to Food

The lack of access to food greatly influences the natural growth and development of children. Key findings about childhood hunger in the United States are as follows[8]:

- About 5.5 million children under 12 years of age are hungry.
- An additional 6.0 million are at risk of hunger.

- Hungry children were 2 to 3 times more likely than children from non-hungry, low-income families to suffer from individual health problems such as unwanted weight loss, fatigue, irritability, headaches, and inability to concentrate in the 6 months prior to the survey.
- Children with a specific health problem are absent from school almost twice as many days as those not reporting specific health problems.

Nutrient Recommendations

To achieve the expected growth and development, children need an array of nutrients on a daily basis. The recommended dietary allowances (RDAs) and dietary reference intakes (DRIs) are the standards used to evaluate the sufficiency of children's total daily food intakes.[9,10] RDAs are set for energy, protein, 10 vitamins, and 7 minerals. Minimum requirements are set for sodium, chloride, and potassium.

Children should have 45-65% of their energy intake from carbohydrates (average of 130 grams each day), 20-35% from fat, and 10-35% from protein. Infants and younger children need 25-40% of energy from fat. Added sugars should comprise no more than 25% of total energy. Major sources of added sugars include soft drinks, fruit drinks, pastries, candy, and other sweets. Protein intake should be 0.95 grams per kilogram of body weight for children between 4 and 14 years of age.

No maximum level is set for saturated fat, cholesterol, or trans fatty acids, as increased risk exists at levels above zero. For cardiovascular health, regardless of weight, children should achieve 1 hour of moderately intense physical activity each day.

Children generally consume about one fourth of their day's energy, fat, and protein intakes and one third or more of their calcium and sodium levels at lunch.[11,12] As many as 20% of adolescent boys and 40% of adolescent girls do not drink milk on a daily basis.[5] Milk is essential for growing children and is their major source of calcium.[13] Chan studied 164 healthy white children and found that those who consumed at least 1,000 mg of calcium per day had a higher bone mineral content than children with intakes of less than 1,000 mg.[14] The higher bone mineral content is especially crucial for girls to prevent osteoporosis later in life.

Cavadini et al examined adolescent food consumption trends in the United States by analyzing dietary intake data from 4 USDA surveys of 12,498 individuals 11-18 years of age. During the 30-year period, shifts occurred in the percentage of energy from total fat (39-32%) and saturated fat (15-12%). Increases were noted for higher fat potatoes and mixed dishes (pizza, macaroni and cheese). Lower fat milks replaced higher fat milks, but total milk consumption decreased by 36% amid an increased intake of soft drinks and noncitrus juices. The high-fat potato intake exceeded the increase in vegetable intake but the number of servings for fruits and vegetables remained below 5 per day. Iron, folate, and calcium intakes were below recommendations for girls.[15]

Boys have higher dietary calcium intakes than girls, especially when compared to adolescent girls ages 13 to 19. On average, most studies show that adolescent girls consume less than 1,000 mg of calcium per day, well below the recommended daily intake of 1,300 mg of calcium for adolescents ages 9 to 18.[16]

The November 1999 American Academy of Pediatrics policy statement encourages pediatricians to recommend milk, cheese, yogurt, and other calcium-rich foods for children's daily diets to help build bone mass and help prevent rickets, a disease that can cause bone deformities.[17] The policy statement recommends children obtain calcium through food first since the eating patterns they develop during childhood are usually the eating patterns they will follow throughout their lives. The Academy recommends that children aim for 800 mg of calcium each day, or the equivalent of approximately three 8-ounce servings of milk or other dairy foods each day. Preteens and adolescents should aim for 1,200 to 1,500 mg of calcium, or the equivalent of at least four 8-ounce servings from the milk group.

The policy states that adequate calcium intake during childhood is necessary for the development of maximal peak bone mass and that low calcium intakes may be an important risk factor for fractures in adolescence. Fifty percent of bone mass is developed during the teen years.[17]

Iron deficiency (less than 3.5 mg%) remains the most common nutrient deficiency among US adolescents. There is an increased demand for iron to compensate for the increased hemoglobin level with growth.[12] National surveys report that adolescent girls 12 to 19 years old have the highest anemia prevalence rates (between 6 and 14%). These adolescents become the mothers of tomorrow.[13]

School-age children 5 to 12 years and adolescent boys 12 to 18 years with a history of iron-deficiency anemia and special health care needs or low iron intake should be screened serially.[18] All nonpregnant girls 12-18 years should be screened for iron-deficiency anemia beginning at adolescence and every 5-10 years throughout their childbearing years. Adolescent girls with the following risk factors for iron deficiency should be screened annually: extensive menstrual or other blood loss, low iron intake, and previous diagnosis of iron-deficiency anemia.

The meals served at school are a major contributor to a child's nutrient intake. These meals are under the direction of a child nutrition professional, but the food service budget and the likes and dislikes of the children dictate what foods are offered and how food is prepared. Parents have more control over the eating environment of younger children, but they control fewer food choices as children age and peers gain more influence. Teachers mediate choices not only by what they say informally, but also by the direct nutrition information they present in the classroom.

The school setting is a unique and appropriate environment for promoting healthy eating behaviors of children. Healthy eating behaviors in childhood serve as the blueprint for encouraging optimal health, growth, and intellectual development.[19] School nutrition professionals (SNPs) who manage the school-based food programs, e.g., the National School Lunch and School Breakfast programs, are encouraged to actively provide nutrition and supporting healthy lifestyles education to students.[20-22] Eating habits learned as a child affect quality of health in childhood and as well as later in life.[23-24]

Schools do not typically incorporate enough nutrition education in the curricula to influence the healthy eating behaviors of children.[25] Researchers found that the majority of school systems do not have a policy for promoting nutrition education in the school setting.[26] How school nutrition professionals perceive their role or level of responsibility in supporting nutrition education for students is unknown.[24]

Many factors influence the implementation of nutrition education in the school setting. One study reported that SNPs identified training in promoting nutrition awareness as one of their highest perceived needs for professional development.[27] Lack of policies at the local, state, and federal levels addressing nutrition education influence the role of the SNP. School administrators and teachers may believe it is their role to deal with the nutrition education issue and not that of the SNP. However, not much is known about whether or not school administrators and teachers support SNPs' effort in providing and reinforcing nutrition education. Researchers found no published research identifying SNPs' perceptions, practices, and barriers concerning their role in supporting and/or reinforcing nutrition education to the school-aged child. A study was designed to compare differences among school nutrition directors, elementary teachers, and principals in elementary students.

Survey Instrument

A validated instrument was randomly distributed to 140 elementary SNPs in Arkansas and Idaho. A 5-point categorical scale was used with strongly disagree, strongly agree, and don't know. Categories were collapsed for reporting purposes into agree, disagree, and don't know. The survey statements were designed to measure practices, perceptions, and barriers to providing nutrition education.

A total of 96 (69%) surveys were returned. Statements were classified into 6 groups: parents, nutrition education, administration, self-assessment, National School Lunch Program (NSLP), and funding. Seventy percent of survey participants indicated that they have adequate training to provide nutrition education; 65% felt it is their role to provide nutrition education; 72% indicated that nutrition education in the classroom is reinforced through the food program. Findings were as follows:

For nutrition education to be successful in the school setting, it has to be implemented in an environment that fosters a team approach. Recommendations are[24]:

- SNPs can take a proactive approach by positioning themselves professionally to promote a nutrition education policy for their school district. If they are not credentialed, they could earn a nationally recognized credential such as the School Foodservice Nutrition Specialist (SFNS) offered by the American School Food Service Association (ASFSA) or the Registered Dietitian (RD) credential from the Commission on Dietetic Registration.
- School officials should give serious consideration to hiring a district-level professional who possesses the knowledge and skills needed to direct a sound school nutrition food program.
- Funding resources to support nutrition education should be actively sought and their availability communicated to all stakeholders involved in providing/reinforcing nutrition education to school-aged children.

Meals Provided by Schools

In 1946, Public Law 79-396 created the National School Lunch Act for the purpose of protecting the health and well-being of the nation's children.[28] The act directs students to pay the full price for lunches but allows local school districts to serve lunch without cost or at a reduced cost to any child who is unable to pay the full cost. Schools use surplus commodities when possible in meal planning and do not discriminate against any child who is unable to pay a full price. Some of the meal ticket systems, however, may label children inappropriately.

The Child Nutrition Act of 1966, Public Law 89-642, authorized the School Breakfast Program as a pilot program; the program was extended to all schools in 1975 using grants-in-aid.[29] During the 1970s, legislation improved the quality of meals, emphasized nutrition education, and enlarged coverage of programming. The Omnibus Budget Reconciliation Act of 1981, Public Law 97-35, targeted benefits based on need and improved program management and accountability at the local (school-site) level.

The Food and Nutrition Service (FNS) of the US Department of Agriculture (USDA) implements programs legislated by Congress. FNS establishes regulations, policies, and guidelines about school foods and monitors program performance. In addition, FNS provides program and administrative funds to states via 7 regional offices. States generally assign the responsibility for program administration to the state educational agency (e.g., the state department of education), which assists local school districts by establishing fiscal recordkeeping systems and monitoring performance. Individual schools are responsible for preparing nutritious meals and serving them to children. A list of federally funded food and nutrition programs is given in Table 8-1.

Schools can serve foods in addition to the requirements at breakfast and lunch at their own discretion. An offer-versus-serve parameter (i.e., they must offer 5 items, but students can select 3) is now extended to all elementary, junior, and senior high students (Public Law 97-35). New FNS regulations allow students to request smaller portions of food items than the amount defined in the 5-item pattern.

School districts receive a reimbursement for meals that are served according to USDA menu standards. Milk yields an additional reimbursement. Schools can choose whether to participate in the School Breakfast Program. However, with hungry and high-risk children slipping through the cracks, schools should ensure that their policies allow access for all children to the School Breakfast Program (SBP), National School Lunch Program (NSLP), and Summer Food Service Program. Congress continually discusses accessibility of school meals and their nutrient composition.

In addition to serving food, the mission of school food service has included nutrition education since the 1940s. A total school program was defined over 60 years ago as one in which students learned the relation between food, nutrition, and health. Public Law 91-248 was enacted in 1970 and was the first federal legislation to specify nutrition education provisions authorizing training school food service workers in nutrition. Public Law 95-166 established the Nutrition Education and Training (NET) program; this program gave new impetus not only to teach children the

Table 8–1 Federally Funded Food and Nutrition Programs in the United States

Program	Provider	Funding/Agency
National School Lunch Program Provides nutritious low-cost lunch to children enrolled in school	All public schools; voluntary in private schools	A/1
School Breakfast Program Provides nutritious breakfast to children in participating schools or institutions	Voluntary by public and private schools	A/1
Special Milk Program Provides milk to school-age children, children in child-care centers, and in schools or institutions where there is no school lunch program	Schools, camps, and child-care institutions not participating in other school nutrition programs	A/1
Summer Food Service Program for Children Provides 1 nutritious meal each day to children as a substitute for the National School Lunch Program and School Breakfast Program during summer vacation	Public and nonprofit private schools; public residential facilities of local, municipal, or county government	A/1-3
Child Care Food Program Provides financial assistance for nutritious food in child-care setting	Licensed child-care centers or family day care homes; Head Start programs	A/1-3
Head Start Program Provides comprehensive health, educational, nutrition, social, and other services to low-income preschool children and their families	Local Head Start program	8/B
Special Supplemental Food Program for Women, Infants, and Children (WIC) Provides supplemental food and nutrition education as an adjunct to health care to low-income pregnant, postpartum, and breastfeeding women and to infants and children at nutritional risk	Health agencies, social services, community action agencies	4/A
Commodity Supplemental Food Program (CSFP) Provides commodity foods to low-income women (pregnant, breastfeeding, or postpartum), infants and children to 6 years of age, and the elderly in certain cases	Public and private nonprofit agencies (community health or social service agencies)	4/A, C/6
Food Stamp Program Provides low-income households with coupons to increase food purchasing power	Local public assistance or social services offices	5/A

continued

TABLE 8–1   continued

Temporary Emergency Food Assistance Program (TEFAP) Provides commodity foods to low-income households through local public or private nonprofit agencies; quarterly distributions by emergency providers	Public and private nonprofit agencies (community action agencies, councils on aging, local health or local school districts)	5/A
Cooperative Extension—Expanded Food and Nutrition Education Program (EFNEP) Provides nutrition education to low-income families and individuals	Local cooperative extension office where program is available	9/A
Food Distribution Program on Indian Reservations (FDPIR) Operates as a substitute for food stamps for eligible needy families living on or near Indian reservations	Local agency	7/A

Key: Funding sources: A = US Department of Agriculture; B = US Department of Health and Human Services; C = Aging Administration.
Administrative agency: 1 = state departments of education, local school districts; 2 = nonprofit, community-based organizations; 3 = for-profit, community-based organizations; 4 = state health agency; 5 = state welfare or social service agency; 6 = state and area aging agencies; 7 = Indian tribal councils; 8 = federal and regional departments of health services; 9 = state and land grant universities.
Source: Adapted from: Kaufman M. Reaching out to those at highest risk. In: *Nutrition in Public Health.* Gaithersburg, Md: Aspen Publishers; 1990:72–82.

value of a nutritionally balanced diet through positive daily lunchroom experience and classroom reinforcement, but also to train teachers and school food service personnel to implement programs.[30] The NET funding is decentralized, with state or regional departments of education directing the award and evaluation of programs.

Child Nutrition Reauthorization Act

The Child Nutrition Reauthorization Act is reauthorized by Congress every 5 years. The federal government invests approximately $16 billion annually in 5 child nutrition programs covered by this act: the School Lunch and Breakfast Programs, the Child and Adult Care Food Programs, Summer School Food Service, the Special Milk Program, and the Special Supplement Nutrition Program for Women, Infants, and Children (WIC).[31]

Initially enacted in 1966, on June 30, 2004, the *Child Nutrition and WIC Reauthorization Act* (S. 2507) was signed into law by President George W. Bush as a bipartisan bill to improve nutritional service programs, promote healthy choices among children, and ensure that free and reduced price lunch benefits apply to children who qualify. Major provisions of the *Child*

Nutrition Improvement and Integrity Act (H.R. 3873), introduced by the House Education and Workforce Committee on March 10, 2004, strengthen the federal programs because they incorporate school wellness policies for healthy school environments. These policies include:

- Promote nutrition education and physical activity at the state and local levels.
- Require local wellness policies with technical assistance available upon request by the school or school district.
- Continue current policy encouraging all children to consume cow's milk; offer a nutritionally equivalent nondairy substitute; and offer several different fat contents.
- Authorize the Fruit and Vegetable Pilot Program, providing free, fresh, and dried produce to 8 states and 3 Indian reservations.
- Ensure food safety by implementing a Hazard Analysis and Critical Control Point (HACCP) system in schools.
- Strengthen partnerships between local farms, school gardens, and child nutrition programs.

To ensure integrity, efficiency, and quality, the School Lunch Program reauthorization will:

- Allow parents to submit a single application for multiple children and electronically file applications to ensure accuracy and result in reduced costs for schools.
- Allow school lunch certifications to be valid for 1 full year.
- Improve accountability by making school districts responsible for the certification process.
- Increase enrollment of eligible children by improving cross-program eligibility without duplicative applications.
- Reduce the stigma among children receiving free and reduced-price meals using technology, such as proposed automated meal card systems that keep students' financial status confidential.
- Train and conduct frequent administrative reviews.

Reauthorization will strengthen program integrity, improve nutrition, and enhance infant formula for the WIC programs as follows:

- Require WIC vendors to purchase infant formula from a list of state-licensed approved wholesalers and distributors approved to distribute infant formula.
- Improve fairness and integrity of the infant formula rebate process.

Info Line

WEB SITE RESOURCES

http://www.frac.org
http://edworkforce.house.gov/issues/108th/education/childnutrition/
    billsummaryfinal.html

- Implement cost containment measures to ensure that WIC food costs and voucher payments are consistent with competitive retail prices for supplemental foods.
- Review WIC supplemental foods for consistency with current nutrition science.

Cross-Sectional Surveys

In cross-sectional surveys among a biracial sample of 10- and 15-year-old children in Bogalusa, Louisiana, school lunch analysis reported 22% and 29% of total energy intake from fat and 20% and 29% from carbohydrate, respectively. Sugar intake represented over one half the total carbohydrate intake. Sodium averaged one third of the recommended daily range.[32] Parcel et al analyzed school lunch aliquots in a cross-sectional sample of schools in Galveston, Texas, and reported that 39% of the day's total fat intake was from lunch.[33]

The School Nutrition Dietary Assessment Study (SNDA-II) collected information from a nationally representative sample of 545 schools and 3,350 students attending 1st to 12th grade in those schools. The schools provided information about the food service operation and all meals served during a 1-week period between February and May 1992.[34] Approximately 3,350 students in 1st to 12th grade completed a 24-hour recall. Parents assisted students in grades 1 and 2, but students in grades 3 to 12 served as their own respondents. The study compared the dietary components from school and other meals with several standards (see Table 8–2).

SNDA data show that the National School Lunch Program is available to 92% of all students in the United States, but only 56% participate. Children whose family income is less than or equal to 130% of the poverty guidelines qualify for free meals, and children whose family income is between 130% and 185% qualify for reduced-price meals. All other children pay full price, but full-price lunches are also federally subsidized.[34]

TABLE 8–2   Dietary Standards Used in the School Nutrition Dietary Assessment Study

Guideline	Standard
National School Lunch Program and School Breakfast Program goals	One third of the RDAs for lunch One fourth of the RDAs for breakfast
Dietary Guidelines for Americans	Limit intake of total fat to 30% or less of calories Limit intake of saturated fat to less than 10% of calories
National Research Council's Diet and Health Recommendations	Limit daily sodium intake to 2,400 mg or less Limit daily cholesterol intake to 300 mg or less Increase daily carbohydrate intake to more than 55% of calories

Source: Adapted from: Burghardt J, Devaney B. *The School Nutrition Dietary Assessment Study—Summary of Findings.* Alexandria, Va: Mathematica Policy Research, Inc; October 1993:3.

The average full price for a school lunch in the 2005-2006 school year was $1.50; average prices ranged from $1.25 in elementary schools to approximately $1.75 in middle and high schools. Many school districts give lunch free to students qualifying for either free or reduced-price lunch.

Approximately 99% of public schools and 83% of all public and private schools participate in the NSLP. Only a small fraction of schools offer neither the NSLP nor another lunch program. Programs with 60% or more of their students qualifying for free or reduced-price lunch receive $0.23 per meal for full-price lunches, $1.86 for reduced-price lunches, and $2.26 for free lunches (Personal communication, Long Beach Unified School District, Long Beach, Calif.).

Characteristics of Participating and Nonparticipating Schools

More than 90 percent of eligible US schools participated in the NSLP in the spring of 1992, with 52% offering only the NSLP and 48% offering the SBP in addition. No schools offered the SBP without also offering the NSLP.[34]

The SBP originally provided breakfast to children in low-income areas and areas where children lived far from school. Since its origination, it has expanded to include non–low-income schools. Schools providing both the NSLP and the SBP generally serve needy students. Schools offering both programs are usually public schools in urban or rural, not suburban areas. Usually, more than 40% of students in these schools are certified to receive free or reduced-price meals.

Schools only offering NSLP are either public or parochial schools in the suburbs. Students are usually white and about 20% of students in these schools are eligible for free or reduced-price meals.[35]

More than 50% of the schools offer a la carte items in addition to NSLP meals. This is much more common in middle and high schools than elementary schools. Cookies and cakes, beverages, frozen desserts, and snack foods are the most commonly offered a la carte items. Nearly 40% of high schools that participate in the NSLP offer at least one a la carte entree (e.g., pizza, cold cut sandwiches, and hamburgers). The following section summarizes data from the SNDA and highlights the NSLP, the SBP, and the overall eating patterns of students.[34]

In the school nutrition environment, student food and beverage choices have included high-fat snacks, a la carte items, and sodas and snacks in vending machines. Researchers in Minnesota reported that availability of a la carte items was inversely associated with both fruit and fruit/vegetable consumption and positively associated with total and saturated fat intake. Snacking from vending machines was negatively correlated with fruit consumption.[36] For 20 secondary schools in Minnesota, the researchers found that approximately 64% and 65% of foods in a la carte areas and vending machines, respectively, did not meet 30% of total energy from fat.[37]

California initiated legislation to create healthier nutrition environments with the Pupil Health and Achievement Act (SB 19) in October 2001. The law established nutritional standards for foods sold at elementary schools, limited availability of carbonated beverages in middle schools, and increased school meal reimbursements. SB 677 became effective in July 2004 and prohibited the sale of carbonated beverages on a phased basis in elementary, middle, and high schools.

Ethnic differences in fast food consumption from previous studies found Latino adolescents more likely than Asians to eat at least 1 meal or snack from a fast food restaurant on any given day.[38] Few studies have found ethnic differences in caffeine intake; however, a study of fourth- and sixth-grade parochial school students reported that Mexican-American children had the highest consumption of soft drinks. Sixth-grade students consumed more soft drinks than their fourth-grade counterparts.[39]

Asian youth in Los Angeles report more vending machine purchases than Hispanic youth.[40] Increased access to vending machines contributes to higher fat snacks and sugar-sweetened beverage choices as snacks. Vending machines at school appear more accessible to Latino (20%) and Asian/other (24%) youths than to white or African-American youths.[41]

Trevino et al reported that Mexican-American children ate more than the recommended number of fat servings and had a higher percentage of energy from fat and saturated fat among the different ethnicities.[42] Among preschool Anglo and Mexican-American children in San Diego, California, Mexican-American preschoolers had significantly lower fat avoidance scores than Anglos.[43]

Data that contrast ethnic differences in fruit/vegetable intake among ethnic groups are limited.[44] Mexican-American children may only consume one half the national daily recommendation for fruit and vegetable intake.[42] CalTEENS reported Latino adolescents having the greatest consumption of fruits and vegetables.[38]

Males were significantly more likely than females to eat 5 or more servings of fruits and vegetables per day. Gender differences in dairy consumption have shown that males are more likely to drink 3 or more glasses of milk per day than females.[45] The tendency is for girls to consume more total servings of fruits and vegetables, fruit and salads, while boys consume more potatoes.[44] CalTEENS reported that girls were significantly more likely to reach their goal of 5 servings a day than boys were able to reach the target of 7 servings a day.[38]

Caffeine intake of boys has been higher than that of girls.[46] Gender differences in fast food intake among children are limited; however, for adults, fast food intake was positively associated with increased energy intake and body mass index for adult women but not for men.[47]

National School Lunch Program

Participation in the NSLP varies with household income, age, gender, and region of the United States. More elementary school students than middle and high school students take part in the program. Generally, more students who are eligible for free and reduced-price meals get NSLP lunches than students who pay full price. More students participate in the program where the full price is comparatively low, and more boys than girls participate.

Info Line

Changing the Scene is the USDA team nutrition umbrella program. Its Web site can be found at www.fns.usda.gov/tn.

More students participate in rural than in urban and suburban schools. Students in the Northeast and West participate less than students in the Southeast, Southwest, and Mountain states. If students are allowed to leave school at lunchtime, NSLP participation declines.[34]

NSLP meals in about 50% of schools include a choice of entree daily; 35% of schools have 2 or 3 entrees, and 8% have 6 or more. High schools and middle schools offer more choices than elementary schools. About half of high schools and 16% of elementary schools have a food bar once a week. Schools must offer whole milk plus 1 type of low-fat, unflavored milk, and a low-fat chocolate milk is common. About 25% of schools offer 4 types of milk. Desserts are not required, but 39% of lunch menus offer dessert.

Lunches provide one third or more of the RDAs for most nutrients. Nutrient intakes that are low in the NSLP meals include iron for 11- to 18-year-old females, zinc for 11- to 18-year-old males, and calories and vitamin B_6 for 15- to 18-year-old males. The average percentage of energy from total fat is 38%, with 15% from saturated fat. A meal's average sodium content is 1,479 mg, which is nearly twice the target of 800 mg or less. Cholesterol in meals averages 88 mg.

Only 1% of schools offer lunches that average 30% or less of calories from fat. Only 1 school in the sample reported having a weekly lunch menu providing an average of less than 10% of calories from saturated fat. Many schools offer at least 1 low-fat lunch choice; 44% offer at least 1 full lunch per week that meets the goal of 30% or less of energy from fat. Low-fat lunches have fewer calories than the average lunches, but they contain similar amounts of protein, vitamins, and minerals. Schools whose average NSLP lunches approach 30% fat employ several menu planning, food purchasing, and food preparation practices to lower the fat content.

Schools that provide lunches with less than 32% of energy from fat offer ground-beef entrees less often and poultry and meatless entrees more often. They offer an extra bread item frequently, in addition to the bread or bread alternate included in an entree (e.g., bread plus rice or spaghetti). They offer fewer vegetables with added fat. Schools that provide low-fat lunches offer fruit and fruit juice more often and offer juice in addition to other items. They serve 2% milk less frequently, with 1% or nonfat milk served often. Salad dressing is served less frequently, but low-calorie dressing is served often. Cakes and cookies are served less frequently than low-fat, high-carbohydrate desserts like yogurt, pudding made from skim milk, and gelatin.

It is important to note that the schools that offer low-fat lunches have 6% lower NSLP participation rates than other schools. Participation rates in schools serving lunches that average 32-35% of calories from fat resemble participation rates of schools with lunches averaging greater than 35%. Schools can modify fat content of lunches without adversely affecting NSLP participation, but fat content below 32% appears to cause a decline in student participation.[34]

School Breakfast Program

The USDA subsidizes school breakfasts with cash reimbursements and commodities if breakfasts achieve one fourth the RDA. In 1992, reimbursement rates were $0.1875 for full-price breakfasts, $0.6450 for reduced-price breakfasts, and

$0.945 for free breakfasts. For severe-need schools, subsidies are $0.8225 for reduced-price breakfasts and $1.1225 for free breakfasts.[34]

The SBP is available to slightly more than 50% of the nation's students, but fewer than 20% participate. Students who are more likely to participate include those certified for free and reduced-price meals, students from low-income families, younger students, male students, African-American students, and students living in rural areas. Average full breakfast price in 1991-1992 was $0.60, and the average reduced price was $0.28. Nearly all SBP breakfasts are provided free or at a reduced price. More than half of all schools participate in the SBP, but rates are higher among elementary and middle schools. Snacks, not breakfast, are especially prevalent in high schools.[34]

In nearly 40% of nonparticipating schools, principals consider joining the program but do not join. They report no need for the program, foresee transportation or scheduling problems, report resource constraints, or have an overall lack of interest or support for the SBP. Many schools serve breakfast after school begins and during the nutrition break, which may increase participation.[34]

About 50% of the breakfasts served do not include a meat or a meat alternate; milk options replicate lunch choices. Breakfasts generally contain breads, ready-to-eat cereals, and orange juice or noncitrus juice. SBP breakfasts provide less than one fourth of the energy RDAs for male students greater than 10 years of age and less than one fourth of the zinc RDA for all ages of boys and girls. Breakfasts average 31% fat and 14% saturated fat.

Forty-four percent of schools offer SBP breakfasts having less than 30% of calories from fat, but only 4% offer breakfasts with less than 10% from saturated fat. The reason that SBP meals have lower fat than NSLP meals is that a meat or meat alternate is not required at breakfast. More than 50% of the SBP breakfasts do not serve a meat item; those with a meat or meat alternate tend to serve sausage, eggs, or cheese. Cholesterol averages 73 mg, and carbohydrate averages 57%. The average sodium content is 673 mg.

Can what your child eats for breakfast affect learning? The cognitive effects of 2 common breakfast foods similar in calories, but different in their macronutrient composition were examined versus no breakfast. Breakfast options for 1 week were instant oatmeal, cold ready-to-eat cereal, or no breakfast. One hour after breakfast consumption, tests of spatial memory, verbal memory, visual perception, short-term memory, visual attention, and auditory attention were conducted. With a sample of 30 boys and girls, aged 6 to 11 years old, the children performed better on a spatial memory task after oatmeal compared to the other breakfasts. Girls recalled more in the short-term memory task after oatmeal than ready-to-eat cereal or no breakfast. For the younger children, auditory attention improved after the oatmeal breakfast. Oatmeal may have provided a slower and more sustained source of energy than ready-to-eat cereal, enhancing performance on cognitive measures.[48]

Many children do not eat breakfast before going to school because of lack of time. They wait until the last minute to get up and parents don't wake them up early enough to eat. A grab' n' go breakfast project in a Pennsylvania middle school was tested for 1 month with participation measured against the prior year's traditional School Breakfast Program rates. The grab' n' go program had food on a cart located as children entered school.

Info Line

> The USDA School Breakfast pilot project allows, in a limited number of schools, nutritious breakfasts free to all students regardless of family income. Project information and application forms are available at http://www.fns.usda.gov.

A t-test assuming unequal variances was used to analyze participation data. As expected, a 2.5 times increase in participation occurred with the grab' n' go breakfast project. CNPs supporting a grab' n' go breakfast say it allows students to start the school day with fuel for mind and body.[49]

Foods Consumed in the Home and Leisure-Time Environment

The home and leisure-time environment of the child may either complement or contradict nutrition knowledge, attitudes, and behaviors learned in the school environment.[2] Parents serve as important role models. Kirk and Gillespie coined 2 new roles of parents that affect children's food choices: the "meaning creator" and the "family diplomat."[50] Previously, mothers functioned as nutritionist, economist, and manager-organizer; today, preparation time, individual preferences, and whether the mother works outside the home influence food choices as much as nutrition. Kids seem to mimic the all-or-nothing attitude of their parents. Many identify foods as "good" or "bad." In fact, 73% of fourth to eighth graders surveyed in a national sample worried about fat and cholesterol. About 85% felt they should avoid all high-fat foods, while 77% felt they should never eat high-sugar foods.

About one half of school-age children eat with their family every day; 89% eat with their family at least 3 times per week. Students who give themselves the best nutrition rating eat more frequently with their families.[51]

Typical Eating Behavior

Describing a typical eating behavior and nutrient intake of children and youth is challenging. USDA Nationwide Food Consumption Surveys (NFCS) profile the intakes of US children and demonstrate that the fat content remains well above recommended levels (see Table 8–3).[5] Typical eating behavior may include skipping meals, dieting, eating fast food frequently, or eating a more vegetarian pattern.

Skipped Meals

Many school-age children skip meals. In a sample of US fourth through eighth graders, more have skipped breakfast (57%) than lunch (41%), followed by dinner (17%).[52] Meal and snack skipping influences dietary adequacy. Of 639

TABLE 8-3   Reported Nutrient Intakes of Youth Compared With Recommended Levels

Dietary Component	National Food Consumption Survey	Recommended
Saturated fatty acids (% energy)	14	< 10
Total fat (% energy)	35-36	Average no more than 30
Polyunsaturated (% energy)	6	Up to 10
Monounsaturated (% energy)	13-14	10-15
Cholesterol (mg/day)	193-296	< 300

Source: Adapted from: Bethesda, MD: National Cholesterol Education Programs; 1990: *NIH Population Panel Report;* 27.

fourth- and sixth-grade students, 9% reported skipping breakfast within the past 24 hours and 5% reported eating nothing the entire morning. The most common reason for missing meals was dislike of particular meals or snacks, lack of time, or forgetting to bring food. Of the respondents, 30% met the recommended number of servings from the 4 food groups, but 44% did not achieve their recommended fruit and vegetable servings. Students who ate breakfast and had a morning snack were 3 times more likely to meet all food group recommendations.[53]

A survey of 146 10th-grade students found that 60% had made a conscious effort to lose weight. In response to the question, "Have you ever tried to lose weight?" 36.5% of the boys said yes, compared with 73.6% of the girls. The survey involved 146 students ranging in age from 13 to 15 years old attending a multiethnic, urban public high school in Los Angeles. Fifteen percent had attempted dieting by age 11 and 84% by age 14. Among girls who had tried dieting, 85% did so by age 13.

Over 40% had dieted by "consciously eating less" than they wanted as an effort to control their weight; 74% of boys, 62% of girls tried to eat or purchase low-fat foods. Other common dieting practices include limiting portion sizes and counting calories. About 44% reported using meal skipping to control their weight.[54]

Breakfast Habits

Breakfast influences behavior and cholesterol level. The breakfast habits and behavior of 382 children in the third and fourth grades revealed that children who ate breakfast exhibited other healthful habits such as brushing their teeth and taking vitamin/mineral supplements. Students who skipped breakfast were significantly more tired and hungry when they arrived at school; however, no significant social and emotional behavior problems or concerns were noted.[55]

Resnicow studied the relationship between breakfast habits and plasma cholesterol in school children 9 to 19 years old. Only 4% reported not eating breakfast regularly, and these children were less likely to believe in the benefits of breakfast. Controlling for age, gender, and body mass index, those who skipped breakfast had significantly higher total cholesterol levels (172 mg%) than breakfast consumers (160 mg%). The ready-to-eat fiber cereal group had lower cholesterol levels than all other breakfast eaters. Those who skipped breakfast reported higher intake of high-fat snacks, and traditional breakfast eaters reported significantly lower intake of high-fiber/low-fat snacks.[56]

Breakfast Affects Behavior

Kleinman and Murphy reported a 1997 study in Pittsburgh, Pensylvania, of children ages 6 to 12, in which they asked their parents to complete a pediatric symptom checklist. Results were correlated with assessments of the hunger status of the children as either "hungry," "at-risk," or "not hungry." The study linked hunger to a large number of behavior problems, especially fighting, stealing, having difficulties with teachers, not acknowledging rules, and clinging to parents.[57] School absences, tardiness, and behavioral problems like hyperactivity were more common in children whose parents reported hunger than in similar low-income children whose parents did not report child hunger.[58]

The first school breakfast study that same year followed 133 students from 1 Philadelphia and 2 Baltimore public schools before and after the start of a universally free School Breakfast Program. All children received free breakfast. The objective was to determine whether a relationship existed between increased participation in the School Breakfast Program and improvements in standardized measures of academic and psychosocial success in school-age children. After the program started, the proportion of students eating at school sometimes or often jumped from about one third of the children to nearly two thirds. Students who increased their school breakfast showed significantly greater gains in math grades and decreased rates of tardiness, absences, hyperactivity, and decreased depression and anxiety compared to students whose school breakfast participation did not increase. The implication is that it is possible to obtain large increases in school breakfast participation, and when school breakfast participation rates go up, student outcome measures improve. A different pilot study in Baltimore in 1997 suggested that feeding children in the classroom produced even higher rates of breakfast participation.[59]

Fat-Avoiding Behaviors

Fat-avoiding behaviors can be observed. In a cross-sectional sample of Mexican-American preschoolers and their parents, significantly higher fat-avoiding behaviors were noted for 143 Anglo-American preschoolers than 198 Mexican-American preschoolers (max score = 7.0, sum score = 4.85 versus 4.35, $p < 0.0001$).[43]

However, the eating pattern of children has predisposed them to a health-risk behavior that illustrates itself in excess weight and high blood cholesterol levels.[15] From an historic perspective, in 1984, a consensus conference by the National Heart, Lung, and Blood Institute adopted the McGovern dietary goals for Americans 2 years and older.[60] Children were included, although studies had only been conducted in adults. Criticism mounted mainly because individuals did not believe that healthy children were at risk for atherosclerosis.[61] From 1972 until 1983 and later in 1986, the American Academy of Pediatrics argued against inclusion of children and recommended a nutritious diet as having 30-40% of energy from fat.[62-64] Some research showed that parents could restrict fat too much, stunting linear growth and sexual maturation; however, research showed that most children returned to normal growth and development when adequate calories are ingested.[65]

The third National Cholesterol Education Program (NCEP) Expert Panel on Blood Cholesterol Levels in Children and Adolescents included children older than 2 years in their recommendations, but effectiveness and safety of the diets for children was lacking.[66] Objections to the application of the guidelines to children continued, however, and the American Academy of Pediatrics endorsed the guidelines in 1998, confirming its acceptance of a diet with 30% of energy from fat with 20-30% of energy from fat when accompanying drug therapy, if warranted.[67] The American Dietetic Association endorsed the low-fat, low-cholesterol diet for children 2 to 11 years.[68]

To support efforts to lower risk for developing CHD, McGill directed a multicenter cooperative study called Pathological Determinants of Atherosclerosis in Youth (PDAY), in which autopsies were performed on 2,876 accident victims, aged 15-34 years, 50% black and 25% women.[69-71] For adolescent boys and girls, aged 15-19 years, fatty streaks made up about 20% of the area of the aorta; plaques accounted for only 0.35%. For adults, 15- to 24-year-olds' increased LDL cholesterol levels correlated with increases in the number of fatty streaks in the aorta in both men and women, but did not appear to affect plaque formation. For 204 Bogalusa Heart Study participants, 2 to 39 years old, fatty streaks appeared after age 10 in the coronary arteries, but no plaques were observed until after age 15 years. Weak correlations were noted between coronary fatty streaks, plaques and intima thickness, and total serum cholesterol or LDL cholesterol.[72-74] Since from birth to 15 years, plaques do not seem to form, Olson[75] suggests that it may take some years after puberty before androgen and estrogen exert their respective effects on atherogenesis.

The Dietary Intervention Study in Children (DISC) was a 6-center randomized trial of 362 boys and 301 girls, 8-10 years who had LDL cholesterol levels between the 80th and 98th percentiles. The intervention group of 334 children received behavioral instruction to promote adherence to an eating plan with 28% of energy from total fat, 8% from saturated fat, up to 9% from polyunsaturated fat, and less than 75 mg cholesterol per 1,000 kcal per day. The usual-care group of 329 children were given pamphlets on heart-healthy eating.[76]

After 3 years, total cholesterol levels among the intervention group declined by −0.43 mmol/L to −0.35 mmol/L, whereas the usual-care group saw a difference of only 1.6%. LDL cholesterol was changed by 1.7%. HDL cholesterol decreased the same in both groups by 7.7%. The results were statistically significant; however, the true biological significance and effect on CVD risk appeared small.[60-61]

As a case in point, the general intent of preventive health guidelines is: "A large number of people exposed to a small risk may generate many more cases than a small number exposed to a high risk" (p 24).[77]

A pediatric population approach may reduce disease risk for a large number of people and thereby affect incidence and mortality rates. Minimal benefit may be acquired by individuals. One important question has been, "Is there evidence that a low-fat diet in childhood will influence preferences for a low-fat diet later in life?"[77]

Research suggests that taste preferences develop in early childhood and low-fat foods in childhood may be retained until early adulthood.[78,79] Birch et al repeatedly exposed children to certain foods and the children learned to accept them. Given this outcome, one could project that the taste of skim milk, vegetables, and other healthful foods may be learned through exposure during childhood. Other studies suggest tracking of eating behaviors occurs such as observed for a cohort of 700 Minnesota students in the 6th through 12th grades. Their eating behaviors tracked, meaning that the relative ranking of a child among peers for more healthful food choices remained constant in the teen years.[80]

The Child and Adolescent Trial for Cardiovascular Health (CATCH) demonstrated new food habits can be learned and retained. After a 3-year, school-based intervention to lower CVD risk by modifying eating, physical activity, and smoking behaviors, students in the intervention condition had a statistically significant lowering in their percentage of energy from total fat and saturated fat, i.e., 33% to 13%, and 30% to 11%, respectively.[81] Nutrient levels were maintained 3 years after the intervention.[82] These studies demonstrate that when children eat low-fat foods and see peers and adults who not only model the behavior in schools, but reinforce the behavior, then if the supportive environment is removed, the behaviors remain. No statistically significant lowering of total serum cholesterol levels occurred for the CATCH students, but the improved dietary behaviors may yield lower lipid levels later in life.[77]

Guidelines to Lower Fat

Krebs and Johnson suggest that the concern for moderate fat and lowering cardiovascular disease shifts to childhood obesity and its comorbidities rather than dwell on certain fat grams.[83] They believe that just hoping that children's innate abilities to self-regulate will be sufficient control without some parental and environmental structure is unrealistic. If internal controls of children were effective, then the increase in childhood obesity even in children less than 5 years old would be less. They suggest constructive guidance for parents and care providers considering children's everyday needs, abilities, and developmental processes. Building realistic expectations alleviates concerns parents have about their children's growth and health and may motivate parents to accept responsibility for the structure of eating and physical activity and to serve as positive role models for healthful living.[83]

Satter states that low fat intakes of children affect their development and health, create problematic relationships between parents and children, and weaken children's lifelong eating attitudes and behaviors.[84]

She reports that people have conflict and anxiety about falling short of eating standards, and US adults are reluctant to change their diets and adhere to dietary recommendations that appear confusing. Low-fat foods are considered less tasty, more difficult and time-consuming to prepare, and more expensive.

On the other hand, commitment to family meals is strong. A consumer survey projected that parents and children eat dinner together an average of 5 times per week. To limit struggles between parents and children regarding eating attitudes, Satter encourages CNPs and other professionals to encourage consistency in feeding children rather than restrictions.[84]

Fruit and Vegetable Intakes

Fruit and vegetable intakes are low. Murphy et al analyzed food group intake from the HHANES data set composed of 3,356 Mexican-American children.[85] Fruits and vegetables were consumed less often than the other food groups. Children chose their calories instead from the meat, dairy, and breads/cereals groups.

The low fruit and vegetable intake of children is common and problematic. About 90% of children participating in a National Heart, Lung, and Blood Institute demonstration/education project called CATCH state that they eat fresh fruit at home most of the time; about three fourths of Anglo-American and African-American children appeared sure they could eat fresh fruit instead of a candy bar. However, of 407 Los Angeles Latinos, 3% consume 4 servings a day, compared with HHANES reporting 5% and 3% of children 6 to 10 and 11 to 15 years eating 4 a day.[86]

Psychosocial and environmental factors influencing consumption of fruit and vegetables among 92 children aged 9 to 11 years were assessed for mothers' diets using a food frequency questionnaire, and for 80 children's diets using 3-day diaries. Macronutrient intake of the children was 37% fat, 50% carbohydrate, and 13% protein. Median fruit, fruit juice, and vegetable intake amounted to about 2.5 servings/day and fiber averaged 12 g/day. Independent predictors of children's fruit intake included mothers' nutritional knowledge (beta = 0.37), mothers' frequency of fruit consumption (beta = 0.30), and mothers' attitude and conviction that increasing fruit and vegetable intake of their children could reduce their risk of developing cancer (beta = 0.27; multiple r^2 = 0.37, p < 0.0001). Children's vegetable consumption was independently explained by the child's liking for commonly eaten vegetables (beta = 0.36) and the mother's belief in the importance of disease prevention when choosing her child's food (beta = -0.27 r^2 = 0.20, p < 0.001). Children's confectionery consumption was predicted by the mother's liking confections (beta = 0.32) and the children's concern for health in choosing what to eat (beta = -0.26 r^2 = 0.16, p < 0.005).[87]

In the Penn State Young Women's Health Study, 86 women 17.1 ± 0.5 y (x ± SD) of age, measured cardiolipoprotein indexes, serum antioxidants, nutrient intakes, aerobic fitness, and percentage body fat. The fifth quintile of oxygen consumption or VO_2 max had significantly lower percentage body fat, higher athletic scores, higher fruit intake, lower total serum cholesterol, and lower ratios of total serum cholesterol to HDL cholesterol than women in the first quintile. Comparing the first and fifth quintiles by percentage body fat, the first quintile had significantly lower weight, lower body mass index, higher estimated VO_2 max, higher athletic scores, lower ratios of total serum cholesterol to HDL cholesterol, and higher fruit, carbohydrate, and fiber intakes. Correlation analyses performed with the data for the entire cohort showed fruit consumption to be positively correlated with VO_2 max and predicted VO_2 max to be positively correlated with circulating beta-carotene and alpha-tocopherol. This study suggests a positive association exists between exercise, fruit consumption, and cardiovascular health of female adolescents.[88]

Student Selections

Students are increasingly responsible for making most of their own food selections. This is true especially by the time children reach the fourth grade. Approximately 65% choose their own breakfast, 46% their lunch, and 74%

their snacks; whereas 73% report that their mother chooses their dinner. Most students (87%) are responsible for cooking or preparing some of their own meals, with 80% making their own breakfast and 57% involved in buying food for meals or snacks.[52]

Research links calcium to weight loss, and reduction of both PMS symptoms and osteoporosis. Intense exercise and vegetarian diets can alter calcium metabolism, suggesting that women should eat more calcium-rich foods, especially since nearly 9 of 10 women do not meet calcium requirements.[89]

Food Allergies

Food allergies are uncommon. If parents think their children's eating habits are unhealthy because they avoid certain foods due to intolerances or hypersensitivities, the avoidance may not be well founded. Although many individuals think they have a food allergy, true food allergies affect only 0.3 to 7.5% of children and fewer than 1% of adults. Food allergies must be verified by a physician using an immunological procedure.[90] If confirmed, 95% of true allergies are caused by 1 of 4 major foods: nuts (43%), eggs (21%), milk (18%), and soy (9%). The remaining 5% are caused by fish and wheat.[91]

Food intolerance is more common and refers to an abnormal physiologic response to a food where the mechanism is unknown or nonimmunologic. Hyperactivity is a different condition, distinguished by signs of developmentally inappropriate inattention occurring in 5-10% of young school children.[92-93] Food allergies do not cause hyperactivity. However, 2 dietary excesses that stimulate the nervous system are caffeine and alcohol (see section on alcohol and caffeine later in this chapter).

RDA Achievement

RDA achievement varies. The SNDA study assessed students' dietary intakes over a 24-hour period and the contribution of NSLP and SBP meals to their intakes. Students eat at least 3 times a day, and more than 50% eat at least 5 times a day. For students of all ages, 88% eat breakfast, 93% eat lunch, and 99% eat dinner. Two thirds have an afternoon snack, and 58% eat an evening snack. Only 15% have a morning snack. Total daily food intake averages 111% of the energy RDAs. Adolescent males consume 17% more calories than the RDA, while females consume 4% more. Students from families below the poverty level average 129% of the energy RDA. Except for adolescent females, vitamin and mineral intake for all age and gender subgroups exceeds the RDAs. Calcium intake is relatively low (80% for 15- to18-year-olds and 87% for 11- to 14-year-olds).[34]

Overall eating patterns average 34% of calories from fat and 13% from saturated fat. Students from low-income families have higher fat intakes than students from higher-income households. Carbohydrate averages 53% of the calories; sodium averages 4,800 mg, and strikingly high intakes are reported for boys.[34]

NSLP participants waste or discard about 12% of the energy in the food they are served. They are more than twice as likely as NSLP nonparticipants to eat cheese, milk, meat, poultry, fish, and meat mixtures than nonparticipants.

The result is that NSLP participants have a higher percentage of energy from fat and saturated fat.

Students who are nonparticipants in the NSLP consume more sweets and sweet drinks. They purchase food from vending machines, the school store, or a la carte from the cafeteria. Nonparticipants consume about 23% of their energy RDA, and less than 20% of the RDAs for vitamin A, vitamin B_6, calcium, iron, and zinc at lunchtime. Students who brought lunch from home met 31% of their energy RDA, but met less than one third of the vitamin A, vitamin B_6, calcium, and zinc RDAs. Students who ate off campus met 34% of their energy RDA, but met one third of the vitamin A, vitamin B_6, calcium, and zinc RDAs.[34]

Students who brought lunch from home or purchased a non-NSLP lunch at school had fewer calories from fat and more from carbohydrate than students who went off campus for lunch. The sodium and fat content of lunches bought off campus is similar to NSLP lunches.

SBP participants' breakfast intakes average 31% of energy from fat (compared with the *Dietary Guidelines* goal of 30% or less) and 13% from saturated fat (compared with the *Dietary Guidelines* goal of less than 10%). Differences in the breakfast consumption of specific types of foods by SBP participants and nonparticipants are consistent with differences in dietary intakes. Although only one half of SBP breakfasts include a meat or meat alternate, SBP participants are 3 times more likely than nonparticipants to consume meat, poultry, fish, or meat mixtures at breakfast. SBP participants are also more likely than nonparticipants to consume milk or milk products at breakfast. The higher proportion of SBP participants consuming foods from these 2 groups explains their higher breakfast intakes of calories, protein, calcium, fat, and saturated fat.[34]

SBP participation is associated with an increased intake of calories over 24 hours. The difference between the 24-hour intakes of SBP participants and nonparticipants is about the same as the calorie difference in their breakfast intake. The effects of SBP participation on the percentage of calories from fat, saturated fat, and carbohydrate eaten at breakfast disappear over 24 hours. The SBP contributes to higher intakes of protein and calcium, both at breakfast and over 24 hours.[34]

Supplements Among US Youth

Supplement use among 423 US adolescents and the association of their supplement use to dietary intake and adequacy was examined using a 2-day, 24-hour recall and supplement assessment questions from the 1994 Continuing Survey of Food Intakes of Individuals (CSFII). Chi-square analysis, weighted percentages, and general linear regression were calculated.[94]

Approximately one third of adolescents reported using supplements, 15.6% reporting a daily use, and 66% used multivitamins. Adolescents using supplements had higher mean dietary intakes of most micronutrients and lowered intakes of total and saturated fat compared to those not using supplements. Vitamins A and E, calcium, and zinc intakes were < 75% of the US RDAs for over one third of the youth. Overall, most youth do not use vitamin or mineral supplements, but among those who do use supplements, intakes are more nutrient dense.[94]

High-Risk Behaviors of Youths

Risk-Taking Behaviors

The National Student Health Survey assessed risk-taking behaviors of a national random sample of 11,319 adolescents, 5,859 8th graders and 5,560 10th graders; 51% were female and 49% were male. All students responded to 11 questions about behaviors related to tobacco, cigarettes, seat belts, illegal drugs, alcohol, exercise, and fried foods.[95-96]

Cigarette smoking, drug use, and alcohol intake were the major behaviors forming a high-risk cluster for 8th- and 10th-grade girls. These 3 behaviors plus chewing tobacco use were the major behaviors forming high-risk behavior for 8th- and 10th-grade boys. Statistically, 27-32% of the variability of the behaviors was explained with these variables.

Each high-risk factor was the outcome variable in a multilinear regression analysis. Significant predictors of the high-risk behavior were identified ($p < 0.05$). Different antecedent behaviors predicted high-risk behavior for girls compared with boys, and for 8th graders compared with 10th graders. Antecedent behaviors that were the major predictors of a high-risk behavior for all 8th graders were mixing alcohol and drugs with swimming and other water sports, using "stay awake" pills, using psychedelic drugs, and believing it is OK for peers to use drugs. Major predictors for all 10th graders were mixing alcohol and drugs with swimming and other water sports, using marijuana, and believing it is OK for peers to use drugs.

For eighth-grade girls, other significant predictors included swimming unsupervised, riding with a driver on drugs or alcohol, and controlling weight by throwing up. Serious thoughts of suicide, thoughts about getting a handgun, and salty snack behavior were significant predictors for 8th-grade boys.

For 10th-grade girls, other significant predictors were riding with a driver on drugs or alcohol, having serious thoughts of suicide, using marijuana, and using diet pills to control weight. Riding with a driver on drugs, using alcohol and drugs within the past month, eating fried foods as snacks, and not warming up before exercise were the major predictors for 10th-grade boys.[96]

These data emphasize the importance of 2 major objectives listed in *Healthy People 2000* for adolescents and young adults: (1) "to reduce the proportion of youth using alcohol, marijuana and cocaine in the past month" and (2) to increase "the individuals 10+ who have discussed with their family these topics in the past month: nutrition, alcohol, physical activity, sexual behavior, tobacco, drug and safety issues."[82] The overall intent of the adolescent and young adult health objectives was to reduce the death rate by 15% to no more than 85 per 100,000 for 15- to 24-year-olds by the year 2000.[97]

Antecedent behaviors that predict high-risk behaviors were identified in this secondary data analysis of the 1987 National Student Health Survey. These behaviors can form the basis of parent, peer, and classroom discussion and education to improve the health and well-being of our youth.

Alcohol and Caffeine Consumption

Alcohol provides calories and energy, but most adolescents drink it for fun and pleasure. Supplanting nutrient-rich foods with alcohol sets a child in a dangerous nutrition and accident-prone track.[1] In Michigan, 45% of white and 48% of Native-American high school students reported using alcohol; almost one half of white, Native-American, and Hispanic male users reported heavy alcohol use.[98] Prevalence may be higher among dropouts.

The Youth Risk Behavior Survey of 9th to 12th graders reported that 88% of youths had consumed alcohol during their lives; 59% reported drinking at least once during the past 30 days. Males were more likely than females (62% and 55%, respectively), and 12th graders were more likely than 9th graders to drink. Of the males, 37% had consumed more than 5 drinks at least once during the past 30 days.[99]

Sarvela et al[100] evaluated drinking habits of rural students in 7th to 12th grade and noted that 39% had ridden in a car with a drinking driver in the past 6 months and 16% had driven after drinking. There was an increased level of both activities as grade level increased.[100]

Caffeine is a nervous system stimulant and not viewed as a negative dietary component. However, caffeine may be of increasing concern as it lowers calcium absorption and increases heart rate and respiration. Arbeit and colleagues reported that caffeine intake per kilogram of body weight of white children 10 to 15 years old was comparable to adults (2.5 versus 2.6 mg/kg). Caffeine sources for children are carbonated beverages, chocolate candy, chocolate pudding and ice cream, and tea.[101]

Inactivity and Obesity

Obesity has been shown to track from childhood into adulthood.[102,103] It is estimated that 40% of children who are obese at 7 years of age carry their obesity into adulthood, and approximately 70-80% of adolescents retain their obesity as adults.[104] Two large surveys of physical activity among US youths—the National Children and Youth Fitness Study (NCYFS I) and the Youth Risk Behavior Survey (YRBS)—profiled physical activity in this population.

NCYFS I reported that if one considers an entire year, typical youths participate in about 1 to 2 hours of moderate to vigorous physical activity per day. However, about 20-30% of students average less than one half hour a day. The YRBS presented physical activity data showing that about 50% of boys and 75% of girls do not have moderate to vigorous activity 3 or more times a week.[105-107] Girls are less active than boys, especially for vigorous activities, and both groups have reduced physical activity with aging.

The President's Council on Physical Fitness and Sports (PCPFS) reports that boys 6 to 15 years old scored an average of 20 seconds lower in 1985 than in 1980 for 6 of 10 age categories. In 1981 and 1985, boys experienced lower scores on pull-ups than in 1979.[108] Girls 12 to 17 years old had lower scores on the 1 mile run in 1979 to 1981 than in 1985.

PCPFS serves as a catalyst to promote activity, fitness, sports, and health for people of all ages, but emphasizes physical activity among youth must include out-of-school programs, the activity levels of teens, school physical education and its importance in a national physical activity promotion effort, the benefits of regular physical education, and its contribution to the promotion of lifetime leisure physical activity and health benefits.

One Surgeon General's Report on Physical Activity and Health[109] outlined the health benefits of physical activity for all ages. Experts emphasize the need for the development of physical activity patterns early in life. Schools remain an obvious place for the development of these patterns.[110] The concern is quality. Surgeon General Dr. David Satcher stated,

> Physical inactivity is a "major epidemic" in the US. . . . I think we've made a serious error by not requiring physical education in grades K through 12. . . . We are paying a tremendous price for this physical inactivity. People pay with pain and suffering and society pays with money and lost productivity.[111]

Elementary and middle school-aged youth are much more likely to participate in regular physical education than high school students. Daily physical education is rare even for the lower grade levels as 1 to 3 days per week is the usual pattern.

In high school, the likelihood of being enrolled in physical education decreases annually with only a few 12th graders likely to be enrolled.[109] Physical education enrollment declines from over 80% of 9th grade boys and girls to 45% and 39% of 12th-grade boys and girls, respectively. Overall enrollment in daily physical education classes has declined among high school students from 42% in 1991 to 27% in 1997.[109] According to recent data,[112] only 48.8% of students in grades 9-12 are enrolled in physical education classes; only 27.4% attend physical education classes daily. Only 73.9% or ¾ of students enrolled in physical education classes, self-report engaging in exercise for at least 20 minutes per average class.

There are other reasons for regular physical education in schools. YRBS[112] data suggest that 60% of high school females and 23% of high school males try to lose weight. Their most commonly used method when attempting to lose or control weight is exercise (51.5%), then dieting (30.4%). Integrating the teaching of nutrition and physical activity in school classes is sensible and an important contributor to decreasing the incidence of obesity. It complements adolescents who are attempting to lose weight but may be using ineffective techniques. Weight-related issues in school-age children are important.[113] Energy balance could offset the rise of obesity.[114-116]

President's Council on Physical Fitness and Sports

One overarching concern is that physical activity has been shown to be inversely associated with adiposity.[107,117] An inactive lifestyle in youth sets the stage for inactivity in adulthood and the propensity for obesity.[118] A number of controlled, primary prevention studies show that by increasing physical activity, one can modestly slow the rise in adiposity among obese youths. Increasing physical activity alone is not as effective as coupling activity with dietary changes and behavior modification. Including parents of obese youths in the combined strategy to change physical activity and eating behavior gives the greatest impact on weight loss.[119,120]

Info Line

The President's Council on Physical Fitness and Sports Research Digest http://www.presidentschallenge.org, www.fitness.gov

Since 1970, the prevalence of obesity among children 6 to 11 years old has increased 54%, and it has increased 39% for 12- to 17-year-olds. Thus, a focus on physical activity and food choices is relevant.[104] Hispanic children are among those experiencing as much as a 120% increase in the prevalence of obesity over the past 20 years. The excess intake of high fat and low complex carbohydrate foods amid minimal physical activity is a major, potential culprit for the obesity trend.[104]

The relationship between consumption of high-fat foods, low physical activity, and obesity was studied using a case-control design for a group of school children with a 30% prevalence of obesity. Of the girls, 35% were obese compared with 26% of the boys. The children who consumed high-fat foods but had low physical activity had a 38% increased risk of obesity compared with children consuming low-fat foods and having high physical activity.[121]

Most cross-sectional data show no significant population increase in the average amount of total calories consumed, but a possible trend toward a lower amount of total fat is noted in the eating patterns of children and the general public.[122] If the trend is real, a concern remains since the percentage of calories from fat still averages more than 35% for boys and girls at all ages.[106,123]

Conditioning and equipping children with skills not only to shift food intakes toward higher fruit and vegetable consumption but also to increase physical activity and reduce television watching is an eating behavior strategy to alter this obesity trend. In a 1991 study by Tucker et al, the amount of television viewing was inversely correlated with amount of exercise in a sample of 4,771 adult females. Women who reported 4 or more hours of watching television each day had twice the prevalence of obesity compared with females who watched less than 1 hour daily. Women who watched 3 to 4 hours of television had almost twice the prevalence of obesity compared to the group that watched less than 1 hour.[124]

Are the television-watching patterns similar for children? Children who watch more television than their peers have greater prevalence of obesity and super-obesity.[125] During prime-time television programs and commercials, references to food focus on low-nutrient beverages and sweets consumed as snacks. Emphasis is on good taste and fresh and natural, with minimal attention given to foods consistent with healthy guidelines for children.[126] Data from NHANES II and III found an increase in the prevalence of obesity by 2% for each additional hour of television viewing. These findings remained after controlling for prior obesity status, region of the United States, season, population density, ethnicity, and socioeconomic status.[127] Table 8-4 gives tips on how parents can reduce the amount of TV time of their children.

The prevalence of obesity among children of military dependents was observed at 2 major medical centers.[128] The prevalence was greater among adolescents than among young children. The percentage of very obese children increased from 5.5% in 1978 to 9.0% in both 1986 and 1990. Children of active duty staff were less frequently obese compared with children of retirees (18% versus 24%), irrespective of age and rank of the parent.

Body Satisfaction

Saarilehto et al investigated dietary counseling for primary prevention of atherosclerosis, i.e., individualized health education and dietary advice aimed at decreasing dietary saturated fat and cholesterol, given repeatedly since

Table 8–4   Tips for TV Time Reduction

Tips

1. Limit children's TV time to 1 to 2 hours daily.

2. Parents should role-model TV practices they want their children to emulate.

3. Prioritize TV time, play time, or other pleasurable activities.

4. Remove the TV from the child's bedroom.

5. Use a TV allowance to mechanically limit television viewing time while permitting it. Allow choices but within allowed time (www.tvallowance.com).

6. Have consistent TV viewing rules for parents and sitters.

7. Turn off the television
   - when nobody is watching it.
   - during family meals.

8. Serve companionship, not snacks, to children during TV time.

9. Keep a TV log for each family member.

Source: Adapted from: Calamaro CJ, Faith MS. Preventing childhood overweight: television viewing. *Nutr Today.* 39(5):194-195.

infancy. They questioned whether it had an effect on prepubertal children's body satisfaction. Using a randomized controlled trial design, participants, 1,062 infants 7 months old, were randomized, 540 to intervention and 522 to control. At 8 years of age, they evaluated body satisfaction of 217 children in the intervention group and 218 in the control group.

When adjusted for relative weight based on measured weight and height, there were no differences in the mean values of estimated current size, desired size, or body dissatisfaction between the girls in the intervention and control groups ($p = 0.62$, $p = 0.72$, and $p = 0.39$, respectively), or between the boys in the intervention and control groups ($p = 0.21$, $p = 0.64$, and $p = 0.53$, respectively). The proportions of children who were satisfied with their size, who wished to be thinner, or who wished to look heavier did not differ between the intervention and control groups in either girls ($p = 0.65$) or boys ($p = 0.85$). Saarilehto et al concluded that long-term, individualized dietary counseling since infancy focusing on dietary fat did not enhance body dissatisfaction or desire to be thinner among 8-year-old children.[129]

Eisenberg et al assessed verbal harassment, such as bullying and hate speech, and its potential harmful effects on young people's psychosocial well-being. They tested the associations of weight-based teasing and body satisfaction on self-esteem, depressive symptoms, and suicidal ideation and attempts among 4,146 middle and high school adolescents in ethnically and socioeconomically diverse communities of Minneapolis/St. Paul. They found 30.0% of adolescent girls and 24.7% of adolescent boys were teased by peers, and 28.7% of adolescent girls and 16.1% of adolescent boys were teased by family members with 14.6% of adolescent girls and 9.6% of adolescent boys teased from both.

Teasing about body weight was associated with low body satisfaction, low self-esteem, high depressive symptoms, and thinking about and attempting suicide, even after controlling for actual body weight. These associations held for adolescent boys and girls across racial, ethnic, and weight groups. Teasing from

2 sources was associated with more emotional health problems than either no teasing or from 1 source. Policy, programs, and education at programs should focus on the harmful effects of teasing and work to reduce this behavior.[130]

Eating Disorders

Approximately 1 million adolescents are affected by anorexia nervosa and bulimia, which are thought to occur for a variety of reasons including pressure to be thin, depression, biological errors, and poor self-concept. As many as 10% of these adolescents may die prematurely as a result of the disorder.

Women are much more likely than their peers to develop anorexia or bulimia if their sisters or mothers already suffer from the eating disorder.[131] Genetic factors may determine susceptibility to eating disorders. Rates of eating disorders among the family members of 323 women, 18 to 28 years old, with anorexia or bulimia were compared with the rates in family members of 181 healthy women the same age. Bulimia nervosa and anorexia nervosa among female relatives of persons with eating disorders was between 4 and 11 times higher compared with the incidence rates among women without relatives with the eating disorder. Rates among male relatives did not appear to be affected by family members' eating disorders. Anorexia and depression have been reported for 4% of 2,100 female twins. Genetic factors may contribute to 58% of the risk for an eating disorder.

Medical and physical signs of disordered eating include amenorrhea or irregular menstrual cycles; abrasions on hands or fingers from purging efforts; changes in hair, skin, and nails; and blood chemistry irregularities in electrolytes, serum iron, serum glucose, and/or cholesterol levels.[132-133]

Early behavioral identification signs of eating disorders are listed in Exhibit 8–1. The American Psychiatric Association delineates diagnostic criteria for 4 types of eating disorders.[93]

Exhibit 8–1 Behavioral Identification Signs of Eating Disorders

Anorexia Nervosa
- restriction of food to safe foods
- excessive rituals around food and its consumption
- intermittent episodes of binge-eating
- exercise taken to an extreme
- compulsive drive for perfection in various areas of life

Bulimia Nervosa
- rigid restriction of food, followed by binges
- binges of high-calorie, sweet, or salty foods
- secretive eating
- leaving for bathroom immediately after meals
- laxative and/or diuretic use and/or vomiting
- frequent mood swings
- erratic behavior such as kleptomania, gambling, substance abuse, compulsive spending, or self-mutilation

Source: Adapted from: Sloan R. Developing an awareness of eating disorders: identifying the high-risk client. *On the Cutting Edge.* 1994;15(6):22.

Anorexia Nervosa

Two subtypes of anorexia nervosa include the *restricting* and the *binge eating/ purging* types. In the binge eating/purging type, the person regularly engages in binge eating or purging behavior such as self-induced vomiting or the misuse of laxatives, diuretics, or enemas. In the restricting type, the person does not regularly engage in these behaviors. Criteria for anorexia nervosa are as follows:

- refusal to maintain body weight at or above a minimal normal weight for age and height (i.e., weight loss leading to maintenance of body weight less than 85% of that expected); or failure to make expected weight gain during periods of growth, leading to body weight 15% below that expected
- intense fear of gaining weight or becoming fat, even though underweight
- disturbance in the way in which one's body weight or shape is experienced, undue influence of body weight or shape on self-evaluation, or denial of the seriousness of the current low body weight
- amenorrhea in postmenarchal women (i.e., the absence of at least 3 consecutive menstrual cycles)

Bulimia Nervosa

Two subtypes of bulimia nervosa exist and include the *purging* and the *nonpurging* types. The purging type regularly engages in self-induced vomiting or the misuse of laxatives, diuretics, or enemas. The nonpurging type does not regularly engage in these behaviors, but uses other inappropriate compensatory behaviors, such as fasting or excessive exercise. Criteria for this classification are as follows:

- recurrent episodes of binge eating where a binge includes both of the following:
  - eating in a discrete period of time, such as 2 hours, an amount of food that is definitely larger than most people would eat during a similar period of time under similar circumstances
  - a sense of lack of control over eating during the episode so that the individual cannot stop eating or control what or how much she or he eats
- recurrent inappropriate compensatory behavior in order to prevent weight gain, such as self-induced vomiting; misuse of laxatives, diuretics, or other medications; fasting; or excessive exercise
- occurrence of binge eating and inappropriate compensatory behaviors, on average, at least twice a week for 3 months
- self-evaluation unduly influenced by body shape and weight
- disturbance does not occur exclusively during episodes of anorexia nervosa

Binge Eating Disorder

This disorder involves recurrent episodes of binge eating and at least 3 of the following:

- eating much more rapidly than normal
- eating until feeling uncomfortably full

- eating large amounts of food when not feeling physically hungry
- eating alone because of being embarrassed by how much one is eating
- feeling disgusted with oneself, depressed, or very guilty after overeating

Criteria also involves marked distress regarding binge eating, which occurs at least twice a week for 6 months. Regular use of purging, fasting, and excessive exercise does not occur.

Eating Disorder Not Otherwise Specified

An eating disorder not otherwise specified is a transient behavior and is characterized by the following criteria:

- All of the criteria for anorexia nervosa are met except the individual has regular menses.
- All of the criteria for anorexia nervosa are met except that, despite substantial weight loss, the individual's current weight is in the normal range.
- All of the criteria for bulimia nervosa are met except binges occur at a frequency of less than twice a week or for a duration of less than 3 months.
- An individual of normal body weight regularly engages in inappropriate compensatory behavior after eating small amounts of food (e.g., self-induced vomiting after the consumption of 2 cookies).
- An individual repeatedly chews and spits out, but does not swallow, large amounts of food.
- Individual meets the criteria for binge eating disorder (recurrent episodes of binge eating in the absence of the regular use of inappropriate compensatory behaviors characteristic of bulimia nervosa).

Onset of Disordered Eating

The age of onset for anorexia seems to peak between 14 and 18 years of age.[132] The precise beginning of anorexia is difficult to discern, as the US population views dieting as a hobby. The mean age of onset for bulimia is about 18 years. If the onset of bulimia occurs after 25 years of age, then chemical dependency problems, suicide attempts, or depression may be linked.[132] Preadolescent and adolescent girls are at high risk for anorexia and bulimia. Youths with insulin-dependent diabetes mellitus are probably more prone to eating disorders than youths with non–insulin-dependent diabetes mellitus.[133]

Eating disorders occur in all population groups, but a culture-bound syndrome may exist.[134] Specific personality and sociocultural factors may predispose certain individuals to the development of eating disorders. Individuals in the middle to upper socioeconomic levels who are high achievers are prone to developing an eating disorder. Situations that promote food restrictions and diet regulating may be antecedents to eating disorders.[135] Youths who are involved in extracurricular activities that stress body form (e.g., ballet or gymnastics) or any highly competitive sport are also at risk.[136]

The Youth Risk Behavior Survey[137] of 9th through 12th graders reports that 69% of male students considered themselves at the right body weight and 17% thought they were underweight; females reported 59% and 7%, respectively. Black students considered themselves less overweight than white or Hispanic students. About 44% of the girls reported that they were trying to lose weight, but only 15% of the boys reported this intent. Even 27% of girls who considered themselves at the right weight reported currently trying to lose weight. Their weight loss methods included exercise, skipping meals, taking diet pills, and inducing vomiting—which they reported significantly more often than boys.

Wrestlers are more weight conscious than nonwrestlers during wrestling seasons, but their feelings and attitudes vacillate.[138] Fifty-six wrestlers in junior high school and 29 in high school completed the eating disorder inventory once during the season and once during the off-season. Seventy-five nonwrestlers were control subjects. Concerns with weight relate entirely to the demands of wrestling and did not appear severe enough to be diagnosed as bulimia nervosa. The number of youth at risk for bulimia nervosa was not significantly different for wrestlers during wrestling season versus nonwrestlers and in wrestlers during wrestling season versus during off-season.[138]

Shisslak implemented a program to educate high school students, staff, and teachers about eating disorders and found more questions about eating disorders answered correctly by participants than by control subjects.[139] Larson reported that 454 white girls, 14 to 19 years old, who responded that their guardians always lectured them about food had significantly higher scores on the drive for thinness and ineffectiveness subscales. Students who responded that their guardians were unaware of their problems also had higher scores on the ineffectiveness and interpersonal distrust subscales.[140]

Info Line

NIGHTMARE ALIVE

We use our filthy hands to feed our hungry hearts.
We stuff our mouths with food we hate and bury guilt inside.
Our bowls are dirty, the plates are too.
Why even bother to clean?
It's on to the next disgusting feast, it's on to the cookies and cream.
We can't seem to stop when we're into a binge and nothing else matters at all.
Our feelings we push down, our anger we hide.
Our lives seem so out of control.
We next rush upstairs to rid all this waste and swear it won't happen again.
We watch as our lives and our souls go around as they flush away into the rot.
And before we know it, it happens again.
We stand at the freezer door impulsively grabbing whatever is there reaching out for the food we crave and the cycle begins all over again until finally this life must end.

Source: Author is an unidentified youth with bulimia.

In another study, 12% of black, low-income adolescents thought they had an eating disorder. Those who were 14 years or older were more likely to think about vomiting to lose weight. Females identified more emotional concerns about being overweight or the need to lose weight. The desire to do everything perfectly was related to eating disorders among middle school students, whereas feeling ineffective as a person was related to eating disorders among high school students. Students who had a self-perceived eating disorder were more often above the 50th percentile for weight for height, and they accurately perceived themselves as such.[141]

Desmond et al administered a 22-item questionnaire on weight perceptions to inner-city black and white adolescent students, 12 to 17 years old. Of the respondents, 40% of heavy black females perceived themselves as overweight, compared to 100% of heavy white females; the trend was similar for heavy males. Black males were more likely to believe that emotions affected eating behavior than white males; black females felt that lack of exercise accounted for their excess weight, and white females felt that eating habits were the cause. Girls obtained their weight control information from television, family, friends, and magazines. Boys used television, family, and athletic coaches for advice.[142]

Important questions about what influences disordered eating behavior and what triggers and perpetuates the condition include the following[143]:

- Do media images control or influence the thinking of youths about their body size? What is the impact of advertising and entertainment media that promote thin bodies on the behavior of young men and women?
- Is there a critical mass of nutrition knowledge that is needed for long-term stability of eating behavior of youths?
- Are specific groups of dieters at greater risk for developing eating disorders?
- Is there an association between physical activity and food restriction in initiating and perpetuating anorexia nervosa?

Community Nutrition Professionals and Eating Disorders

Community nutrition professionals, often registered dietitians, are part of the healthcare team working with anorexic and bulimic youth. They must recognize and treat these behaviors. Individual and group sessions with clients can focus on nutritional concerns and restoration of normal eating patterns.[144]

Another alternative is employing medical nutrition therapy in a 2-phase approach as recommended by the American Dietetic Association.[145] The education phase consists of collecting relevant information; establishing a collaborative relationship; and defining and discussing relevant principles and concepts of food, nutrition, and weight regulation. Other objectives are to present examples of hunger patterns, typical food intake patterns, and the total energy intake of an individual who has recovered from an eating disorder, and to educate the family, thereby decreasing their frustrations while supporting the recovery process. In addition, attention should be given to separating food- and weight-related behaviors from feelings and psychological issues; changing food behaviors in an incremental manner until the food intake pattern is normalized; slowly increasing or decreasing body weight; learning to maintain a weight that is healthful for that individual; and learning to be comfortable in social eating situations.

The success rate of recovery from bulimia nervosa is greater when the individual has positive self-image and body image, strong relationships with others, and maintenance of an ideal body weight. The outcome is highly variable and ranges from chronic symptoms and relapses to full remission at follow-up.[146] Rates of recovery can be as low as 13% at follow-up among hospitalized bulimia nervosa patients, to over two thirds of patients at follow-up.[147-149]

Teen Pregnancy

Approximately one million teens become pregnant each year in the United States. This results in approximately 520,000 births, 405,000 abortions, and 80,000 miscarriages. More than 10% of this total is in the state of California (approx 61,000 in 1997), and 10% of the California total (approximately 4,800 births) is in Orange County.[150,151]

California has the second highest teen pregnancy rate in the nation. One hundred twenty-five pregnancies per 1,000 women aged 15-19 occurred in 1997. The national rate is 97 per 1,000 women. Although the rate of increase in both percentage and absolute numbers rose dramatically in the 1970s and 1980s, the numbers have stabilized or dropped slightly.[151]

In 2005, the birth rate among adolescents 10-14 years old had fallen to the lowest level since 1946. Although there were 137,000 mothers 10-14 years old delivering a live birth between 1990 and 2002,[133] there were 12,901 births in 1994 compared to 7,315 births in 2002 for this age group. This was a 43% decline. The 2002 rates remain the highest among non-Hispanic black (1.9 per 1,000) and Hispanic adolescents (1.4 per 1,000). The rates for Asian-Pacific Islander or non-Hispanic young white teens is the lowest at 0.3 and 0.2 per 1,000, respectively.[152]

Birth rates of the youngest teenagers in 2000-2002 ranged from the national low of 0.2 per 1,000 in Maine to a high of 2.0 in Mississippi and the District of Columbia. Infants born to moms 10-14 years old are more likely to be preterm, low birth weight, and 3 times as likely to die during their first year—15.4 per 1,000 versus 6.1 per 1,000.[152]

Unless the adolescent's growth at the time she conceives is completed, there will be a greater demand for food energy and nutrients.[153,154] Most adolescents who become pregnant after age 16 do not have an increased nutrient need for growth. However, eating patterns of adolescents reflect a high consumption of fast foods, frequent snacking, independence of food choice, dieting, and skipping of meals, with a preoccupation with physical appearance and peer influence. A study of 1,268 adolescents 13 to 19 years of age showed that 69% of the teens had previously dieted; 33% were dieting at the time of the inquiry, and 14% were considered chronic dieters.[155]

Community nutrition professionals can teach pregnant adolescents skills for healthy eating. These skills might include learning to read food labels, analyzing their own intake and showing the difference between what they eat and what they should eat, and practicing food preparation methods for nutrient-dense foods and snacks they like.

Important research questions that need to be asked on this topic include the following:[143]

- Is there an optimal weight gain for pregnant adolescents at different ages? (see Chapter 9)
- Are the nutrient needs of pregnant adolescents at different ages based on data from pregnant adolescents at different ages?
- What are predisposing cultural factors that can influence the incidence of pregnancy in adolescence?
- Do effective methods exist to teach and to train pregnant adolescents how to modify their eating patterns for the health of their babies and themselves?
- Is breastfeeding harmful to adolescent mothers' bones? (see Chapter 9)

Current Challenges and Major Nutrition Initiatives to Achieve *Healthy Youth 2010* Goals

Primary prevention efforts are more effective if children over 2 years old who are at high risk for chronic disease are identified. Lifestyle changes early in life can affect the course of disease. It is assumed that changes may be more readily achievable at young ages, before lifelong habits are established.

Anatomical data have become available to strengthen the argument for a low-fat eating pattern in youth. No information was available regarding associations between serum lipid or lipoprotein levels and atherosclerosis in youth until data from the Bogalusa Heart Study were published. This study reported an association between low-density lipoprotein (LDL) cholesterol concentrations and aortic lesions in 44 deceased adolescents in Bogalusa, Louisiana.[156,157] About the same time, in 1983, a group of pathologists and scientists organized the Pathobiological Determinants of Atherosclerosis in Youth Study. They focused on atherosclerosis among individuals 15 to 34 years old who were victims of violent death. The data involved 390 young men.[158]

Pathologists at central laboratories graded the arteries for atherosclerotic lesions. Serum total lipoprotein cholesterol and thiocyanate concentrations were measured. The percentage of intimal surface having atherosclerotic lesions in both the aorta and the right coronary artery had a positive association with serum very-low-density lipoprotein plus LDL cholesterol concentration. The percentage was negatively associated with serum high-density lipoprotein (HDL) cholesterol concentration.

Smoking was measured indirectly with serum thiocyanate concentration. It was strongly associated with prevalence of raised lesions, especially in the abdominal aorta. Lipoprotein levels did not explain the effect of smoking. Even after adjusting for lipoprotein cholesterol levels and smoking, black children had more extensive total surface involvement of the aorta than white children. These associations clarify the role of serum lipoprotein cholesterol concentrations and smoking on the early stages of atherosclerosis among youths and young adults.[158]

The arteries of 760 young people 30-34 years old dying of suicide, homicides, and accidents were examined and one fifth of the young men had advanced plaques or deposits of fat in their coronary arteries, suggesting future heart attacks and strokes. Males were more than twice as likely to have the plaques than women of the same age range. Major risk factors for clogged arteries were obesity and a high level of low-density lipoprotein or LDL. Those with LDL levels above 160 milligrams per deciliter were $2^1/_2$ times more likely to have advanced plaques. Smoking, high blood pressure, and a low level of high-density lipoprotein, or HDL, places people at a slightly higher risk of artery blockage.

Young men 20-30 years old with high cholesterol are 2 to $3^1/_2$ times more likely to die of heart disease, and have 4 to 9 less years of life expectancy than men with healthier cholesterol levels. These research studies suggest that people in their early 20s should have cholesterol testing as recommended by the National Cholesterol Education Project.[66]

Primary prevention efforts are fueled by the important finding that risk factors for cardiovascular disease tend to remain or track in the same relative rank within a population. Children with high levels of cardiovascular risk are earmarked for adult disease. The concept of tracking yields 2 major implications: (1) that a relative ranking of an individual with respect to his peers can be maintained, and (2) that the potential exists for identification of risk.

Several studies demonstrated an association of cardiovascular risk factor variables within school-age children as they age. These studies were conducted in Bogalusa, Louisiana; Muscatine, Iowa;[7,159-162] and San Diego,[163] and within young adults in the Naval Aviator Study,[164] the Evans County Study,[165] and the Tecumseh Study.[166]

In the Bogalusa Heart Study, tracking of serum total cholesterol, anthropometric measures, and blood pressure were noted early in the longitudinal observations as follows:[161]

- *Anthropometric measures:* Pearson product moment correlation coefficients for height were the lowest due to changes noted for growth. For weight, coefficients between readings 3 years apart were 0.82 to 0.91 across all age groups of children ($p < 0.0001$); readings 4 years apart ranged from 0.70 to 0.85 ($p < 0.0001$). Right triceps skinfolds tracked with correlations from 0.72 to 0.83 for a 3-year span and 0.64 to 0.77 for a 4-year span.
- *Blood pressure:* The Pearson product moment correlation coefficient for systolic blood pressure for a 3-year span was 0.57 and for a 4-year span was 0.50 (for both, $p < 0.0001$). Diastolic pressure correlations were 0.40 ($p < 0.001$) and 0.38 ($p < 0.0001$), respectively.
- *Serum total cholesterol:* For the 3- and 4-year spans, a 0.64 and 0.61 correlation coefficient were observed (for both, $p < 0.0001$). LDL cholesterol yielded correlation coefficients of 0.70 and 0.67 (for both, $p < 0.0001$).

These tracking data indicate that specific children who will continue to have abnormal levels of risk factors can be identified. Specific primary preventive measures can be taken to meet the needs of individual children.

Dietary Recommendations for Children Over 2 Years of Age

Several objectives in *Healthy People 2010* set the nutrition agenda for school-age children.[21] The Pediatric Panel Report of the National Cholesterol Education Panel (NCEP) underscores these objectives for all children 2 years and older by recommending maintenance of a healthy body weight and an eating pattern with less than 30% of total energy as fat, 10% as saturated fat, and less than 300 mg of cholesterol per day.[167] This is called the Step 1 eating pattern.

Step 1 Eating Pattern

The preferred eating pattern for all children aged 2 and older requires a high complex carbohydrate intake to reach the lower fat composition and to achieve adequate calories for growth and development of children. If children are identified to have an elevated LDL level greater than or equal to 130 mg/dL, then the Step 1 pattern should definitely be followed. If LDL level is not reduced after 3 to 6 months, then Step 2 is recommended by NCEP.

Step 2 Eating Pattern

In the Step 2 eating pattern, fat provides 30% or less of total energy intake, saturated fat is lowered to 8-9% of total energy, and dietary cholesterol is decreased to less than 150 mg per day. A 5-15% reduction in the LDL cholesterol level has been noted with the Step 2 eating pattern. A 23% decrease has been reported when oat bran, psyllium, or lotus bean gum has been added as a supplement to a low-fat eating pattern. Even a 10-15% reduction in LDL cholesterol has been noted when psyllium is added to a Step 1 pattern, but the research data are not consistent.

Fiber

A fiber recommendation for all children is needed for a healthy gastrointestinal tract, yet a broad-based recommendation remains speculative at this time. Fiber intake of 10-year-old Bogalusa Heart Study children from 1973 to 1982 averaged 4 to 5 grams. Fiber data were compared from several nationwide food consumption surveys and showed that the total average dietary fiber intake of children is low. Vegetables and fruits are usually the major source of dietary fiber for children aged 2 to 11, bread and cereal have become the 2 major dietary fiber sources. Children who eat breakfast consume more fiber than children who do not.[12,168]

Wynder et al have suggested a 25/25 standard: 25% of the total energy intake for children as fat and 25 grams of fiber per day.[169] An increase in complex carbohydrate to achieve a fat intake of 30% or less creates a high-fiber eating pattern. In 1994, The American Health Foundation convened child nutrition researchers to explore support for a fiber recommendation for children. Based on the current state of the science, a 0.5 gram per kilogram recommendation appears unrealistic, especially for large 18-year-old boys; the 10 grams per 1,000 kcal creates high intakes for very young children.

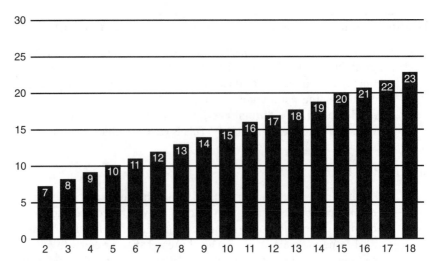

FIGURE 8–2 American Health Foundation recommended fiber intake for children: "Age of Child Plus 5 Rule."
Source: American Health Foundation, New York; 1994.

A new, age-sensitive formula was proposed to determine children's dietary fiber needs. It is called the "Age of Child Plus 5 Rule" (see Figure 8–2). The formula is proposed to ensure that children from 3 to 18 years grow into their fiber requirements as a natural way of eating, with an annual increase in fiber above their basal needs. An objective of the recommendation is to introduce a consensus of thinking about fiber and encourage all healthcare groups and professional organizations to use the guide in their programs and materials.[170]

General Eating Pattern Guide for Children

To achieve a healthy eating pattern, children and adults who prepare food for children can use the 2005 Food Guide Pyramid as the planning blueprint.[171] The pyramid is the visual presentation of the *Dietary Guidelines.*[172] (See Chapter 2.)

California Assembly Bill 2109 mandated the California Department of Education to develop nutrition guidelines for all food and beverages sold on school campuses in California.[173,174] The Nutrition Guidelines for California School Foods that resulted represented a 3-tiered approach to dietary modification of lunch and breakfast menus. Each level reduces the fat content and increases the fiber content through the increase in whole-grain foods, fruits, and vegetables:

- Tier 1 has the least change with modification primarily in the quality of the food that children receive. For example, this includes serving a fresh fruit rather than a canned one, or serving whole-grain bread rather than plain white bread.
- Tier 2 decreases the quantities of certain foods and replaces them with increased quantities of other foods to maintain the calories children

need for energy and growth. For example, butter, gravies, and rich desserts—which all add calories primarily in the form of fat—are served less frequently. Instead, the lower-fat forms of meat, cheese, milk, and desserts are used, and calories are increased by adding servings of bread and bread alternates, fruits, and vegetables.

- Tier 3 has the greatest change. It is the last step for increasing servings of beans, fruits, and vegetables. All high-fat desserts are replaced with fresh fruits; whole-grain breads are served, and minimal fat is added in cooking. Reaching this tier achieves the nutrition guidelines for child nutrition programs. Nutrient content reflects 30-35% of the total calories as fat and one third of the RDAs for vitamins and minerals with moderation of sodium and sugar.

The eating pattern identified in California's school nutrition guidelines is based on the original *California Daily Food Guide*,[174] currently used by California for all nutrition programs. These guidelines could be used for all snacks and meals planned for children throughout the United States. The *California Daily Food Guide* provides quantitative, life-cycle dietary recommendations with ethnic-, age-, and gender-specific food guides. The importance of these guidelines is the continuity they provide for programs and for the public. If the pattern is followed in childhood, then continuing the pattern into adolescence and adulthood is easier and probable.

Child Nutrition as a Component of Comprehensive School Health

Comprehensive school health education is a primary prevention strategy for teaching disease prevention and health promotion life skills to children, parents, and future parents.[175-177] Comprehensive school health education is based on a planned, sequential pre-K through 12th-grade curriculum that addresses the physical, mental, emotional, and social dimensions of children.[178]

Health education has evolved from emphasizing dissemination of knowledge to emphasizing modification of health behavior.[179] Table 8-5 contrasts traditional health education with health instruction that emphasizes health-promoting behaviors. Several theoretical models explain health behavior, including the Health Belief Model, Theory of Reasoned Action, Multiattribute Utility Theory, and Social Learning Theory.[180]

Critical factors influencing an individual's health behavior include the following[181]:

- knowledge about the disease
- perceived threat of illness
- attitudes about health care
- social interaction
- social norms
- social structure
- accessibility of health services
- demographic factors

Table 8–5   Traditional Health Education Versus Health Instruction in a Health-Promoting School

Traditional Health Education	Health Instruction in a Health-Promoting School
Emphasizes knowledge and attitude changes predisposing to behavior change.	Applies multiple theories and models to development and intervention designed to promote health-enhancing behaviors.
Organizes the health instruction program around 10 content areas.	Focuses on 6 priority health behaviors within the 10 content areas.
Views the school health program as instruction, health services, and a healthful school environment.	Expands the program to include health promotion regarding food services, physical education, guidance, work site, and integration of school and community.
Considers health instruction as the focal intervention strategy.	Replaces the health instruction model with a health promotion model that employs multiple strategies.
Considers health education only in limited classroom terms.	Coordinates health promotion activities with community programs and infuses health content throughout the curriculum.
Promotes coordination of the health education program via a school health advisory council.	Promotes coordination of the school health program within the school through interdisciplinary and interagency teams.
Concentrates on didactic, teacher-led health instruction and acquisition of facts.	Promotes active student participation matching teaching techniques with instruction.
Tends to respond to a series of problems or crises one by one.	Includes common skills in the curriculum.
Considers the adoption of health-promoting behaviors a result of health instruction.	Develops caring schools and communities with high expectations for pupil success.
Does not routinely involve parents actively in the school health program.	Considers family support and involvement in health and development of the total school health program as the nucleus of the health-promoting school.

Source: From "Encouraging Parental Involvement in School" by IM Young in *Young Health Promotion: From Theory to Practice in School and Community,* by D Nutbeam, et al. London: Forbes Publication Ltd, 1991: 218-232. Reprinted with permission of Ian M. Young.

Health status and health risk result from multiple factors. Therefore, researchers believe that multiple interventions are needed to effect behavioral, environmental, or social changes.[182-187]

The 10 content areas essential for a comprehensive program are community health, consumer health, environmental health, family life, growth and development, nutrition, personal health, prevention and control of disease, safety and accident prevention, and substance use and abuse. Common content areas required by state mandates include drug and alcohol abuse prevention (required in 29 states), tobacco use prevention (required in 20 states), and nutrition (required in 19 states).[188-189]

The Public Health Service identified 4 major factors that contribute to premature illness and death in the general population.[190] They include heredity (20%), environment (20%), healthcare delivery system (10%), and unhealthy lifestyle (50%). The Centers for Disease Control and Prevention targeted education for behavior change in 6 areas as critical to reducing premature illness and death among adolescents: nutrition, physical activity, intentional and unintentional injury, alcohol and other drug use, smoking, and reproductive health.[191] These priority behaviors complement objectives from *Healthy People 2010*, one third of which focus on children and youth.

Two of the six education goals set by the Centers for Disease Control and Prevention would be difficult to attain without implementation of an effective school health program—readiness for learning and a safe, disciplined, drug-free, and violence-free environment.

Child nutrition and food services is one of the 10 components of comprehensive school health. School cafeterias are a primary prevention arena—a potential learning laboratory for children and campus food sales where demonstration and education studies can be conducted to evaluate menu changes and acceptability to students.[192-194] With national efforts to legislate comprehensive school health programs, support for a comprehensive approach strengthens each component (e.g., child nutrition or physical education and their respective programs). Appendix 8–B outlines strategies to promote 5 A Day messages in a comprehensive school health program.

Coordination of Food Service With Classroom Education

School nutrition directors acknowledge the need for nutrition education for schoolchildren, but given the daily priority of feeding millions of hungry students, nutrition education falls to the back burner. The cafeteria, the classroom, and support from parents and the community are essential for success in improving eating habits.[195]

To continue an emphasis on nutrition education, CNP professionals should[195]:

1. Identify the nutrition education needs of the students, teachers, and parents.
2. Clearly define objectives.
3. Evaluate health education models.
4. Develop relationships with allies and industry partners.
5. Test pilot projects and programs that address assessed needs.
6. Lobby for adequate funding to meet assessed needs.

A relatively newly defined role for community nutrition professionals is nutrition education in schools. Even though nutrition education has been taught for decades in the classroom as part of health, science, and home economics, the past 2 decades have seen an increase in specific professional positions of school nutrition and child nutrition educators and specialists. Placement of child nutrition specialists on the school campus to coordinate food service activities with classroom instruction strengthens the role of nutrition in health and in comprehensive school health education. Creative approaches to nutrition education in the classroom are needed.

In a survey of 407 students in the 4th to 8th grade, 94% thought that the food they eat can affect their future health. Of the respondents, 99% understood the importance of exercise for good health; 80% could identify 3 of the 4 food groups; and 98% recognized the importance of eating plenty of fruits, vegetables, and high-fiber foods.[196]

Simply knowing about fruits, vegetables, and fiber is not enough to make individuals eat more. Because students report that their primary sources of nutrition information are schools (95%), parents (86%), and health professionals (73%), it behooves schools to be actively involved in nutrition education. Surveys support nutrition education as an acceptable method for reducing population risk factors for chronic disease, and nutrition education provides a more inexpensive approach compared to medical and clinical strategies.[197] Roper surveys have identified nutrition at a consistently high level of interest in the United States since the mid-1970s. Almost all individuals from 1976 to 1985 reported that the nutritional value of food (90% reported) and their specific diets (60% reported) were very important to their health.[198]

The Food for Thought, All About Nutrition and You! program in the Palm Beach (Florida) School District revealed that 10% of children were either underweight or overweight. Age-appropriate nutrition education activities were placed in the curriculum, and students prepared healthy snacks in the classroom. An increased acceptance of vegetables, skim milk, and other foods that had been used during class were noted by the child nutrition employees in the cafeteria. The majority of teachers, principals, and students wanted to continue the program the following year, and test packets were distributed to other district schools.[199]

Each of the 6 lessons in the Stanford Nutrition Action Program (SNAP) curriculum to lower dietary fat included role modeling, goal setting, problem solving, group activities, and skills-building tasks.[200] Videotapes, food demonstrations, and posters that enhanced group discussions were frequently added to increase interest and appeal of the multiethnic population. All printed materials were written at or below the 5th-grade reading level. The curriculum combined interactive teaching techniques and behavior change methods to aid participants to overcome barriers to reducing fat. Self-assessment of current eating patterns involved completing a SNAP Quick Check worksheet (see Figure 8–3).

It appears that the earlier nutrition education is integrated into the classroom, the more likely students will practice healthy eating behaviors. The FUN Kit provides nutrition education for preschoolers with puppets, music cassettes, and stickers.[201] Liang developed nutrition lessons using musical compositions about my body, my friends (see Figure 8–4).[202] The International Food Information Council and the National Center for Nutrition and Dietetics have developed classroom posters and materials that present nutrition as fun and something children will want to do. The American Heart Association, the American Cancer Association, and the National Dairy Council are only a few

Source: Albright CL, Bruce B. Development of a curriculum to lower dietary fat intake in a multiethnic population. <u>Nutr Education.</u> July/August 1997; 29, 4: 215-223.

Do you:		Circle your answer	
• Eat eggs, bacon, or sausages (like chorizo)?	Not often/Never	or	Often
• Eat hot dogs or lunch meat like bologna or salami?	Not often/Never	or	Often
• Eat beef (including hamburger), pork, or ham?	Not often/Never	or	Often
• Eat chicken with skin?	Not often/Never	or	Often
• Eat fried chicken or fried fish?	Not often/Never	or	Often

Do you:		Circle your answer	
• Drain the fat off of cooked meat?	Often	or	Not often/Never
• Cut the fat off beef, pork, or chicken?	Often	or	Not often/Never
• Have meals with only a small amount of meat?	Often	or	Not often/Never
• Have a main meal with no meat or eggs?	Often	or	Not often/Never
• Buy lean meats or meats with less fat?	Often	or	Not often/Never

My goals for the week:

I, _____, will_____

To accomplish this, I will:

1._____

2._____

3._____

4._____

5._____

FIGURE 8–3   SNAP Quick Check
Source: Albright CL, Bruce B. Development of a curriculum to lower dietary fat intake in a multiethnic population. *Nutrition Education.* July/August 1997;29(4):215-223.

of the many nonprofit groups that have developed numerous curricula for all ages of schoolchildren. Each of these organizations has developed nutrition education materials that are generally available at a minimal cost, such as Changing the Course, Early Start, and Heart Works. These organizations

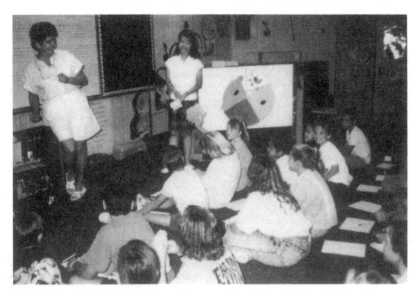

FIGURE 8–4 A creative, age-sensitive nutrition education curriculum for upper elementary children.
Source: Reprinted with permission of Liang T, Frank G. Hello my friend—what did you eat today? *J Nutr Education.* 1994;26:205B-206B.

support community outreach and training of CNPs and allied health and education professionals. Working collaboratively with these organizations and volunteers can be advantageous to schools with budget restrictions. Continuing education hours can be accrued for teachers and child nutrition employees. Additionally, complete up-to-date and effective curricula from these organizations can link classroom education with the cafeteria and parents and tap community resources.

Team Nutrition is the implementation tool for USDA's School Meals Initiative for Healthy Children. It aims to leverage government resources through public-private partnerships and promotes food choices for healthful eating among children. The goal is to empower schools to serve meals that meet and motivate pre-K through 12th-grade children to make healthy food choices. Team Nutrition focuses on variety, fruits, vegetables, grains, and low-fat choices.

Two major components are Nutrition Education and Technical Assistance and Training. Technical Assistance supports school food service personnel and gives them tools and skills to achieve the School Meals Initiative for Healthy Children. Nutrition Education links schools, the media, homes, and the community to motivate and empower children with science-based, kid-friendly nutrition messages. Even at the beginning of the new millennium, a dim picture exists about US kids, food, and fitness, since 35% of elementary school-age children eat no fruit, and 20% eat no vegetables on a given day; 27% of children 6-11 are considered obese, and 90% of children consume fat above the recommended level.[203]

Four of the leading causes of adult death—heart disease, cancer, stroke, and diabetes—have a diet relationship. About $250 billion/year is spent in the resulting medical costs and lost productivity. Team Nutrition is directing dietary behavior change of youth toward healthy patterns to reduce risk factors of these diseases early in life.[203]

The great purple Power Panther is the USDA's new mascot to encourage children and their families to eat healthy and exercise. A national campaign is designed to reach school-aged children (age 2 to 18 years) and their caregivers through materials and activities that incorporate the Power Panther and its message, "eat smart, play hard." Caregivers include parents, guardians, child-care providers, after-school providers, and teachers.[203]

In the year 2000, the Senate Agriculture Appropriations Subcommittee recommended that the USDA develop recommendations for a comprehensive, integrated approach to nutrition education. The recommendations may highlight current programs such as Team Nutrition, the Nutrition Education and Training Program (NET), and other school-based nutrition programs. The report will identify gaps in current programs and potential funding approaches. It will be developed in close consultation with other government agencies such as the Department of Education, the Department of Health and Human Services, and the Centers for Disease Control and Prevention. The American Dietetic Association, the Society for Nutrition Education, the National Association of State NET coordinators, and the American School Food Service Association will be actively involved. Improving coordination and integration are the broad goals. The specific goals are:

- Create opportunities for better coordination and integration of nutrition education within and across programs.
- Identify needed improvements in the overall approach to nutrition education for the Food and Nutrition Service target populations.
- Focus on barriers to implementing the improvements or capitalizing on opportunities.
- Develop ideas for practical, innovative solutions.

Action for Healthy Kids (AFHK) was launched at the national 2002 Healthy Schools Summit as a national nonprofit organization (see www .actionforhealthykids.org).[204] It addresses the epidemic of overweight, undernourished, and sedentary youth by focusing on changes at school and by improving nutrition and physical activity in schools to enhance children's

Info Line

Team Nutrition Headquarters Office:
USDA Team Nutrition
3101 Park Center Drive, Room 802; Alexandria, VA 22302
Phone: (703) 305-1624; Fax: (703) 305-2148;
Web site: http://www.usda.gov/fcs/team/htm.

readiness to learn. The school environment was listed in former US Surgeon General David Satcher's 2001 report, *Call to Action to Prevent and Decrease Overweight and Obesity.*

Over 40 national organizations and agencies representing education, physical activity, health, and nutrition guide and support the organization. The partners develop shared resources, facilitate information exchange, raise public awareness, and evaluate efforts to identify and disseminate best practices. AFHK created 51 state teams made up of volunteers, including school administrators, educators, and health professionals. For example:

- Alabama—conducted a school vending machine survey of 1,400 school principals and distributed *A Guide to Healthy Vending* to all Alabama principals.
- Indiana Team—provided all superintendents with a position paper on the relationship of recess and academic performance. A Healthy Hoosier award is given for outstanding efforts such as actively promoting fruits/vegetables and low-fat/nonfat dairy products.
- Texas—established school health-advisory groups in a majority of districts.
- Kansas—awarded mini-grants to schools to form school health councils for improving healthy food and beverage choices and for increased physical activity during and after school.

Action Plan—Targeting Success

To create or adapt child nutrition programs to achieve *Healthy People 2010* objectives, any action plan should include the 2005 Dietary Guidelines for Americans, the 2005 Food Guide Pyramid, and the National Cholesterol Education Panel recommendations. If achieved, these objectives collectively have the potential to reduce eating disorders, promote healthy weight management, and reduce nutrient imbalance. They enhance nutrition education in the classroom and assist students with skills such as making healthy food choices during leisure eating time. In addition, they promote healthy and acceptable meal planning in schools.

The Predisposing, Enabling and Reinforcing, or PRECEDE, model for school health intervention can serve as a blueprint for developing a nutrition education and food service management action plan. PRECEDE addresses predisposing, enabling, and reinforcing factors in schools.[205]

- *Predisposing factors* are the demographic and population norms often beyond the scope of a program and are usually nonmodifiable. However, increasing fruit and vegetable intake to 5 a day in the population would establish a new, preferred norm.
- *Enabling factors* concern availability and accessibility in the school, such as the cafeteria, vending machines, and campus stores.
- *Reinforcing factors* address attitudes and behaviors of peers, parents, teachers, administrators, and media that either support or discourage behavioral change.

Community nutrition professionals can structure their action plans based upon this framework and reduce unknowns, thereby focusing their energies and budgets on specific modifiable factors. In addition to action plans directed toward comprehensive school health, the health and nutrition plight of many children must be curtailed. Direct health services are essential in some settings to complement meals and education at school.

The Healthy Start Initiative in California provides immediate care clinics on school grounds for high-risk populations. This approach is a template for a national mandate. Nutrition services in the form of the School Breakfast Program should be visible and be incorporated at the beginning of each Healthy Start program as a direct service. This is a priority when obesity, anorexia nervosa, iron deficiency anemia, lead poisoning, hunger, and nutrient imbalances are prevalent among youth. In addition, each district should work to increase its reimbursement rate by offering nutritious meals and promoting participation of all students in the School Breakfast Program and National School Lunch Program through marketing to the community, school boards, parents, teachers, and students.

As changes are made, action plans must be monitored to identify what works and what does not work. Often community nutrition programs lack sufficient evaluation. Evaluation is crucial if major issues are to be corrected and if successful program components are identified for generalizability to other locations and situations.

Implementation and process evaluation may include questionnaires and observational measures to assess readiness of the students and faculty prior to the program implementation. Outcome evaluation may include questionnaires and observational measures to assess program effects on food consumption and nutrient outcome. Evaluation tools can include instruments for staff, as well as for students. Examples of evaluation tools include:

- *Meal quality assessment instrument:* A checklist that can be used by school nutrition staff to address food preparation and menu planning consistent with dietary guidelines for schoolchildren. It might require 15 to 20 minutes of direct observation, marking observations on a Scantron form. The assessment tracks qualitative changes in menus.
- *Pre-/posttest:* 5 to 10 items that can be used at a training class to establish baseline knowledge of employees or teachers.
- *Basic nutrition knowledge questionnaire:* May contain 10 to 25 items directed toward general information students should have (e.g., ability to identify foods by specific food group, the role of foods in chronic disease prevention, food misconceptions, and nutrition message in the media).
- *Attitudinal questionnaire:* May focus on student likes and dislikes, such as fruits and vegetables or high-fat and protein foods. Scales using facial expressions are helpful when assessing attitudes of younger children.
- *Behavioral questionnaires:* Behavior can be measured with 1- to 3-day food records, a specific instrument such as the Fat/Cholesterol Avoidance

Scale, or a food frequency questionnaire set up specifically for adolescents that can measure actual food and nutrient intakes.[43]

- *School self-assessment:* A team approach is recommended for districts to assess standards of practice, to identify both strengths and areas for improvement, and to promote a vested interest by all so that the program can progress toward nutrition integrity.[206]

Who Is Responsible for Sound Nutrition in Schools?

Schools have 2 major child nutrition responsibilities: (1) to protect the health and well-being of students with wholesome foods, and (2) to provide an enjoyable environment that makes healthful foods accessible to all children. To achieve these responsibilities, coordinating classroom learning with cafeteria decision making and supporting in-service training for child nutrition employees and teachers are paramount.

The key national players are the USDA and its Nutrition Education and Training Program, National School Lunch Program, breakfast and commodity programs, the American School Food Service Association,[207] the School Nutrition Services Dietetic Practice Group of the American Dietetic Association, state child nutrition directors, and numerous food manufacturers. These groups and organizations such as the Society of Nutrition Education and Behavior and the American Public Health Association are likewise responsible for informing legislators of the needs and priorities for effective and efficient school nutrition programs across the United States. As school nutrition is integrated with comprehensive school health, the Centers for Disease Control and Prevention and other national survey and professional organizations gain importance.

The School Meals Initiative for Healthy Children took effect in 1998-1999 after a series of public hearings and roundtables. The USDA considered the suggestions and insights of school food service, nutrition, health, medical, and education professionals and the general public to update the nutrition standards for meal planning dramatically. Three specific components remain today[208]: (1) Nutrient Standard Menu Planning (NuMenuS) to provide a 1-week assessment of meals to reflect nutrient content; (2) the nutrient composition of commodities, variety among the commodities; and new product development; and (3) reduction of administrative paperwork for the claims process and the review/certification process.

School food service planners and directors must ensure that lunches offered to schoolchildren (aged 2 years and older) meet nutrient standards. School districts can use a nutrient-standard computerized menu planning procedure or an assisted nutrient-standard menu planning process available through the USDA. Breakfast and lunch must provide one fourth and one third of the RDA, respectively, for a child as a minimum standard for planning meals and the 2005 *Dietary Guidelines for Americans* must be achieved (i.e., < 30% of energy from total fat and < 10% of energy from saturated fat).

The American School Food Service Association has led the challenge to postpone implementation because school districts do not have the resources needed to computerize their menus. The association does not believe that the administrative controls have been streamlined sufficiently. USDA plans to launch a nationwide nutrition education campaign aimed at the lunchroom and the classroom to introduce children, food service staff, classroom teachers, and parents to an improved way to plan meals and make improved meal planning a part of their lifestyle.[208]

Targeting Change in the School Eating Environment

Specific ways to target change in the eating environment of schools are presented below.[209]

Time Allocation for Meals

Students may have 12 to 25 minutes for lunch. This includes obtaining their meal, finding a place to sit, eating, socializing, and discarding waste. This rushed environment decreases chances for optimal food intake. Children probably need a minimum of 15 to 20 minutes from the time they are seated to eat, talk a little, and experience lunch without rushing.

Meal monitors are employed in some schools as traffic controllers and time keepers. If their efforts are positive and not demeaning for students, a receptive environment occurs. Some schools even present lunch as a pleasant social time with music and citizenship awards for cleanup and manners.

Acceptability of Menus

Student meal acceptance has usually been based on plate waste. To lower plate waste, menu planners have developed potato, salad, and sandwich bars. High school youth advisory groups have been devised by the American School Food Service Association to bring students into the planning, tasting, and decision-making process.[209] Upper elementary students should be given similar choices to build their food decision-making skills.

The multicultural environment found in many schools today requires school foods that are diverse in taste and enhance the cultural pride of the students. To increase acceptability, cultural foods should be incorporated. However, with westernization, the benefits of nutritious foods from different cultures have been lost (e.g., tofu has been deleted from Asian dishes and high-fiber ingredients have been left out of salads and vegetables of the Middle East). Individual student tastes and cultural practices have been shaped by societal norms and food preferences of the West.

Hong et al identified the top 5 school lunch entrees for 5th- and 6th-grade students in the ABC Unified School District in Los Angeles County.[210] The 172 students were 30% Hispanic; 30% Asian; 30% White, and 10% Portuguese, East Indian, and other. A significant correlation was noted between the acceptance and the frequency of eating the routine entrees and acceptance of a new recipe for a tofu (low-fat) Chinese meat bun: nacho beef and cheese, $r = 0.739$; pepperoni pizza, $r = 0.753$; spaghetti, $r = 0.739$; chicken chunks, $r = 0.717$; diced turkey, $r = 0.786$; Chinese meat bun, $r = 0.850$ (for all, $p < 0.001$). When given culturally diverse foods, culturally diverse children select and eat them.

Healthful Content of Menus

Several education/demonstration studies have successfully reduced the fat and saturated fat content of school recipes. The Go for Health program focused on influencing the student environment by enhancing physical activity classes and by lowering the fat content of school lunches (saturated fat from 16% to 10%, and total fat from 32% to 19%). Dietary recalls of students indicated that they consumed fewer calories, less total fat, and less sodium than students who were not offered the modified menus.[211]

The Heart Smart program developed a complementary approach for cardiovascular health promotion. The school cafeteria and classroom were effective vehicles to translate reduced fat, sodium, and sugar content of menus into acceptance foods.[193,194]

The American School Food Service Association initiative called Healthy EDGE (Eating, the Dietary Guidelines and Education) focuses on team building in schools and communities to work together to make the *Dietary Guidelines for Americans* a part of school policy and on activities that will effectively improve the nutritional health of students.[207] This initiative is the impetus for child nutrition employees to practice healthy menu planning for schoolchildren.

Chicago Charter School, *Namaste*—Innovation With Education

In fall 2005, 90 kindergarten and first-grade students began classes at Chicago's newest charter school, Namaste, which takes a unique approach to teaching. The novel approach is blending education with health in the school meal environment in the early elementary years among inner-city children. Nearly 1 in every 4 of Chicago's kindergarten-aged children is overweight; more than twice the national rate, which, unfortunately, paved the way for Namaste's funding from the Chicago Public School District this year.[212]

The founders of Namaste, Allison Slade and Katie Graves, spent 2 years teaching in low-income areas around the country with the nonprofit organization Teach for America and found the experience very rewarding. Their long-term commitment is to improve the quality of education and life for all young people. Namaste, which literally means, *my inner light salutes your inner light,* integrates physical fitness and nutrition as core components of the curriculum to provide a learning environment that is often difficult to attain, particularly in low-income schools. This approach breaks the barriers to good health and increases opportunities for high academic achievement.

Namaste's physical education program includes 60 minutes of physical education each day with an emphasis on developing health-related fitness, physical competence, and cognitive understanding about physical activity. The curriculum includes yoga, martial arts, and other activities that aren't focused on competition. Each Friday, Namaste hosts a family breakfast for parents and students to eat a healthy breakfast together and listen to a speaker discuss health, nutrition, and other educational topics (see Figure 8–5). A walking program for parents emphasizing walking their kids to school and family nutrition journals were planned. A special nutrition education curriculum for the school complements hot meals and selections from the salad bar for every meal. Namaste has also formed a collaborative with the Center for

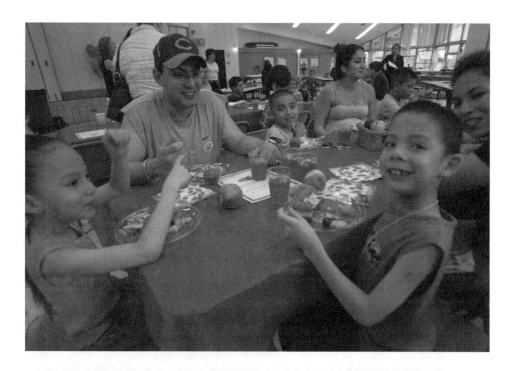

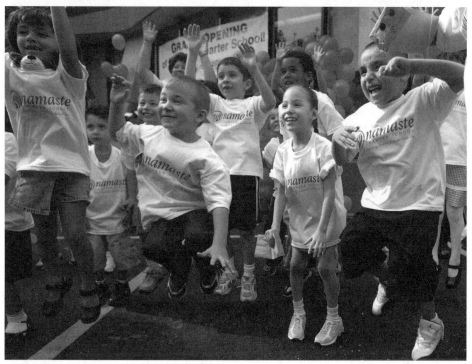

FIGURE 8–5 Physical fitness and nutrition are at the core of Namaste Charter School's curriculum in Chicago; 2005.
Source: Janet Helm.

Obesity Management and Prevention at Children's Memorial Research Center for evaluation and future programs. Namaste is located in McKinley Park, at 3540 S. Hermitage Avenue. Its phone number is (773) 715-9558. Its Web site is at www.namastecharterschool.org.

Trained Food Service Personnel

The American School Food Service Association has a strong commitment to continuing education that addresses sanitation, safety, meal planning, and meal preparation for health promotion in schools. School districts should support the food service staff and share expenses in training and upgrading this aspect of the school environment. Often child nutrition employees are at the low end of pay scales; their work may be seen as tertiary to education and physical fitness. This is demeaning and unnecessary: no hungry or malnourished child can think, concentrate, or participate at his or her fullest potential.

In California, Frank and Adsen[213] conducted a statewide census of training needs, querying 547 directors and 1,266 managers. Respondents indicated that training programs was the number 1 factor in influencing their personal career development and retention. Food preparation and healthy menu planning were the 2 courses they felt would be most helpful in their daily work. On-the-job-training was the most common form of training, and respondents preferred either their school site or their district office for training.

To train child nutrition employees in healthy menu planning, Shaping Healthy Meals for School Children was developed as a 10-lesson curriculum to be taught in a train-the-trainer format.[214] Shaping Healthy Meals uses the California Daily Food Guide (CDFG) and has been approved for continuing education units by the California School Food Service Association. The curriculum integrates several worksheets from the American Cancer Society's cafeteria training manual, *Changing the Course*, mentioned earlier. This is one of several excellent hands-on curricula and model programs that blend multiple materials with the immediate need in schools for relevant training about low-fat, tasty, and nutritionally adequate foods.

Cafeteria intervention in the form of in-service education training can follow a population-based approach and be given to all participating schools in a district or to multiple districts in a county. Training in most school districts is not but should be formalized in a consistent, sequential manner on a monthly or bimonthly basis. A train-the-trainer format, which identifies employees who are trained and then become trainers for their peers, strengthens the likelihood that school districts will sustain the program.

Food Service Delivery System

The ability of school cafeterias to link with classroom education is often influenced by the skills of child nutrition employees, the type of food service delivery system, and the degree to which the teachers are aware of the food service system.

A *centralized service* is a food service system in which all food is prepared in a central kitchen. Such a service often uses a cook-chill process—transporting the food daily to specific school sites, refrigerating, and then heating it before serving it. This system provides an opportunity to train a kitchen staff and influence thousands of meals daily prior to distribution. The major concerns are that foods are often purchased preportioned and that cooking equipment is automated in an assembly line. Menu changes must fit into the equipment and production process and the food specifications required of food companies.[215]

The *decentralized service* is a food service system in which all food is prepared on each school campus under the supervision of a site manager. This type of service creates a sense of ownership by the staff, who feel very responsible for their kids. Training at the site involves identifying the readiness of each employee, who may be responsible for only single types of foods (e.g., the baker, the main entree cook, etc.). For this type of service, training is directed toward skill development of the different preparation positions.[1]

For either delivery system, training food service staff in the use of point-of-choice nutrition information is a basic marketing effort. Nutrition information can be placed adjacent to foods to complement classroom education. For example, a label could read, "tossed salad with flaked tuna, 1½ cups: 144 calories, 241 retinol equivalents (RE) vitamin A, 36 mg vitamin C," or "hamburger on whole-wheat bun: 266 calories, 41% fat, 362 mg sodium." Point-of-choice nutrition information has been used to guide individuals in making healthy food choices with comparisons, nutrient information, and color coding like a stop light.[216-217]

Because school menus are increasingly being evaluated by a nutrient standard, computerized databases are being used by employees. Increasing the technical skills of child nutrition employees can be accomplished by integrating the computer training into routine procedures.

Many programs are available, such as Computrition, Inc, DINE Systems, and NutriKids.[218-221] Each system has unique characteristics—ranging from extensive food production, purchasing, and inventory programs on Computrition to evaluation by USDA meal components on NutriKids. NutriKids is a food database designed specifically for child nutrition programs. It contains over 1,100 common ingredients and 200 recipes. DINE has over 7,200 foods and produces a printout with an overall menu score based on consensus dietary recommendations (e.g., less than 30% fat and less than 3,300 mg of sodium[219-221]) (see Chapter 9).

High-Risk Youth Programs

Part of the solution to the problem of obesity is school involvement in secondary prevention programs. Schools can develop goals and plans to provide low-fat food choices matched with ample opportunities for continuous physical activities and sports participation. Dedicated school staff and faculty must be identified to champion the cause. Parental involvement in the program should be garnered to build self-esteem, reinforce positive behavior change, and identify depression among youth and their families.

The SHAPEDOWN program is a secondary prevention program for obese adolescents, which has produced significant long-term outcomes. It is transferable to various settings and may provide the foundation for a school-based program.[222]

Partnership With the Community

Developing a partnership with the community is a growing trend for child nutrition directors. A community advisory group of 8 to 12 individuals can consist of a community leader, a local pediatrician or family practice physician, a grocery store owner, a restaurant owner, an American Cancer Society representative, an elementary school teacher, a newspaper/radio or television reporter, a member of the clergy, a health agency representative, a local nutritionist, and/or a popular personality. The advisory group can respond to a program's philosophy, needs, progress, and any changes in format. This group can reinforce and publicize positive efforts occurring in child nutrition programs.

At the same time, child nutrition directors and the nutrition education specialists they employ can serve as nutrition resources for the media and community health efforts. For example, a concern is that only 8% of child nutrition directors employ such a specialist, often due to lack of funds.[213]

USDA established the National Food Service Management Institute at the University of Mississippi with the Child Nutrition and WIC Reauthorization Act of 1989. The institute aims to build the future through child nutrition and designs and conducts activities to improve the operation and quality of child nutrition programs. The institute, which is a national resource center for all child nutrition programs, has 3 divisions:

1. *Development and Applied Research:* conducts research designed to provide appropriate management tools that ensure cost-effectiveness, quality, nutritious food service, and employee performance standards.
2. *Education and Training:* designs and develops competency-based training modules and materials for child nutrition program employees and provides technical assistance.
3. *Technology Transfer:* acts as a clearinghouse and information center for all areas of relevant research and information and collects, evaluates, and disseminates materials.

Participation in Professional Organizations

The American School Food Service Association (ASFSA) and state chapters support a national membership of more than 65,000. ASFSA is the mouthpiece for child nutrition professionals and has active lobbying efforts in Congress. Legislative efforts are directed toward universal feeding and challenging block grants to fund the National School Lunch Program, the School Breakfast Program, and the Summer Food Service Program.

Info Line

The National Food Service Management Institute is authorized by the US Congress and administered by the US Department of Agriculture. For information write to PO Drawer 188, University, MS 38677-0188. Telephone: (662) 915-7658 or 1-800-321-3054. E-mail nfsmi@olemiss.edu. Web site: http://www.nfsmi.org.

Info Line

In 2003 the Arkansas General Assembly and Governor Mike Huckabee passed Act 1220, "An act to create a child health advisory committee to coordinate statewide efforts to combat childhood obesity and related illnesses; to improve the health of the next generation of Arkansans." Beginning in 2003, all Arkansas schoolchildren have an annual body mass index (BMI) test and the data is given confidentially to the students' parents. Suggestions are included for treatment if the child is obese or at risk of becoming obese.

Interacting factors and stakeholders are students and their teachers, coaches, museum educators, parents, and primary healthcare providers, all of whom need basic knowledge of human nutrition, obesity, and BMI.

To further the statewide educational approach for pre-K to 12th-grade students in Arkansas, the following 2 major strategies are being considered: (1) training teachers, museum educators, cooperative extension service specialists, coaches, school nurses and counselors, parents, physicians, pharmacists, nurses, and physician assistants; and (2) delivering interactive television (ITV) instruction to middle school students. The first strategy will merge with an established educational program for pre-K through 12th-grade health science teachers and students called the Partners in Health Sciences (PIHS). This program has existed at the University of Arkansas for Medical Sciences (UAMS) since 1991 and has trained over 16,000 participants totaling 60,069 hours of training/education.[223]

The American Dietetic Association (ADA) and the School Food Services Dietetic Practice Group are major professional organizations of registered dietitians (RDs) employed in school systems. The ADA collaborates with other national organizations to produce nutrition education materials for school-age children. In addition, many food companies employ RDs who manage complete healthcare lines and specialty lines for schools (e.g., US Foodservice, Arrow-Sysco, and ConAgra). Child nutrition directors and managers work directly with the food companies to achieve products lower in fat, sodium, and sugar for their menus.

The Association of State School Nutrition Directors and Supervisors meets annually to update programs on USDA guidelines and pending federal legislation affecting school meals, to discuss innovations, and to provide continuing education. These directors oversee all USDA food programs in schools and day care facilities in their respective states.

Guidelines for Adolescent Preventive Services

A major area of concern is the current adolescent morbidity and mortality. This toll on young lives creates a health crisis for today's youths. Problems include unplanned pregnancy, sexually transmitted disease, including human immunodeficiency virus (HIV), alcohol and drug abuse, and eating disorders.[204] Adolescence is a period of experimentation and risk taking. The resulting behaviors of youths threaten their current health and may have long-term consequences on their adult functioning. In addition, youths should be screened for substance abuse and certain behavioral and biomedical conditions. Vaccinations to protect youths from infectious diseases such as measles and rubella are also an important part of primary care.

The American Medical Association (AMA) focuses on the adolescent population through *Healthy Youth 2010*, supporting 21 critical adolescent objectives. Its effort is based on attaining 21 critical objectives among 10- to 24-year-olds (see Table 8–6).

Table 8–6   Critical Health Outcomes Among 10- to 24-Year-Olds

Healthy People 2010 Objective No.	Objective
Mortality and overall health	
16-03	Reduce deaths of adolescents and young adults who are: 10 to 14 years, 5 to 19 years, and 20 to 24 years
15-15	Reduce deaths caused by motor vehicle crashes (also a leading health indicator)
26-01	Reduce deaths and injuries caused by alcohol- and drug-related motor vehicle crashes
18-01	Reduce the suicide rate
15-32	Reduce homicides for those who are 10 to 14 years of age and for those who are 15 to 19 years of age (also a leading health indicator)
09-07	Reduce pregnancies among adolescent females
13-05	Reduce the number of cases of HIV infection among adolescents and adults
25-01	Reduce the proportion of adolescents and young adults with *Chlamydia trachomatis* infections
19-03	Reduce the proportion of children and adolescents who are overweight or obese (also a leading health indicator)
Behaviors that substantially contribute to important health outcomes	
15-19	Increase use of safety belts
26-06	Reduce the proportion of adolescents who report that they rode, during the previous 30 days, with a driver who had been drinking alcohol
18-02	Reduce the rate of suicide attempts by adolescents
15-38	Reduce physical fighting among adolescents
15-39	Reduce weapon carrying by adolescents on school property
06-02	Reduce the proportion of children and adolescents with disabilities who are reported to be sad, unhappy, or depressed
18-07	Increase the proportion of children with mental health problems who receive treatment

TABLE 8–6   continued

Leading health indicators

26-11	Reduce the proportion of persons engaging in binge drinking of alcoholic beverages
26-10	Reduce past-month use of illicit substances
25-11	Increase the proportion of adolescents who abstain from sexual intercourse or use condoms if currently sexually active
27-02	Reduce tobacco use by adolescents
22-07	Increase the proportion of adolescents who engage in vigorous physical activity that promotes cardiorespiratory fitness 3 or more days per week for 20 or more minutes per occasion

Objectives that address both critical health outcomes and the leading health indicators

15-15	Reduce deaths caused by motor vehicle crashes
15-32	Reduce homicides for those who are 10 to 14 years of age and for those who are 15 to 19 years of age
19-03	Reduce the proportion of children and adolescents who are overweight or obese

Source: Towey K, Fleming M. *Healthy Youth 2010—Supporting the 21 Critical Adolescent Objectives.* Chicago, Ill: American Medical Association; 2004.

The AMA has developed the Guidelines for Adolescent Preventive Services (GAPS), a comprehensive set of recommendations for community organizations that can serve as the potential content of preventive health services. These recommendations address problems common to youths of all ethnic groups (e.g., suicide, unplanned pregnancy, sexually transmitted disease), and they are directed to primary and secondary prevention. Because schools and community organizations have increased health education programs, and primary care physicians and other health care providers including community nutrition professionals are bringing preventive services into their clinical practice, GAPS provides a blueprint for the delivery of services.[224]

The GAPS guidelines emphasize health guidance and prevention of behavioral and emotional disorders. Health guidance includes health education, health counseling, and anticipatory guidance. Because adolescence is a time of experimentation and risk taking, the resulting behaviors may threaten current health or may have long-term consequences. Four types of services are identified: healthcare delivery, health guidance, screening for specific conditions, and immunizations for the primary prevention of selected infectious disease.[224]

Developing healthy eating patterns is the health promotion focus to prevent high blood cholesterol, alcohol abuse, and depression. In addition, a series of annual health visits between the ages of 11 and 21 years is recommended for all youths. Adolescents who have initiated health-risk behaviors can be identified. If they are at early stages of physical or emotional disorders, opportunities for communication and support can be formed. The recommended frequency of specific GAPS preventive services is outlined in Exhibit 8–2. These services can reinforce health promotion messages for adolescents and their parents.

Exhibit 8–2   Recommendations Developed for Guidelines for Adolescent Preventive Services (GAPS)

1. From age 11 to 21, all adolescents should have an annual preventive services visit.
2. Preventive services should be age and developmentally appropriate, and should be sensitive to individual and sociocultural differences.
3. Physicians should establish office policies regarding confidential care for adolescents and how parents will be involved in that care. These policies should be made clear to adolescents and their parents.
4. Parents or other adult caregivers should receive health guidance at least once during their child's early adolescence, once during middle adolescence, and, preferably, once during late adolescence.
5. All adolescents should receive health guidance annually to promote a better understanding of their physical growth, psychosocial and psychosexual development, and the importance of becoming actively involved in decisions regarding their health care.
6. All adolescents should receive health guidance annually to promote the reduction of injuries.
7. All adolescents should receive health guidance annually about dietary habits, including the benefits of a healthy eating pattern and ways to achieve it and safe weight management also.
8. All adolescents should receive health guidance annually about the benefits of exercise and should be encouraged to engage in safe exercise on a regular basis.
9. All adolescents should receive health guidance annually regarding responsible sexual behaviors, including abstinence. Latex condoms to prevent sexually transmitted diseases (STDs), including HIV infection, and appropriate methods of birth control should be made available, as should instructions on how to use them effectively.
10. All adolescents should receive health guidance annually to promote avoidance of tobacco, alcohol, other abusable substances, and anabolic steroids.
11. All adolescents should be screened annually for hypertension according to the protocol developed by the National Heart, Lung, and Blood Institute Second Task Force on Blood Pressure Control in Children.
12. Selected adolescents should be screened to determine their risk of developing hyperlipidemia and adult coronary heart disease, following the protocol developed by the Expert Panel on Blood Cholesterol Levels in Children and Adolescents.
13. All adolescents should be screened annually for eating disorders and obesity by determining weight and stature and by asking about body image and dieting patterns.
14. All adolescents should be asked annually about their use of tobacco products, including cigarettes and smokeless tobacco.
15. All adolescents should be asked annually about their use of alcohol and other abusable substances, and about their use of over-the-counter or prescription drugs for nonmedical purposes, including anabolic steroids.
16. All adolescents should be asked annually about involvement in sexual behaviors that may result in unintended pregnancy and STDs, including HIV infection.
17. Sexually active adolescents should be screened for STDs.

continued

Exhibit 8–2 continued

18. Adolescents at risk of HIV infection should be offered confidential HIV screening with the enzyme linked immunosorbent assay (ELISA) and confirmatory test.
19. Female adolescents who are sexually active or any female 18 or older should be screened annually for cervical cancer by use of a Pap test.
20. All adolescents should be asked annually about behaviors or emotions that indicate recurrent or severe depression or risk of suicide.
21. All adolescents should be asked annually about a history of emotional, physical, and sexual abuse.
22. All adolescents should be asked annually about learning or school problems.
23. Adolescents should receive a tuberculin skin test if they have been exposed to active tuberculosis, have lived in a homeless shelter, have been incarcerated, have lived in or come from an area with a high prevalence of tuberculosis, or currently work in a healthcare setting.
24. All adolescents should receive prophylactic immunizations according to the guidelines established by the federally convened Advisory Committee on Immunization Practices.

Source: Adapted from: American Medical Association. *Guidelines for Adolescent Preventive Services.* Chicago, Ill: American Medical Association; 1992:1-9.

Rapid behavioral changes occur during adolescence. Frequent visits that screen youth for health risk behaviors can provide health guidance and ensure that accurate information is recorded. Because the clients are adolescents, GAPS recommend that all information given by adolescents during the medical visit should remain confidential to build a medical bond and promote future contact.

The Public Health Service conducted a cross-sectional review of progress on *Healthy People* objectives related to adolescents and young adults. Sixty objectives target youth as outlined in Table 8–6, with several pertaining to tobacco, alcohol, and other drugs. Some reductions in tobacco and substance abuse have occurred among young people.

The lack of adequate access to appropriate health services and the selective approach of certain existing programs are barriers to quality health care for adolescents and young adults. Action items for achieving the objectives for adolescents and young adults include[225]:

- reevaluating the targets and strategies for sexual activity
- identifying and supporting catalyst agencies to help move strategies from a categorical to a broader life view
- assessing the impact and periodicity for clinical preventive services proposed for adolescents

Outcomes for Children and Youth

Outcomes advocated by most research on youth include development, resiliency, protective factors, and developmental assets. The major aims of youth programs are to enhance youngsters' opportunities, their motivations, and capability to develop appropriately and to function effectively. A broader goal may be building a personal base for youth from the following domains:

1. *Academics* including school engagement; motivation and ability to work and relate at school; motivation for self-learning and enhancement of literacy; feelings of academic competence.
2. *Healthy and safe behavior* including the ability to make good decisions about diet, hygiene, health care, involvement in activities; ability to solve interpersonal problems and resolve conflicts; ability to delay gratification and resist impulses and inappropriate social pressures.
3. *Social-emotional functioning* including the ability to relate socially and in working relationships with others encompassing cultural competencies and understanding behavioral norms; ability to handle and reduce stress; ability to express and manage feelings; positive feelings about self and others; feelings of social-emotional competence and connection with significant others; a resilient temperament.
4. *Communication*—verbal and nonverbal—including basic language skills and the ability to read and interpret social cues and understand the perspectives of others.
5. *Character/values* including personal, social, and civic responsibility; integrity; self-regulation, sense of purpose; and feelings of hope for the future.
6. *Self-direction* including ability to make and follow through on good decisions for oneself; feelings of autonomy/self-determination.
7. *Vocational and other adult roles* including knowledge, skills, and attitudes for acquiring and maintaining employment, initiating and maintaining intimate adult relationships, and providing effective parenting.
8. *Recreational and enrichment pursuits,* including the ability to engage in venues for enhancing quality of life and creativity and for reducing stress.

Primary Prevention—California Adolescent Nutrition and Fitness Program

The California Adolescent Nutrition and Fitness Program (CANFit) provides $5,000 to $50,000 grants for nutrition education and fitness intervention. This initiative is the first of its kind to fund outreach directly to community-based organizations serving 10- to 14-year-old African-American, Latino, Asian, and American Indian Youths.[226] CANFit questioned and learned the following:

- *Why Nutrition and Fitness?* Among low-income, multiethnic California adolescents, > 49% are overweight, only 21% meet minimum fitness standards, and more than 28% have blood values consistent with iron deficiency anemia. CANFit believes these results are the consequences of a lack of regular exercise; inconsistent eating patterns; high consumption of fat, sugar, cholesterol, sodium, and calories; and low consumption of essential nutrients, including fruits and vegetables.
- *Why Adolescents?* Adolescents spend about 40% of the family food dollar, prepare 13 meals per week for themselves and/or their families, need

the proper nutrients to sustain their rapid growth, and form eating and physical activity habits that will last a lifetime.

- *Can CANFit Fill a Community Need?* Adolescents are among the most poorly nourished Americans. Changes in the American diet, cutbacks in school health and physical education programs, and relatively inactive lifestyles contribute to increased obesity and declining fitness levels. These negative events occur when adolescent bodies are undergoing extensive growth and development.

CANFit targets low-income, multiethnic adolescents as these groups tend to have the greatest unmet nutrition and physical activity education needs. CANFit provides training, technical assistance, and other resources to organizations that can provide nutrition, physical activity, and leadership skills to these youths (see Figure 8-6).

Planning grants focus on assessment of needs, development of specific action plans, and defining the intrastructure to implement those plans. Intervention grants implement-specific programs within community-based organizations among high-risk youths. The content of the grants reflect youth-driven programs, capacity-building activities for the member organizations, and process and impact evaluations.[226]

To further its mission to seed nutrition and fitness programs for the youth in California, CANFit awards about 10 $1,000 scholarships annually to minority college students majoring in nutrition or physical education at California colleges and universities. Applicants submit competitive essays entitled, "The Three Most Important Nutrition or Fitness Challenges Facing California's Adolescents . . . and Here's What I Would Do." The program provides a unique model that could be replicated in other states and communities.

In 2002, CANFit launched the Promoting Healthy Activities Together (PHAT) campaign to improve the nutrition and physical activity knowledge, attitudes, skills, and behaviors of African-American 10- to 14-year-olds attending after-school programs in the San Francisco Bay area.[227]

Using a community-based approach, the PHAT campaign embraced music, dance, emceeing, and other elements of hip-hop culture to deliver important messages about healthy eating and physical activity. Organized settings were community centers and after-school programs. Over 2 months, more than 80 youth worked weekly with local hip-hop talent. The goal was to develop personal nutrition and fitness messages as raps, artwork, and hip-hop dance routines. These were featured at the PHAT Community Health and Hip-Hop Showcase, and in a PHAT video.

Recommendations from the PHAT campaign are:[227]

1. *Keep it real and stay focused*—Determine focus and try not to include multiple nutrition and physical activity messages. Determine single behaviors, attitudes, or knowledge for participants to adopt. Reinforce messages in all parts of the campaign. Connect youth messages with health messages. The title "PHAT" was appealing to youth. The healthy activities promoted in the art were clear and included increasing water consumption, decreasing consumption of fast food and sodas, and increasing physical activities.
2. *Involve youth in the planning*—Solicit ideas from youth to keep things real. Involve youth in the decision making from title to promotional materials and incentives. Have volunteers who can walk the walk and talk the talk.

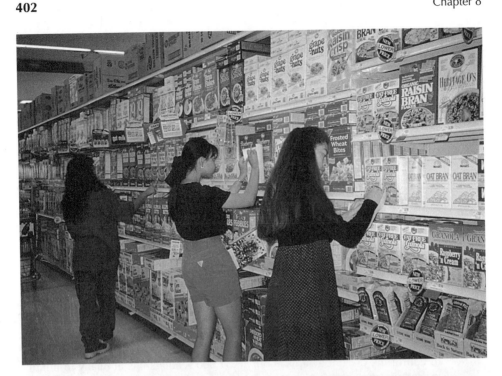

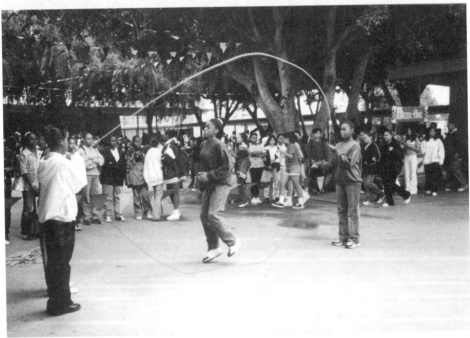

FIGURE 8–6 Youth receive nutrition education such as food label reading at Escondido Community Health Center and physical education instruction and skill development at Culver City Youth Health Center. Both are CANFit program sites.
Source: Arnell Hinkle, Ex. Dir., California Adolescent Nutrition & Fitness Program.

Info Line

CANFIT MISSION

The CANFit program is a unique state-wide organization whose mission is to engage communities and build their capacity to improve the nutrition and physical activity of California's low-income, African-American, American Indian, Latino, and Asian/Pacific Islander youth between the ages of 10 and 14. The program supports local projects that build community leadership and stimulate change at multiple levels, from individual behavior to public policy, in the area of nutrition education and physical activity. The projects should integrate the cultural, linguistic, social, and demographic characteristics of youth, change social and community norms, identify and incorporate into the intervention the ethnic specific messages likely to motivate behavior change, address the multiple influences, e.g., mass media, environment, peers, family, etc., affecting adolescent eating and physical activity behaviors, employ individuals who are highly credible and respected by the targeted groups to deliver the program, improve eating and exercise habits, increase nutrition and physical activity skills, improve critical thinking skills, set policies that support healthy eating and physical activity behaviors in communities and organizations, and improve access to quality food and safe recreational facilities. Their Web site is at www.canfit.org.

3. *Collaborate with credible professionals*—Employ community people who are not only involved with hip-hop culture (choreographers, emcees, graphic artists), but have experience working with young people and a desire to improve their nutrition and fitness.
4. *Maintain variety, structure, and accountability*—Offer various appealing activities. Tell youth what they will be doing if they choose to participate, what is expected of them, and how long they will have to sustain the activity.
5. *Create incentive*—Use incentives and prizes to initiate interest. Then incorporate elements of hip-hop culture that they enjoy, and expose them to positive role models.

National Institutes of Health Interventions

Several major intervention studies have been funded by the National Institutes of Health to alter the high-risk status of certain children. Results may have implications for future health policy and medical practice. A brief description of 3 of these studies follows.[228]

NHLBI Growth and Health Study

The National Heart, Lung, and Blood Institute Growth and Health Study began in September 1985 to assess the occurrence of obesity in young women, factors that could predict and correlate with the transition to obesity, and the association of obesity with various risk factors for heart disease. The study population includes both African-American and white girls, 9 to 10 years old at entry. The group is 51% African-American. Dietary and physical activity, socioeconomic status, and lifestyle variables are assessed.

Child and Adolescent Trial of Cardiovascular Health

This trial began in 1987 to measure and to compare the effects of school-based interventions to promote lifelong behavior among elementary schoolchildren and adolescents to reduce cardiovascular risk. About 12,000 girls and boys in the third, fourth, and fifth grades and from all major US ethnic groups are involved. Total serum cholesterol is the primary outcome measure. Interventions include classroom curricula, family-focused dietary modifications, physical activity, and tobacco use.

Framingham Heart and Offspring Studies

This study has been identified as the landmark longitudinal study of risk factors associated with the development of cardiovascular disease. The Framingham Study began in 1948 and provides surveillance of adults in Framingham, Massachusetts. The Framingham Offspring Study began in 1971 with 5,135 participants, of which 3,555 were offspring of the original cohort. Endpoints for both studies are coronary heart disease, stroke, hypertension, congestive heart failure, and peripheral arterial disease.

The most well-known finding from the Framingham Study was that high blood cholesterol, high blood pressure, and cigarette smoking were identified as the 3 major risk factors for heart disease. In addition, smoking was listed as a significant independent variable contributing to the risk of stroke, and specifically brain infarction. Obesity was identified as a major independent risk factor.

The Framingham Offspring Study reports that offspring have slightly lower blood cholesterol and blood pressure levels than their parents. Children of parents with hypertension have higher blood pressures than other children. Smoking among men has decreased to half that of their fathers, but women smoke more than their mothers. Heart disease mortality has declined, but the reason remains unclear.

President's Council on Physical Fitness and Sport

Prior US President Bill Clinton appointed a diverse group of 15 physical fitness, sports, health, and community leaders to serve on the President's Council on Physical Fitness and Sport. These appointees are from the fields of medicine, professional and amateur sports, physical education, and training and advocacy for physically disabled persons. The council supports activities throughout the United States to energize Americans to become more physically active, healthier, and more physically fit.[229]

School-age youth can participate in the President's Council annually via the physical education department at their schools. Planned activities commonly comprise routine evaluation of the fitness level of youths. Standards are set and awards are given for students who meet and/or exceed the criteria for several measures.

Children Around the World

Japan

Matsui et al measured the anthropometrics, serum lipids, fasting serum insulin (FSI), food intake, and physical activity in 1,330 children in 3 age groups (6 to 7, 9 to 10, and 12 to 13) in Nagao, Japan, during 1994-1996. Serum total cholesterol (TC) and high-density lipoprotein cholesterol (HDL-C) levels were positively correlated, and HDL-C and TG were negatively correlated in all age groups. FSI was significantly higher in older children and for girls, and it was positively correlated with the body mass index (BMI) and triceps skinfold thickness in ages 9 to 10 and 12 to 13. No significant correlation was noted with waist:hip ratio. At 12 to 13 years, FSI was positively correlated with TC and TG and negatively correlated with HDL-C. Children with high FSI (> 11.4 µU/mL) and 12- to 13-year-old had > 30% energy from fat, less physical activity, high triceps skinfold, and a nonsignificant, positive correlation between TC and HDL-C. Matsui et al concluded that a high-fat diet, low physical activity, and high body fat influence the FSI and serum lipid levels.[230]

United Kingdom

Since serum lipid and lipoprotein cholesterol levels track from childhood and are associated with risk of coronary heart disease, research continues to explore whether they are influenced by dietary intake and exercise. A cohort of 119 British children 12 to 15 years old completed a dietary and exercise questionnaire. The ratio of total to high-density lipoprotein cholesterol fell with increasing fiber intake, but after adjustment for age, body mass index, sex, and other dietary factors, it was not statistically significant. Children exercising at least once a day had significantly lower serum total cholesterol and low-density lipoprotein cholesterol levels than those exercising less frequently, even after adjusting for dietary fiber.[231]

Netherlands

The Amsterdam Growth and Health Study is an observational longitudinal study of 6 repeat measures over 15 years on 181 youth aged 13 years at entry. For diastolic blood pressure no significant relationships were found. High risk for systolic blood pressure was inversely related to smoking habits (OR = 0.52; $p = 0.01$) where OR is odds ratio and p is statistical probability. No significant relationships were found for TC; high HDL was positively related to the intake of carbohydrates (OR = 1.2; $p = 0.02$) and to smoking habits (OR = 1.6; $p = 0.04$); high TC:HDL ratio was positively related to the intake of carbohydrates (OR = 1.3; $p = 0.01$). High subscapular skinfold (SSE) was positively related to the intake of protein (OR = 1.5; $p = 0.01$) and smoking habits (OR = 1.8; $p = 0.01$) and inversely related to daily physical activity (OR = 0.81; $p = 0.01$). High VO_2 max was inversely related to daily physical activity (OR = 0.67; $p = 0.01$).[232]

Method Alert

Often researchers conduct extensive dietary analysis and make strong recommendations based on a 1-day food record or recall that they assume is usual for the participant. Craig et al conducted a secondary analysis after evaluating actual research data and conducting hypothesis tests to understand how days with atypical food intake affect estimates of usual nutrient intake from 2,560 4-day food records.[233] Records from 1,090 participants, 50-79 years, who participated in the Women's Trial Feasibility Study in Minority Populations, a randomized dietary intervention trial, were analyzed. Food records were classified as atypical if 1 or more days were marked as more than usual or less than usual. Total amounts and nutrient densities were examined for all macronutrients, fiber, vitamin C, beta carotene, and calcium. Analyses included associations of demographic characteristics with the likelihood of completing a 4-day food record with atypical intake days, testing whether nutrient intake differed among records with and without atypical days, and identification of any differences in total energy and percent energy from fat among typical and atypical intake days.[233]

Approximately 16% of records included at least 1 atypical day. A greater frequency of less-than-usual intake was associated with younger age, higher income, and higher body mass index. Black women were less likely to report more-than-usual intake than both white and Hispanic women. Records with less-than-usual intake had lower intakes of all nutrients analyzed except alcohol. No differences in nutrient densities were noted for the different records. Records with more-than-usual intake had higher intakes of alcohol and all nutrients except beta carotene and vitamin C and higher nutrient density measures of alcohol and decreased nutrient density measures of protein, vitamin C, and fiber. Atypical intake days are common in 4-day food records and can have a large effect on mean total intakes. Researchers should address the role of atypical intake days when analyzing and interpreting research results.[233]

Healthy People 2010 Actions

Nutrition-related objectives are outlined for school-age children in Exhibit 8–3. Obesity and dental caries are major concerns. Alcoholic beverage consumption, high fat intakes, and low calcium and complex carbohydrate intakes are the focus of specific directives. Community nutrition professionals have a new frontier and opportunity for their services. Attention to adolescent health gained prominence during the 1990s. Nutrition services need to be integrated and clearly defined to effect positive change in the lives of the newest generation of young adults. Table 8–7 contrasts *Healthy People 2010* goals for adolescents with the 1991, 1992, and 2000 targets.

Strategies to achieve nutritionally healthy and fit youths include embellishing efforts for comprehensive school health education for all children; enhancing complementary physical activity and child nutrition programs at schools; assessing the readiness of students and faculties for change before programs are planned and implemented; developing youth-driven programs; and incorporating the family, the various living and eating environments of adolescents, and the community.[234-236]

Exhibit 8–3 DATA 2010. The Healthy People 2010 Database–November 2000, Focus Area: 22–Physical Activity and Fitness

Objective Number	Objective	Baseline Year	Baseline	Target 2010
07-02f	School health education–Alcohol and other drug use (provided by middle, junior high, and senior high schools)	1994	90	95
07-02h	School health education–Unhealthy dietary patterns (provided by middle, junior high, and senior high schools)	1994	84	95
07-02i	School health education–Inadequate physical activity (provided by middle, junior high, and senior high schools)	1994	78	90
09-07	Adolescent pregnancy–Among adolescent females (rate per 1,000 females aged 15 to 17 years)	1996	68	43
	American Indian or Alaska native	1996	UK	43
	Asian or Pacific Islander	1996	UK	43
	Asian	1996	UK	43
	Native Hawaiian and other Pacific Islander	1996	UK	43
	Black or African American	1996	124	43
	White	1996	58	43
	Hispanic or Latino	1996	105	43
	Not Hispanic or Latino	1996	62	43
16-02b	Child deaths (rate per 100,000 children aged 5 to 9 years)	1998	17.7	12.3
16-03a	Adolescent and young adult deaths–Adolescents aged 10 to 14 years (rate per 100,000)	1998	22.1	16.8
16-03b	Adolescent and young adult deaths–Adolescents aged 15 to 19 years (rate per 100,000)	1998	70.6	39.8
16-03c	Adolescent and young adult deaths–Young adults aged 20 to 24 years (rate per 100,000)	1998	95.3	49.0

continued

Exhibit 8–3   continued

Objective Number	Objective	Baseline Year	Baseline	Target 2010
19-03b	Overweight or obesity in children and adolescents–Adolescents (adolescents aged 12 to 19 years)	1988-1994	11	5
	American Indian or Alaska native	1988-1994	UK	5
	Asian or Pacific Islander	1988-1994	UK	5
	Black or African American	1988-1994	13	5
	White	1988-1994	11	5
	Hispanic or Latino	1988-1994	UK	5
	Mexican American	1988-1994	14	5
	Not Hispanic or Latino	1988-1994	10	5
	Female	1988-1994	10	5
	Male	1988-1994	11	5
	Lower family income level (< 130% of poverty threshold)	1988-1994	16	5
	Higher family income level (> 130% of poverty threshold)	1988-1994	8	5
19-15	Meals and snacks at school–Children and adolescents	UK	UK	UK
22-06	Moderate physical activity in adolescents (grades 9-12)	1999	27	35
22-07	Vigorous physical activity in adolescents (grades 9-12)	1999	65	85
22-08a	Physical education requirement in schools (middle and junior high schools)	1994	17	25
22-08b	Physical education requirement in schools (senior high school)	1994	2	5
22-09	Daily physical education in schools (grades 9-12)	1999	29	50
22-10	Physical activity in physical education class (grades 9-12)	1999	38	50
22-11	Television viewing–Children and adolescents (grades 9-12)	1999	57	75

22-14b	Community walking—Trips to school of 1 mile or less (age adjusted, children and adolescents aged 5 to 15 years)	1995	31	50
22-15b	Community bicycling—Trips to school of 2 miles or less (age adjusted, children and adolescents aged 5 to 15 years)	1995	2.4	5.0
26-10a	Adolescent and adult use of illicit substances			
	Adolescents—No alcohol or illicit drug use in past 30 days (adolescents aged 12 to 17 years)	1998	79	89
	American Indian or Alaska native	1998	72	89
	Asian or Pacific Islander	1998	87	89
	Asian	1998	UK	89
	Native Hawaiian and other Pacific Islander	1998	UK	89
	Black or African American	1998	82	89
	White	1998	77	89
	Hispanic or Latino	1998	79	89
	Not Hispanic or Latino	1998	79	89
	Female	1998	79	89
	Male	1998	79	89
	Poor	1998	78	89
	Near poor	1998	75	89
	Middle/high income	1998	80	89
26-11a	Binge drinking—High school seniors	1998	32	11
	American Indian or Alaska native	1998	UK	11
	Asian or Pacific Islander	1998	UK	11
	Asian	1998	UK	11
	Native Hawaiian and other Pacific Islander	1998	UK	11
	Black or African American	1998	12	11
	White	1998	36	11

continued

Exhibit 8-3   continued

Objective Number	Objective	Baseline Year	Baseline	Target 2010
26-11a	Binge drinking—High school seniors			
	Hispanic or Latino	1998	28	11
	Not Hispanic or Latino	1998	UK	11
	Female	1998	24	11
	Male	1998	39	11
	Poor	1998	UK	11
	Near poor	1998	UK	11
	Middle/high income	1998	UK	11

UK = unknown

Source: Adapted from: US Department of Health and Human Services. DATA 2010—the *Healthy People 2010* Database. *CDC Wonder*. Atlanta, Ga: Centers for Disease Control; November 2000.

Table 8–7 Progress Report on Health Objectives for Adolescents

Objective No.	Objective	1987 Baseline	1991	1992	Year 2000 Target	2010
3.5	Reduce initiation of smoking by children and youths so no more than 15% are regular smokers by age 20	30%	24%	—	15%	17%
3.5a	Lower socioeconomic status youth	40%	31%	—	18%	18%
3.9	Reduce smokeless tobacco use by males aged 12 through 24					
	Males aged 12-17	6.6%	5.3%	—	4%	4%
	Males aged 18-24	8.9%	9.9%	—	4%	4%
3.9a	American Indian/Alaskan native youths	18-64%	19.7%	—	10%	10%
4.1b	Reduce deaths among youths aged 15-24 caused by alcohol-related motor vehicle crashes	21.5	14.1	—	18.0	4%
4.5	Increase by at least 1 year the average age of first use of:					
	cigarettes	11.6%	—	11.5%	12.6%	—
	alcohol	13.1%	—	12.6%	14.1%	16.1%
	marijuana	13.4%	—	13.5%	14.4%	17.4%
4.6	Reduce substance use in the last month					
	Alcohol: 12- to 17-year-olds	25.2%	—	15.7%	12.6%	11%
	18- to 20-year-olds	57.9%	—	50.3%	29.0%	50%
	Marijuana: 12- to 17-year-olds	6.4%	—	4.0%	3.2%	0.7%
	18- to 25-year-olds	15.5%	—	11.0%	7.8%	11%
	Cocaine: 12- to 17-year-olds	1.1%	—	0.3%	0.6%	0.6%
	18- to 25-year-olds	4.5%	—	1.8%	2.3%	2.0%
4.7	Reduce heavy drinking of alcoholic beverages in past 2 weeks among:					
	High school seniors	33%	—	27.9%	28%	11%
	College students	41.7%	—	41.4%	32%	20%

Source: Adapted from: American Medical Association. *Target 2000.* Chicago, Ill: American Medical Association; Fall 1994:6.

The National Commission on the Role of the School and the Community in Improving Adolescent Health has called the nation to action to address the problems of youth. In *CODE BLUE: Uniting for Healthier Youth*, the commission states that the situation is an emergency and that life-threatening events are occurring in the lives of US youths. These events threaten the very survival and healthy functioning of adolescents, the future of the children birthed by adolescents, and the viability and competitiveness of the American workforce in general. All sectors of society are involved, and their dedication is needed to redirect the future of this generation.[237]

References

1. Frank GC. Nutrition issues. In: Cortese P, Middleton K, eds. *The Comprehensive School Health Challenge.* Santa Cruz, Calif: ETR Assoc; 1994:373-411.
2. Frank GC. Assessing diets of children: environmental influences on dietary data collection methods with children. *Am J Clin Nutr.* Special issue: First International Conference on Dietary Assessment Methods. 1994;59(suppl):207s-211s.
3. Frank GC. Nutrition for teens. In: Henderson A, Champlin S, eds. *Promoting Teen Health.* Thousand Oaks, Calif: Sage Publications; 1998: 28-45.
4. Sikand G, Kris-Etherton P, Frank-Spohrer G. Nutritional guidelines for the prevention of cardiovascular disease. In: Wong N, ed. *Primary Prevention of CVD.* New York, NY: McGraw-Hill; 2000.
5. Prevalence of overweight among children and adolescents: US 1999-2000. Centers for Disease Control and Prevention, National Center for Health Statistics. Available at: http://www.cdc.gov/nchs/products/pubs/pubd/hestats/overwght99.htm. Accessed March 9, 2004.
6. Frank GC. The obesity problem among children—what can pediatricians do? *California Pediatrician.* Spring 2000;16(1):35-36.
7. Berenson GS, McMahan CA, Voors AW, et al. *Cardiovascular Risk Factors in Children—The Early Natural History of Atherosclerosis and Essential Hypertension.* New York: Oxford University Press; 1980.
8. Food Research and Action Center. *Community Childhood Hunger Identification Project.* Washington, DC: Food Research and Action Center; 1991.
9. Food and Nutrition Board, National Academy of Sciences, National Research Council. *Recommended Dietary Allowances.* 10th ed. Washington, DC: National Academy Press; 1989.
10. National Academy of Sciences, Institute of Medicine (IOM). *Dietary Reference Intakes for Energy, Carbohydrate, Fiber, Fat, Fatty Acids, Cholesterol, Protein, and Amino Acids.* Washington, DC: National Academy Press; Released September 5, 2002. Available at http://www.IOM.edu/. Accessed December 14, 2006.
11. Frank GC, Berenson GS, Schilling PE, et al. Adapting the 24-hour dietary recall for epidemiologic studies of school children. *J Am Diet Assoc.* 1977;71:26-31.
12. Frank GC. Dietary studies of infants and children. In: Berensox GS et al. *Cardiovascular Risk Factors in Children—The Early Natural History of Atherosclerosis and Essential Hypertension.* New York: Oxford University Press; 1980:289-307.

13. Wotecki CE. Nutrition in childhood and adolescence—Parts 1 and 2. *Contemporary Nutr.* 1992;17(2):1-2.

14. Chan GM. Dietary calcium and bone mineral status of children and adolescents. *Am J Dis Children.* 1991;145:631-634.

15. Cavadini C, Siega-Rizb A, Popkin B. US adolescent food intake trends from 1965 to 1996. *West J Med.* Dec 2000;173(6):378-383.

16. Iuliano-Burns S, Whiting SJ, Faulkner RA, Bailey DA. Levels, sources, and seasonality of dietary calcium intake in children and adolescents enrolled in the University of Saskatchewan pediatric bone mineral accrual study. *Nutr Res.* 1999;19(10):1471-1483.

17. American Academy of Pediatrics. Calcium requirements of infants, children and adolescents. *JAAP.* 1999;104:1152-1157.

18. CDC, US Department of Health and Human Services. Recommendations to prevent and control iron deficiency in the United States. *MMWR.* 1998;46(No RR-3):1-29.

19. Wechsler H, Brener N, Kuester S, Miller C. Foodservice and foods and beverages available at school: results from the school health policies and programs study 2000. *J Sch Health.* 2001;71(7):313-324.

20. United States Department of Education (USDE), National Center for Education Statistics. *Nutrition Education in Public Elementary School Classrooms.* Washington, DC: US Dept of Education; 2000. NCES 2000-040.

21. Healthy People 2010. Schools, worksites, and nutrition counseling, 19-15. Available at: http://www.healthypeople.gov/document/HTML/volume2/19Nutrition.htm. Accessed December 14, 2006.

22. US Department of Agriculture (USDA), Food and Nutrition Services (FNS). *Promoting Healthy Eating: An Investment in the Future. A Report to Congress.* Alexandria, Va: US Dept of Agriculture; December 1999.

23. Celebuski C, Farris E. Nutrition education in public elementary school classrooms, K-5. *Education Statistics Q.* 2000;2(1):66-69.

24. Carr D, Lamber L. How do school nutrition directors feel about providing nutrition education in the elementary setting? *Nutrition Link.* 2004; 29(1):6-7.

25. Auld GW, Romaniello C, Heimendinger J, Hambidge C, Hambidge M. Outcomes from a school-based nutrition education program alternating special resource teachers and classroom teachers. *J Sch Health.* 1999; 69(10):403-408.

26. Meyer MK, Conklin MT, Lewis JR, et al. Barriers to healthy nutrition environments in public middle grades. *J Child Nutr Manage.* 2001; 2:66-71.

27. Sullivan K, Harper M, West CK. Professional development needs of school foodservice directors. *J Child Nutr Manage.* 2001;25:89-95.

28. United States of America. Congressional Record. Public Law 79-396, 60 Stat 231. 1946.

29. United States of America. Congressional Record. Public Law 89-642, 80 Stat. 1966.

30. United States of America. Congressional Record. Public Law 95-166, 91 Stat 1325. 1977.

31. Edwards H. Child nutrition reauthorization update. *PNPG Post.* 2004; 15(1):1-2.

32. Frank GC, Farris RP, Cresanta JL, et al. Dietary intake as a determinant of cardiovascular risk factor variables: observations in a pediatric population. In: Berenson GS, ed. *Causation of Cardiovascular Risk Factors in Children: Perspectives on Causation of Cardiovascular Risk in Early Life.* New York: Raven Press; 1986:254-291.

33. Parcel GS, Simmons-Morton BG, O'Hara NM, et al. School promotion of healthful diet and exercise behavior: an integration of organizational change and social learning theory interventions. *J School Health.* 1987;57:150-156.

34. Burghardt J, Devaney B. *The School Nutrition Dietary Assessment Study—Summary of Findings.* Princeton, NJ: Mathematica Policy Research, Inc; 1993:3-24.

35. USDA Food and Nutrition Services. *Characteristics of National School Lunch and School Breakfast Program Participants* [executive summary]. Updated July 13, 2004. Available at: www.fns.usda.gov/OANE/MENU/Published/CNP/FILES/NSCPchar.htm. Accessed December 14, 2006.

36. Kubik MY, Lytle LA, Hannan PJ, Perry CL, Story M. The association of the school food environment with dietary behaviors of young adolescents. *Am J Public Health.* 2003;93(7):1168-1173.

37. French SA, Story M, Fulkerson JA, Gerlach AF. Food environment in secondary schools: a la carte, vending machines, and food policy and practices. *Am J Public Health.* 2003;93(70):1161-1167.

38. Foerster SB, Fierro MP, Gregson J, Hudes M, Oppen M, Sugarman S. 1998 California teen eating, exercise, and nutrition survey: also profiling body weight and tobacco use—media highlights. 2000. Available at: http://www.phi.org. Accessed October 26, 2002.

39. Cullen KW, Ash DM, Warneke C, de Moor C. Intake of soft drinks, fruit-flavored beverages, and fruits and vegetables by children in grades 4 through 6. *Am J Public Health.* 2002;92(9):1475-1478.

40. Tayag N. *Ethnic Gender Differences in Eating Among Youth* [master's thesis]. Long Beach: California State University; 2004.

41. Public Health Institute. *A Special Report on Policy Implications from the 1999 California Children's Healthy Eating and Exercise Practices Survey (CalCHEEPS).* 2000. Available at: http://www.calendow.org. Accessed June 25, 2001.

42. Trevino RP, Marshal RM, Hale DE, Rodriquez R, Baker G, Gomez J. Diabetes risk factors in low-income Mexican-American children. *Diabetes Care.* 1999;22(2):202-207.

43. Frank GC, Zive M, Nelson J, et al. Fat and cholesterol avoidance among Mexican American and Anglo preschool children and parents. *J Am Diet Assoc.* 1991;91:954-961.

44. Reynolds KD, Baranowski T, Bishop DB, et al. Patterns in child and adolescent consumption of fruit and vegetables: effects of gender and ethnicity across four sites. *J Am Coll Nutr.* 1999;18(3):248-254.

45. Centers for Disease Control and Prevention. Youth Risk Behavior Surveillance System: 2001 results. 2001. Available at http://www.cdc.gov/nccdphp/dash/yrbs/index.htm. Accessed October 26, 2002.

46. Skinner JD, Carruth BR, Houck KS, Morris M, Moran J, Coletta F. Caffeine intake in young children differs by family socioeconomic status. *J Am Diet Assoc.* 2000;100(2):229-231.

47. Jeffrey RW, French SA. Epidemic obesity in the United States: are fast foods and television viewing contributing? *Am J Public Health.* 1998;88:277-280.

48. Busch CR, Taylor HA, Kanarek RB, Samuel P. The effects of breakfast content on cognition in children. *Am J Clin Nutr.* 2002;75(2s):158.

49. Conklin M, Bordi P, Schaper M. Grab' n' go breakfast increases participation in the School Breakfast Program. *J Child Nutr Manage.* 2004;1.

50. Kirk MC, Gillespie AH. Factors affecting food choices of working mothers with young families. *J Nutr Education.* 1990;22:161-168.

51. National Center for Nutrition and Dietetics and International Food Information Council. *Where Do Kids Get Nutrition Information?* Chicago, Ill: American Dietetic Association; 1991.

52. National Center for Nutrition and Dietetics and International Food Information Council. *Kids at the Table: Who's Placing the Orders?* Chicago, Ill: American Dietetic Association; 1991.

53. Bidgood BA, Cameron G. Meal/snack missing and dietary adequacy of primary school children. *J Can Diet Assoc.* 1992;53:164-168.

54. American Dietetic Association. Dieting practices among high school students. *ADA Times.* 2004;2(1):3.

55. Lindeman AK, Clancy KL. Assessment of breakfast habits and social/emotional behavior of elementary schoolchildren. *J Nutr Ed.* 1990;22:226-231.

56. Resnicow K. The relationship between breakfast habits and plasma cholesterol levels in schoolchildren. *J School Health.* 1991;61:81-85.

57. Kleinman RE, Murphy JM, Little M, et al. Hunger in children in the United States: potential behavioral and emotional correlates. *Pediatrics* [serial online]. 1998;101:E3.

58. Simeon DT, Grantham-McGregor S. Effects of missing breakfast on the cognitive functions of school children of differing nutritional status. *Am J Clin Nutr.* 1989;49:646-653.

59. Pollitt E. Does breakfast make a difference in school? *J Am Diet Assoc.* 1995;95:1134-1139.

60. NIH Consensus Development Conference Statement. Lowering blood cholesterol. *JAMA.* 1985;253:2080-2086.

61. Olsen RE. Mass intervention vs screening and selective intervention for the prevention of coronary artery disease. *JAMA.* 1986;255:2204-2207.

62. American Academy of Pediatrics Committee on Nutrition. Cholesterol in childhood. *Pediatrics.* 1998;101(1):141-147.

63. American Academy of Pediatrics Committee on Nutrition. Toward a prudent diet for children. *Pediatrics.* 1983;71:78-80.

64. American Academy of Pediatrics Committee on Nutrition. Prudent lifestyle for children: dietary fat and cholesterol. *Pediatrics.* 1983;78:521-525.

65. Pugliese MT, Lifshitz F, Grad G, Marks-Katz M. Fear of obesity: a cause of short stature and delayed puberty. *N Engl J Med.* 1983;309:513-518.

66. National Cholesterol Education Program (NCEP). Report of the expert panel on blood cholesterol levels in children and adolescents. *Pediatrics.* 1992;89(suppl):525-584.

67. American Academy of Pediatrics Committee on Nutrition. Cholesterol in childhood. *Pediatrics.* 1998;101:141-147.

68. The American Dietetic Association. *On the Pulse.* Chicago, Ill: ADA; 1999.

69. Pathological Determinants of Atherosclerosis in Youth Research Group. A preliminary report on the relationship of atherosclerosis in young men to serum lipoprotein cholesterol concentrations and smoking. *JAMA.* 1990;264:3018-3024.

70. McGill HC Jr, McMahan CA, Malcolm GT, Oalmann MC, Strong JP, for the PDAY Research Group. Effect of serum lipoproteins and smoking on atherosclerosis in adolescents and young adults: implications for prevention from the pathobiological determinants of atherosclerosis in youth studies. *JAMA.* 1999;281:727-735.

71. Strong JP, Malcome GT, McMahan CA, et al, for the PDAY Research Group. Prevalence and extent of atherosclerosis in adolescents and young adults: implications for prevention from the pathobiological determinants of atherosclerosis in youth studies. *JAMA*. 1999;281: 727-735.

72. Berenson GS, Wattigney WA, Tracy RE, et al. Atherosclerosis of the aorta and coronary arteries and cardiovascular risk factors in persons aged 6 to 30 years and studied at necropsy (the Bogalusa Heart Study). *Am J Cardiol*. 1992;70:851-858.

73. Tracy RE, Newman WP, Wattigney WA, Srinivasan SR, Strong JP, Berenson ES. Histologic features of atherosclerosis and hypertension from autopsies of young individuals in a defined geographic population: the Bogalusa Heart Study. *Atherosclerosis*. 1995; 116:163-179.

74. Berenson GS, Srinivasan SR, Bao W, Newman WP, Tracy RE, Wattigney WA, for the Bogalusa Heart Study. Association between multiple cardiovascular risk factors and atherosclerosis in children and young adults. *N Engl J Med*. 1998;338:1650-1656.

75. Olsen RE. Is it wise to restrict fat in the diets of children? *JADA*. 2000;100(1):28-32.

76. DISC Collaborative Research Group. Dietary Intervention Study in Children (DISC) with elevated low-density lipoprotein: design and baseline characteristics. *Ann Epidemiol*. 1993;3:393-402.

77. Lytle LA. In defense of a low-fat diet for healthy children. *JADA*. 2000; 100(1):39-41.

78. Birch LL, Marline DW. I don't like it; I never tried it: effects of exposure to food on two-year-old children's food preferences. *Appetite*. 1982; 4:353-360.

79. Birch LL, Fisher JO. Development of eating behaviors among children and adolescents. *Pediatrics*. 1998;101(suppl):539-549.

80. Kelder SH, Perry CL, Knut-Inge K, Lytle LA. Longitudinal tracking of adolescent smoking, physical activity, and food choice behaviors. *Am J Public Health*. 1994;84:1121-1126.

81. Luepker RV, Perry DL, McKinlay SM, et al. Outcomes of a field trial to improve children's dietary patterns and physical activity: the Child and Adolescent Trial for Cardiovascular Health (CATCH). *JAMA*. 1996;275: 768-776.

82. Nader PR, Stone EJ, Lytle LA, et al. Three-year maintenance of improved diet and physical activity: the CATCH cohort. *Arch Pediatr Adolesc Med*. 1999;153:695-704.

83. Krebs NF, Johnson SL. Guidelines for healthy children: promoting eating, moving, and common sense. *JADA*. 2000;37-38.

84. Satter E. A moderate view on fat restriction for young children. *JADA*. 2000;100(1):32-36.

85. Murphy SP, Castillo RO, Martorell R, et al. An evaluation of food group intakes by Mexican-American children. *J Am Diet Assoc*. 1990;90: 388-393.

86. Palmer R, Johnson A. Los Angeles County Unified School District data. Los Angeles: University of Southern California; 1991.

87. Gibson EL, Wardle J, Watts CJ. Fruit and vegetable consumption, nutritional knowledge and beliefs in mothers and children. *Appetite*. October 1998;31(2):205-228.

88. Lloyd T, Chinchilli VM, Rollings N, et al. Fruit consumption, fitness, and cardiovascular health in female adolescents: the Penn State Young Women's Health Study. *Am J Clin Nutr*. 1998;67(4):624-630.

89. National Dairy Council. Calcium close up: an inside look at nutrition research especially for women. *Nutrition and Health-News Alert.* November 11, 1999:1-2.

90. Sampson H, Buckley R, Matcalf D. Food allergy. *JAMA* 1987;258: 2886-2903.

91. May CD. Food allergy: perspective, principles, practical management. *Nutr Today.* November-December 1980:28-31.

92. American Psychiatric Association. *Diagnostic and Statistical Manual (DSM III).* 3rd ed. Washington, DC: American Psychiatric Association; 1980.

93. American Psychiatric Association. *Diagnostic and Statistical Manual (DSM IV).* 4th ed. Washington, DC: American Psychiatric Association; 1994.

94. Stang J, Story M, Harnack, L, Neumark-Sztainer D. Relationships between vitamin and mineral supplement use, dietary intake, and dietary adequacy among adolescents. *JADA.* 2000;100:905.

95. American School Health Association. *The National Adolescent Student Health Survey: A Report on the Health of American's Youth.* Kent, Ohio: American School Health Association; 1989.

96. Frank GC, Deeds S, Cox S, et al. Clusters count—multi-risk taking behaviors of adolescents. Presented at the annual meeting of the American Alliance for Health, Physical Education, Recreation and Dance; April 3-7, 1991; San Francisco, Calif.

97. US Department of Health and Human Services. DATA2010—the *Healthy People 2010* Database. *CDC Wonder.* Atlanta, Ga: Centers for Disease Control; November 2000.

98. Bachman JG, Wallace JM, O'Malley PM, et al. Racial/ethnic differences in smoking, drinking, and illicit drug use among American high school seniors, 1976-89. *Am J Public Health.* 1991;81:372-377.

99. Centers for Disease Control and Prevention. Alcohol and other drug use among high school students—United States. *JAMA.* 1991;266: 3266-3267.

100. Sarvela PD, Pape DJ, Odulana J, et al. Drinking, drug use, and driving among rural midwestern youth. *J School Health.* 1990;60:215-219.

101. Arbeit ML, Nicklas TA, Frank GC, et al. Caffeine intakes of children from a biracial population: the Bogalusa Heart Study. *J Am Diet Assoc.* 1988;88:466-470.

102. Charney E, Goodman HC, McBride M, et al. Childhood antecedents of adult obesity—do chubby infants become obese adults? *N Engl J Med.* 1976;295:6-9.

103. Garn SM, LaVelle M. Two decade follow-up of fatness in early childhood. *Am J Dis Children.* 1985;139:181-185.

104. Kolata G. Obese children: a growing problem. *Science.* 1986;232:20-21.

105. Ross JG, Gilbert GG. The national children and youth fitness study: a summary of findings. *J Phys Ed Rec Dance.* 1985;56:45-50.

106. US Centers for Disease Control and Prevention. Vigorous Physical Activity Among High School Students—1990. *MMWR.* 1992;41(3):33-35.

107. Pate RR, Dowda M, Ross G. Associations between physical activity and physical fitness in American children. *Am J Dis Children.* 1990;144:1123-1129.

108. US Department of Health and Human Services. *President's Council on Physical Fitness and Sports Youth Fitness Survey.* Washington, DC: US Government Printing Office; 1986.

109. *Physical Activity and Health: A Report of the Surgeon General.* Atlanta, Ga: US Dept of Health and Human Services, Centers for Disease Control

and Prevention, National Center for Chronic Disease Prevention and Health Promotion; 1996.

110. Sallis JF, McKenzie TL, Kolody B, Lewis M, Marshall S, Rosengard P. Effects of health-related physical education on academic achievement: project SPARK. *Research Q Exercise Sport.* 1999;70,127-134.

111. NASPE. *Surgeon General Nominee Promotes Physical Education.* Reston, Va: American Alliance for Health Physical Education, Recreation and Dance; winter 1998:6.

112. YRBS. *Youth Risk Behavior Surveillance—United States, 1997.* Atlanta, Ga: US Dept of Health and Human Services and Centers for Disease Control and Prevention; 1998.

113. Freedman DA, Dietz WH, Srinivasan SR, Berenson GS. The relation of overweight to cardiovascular risk factors among children and adolescents: the Bogalusa Heart Study. *Pediatrics.* 1999;103: 1175-1182.

114. Andersen RE, Crespo CJ, Bartlett SJ, Cheskin LJ, Pratt M. Relationship of physical activity and television watching with body weight and level of fatness among children: results from the third National Health and Nutrition Examination Survey. *JAMA.* 1998;279,938-942.

115. Beunen G, Malina RM, Lefevre J, et al. Size, fatness and relative fat distribution of males of contrasting maturity status during adolescence and as adults. *Int J Obes.* 1994;18:670-678.

116. Gidding SS, Leibel RL, Daniels S, Rosenbaum M, Van Horn L, Marx GR. Understanding obesity in youth: a statement for healthcare professionals from the Committee of Atherosclerosis and Hypertension in the Young of the Council on Cardiovascular Disease in Young and the Nutrition Committee, American Heart Association. *Circulation.* 1996;94:3383-3387.

117. Suter E, Hawes MR. Relationship of physical activity, body fat, diet, and blood lipid profile in youths 10-15 years old. *Med Sci Sports Exercise.* 1993;25:748-754.

118. Pate RR. Physical activity in children and youth: relationship to obesity. *Contemporary Nutr.* 1993;18(2):1-2.

119. Sasaki J, Shindo M, Tanaka H, et al. A longterm aerobic exercise program decreases the obesity index and increases the high density lipoprotein cholesterol concentration in obese children. *Int J Obes.* 1987;11:339-345.

120. Epstein LH, Valoski A, Wing RR, et al. Ten year followup of behavioral, family-based treatment for obese children. *JAMA.* 1990;264:2519-2523.

121. Muecke L, Morton-Simons B, Huang IW, et al. Is childhood obesity associated with high-fat foods and low physical activity? *J School Health.* 1992;62:19-23.

122. Stephen A, Wald N. Trends in individual consumption of dietary fat in the United States, 1920-1984. *Am J Clin Nutr.* 1990;52:457-469.

123. Schlicker SA, Borra ST, Regan C. The weight and fitness status of US children. *Nutr Rev.* 1994;52(1):11-17.

124. Tucker LA, Bagwell M. Television viewing and obesity in adult females. *Am J Public Health.* 1991;81:908-911.

125. Gortmaker SL. Increasing pediatric obesity in the US. *Am J Dis Children.* 1987;141:535-541.

126. Story M, Faulkner P. The prime time diet: a content analysis of eating behavior and food messages in television program content and commercials. *Am J Public Health.* 1990;80:738-740.

127. Dietz WH Jr, Gortmaker SL. Do we fatten our children at the television set? Obesity and television viewing in children and adolescents. *Pediatrics.* 1985;75:807-812.

128. Tiwary CM, Holgiun A. Prevalence of obesity among children of military dependents at two major medical centers. *Am J Public Health.* 1992;82:354-357.

129. Saarilehto S, Lapinleimu H, Keskinen S, Helenius H, Simell O. Body satisfaction in 8-year-old children after long-term dietary counseling in a prospective randomized atherosclerosis prevention trial. *Arch Pediatr Adolesc Med.* 2003;157:753-758.

130. Eisenberg ME, Neumark-Sztainer D, Story M. Associations of weight-based teasing and emotional well-being among adolescents. *Arch Pediatr Adolesc Med.* 2003;157:733-738.

131. Mundell EJ. Eating disorders may cluster in families. *Am J Psychiatry.* 2000;157:393-401,469-471.

132. Hsu LK. Clinical features. In: *Eating Disorders.* New York: Guilford Press; 1990:22-24.

133. Sloan R. Developing an awareness of eating disorders: identifying the high-risk client. *On the Cutting Edge.* 1994;15(6):21-22.

134. Halmi HK, ed. *The Psychology and Treatment of Anorexia Nervosa and Bulimia Nervosa.* Washington, DC: American Psychiatric Press; 1992.

135. Hsu LK. Epidemiology. In: *Eating Disorders.* New York: Guilford Press; 1990:71.

136. Druss RG, Silverman JA. Body image and perfectionism of ballerinas. *Gen Hosp Psychiatry.* 1979;2:115-121.

137. Centers for Disease Control and Prevention. Body weight perceptions and selected weight-management goals and practices of high school students—United States. *JAMA.* 1991;266:2811-2812.

138. Dale KS, Landers DM. Weight control in wrestling: eating disorders or disordered eating? *Med Sci Sports Exercise.* 1999;31:1382-1389.

139. Shisslak CM, Crago M, Neal ME. Prevention of eating disorders among adolescents. *Am J Health Promotion.* 1990;5:100-106.

140. Larson B. Relationship of family communication patterns to eating disorders inventory scores in adolescent girls. *J Am Diet Assoc.* 1991;91:1065-1067.

141. Balentine M, Stitt K, Bonner J, et al. Self-reported eating disorders of black, low-income adolescents: behavior, body weight perceptions, and methods of dieting. *J School Health.* 1991;61:392-396.

142. Desmond SM, Price JH, Hallinan C, et al. Black and white adolescents' perceptions of their weight. *J School Health.* 1989;59:353-358.

143. Dodd JM, Bessinger C. Societal issues and nutrition [ADA Research Conference proceedings]. *J Am Diet Assoc.* 1993;93:77-85.

144. Mitchell JE, Eckert ED. Scope and significance of eating disorders. *J Consult Clin Psychol.* 1987;55:628-634.

145. American Dietetic Association. Position of the ADA: nutrition intervention in the treatment of anorexia nervosa, bulimia nervosa, and binge eating. *J Am Diet Assoc.* 1994;94:902-907.

146. Rorty M, Yager J, Rossotto E. Why and how do women recover from bulimia nervosa? The subjective appraisals of 40 women recovered for a year or more. *Int J Eating Disorders.* 1993;14:249-260.

147. Vandereycken W, Depreitere L, Probst M. Body-oriented therapy for anorexia nervosa patients. *Am J Psychotherapy.* 1987;41:252-259.

148. Herzog DB, Sacks NR, Keller MB, et al. Patterns and predictors of recovery in anorexia nervosa and bulimia nervosa. *J Am Acad Child Adolesc Psychiatry.* 1993;32:835-841.

149. Reiff DW, Reiff KKL. *Eating Disorders—Nutrition Therapy in the Recovery Process.* Gaithersburg, Md: Aspen Publishers, Inc; 1992.

150. National Center for Health Statistics, Vital Statistics Report. The Alan Guttmacher Institute, Centers for Disease Control. Besharov D, Gardiner, K. Teen sex. *The American Enterprise.* January/February 1993;4(1):52-59.

151. Centers for Disease Control. *Natality & Teenage Pregnancy Reports.* September 21, 1995. Available at: http://www.cdc.gov/nchs/pressroom/ 95news/nr44_3s.htm. Accessed December 14, 2006.

152. Centers for Disease Control. Births to 10-14 year-old mothers, 1990-2002: trends and health outcomes. PHS 2005-1120. *NVSR.* 2004;53(7). Available at: http://www.cdc.gov/reproductivehealth/GISATLAS/index.htm. Accessed December 14, 2006.

153. Ventura SJ, Taffel SM, Mosher WD. Monthly Vital Statistics Report. Trends in pregnancies and pregnancy rates: estimates for the United States, 1980-1992. *MVSR.* 1995;43:11(S).

154. Story M. Nutrient needs during adolescence and pregnancy. In: Story M, ed. *Nutrition Management of the Pregnant Adolescent: A Practical Reference Guide.* Washington, DC: National Clearinghouse; 1990:21-28.

155. Story M. Eating behaviors and nutritional implications. In: Story M, ed. *Nutrition Management of the Pregnant Adolescent: A Practical Reference Guide.* Washington, DC: National Clearinghouse; 1990:29-35.

156. Newman WP III, Freedman DS, Voors AW, et al. Relation of serum lipoprotein levels and systolic blood pressure to early atherosclerosis: the Bogalusa Heart Study. *N Engl J Med.* 1986;314:138-144.

157. Freedman DS, Newman WP III, Tracy RE, et al. Black-white differences in aortic fatty streaks in adolescence and early adulthood: the Bogalusa Heart Study. *Circulation.* 1988;77:856-864.

158. Wissler RW, Robertson AL, Cornhill JF, et al. Relationship of atherosclerosis in young men to serum lipoprotein cholesterol concentrations and smoking. *JAMA.* 1990;264:3018-3024.

159. Frerichs RR, Webber LS, Voors AW, et al. Cardiovascular disease risk factor variables in children at two successive years—the Bogalusa Heart Study. *J Chronic Dis.* 1979;32:251-262.

160. Voors AW, Webber LS, Berenson GS. Time course study of blood pressure in children over a three-year period—the Bogalusa Heart Study. *Hypertension.* 1980;2(suppl 1):102-108.

161. Webber LS, Cresanta JL, Voors AW, et al. Tracking of cardiovascular disease risk factor variables in school-age children. *J Chronic Dis.* 1983;36:647-660.

162. Clarke WR, Schrott HG, Leaverton PE, et al. Tracking of blood lipids and blood pressure in school age children: the Muscatine Study. *Circulation.* 1978;58:626-634.

163. Zive MM, Frank-Spohrer GC, Sallis JF, et al. Determinants of dietary intake in a sample of white and Mexican-American children. *J Am Diet Assoc.* 1998;98(11):1282-1289.

164. Oberman A, Lane NE, Harlan WR, et al. Trends in systolic blood pressure in the Thousand Aviator Cohort over a 24-year period. *Circulation.* 1967;36:812-822.

165. Heiss G, Tyroler HA, Hames C. Cholesterol tracking: prediction over time of serum cholesterol in Evans County, GA. *Advances Exper Med Biol.* 1977;82:112-114.

166. Higgins MW, Keller JB, Metzner HL, et al. Studies of blood pressure in Tecumseh, Michigan—II. Antecedents in childhood of high blood pressure in young adults. *Hypertension.* 1980;2(suppl 1):117-123.

167. National Cholesterol Education Program. National Heart, Lung, and Blood Institute. *Population Panel Report. Pediatric Panel Report.* Bethesda, Md: National Institutes of Health; April 1991.

168. Carroll MD, Abraham S, Dresser CM. *Dietary Intake Source Data: United States 1976-1980.* Washington, DC: National Center for Health Statistics; March 1983. Vital and Health Statistics Series II, 231 USDHHS, PHS, NCHS, DHHS pub. 83-1681.

169. Wynder EL, Weisburger JH, Ng SK. Nutrition: the need to define "optimal" intake as a basis for public policy decisions. *Am J Public Health.* 1992;82:346-350.

170. Fulgoni VL, Mackey MA. Total dietary fiber in children's diets. In: Williams CL, Wynder EL, eds. Hyperlipidemia and the development of atherosclerosis. *Ann NY Acad Sci.* 1991;623:369-379.

171. *The Pyramid Plan.* Washington, DC: US Department of Agriculture, Human Nutrition Information Service; April 2005. Available at: www.mypyramid.gov. Accessed December 14, 2006.

172. *Dietary Guidelines for Americans.* Washington, DC: US Dept of Agriculture and US Dept of Health and Human Services; 2005.

173. State of California. 1989. Assembly Bill 2109, J Speier.

174. California Department of Health Services. *California Daily Food Guide.* Sacramento, Calif: California Department of Health Services; 1990. F-89-559.

175. Gold R, Parcel G, Walberg H, et al. Summary and conclusions of the THTM evaluation: the expert work group perspective. *J School Health.* 1991;61(1):39-42.

176. Harris L. *An Evaluation of Comprehensive Health Education in American Public Schools.* New York: Metropolitan Life Foundation; 1988.

177. Roper WJ. Preface to the Teenage Health Teaching Modules Evaluation. *J School Health.* 1991;61(1):19.

178. Allensworth DD, Kolbe LJ. The comprehensive school health program: exploring an expanded concept. *J School Health.* 1987;57(10):31.

179. Elder JP. From experimentation to dissemination: strategies for maximizing the impact and spread of school health education. In: Nutbeam D, Haglund B, Farley P, et al, eds. *Youth Health Promotion: From Theory to Practice in School and Community.* London, England: Forbes Publications Ltd; 1991:22-32.

180. Glanz K, Lewis FM, Rimer BK. *Health Behavior and Health Education.* San Francisco, Calif: Jossey-Bass Publishers; 1991.

181. Cummings K, Becker M, Maile M. Bringing the models together in an empirical approach to combining variables used to explain health actions. *J Behav Med.* 1980;3:123-145.

182. Pentz M, Dwyer J, MacKinnon D, et al. A multicommunity trial for primary prevention of adolescent drug abuse: effects on drug use prevalence. *JAMA.* 1989;261:3259-3266.

183. Dhillon HS, Tolsma D. *Meeting Global Health Challenges: A Position Paper on Health Education.* Geneva, Switzerland: World Health Organization; 1991.

184. Dryfoos J. *Adolescents at Risk: Prevalence and Prevention.* New York: Oxford University Press; 1990.

185. Green LW, Krueter MW. *Health Promotion Planning: An Educational and Environmental Approach.* Toronto, Ontario, Canada: Mayfield Publishing; 1991.

186. Perry C. Conceptualizing community-wide youth health promotion programs. In: Nutbeam D, Haglund B, Farley P, et al, eds. *Youth Health*

Promotion: From Theory to Practice in School and Community. London, England: Forbes Publications Ltd; 1991;1-22.

187. Benard B. *An Overview of Community Based Prevention. OSAP Prevention Monograph 3: Prevention Research Findings, 1988.* Washington, DC: US Dept of Health and Human Services; 1990. Publication (ADM) 89-1615.

188. National Health Education Organizations. The limitations to excellence in education. *J School Health.* 1984;54:256-257.

189. Lovato CY, Allensworth DD, Chan FA. *School Health in America: An Assessment of State Policies to Protect and Improve the Health of Students.* 5th ed. Kent, Ohio: American School Health Association; 1989.

190. Kolbe LJ. An epidemiological surveillance system to monitor the prevalence of youth behaviors that most affect health. *Health Ed.* 1990;21(6):40-43.

191. Novello AC, DeGraw C, Kleinman DV. Healthy children ready to learn: an essential collaboration between health and education. *Public Health Rep.* 1992;107W:3-14.

192. Frank GC, Vaden A, Martin J. School health promotion: child nutrition programs. *J School Health.* 1987;57:451-460.

193. Frank GC, Nicklas T, Forcier J, et al. Cardiovascular health promotion of children: the Heart Smart School Lunch Program, Part I. *School Food Serv Res Rev.* 1989;13:130-136.

194. Frank GC, Nicklas T, Forcier J, et al. Cardiovascular health promotion of children: student behavior and institutional foodservice change, Part II. *School Food Serv Res Rev.* 1989;13:137-145.

195. Gordon R. One perspective: needed nutrition education. *Nutrition Link.* September 2000:5.

196. National Center for Nutrition and Dietetics and International Food Information Council. *Kids Earn Good Marks for Nutrition Knowledge.* Chicago, Ill: American Dietetic Association; 1991.

197. Levy SR, Iverson BK, Walberg HJ. Nutrition education research: an interdisciplinary evaluation and review. *Health Education Q.* 1980;7:107-126.

198. *Children's Eating Habits.* Roper Survey Incorporated; 1985.

199. Dubinsky LD, Bodner JH. Food for thought: starting a K-3 nutrition education program. *J School Health.* 1991;61:181-183.

200. Albright CL, Bruce B. Development of a curriculum to lower dietary fat intake in a multiethnic population. *J Nutr Education.* July/August 1997;29(4):215-223.

201. Portland Public Schools. *Fundamental Understanding of Nutrition (FUN) Program. A Comprehensive Nutrition Education Program for Grades K-3.* Portland, Ore: Nutrition Services; 1989.

202. Liang T, Frank GC. Songs to teach nutrition. *J Nutr Education.* 1994;26:87-92.

203. US Department of Agriculture. *Team Nutrition.* Alexandria, Va: Food and Nutrition Service, 1999.

204. US Department of Health and Human Services. *Action for Healthy Kids.* 2002 Health Schools Summit. Washington, DC; 2002. Available at: www.actionforhealthykids.org. Accessed December 14, 2006.

205. Green LW, Kreuter MW, Deeds SG, et al. *Health Education Planning—A Diagnostic Approach.* Palo Alto, Calif: Mayfield Publishing Co; 1980:142-158.

206. Sneed J, Scheule B, Gregoire M. Implementing nutrition integrity in child nutrition programs: implications for dietetic practitioners and educators. *Top Clin Nutr.* 1999;15(1):1-9.

207. American School Food Service Association. The healthy EDGE in schools. *J Am School Food Service Assoc.* March 1991;45(suppl):8.

208. American School Food Service Association. New CN program regs proposed. *J Am School Food Service Assoc.* August 1994;48: 12-13.

209. American School Food Service Association. *Youth Advisory Council—At the Starting Line.* Alexandria, Va: American School Food Service Association; 1990.

210. Hong Li-Tsu, Frank GC, Toma R, et al. The nutrient analysis and sensory evaluation of a new recipe for school lunch—modified Chinese meat bun. Abstract presented at the California Dietetic Association, April 1992; Los Angeles, Calif.

211. Simons-Morton BG, Parcel GS, Baranowski T, et al. Promoting physical activity and a healthful diet among children: results of a school-based intervention study. *Am J Public Health.* 1991;81:986-991.

212. Slade A, Graves K. *Namaste Charter School.* Chicago Public School System. Chicago, Ill: Weber Shandwick Communications; 2005. Available at: www.namastecharterschool.org. Accessed December 14, 2006.

213. Frank GC, Adsen MA. *Technical Report: California Statewide Census of Child Nutrition Program Employees.* Long Beach: California State University–Long Beach, Child Nutrition Program Management Center; 1992:1-132.

214. Frank GC, Desai S. Shaping healthy meals for school children: food service employee training curriculum. Long Beach: California State University-Long Beach; 1992:32.

215. Cinciripini PM. Changing food selections in a public cafeteria. *Behavior Mod.* 1984;8:522-539.

216. Schmitz MF, Fielding JE. Point-of-choice nutritional labeling: evaluation in a worksite cafeteria. *J Nutr Ed.* 1986;18:S65-S68.

217. Anderson J, Haas MH. Impact of a nutrition education program on food sales in restaurants. *J Nutr Ed.* 1990;22:232-238.

218. Luros E. Computrition, Inc. 1992. Chatsworth, Calif.

219. Dennison D, Dennison KF, Frank GC. The DINE evaluation process: improving food choices of the public. *J Nutr Ed.* 1994;26(2):87-93.

220. LunchByte Systems, Inc. *NutriKids.* Rochester, NY: LunchByte Systems, Inc; 1992.

221. Frank GC. Nutrient profile on personal computers—a comparison of DINE with mainframe computers. *Health Education.* 1985;16:16-19.

222. Mellin LM, Slinkard LA, Irwin CE. Adolescent obesity intervention: validation of the SHAPEDOWN program. *J Am Diet Assoc.* 1987; 87:333-338.

223. Burns ER. Anatomy of a successful K-12 educational outreach program in the health sciences: eleven years experience at one medical sciences campus. *Anatomical Record.* 2002;269:181-193.

224. American Medical Association. *Guidelines for Adolescent Preventive Services.* Chicago, Ill: American Medical Association; 1992:3.

225. American Medical Association. *Target 2000.* Chicago, Ill: American Medical Association; Fall 1994.

226. Hinkel A. *California Adolescent Nutrition and Fitness.* Berkeley, Calif: CANFit, 2005.

227. CANFit: affecting environmental change through appropriate programs for minority audiences. *The Digest.* 2004;1,3-6.

228. Lytle L. Nutrition education for school-aged children. *J Nutr Education.* 1995;27:298-311.

229. US Department of Health and Human Services. The President's Council on Physical Fitness and Sports. *The President's Council on Physical Fitness and Sports Newsletter.* 1994;94(1):1-8.

230. Matsui I, Nambu S, Baba S. Evaluation of fasting serum insulin levels among Japanese school-age children. *J Nutr Sci Vitaminol.* 1998;44(6):819-828.

231. Morley R, Baker BA, Greene LC, Livingstone MB, Harland PS, Lucas A. Dietary fibre, exercise and serum lipids and lipoprotein cholesterols in 12 to 15 year olds. *Acta Paediatr.* 1998;87(12):1230-1234.

232. Twisk JW, Kemper HC, van Mechelen W, Post GB. Which lifestyle parameters discriminate high- from low-risk participants for coronary heart disease risk factors. Longitudinal analysis covering adolescence and young adulthood. *J Cardiovasc Risk.* 1997;4(5-6):393-400.

233. Craig MR, Kristal AR, Cheney CL, Shattuck AL. The prevalence and impact of 'atypical' days in 4-day food records. *J Am Diet Assoc.* 2000;100:421-427.

234. Jackson SA. Comprehensive school health education programs: innovative practices and issues in standard setting. *J School Health.* 1994;64:177-179.

235. Allenworth DD. The research base for innovative practices in school health education at the secondary level. *J School Health.* 1994;64:180-187.

236. Cortese P, Middleton K, eds. *The Comprehensive School Health Challenge: Promoting Health through Education.* Santa Cruz, Calif: ETR Associates; 1993. 95061-1830.

237. National Commission on the Role of the School and the Community in Improving Adolescents' Health. *CODE BLUE: Uniting for Healthier Youth.* Alexandria, Va: National Association of State Boards of Education; 1990.

ADULTS AND THEIR NUTRITIONAL NEEDS

Learning Objectives

- Describe the major chronic diseases of adult men and women.
- Identify major research initiatives undertaken to evaluate primary and secondary prevention approaches for breast and colon cancer, heart disease, and osteoporosis among women.
- List the major primary and secondary prevention strategies to educate and to interest men in nutrition and eating behavior programs for improved health and wellness.
- Detail community-based nutrition programs that target adults and their health needs.

High Definition Nutrition

Aerobics—exercise that increases the body's ability to use oxygen and improves endurance.

Body work—any type of regularly practiced physical activity (e.g., a sport, a special exercise program, or a hobby involving body movement).

Certified lactation educator (CLE)—the individual who completes basic lactation courses successfully and qualifies for a lactation educator certificate. This designation enables the individual to teach breastfeeding education classes to parents and provides healthcare professionals with a basic understanding to help mothers breastfeed. This provides the foundation for the lactation consultant courses.

Certified lactation specialist (CLS)—an individual who has completed the degree program or the lactation certificate program for those who hold previous master's or doctoral degrees. A lactation specialist is qualified clinically and academically to assist mothers with breastfeeding problems and to teach professionals about breastfeeding (*Source:* The Lactation Institute and Breastfeeding Clinic, 16430 Ventura Blvd, Suite 303, Encino, CA 91436).

Fitness—having adequate muscular strength and endurance to accomplish individual goals, reasonable joint flexibility, an efficient cardiovascular system, and a body composition that falls within the normal range of body weight and percent body fat.

Lactose—sugar found naturally in all mammalian milk and in most products derived from it.

Lactose maldigestion—the incomplete breakdown of lactose in the intestinal tract due to low levels of the enzyme lactase.

Lactose intolerance—the occurrence of symptoms in a person with lactose maldigestion.

Milk protein allergy—a reaction to one or more of cow's milk proteins mediated by the body's immune system.

Strength training—training that enhances size and strength of particular muscles and body regions.

Introduction

The living arrangements of adult men and women vary from single adults living alone or together to adults who are the head of the household or are a member of a nuclear or extended family. The adult years encompass 4 decades (from 18 to 45 years of age) and, for some individuals, these years are marked by maturity, financial acumen, community service, and a potential increasing awareness of global issues and their own health.

Over a 7-month interval in 1999, about 17 million US adults surfed the Internet and the number exceeds 30 million currently. Health-related information is the second most popular category on the Web.[1]

The adult years may reflect single parenting, the onset of chronic disease symptoms, unemployment, or reduced economic independence. There may be an effect of husbands' education on fatness of their wives. Data were obtained on 588 healthy, occupationally active, married Polish women, age 21 to 62 years, with 12 years of education. Analysis of 2 socially different groups, i.e., those moving up and moving down the social scale, showed that women with secondary schooling who married up socially were consistently leaner than women who married down socially. Fat distribution followed a similar pattern. Women moving down the social scale had more abdominal body fat compared to women moving up the social scale.[2]

Women during the childbearing years from 20 to 50 often demonstrate a need to remain youthful in appearance, attractive, and vital in the family day-to-day functioning. Personal health and nutrition may not be priorities. Young adult men generally continue with established sports and athletic interests either from the vantage point of the sports field or from in front of the television. For individuals entering the adult years, fitness and a wellness approach to living as part of primary prevention of disease generate more interest than in prior decades. However, disease prevention remains a future and somewhat distant frontier for many of today's adults.

Obesity drives most of the negative health conditions that adults experience. Between 1971 and 2000, the prevalence of obesity in the United States increased from 15 to 31%.[3] Unhealthy diets and sedentary behaviors are considered the primary causes of deaths attributable to obesity.[4] The CDC analyzed data from 4 National Health and Nutrition Examination Surveys (NHANES): NHANES I (conducted during 1971-1974), NHANES II (1976-1980), NHANES III (1988-1994), and NHANES V (1999-2000). Between 1971 and 2000, mean energy intake in kcals increased, mean percentage of kcals from carbohydrate increased, and mean percentage of kcals from total fat and saturated fat decreased.[5]

Between 1971 and 2000, a statistically significant increase in average energy intake occurred. For men, average energy intake increased from 2,450 kcals to 2,618 kcals ($p < 0.01$) where p is the statistical probability, and for women, from 1,542 kcals to 1,877 kcals ($p < 0.01$). For men, the percentage of kcals from carbohydrate increased between 1971-1974 and 1999-2000 from 42 to 49% ($p < 0.01$), and for women, from 45 to 52% ($p < 0.01$). The percentage of kcals from total fat decreased from 37 to 33% ($p < 0.01$) for men and from 36 to 33% ($p < 0.01$) for women. The percentage of kcals from saturated fat decreased from 14 to 11% ($p < 0.01$) for men and from 13 to 11% ($p < 0.01$) for women. A slight decrease was observed in the percentage of kcals from protein, from 17 to 16% ($p < 0.01$) for men and from 17 to 15% ($p < 0.01$) for women.[5]

Although a decrease in the percentage of kcals from fat occurred during 1971-1991, an increase in total kcals also occurred; absolute fat and carbohydrate intakes in grams increased.[6,7] A 62-gram increase occurred among women ($p < 0.01$) and a 68-gram increase occurred among men ($p < 0.01$). Total fat intake in grams increased among women by 7 g ($p < 0.01$) and decreased among men by 5 g ($p < 0.01$).[5]

The increase in caloric intake reflects previously reported trends in dietary intake in the United States. USDA survey data for 1977-1996 suggested the increase in energy intake was primarily from consumption of food away from home, increased energy consumption from salty snacks, soft drinks, and pizza,[8] and increased portion sizes.[9]

The 15 leading causes of death in 2003 for men and women were as follows: (1) diseases of the heart, (2) malignant neoplasms, (3) cerebrovascular diseases, (4) chronic lower respiratory diseases, (5) accidents (unintentional injuries), (6) diabetes mellitus, (7) influenza and pneumonia, (8) Alzheimer's disease, (9) nephritis, nephrotic syndrome, and nephrosis, (10) septicemia, (11) intentional self-harm (suicide), (12) chronic liver disease and cirrhosis, (13) essential (primary) hypertension and hypertensive renal disease, (14) Parkinson's disease, and (15) pneumonitis due to solids and liquids.[10]

The Adult Female and Her Nutrition Needs

Pregnancy

The birth rate for women aged 40 to 44 years increased in 2003 while the rate for women aged 45 to 54 years remains unchanged. Birth rates for women aged 40 to 44 years rose 5% between 2002 and 2003 from 8.3 to 8.7 births per 1,000 women. The rate for women aged 45 to 54 years remained unchanged at 0.5. The birth rate for women aged 40-44 years has more than doubled since 1981. For other groups, birth rates for women aged 30-34 years increased by 4% from 2002 to 2003, while the rate for women aged 35-39 years rose 6%.[11]

The United States has been ranked 28th among 37 countries in the world in infant mortality. This relatively low ranking is due to various reasons, including lack of nutrition education and prenatal care of women during pregnancy. In fact, inadequate nutrition during pregnancy is linked to the following conditions[12,13]:

- iron deficiency anemia, which creates low levels of hemoglobin and endangers the health of mother and baby
- gestational diabetes, seen in increased blood sugar levels during pregnancy that may predispose the woman to abnormal blood sugar levels later in life
- toxemia or preeclampsia symptoms of increased blood pressure; swelling in face, hands, and feet; and convulsions
- stillbirths
- birth defects

Current recommendations are that each pregnant woman's eating pattern should be reviewed, designed, and monitored by a registered dietitian (RD) to ensure that individual needs are being met.[14]

Pre-Conception Nutrition

Future mothers need a watchful approach not only to their eating patterns during pregnancy, but also to their food choices at least 3 months before conception. Studies of the eating patterns of nonpregnant women of child-bearing age reveal possible inadequacies in vitamins and minerals important to a healthy pregnancy.

Women's nutritional status before pregnancy can greatly affect the fetus. Inadequate maternal nutrient stores can prevent the placenta from growing to an adequate size, resulting in a small or a malnourished infant. Pregnant adolescents are at high risk, simply because they are still growing and need extra stores of iron, calcium, and zinc.

Supplements During Pregnancy

The National Academy of Science's Institute of Medicine recommends individual assessment of dietary practices for all pregnant women. A well-balanced eating pattern is generally sufficient for optimal nutrition. Table 9-1 details nutrient needs for young girls and women whether pregnant or not, and the additional needs during pregnancy or lactation. Dietary supplements should not replace food. In fact, iron is the only supplement often required during normal pregnancy. Larger amounts are needed in the second and third trimesters, especially for the oldest and the youngest women. The fetus may exhaust the mother's body stores of iron and cause her to become anemic. A low-dose supplement of 30 mg is generally sufficient to provide the extra iron needed.[13]

Calcium Needs

The current recommended dietary allowance (RDA) for calcium during pregnancy and lactation is 1,300 mg/day for those less than 18 years old and 1,000 mg/day for those more than 19 years. During lactation these calcium intakes remain (see Table 9–1). Pregnancy creates a significant physiologic stress on maternal skeletal homeostasis. Full-term infants accumulate approximately 30 g of calcium during gestation, mainly during the third trimester. Data suggest that no permanent decline in body calcium occurs with pregnancy if recommended dietary calcium intake is achieved. No association is observed between parity and bone mass, and no evidence has surfaced to support changing the current recommendation of calcium intake for well-nourished, pregnant adolescent and adult women.[13,15]

About 160 to 300 mg/day of maternal calcium is lost in breast milk. Longitudinal studies show that healthy women have an acute bone loss during lactation, but this is followed by rapid restoration of bone mass after weaning and return of menses. Data are not definitive to show whether calcium requirements differ for pregnant women with closely spaced pregnancies or at the extremes of reproductive years. Calcium intakes in 82 pregnant women ages 18 to 35 was assessed during their third trimester. Women who consumed more than the amount of calcium in 3 glasses of milk had lower blood pressure than those who consumed less. An average 7.3% suffered from high blood pressure.[16]

Prenatal Weight Gain

The prepregnancy weight dictates the recommended weight gain during pregnancy. The prepregnancy weight, concomitant body mass index (BMI), and recommended weight gain are as follows:

- If underweight (e.g., BMI < 19.8), then 28 to 40 pounds is recommended.
- If normal weight (e.g., BMI > 19.8 and < 26), then 25 to 35 pounds is recommended.
- If overweight (e.g., BMI is 26 to 29), then 15 to 25 pounds is recommended.
- If obese (e.g., BMI > 29), then at least but not more than 15 pounds is recommended.

Weight gain during pregnancy should be gradual, with 25% of the total weight gain during the first trimester (4 to 6 pounds) and 75% during the second and third trimesters (approximately one half to one pound a week).[14] Overall rate of gain should remain relatively constant during the last two thirds of gestation. During the second trimester, weight gain reflects expansion of maternal fluids and tissues. Weight gain during the third trimester represents growth of the fetal compartment (see Figure 9–1).[17]

Adolescents and young African-American women generally are at high risk for low-birth-weight babies. They should gain at the upper end of the recommended weight gain ranges. Nutrition supplementation during a high-risk pregnancy is advised for iron at 30 mg ferrous iron daily during the second and third trimesters. Folate at 300 mg daily may be needed if dietary

TABLE 9–1 Recommended Dietary Allowances*† for Adolescents and Women Daily During Pregnancy and Lactation

Life Stage Group‡	Energy (kcal)	Protein (g)	CHO (g)	Vitamin A (µg RE)§	Iron (mg)	Zinc (mg)	Iodine (µg)	Calcium (mg)	Folate (µg)
Females									
9-13	2,071	0.95	130	600	15	8	120	1,300	300
14-18	2,368	0.85	130	700	18	9	150	1,300	400
19-30	2,403	0.8	130	700	18	8	150	1,000	400
31-50	2,403	0.8	130	700	8	8	150	1,000	400
> 51	2,403	0.8	130	700	8	8	150	1,300	400
Pregnancy									
14-18, 1st trimester	2,368	1.1	175	750	27	13	220	1,300	600
2nd trimester	2,708	1.1	175	750	27	13	220	1,300	600
3rd trimester	2,820	1.1	175	750	27	13	220	1,300	600

continued

19-50, 1st trimester	2,403	1.1	175	770	27	220	11	1,000	600
2nd trimester	2,743	1.1	175	770	27	220	11	1,000	600
3rd trimester	2,855	1.1	175	770	27	220	11	1,000	600
Lactating									
14-18, 1st 6 mo	2,698	1.1	210	1,200	10	290	14	1,300	500
2nd 6 mo	2,768	1.1	210	1,200	10	290	14	1,300	500
19-50, 1st 6 mo	2,733	1.1	210	1,300	9	290	12	1,000	500
2nd 6 mo	2,803	1.1	210	1,300	9	290	12	1,000	500

*The allowances, expressed as average daily intakes over time, are intended to provide for individual variations among most normal persons as they live in the United States under usual environmental stresses. Diets should be based on a variety of common foods in order to provide other nutrients for which human requirements have been less well defined.

†This table does not include nutrients for which dietary reference intakes have recently been established (see Dietary Reference Intakes for Calcium, Phosphorus, Magnesium, Vitamin D, and Fluoride [1997], Dietary Reference Intakes for Thiamin, Riboflavin, Niacin, Vitamin B_6, Folate, Vitamin B_{12}, Pantothenic Acid, Biotin, and Choline [1998], and Dietary Reference Intakes for Vitamin E, Vitamin C, Selenium, and Carotenoids [2000]).

‡Weights and heights of reference adults are actual medians for the US population of the designated age, as reported by NHANES II. The median weights and heights of those under 19 years of age were taken from Hamill PW, Drizd TA, Johnson CL, et al. Physical Growth: National Center for Health Statistics Percentiles: Development of a Research Child Growth Preference. AMJ Cl Nutr 1979;32:607-629. The use of these figures does not imply that the height-to-weight ratios are ideal.

§Retinol equivalents 1 retinol equivalent = 1 μg retinal or 6g β-carotene.

Source: Adapted from: Monsen ER. Dietary Reference Intakes for the antioxidant nutrients: vitamin C, vitamin E, selenium, and carotenoids. J Am Diet Assoc. 2000;100:637-640.

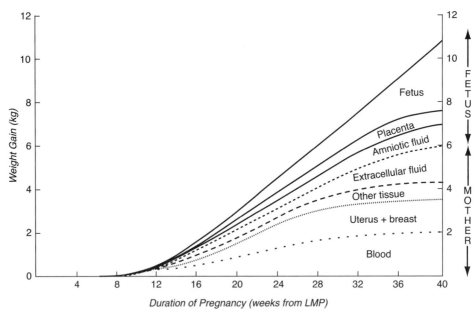

FIGURE 9–1 Pattern and distribution of weight gain: constant gain during second and third trimesters, but different distribution (second trimester to mother and third trimester to fetus). *Source:* Reprinted from Pitkin R. *Nutrition During Pregnancy.* Los Angeles, Calif: Nutritional Medicine in Medical Practice Symposium; 1993.

folate intake is inadequate. Pregnant women who do not have an adequate eating pattern, are expecting multiple births (twins, triplets, etc.), smoke, or abuse alcohol or other drugs may need a multivitamin supplement. The supplement should contain 300 mg folate, 30 mg ferrous iron, 15 mg zinc, 2 mg copper, 250 mg calcium, 2 mg vitamin B_6, 50 mg vitamin C, and 5 mg vitamin D. A 600-mg calcium supplement seems to be appropriate for women under 25 years whose dietary intake is less than 600 mg daily. Zinc at 15 mg and 2 mg of copper should be provided when therapeutic levels of iron are given to treat anemia. Preconceptional administration of folate may be effective in reducing the risk of neural tube defect in the fetus.[17]

Docosahexaenoic acid (DHA) is vital to infant neurological and visual development; in fact, neither the mother nor her developing fetus/infant can make adequate quantities of DHA to support proper central nervous system development in infants. A National Institute of Health and International Society for the Study of Fatty Acids and Lipids (NIH/ISSFAL)–sponsored workshop recommended 300 mg DHA/day for pregnant and lactating women.[18]

The typical American diet provides many women with 100 mg DHA/day or less. Primary dietary sources of DHA are fish (including anchovies, salmon, herring, mackerel, tuna, and halibut) and organ meat. Small amounts are also found in poultry and egg yolks. DHA is a long-chain polyunsaturated fatty acid that is a major structural component in the gray matter of the brain and the retina of the eye. It is an omega-3 fatty acid that occurs naturally in breast milk and is essential for normal brain and eye development. DHA is important throughout pregnancy and lactation for the health of the mother and her fetus/infant. In a study of lactating women, infants of those who received DHA supplements during 4 months of nursing had significantly improved psychomotor development, such as eye-hand coordination, at 2.5 years of age compared to infants of women who received placebo.[19]

There are several reasons a woman's DHA levels may be low. These include:

- low dietary intake of fish and organ meat in Western societies, because women observe warnings to avoid fish during pregnancy and lactation due to possible contamination from mercury and polychlorinated biphenyls (PCBs)[20]
- transference of DHA from maternal fat stores to the fetus, especially during the third trimester of pregnancy[21]
- closely spaced pregnancies after the first pregnancy[22]
- multiple births rather than 1 birth[23]
- cigarette smoking, which reduces DHA content of breast milk[24]
- a vegan or vegetarian diet low in DHA[25]

A healthy eating plan for pregnant women includes the following[14]:

- 5 servings of fruits and vegetables (1 high in vitamin A [such as apricots, carrots, broccoli] and 1 high in vitamin C [oranges, grapefruit, tomatoes])
- 7 servings of breads and cereals (4 whole grain) (1 serving equals 1 slice of bread, $1/2$ bun, $1/2$ cup cooked cereal, $3/4$ cup dry cereal)
- 3 servings of milk and milk products (1 serving equals 8 ounces milk or yogurt, $1/2$ cup grated cheese, 2 cups cottage cheese)
- 7 one-ounce servings of cooked meat, fish, poultry, or other protein foods such as beans, eggs, tofu, and peanut butter
- 3 teaspoons unsaturated fats, margarine, salad dressing
- 1 serving of foods rich in folate, such as dark green leafy vegetables, orange juice, liver, dried beans, or peas

Women often experience nausea and vomiting in the first trimester. The following practices may reduce the discomfort[14]:

- Eat small, frequent meals at 2- to 3-hour intervals; supplement meals with nutritious between-meal snacks like whole-grain breads or cottage cheese.
- Drink at least 10 glasses of fluid each day, but not during meals.
- Eat dry crackers immediately upon feeling nauseous.
- Do not skip meals, as this may cause illness due to a lack of adequate blood sugar.
- Avoid or limit greasy, fried, or spicy foods and caffeinated drinks.
- Eat foods slowly.
- Avoid very hot or very cold foods.
- Do not resort to home remedies or over-the-counter medications without consulting the obstetrician.

Caffeine

Caffeine-containing foods or beverages consumed in moderation do not appear to affect fertility or create adverse health effects for the mother or fetus.[26] Although studies differ in design and variables examined, the general consensus is that caffeine consumption does not affect the reported time to conceive. One study compared 2,800 women who delivered babies with 1,800 women diagnosed as infertile. Researchers reported that caffeine intake had little or no effect on the reported time to conceive. A Canadian study of 40,000 women reported adverse effects of cigarettes and alcohol intake on pregnancy. Nonsmokers did not experience delayed conception, regardless of whether they were high or low caffeine consumers.[27]

The data regarding caffeine and miscarriages vary. Research at McGill University reported an association between the 2. However, a study in the United States controlling for nausea, smoking, alcohol intake, and age of the mother reported no association. Moderate caffeine consumption (i.e., about three 8-ounce cups of coffee, tea, or carbonated beverage) has not been shown to cause either early birth or low-birth-weight babies, nor to influence motor development of the infant later in life.[28]

Caffeine transfers into breast milk, but an intake limited to 2 or 3 cups of coffee a day does not appear to give a significant amount in breast milk. The American Academy of Pediatrics Committee on Drugs supports this recommendation as an acceptable and safe level.[26,29,30]

Herbs in Pregnancy and Lactation

Marketing directly to pregnant and lactating women has surfaced in the supplement industry. Issues such as postpartum blues, milk production, and low iron are addressed but validity of products is unknown (see Table 9–2), and such marketing should be received with caution.

Aspartame in Pregnancy

Aspartame, which is sold as NutraSweet brand sweetener, provides the sweet taste of sugar at 4 calories per individual pack. Aspartame is composed of the amino acids aspartic acid and phenylalanine.

Since its discovery in 1965, aspartame has been thoroughly reviewed by numerous regulatory agencies and scientific organizations and found safe for consumption by pregnant women and teens. An 8-ounce glass of milk has 6 times more phenylalanine and 13 times more aspartic acid than an equivalent amount of carbonated beverage sweetened with NutraSweet. An 8-ounce glass of fruit juice contains 3 to 5 times more methanol than an equivalent amount of soda sweetened with NutraSweet.[31]

Individuals with phenylketonuria (PKU) cannot properly metabolize phenylalanine and must monitor their intake of this amino acid from all foods. Infants are routinely screened for PKU within 28 days of birth. Foods should contribute nutrients via a variety of foods and beverages. Foods sweetened with aspartame satisfy one's taste for sweets but may not provide a full array of nutrients to support growth of both the fetus and the mother.

Choline in Pregnancy

Choline may enhance fetal brain development and memory later in life. One large egg provides 215 mg of dietary choline, a little less than half of the daily intake recommended for pregnant women (450 mg).[32] Choline content claims are approved on the labels of foods rich in this important nutrient.

TABLE 9–2 Herbal Supplements Marketed to Pregnant and Nursing Moms

Product	Claim
More Milk Nettles, Blessed Thistle, Fennel Seed	Increase breast milk production. Blessed Thistle is contraindicated during pregnancy.
Fenugreek Seed Tincture Fenugreek Seed	Increase breast milk production. Do not use during pregnancy.

Breast Compress
   Mullein Leaf, Chamomile Flower,
   Burdock Root, Calendula Flower,
   Yarrow Flower
	Externally to relieve breast tenderness, mastitis, breast engorgement, and plugged ducts.

Relax and Rebuild Tincture
   Milky Oatseed, Scullcap, Chamomile,
   Raspberry Leaf, Nettles
	Helps nursing moms get back to sleep. Chamomile may promote menstruation; caution for use during pregnancy.

Raspberry Leaf Tincture Raspberry Leaf	At postpartum to slow bleeding and regain uterine tone.

Boost Tincture
   Yellowdock Root, Dandelion Root,
     Nettles
	For low iron.

Up-Lift Tincture
   St. John's Wort, Motherwort, Scullcap,
   Lemon Balm, Nettle, Milky Oatseed
	For postpartum depression.

Crampbark Complex Crampbark, Motherwort, Raspberry Leaf	Relieves cramps and postpartum emotions.

Source: PHNPG. The use of herbs during lactation. *The Digest.* Fall 1999:16-17.

Foods that contain over 110 mg of choline per serving, including eggs and beef liver, include a claim that they are an excellent source of choline and those with over 55 mg, a good source.[32]

DHA in Pregnancy

Both observational and intervention studies have illustrated the potential role of n-3 fatty acids in gestational length.[33] In observational studies, polyunsaturated fatty acids were quantified in maternal erythrocytes obtained within 2 days of delivery from randomly selected groups of 62 Faroese and 37 Danish women.[34] Gestational age was an average of 2 days longer ($p = 0.3$) and birth weight averaged 140 g more ($p = 0.1$) in the Faroese group.[34] A 20% increase in n-3 fatty acids was associated with an increase in 5.7 days of pregnancy within 40 weeks of gestation in Danish women (95% confidence interval 1.4 to 10.1 days; $p = 0.02$) after controlling for potential confounders.[34]

Essential fatty acid deficiencies were significantly higher among preterm infants ($p < 0.005$).[35] Concentration of n-6 and n-3 fatty acids were significantly lower in the artery phospholipids of preterm infants ($p < 0.005$). No significant correlations were observed with anthropometric parameters, but positive correlations were noted for DHA arterial wall concentration, birth weight, and length.[35]

The maternal percentage of total arachidonic acid (AA, 20:4n-6) in erythrocytes and plasma was significantly increased by 70% in preterm cases versus control cases ($p < 0.05$) at delivery, which directly corresponded to a lower n-3:n-6 ratio in preterm cases ($p < 0.009$).[17] DHA deficiency was significantly higher in preterm maternal erythrocytes and amnion ($p < 0.001$). These women also exhibited significantly lower levels of DHA.[36]

Fish oil may affect pregnancy duration, birth weight, and birth length. Five hundred thirty-three Danish women in their 30th week of pregnancy were randomized, in a ratio of 2:1:1, to receive either 4 g fish oil (2.7 g n-3 fatty acids; 32% EPA, 23% DHA) daily, 4 g olive oil, or no supplement.[37] A food frequency questionnaire determined baseline fish consumption. At delivery, side effects and complications, including blood loss, were evaluated. No significant differences were reported between groups, except for significant gastrointestinal belching and unpleasant taste among fish oil recipients. Among women in the n-3 fatty acid group, pregnancy duration averaged 4.0 days longer than in the olive oil group (95% confidence interval 1.5-6.4, $p < 0.005$) and infants averaged 107 g ($p < 0.05$) more weight at birth. This effect was strongest in women with an initial low fish consumption.[37]

In a randomized, placebo-controlled pilot study, maternal third trimester DHA status and infant DHA status were compared for 53 women divided into 3 groups: (1) 4 eggs weekly (low egg group, 16 women); (2) up to 12 eggs weekly (regular egg group, 19 women); (3) up to 12 high-DHA eggs weekly (high-DHA egg group, 18 women).[38] Written records and biweekly telephone interviews verified intake.

After delivery, the cord blood, placenta weight, body length, and head circumference were measured. Regression analysis demonstrated that the high-DHA group had fewer low-birth-weight (0% vs 13 and 26%) and fewer preterm (6% vs 25 and 26%) infants, and larger placentas (760 g vs 658 g and 663 g).[38]

Potential Mechanisms.   Prostaglandins have an important physiological role in human parturition, being involved in the mechanisms of both uterine contractions and cervical ripening.[33] $PGF_{2\alpha}$ and PGE_2 increase uterine contractility at all stages of pregnancy, while $PGF1_2$ may inhibit myometrial contractility. Maintenance of pregnancy, and thereby the length of the gestation period may be determined by a balance between stimulatory and inhibitory prostaglandins. The type and amount of polyunsaturated fatty acids in foods can modify endogenous prostaglandin production. Higher levels of n-3 fatty acids can exert their effects through competing with AA and thus limiting its effectiveness as a stimulatory prostaglandin precursor. Effectively modifying the n-3:n-6 fatty acid ratio can influence the production of prostaglandins and affect the onset of parturition.

The effects of n-3 fatty acids on prostaglandin synthesis were evaluated to determine if n-3 fatty acids would prevent or delay the switch from myometrial contractions.[39] These occur throughout pregnancy and finally build to expulsive labor contractions. Researchers placed myometrial electrodes, and uterine, jugular, and carotid catheters in the fetal jugular vein, carotid artery, and the amniotic cavity of 12 ewes to deliver a 20% n-3 fatty emulsion or a control emulsion from day 124 of gestation until the end of pregnancy. On day

125, premature labor was induced and achieved when myometrial contractions switched to expulsive contractions. The onset of labor and the time of delivery were significantly different between n-3 fatty acid-infused ewes (53 and 68 hours) and control ewes (20 and 30 hours), suggesting an alteration in the prostaglandin production of the pregnant ewes, resulting in a delay of labor.[39]

N-3 fatty acids may delay premature delivery in sheep and could be extended to humans. Preterm birth remains one of the most common causes of infant morbidity and mortality in modern society. Cause and cure require uncovering the exact mechanisms. N-3 fatty acids affect prostaglandin production and metabolism and may extend gestation toward term delivery.[39]

Quality Assurance in Prenatal and Postpartum Nutrition

Quality assurance/quality improvement criteria for nutritional well-being of prenatal women and adolescents were developed by the Public Health Nutrition Practice Group of the American Dietetic Association[40] (see Appendix 9-A). The criteria are synonymous with clinical indicators and include women and adolescents at their first postpartum visit and breastfeeding women and adolescents with no chronic medical conditions. Preconception nutrition care does not fall within the scope of the criteria list.

The criteria are based on several sources.[41-43] They were field tested at 6 sites that served various cultural and geographic populations. A 75% achievement level at a minimum of 1 test site was required for retention as a final criteria. Implementation of the criteria requires a careful and thorough training of the monitoring staff and the employment of certified lactation educators and specialists.

Women, Infants, and Children (WIC) Program

WIC Facts

The Special Supplemental Nutrition Program for Women, Infants, and Children (WIC) is a short-term intervention program designed to influence lifetime nutrition and health behaviors in a targeted, high-risk population. WIC strengthens health and nutrition for families. It provides quality nutrition education and services, breastfeeding education and support, monthly supplemental nutritious foods, and access to prenatal and pediatric health care services. WIC serves more than 7.4 million pregnant women, new mothers, infants, and preschool children through 10,000 clinics nationwide. WIC requires income level of 185% of poverty or less, or enrollment in Medicaid and nutrition risk verified by a healthcare professional.

Each WIC dollar produces $1.92 to $4.21 in Medicaid savings for newborns and their mothers. It costs $22,000 per pound to raise a low- (less than 5.5 pounds) or very low-birth-weight (less than 3.25 pounds) infant to normal weight (7 pounds). It costs $40 per pound to provide WIC prenatal benefits. Medicaid costs were reduced on average $12,000 to $15,000 per infant for every very low-birth-weight birth prevented. A description of the nutritional management and data collection of WIC participants is outlined in Exhibit 9-1.

WIC is streamlined and effectively managed. WIC managers have developed strategies to reduce costs, stretch resources, and provide efficient,

Exhibit 9-1 Managing WIC Participants

Nutrition history and assessment is a process. After obtaining history and nutrition information, participants are interviewed and a nutritional care plan is developed based on individual participant needs.

Subjective Information
Subjective information is obtained for each participant. Nutrition question-naires are completed by each participant prior to their counseling session. Each questionnaire administered asks a series of nutrition-related questions and then asks for the participant to recall everything eaten and drunk the previous day for a 24-hour recall. The participant is then counseled according to the infor-mation she provides.

The prenatal nutrition questionnaire asks questions like:

- Are you on a special diet?
- Have you ever breastfed or tried to breastfeed?
- How will you feed your baby: breastfeed, formula, breast and formula, or not sure?
- Do you take prenatal vitamins, iron pills, herbs, antacids, and/or laxatives?
- Do you have any of these problems: nausea, vomiting, heartburn, and/or constipation?
- Do you have a refrigerator, stove, hot plate, microwave, and/or running water?
- How many times a day do you usually eat?

The breastfeeding/postpartum woman and newborn infant questionnaire includes questions like:

- Do you often skip meals?
- Are you employed or going to school?
- What method of birth control are you using?
- How many times does your baby nurse or get a bottle in 24 hours?
- Do you have any concerns about breastfeeding?
- What brand of formula do you give your baby (if formula is used)?
- What else do you give your baby—juice, sugar water, tea, cereal, baby food, other?

The infant nutrition questionnaire asks questions like:

- How do you feed your baby: breast, breast and bottle, bottle?
- Does your baby drink a bottle in bed?
- What baby foods do you give your baby?
- What finger foods do you give your baby?

The child nutrition questionnaire includes questions such as:

- Does your child feed himself/herself?
- Is your child allergic to any foods?
- Does your child eat things like plaster, dirt, clay, or paint chips?
- Does your child use a bottle, cup, spoon, and/or fork?

Objective Information
Objective information is obtained, discussed, and integrated into the care plan. Objective data include:

- routine medical checkups to remain on the WIC program. Information gathered includes height, weight, hemoglobin, hematocrit, and basic physical exam results. Height and weight can also be measured at the WIC site. Growth charts are utilized to assess growth rate for the children.

- physician recommendations for alternate infant formulas when an infant is not tolerating a standard formula provided by WIC.
- participants' income and address verification, which determines eligibility for participation.
- documentation if a participant uses drugs, alcohol, or cigarettes, warranting referrals to other community programs.
- background information, such as a new address, phone number, grocery store, and changes to be entered in the computer system.
- in cases where participants speak Spanish, Chinese, or another language other than English, translators would assist. Foods a participant ate and drank the previous day are analyzed according to the Food Guide Pyramid

Food Guide Pyramid

- Insufficiencies are addressed and discussed.
- Visual aids (food models and handouts) enhance the information presented.
- One nutritional goal to practice at home is selected. It is important that the participant selects the goal and that it is attainable and realistic. If the goal is to stop putting juice in the baby's bottle, then problems associated with juice in the bottle are explained, such as the risk of baby bottle tooth decay, anemia, obesity, and ear infections.

Closure

Concerns and questions are addressed as the counseling session closes, and a follow-up appointment is made. Participant problems/concerns are documented in the Integrated Statewide Information System (ISIS) computer system, making it simple for the staff member to review and discuss during the next appointment. The counselor completes either a problem, intervention, and goal (PIC) note or a source of information, assessment, and plan (SAP) note, entering it into the computer.

Summary

The process of counseling WIC participants is thorough because information is gathered from medical exams, doctor recommendations, nutrition questionnaires, and participant interviews. The nutritional care plan and goals are directed standards for good health and decisions of the participant. This process helps to ensure that the goals are realistic and obtainable, and overall health is strengthened by making referrals to other community programs when appropriate.

Examples of Nutritional Assessments and Care Plans

WIC Participant Maria J.

1. Subjective/Objective:
   - 24-year-old Hispanic pregnant female
   - ht/wt: 61"/137 lb, BMI = 25.9 (prepreg), no weight gained at 10 weeks' gestation
   - 3-lb weight gain expected
   - experiencing nausea/vomiting, decreased appetite
   - mild lactose intolerance
   - no HGB/HCT available
   - 24-hour diet recall—low in milk, low in breads, grains
   - takes prenatal vitamins
   - breastfed baby 3 years ago

Exhibit 9–1   continued

2. Assessment:
- below normal weight gain
- recommend (Rx) guidelines for nausea/vomiting during pregnancy
- Rx alternative calcuim sources due to lactose intolerance
- Rx HGB/HCT at next MD visit
- Rx breastfeeding

3. Plan
- discuss recommended weight gain during pregnancy
- discuss handout *Relief for Common Problems During Pregnancy*
- discuss alternative sources for calcuim
- review FGP and Rx intakes during pregnancy
- suggest HGB/HCT at next MD appointment
- discuss breastfeeding
- follow up at next trimester appointment

WIC Participant Christina S.

1. Subjective/Objective:
- 23-year-old pregnant Hispanic female
- ht/wt: 62"/134 lb, BMI = 20 (prepreg), 19-lb wt gain at 34 weeks' gestation
- 20- to 28-lb weight gain expected
- HGB/HCT in normal range
- no reports of nausea/vomiting
- 24-hour recall: low in vitamin A fruit/vegetables; low in milk
- plans to breastfeed and formula feed

2. Assessment:
- adequate weight gain
- Rx 1 vitamin A fruit/vegetable daily
- Rx 3 servings dairy products daily
- Rx breastfeeding

3. Plan:
- discuss Food Guide Pyramid and Rx intakes for pregnancy
- provide handout *Give Your Baby a Healthy Start*
- discuss vitamin A sources
- discuss dairy sources
- discuss plan to breastfeed
- schedule follow-up at postpartum/infant enrollment appointment

effective services. Cost-containment efforts include competitively bid manufacturer rebates; competitive purchase of WIC foods; WIC food price, brand, and container-size restrictions; and competitive WIC store prices. Many of these efforts have occurred through multiple state collaboratives. WIC programs have harnessed computer technology to more efficiently manage WIC benefits and detect potential fraud and abuse. WIC managers continue to explore means to reduce costs and increase accountability.[44]

WIC Participants in 2002

In April 2002, 8,016,918 women, infants, and children were enrolled in the WIC program. Fifty percent of WIC participants were children. Infants accounted for 26% and women 24% of WIC participants.[45]

Women were further divided into groups labeled pregnant (11%), breastfeeding (6%), and postpartum (8%). The percentage of breastfeeding women has risen steadily from 4% in 1994 to 6% in 2002. Most (85%) of the pregnant women participating in WIC are between the ages of 18 and 34 as are 85% of breastfeeding and 86% of postpartum women. Only 7% of women WIC clients are age 17 or younger, continuing a decline from 9% reported in 1998. The 2002 data show sustained increases in WIC coverage of pregnant women in their early stages of pregnancy. In 2002, more pregnant WIC participants enrolled in the program during their first than second trimesters, with 48% in the first trimester and 40% in the second. Only 11% enrolled in the third trimester, down from 12% reported in 1998.

In the 2002 report, for the first time, Hispanics made up the largest ethnic group of WIC participants (38%). Non-Hispanic whites were next largest (36%), followed by non-Hispanic blacks (20%), Asian or Pacific Islanders (4%), and American Indian or Alaska natives (1%). The average annualized income of families/economic units of persons enrolled in the WIC program in April 2002 was $14,550.[45]

Women's Health Issues

Cardiovascular disease is the major cause of death for US women. It kills approximately 500,000 more women than men each year, with most deaths occurring in the fifth decade.[46] The major risk factors for cardiovascular disease in women are prevalent and modifiable among all ethnic groups but differences in chronic disease risk exist (see Table 9–3). Lung cancer and breast cancer are the top 2 causes, respectively, of cancer death among women.[47] Osteoporosis is more common among women than men, causing over 1.5 million bone fractures annually.[48] Mortality rates differ among women in various ethnic groups related to risk and access-to-health care issues.

Women's perceptions of their health risks may differ from reality.[49] For example, women of all ethnic groups may carry excess body weight and feel fat but not think their weight carries a health risk. African-American women might not participate in cancer screenings and might not practice breast self-exams or think of themselves at high risk for breast cancer. Many women do not make the connection between illness or morbidity and mortality. They do not view themselves as a potential statistic. Nor do they think their eating behavior is poor, since they see no immediate adverse effect. However, women of all ethnic groups face major health issues.

Women's Health Initiative

Cardiovascular diseases, cancer, and osteoporosis have become the most common causes of mortality, disability, and impaired quality of life among postmenopausal women. They respond to primary prevention efforts with dietary, behavioral, and drug interventions. In 1992, under the leadership of

TABLE 9-3   Differences in Chronic Disease Risk Among Women of Color

Target Group	Demographic and Health Characteristics
Women of color more likely to be negatively affected by numerous chronic diseases including: • Cancer • Coronary heart disease • HIV/AIDS • (PID) and other sexually transmitted infections (STIs) • Pelvic inflammatory disease (PID) • Diabetes • Gall bladder disease: renal disease	

African American	• 12% of the US population
	• 16.4 million African-American women
	   31.9% and 35.5% of all black Americans and black women were in poverty, respectively
	   48% of all black female-headed families had incomes below the poverty level
	   75% of the 2 million black families in poverty were headed by women
	   16% of the uninsured were black in 1992 (20%), only 51% of African Americans were uninsured
	   75% of Anglos had private insurance; blacks make up 40% of Medicaid enrollees
	• Life expectancy
	   Black females 74 years vs 80 years Anglos
	   Black males 65 years vs 73 years Anglos
	   African-American women are at 2.2 times greater risk of death for any cause than white women
	• Single-parent female-headed families
	   48% of single-parent families in the United States are headed by African-American women
	   Over 40% of men in jail are black Americans and have responsibility for family survival

Asian/Pacific Islanders
- Fastest growing minority group
  Between 1980 and 1990, a 108% growth
  36% are females over the age of 20 (average age = 31.8)
  27 different Asian American and 30 PI groups immigrants from 20 Asian countries
  70% of the population resides in 7 states
  11.9% of families live below the poverty level compared to 10.3% of total population
  65.6% are foreign born and 75.4% speak a language other than English
- 12% of households are female headed
  26.2% of Cambodian households
- 74% of women have high school diploma
- 31.8% have at least a bachelor's degree
  19%, 25.3 %, and 29.8% of Hmong, Cambodian, and Laotians have high school diploma, respectively
- Labor force participation (56.8% total)
  60% Asian and 62.5% Pacific Islander, 19.9% Hmong, 37.3% Cambodian, and 49.5% Laotians
- Distinct experiences and cultures

Native American/Alaskan native
- 1.9 million total (less than 2% of United States population)
- Estimated 400 tribal nations
- Approximately 200 languages or dialects spoken
- Over 1/2 are under 24 years of age
- Close to 50% of urban women earn under $10,000, which is their total household income
- 1/2 report some kind of health insurance coverage but less likely to receive Medicaid

Arab Middle Eastern
- The Arab Middle East includes:
  North Africa, Nile Valley/African Horn, Fertile Crescent, and Gulf and Arab Peninsula
- 1 million to 3 million total in the United States
  US Census 716,391 first generation and 154,347 second generation (from 20 countries)
- 86% speak English well and 50% have some higher education

NIH director Bernadine Healy, NIH initiated the Women's Health Initiative (WHI). The 12-year clinical trial ended in September 2005. The WHI had 3 major components: a randomized controlled trial of promising but unproven approaches to prevention, an observational study to identify predictors of disease, and a trial of community approaches to develop healthful behaviors. A symbol was adopted to identify the trial approach for a multicultural representation (see Figure 9–2).[50]

The randomized, controlled clinical trial of the Women's Health Initiative enrolled 60,000 postmenopausal women 50 to 79 years of age between 1993 and 1996. This trial had 3 interventions, and women enrolled in 1 or more of the components. One intervention evaluated the effect of a low-fat dietary pattern on prevention of breast and colon cancer and coronary heart disease. A second intervention examined the effect of hormonal-replacement therapy on prevention of coronary heart disease, osteoporosis, and/or increased risk

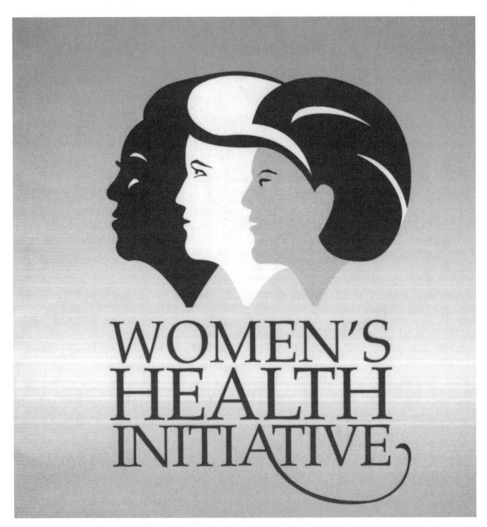

FIGURE 9–2   Women's Health Initiative emblem used on all communications. *Source:* National Institutes of Health. Bethesda, Md; 1995.

of breast cancer. The third intervention evaluated the effect of calcium and vitamin D supplementation on prevention of osteoporosis and colon cancer. Primary, secondary, and tertiary outcomes were tested for the various arms of the trial and are outlined in Table 9-4.

The trial required 4 years for protocol development and recruitment and 9 years of follow-up to achieve the goals. The first participants were enrolled in September 1993 and close-out appointments ended in March 2005. Women who were ineligible or unwilling to participate in the trial enrolled in a long-term, 9- to 11-year observational study that identified new risk factors and biological markers for diseases in women. About 100,000 women participated in this part of the study for a total of 160,000 women.

WHI studies were performed at 40 clinical centers located throughout the United States. The coordinating center, the Fred Hutchinson Cancer Research Center in Seattle, Washington, managed data collection and analysis. Each of the 40 clinical centers recruited a minimum of 3,490 postmenopausal women over a 3-year period for the clinical trial and observational study. The broad geographic distribution of the clinical centers allows recruitment of medically underserved areas or target minority populations and gives a representative cross-sectional sample of the US population (see Figure 9-3). Ten of the clinical centers recruited primarily minority populations—African Americans, Hispanics, and Native Americans.

The final sample size for WHI randomizations and enrollments by study component were 27,348 women in hormone replacement theraphy (HRT), 48,837 undergoing dietary modification (DM), 36,282 taking calcium/vitamin D (CaD), 68,135 in the clinical trial (CT) total, and 93,720 in the observational study (OS). The WHI total was 161,855. The age distribution for DM is 6,958 age 50 to 54, 11,042 age 55 to 59, 22,714 age 60 to 69, and 8,123 age 70 to 79. The ethnicity distribution for the clinical trial that combines HRT, DM, and CaD was 12,609 minority women and 55,626 nonminority.

Managing Community-Based Clinical Trials

In March 2000, early study results surfaced for participants in the WHI hormone study. All HRT participants were informed that the trial was stopped. The news did not affect any other WHI study components.[51] However, there were important reasons why 1 of the trials ended early.

- Hormone replacement therapy (HRT) was being prescribed to over 20 million women in the United States alone in the year 2000 and had been used for decades to relieve menopausal symptoms.
- Many studies involving large numbers of postmenopausal women observed that women who used HRT over long periods had less heart disease than women who did not.
- The hormone users in these studies differed from the nonusers in many other ways; besides their hormone use, e.g., the hormone users had healthier lifestyles and saw physicians more often, which alone could explain why hormone users had fewer heart diseases.
- To determine how HRT affected health outcomes, randomized, controlled clinical trials in which hormone users were similar to nonusers in all respects except for their use of hormones were needed.

TABLE 9–4 Primary, Secondary, and Tertiary Outcomes for the Women's Health Trial, NIH, 1994–2005

Outcome	Hormone Replacement	Dietary Modification	Vitamin D/Calcium Supplementation	Observational Study
Cardiovascular	a	b	c	c
Coronary heart disease	b	b	c	c
Stroke	b	b	c	c
Congestive heart disease	b	b	c	c
Angina	b	b	c	c
Peripheral vascular disease	b	b	c	c
Coronary revascularization	b	b	c	c
Total cardiovascular	b	b	c	c
Cancer				
Breast cancer	b	a	b	c
Endometrial cancer	b	b	c	c
Colorectal cancer	c	a	b	c
Ovarian cancer	b	b	c	c
Total cancers	b	b	b	c
Fractures				
Hip	b	c	a	a
Other fractures	b	c	b	a
Total fractures	b	c	b	a
Venous thromboembolic disease				
Pulmonary embolism	b	c	c	a
Deep vein thrombosis	b	c	c	a
Diabetes mellitus requiring therapy	b	b	c	a
Death from any cause	b	b	b	a

Note: a = primary; b = secondary; c = tertiary end point.
Source: Adapted from: National Institutes of Health. *Women's Health Initiative.* 1995;1(Section 2):2-22.

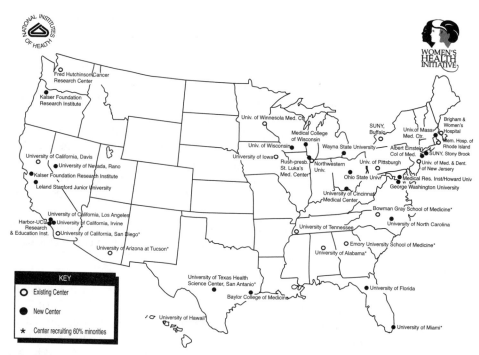

FIGURE 9–3 Location of Women's Health Initiative clinical centers, National Institutes of Health.
Source: Reprinted from National Institutes of Health, *Women's Health Initiative,* 1994.

- WHI was designed to determine the benefits and risks of long-term hormone use in women taking HRT. WHI was originally designed to be the first trial large enough and long enough to answer the question.

HRT Enrollment Status

- Between 1993 and 1998, 27,348 women (ages 50 to 79) were enrolled in the WHI-HRT study.
- Sixty percent (16,609) had a uterus and were randomized to either inactive (placebo) pills or pills containing estrogen combined with progestin estrogen replacement therapy (PERT).
- Forty percent (10,739) had a hysterectomy and were randomly assigned to either placebo pills or pills containing estrogen only for estrogen replacement therapy (ERT).
- The primary question to be answered was whether HRT reduced heart disease over the course of the study, which averaged 8.4 years for the entire study group, even though some women took study pills for up to 11.5 years by the end of the study.
- Additional questions assessed whether HRT reduced bone fractures, increased breast cancer, affected memory, or resulted in other health benefits or risks for postmenopausal women.

Data from the WHI Hormone Study suggested that there was a small increase in the number of heart attacks, strokes, and blood clots in the legs and lungs of women taking active hormone pills compared to placebo pills in the initial years of the trial. The longer on HRT, the lower the risk.

The actual numbers of WHI women who had any of these cardiovascular events was lower than expected and seen in the general population. Very few women had a cardiovascular event. Heart attacks, strokes, or blood clots each affected less than 1% of the women, whether they took placebo pills or active hormones (estrogen alone or estrogen combined with progestin).

Data from national sources indicated that between 0.2 and 1% of WHI women would have a cardiovascular event each year. Younger women tended to have fewer events and older women tended to have more events. Overall, WHI women experienced fewer cardiovascular disease (CVD) events than expected during the initial years. However, WHI women on active HRT experienced a somewhat greater rate of CVD events in the first 2 years than women on placebo. Original estimates were that for every 1,000 women taking active hormones, 5-10 fewer may have heart attack over the course of the study compared to women taking placebo pills.[51]

When WHI began, information was lacking on the effects of hormones on heart disease during the initial years of hormone use. An independent group of medical experts, the Data and Safety Monitoring Board (DSMB), reviewed study data every 6 months for the purpose of evaluating the safety of participants in both groups. The DSMB focused on the major health outcomes that were investigated, i.e., heart diseases, bone fractures, and breast and other cancers. In 2000, the DSMB recommended that WHI break the blind and provide this information to all HRT participants.[51]

The Heart and Estrogen-Progestin Replacement Study (HERS) was the first published trial to study the effect of hormones on actual heart disease events. It studied 2,764 women with preexisting heart disease for an average of 4.1 years. HERS did not collect the number and kind of blood samples from participants as done in WHI and the investigators could not explain the increase in heart attacks (fatal and nonfatal) during year 1. HERS had been the only published clinical trial with enough women to evaluate the effects of hormones on heart attacks, strokes, and blood clots beyond 2 years. All HERS women had a prior history of heart disease, so it is unknown how the long-term results from HERS relate to WHI women with no history of heart disease. In HERS:

- Heart attacks were higher in the first year only (predominantly in the first 4 months), and then decreased over time. Women on active hormones had fewer heart attacks in years 3 and 4 compared to women on placebo. By the end of the study, there were no differences between women taking active versus inactive pills in the total number of heart attacks.
- Blood clots remained elevated over the 4-year study, but declined somewhat during the study.

Although 1 part of the HRT ended early, the DSMB recommended that all other WHI hormone trial components continue. The board would not have recommended this action if the differences between women taking active hormones and those taking placebo pills were large enough to suggest that it is unsafe to continue pill studies. Recent studies were reported in the media showing that the risk of breast cancer while on hormones was absent or

Info Line

Dr. Bernadine Healy posed an interesting question to the public, which was, "So what to do now, ladies?" Data from WHI reduced by one half the number of women using HRT.[52] Why? First, hormone therapy is not a public-health potion. To be so, benefits would have to vastly exceed risks for the majority of the population, and that's just not the case. Second, hormones should not be initiated in older women, a regular practice of the past. They are more stroke-prone and more likely to have underlying blood vessel disease, which can be exacerbated by hormone treatment. Third, women who have had hysterectomies should feel reassured. For them, years of estrogen alone bring little harm, particularly with regard to breast cancer. As for stroke, it appears that patches, which don't cause blood clotting the way oral doses do, are a logical consideration for lowering risk. A final important message for an individual woman really troubled by menopausal symptoms or fearful about osteoporosis is that the risk of HRT is tiny (less than 1 serious event problem per 1,000), especially with the lower doses now available.[52]

lower than that seen in the general population at the beginning of WHI. The risk of taking estrogen combined with progestin was about the same. These recent studies were not randomized trials, and most of the women did not use the form or dose of hormone replacement used in WHI. Neither study provided direct evidence that continuous (daily, low dose) progestin, as used in WHI, was associated with increased risk. Neither HERS nor WHI, which uses continuous progestin, show an increased risk of breast cancer.[51]

Many hypotheses have been generated regarding hormones, e.g., changes in specific proteins involved in blood clotting and increases in the fats in the blood known as triglycerides. This is seen in an increase in proteins associated with inflammation of the arterial walls, e.g., C-reactive protein. Questions remain about selective estrogen receptor modulators (SERMS) and phytoestrogens. SERMS such as raloxifene and tamoxifen have been reported to increase blood clots; but no definitive data exists on whether heart attacks or strokes increase when one takes SERMS.

Oral contraceptive hormones may increase a person's risk for stroke. Birth control pills have much higher amounts of estrogens and progestins than are found in HRT pills. Strokes were only slightly increased in HERS participants taking active hormones. WHI is showing a small increase in the number of strokes in women using active hormones compared to inactive pills.

The *Nurses' Health Study* reported that HRT users have less heart disease than nonusers. The study sample is 121,700 women originally 42 to 67 years old. Most of observational studies have reported that the women who were taking hormones for any extended period differed from those who were not using hormones in many other ways besides their hormone use. Estrogen users in these studies were less likely to be obese and to smoke, more likely to be physically active, more likely to see physicians regularly, and more highly educated. These differences could explain why hormone users had less

heart disease in these studies. Other interesting findings from the *Nurses'
Health Study* include the following: reproductive experience (number of
births, age at menarche, and age at first birth) had no important association with heart disease risk, and for middle-aged women, moderate alcohol
consumption appeared to decrease the risk, of heart disease and ischemic
stroke and increase the risk of subarachnoid hemorrhage. Mild to moderate
overweight status increased the risk of heart disease in middle-aged women.

Other studies are being conducted or have recently concluded with findings forthcoming.

The Women's International Study of Long-Duration Oestrogen after
Menopause *(WISDOM)* is a 10-year study of 34,000 women—18,000 from the
United Kingdom and the remainder from other countries. The study is conducted by the Medical Research Council of the United Kingdom. It is similar
to WHI because most of the WISDOM women do not have preexisting heart
disease. Women with uteruses are being randomized to the same estrogen and
progestin pills or inactive pills that are being used in WHI. However, women
with hysterectomies are being randomized not only to the same estrogen-only
and inactive pills, but also to the estrogen and progestin combination pills
used in WHI.

The Postmenopausal Estrogen-Progestin Interventions *(PEPI)* trial studied the effects of estrogen only versus 3 different estrogen and progestin
combinations compared to placebo among women with no known heart
disease. PEPI evaluated risk factors for heart diseases, including blood cholesterol, blood pressure, factors that regulate blood glucose, and blood clotting factors in 875 women over a period of 3 years.

The Estrogen Replacement and Atherosclerosis Study *(ERA)* presented
findings in March 2000. The trial included 309 women with preexisting heart
disease who were randomized to active estrogen or estrogen-progestin pills
or placebo pills used in WHI whether the women had a uterus or not. After
3 years, the rate of progression of atherosclerotic plaques in the blood vessels
of the heart was similar in both active hormone and placebo groups. This
suggests that hormone neither provided benefit against nor increased risk of
heart disease within 3 years.

Three other angiographic trials of hormones for postmenopausal women
with preexisting heart disease use the degree of narrowing of the coronary
arteries over time as the primary study endpoint, rather than actual heart attacks or other cardiovascular outcomes. All 3 are of relatively short duration
(< 4 years) with few women. They include:

- The Women's Estrogen/Progestin Lipid Lowering–Hormone Atherosclerosis Regression Trial *(WELL-HART)* is a 3-year trial that randomized
  226 women with and without hysterectomies to placebo or estrogen
  (estradiol 1 mg/d, with or without a cyclic progestin, MPA 5 mg/d for
  12 days/month). All women were offered lipid-lowering therapy.
- The Women's Angiographic Vitamin and Estrogen Study *(WAVE)* is a
  2 to 4 year study that randomized 423 women to either placebo pills or
  the same estrogen and progestin combination as in WHI if they have a
  uterus. If they have had a hysterectomy, women were randomized to the
  WHI estrogen. All women were also randomized to either antioxidant
  vitamins (vitamin E 400 IU bid + vitamin C 500 mg bid) or placebo.

Info Line

Women do face blood clots and major health conditions such as heart attacks and strokes. *Blood clots in the legs and lungs* occur in the veins, which are blood vessels that bring blood back to the heart from the tissues. Unlike the blood in the arteries, which has pressure imparted on it from the pumping of the heart, venous blood has low pressure and flows slowly. If blood flow is slowed or obstructed, or if there is an injury to the vein, clotting can occur. Risk factors include prolonged immobilization, surgery, pregnancy, blood diseases, some kinds of cancer, and some genetic disorders. Birth control pills increase risk of blood clots, especially among smokers. HRT increases the risk of blood clots. There are many proteins involved in determining whether blood will clot or not and it is unclear which factors may be affected by estrogen and/or progestins.

Heart attack occurs when the arteries that supply the blood to the heart are blocked. The heart muscle does not receive adequate oxygen and is damaged. Blockage of arteries is generally caused by the rupture of a plaque (fatty deposit) in the wall of the artery, which may cause a blood clot to form. A number of heart disease risk factors are known to contribute to plaque formation; they include high blood cholesterol, high blood pressure, smoking, diabetes, and possibly an inflammation of the arterial wall or a tendency to form blood clots. Most research to date have suggested that hormones decrease the chance of arterial disease with each passing year of use.

A *stroke* (cerebrovascular accident) is the death of brain tissues (cerebral infarction) because of a lack of blood flow to the brain. Strokes are caused by underlying problems similar to those described for heart attacks. In an ischemic stroke, the blood supply to part of the brain is cut off because either atherosclerosis (fatty deposits) or a blood clot has blocked a blood vessel. In hemorrhagic stroke, a blood vessel in the brain bursts and prevents normal blood flow and allows blood to leak into the brain.

- The Estrogen and Graft Atherosclerosis Research *(EAGAR)* Study randomized 160 women to an estrogen combined with continuous progestin (MPA) for an average of 3.5 years.

The Physicians' Health Study showed that aspirin can prevent heart disease in men, but the study didn't include women; the Women's Health Study is analyzing its data to answer this question in women. A recent study reported that women who took low-dose aspirin regularly were less likely to have a first heart attack than women who did not take aspirin.[34]

The Future for Women

Strategies to enhance adoption of healthful behaviors are needed. Studies will mobilize community resources to enhance adoption of these behaviors by providing education, removing barriers, and improving social support. Many behaviors target national goals described in *Healthy People 2010*.[53] As noted previously, some clinical research centers focus on minority women and the medically underserved because these groups have not received sufficient attention and have lagged in adoption of preventive behaviors.

The Women's Health Initiative will provide important, scientific, valid information for women, their healthcare providers, and their communities. Data will indicate the benefits and risks of preventive approaches and the means of achieving successful adoption of these behaviors.[50]

The American Dietetic Association initiated the Nutrition and Health Campaign for Women, which includes research, public policy, industry, media, and grassroots efforts. The campaign recognizes that for each of these efforts, attention must be given to ethnic diversity, special needs of women, low-income women, young girls and teens, older women, and women with disabilities.[54]

Three key messages form the basis of the campaign:

1. Nutrition has a critical role in fitness and prevention of disease.
2. A low-fat diet is a preventive approach to high cholesterol and breast cancer. Regular exercise can enhance the effects.
3. Calcium can help prevent osteoporosis if girls between the ages of 8 and 18 years and older women consume adequate calcium.

For more information, see the Department of Health and Human Services Office of Women's Health (OWH) Web site at www.4woman.gov.

A Prospective Study of Diet Quality and Mortality in Women

Many diet and health studies focus on the association of single nutrients, foods, and food groups and disease prevention or promotion. Few studies evaluate dietary patterns involving complex foods, many nutrients, and components.

To examine the association of mortality with a multifactorial diet quality index, data from the Breast Cancer Detection Demonstration Project were examined. Women had a median follow-up of 5.6 years. The sample was 42,254 women, mean age, 61.1 years who completed the food frequency questionnaire portion of the survey. The main outcome measure was all-cause mortality compared by quartile of a recommended food score (RFS). The RFS was the sum of the number of foods recommended by current dietary guidelines, i.e., fruits, vegetables, whole grains, low-fat dairy, and lean meats and poultry that were consumed at least once a week. The maximum score was 23. There were 2,065 deaths from all causes. The RFS was inversely associated with all-cause mortality. This meant those in the upper quartiles of the RFS had relative risks (rr) for all-cause mortality of 0.82 (95% confidence interval [CI], 0.73-0.92), compared to an rr = 0.71 (95% CI, 0.62-0.81) and 0.69 (95% CI, 0.61-0.78) for the next 2 quartiles. All were adjusted for education, ethnicity, age, body mass index, smoking status, alcohol use, level of physical activity, menopausal hormone use, and history of disease (χ^2 for trend = 35.64, $p < 0.001$ for trend where p is statistical probability). These data suggest that achieving current dietary guidelines may decrease risk of mortality in women.[55]

Info Line

E-sources for women's health issues are available:

National Women's Health Information Center (NWHIC)
US Department of Health and Human Services, (800) 994-WOMAN (9662)
www.4woman.gov
　　Steps to Healthier Woman aims to improve women's health by providing
information on chronic diseases, physical activity, tobacco use, and steps
women can take to reduce illness and death. *Frequently Asked Questions
About Menopause* explains symptoms, hormone therapy, safety and effectiveness of herbal products, and health risks associated with menopause.

Purdue University
Purdue Extension—1140 AGAD
West Lafayette, IN 47907-1140
www.ces.purdue.edu/extmedia/CFS/CFS-608-W.pdf
　　This document discusses key nutritional links to heart disease, breast
cancer, osteoporosis, anemia, weight management, premenstrual syndrome
(PMS), pregnancy, and breastfeeding. Provides a sample meal plan and a list
of foods that are good sources of iron, vitamin C, and folate.

American Heart Association Circulation
www.circ.ahajournals.org/cgi/reprint/109/10/e158
　　Circulation—Heart Disease Prevention in Women summarizes guidelines
for preventing heart disease in women. It helps patients assess their risk,
makes recommendations on lifestyle changes and other interventions, and
discusses drug therapies for women at high risk.

Weight-Control Information Network (WIN)
1 Win Way
Bethesda, MD 20892-3665
(202) 828-1025 or (toll free) (877) 946-427
www.niddk.nih.gov/publications/myths.htm
　　Information provided clarifies myths such as: starches are fattening,
grapefruit burns fat, and skipping meals is a good way to lose weight.

National Women's Health Information Center (NWHIC)
US Department of Health and Human Services, (800) 994-WOMAN (9662)
www.4woman.gov
　　Tips for Health Care Providers was designed for use when screening for
eating disorders and alerts one to questions to ask adolescent patients and
their parents. Available at: www.4woman.gov/BodyImage/Bodywise/bp/Body
Wise.pdf.

National Heart, Lung, and Blood Institute Health Information Center
PO Box 30105
Bethesda, MD 20824-0105
Attn: The Heart Truth
(301) 592-8573
www.nhlbi.nih.gov/health/hearttruth

The Heart Truth is a national awareness campaign for women about heart disease. An online tool kit contains information and materials to plan a Heart Truth event.

Office of Dietary Supplements
National Institute of Health
6100 Executive Blvd, Room 3B01, MSC 7517
Bethesda, MD 20892
(301) 435-2920
http://ods.od.nih.gov/factsheets/BlackCohosh.asp
    Question and Answer fact sheet provides an overview of the use of black cohosh for menopausal symptoms, reviews clinical studies and effects on hormone levels, and addresses safety concerns.

American Dietetic Association
120 South Riverside Plaza, Suite 2000
Chicago, IL 60606-6995
(800) 877-1600 Ext. 500
    Women's Health and Nutrition—Position paper of the American Dietetic Association and Dietitians of Canada. *J Am Diet Assoc.* 2004;104:984-1004. Available online at: www.eatright.org.

Women's Health and Reproductive Nutrition Dietetic Practice Group
www.whrndpg.org

Source: Forman A. Focus on resources–women's health issues. *Networking News.* 2005; 27(1):1,6.

Osteoporosis

Osteoporosis affects more than 25 million people in the United States, resulting primarily in bone fractures among postmenopausal and elderly women. In the absence of primary prevention during the next decades, women over 45 years old will experience 5.2 million fractures and incur $45.2 billion in healthcare costs.

There are about 195,000 vertebral fractures in the United States annually. At 50 years of age, a US white woman has a 32% chance of a vertebral fracture, 16% chance of a hip fracture, and 15% chance of a wrist fracture.[56] Peak bone mass achieved in the first 30 years of life and the rate at which bone is lost later in life are the major predisposing factors for osteoporosis. Adequate calcium intake, hormones, and lifestyle (mainly exercise) are critical to the process (see Chapter 16).

Low-dose hormone replacement therapy combined with increased intakes of calcium and vitamin D may prevent bone loss as much as higher doses of HRT and do so with minimal side effects. Postmenopausal women > 65 years old with low bone mass received low doses of HRT and adequate intakes of calcium (1,200 mg/day) and vitamin D. They had a 5% increase in bone density at the spine, and increases in total body bone mineral content. The treatment is similar or superior to higher-dose treatments and is well tolerated.[57]

Obesity

More than one third of US adults are considered obese. Approximately 35% of white females, 49% of African-American females, and 47% of Hispanic females are overweight or obese.[54] Excess weight is linked to 5 of 10 leading causes of death in the United States: coronary heart disease, some cancers, diabetes, stroke, and atherosclerosis.

Studies have examined women's body weights and their personal values about their body size. One study reported the results of an open-ended interview completed by 36 white and 31 black women of varying socioeconomic status (SES).[58] The women's body size values and body mass index were assessed. Black women of lower SES were heavier, perceived themselves as heavier, and perceived attractive body size as heavier than black women of higher SES and white women of all SES levels. The body weight they considered overweight was considerably higher for black women of lower SES than for other cohorts.

Over one third of black women perceived themselves as thinner than their actual size. White and black women at a higher SES reported more pressure to be thin because of lifestyle and their environment, especially the media. Black women tend to view obesity as the result of their capacity and opportunity for physical activity, and not a function of their eating behavior. Black women do believe obesity places them at risk for health problems. White women see obesity as a major threat to their self-esteem and social acceptance.[58]

It appears that black women of lower SES have a wider range of perceptions about normal and attractive body size. Their ideas of normal weight versus excess weight are more affected by social status, family, and peers when compared to white women and black women at higher SES, who are affected by images in the media. This type of study needs to be extended to larger samples of women in various ethnic groups. Diverse approaches to weight management require an understanding of the meaning of weight for individuals and their social context[58] (see Chapter 15).

Clinical guidelines on the health risks of obesity use body mass index (BMI; calculated as weight in kilograms divided by the square of height in meters) and waist circumference, but the waist:hip ratio may provide independent information.[59] To assess the associations of BMI, waist circumference, and waist:hip ratio with multiple disease end points, Folsom et al conducted a prospective cohort study in 1986 of 31,702 Iowa women, 55 to 69 years old, and free of cancer, heart disease, and diabetes. Random sampling and mail survey was used. Study end points were total and cause-specific mortality, incidence of site-specific cancers, self-reported diabetes, hypertension, and hip fracture over 12 years. Comparing quintile 5 to 1, the waist:hip ratio was the best anthropometric predictor of total mortality, rr = 1.2 (95% confidence interval, 1.1-1.4); rr 0.91 (95% confidence interval, 0.8-1.0) for BMI and 1.1 (95% confidence interval, 1.0-1.3) for waist circumference. Waist:hip ratio was associated positively with mortality from coronary heart disease, other cardiovascular diseases, cancer, and other causes. The waist:hip ratio was associated less consistently than BMI or waist circumference with cancer incidence. All anthropometric indexes were associated with incidence of diabetes and hypertension. Women in both the highest quintiles of BMI and waist:hip ratio had a relative risk of diabetes of 29 (95% confidence interval, 18-46) versus women in the lowest combined quintiles. The waist:hip ratio offers additional prognostic information beyond BMI and waist circumference.[59]

Stettler et al[60] identified risk factors in an African-American population, which are present at birth and predispose individuals to adiposity defined as BMI > 85 percentile. Anthropometric and socioeconomic variables were collected at birth for 447 African-American individuals who were followed until young adulthood, when skinfold thickness was measured. Three variables measured at birth were independently associated with adiposity in young adulthood, explaining 12% of the variance. The variable, odds ratios, and 95% CIs were 2.7 (1.2, 6.2) for female sex, 4.0 (14, 11.2) for first-born status, and 1.15 (1.06, 1.25) for each unit increment in maternal prepregnancy BMI. After adjustment for these variables, birth weight for gestational age and socioeconomic variables were not associated with adiposity.

Hypertension

Hypertension, a major risk factor in cardiovascular disease, is 2 to 3 times more common in women than in men, and is highest among African-American women.[54] Hypertension occurs nearly 3 times more frequently among overweight adults than normal-weight adults, and data suggest that one third of all cases are caused by excess weight. Likewise, elevated blood pressure in overweight adults leads to an increased rate of stroke.

The National Health and Nutrition Examination Survey (NHANES) III data show a decline in the age-adjusted prevalence of hypertension for women 20 to 74 years of age, from 34% (NHANES II) to 20% (NHANES III). The age-adjusted prevalence rate of hypertension is 31% among African-American women and 19% among white women (see Chapter 14).

Diabetes

Diabetes mellitus, or high blood glucose, is a serious disorder that increases the risk of coronary heart disease. Diabetes is often called a woman's disease because, after age 45, about twice as many women as men develop diabetes. Over 80% of individuals with diabetes die of some type of cardiovascular disease (e.g., myocardial infarction). The risk of death from coronary heart disease is twice as common among women than men with diabetes. Compared with nondiabetic women, diabetic women tend to experience more hypertension and dyslipidemia. Untreated diabetes can also contribute to the development of kidney disease, blindness, problems in pregnancy and childbirth, neuropathy, and gangrene. For unknown reasons, the risks of heart disease and heart-related death are higher for diabetic women than for diabetic men. Non–insulin-dependent diabetes mellitus, or type 2 diabetes, develops in adulthood and is the most common form of the disease. Of all individuals with non–insulin-dependent diabetes mellitus, 85% are at least 20% overweight.

A prospective cohort of 75,521 US women 38 to 63 years old without previous diagnosis of diabetes mellitus, coronary heart disease, stroke, or other CVDs in 1984 completed detailed food frequency questionnaires (FFQs) in 1984, 1986, 1990, and 1994.[61] The 12-year follow-up was part of the Nurses' Health Study. A higher intake of whole grain foods was associated with a lower risk of ischemic stroke.

Coronary Heart Disease and Cancer

Women with high total cholesterol and high LDL (low-density lipoprotein) cholesterol levels have significantly higher heart disease rates. Low HDL (high-density lipoprotein) cholesterol is associated with a high risk for heart disease; each milligram percent decline in HDL cholesterol produces a 2 to 3% increase in coronary disease risk. The National Cholesterol Education Panel recommendation is greater than 50 mg% HDL; less than 35 mg% HDL is a strong risk factor for coronary heart disease (CHD). With this backdrop, women seek to raise or to sustain their HDL levels beyond the impact of genetics. Weight loss, exercise, alcohol, and estrogen replacement enhance HDL cholesterol. Every pound of weight loss increases HDL cholesterol by one half of a percent. Moderate, consistent exercise increases HDL cholesterol by 10%.[62]

The placement of body fat influences disease risk. A waist:hip ratio greater than 1.0 increases a women's risk for CHD, cancer, and other chronic diseases. It appears that stability of weight, especially in peri- and postmenopausal years, is associated with increased breast cancer risk. Several large cohort studies in the United States (89,494 nurses 34 to 59 years old) and in the Netherlands (62,573 women 55 to 69 years old) did not report significant associations between risk of breast cancer and fat intake.[62] It is thought that the vast majority of these women had a consistently high fat intake. A true test of the effect of low-fat eating behaviors on cancer risk with a sufficiently large sample has not been conducted, but will be addressed in the WHI.

Alcohol, omega-3 fatty acids, vitamins and minerals, and aspirin are being investigated for their role in cancer and CHD risk. Alcohol intake increases risk of breast cancer; but moderate alcohol intake of 2 servings a day increases HDL cholesterol levels, which may lower overall CHD risk. The alcohol and breast cancer association appears to be dose related, beginning with as few as 2 drinks a day.

There are benefits to eating tree nuts, for example, walnuts and other nuts grown on trees, e.g., almonds, pecans, pine nuts, and hazelnuts contain good fats: 88% of the fat in walnuts is mono- or polyunsaturated and walnuts are a good source of omega-3 fatty acids. A 12.4% decrease in LDL cholesterol levels was reported for men who ate walnuts daily for a 4-week period. A study in Spain in 2000 concluded that daily consumption of just a handful of walnuts lowers the risk of coronary heart disease by 11% for both men and women, corroborating the earlier findings.[63]

Info Line

Up-to-date information on new foods appearing on grocery shelves is available at www.supermarketsavvy.com/supermarket_savvy.asp.

Vitamins A, C, and E and selenium are being examined for their role in breast cancer risk, whereas the role of vitamins in CHD has resulted in recommendations for behavioral changes. For example, vitamin E supplementation for more than 2 years gave healthy women a relative risk for major coronary disease of 0.59 (95% CI; 0.38 to 0.91) after adjusting for age, smoking status, and use of other antioxidants.[64]

Lactose Intolerance

A condition that is not life threatening, but a discomfort, is lactose intolerance. Ethnic difference in prevalence is evident. Prevalence of lactose maldigestion in the United States is about 15% among whites, 53% among Mexican Americans, 80% among African Americans, and 90% among male and female Asian Americans, totaling about 30-50 million Americans.[65,66] The proportion who experience symptoms, i.e., lactose intolerance, is about one-third,[67] and the extent of symptoms depends on a variety of biological, psychological, and dietary factors. Transient lactose intolerance, caused by mild viral infections, may result in a shutdown of lactase production for a few weeks. True milk protein allergies affect only about 1-3% of the pediatric population,[68,69] with a lower prevalence in adults. Most children outgrow milk allergies by 3 years of age. Table 9–5 gives recommendations for lactose symptoms.

Physical Activity

The National Health Interview Survey data revealed that 37.7% of women at least 18 years of age exercise regularly. White women exercise more often than African-American women (39% versus 28%). As age increases, irrespective of race, fewer women report exercising regularly.[59]

People of all ages can improve the quality of their lives through a life-long practice of moderate physical activity creating a body work ethic. The value premise of the document is that a regular, preferably daily regimen of at least 30-45 minutes of brisk walking, bicycling, or even working around the house or yard can lower a man's or woman's risks of developing coronary heart disease, hypertension, colon cancer, and diabetes. Regular physical activity greatly reduces the risk of dying from coronary heart disease, the leading cause of death in the United States. Physical activity reduces the risk of developing diabetes, hypertension, and colon cancer; enhances mental health; fosters healthy muscles, bones, and joints; and helps maintain function and preserve independence in older adults.

TABLE 9–5   Nutrition Therapy Key Recommendations for Clients With Lactose Intolerance Symptoms

---

- Consume dairy foods in smaller amounts and with food.
- Try flavored milks such as chocolate—these may be better tolerated.
- Try yogurt and hard cheeses (cheddar, Monterey Jack, mozzarella)— these contain less lactose.
- Increase consumption of dairy products gradually, to rebuild the ability to digest lactose.
- Consider a commercial lactase preparation such as Lactaid or Dairy Ease to help digest the lactose in dairy products.
- Use lactose-reduced or lactose-free milk.
- Consume other good food sources of calcium like broccoli, kale, almonds, and fortified foods to help meet calcium requirements.

Source: Dairy Council of California. What to tell your clients about lactose intolerance: separating myth from reality. *California Nutrition Council Newsletter.* Summer 2000:10-11.

Concerns exist because:

- at least 60% of Americans are not regularly active.
- 25% are not active at all.
- ¼ of young people walk or bicycle.
- 14% of young people report no recent vigorous or light-to-moderate physical activity.
- physical activity declines dramatically during adolescence.

Families, health professionals, businesses, community leaders, schools, and the media and entertainment industries need to create a demand for physical activity in the lives of all Americans. Physical activity must be an essential health objective, like sound nutrition, the use of seat belts, and the prevention of adverse health effects of tobacco. People can benefit from even moderate levels of physical activity. Americans can substantially improve their health and quality of life by including moderate amounts of physical activity in their daily lives. Health benefits appear to be proportional to amount of activity; thus, every increase in activity adds some benefit.

Endurance Versus Resistance Exercise

Endurance-type physical activity involves repeated use of large muscles, such as in walking or bicycling, and it gives health benefits. Resistance exercise, which increases muscle strength by lifting weights, preserves and enhances muscular strength and endurance, prevents falls, and improves mobility in the elderly.

The concern for our youth is that nearly half of youth from 12 to 21 years of age are not vigorously active on a regular basis. Moreover, physical activity declines dramatically during adolescence. Daily enrollment in physical education classes has declined among high school students from 42% in 1991 to 25% in 1995.

School-based interventions for youth are promising, not only to reach young people between the ages of 6 and 16 years, but also for the potential impact on lifelong habits. Childhood and adolescence may be pivotal times for preventing sedentary behavior among adults by maintaining the habit of physical activity throughout the school years.

Two future challenges include identifying key determinants of physically active lifestyles among the diverse populations in the United States including special populations, women, and young people and using this information to design and disseminate effective programs.

A major concern about physical activity programs for women is that the programs generally offer approaches for women already physically active. Marcus and Stanton[70] recommend a theoretical model to develop appropriate exercise programs. Their model links stages of change with stages of readiness to adapt a new behavior such as a physical activity program. In the Imagine Action model, individuals can be classified in one of several stages, as follows:

- *Precontemplator:* Individual is not thinking about change. Common comment is, "Do I need this?"
- *Contemplator:* Individual is thinking but not doing. Common incentive is, "Try it, you'll like it!"
- *Preparer:* Individual is participating but not regularly. Common comment is, "I'll try it once."

- *Person in action:* Individual is regular participant. Common incentive is, "Keep it going."
- *Maintainer:* Physical activity has become a regular part of lifestyle. Common response is, "I won't stop now."

This model has been used to define and to tailor exercise programs to meet people at their level of need. For example, low-impact aerobics are suitable for individuals who have never exercised and don't wish to show their lack of activity.[70] Women with hypertension, type 2 diabetes mellitus, or any joint disease may also benefit from low-impact aerobics.

Average energy expenditure during various types of physical activities is shown in Table 9–6.[71] Women are encouraged to select physical activities they enjoy and can place into their lifestyle. Consistent, frequent participation in activities women enjoy has a positive influence on their long-term adherence.

Individuals should strive for a minimum of 3 exercise sessions each week. If they find a particular week's pattern tiring, they should repeat it before moving to the next pattern. A walking program does not have to be completed in 12 weeks.

Individuals should check their pulse periodically to see if they are exercising within a target zone (see Table 9–7). As individuals become more physically fit, they should try exercising within the upper range of the target zone. Encourage individuals to increase their brisk walking time gradually from 30 to 60 minutes, 3 or 4 times a week. Remind them that their goal is to acquire both cardiovascular benefits and enjoyment.

TABLE 9–6   Relative Energy Expenditure of 14 Common Physical Activities

Physical Activity	Energy Expenditure*
Bicycling 6 mph	240 cals/hr
Bicycling 12 mph	410 cals/hr
Cross-country skiing	700 cals/hr
Jogging 5$1/2$ mph	740 cals/hr
Jogging 7 mph	920 cals/hr
Jumping rope	750 cals/hr
Running in place	650 cals/hr
Running 10 mph	1280 cals/hr
Swimming 25 yds/min	275 cals/hr
Swimming 50 yds/min	500 cals/hr
Tennis—singles	400 cals/hr
Walking 2 mph	240 cals/hr
Walking 3 mph	320 cals/hr
Walking 4$1/2$ mph	440 cals/hr

*Energy expended varies in proportion to body weight; a 100-pound person burns one third fewer calories (i.e., multiply the number of calories by 0.7); for a 200-pound person, multiply by 1.3. A preferred way to increase calories per activity is to increase the time spent per activity.

Source: Adapted from: *Exercise and Your Heart.* National Heart, Lung, and Blood Institute/American Heart Association; August 1993. NIH Publication No. 93-1677.

TABLE 9–7 Target Heart Rate Zone by Age for Men and Women

Age	Target Heart Rate Zone (Beats/Minute)
20 years	100-150
25 years	98-140
30 years	95-142
35 years	93-138
40 years	90-135
45 years	88-131
50 years	85-127
55 years	83-123
60 years	80-120
65 years	78-116
70 years	75-113

Source: Reprinted from *Exercise and Your Heart.* Bethesda, MD, National Heart, Lung, and Blood Institute/American Heart Association; August 1993. NIH Publication No. 93-1677.

Use the following method to check if an individual is within target heart rate zone:

1. Immediately after exercising stops, have the individual take his or her pulse. He or she should place the tips of the first 2 fingers lightly over one of the blood vessels on the neck, just to the left or right of the Adam's apple. Or the individual could try the pulse spot inside the wrist just below the base of the thumb.
2. The individual should count the pulse for 10 seconds and multiply the number by 6.
3. The person should compare the number to the target heart rate in Table 9–7. He or she should look for the age grouping that is closest to the individual's age and read the line across. For example, if the person is 43, the closest age on the chart is 45; the target zone is 88-131 beats per minute.

FIT or FITT?

FIT is an acronym signifying frequency, intensity, and time for an exercise prescription. Developed in the 1970s, it was used primarily to assist those interested in knowing how much aerobic exercise to perform for optimal benefit. The formula for aerobic exercise historically has suggested 20-minute periods of physical activity at least 3 days a week at designated target heart rate intensities.[72]

A new acronym, frequency, intensity, time, and type (FITT), delineates the different *types* of exercise prescription common in the new millennium.[73] The physical activity pyramid illustrates the FIT formula for 6 different types or levels of physical activity, each with its own FIT formula and each with its own unique benefits.

Level 1: Lifestyle Physical Activity

> At the base of the physical activity pyramid is lifestyle; includes physical activities that people can do as part of their regular everyday work or daily routine.

Level 2: Active Aerobics

> The second level of the pyramid includes active aerobic activities, or those performed at a pace for which the body can supply adequate oxygen to meet the demands of the activity.

Level 2: Active Sports and Recreational Activities

> Within the second level of the physical activity pyramid are active sports and recreational activities.

Level 3: Flexibility Exercises

> Flexibility exercises are included at the third level of the pyramid and refer to exercises done specifically to give joints a full range of motion as a result of having long muscles and elastic connective tissues.

Level 3: Muscle Fitness Exercises

> Muscle fitness includes strength and muscular endurance. The American College of Sports Medicine (ACSM)[72] recommends that muscle fitness exercises be completed at least 2 days a week. Exercises for several different muscle groups (8 to 10) should be done using a percentage of the maximum weight the individual can lift. The percentage (intensity) depends on the type of muscle fitness to be developed. Each exercise should be performed 8 to 12 times (a set). More frequent training and additional sets or repetitions can increase strength, but the additional improvement is relatively small.

Level 4: Inactivity

> The top of the pyramid identifies inactivity as an important stage when adequate amounts of sleep and rest are necessary after vigorous exercise.

Exercise Benefits

> Exercising reduced breast cancer risk in more than 121,000 middle-aged women followed for 16 years. Women who walked, biked, and did aerobics for 7 or more hrs/wk were at nearly 20% less risk for breast cancer than women who exercised < 1 hr/wk. Physical activity may reduce circulating estrogens, which stimulate growth of cancer cells.[74]

> Moderate physical activity can cut the risk of type 2 diabetes by ~ 50% as observed for more than 70,000 middle-aged women followed for 8 years. Brisk walking for 1 hr/day or other leisure activity of moderate intensity lowered the risk of type 2 diabetes by 46% compared to those who exercised the least. Physical activity improves insulin sensitivity and assists with weight loss.[75]

Info Line

Three reproducible fact sheets, developed by the National Heart, Lung, and Blood Institute and the Indian Health Service, are designed for American Indian and Alaska native women.

- "Keep the Harmony Within You—Check Your Blood Pressure" offers useful tips for people who have high blood pressure.
- "Treat Your Heart to a Healthy Celebration" emphasizes that native foods and traditional ways of preparing foods can help people stay healthy. Tips for making healthy food choices are offered.
- "Give Your Heart a Workout" stresses the importance of tobacco being a gift of the earth; it should be used to show respect and honor and should not be abused. The harmful effects of tobacco are described.

Free fact sheets are available at NHLBI Information Center, PO Box 30105, Bethesda, MD 20824-0105.

Recreational activity significantly cut the risk of gallbladder surgery in more than 60,000 middle-aged women. An average of 2-3 hours/week of biking, jogging, and running reduced surgery risk by about 20%. Studies with men replicate the findings, but the mechanism creating this beneficial effect is not clear.[76]

In Part III of this book, separate chapters address different chronic diseases. Issues relevant to both women and men are included.

The Adult Male and His Nutrition Needs

Significant changes in the roles of men and women during the last decade have led to new challenges regarding health and nutrition of men. More than 75% of men stated in a Gallup Poll that they are concerned about the effect of eating on their health. The strange twist was that only 23% of the men could name the major food groups. Men appear to have ideas or assumptions about the components of healthy eating, but they have limited knowledge to help them make informed food choices.[77]

Men have many of the same risk factors as women for chronic disease, but some differences exist. Due to a greater muscle mass, men have higher metabolic rates, which result in a higher calorie expenditure than women for the same activity. Men accumulate fat in their midsection rather than in the upper or lower body as observed for women. The midsection location for fat deposition increases a man's waist:hip ratio and his risk for cardiovascular disease, hypertension, and diabetes. Conversely, men appear to be more successful than women at losing weight; however, their lifestyle and work habits may invite excess weight gain.[77]

Eating on the run and choosing high-fat and high-sugar baked products adds excessive fat calories. Approximately 30% of a man's energy and fat intake is ingested outside his home. This includes snacks that come from vending machines, snack bars, and airport terminals. Business meals, entertaining, and relaxing after work often include alcoholic beverages, which increase the total number of calories ingested, stimulate insulin, and promote weight gain. High-fat food selections at meals and snacks instead of abundant carbohydrate foods promote a higher weight gain.

Men who consistently participate in a physical activity, fitness program, or team sports may demonstrate a keener sense about food selections to enhance performance. The desire to remain physically fit opens the door for focused nutrition education and primary prevention efforts.[77]

Researchers placed 39 normal-weight young adult college students into a group to earn points for snack foods or fruits and vegetables (f/v); or to earn points for snack foods or sedentary activities. Snack foods included candy bars, cookies, potato chips, and corn chips. Healthy foods included grapes, pineapple, oranges, and carrots. Sedentary activities included computer games, television, music videos, games and puzzles, and magazines.[78]

Researchers determined how hard participants worked to access snack foods compared to alternatives. Results showed that participants shifted from snack foods to f/v and then to nonfood activities when access to snack foods was decreased.

In addition, the researchers found that 3 changes increased the choice of f/v: (1) Increasing access to f/v or alternative activities by modifying the environment to reduce availability of high-fat snack foods; (2) adjusting food prices of high-fat snacks, and (3) decreasing the cost of f/v in vending machines.[78]

Research Regarding Prostate Cancer and Dietary Components

During the past 15 years, an increasing body of knowledge has identified a potential role for dietary fat, especially animal fat, in the etiology of prostate cancer. In 1995, Whittemore et al reported an increased energy intake with increased prostate cancer risk among 3 racial groups. The association was due primarily to saturated fat. The association between adult stature and body weight and prostate cancer has been explored; however, current research does not support a link between high body mass and the risk of prostate cancer.

Although the results from several large cohort studies are inconsistent, a few international ecological studies have reported positive correlations between the per capita intake of fat and prostate cancer mortality; $r = 0.6$-0.7 (r = Pearson product moment correlation coefficient). Strength of association is highest for the subclassification of saturated and animal fat. Future studies must clarify the role of the subclassifications to differentiate among the predisposing factors.

Soy Changes Mood of Men

Soy is the most widely used botanical by pre- and postmenopausal women, but its use by men increases as research shows the benefits on heart health. Soy sales in the United States have increased from $940 million in 1990 to about $4 billion in 2004. Isoflavones, a naturally occurring plant estrogen in soy protein, may reduce the risk of prostate cancer.[79]

Researchers from Wake Forest University Baptist Medical Center summarized soy research stating potential beneficial effects of isoflavones in reducing the risk of various cancers, osteoporosis, cardiovascular disease, and postmenopausal symptoms have been identified, but knowledge of neurobehavioral effects have not been researched sufficiently. Dose and gender of individuals also have an influence.

Long-term consumption of an isoflavone-rich diet made male monkeys prone to aggression and impacted their social behavior. Research suggests that it could have an adverse effect on the behavior of men. The study is consistent with emerging literature showing that soy can have a negative impact on the behavior of male rodents. Previous studies have shown no difference in aggression in females given large doses of soy.

For the 15-month study, researchers divided adult male monkeys into 3 groups and fed them different amounts and types of protein. One group had about 125 mg of isoflavones a day. The second group had half that amount, and the third group's protein came from milk and animal sources. Those on the highest dose were markedly more aggressive, yet at times more isolated, showing extreme behaviors.

Isoflavone levels of 125 mg per day are higher than amounts consumed by many Asians, who typically eat more soy than other populations. But the isoflavone levels are comparable to levels found in many dietary supplements sold in the United States. Further research is needed to understand the balance for soy to provide a beneficial rather than a negative effect.[79]

Male Fatigue and Testosterone

The number of men taking testosterone replacement therapy (TRT) increased 29% from 2001 to 2002, when nearly 2 million prescriptions were written. This occurred when there was no clear proof that TRT combats fatigue, depression, or low sex drive in healthy men. Little proof exists that there are benefits or risks of supplemental testosterone, because no large, long-term studies have been done.[80]

Extra testosterone could be life-threatening, as the major concern is prostate cancer. Suppressing testosterone slows both prostate cancer and benign prostatic hyperplasia, and about half of men over age 50 have undetected cancer cells in their prostate glands. Increasing testosterone may enhance the risk of stroke-causing blood clots, cardiovascular disease, and sleep apnea.

An Institute of Medicine panel called for more research on testosterone therapy while posing with extreme caution in using it until the research was completed. Research should first involve frail men over 65 with clear testosterone deficiencies who would benefit the most. Studying the larger cohort of healthy men, 50 years and older, who might be interested in using testosterone to fight symptoms of aging would be controversial, because potential long-term risks would be greater than anticipated benefits.

Men's testosterone levels decline about 1% a year beginning at 30 years of age even though men in their 70s father children. Clinical testosterone deficiency, or hypogonadism, affects 2 million to 4 million US men. Serum testosterone level < 200 is deficient but 400 is the average at age 80. Andropause is reflected in decreased sex drive, fatigue, loss of strength and muscle mass, and difficulty concentrating.[80]

Reducing CHD Risk

Once men have been diagnosed with a chronic disease (e.g., hypertension or diabetes) or identified as having a risk factor for coronary heart disease (CHD) (e.g., hyperlipidemia), they may be more receptive to dietary instruction and behavioral change. Data from numerous randomized clinical trials have shown that lowering cholesterol levels among men at high risk for CHD reduces the incidence of CHD. These are summarized as follows[81]:

- The *Lipid Research Clinics Coronary Primary Prevention Trial* showed a 19% lower incidence of CHD among men in the cholestyramine and diet arm of the trial versus those in the placebo and diet group. Total plasma cholesterol and LDL cholesterol were 8% and 12% lower, respectively, in the cholestyramine and diet group compared with the placebo and diet group.[82,83]
- In the *Multiple Risk Factor Intervention Trial,* the effect of a multifactor intervention over 7 years on mortality from CHD was observed in 12,866 high-risk men, aged 35 to 57. The men were randomized into either (1) special intervention, including stepped-care hypertension reduction, nutrition modification to reduce serum total cholesterol, and smoking cessation; or (2) the usual care from their own physicians. A 7.1% decrease in mortality (which was not significant) was observed in the special-intervention group compared to the usual-care group. CHD mortality was 17.9 per 1,000 in the special-intervention group and 19.3 per 1,000 in the usual-care group.[84]
- The *Cholesterol-Lowering Atherosclerosis Study* assessed the effects of decreasing LDL cholesterol and increasing HDL cholesterol on the growth of atherosclerotic lesions. Participants included 162 eligible men who had coronary bypass surgery; they were randomized into a treatment or control group. The 80 treatment group participants received colestipol-niacin and instruction for a low-fat diet (i.e., 22% calories from fat; 10% as poly-unsaturated, 4% as saturated, and 125 mg of cholesterol a day). The 82 members of the control group received placebo pills and instruction on a low-fat diet comprised of 250 mg of cholesterol per day, 26% calories from fat, 10% as polyunsaturated and 5% as saturated. For the colestipol group, plasma total cholesterol and LDL cholesterol were lowered by 26% and 43%, respectively, and HDL cholesterol was increased by 37% within 2 years. This is in contrast to the placebo group, whose total cholesterol and LDL cholesterol were lowered by 4% and 5%, respectively. The colestipol group had significantly less lesion progression and new atheroma development in the native coronary arteries. Atherosclerotic regression was noted in 16.2% of the colestipol men versus 2.4% in the placebo group.[85]
- In the *Veterans Administration Cooperative Study Group on Antihypertensive Agents,* a positive benefit was noted when blood pressure was controlled. For middle-aged men with an average diastolic level of 115-129 mm Hg, a 93% reduction in the rate of nonfatal CHD was noted. If their diastolic blood pressure was 105-114 mm Hg, the reduction was 69%. For most of the clinical trials with antihypertensive drugs, the men who received the drug had a significant reduction in the incidence of stroke.[86]

Data show that the incidence of CHD morbidity and mortality can be reduced in men at high risk for CHD, and also that primary and secondary prevention efforts are effective in reducing CHD mortality. The incidence of recurrent myocardial infarction and death due to CHD can be reduced. Lowering plasma total cholesterol levels and LDL cholesterol levels (e.g., by a fat-modified eating pattern) can lower the incidence of CHD among men either with or prior to a diagnosis of CHD.[81]

The extent of the reduction in CHD has been defined by baseline serum cholesterol level. That is, individuals in the 250 to 300 mg/dL range can expect for each 1% reduction in the serum cholesterol level a 2% reduction in the incidence of CHD. This means that a 10-15% reduction in the serum cholesterol level can reduce CHD risk by 20-30%. Men who smoke or have hypertension can greatly benefit from cholesterol lowering.[84]

Intervention and longitudinal studies demonstrate a benefit of both minimal and average increases in HDL cholesterol levels. Every 1 mg/dL increment in baseline HDL cholesterol produced a 3.5-5.5% decrease in CHD as noted in the Lipid Research Clinic's Coronary Primary Prevention Trial, the Lipid Research Clinic's Prevalence Study, and the Framingham Study. Specifically, each 1 mg/dL increase in HDL cholesterol from baseline equaled a 4.4% reduction in CHD risk.[84]

For men who stop smoking, overall CHD risk status improves. Stopping after one or more myocardial infarctions also improves the prognosis of fatal and nonfatal CHD.[85] Further, the Physician's Health Study, with 22,071 men, observed that taking 1 aspirin every other day can lower heart disease risk. In addition, the Baltimore Longitudinal Study of Aging has yielded important data regarding the natural aging process (see Chapter 10).[81]

Adult men do experience osteoporosis and fractures of the hip and vertebrae but at a lower frequency than women. Calcium intake, exercise, and overall eating pattern is as important for men as for women. The recommended adequate intake, or AI, for males is 1,300 mg per day in adolescence, declines to 1,000 mg per day for men aged 19 to 50 years of age, and increases to 1,200 mg per day for men 51 years of age and older.[13]

High cholesterol can be treated by diet and cholesterol-lowering medications, such as statins, which alter cholesterol synthesis, and newer, over-the-counter products, such as Benecol and Take Control, which contain plant sterols. These interfere with the absorption of cholesterol from the intestines.[87]

Martinez-Gonzalez studied lifestyle characteristics that may predict changes in total serum cholesterol and high-density lipoproteins (HDL cholesterol). The 3-year study followed a sample of 980 healthy Spanish male and female employees. All workers participated in a multifactorial program to prevent cardiovascular disease. The association between lifestyle factors and lipid changes was controlled for dietary modifications. In a multivariate analysis, decreases in body mass index and in alcohol consumption were associated with significant reductions in total serum cholesterol. Maintaining sports at posttest or starting to practice them was significantly and independently associated with favorable changes in serum cholesterol. Leisure-time exercise ($p = 0.002$) and giving up smoking ($p = 0.06$) were each associated with increased HDL cholesterol where $p =$ statistical probability.[88]

Issues in Men's Health

- Resistance training offers free-radical protection because lifting boosts both levels of free radicals and the levels of enzymes that combat them to increase antioxidant defenses.
- Selective apoptotic antineoplastic drugs (SAAND) turn cancer cells off and reduce prostate cancer progression.

- Levels of hostility and homocysteine in 64 healthy people have been found highly correlated and both damage the inside of arterial wall, leading to plaque formation and higher CHD risk.
- Surgeons at the University of Alberta in Edmonton transplanted pancreatic islet cells into 8 type 1 patients, resulting in perfect sugar control.[89]
- Stanol spreads, e.g., Benecol taken 3×/day, lowered LDL cholesterol by 17% over 8 wks of intervention.[87,90]
- Attempted weight loss for most men involves 2.4 days of diet and then a return to burgers, fries, and shakes. Successful approaches are[90]:
    1. Add fat, such as monounsaturated olive and peanut oil to foods and cooking.
    2. Add snacks with a low glycemic index, e.g., low-fat chocolate milk, peanuts, and low-fat yogurt.
    3. Add carbohydrates since they induce serotonin. Carbohydrates are the so-called feel-good chemicals and include light popcorn, bagels, pasta, and oven-baked potatoes.
- Vitamin E supplements given to men produced a 20% lower risk of prostate cancer; daily zinc supplements produced 45% less risk, and selenium (55 micrograms/day or the RDA) produced a 60% reduction in prostate cancer. Wheat germ is a good source of zinc and selenium.[91]

Obesity and Healthy Body Weight

The risk of diabetes increases about twofold in people who are mildly overweight, fivefold in those who are moderately overweight, and tenfold in those who are obese. Medical professionals strongly recommend achieving a healthy weight, which is considered the single most important strategy for adults to improve their health status. A 10% weight loss promotes positive health benefits. Overweight people who lose only 2 pounds can lower blood cholesterol, and a 7-pound weight loss can lower high blood pressure to normal.

The *2005 Dietary Guidelines for Americans* contain a suggested healthy body weight range based on an individual's height.[92] It is recommended that women attain the lower weight in a range unless they are physically active, in which case they are recommended to attain the higher weight in a range.

Millions of men and women in the United States strive to control their body weight. One of the most controversial weight-loss methods is the very-low-calorie diet (VLCD), a diet containing no more than 800 kcal per day

Info Line

A quick way to estimate healthy body weight for women, 18 to 25 years old, is to use the formula of 100 pounds plus 5 pounds for every inch over 5 feet. For example, a woman who is 5 feet 7 inches would have a healthy body weight of 135 pounds. The weight range is ± 10%, and for each year under 25, subtract 1 pound. For men, the formula is 110 pounds at 5 feet plus 5 pounds for every inch over 5 feet.

Source: Sizer F, Whitney EN. *Nutrition: Concepts and Controversies.* 8th ed. Belmont, Calif: Wadsworth/Thomson Learning; 2000. Available at: www.wadsworth.com.

or no more than 12 kcal per kg of ideal body weight per day. The VLCD is designed to promote significant short-term weight loss rapidly, while avoiding the risks of total fasting.[93]

Very-low-calorie diets are provided in the context of comprehensive treatment programs, in the course of which the patient's usual intake is totally replaced by specific foods or liquid formulas. Weight loss on a VLCD averages 1.5 to 2.5 kg/week, with total losses averaging 20 kg after 12 to 16 weeks of treatment. In contrast, standard low-calorie diets that provide 1,200 kcal/day produce losses of 0.4 to 0.5 kg/week and an average total loss of 6 to 8 kg. There is little evidence that an intake of less than 800 kcal/day leads to even greater weight loss. To preserve lean body mass, it appears necessary to provide protein of high biological value in an amount of at least 1 g/per kg of ideal body weight per day. Serious complications are infrequent with modern VLCDs; the most common complication is cholelithiasis.[81]

It appears that modern VLCDs are generally safe under proper medical supervision. They may be used with adults who are moderately or severely obese, and they may be expected to promote significant short-term weight loss and to improve obesity-related disorders. Long-term weight loss, however, is not very impressive. It appears helpful to accompany a VLCD with behavioral measures and physical activity.[81]

The Consumer in the Health and Fitness Market

When individuals accept a personal responsibility for their health, they often find their participation in aerobic exercise and physical conditioning more likely if they can work amid family and friends. Many of today's health-conscious consumers consider joining a health club as important as paying for medical services. There are a variety of facilities from private club memberships with fitness rooms, to fitness centers for families, to facilities located in large business centers. The location and hours of operation often influence attendance. The extent of programs offered (e.g., aerobics and child care) may determine whether women participate.

Facilities may have highly automated equipment in addition to free weights, stationary exercise bikes, treadmills, stair climbers, and rowing machines. Qualifications of personnel determine the level of counseling, instruction, and follow-up to defined programs. Personal trainers are generally available to assist clients with programs. Promotion of fuel in the form of energy bars is common but not without risk. Over 800 deaths were linked to energy bars containing *Ephedra*—a popular weight-loss and energy-boosting product.[94]

Most fitness centers require monthly or annual contracts; special reduced entrance fees are often available 2 or 3 times a year. Membership may include a trial period or the opportunity to add additional services to a basic membership packet. This may include racquetball or aerobic exercise fees.

Passive exercise devices and techniques are still available in most facilities for strength training (e.g., barbells, dumbbells, and exercise machines). Isometric training requires a person to push against an immovable object. Vibrating equipment and rubberized inflatable suits do not cause the body to expend appreciable energy. Strength training has a small impact on cardiovascular fitness and only expends about 4 calories per minute.[95] Other equipment available includes motion machines, motor-driven exercise bikes, vibrating belts, rowing machines, rubberized inflatable suits, and electrical stimulation devices. Cosmetic additions to health clubs may include spas, steam baths, massages, and saunas. Tanning beds may be available, but their use is a concern due to the exposure to 2 types of ultraviolet radiation, ultraviolet B (UVB) and ultraviolet A (UVA). The light is similar to sunlight but is more intense and can produce an effect in a relatively short period of time. Because tanning booths are not inspected, users should take caution.

The overall purpose of regular physical activity is to condition the heart and blood vessels. Other benefits include the following[95]:

- maintaining normal blood pressure or reducing blood pressure in people with hypertension
- maintaining a healthy body weight
- preventing or reducing chronic low-back pain
- improving sleep habits
- reserving energy for work and leisure
- increasing ability to cope with illness or accidents
- reducing fatigue

Both women and men have a greater chance of dying from heart disease, cancer, and several other causes when they have sedentary lifestyles than when they have a modest amount of activity. Greater longevity is associated with a daily brisk walk lasting 30 to 60 minutes. Strength training generally is not aerobic, but isometric. What is important to note is that strenuous exercise, such as long-distance running, is not required for good health.[95] Persistent and consistent aerobic exercise can create a training effect or real physiologic changes, but a sufficient amount and duration of exercise is required for a training effect (see Table 9–8).[96]

Info Line

READY TO CHANGE?

To begin lifestyle changes, check this Web site: http://www.americanheart.org/ and search for CAP. It offers facts, tips, and tools for developing an eating plan, starting an exercise program, and keeping track of your medications. Risk factors for coronary heart disease and stroke are listed.

Selecting appropriate clothing and shoes for exercise is important. Cotton clothing for comfort is needed for exercise in hot, humid weather. Sufficient clothing is needed for exercise in cold weather to retain the body heat without creating excess sweat. Shoes should be selected to provide ample support and a comfortable fit during activities such as running, jogging, biking, etc.

During pregnancy, the major concern regarding exercise is whether there is a possibility of injury to the fetus or to the mother. During the first trimester, a possible teratogenic effect of high maternal body temperature can occur. Keeping a core body temperature is important. It is not known if certain exercises are potentially more harmful or if a threshold of intensity of an exercise is an issue.[97]

TABLE 9–8 Popular Aerobic Activities and Fitness Points Achieved

Points	Exercise	Amount	Duration
11	Walking/running	3.0 miles	30-36 minutes
10.5	Swimming	1,000 yards	17-25 minutes
10	Walking/running	1.5 miles	Under 9 minutes
9	Running in place	100-110 steps/minute	15-17 minutes
9	Cycling	6 miles	Less than 18 minutes
9	Rope skipping	—	30 minutes
8	Rowing	20 strokes/minute	36 minutes

Source: Data from Cooper K. *The New Aerobics.* New York: Bantam Books; 1970.

Health Beliefs, Eating Patterns, and Vitamin/Mineral Supplementation

Health beliefs, self-reported health status, and vitamin/mineral supplementation were assessed with a random sample of 1,730 adults in 7 western US states.[98] Chi-square analysis was used on pooled data to evaluate significant differences in demographic and personal characteristics across frequency of vitamin/mineral supplement use. Three frequency categories were nonuser, regular user, and occasional user. Health status was a self-reported measure, described as excellent, very good, good, fair, or poor.

Of the respondents, 35% reported their health as very good, 21% responded excellent, 8% said fair, and 3% said poor. A significant difference was noted in eating patterns for different ethnic groups and different educational levels. More whites considered themselves in better health ($p < 0.001$). Adults with a higher education reported having better health ($p < 0.01$) where p = statistical probability. A significant difference was noted in reported health status by income and marital status. Married adults and individuals at higher income categories reported a higher health rating ($p < 0.01$ and $p < 0.001$, respectively). A positive association was found between vitamin/mineral supplement users and perception of reduced susceptibility and/or severity of health problems ($p < 0.01$). Specific illnesses cited were stress, colds, skin problems, heart attacks, and cancer.

Findings from this study are consistent with earlier findings. Supplement use was common among individuals who followed an exercise regimen or believed that supplement use provided a health benefit.[99-101] In fact, taking a vitamin supplement may fulfill the general public's need to be proactive about their health. Exhibit 9–2 demonstrates the role of B-vitamins and readily available food sources.

The Dietary Supplement Health and Education Act of 1995 (DSHEA) expanded the definition of dietary supplements beyond essential nutrients and distinguished them from drugs or food additives. A less restrictive regulatory environment for supplements draws the following implications:

- Claims may be made by manufacturers, retailers, and others regarding popular nonvitamin, nonmineral (NVNM) supplements.
- Usage prevalence and trends by consumers may not be monitored.

- Inconsistent classification may occur.
- Limited data on actual use may be published.

Garlic and ginseng are the most popular supplements. The third National Health and Nutrition Examination Survey reported highest supplement intake for garlic and lecithin.[102] NVNM supplement use increases with age, more healthful lifestyles, higher alcohol consumption, and obesity. Associations with education, income, region, and urbanization are not strong.[103] Radimer et al recommend standardized survey procedures include phrasing of questions, reference time, supplement categories, and representative use. Standardization can improve our ability to assess supplement use, prevalence, and trends.[103]

Exhibit 9-2   B-Vitamins, Function, Deficiency, Sources

Folate (Folic Acid or Folacin)

Functions
- Folate plays an essential role in making new body cells by helping to produce DNA and RNA, the cell's master plan for cell reproduction.
- Works with vitamin B_{12} to form hemoglobin in red blood cells.
- Eating plans rich in folate may help protect against heart disease.
- Can help women lessen risk of delivering a baby with neural tube defects, like spina bifida.

Deficiency
- A deficiency affects normal cell division and protein synthesis, especially impairing growth.
- Anemia, caused by malformed blood cells that can't carry as much oxygen, may be the result of folate deficiency.
- Pregnant women who don't get enough folate, especially during the first trimester, have a greater risk of delivering a baby with neural tube defects such as spina bifida. Dietitians recommend all women of childbearing age consume adequate amounts of folate in their eating plans.

Sources
Leafy vegetables, some fruits, legumes, liver, yeast breads and wheat germ, and some fortified products like cereals, juices, rice, or pastas are good sources. Most enriched grain products—bread, flour, corn grits, cornmeal, farina, rice, macaroni, and noodles—must be fortified with folate according to law.

Food	Folate (mcg)
Spinach (1/2 cup)	130
Navy beans, boiled (1/2 cup)	125
Wheat germ (1/4 cup)	80
Avocado (1/2)	55
Orange (1 medium)	45
Slice of bread (fortified)	40
Peanuts (dried, one ounce)	40

Vitamin B$_{12}$ (Cobalamin)

Function
- Works closely with folic acid to make red blood cells.
- Helps your body use fatty acids and amino acids.
- Serves as a vital part of many body chemicals and so occurs in every body cell.

Deficiency
- A deficiency may result in anemia, fatigue, nerve damage, a smooth tongue, or very sensitive skin. Deficiencies can be masked—even progress—if extra folic acid is taken to treat or prevent anemia.
- Strict vegetarians, who eat no animal products, and their infants are at risk for developing a vitamin B$_{12}$ deficiency. This could cause severe anemia and irreversible nerve damage. For these groups, as well as some elderly people, including fortified foods or a dietary supplement can prevent these problems.

Sources
Animal products—meat, fish, poultry, eggs, milk, and other dairy foods. Some fortified foods have vitamin B$_{12}$ as well.

Food	Vitamin B$_{12}$ (mcg)
Salmon, cooked (3 oz)	3.0
Beef tenderloin, lean, broiled (3 oz)	2.2
Yogurt, skim (1 cup)	1.4
Shrimp, cooked (3 oz)	1.3
Milk (1 cup)	0.9

Thiamin (Vitamin B$_1$)

Function
- Helps produce energy from carbohydrates in all the cells of your body.

Deficiency
Because most Americans consume many grain products, a thiamin deficiency is rare today, with one exception: chronic alcoholics.

Sources
Whole-grain and enriched grain products, such as bread, rice, pasta, tortillas, and fortified cereals, provide much of the thiamin we eat. Pork, liver, and other organ meats provide significant amounts too.

Riboflavin (Vitamin B$_2$)

Function
- Helps produce energy in all cells of your body
- Helps change the amino acid called tryptophan in your food into niacin (protein is made of many different amino acids)

Deficiency
Except for people who are severely malnourished, a deficiency isn't likely. Contrary to popular myth, riboflavin doesn't cause hair loss.

Sources
Milk and other dairy foods are major sources of riboflavin. Some organ meats—liver, kidney, and heart—are excellent sources. Enriched bread and other grain

continued

Exhibit 9–2   Continued

products, eggs, meat, green leafy vegetables, and nuts supply smaller amounts. Ultraviolet light, such as sunlight, destroys riboflavin. That's why milk is packed in opaque plastic or cardboard containers, not clear glass.

Food	Riboflavin (mg)
Beef liver, braised (3 oz)	3.5
Yogurt, skim (1 cup)	0.4
Milk, skim (1 cup)	0.4
Enriched corn tortilla	0.2
Egg, one large	0.2

Niacin

Function
• Helps your body use sugars and fatty acids.
• Helps enzymes function normally in your body.
• Helps produce energy in all the cells in your body.

Deficiency
For people who consume adequate amounts of protein-rich foods, a niacin deficiency isn't likely. Pellagra is caused by a significant niacin deficiency– symptoms include diarrhea, mental disorientation, and skin problems.

Sources
Foods high in protein are typically good sources of niacin: poultry, fish, beef, peanut butter, and legumes. Niacin is also added to many enriched and fortified grain products.

Food	Niacin (mg NE)
Turkey breast, roasted (3 oz)	6.0
Peanut butter (2 TBSP)	4.0
Enriched spaghetti, cooked (1/2 cup)	2.5
Enriched corn tortilla (1)	1.0
Black-eyed peas, frozen, cooked (1/2 cup)	0.5

Pyridoxine (Vitamin B$_6$)

Function
• Helps your body make nonessential amino acids, or proteins, which are then used to make body cells.
• Helps produce other body chemicals, including insulin, hemoglobin, and antibodies to fight infection.
• Helps turn the amino acid called tryptophan into 2 important body substances: niacin and serotonin (a messenger in your brain).

Deficiency
A deficiency can cause mental convulsions among infants, depression, nausea, or greasy, flaky skin. For infants, breast milk and properly prepared infant formulas contain enough.

Sources
Chicken, fish, pork, liver, and kidney are the best sources. Whole grains, nuts, and legumes also supply reasonable amounts.

Food	Pyridoxine (Vitamin B$_6$) (mg)
Chicken, light meat (3 oz)	0.5
Pork, loin (3 oz)	0.5
Peanut butter (2 Tbsp)	0.1
Black beans, boiled (1/2 cup)	0.1
Almonds (1 oz)	< 0.1

Biotin

Function
Helps your body produce energy in your cells and helps metabolize (use) protein, fat, and carbohydrate from food.

Deficiency
It's rarely a problem for healthy people who eat a variety of foods. In those rare cases, symptoms may appear, including depression, fatigue, appetite loss, and heart abnormalities.

Sources
Biotin is found in a wide variety of foods, including eggs, liver, yeast breads, and cereals.

Pantothenic Acid

Function
Helps your body produce energy in your cells and helps metabolize (use) protein, fat, and carbohydrate from food.

Deficiency
It's rarely a problem for people who eat a variety of foods. Consuming too much may result in occasional diarrhea and water retention.

Sources
Meat, poultry, fish, whole-grain cereals, and legumes are among the better sources. Milk, vegetables, and fruits also contain varying amounts.

Choline
Recommendations for choline are available, but no nationally representative estimates of the intake of choline from food or from food supplements exist. Choline is produced by the body and found in a variety of foods. Choline deficiency is not a problem for most Americans.

Source: The American Dietetic Association. *Complete Food & Nutrition Guide.* Hoboken, NJ: Chronimed Publishers; 1996.

The American Dietetic Association's Survey of American Dietary Habits explored US eating patterns and attitudes about eating to influence health.[104] Three population subgroups were identified: Group A—"I'm doing it" (26%); Group B—"I know, but" (38%); and Group C—"Leave me alone" (36%).

Individuals in Group A believe nutrition and foods are important but tend to have misconceptions about the interactions; 93% of this group feel they are doing all they can. In Group B, only 32% of members are willing to give up favorite foods. For Group C, 83% are adamant about not giving up their favorite foods.

In another study, women who ate breakfast had daily fat intakes with ≤ 30% energy from fat compared to the women who skipped breakfast (40% vs 28%; $p < 0.001$).[105] For both genders, the breakfast meal contained the lowest mean percent energy from fat compared to other eating occasions ($p < 0.05$). Adults under 30 years were more likely to skip breakfast than were older adults and only 75% of adults consumed breakfast regularly in 1991.[106]

A consumer profile study on produce use revealed that people tried a new type of produce for the following reasons: a friend recommended it (29%), a household member requested it (21%), it was needed for a recipe (18%), and they heard or read about it in a magazine (16%).[107]

To identify regional and sociodemographic differences in fruit and vegetable intake, a 7-item food frequency questionnaire (FFQ) was given to 15,060 individuals from 48 schools, 60 work sites, 50 churches, and 15 WIC clinics. Mean daily intake was 3.6 servings of fruits and vegetables, but significant differences were found among the regional study centers (low of 3.0 to high of 4.1) and by age (< 30 years = 3.7 servings per day; 30 to 49 years = 3.4; > 50 years = 3.7), education (< high school = 3.4 servings per day; high school graduate = 3.4; some college = 3.5; college graduate = 3.9), ethnicity (black = 3.7 servings per day; Hispanic = 3.0; white = 3.6; other = 3.7), marital status (married = 3.6 servings per day; single = 3.5), and food-shopping responsibilities (little = 3.2 servings per day; about half = 3.6; most = 3.8). Only 17% of respondents ate 5 or more servings of fruits and vegetables per day.[108]

Cholesterol and fat content of foods continue to be major concerns of the US consumer. Vitamins and minerals rank high. Although balance, variety, and moderation are key concepts that Americans believe influence the health quality of their eating pattern, two thirds of Americans choose food based on a good or bad perception. Overall, 80% of US adults are concerned about the effect of what they eat on their future health.[104]

Men eat out slightly more often than women. The average number of meals eaten away from home in a week increases for men after 24 years of age and as the family income increases. Lunch is the most common commercially prepared meal; breakfast is the most frequently skipped meal. About 54% eat one or more dinner meals away from home each week.[109]

Fast food consumption of US adults does impact their energy and nutrient intakes and overweight status. The diet quality and overweight status of free-living adults, ages 20 years and older, were compared after they were grouped by their fast food intake status.[110-111] The 1994 to 1996 Continuing Survey of Food Intakes by Individuals (CSFII 1994-1996) provided the data.[112] Preliminary analysis of USDA's 1989-1991 Continuing Survey of Food Intakes by Individuals (CSFII 1989-1991) showed that 16% of adults, ages 20 years and older, reported consuming fast food on day 1 of the survey.

The new analysis focused on: (1) effect of fast food on diet quality of males and females based on day-1 data; (2) comparison of dietary and overweight status of adults who ate fast food on 1, 2, or none of the survey days; and (3) within-person analysis comparing energy and macronutrient intakes of adults who ate fast food on 1 of the 2 survey days. Sample size was 9.872 adults 20+ years of age. The main results were as follows:

- At least 1 in 4 adults reported eating fast food.
- The diet of males and females eating fast food was high in energy and energy density.
- Fast food provided more than one third of the day's energy, total fat, and saturated fat; and was high in energy density.
- Very small amounts of milk and fruits, but substantially large amounts of nondiet carbonated soft drinks were consumed at fast-food restaurants (FFR).
- Controlling for age, gender, socioeconomic and demographic factors, energy and energy density increased and micronutrient density decreased with frequency of fast food consumption.
- Adults eating fast food on at least 1 survey day had higher mean body mass index values than those who did not eat fast food on either survey day.
- There was a small, but significant, positive association between fast food consumption and overweight status of the adults.
- Within-person comparisons showed that energy intakes were higher on a fast food day than on a non-fast food day.

In other research, 2 algorithms classified 101 Singaporean Chinese (mean age = 38.7; 51% men) out of 716 respondents by stage of change for consuming the recommended servings of grains, primarily cereals, fruit, and vegetables.[113] An objective self-administered FFQ followed by a brief telephone interview assessed intentions and were used to determine stage of readiness. Validity was established using three 24-hour dietary recalls. Significant increases across the stages occurred for mean intake of grains. For grain intake, algorithms classified 89% of participants with inadequate intakes into the preaction stages, and 75% of those having adequate intakes into the action or maintenance stages. For fruit and vegetable intake, 93% having inadequate intakes were classified into the preaction stages, and 76% of those having adequate intakes were classified into the action or maintenance stages. It appears that algorithms can assess stages of change for food-based goals and project successful approaches for people.

In the book *Intuitive Eating*, Tribole and Resch[114] identify various types of eaters, i.e., careful, unconscious, chaotic unconscious, refuse-not unconscious, waste-not unconscious, and emotional unconscious, professional, or intuitive. By clarifying the individual's eating style, the movement toward an intuitive eater is smoother. In the hospital, registered dietitians (RDs) do not have time to obtain detailed food diaries or to discuss emotions each time the person eats a meal or snack. Inadequate counseling skills often deter RDs from exploring the emotional issues related to the clients' food. Rudimentary guidelines are often the end points of a hospital diet instruction.

In the book, 10 principles of intuitive eating guide the reader toward becoming an intuitive eater. For example, principle 3, make peace with food, suggests, "Give yourself unconditional permission to eat," which is in contrast to counseling in a clinical setting. Principle 4, challenge the food police, counters the guilt resulting from categorized foods and food lists from professionals. Counseling in hospitals usually focuses on avoidance or missing nutrients/food groups and not on fullness, which is principle 5, feel your fullness, and on satiety, explored in principle 6, discover the satisfaction factor. The authors believe registered dietitians focus on servings and calorie requirements, total carbohydrate, protein, and fat intakes. They believe intuitive eaters practice a gentle approach to nutrition as shown in principle 10, honor your health-gentle nutrition. *Intuitive eating* focuses on attention to one's body by listening to its clues rather than battling its biological urges or following a strict meal plan. Identifying, coping, and understanding the emotions linked with food eliminates the win or lose mentality. Continual self-improvement is likely to occur.[114]

An additional competency is required for RDs counseling clients with eating disorders, i.e., experience in counseling and a multidisciplinary approach. Clients with disordered eating have specific psychological issues, e.g., distorted body image, food preoccupation, family or societal pressure, depression, and anxiety. A nonjudgmental approach and the ability to understand the client's needs, assess a client's nutritional status, interpret lab results and request them, as well as having a knowledge of specific food-drug and drug-drug interactions, is essential.

Community-Oriented Programs

Several community-based organizations provide direct service to adults on a national basis. Only 3 of the programs are described here—the Cooperative Extension System, the Consumer Program, and the Expanded Food and Nutrition Education Program (EFNEP).

The Cooperative Extension System

The Cooperative Extension (CE) System is a nationwide, tax-supported, educational program that enables people to make practical decisions in life. The CE mission is to help people improve their lives through an educational process using scientific knowledge focused on issues and needs. The CE System is based on a funding partnership of federal, state, and county governments. The Smith Lever Act of 1914 established a partnership between the US Department of Agriculture (USDA) and land grant universities. Legislation in various states allowed governments or organized groups at the county level to become a third legal partner.[115]

This educational system includes professionals in each US land grant university, at Tuskegee University, and in American Samoa, the District of Columbia, Guam, Micronesia, Northern Marianas, Puerto Rico, and the US Virgin Islands. The land grant universities are listed in Appendix 9–B.

Basic programs of the CE System include the following:

- agriculture competitiveness and profitability
- community resources and economic development
- family development and resource management
- 4-H and youth development
- leadership and volunteer development
- natural resources and environmental management
- nutrition, diet, and health

From these basic programs and with strategic planning, national initiatives are developed every 5 years. The current national initiatives are:

- food safety and quality
- international marketing
- plight of young children
- revitalizing rural America
- sustainable agriculture
- waste management
- water quality
- youth at risk

In most states, the CE System is the university's service window to each county. Research information flows from the university to help a diversified audience to (1) improve the quality of their lives, (2) develop problem-solving skills, (3) become more competent consumers, (4) conserve and wisely use the natural resources, and (5) build better communities.

Resident professional researchers and educators are located in county offices. These professionals include farm advisors, home economists, and 4-H youth development advisors. The county-based advisors link with land grant university research programs through CE specialists who are faculty.

Cooperative Extension programs differ from most programs offered by universities and community-based organizations in 3 important ways[115]:

1. All of CE training activities and programs are offered free or for a small fee to cover the cost of materials used in the program.
2. Most of CE's educational programs do not offer college credit.
3. CE programs are held at off-campus locations throughout the county, at times and places convenient to the clientele.

Besides offering workshops, seminars, and field days, CE publishes information on various topics of interest to consumers, homemakers, business people, farmers, educators, and researchers. Businesses and industries receive CE information and training principally in the areas of agronomy and range management, environmental horticulture, and consumer marketing.

Major programs in CE include the Adult and Youth Expanded Food and Nutrition Education Program, the Home Economics Program, the Environment Horticulture Program, the 4-H Youth Development Program, and the Urban Horticulture Program.

Consumer Program

The Consumer Program responds to consumer needs for sound, objective information on food safety, food fads, prenatal and infant information, food quality, and childhood obesity. Consumers receive information on financial planning and management skills through MONEY SENSE programs. New parents and parents of school-age children benefit from age-appropriate home-learning programs such as Parent Express and the Caring series.

Expanded Food and Nutrition Education Program (EFNEP)

The EFNEP was established in 1969 when the federal government officially realized that hunger existed in the United States. The program's mission is to improve the dietary well-being of low-income families. The goal of EFNEP is to help low-income families, especially those with young children, to acquire the knowledge, skills, attitudes, and behavior changes necessary to improve their food intake. The target audience includes low-income families living in rural or urban areas and, specifically, family members who are responsible for planning and/or preparing their family's meals. Nutrition education assistants are recruited from the community and receive a 6-week training session before placement in an assigned work area. They receive training in basic nutrition, food purchasing, budgeting, menu planning, and community resources, and they receive monthly in-service training as needed.

Working with small groups of 6 to 8 people, EFNEP makes serial presentations to introduce basic nutrition, meal planning, food preparation, sanitation, food storage, food preservation, and food buying to participants (see Figure 9–4). Food demonstrations and food sampling help participants learn additional key nutritional concepts and practices. Six to eight class sessions are held, with the last session consisting of a visit to a local supermarket to practice wise shopping (see Figure 9–5). Upon completion of 6 to 8 group sessions, a certificate of participation is presented to each participant.

Since 1986, EFNEP has expanded to include training in local emergency food distribution systems. Training is also available for staff and volunteers in related agencies that work with low-income groups. EFNEP has developed a creative media approach that includes a food stamp hotline, a Spanish language radio program, and videotapes to disseminate nutrition information.

In 1970, a youth component of EFNEP was implemented to instill positive behaviors in children at an earlier age. The youth component of EFNEP operates under the 4-H Youth Development Program. The target audience includes youths, 5 to 18 years old, who live in low-income geographic areas; youths from families participating in adult EFNEP; youths who receive free or reduced-price school lunch and free breakfast; youths from families receiving Aid to Families with Dependent Children (AFDC); and youths from families enrolled in other low-income programs.

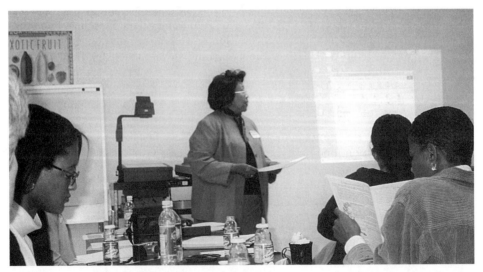

FIGURE 9–4 Edwina Williams, RD, MSHA, Adult Education Coordinator, Expanded Food and Nutrition Program, trains community outreach staff in a new program for low-income adults in Los Angeles, CA.

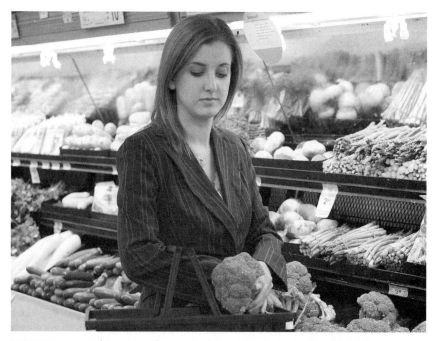

FIGURE 9–5   Making wise choices in the grocery store. Image copyright Shutterstock, Inc.

The CE staff provide an educational curriculum that reflects the nutritional needs and cultural heritage of the audience. The curriculum also includes information on food safety, shopping, and developing job skills. The programs can be tailored to meet special educational needs, such as the needs of developmentally disabled children; soon-to-be emancipated foster children; low-literacy youths; pregnant adolescents; and immigrant children. Programs are also delivered via summer day camps and after-school programs. Volunteers and extenders for the programs include parents, teachers, agency staff, college and university students, and recreation leaders.[115]

Federally Funded Research on US Adults

In the United States, the National Heart, Lung, and Blood Institute funds various programs in adult research. Projects address major health concerns. The currently funded investigations are described briefly next.[59]

Atherosclerosis Risk in Communities

Initiated in July 1985, the Atherosclerosis Risk in Communities Study measures the association of CHD risk factors with both atherosclerosis and new CHD. The target population is a representative cohort from 4 diverse communities. The study population comprises men and women, ages 35 to 74, residing in 4 communities, each with a cohort of 4,000 participants; 1 community cohort is only African-American participants. Hospital records, death certificates, and out-of-hospital deaths are compiled.

Method Alert

An interactive heart health assessment tool called Method Alert allows assessment of health and determination of appropriate behavior changes. The Office on Women's Health in the Department of Health and Human Services worked with the American Heart Association to expand services of the National Women's Health Information Center (NWHIC). Its Web site is http://www.4woman.gov; it can be reached by phone at: (800) 994-WOMAN.

USDA's Interactive Healthy Eating Index (IHEI), available at http://www .usda.gov/cnpp, allows comparison of eating habits of men and women with the *US Dietary Guidelines.*

Healthy People 2010 Actions

The major objectives to promote health among adults include several diet-related behaviors (see Exhibit 9–3). These include reducing weight; lowering sodium intakes; increasing complex carbohydrates; and reducing total fat, alcohol, and saturated fat. To achieve these objectives, worksite wellness programs, as well as drug and alcohol policies, are necessary. Education and access to programs ranging from breastfeeding promotion to dental health must be available to individuals from all ethnic groups. Community nutrition professionals have an important role in the transfer of nutrition knowledge and the integration of positive nutrition behaviors into the daily lives of adults, especially pregnant and lactating women[116] (see Exhibit 9–4 for model nutrition objectives).

Exhibit 9–3 Healthy People 2010 Objectives for Adults

Objective Number		Baseline 1997	Target 2010
04-01	End-stage renal disease per 100,000,000		
	20 to 44 years	109	217
	45 to 64 years	545	217
07-03	Health-risk behavior information for college and university students	6%	25%
07-05 a	Worksite health promotion < 50 employees	UK	UK
b	... 50+ employees	34%	75%
c	... 50-99 employees	33%	75%
d	... 100-249 employees	33%	75%
e	... 250-749 employees	38%	75%
f	... 750+ employees	50%	75%
07-07	Patient and family education	UK	UK
09-11	Pregnancy prevention		
	Females 18-24 years	64%	90%
16-19a	Increase to at least 75% the proportion of mothers who breastfeed their babies in the early postpartum period and to at least 50% the proportion who continue breastfeeding until their babies are 5 to 6 months old. (Baseline: 64% at discharge from birth site and 29% at 5 to 6 months in 1998.)		

continued

16-06a	Increase to at least 90% the proportion of all pregnant women who receive prenatal care in the first trimester of pregnancy. (Baseline: 83% of live births in 1998.)		
16-06b	Proportion of pregnant women receiving early and adequate prenatal care	1998 Baseline	2010 Target
	Black women	67*	90*
	American Indian/Alaska native women	57*	90*
	Hispanic women	66*	90*
	White women	76	90
	Asian/Pacific Islander women	74	90
*Percentage of live births.			
17-04	Receipt of useful information about prescriptions from pharmacies	UK	UK
19-16	Worksite promotion of nutrition education and weight management classes at worksite, 50+ employees	28%	85%
	... at worksite or health plan 50+ employees	55%	85%
	... at health plan only	39%	85%

Source: Adapted from: US Department of Health and Human Services. DATA2010–the *Healthy People 2010* Database. *CDC Wonder.* Atlanta, Ga: Centers for Disease Control; November 2000.

Exhibit 9–4 Model Nutrition Objectives for Reduced Risk Factors

By 20__, ____% of pregnant women will avoid the harmful substance [*tobacco, alcohol, drugs, caffeine*] during pregnancy.

By 20__, ____% of women will breastfeed upon hospital discharge and ____% will continue breastfeeding for ____ months.

By 20__, ____% of [*pregnant women, lactating women, infants, women of childbearing age, adults*] will consume a nutritionally adequate and prudent diet consistent with established state or federal recommendations.

Source: Model State Nutrition Objectives. Association of State and Territorial Public Health Nutrition Directors, June 1988. Adapted from: Kaufman M. *Nutrition in Public Health–A Handbook for Developing Programs and Services.* Gaithersburg, Md: Aspen Publishers, Inc; 1990:570.

References

1. Sutherland L. Nutrition professionals in cyberspace: getting wired for the new millennium. *JADA.* 1999;11:1365-1366.
2. Lipowicz A. Effect of husbands' education on fatness of wives. *Am J Hum Biol.* 2003;15(1):1-7.
3. Flegal KM, Carroll MD, Ogden CL, Johnson CL. Prevalence and trends in obesity among US adults, 1999-2000. *JAMA.* 2002;288:1723-1727.
4. US Department of Health and Human Services. The Surgeon General's call to action to prevent and decrease overweight and obesity. Rockville, Md: US Dept of Health and Human Services, Public Health Service, Office of the Surgeon General; 2001.

5. Wright JD, Kennedy-Stephenson J, Wang CY, McDowell MA, Johnson CL. Trends in Intake of Energy and Macronutrients—United States, 1971-2000. MMWR Weekly National Center for Health Statistics, CDC; February 6, 2004;53(04):80-82.

6. Ernst ND, Obarzanek E, Clark MB, Briefel RR, Brown CD, Donato K. Cardiovascular health risks related to overweight. *J Am Diet Assoc.* 1997;97(suppl):S47-S51.

7. Chanmugam P, Guthrie JF, Cecilio S, Morton JF, Basiotis PP, Anand R. Did fat intake in the United States really decline between 1989-1991 and 1994-1996? *J Am Diet Assoc.* 2003;103:867-872.

8. Nielsen SJ, Siega-Riz AM, Popkin BM. Trends in energy intake in US between 1977 and 1996: similar shifts seen across age groups. *Obes Res.* 2002;10:370-378.

9. Nielsen SJ, Popkin BM. Patterns and trends in food portion sizes: 1977-1998. *JAMA.* 2003;289:450-453.

10. Hoyert DL, Kung H, Smith BL. *National Vital Statistics Report—Deaths: preliminary data for 2003.* Atlanta, Ga: Centers for Disease Control. Division of Vital Statistics; 2005;53(15).

11. CDC/NCHS. Births: preliminary data for 2003. *NVSR.* 2004;53(9).

12. Harvard School of Public Health. US infant mortality rates up. Boston, Mass: HPH-Now; December 10, 2004.

13. Food and Nutrition Board. National Research Council, Committee on Dietary Allowances. *Recommended Dietary Allowances.* 10th ed. Washington, DC: National Academy Press; 1989.

14. *Eating for Two: Pregnancy and Nutrition Guidelines From the California Dietetic Association.* San Diego, Calif: California Dietetic Association; 1993.

15. National Academy of Science. Institute of Medicine. *Consensus Development Conference Statement: Optimal Calcium Intake.* Bethesda, Md: June 6-8, 1994.

16. Ortega RM, Martinez RM, Lopez-Sobaler AM, Andres P, Quitas ME. Influence of calcium intake on gestational hypertension. *Ann Nutr Metab.* 1999;43(1):37-46.

17. Pitkin R. Nutrition during pregnancy. Nutritional Medicine in Medical Practice Symposium. 1993; Los Angeles, Calif.

18. Martek Bioscience Corporation. *The importance of DHA for women and their babies.* Columbia, Md: Martek; 2004.

19. Jensen CL, Frager TC, Zou Y, et al. Effects of maternal docosahexaenoic acid (DHA) supplementation on visual function and neurodevelopment of breast-fed infants. *Pediat Res.* 2001;49:448A.

20. Kris-Etherton PM, Harris, WS, Appel LJ. Omega-3 fatty acids and cardiovascular disease: new recommendations from the American Heart Association. *Arterioscler Thromb Vasc Biol.* 2003;23:151-152.

21. Otto SJ, Houwelingen AC, Antel M, et al. Maternal and neonatal essential fatty acid status in phospholipids: an international comparative study. *Eur J Clin Nutr.* 1997;51(4):232-242.

22. Al MD, Houwelingen AC, Hornsha G, et al. Relation between birth order and the maternal and neonatal docosahexaenoic acid status. *Eur J Clin Nutr.* 1997;51:548-553.

23. Zeijdner EE, Houwelingen AC, Kesder AD, et al. Essential fatty acid status in plasma phospholipids of mother and neonate after multiple pregnancy. *Prostaglandins Leukot Essent Fatty Acids.* 1997;56(5):395-401.

24. Agostoni C, Marangoni F, Giovannini M. Long chain polyunsaturated fatty acids, infant formula, and breast feeding. *Lancet.* 1998;352:1703-1704.

25. Conquer JA, Holub BJ. Dictary docosahexaenoic acid (omega-3), and vegetarian nutrition. *Vegetarian Nutr: Int J.* 1997;1/2:42-49.

26. Infante-Rivard C, Fernandez A, Gauthier R, et al. Fetal loss associated with caffeine intake before and during pregnancy. *JAMA.* 1993;270:2940–2943.

27. Olsen J. Cigarette, tea and coffee drinking and subfecundity. *Am J Epidemiol.* 1991;133(7):734-739.

28. Barr HM, Streissguth AD. Caffeine use during pregnancy and child outcome: a 7-year prospective study. *Neurotoxicol Teratol.* 1991;13:441-448.

29. American Academy of Pediatrics' Committee on Drugs. The transfer of drugs and other chemicals into human milk. *Pediatrics.* 1994;93:137-150.

30. Mills JL, Holmes LB, Aarons JH, et al. Moderate caffeine use and the risk of spontaneous abortion and intrauterine growth retardation. *JAMA.* 1993;269:595-597.

31. American Dietetic Association. National Center for Nutrition and Dietetics. *Aspartame in Pregnancy* [nutrition fact sheet]. Chicago, Ill: ADA; 1994.

32. Zeisel SH. Nutritional importance of choline for brain development. *AJCN.* 2004;23:621-626.

33. The role of DHA in pregnancy outcomes [editorial]. *Research Communique.* 2000:1-4.

34. Olsen SF, Hansen HS, Sommer S, et al. Gestational age in relation to marine n-3 fatty acids in maternal erythrocytes: a study of women in the Faroe Islands and Denmark. *Am J Obstet Gynecol.* 1991;164:1203-1209.

35. Foreman-van Drongelen MM, Al MD, van Houwelingen AC, Blanco CE, Hornstra G. Comparison between the essential fatty acid status of preterm and full-term infants, measured in umbilical vessel walls. *Early Hum Dev.* 1995;42:241-251.

36. Reece MS, McGregor JA, Allen KGD, Harris MA. Maternal and perinatal long-chain fatty acids: possible roles in preterm birth. *Am J Obstet Gynecol.* 1997;176:907-914.

37. Olsen SF, Sorensen JD, Secher NJ, et al. Randomized controlled trial of effect of fish-oil supplementation on pregnancy duration. *Lancet.* 1992;339:1003-1007.

38. Borod E, Atkinson R, Barclay WR, Carlson SE. Effects of third trimester consumption of eggs high in docosahexaenoic acid on docosahexaenoic acid status and pregnancy. *Lipids.* 1999;34:S231.

39. Baguma-Nibasheka M, Brenna JT, Nathanielsz PW. Delay of preterm delivery in sheep by omega-3-long-chain polyunsaturates. *Biol Reprod.* 1999;60:698-701.

40. Caldwell M, ed. *Quality Assurance/Quality Improvement Criteria for Nutritional Care of Pregnant and Postpartum Women and Adolescents.* Public Health Nutrition Practice Group of the American Dietetic Association, and USDHHS, DHS, CDC, NCCDPHP, ADA, Division of Nutrition. September 1993.

41. Mitchell MC, Lerner E. Weight gain and pregnancy outcome in underweight and normal weight women. *J Am Diet Assoc.* 1989;89:634-638.

42. *Nutrition During Pregnancy, Part I Weight Gain, Part II Nutrient Supplements.* Washington, DC: Institute of Medicine, National Academy Press; 1990.

43. *Primer on Indicator Development and Application. Measuring Quality in Health Care.* Oakbrook Terrace, Ill: Joint Commission on Accreditation of Health Care Organizations; 1990.

44. National Association of WIC Directors. *1999 Legislative Agenda.* Washington, DC. Available at: www.fns.usda.gov/WIC/lawsandregulations/. Accessed December 15, 2006.

45. Kresge J. *WIC Participant and Program Characteristics—PC2002.* Washington, DC: Office of Analysis, Nutrition, and Evaluation, Food and Nutrition Service, USDA; September 2003.

46. American Heart Association. *1993 Heart and Stroke Statistics.* Dallas, Tex: American Heart Association; 1992.

47. American Cancer Society. *Cancer Facts and Figures.* Atlanta, Ga: American Cancer Society; 1994.

48. Avioli LV. Significance of osteoporosis: a growing international health care problem. *Calcif Tissue Int.* 1991;(suppl 5B):25-45.

49. The Gallup Organization. *Women's Knowledge and Behavior Regarding Health and Fitness.* Survey conducted for the American Dietetic Association and Weight Watchers International; June 1993.

50. National Institutes of Health. *Women's Health Initiative.* 1993; (Section 1):1-58.

51. National Institutes of Health. *Women's Health Initiative* [activity reports]. 2000.

52. Healy B. So what to do now, ladies? *US News & World Report.* March 2004:68.

53. *Healthy People 2000: National Health Promotion and Disease Prevention Objectives.* Washington, DC: US Dept of Health and Human Services; 1991. DHHS (PHS) publication 91-50212.

54. Finn S. 1993. ADA's nutrition and health campaign for women promotes research and behavioral change. *Perspect Appl Nutr.* Winter 1993;1(3):3-7.

55. Kant AK, Schatzkin A, Graubard BI, Schairer C. A prospective study of diet quality and mortality in women. *JAMA.* 2000;283:2109-2115.

56. Black DM, Cummings SR, Genant HK, et al. Axial and appendicular bone mineral and a woman's lifetime risk of hip fracture. *J Bone Min Res.* 1992;7:633-638.

57. Recker RR, Davies KM, Dowd RM, Heaney RP. The effect of low-dose continuous estrogen and progesterone therapy with calcium and vitamin D on bone in elderly women. *Ann Intern Med.* 1999;130:897-904.

58. Allan JD, Mayo K, Michel Y. Body size values of white and black women. *Res Nurs Health.* 1993;16:323-333.

59. Folsom A, Kushi L, Anderson K, et al. Associations of general and abdominal obesity with multiple health outcomes in older women—the Iowa Women's Health Study. *Arch Intern Med.* 2000;160:2117-2128.

60. Stettler N, Tershakovec A, Zemel B, et al. Early risk factors for increased adiposity: a cohort study of African American subjects followed from birth to young adulthood. *Am J Clin Nutr.* 2000;72:378-383.

61. Liu S, Manson JE, Stampfer MJ, et al. Whole grain consumption and risk of ischemic stroke in women. *JAMA.* 2000;284(12):1534-1540.

62. National Cholesterol Education Program. *Report of the Expert Panel on Detection, Evaluation, and Treatment of High Blood Cholesterol in Adults.* Bethesda, Md: US Dept of Health and Human Services, Public Health Service, National Institutes of Health, National Heart, Lung, and Blood Institute; January 1988. NIH Pub. No. 88-2925.

63. *Supermarket Savvy. Benefits of Tree Nuts.* Linda McDonald Associates, Inc., Houston, Tex; July/August 2000.

64. Stampfer MJ, Hennekens CH, Manson JE, Golditz GA, Rosner B, Willett WC. Vitamin E consumption and the risk of coronary disease in women. *N Engl J Med.* 1993;328:1444-1449.

65. National Digestive Diseases Information Clearinghouse. *Lactose Intolerance.* Bethesda, Md: National Institutes of Health; April 1994. NIH Publ. No. 94-2751.

66. Sahi T. Genetics and epidemiology of adult-type hypolactasia. *Scand J Gastroenterol.* 1994;202(suppl):7-20.

67. Carroccio A, Montalto G, Cavera G, Notarbatolo A. Lactose intolerance and self-reported milk intolerance: relationship with lactose maldigestion and nutrient intake. Lactase Deficiency Study Group. *J Am Coll Nutr.* December 1998;17(6):631-636.

68. Bock SA. Prospective appraisal of complaints of adverse reactions to foods in children during the first 3 years of life. *Pediatrics.* May 1987; 79(5):683-688.

69. Hill DJ, Hosking CS. The cow milk allergy complex: overlapping disease profiles in infancy. *Eur J Clin Nutr.* 1995;49(S1):1-12.

70. Marcus BH, Stanton AL. Evaluation of relapse prevention and reinforcement to promote exercise. *Res Q Ex Sp.* 1993;64(4):447-452.

71. US Department of Health and Human Services and the American Heart Association. PHS. *Exercise and Your Heart.* Bethesda, Md: National Institutes of Health; August 1993. NIH publication No. 93-1677.

72. American College of Sports Medicine. *ACSM's Guidelines for Exercise Testing and Prescription.* 5th ed. Baltimore, Md: Williams & Wilkins; 1995.

73. Pangrazi R, Corbin C. The physical activity pyramid. *Top Clin Nutr.* 1999;14(3):53-61.

74. Rockhill B, Willett WC, Hunter DJ, Manson JE, Hankinson SE, Colditz GA. A prospective study of recreational physical activity and breast cancer risk. *Arch Intern Med.* October 25, 1999;159(19):2290-2296.

75. Hu FB, Sigal RJ, Rish-Ewards JW, et al. Walking compared with vigorous physical activity and risk of type 2 diabetes in women: a prospective study. *JAMA.* October 20, 1999;282(15):1433-1439.

76. Research roundup. *Environ Nutr.* December 1999;22(12):8.

77. American Dietetic Association. *Men's Health Campaign.* Chicago, Ill: American Dietetic Association; 1991.

78. Goldfield GS, Epstein LH. Fruit and vegetable research. *Health Psychol.* 2003;21(3):229-303.

79. Kaplan J. Hormones and behavior. *Food Navigator: News & Analysis.* April 5, 2004;45(4):278-284.

80. Shute N. What about men? *US News & World Report.* March 15, 2004; 64-66.

81. Kris-Etherton P, ed. *Cardiovascular Disease: Nutrition for Prevention and Treatment.* Chicago, Ill: American Dietetic Association; 1990:98-107.

82. Lipid Research Clinics Program. The Lipid Research Clinic's Coronary Primary Prevention Trial results, I: reduction in incidence of coronary heart disease. *JAMA.* 1984;251:351-364.

83. Lipid Research Clinics Program. The Lipid Research Clinic's Coronary Primary Prevention Trial results, II: the relationship of reduction in incidence of coronary heart disease to cholesterol lowering. *JAMA.* 1984;251:365-372.

84. Multiple Risk Factor Intervention Trial Research Group. Multiple Risk Factor Trial, Risk factor changes and mortality result. *JAMA.* 1982;248:1465.

85. Illingworth DR Meninolin plus colestipol in therapy for severe heterozygous familial hypercholesterolemia. *Ann Intern Med.* 1984;101:598-604.

86. Veterans Administration Cooperative Study Group on Antihypertensive Agents. Effects of treatment on morbidity in hypertension, II: results in patients with diastolic blood pressure averaging 90 through 114 mm Hg. *JAMA*. 1970;213:1143.

87. Blair SN, Capuzzi CM, Gottlieb SO, Nguyen T, Morgan JM, Cater NB. Incremental reduction of serum total cholesterol and low-density lipoprotein cholesterol with the addition of plant stanol ester-containing spread to statin therapy. *Am J Cardiol*. July 1, 2000;86(1):46-52.

88. Martinez-Gonzalez MA, Fernandez-Garcia J, Sanchez-Izquierdo F, Lardelli-Claret P, Jimenez Moleon J, Galvez-Vargas R. Life-style factors associated with changes in serum lipids in a follow-up study of cardiovascular risk factors. *Eur J Epidemiol*. 1998;14(6):525-533.

89. Toso C, Morel P, Bucher P, et al. Insulin independence after conversion to tacrolimus and sirolimus-based immunosuppression in islet-kidney recipients. *Transplantation*. October 15, 2003 76(7):1133-1134.

90. Good B. Dinner with all the fixin's. *Men's Health*. November 2000: 82-90.

91. Lonn E, Bosch J, Yusuf S, et al. Effects of long-term vitamin E supplementation on cardiovascular events and cancer: a randomized controlled trial. *JAMA*. 2005;293(11):1338-1347.

92. *Dietary Guidelines for Americans*. Washington, DC: US Dept of Agriculture and US Dept of Health and Human Services; 2005.

93. Schapell DS. A critical evaluation of popular low calorie diets in America: part I. *Top Clin Nutr*. 1988;3:36-40.

94. Kurtz C. Ephedra: a weight loss supplement. *California Council Newsletter*. Summer 2000:12-13.

95. Edlin G, Golanty E. *Health and Wellness—A Holistic Approach*. 4th ed. Sudbury, Mass: Jones and Bartlett Publishers; 1992:111-112.

96. Cooper K. *The New Aerobics*. New York: Bantam Books; 1970.

97. Drury TF, ed. Assessing physical fitness and physical activity in population-based surveys. Washington, DC: National Center for Health Statistics; 269. DHHS Pub. No. (PHS) 89-1253;1989.

98. Read MH, Bock MA, Carpenter K, et al. Health beliefs and supplement use: adults in seven western states. *J Am Diet Assoc*. 1989;89(12):1812-1813.

99. Gray GE, PagniniHill A, Ross RK, Henderson BE. Vitamin supplement use in a southern California retirement community. *J Am Diet Assoc*. 1986;86:800.

100. Levy AS, Schuchez RE. Patterns of nutrient intake among dietary supplement users: attitudinal and behavioral correlates. *J Am Diet Assoc*. 1987;87:754.

101. Ranno BS, Wardlaw GM, Geiger CJ. What characterizes elderly women who overuse vitamin and mineral supplements? *J Am Diet Assoc*. 1988;88:347.

102. National Center for Health Statistics. *Third National Health and Nutrition Examination Survey (NHANES III), 1988-94*. NHANES III Vitamin and Mineral Supplements Data File Documentation. April 1998. Series 11, No. 2A.

103. Radimer KL, Subar AF, Thompson FE. Nonvitamin, nonmineral dietary supplements: issues and findings from NHANES III. *J Am Diet Assoc*. 2000;100:447-454.

104. American Dietetic Association. *Survey of American Dietary Habits*. Chicago, Ill: American Dietetic Association; October 1991.

105. Huang Y, Hoerr S, Song W. Breakfast is the lowest fat meal for young adult women. *JNE*. 1997;29:184-188.

106. Haines P, Guilkey D, Popkin B. Trends in breakfast consumption of adults between 1965 and 1991. *J Am Diet Assoc.* 1996;96:1-7.

107. Fresh trends 92: a profile of fresh produce consumers. *The Packers Focus.* 1992.

108. Thompson B, Demark-Wahnefried W, Taylor G, et al. Baseline fruit and vegetable intake among adults in seven 5 a day study centers located in diverse geographic areas. *J Am Diet Assoc.* October 1999; 99(10):1241-1248.

109. National Restaurant Association. *Meal Consumption Behavior.* Washington, DC: National Restaurant Association; 1991.

110. US Department of Labor, Bureau of Labor Statistics. *Average Annual Expenditures and Characteristics of All Consumer Units, Consumer Expenditure Survey, 1993-2001.* Available at: http://www.bls.gov/ cex/2001/standard/multiyr.pdf.

111. Bowman SA, Vinyard BT. Fast food consumption of US adults: impact on energy and nutrient intakes and overweight status. *J Am College Nutr.* 2004;23(2),163-168.

112. US Department of Agriculture, Agricultural Research Service, Food Survey Research Group. *The Continuing Survey of Food Intakes by Individuals and the Diet and Health Knowledge Survey, 1994-96* [CD-ROM data]. Washington, DC: USDA; 1996.

113. Ling AM, Horwath C. Defining and measuring stages of change for dietary behaviors: readiness to meet fruit, vegetable and grain guidelines among Chinese Singaporeans. *J Am Diet Assoc.* 2000;100:898.

114. Tribole E, Resch E. *Intuitive Eating: A Recovery Book for the Chronic Dieter/Rediscover the Pleasures of Eating and Rebuild Your Body Image.* NewYork, NY: St. Martin's Paperbacks; 1995.

115. US Department of Agriculture. *Cooperative Extension System.* Washington, DC: USDA; 1994.

116. Kaufman M. *Nutrition in Public Health—a Handbook for Developing Programs and Services.* Gaithersburg, Md: Aspen Publishers, Inc; 1990:570.

OLDER ADULTS

Learning Objectives

- Characterize the nutritional needs of older adults in the United States.
- Describe the nutrition program components of Title IIIC of the Older Americans Act.
- Outline the qualifications of a community nutrition professional who functions in a congregate food service setting.
- Specify primary, secondary, and tertiary intervention for older adults at different stages of health.
- List the reasons for expanding the recommended dietary allowances for the decades of life after 50 years of age.
- Describe the Nutrition Screening Initiative and the different levels of screening.
- Discuss compressed morbidity, syndrome X, and ageism.

High Definition Nutrition

Ageism—the feelings of prejudice that result from misconceptions and myths about older people. This prejudice generally evolves from beliefs that aging makes people senile, unattractive, asexual, weak, and useless.

Compressed morbidity—a few years of major illness among the very old.

Old-old—age 75 to 84.

Oldest-old—age 85 and over.

Social gerontologists—professionals who study how the older population and the aging process are affected by and affect the social structure.

Social gerontology—the area of gerontology concerned not only with the impact of social and sociocultural conditions on the process of aging but also with the social consequences of this process.

Young-old—age 65 to 74.

Older Adults in the United States

Members of the newest generation of older adults have broken out of the rest home image and generated some unrest of their own by their desire to remain healthy and vital into their 90s and 100s. Over 40,000 older adults (or elders, as many prefer being called) have reached their 100th birthday. This growing and graying portion of our population has far from a rest home mentality. With an estimated 22% of the US population at age 65 or older by 2050, the upper limit for being old has increased.[1]

History will be made by the way the United States cares for its older adult population. The stage has been keenly described by Daniel Perry, executive director of the Alliance for Aging Research:

> The US cannot afford to find itself in the 21st century with vastly larger populations of older persons but without a much higher level of knowledge about the biology of aging and health than we have in the 1990s. The senior citizens of 2020 and beyond—today's "Baby Boomers"—must benefit from as-yet-undiscovered insights in health, medicine, and nutrition. Otherwise the future may be marked by excessive demand for long-term nursing care and severe rationing of medical care.
>
> A more positive alternative future, one marked by improved health, vitality, and personal independence for older Americans, is an achievable goal. Already nursing home admissions are falling relative to the growing numbers of people in their 70s, 80s, and 90s. The newest figures show that the dependency rate among the very old declined in the 1980s, catching even professional demographers by surprise. Among the reasons cited: a higher level of education among those now entering old age, higher economic status, the applications of new technologies such as joint replacements and cataract surgery, and better nutrition than that experienced by the elderly in the past.
>
> If we are to achieve healthy and successful aging on a mass scale in our society, the role of good nutrition will be a key to success.[2]

Social gerontologists view aging in terms of 4 distinct processes:

- *Chronological aging* is aging on the basis of a person's years from birth. Ages of individuals are defined as the "young-old," the "old-old," and the "oldest-old."[1]
- *Biological aging* refers to the physical changes that reduce the efficiency of organ systems such as the lungs, heart, and circulatory system.
- *Psychological aging* includes the changes that occur in sensory and perceptual processes and mental functioning involving memory, learning, and intelligence. Changes in adaptive capacity, personality, drives, and motives also demonstrate psychological aging.
- *Social aging* refers to an individual's changing roles and relationships in the social structure. These roles and relationships involve interactions with family and friends; with the working world; and within religious, professional, and political organizations.

Senescence is the period of life generally beginning after age 30 when changes that reflect normal declines in all organ systems occur. It occurs gradually throughout the body, ultimately reducing the viability of different body systems and increasing their vulnerability to disease. This is the final stage in the development of an organism.

Gerontologists study the ability of older adults to remain independent and to maintain their competence. Competence is considered the theoretical upper limit of an individual's abilities to function in the areas of health, social behavior, and cognition.[3] Some of the abilities needed to adapt to environmental pressure and change include problem solving and learning; performing on the job; and managing the basic activities of daily living such as dressing, grooming, and cooking.[3,4]

A rapid increase occurred in the median age of the US population from 1970 to 1990: it increased from 28 to 33 years of age. This 5-year increase in the median age during a 20-year period is a noteworthy demographic event.[5] Key factors creating this rise include a steep decline in the birth rate after the mid-1960s, coupled with high birth rates from 1890 to 1915 and just after World War II, which yielded the baby boomers. Additional factors include the large number of immigrants entering the United States via Ellis Island, New York, before the 1920s.

A dramatic demonstration of the changing US age distribution is the shift in the proportion of older adults compared to young persons. In 1970, about 4% of the US population was 65 or more years of age. Young persons 0 to 17 years of age comprised 40% of the population. By 1980, the reduced birth rates of the 1970s created a decline of young persons to 28% percent of the population. By 2030, there will be an almost equal proportion of young persons 0 to 17 years compared with elderly (22% and 21%, respectively).[6] After 2030, current trends will create a death rate that is greater than the birth rate.

The population aged 85 and older is called the oldest-old.[7] This group has grown more rapidly than any other age group in the United States. In 1990, of the 31.2 million persons aged 65 and over in the United States, 32% were age 75 to 84, and 10% were age 85 and over.[8] Mortality rates among adults have declined significantly since the mid-1940s. The result is an unprecedented number of individuals reaching advanced old age and requiring health and social services.[7] The population of oldest-old Americans has thereby increased 23 times, compared to a 12 times growth in the 75 to 84 age group and an eightfold increase among individuals 65 to 74 years of age. The number of individuals over 85 years of age increased by 300% from 1960 to 1990.[6] This age group reached 4.6 million in 2000 and is expected to reach 8 million in 2030 before the baby boomers reach old age. The baby boomers will not begin to turn 85 until after 2030.

A Population That Is Older, Healthier, and Wealthier

Older Americans are healthier, wealthier, and better educated than ever before, but many older Americans fall through the cracks. Within 30 years, 1 in 5 Americans—70 million people—will be 65 or older, and almost 400,000 could be 100, as baby boomers born between 1946 and 1964 reach retirement age. Older Americans 2000: Key Indicators of Well-Being broke the fading myth that the growing legions of elderly are living in poverty and ill health. American women could only hope to live to the age of 51 in 1900; today, they can expect to celebrate their 80th birthdays. Men have also seen their life expectancy soar from 48 to 78.[9]

Fewer elderly people than children live below the poverty line. The proportion of seniors living in poverty declined from 35% in 1959 to 11% in 1998. That is because of better Social Security and pensions, improved health care, and higher levels of education. About 72% of non-Hispanic whites aged 65 and older had finished high school, compared with 44% of older blacks and 29% of elderly Hispanics. Many older blacks have fewer assets and more debts than older whites. Although the median net worth in households headed by people 65 and older increased by 69% between 1984 and 1999, half of older black households were worth less than $13,000 in 2003, once debts were subtracted from the value of real estate, stocks, bonds, and other assets. That can be compared with a median net worth of $181,000 in older white families. Many older blacks do not own their own homes, have little savings, and have not bought stocks. While the situation improved between 1984 and 1994, it deteriorated sharply between 1994 and 1999.

The economic gap is partially blamed for a greater incidence of chronic diseases such as arthritis and diabetes among blacks. In 1995, 67.2% of blacks aged 70 and older suffered from arthritis, compared with 57.9% of non-Hispanic whites. More than 20% of blacks in that age group had diabetes, nearly double the rate for non-Hispanic whites. The upcoming generations of younger African Americans and Hispanics may be destined for the same fate.

Due to the graying of the nation, new studies focusing on social gerontology seek to identify the processes that promote successful aging and keep aging adults independent and functional. Characteristics of normal aging are listed in Exhibit 10–1. Almost 43% of the remaining years of men and women currently between the ages of 65 and 69 will be spent depending on others. Their dependence will involve activities of daily living including rising from bed or a chair, bathing, dressing, and eating (see Table 10–1). A decrease in functional capacity corresponds to the time when the most drastic reductions in muscle mass and strength are observed. Further, there is a strong association between functional dependency and nutritional status in elders with chronic illness.[10]

Framingham Study data indicate that 40% of women from 55 to 64, 45% from 65 to 75, and 65% from 75 to 84 could not lift 4.5 kg, and a similar percentage could not perform heavy household work.[11] This decreased capacity places older persons at increased risk of dependence and institutionalization.

Among the very old, muscle strength is highly related to function and significantly and positively correlated to normal walking speed for males and females. Among very frail, institutionalized men and women, muscle strength is associated with walking speed, chair stand time, and the ability to climb stairs.

Nursing home residents classified as "fallers" are significantly weaker in the knees and ankles. Of a sample of 1,042 home-dwelling men and women over 60 years of age living in their own homes, 365 (35%) reported 1 or more falls in the prior year. Factors that separated fallers from nonfallers were polypharmacy (the practice of taking multiple medications), leg muscle power, arthritis, and handgrip strength of the dominant hand. Handgrip strength was the most important factor and can be predictive of lower-extremity strength.[12]

Because age-related loss in muscle mass may be an important determinant in the reduced maximal aerobic capacity seen in elderly men and

Exhibit 10–1   Characteristics of Normal Aging

Individuals age at very different rates. Even for 1 person, organs and organ systems have different rates of decline. Data from the Baltimore Longitudinal Study of Aging suggest these general changes:

- *Heart*: The heart grows slightly larger with age. Maximal oxygen consumption during exercise declines in men by about 10% with each decade of adult life, and in women by about 7.5%. Cardiac output remains basically the same, even with increased efficiency of the heart.

- *Lungs*: Maximum vital capacity declines by about 40% between 20 and 70 years of age.

- *Brain*: The brain loses neurons but increases connections between cell synapses and regrows branch-like extensions called dendrites and axons, which transmit brain messages.

- *Kidneys*: The kidneys lose efficiency extracting wastes from the blood; this is accompanied by a decline in bladder capacity. Urinary incontinence occurs with tissue atrophy.

- *Body fat*: The body redistributes fat from under the skin to deeper parts of the body. Women tend to store fat in the hips and thighs, whereas men store fat in the abdominal area.

- *Muscles*: Muscle mass decreases by about 22% for women and 23% for men between 30 and 70 years of age.

- *Sight*: Vision acuity and difficulty focusing begin in the 40s. Susceptibility to glare and difficulty seeing at low levels of illumination increase with aging.

- *Hearing*: Hearing declines more quickly in men than in women, with an additional decline in the ability to hear higher frequencies.

- *Personality*: Personality is consistent unless it is altered by a disease process.

Source: Adapted from: National Institutes of Health, National Institute on Aging. What is normal aging? *In Search of the Secrets of Aging.* Washington, DC: National Institutes of Health, National Institute on Aging; 1993:25. Publication No. 93–2756.

women, researchers have applied muscle strengthening and training programs to frail, institutionalized, elderly men and women. One program involved 10 individuals whose mean age was 90 ±3 years (range 86 to 96 years).[12] Muscle strength increased by almost 180%, and muscle size increased by 11% after 8 weeks of training. Increased muscle strength promoted gait, speed, and balance. Significant muscle hypertrophy was observed. Aging does not decrease the ability to adapt to a progressive resistance training program, if the training has sufficient intensity to elicit significant gains in strength and muscle mass. Sufficient intensity is defined as above 60% of maximal lifting capacity.

Assessing and correcting any nutritional deficiencies are essential because specific nutritional deficiencies can place older adults at risk or decrease their

TABLE 10–1   Range of Functional Status of Older Adults

Activities	Independent	Dependent
Personal Activities		
Bathing	Bathes self completely or requires help with hard-to-reach parts (i.e., back).	Does not bathe self; requires assistance with more than one body part; requires help getting into or out of bath or shower.
Dressing	Dresses self including getting clothes from closet or drawers and manages fasteners.	Does not dress self.
Toileting	Manages toileting and hygienic activities by self.	Needs assistance getting to and using toilet or uses commode or bedpan.
Transferring	Gets in and out of bed and chair without assistance.	Needs assistance getting in and out of bed or chair.
Continence	Self-controlled.	Partial or total.
Feeding	Gets food from plate to mouth.	Needs assistance eating or is dependent on tube or parenteral feeding.
Instrumental Activities		
Telephone use	Finds and dials numbers.	Cannot use telephone.
Shopping	Manages shopping for needs.	Unable to shop.
Food preparation	Plans, prepares, and serves meals.	Requires meals prepared and served by someone else.
Housekeeping	Can maintain living quarters alone.	Does not perform housekeeping tasks.
Laundry	Does own laundry.	Needs laundry done by others.
Transportation	Travels independently by public transportation or car.	Does not travel at all.
Medications	Manages dose and time of medications.	Cannot manage medications.
Finances	Manages all financial matters.	Cannot handle money.

Source: Adapted from: Chernoff R. Meeting the nutritional needs of the elderly in the institutional setting. *Nutrition Reviews.* 1994;52(4):133.

ability to respond to the exercise. Dehydration, due to a decreased sensation of thirst and a decreased ability to concentrate urine, affects muscle response. Vitamin D deficiency due to decreased exposure to the sun and decreased consumption of milk is likewise associated with decreased muscle strength.

Undernutrition of older adults has been shown to have a positive association with dysphagia, slow eating, low protein intake, poor appetite, the presence of a feeding tube, and chronological age. Overnutrition, commonly seen as excess food intake, has been shown to be inversely associated with poor appetite, number of feeding impairments, protein intake, and mental state.[13]

Chronic diseases may predispose older adults to impaired mobility and falls. The reduced physical activity linked with institutionalization may increase their functional impairment. However, increased levels of physical activity through walking and/or strengthening exercises may reverse the effects of a very sedentary life.[12]

Based on current mortality rates, a 65-year-old person in 1997 could expect to live to be nearly 83 years old. Most older persons are not severely limited in their daily activities, despite living with chronic conditions. Fewer than 10% of noninstitutionalized persons 70 years old are unable to perform one or more activities of daily living (bathing, dressing, etc.). This disability increases with age from close to 5% among 70- to 74-year-olds to nearly 22% among those 85 years and older. Nearly 22% of noninstitutionalized persons 85 years of age or older are unable to perform one or more activities of daily living (bathing, dressing, using the toilet, etc.). Seven out of 10 nondisabled persons 65 years of age and over participate in some form of exercise at least once every 2 weeks, but only about one third achieve recommended exercise levels.[14]

Theories of Aging

Theories of aging range from programmed theories to error theories about the process.[13] Programmed theories propose that aging progresses through a biological timetable, perhaps continuing the one that regulates childhood growth and development. Error theories emphasize environmental damage to body cells, organs, and systems, which gradually causes them to function inadequately. These theories overlap, have unique characteristics, and are discussed in the following sections.[15,16]

No single theory explains all the changes accompanying aging. Aging involves many processes, interactive and interdependent, that influence life span and health. Gerontologists are studying the multitude of factors that may be involved, including environmental factors that affect aging cells, tissues, and organs, and the body's genetic response to such factors.[17]

Programmed Theories

The *programmed senescence theory* views aging as the result of the sequential switching on and off of certain genes. Senescence becomes the time when age-associated deficits are manifested. The *endocrine theory* proposes that biological clocks controlled by hormones set the pace of aging. *Immunological theory* suggests sequential decline in immune system functions, leading to an increased vulnerability to infectious disease, aging, and death.

Error Theories

The *wear and tear theory* proposes that cells and tissues have vital parts that wear out, whereas the *rate of living theory* suggests that the greater an organism's rate of oxygen basal metabolism, the shorter its life span. The *cross-linking theory* proposes that an accumulation of cross-linked proteins damages cells and tissues, thereby slowing bodily processes. The *free radicals theory* suggests that accumulated damage caused by oxygen radicals causes cells and then organs to stop functioning. The *error catastrophe theory* links damage to mechanisms that synthesize proteins, resulting in faulty proteins that accumulate and cause catastrophic damage to cells, tissues, and organs. The *somatic mutation theory* proposes that genetic mutations occur and accumulate with increasing age, which causes cells to deteriorate and malfunction.[18]

Aging Processes

Aging processes can be divided into 3 general categories: genetic, biochemical, and physiological.[17]

Genetic Processes

The proteins produced by genes have many functions in each cell and tissue in the body. Some of their actions relate to aging. Antioxidants appear to prevent damage to cells, and some proteins may repair damaged DNA or help cells respond to stress. Some proteins appear to have direct control of cell senescence.

Cell senescence can be visually observed. Inside a cell, threadlike pairs of chromosomes float in cytoplasm along with other tiny organelles that perform the cell's work. The cell is surrounded by a membrane whose surface sends and receives messages from other cells. The chromosomes are rodlike structures that divide into 2 chromosomes, which migrate to opposite sides of the cell and form a nucleus. The entire process repeats itself over and over.[19]

This process of mitosis or asexual cell division occurs in nearly all of the 100 trillion or so cells composing the human body. However, after a certain number of divisions, cells experience a state of cell senescence and they do not divide or proliferate. DNA synthesis is blocked.[20] An example is the young human fibroblasts or collagen-producing cells, which divide about 50 times and then stop. This phenomenon has been named the *Hayflick limit*, after Leonard Hayflick.[21]

Gerontologists have found links between senescence and human life spans based on the Hayflick limit. Fibroblasts taken from 75-year-olds have fewer divisions remaining than cells from children, and the longer the life span of a species, the higher its Hayflick limit. (For example, human fibroblasts have a higher Hayflick limit than mice fibroblasts.)

Biochemical Processes

The biochemistry of aging remains fascinating and involves research about the damage of cells by oxygen radicals, glucose cross-linking of proteins, and even the differing role of proteins (e.g., heat shock proteins, hormones, and growth factors).

Oxygen Radicals

Oxygen radicals demolish proteins and damage nucleic acids in cells. The free radical theory of aging suggests that damage caused by oxygen radicals is responsible for many of the bodily changes that come with aging, as well as for degenerative disorders (including cancer), atherosclerosis, cataracts, and neurodegeneration.[22]

Glucose Cross-Linking

Blood sugar or glucose is also suspected as a cause of cellular deterioration. During glycosylation, glucose molecules attach themselves to proteins and initiate a chain of chemical reactions that results in proteins binding together or cross-linking. This alters their biological and structural roles. Cross-links, which have been termed advanced glycosylation end products, appear to toughen tissues and are linked to stiffening connective tissue (collagen), hardened arteries, clouded eyes, reduced nerve function, and inefficient kidneys.

These deficiencies often accompany aging and appear at younger ages in people with diabetes. Thereby, much research has focused on the relationship of cross-linking to diabetes and aging.[17]

DNA Repair

In the normal life of a cell, DNA undergoes continual damage from oxygen radicals, ultraviolet light, and other toxic agents. Damage involves deletions or destroyed sections, mutations, or changes in the sequence of DNA bases comprising the genetic code. Biologists suggest that the DNA damage accumulates and deteriorates tissues and organs. Heat-shock proteins are produced when cells are exposed to various stressors including heat, toxic heavy metals, chemicals, and behavioral and psychological stress.

Hormones

At the Veterans Administration hospitals in Milwaukee and Chicago, a small group of men 60 years and over received recombinant human growth hormone injections 3 times a week. These injections dramatically reversed some signs of aging and increased their lean body mass, reduced excess fat, and thickened their skin. Signs of aging returned when the injections stopped.[17]

Hormone replacement using estrogen alleviates the discomforts of menopause. Estrogen lessens the accelerated bone loss and may contribute to a decrease in cardiovascular disease among older adults. Testosterone replacement may benefit aging men by increasing bone mass, muscle mass, and strength. Hormones are affected by growth or trophic factors, such as insulin-like growth factor (IGF-1) and the growth hormone, which modulate cell activities.[17]

Physiological Processes

Many answers to questions about normal aging are coming from the Baltimore Longitudinal Study of Aging. This longitudinal study began in 1958, and the researchers are studying the aging process in more than 1,000 people (primarily men) from age 20 to beyond age 90.[23]

Researchers have found that variations in human development increase as people age and that organ systems within a single individual can change at different rates. These findings suggest that aging is a multifactorial process that is influenced by genetic factors, lifestyle, and disease processes.

The National Institute of Aging's Biomarkers of Aging project began in 1987. It is a 10-year project to identify key biological signs that characterize the aging process. Researchers believe that biomarkers are a better measure of an organism's aging status than chronological age. Biomarkers improve the ability to study normal aging, diseases, and antiaging interventions. Two organ systems, the endocrine system and the immune system, are the focus of much of the physiological research on aging.[17-24] Other factors include energy consumption and behavioral factors.

The Immune System

Many cells, substances, and organs compose the immune system. The thymus, spleen, tonsils, bone marrow, and lymphatic system produce, store, and transport B lymphocytes and T lymphocytes, antibodies, interleukins, and interferon. White blood cells are lymphocytes that fight invading bacteria and other foreign cells.

Lymphocytes are classified as either B cells or T cells. B cells mature in the bone marrow. One of their functions is to secrete antibodies in response to infectious agents or antigens. T cells develop in the thymus and are classified as cytotoxic T cells and helper T cells. Cytotoxic T cells attack infected or damaged cells. Helper T cells produce chemicals called lymphokines, which mobilize other immune system substances and cells.[24]

The Endocrine System

The thymus shrinks in size as people age. The number of T cells remains fairly constant, while the proportion of proliferation and function declines. In older adults, T cells destroyed by trauma (such as decubitus ulcers) take longer to renew than they do in younger people.

The interleukins are 1 group of T-cell products that relay signals regulating the immune response. Interleukin-6, which increases with age, may interfere with the immune response. Interleukin-2 stimulates T-cell proliferation but declines as people age.

Energy Restriction

Mice fed diets with all essential nutrients but 30–60% fewer calories survive several months longer than mice on a normal feeding schedule. Energy restriction has been shown to increase the life spans of nearly every animal species, including protozoa, fruit flies, mice, rats, and other laboratory animals. Primates are currently being studied.[17]

Behavioral Factors

Other aspects of eating and exercise influence changes commonly seen with aging. High blood lipid levels, alteration of blood glucose and insulin, obesity, and increased body fat at the waist and abdomen are common among older people. This constellation has been given the name *syndrome X* (see Chapter 17). The relationship of syndrome X to heart and other cardiovascular diseases is being studied.[24]

Syndrome X may be prevented with low-fat and low-cholesterol eating patterns and physical activity regimens. Overall nutrient intake, such as calcium and vitamin D, slows the thinning of bones that is common with aging in older women that predisposes them to osteoporosis. Vitamin E may be important to the immune system, and beta-carotene, vitamin C, and vitamin E may retard oxidative damage.[24]

What is startling to many experts is the finding that most older people are not getting the recommended dietary allowances (RDAs) for some nutrients. The Baltimore Longitudinal Study on Aging found deficiencies among elderly people in calcium; zinc; iron; magnesium; vitamins B_6, B_{12}, D, and E; and folic acid.[23] The US Department of Agriculture (USDA) Human Nutrition Research Center on Aging confirmed the finding; however, it is compounded by the fact that RDAs are just now expanding to encompass older people. RDAs have generally been identified as a composite for adults 51 years of age and older.[25]

Ethnic Minorities and Older Adults

Ethnic minorities comprise 14% of the US population over 65 years of age. Ethnic minorities include a smaller proportion of elderly and a larger proportion of younger adults than the white population. In 1990, 13% of whites, 8% of African Americans, and 5% of Hispanics were 65 years of age or older. Higher fertility and mortality rates exist for the nonwhite population under age 65 compared to the white population under 65 years of age. In the year 2000, the proportion of older persons increased at a higher rate for the nonwhite population than for the white population. This is in part due to the large proportion of children in comparison to their parents and especially their grandparents, who will reach old age. By 2020, 22% of the older population will be nonwhite; by 2050, 32% will be nonwhite.[26,27]

African-American Older Adults

The young outnumber the old among this ethnic group because of the higher fertility rates and higher mortality rates at midlife. The median age of African Americans is 24.9 years, which is almost 7 years younger than the median age for whites. Mortality rates in childhood and youth for African Americans are higher than for whites. The fastest-growing segment of the African-American population is individuals over 65 years of age. The life expectancy for black men and women was 68.9 and 75.7 years in 2002, respectively; this is in contrast with the life expectancy of 75.3 years for white men and 80.3 years for white women. There is only 1.5–2.0 years difference between these ethnic groups in life expectancy after age 65.[27]

Hispanic-American Older Adults

After African Americans, Hispanic Americans are the next largest ethnic minority population. Over 85% live in metropolitan areas. Hispanic Americans are the fastest-growing population group in the United States.[28,29] During the 10-year period from 1970 to 1980, older Hispanics in the United States increased by

74%, while there was only a 25% increase among all older adults. Hispanic Americans represent many different groups, and each group has its own distinct national and cultural heritage. These groups include Mexicans, Puerto Ricans, Cubans, Central or South Americans, and the US-born Mexican-American (Chicano) population. The Chicano population has a history in the United States that predates the entrance of English-speaking groups.

These Hispanic groups are bonded by a common language but differ substantially in terms of geographic concentration, income, and education. Mexican Americans are the largest yet poorest group. They constitute 64% of the Hispanic population. Cubans represent the wealthiest and most educated Hispanic group. They have the largest proportion of foreign-born older adults among the 3 major Hispanic groups. The largest populations of Puerto Ricans and Cubans live in New York City, New Jersey, and Florida. The Hispanic populations are concentrated in California, Texas, and Florida.[30]

The median age of the Spanish-speaking population is 23.2 years, which is 7 years younger than the US median age.[31] Only 3.5% of the Spanish-speaking population is 65 years of age and over. This percentage has remained stable over the past decade.[32]

Pacific-Asian Older Adults

About 6% of the Pacific-Asian population is 65 years of age and older. This group increased rapidly between 1965 and 1975 because of the 1965 repeal of quotas based on race and nationality and the immigration of Southeast Asians in the 1970s.[30] Asian Americans have a diversity of language, culture, acculturation to the United States, and socioeconomic status. Due to previous immigration patterns, many Japanese-American and Chinese-American elders have lived in this country for 40 to 50 years. This contrasts with older adults from Vietnam, Cambodia, and other Southeast Asian countries who immigrated after the Vietnam war. The Vietnam war immigrants tend to be less acculturated and have lower income levels than earlier immigrants.

In contrast to other ethnic minority groups and to white older adults, Pacific Islanders have a larger percentage of men living alone. This is due to a high male immigration in the early 1900s, coupled with previous restrictions on female immigration. It is not due to a higher life expectancy for Asian-Pacific men.

Demographic Characteristics

Older adults live in every US state, but they are not evenly distributed. In 1988, 31% of the older population lived in cities, 43% in suburbs, and 26% in rural areas. The Northeast is home to the oldest population of adults over 65, represented by 13.6% of its population. This contrasts with 12.6% for the total United States.[33] Florida has the highest median age in the United States (36.4 years) and Utah the lowest (25.7 years).

Change of residence is relatively rare for older people in the United States. Of the older population, 23% moved between 1975 and 1980, compared with 48% of individuals under 65 years of age. When older Americans move, they tend to move to a similar environment, such as rural to rural or large town to large town.[34]

For whites 65 years of age and older in 1988, the median level of education was 12.2 years; for African Americans it was 8.4 years, and for Hispanic Americans it was 7.5 years.[5] A disproportionate ratio of older minorities today have less than a high school education. Educational level is closely associated with economic well-being, and ethnic differences in education have a major impact on poverty levels of older adults.

Due to past mandatory retirement practices and incentives of early retirement, only 16% of men and 7% of women over age 65 are in the labor force. Part-time work is popular, and more than 50% of retired workers are employed in part-time or temporary jobs. Social Security remains the major source of income for older Americans. Increases in Social Security benefits with annual cost-of-living adjustments have improved the economic status of older Americans. Approximately 12% of senior citizens live on incomes below the poverty level, compared to 35% living below poverty level in the late 1950s.[32]

Nutritional Status of the Elderly Living Independently and in Long-Term Care

About 1.5 million US residents over 65 years of age (5%) live in one of the 20,000 nursing homes across the country. Nutritional status of older Americans, whether residing in an institution or living independently, has been profiled using various study designs. Results of these studies indicate energy intakes below the RDAs for about one third of elders, and vitamin and mineral intake below the RDAs for as many as 50% with 10–30% confirmed by serum analysis.[35-37] A fairly consistent picture of low energy and protein intake among institutionalized older adults and over 50% at high nutritional risk due to physical and serum measures have been noted.[37-39]

A prospective study of older adults in the North Chicago Veterans Affairs Medical Center included a 67-item clinical database. In univariate analysis, 7 items were significant predictors of death among the 55 men who died: age, functional level, triceps skinfold, midarm circumference, albumin, cholesterol, and hematocrit. A threshold level was defined for each variable. That is, a significant increase in mortality occurred when the level fell below the threshold. For albumin, cholesterol, and hematocrit, the threshold was within generally acceptable limits (albumin concentration of less than 4.0 g/dL, total serum cholesterol level below 160 mg/dL, and hematocrit less than 41%). Similar results have been reported by others.[40,41] An additional multivariate analysis identified serum total cholesterol and hematocrit as the strongest primary and secondary predictors of mortality, respectively.

This study recommended reformulating nutritional status indicators of older adults at different decades of life after 50 and considering their major residence. The nursing home environment may not be conducive to the maintenance of nutritional status above nonthreatening levels.[37] Two major categories of factors that predispose institutionalized older adults to a nutritional risk status have been identified as follows[37]:

1. factors causing inadequate intake
   - psychosocial setting
   - sensory perception—taste, smell, cognition, attention, manual dexterity
   - ability to chew and swallow (30–80% of nursing home residents are edentulous,[42] and 20–40% have dysphagia)[43,44]

- mood (33% of nursing home residents have depression)[45,46]
- appetite
- inability to feed self and lack of assistance with eating
2. factors causing increased nutritional requirements
    - hyperactivity such as Parkinson's disease
    - infection (15–20% experience active urinary, respiratory, skin, or eye infection)
    - fever
    - wounds
    - anorexia

Frequency and Indicators of Undernutrition in the Elderly

Vitamin, mineral, and protein-energy undernutrition of the elderly exists.[47] For example:

- 50% consume less than the RDAs for minerals and vitamins
- 10–30% have subnormal levels of minerals and vitamins
- 16–18% of the elderly in community living consume less than 1,000 calories a day
- 54% of nursing home residents are undernourished
- 10% of the patients lose 5% of their weight in 30 days or 10% of their weight in 180 days or less
- 43% have serum albumin levels of 3.5 mg/dL
- 63% have pyridoxine deficiencies
- 18% have thiamine deficiencies
- 2% have ascorbic acid deficiencies

Within the next decade, 20–50% of all deaths in hospitals will be related to cachexia resulting from that disease being treated instead of treating the nutritional problems. Dramatic insight into the importance of nutritional care reflects the GAIN Registry Survival Curve of weight loss trends of 1,000 nursing home residents in the United States between Florida and Washington. The residents were losing weight over a 6-month period. The residents were observed over another 6 months to see what would happen if weight changed. In the residents who continued to lose weight, one third of them died within 6 months. Of those who maintained their weight, 25% died within the next 6 months. Of those who gained weight, only 1 in 10 died in the next 6 months.[47]

Underutilization of Calcium and Vitamin D Supplements in an Academic Long-Term Care Facility

A cross-sectional chart review study of 177 elderly residents in an 899-bed academic long-term care facility was conducted. Calcium and vitamin D supplements were prescribed for only 9–12% of seniors. Of the 12 who were osteoporotic, 66% were prescribed calcium and 58% were prescribed vitamin D supplements. Of the 8 who had hip fractures, only 25% were prescribed calcium and a similar percentage were prescribed vitamin D supplements. Female residents were more likely than male residents to receive calcium ($p < 0.05$) and vitamin D supplements ($p = 0.08$).[48]

Protein-calorie undernutrition has been frequently observed among institutionalized older adults. Modifiable causes, a means to identify the cause, and corrective actions have been enumerated[37] (see Table 10-2). Aggressive but often simple forms of medical nutrition therapy may tilt the nutritional status of institutionalized elders in a positive direction. Taste-free supplements

TABLE 10–2 Fourteen Modifiable Causes of Protein-Calorie Undernutrition in an Institutional Environment

Cause	Method of Identification	Corrective Action
Staff unawareness	Lack of documentation in chart by MD, RN, or RD	Staff education
Inappropriate use of restricted diets	Patient receiving a restricted diet no longer indicated	Replace by ad lib diet
Use of drugs that impair desire or ability to eat	Review of medications	Discontinue or replace offending drug
Unmet need for eating assistance or self-help eating devices	Observation and calorie count	Provide assistance or devices
Suboptimal technique of assistance	Observation	Retrain the nursing aide
Suboptimal dining environment	Observation	Improve the environment
Prescription of maintenance instead of repletion dietary intakes (oral or enteral)	Less than 1.5× RDA of calories and protein prescribed*	Increase prescription to 1.5× RDA calories and protein
Inadequate nutritional support during intercurrent illness	Weight and/or albumin decline during illness; inadequate nutrition support	Project MD will consult on each patient during intercurrent illness
Unrecognized febrile illness	Daily temperatures reveal elevations	Identify and treat infections
Unmet need for modified diet	Clinical review	Prescribe indicated modified diet
Inadequate management of tube-feeding complication	Prescribed tube-feeding volume not being administered or absorbed	Correct management of complication
Poor dental status	Oral examination	Prompt dental care
Unmet need for dysphagia workup	Clinical signs suggest dysphagia; workup not requested	Consult speech pathology for swallowing evaluation
Suboptimal treatment of dysphagia	Recommendations of speech pathology not being followed	Speech pathologist retrains ward staff

*RDAs are the standards used to calculate an adequate eating pattern for an individual; the standards, however, are more accurately used to evaluate intake of groups.
Source: Reprinted from Abbasi AA, Rudman D. Undernutrition in the nursing home: prevalence, consequences, causes and prevention. *Nutr Rev.* 1994;52(4):119.

and calorie-dense foods such as chocolate and candy have been used to improve the overall energy intake and nitrogen balance of institutionalized elders.[49] The community nutrition professional may find these observations and results instructive when designing and implementing nutrition programs for older adults who live independently.

Due to gaps in the science, future research should have a twofold purpose for elderly in long-term care: first, to support quality nutritional management in long-term care, and second, to educate the interdisciplinary team to integrate their prevention and treatment strategies toward unintentional weight loss of the elderly. The goal is that no patient shall be left behind as a result of failed nutritional status. A Patient Nutrition Bill of Rights has been proposed for every hospital in America, so that every patient can be informed of their nutritional status or have family members know their nutritional status.[47]

Screening for Undernutrition in At-Risk Residents

The "MEALS" mnemonic (i.e., Medication, Emotional problems [depression], Anorexia tardive [nervosa], Liquor use [alcoholism]) reflects areas of screening.[50] Technique for early detection is to weigh residents weekly. Drugs may cause gastric distress, constipation, diarrhea, nausea, metallic taste, etc. Almost every classification of drug can contribute to anorexia.

Normal regulation of food intake is influenced by sociological, psychological, and physiological factors. *Sociological* relates to the eating environment and interaction. *Psychological* relates to choices and confidence allowing independence rather than an ordered/artificial schedule for eating. *Physiological* relates to what seniors smell, taste, and see.

Protocols should define what the first intervention should be and the monitoring steps to ensure negative conditions are arrested. This requires a team approach with community nutrition professionals as active members.

Community Nutrition Professionals in Home Care

Home care is an acceptable alternative to care and rehabilitation received within a hospital or medical environment. Services may include personal hygiene, assistance with homemaking and shopping, technical care including dialysis, and medical nutrition therapy (e.g., parenteral nutrition). This type of service has been one of the fasting growing sectors of the healthcare system.[51–53]

Tailored medical nutrition therapy at home may involve older adults with gastrointestinal disorders (e.g., Crohn's disease, short bowel syndrome, and ischemic bowel disease), HIV, cancer, end-stage renal disease, or amputation from diabetes. Using home visits, screening, and monitoring, community nutrition professionals can identify problems associated with an individual's inability to receive the required daily food pattern. The feedback, status, and care plan to rectify any problems can be directed back to the physician for continuity and efficient delivery of the medical nutrition therapy.

Community nutrition professionals who are registered dietitians (RDs) may receive reimbursement from some insurance companies if the following occurs[54]:

- The RD is employed by the physician.
- The RD services are medically supervised.
- The RD services are medically necessary.

With the blossoming of the home health industry, it is imperative to blend the skill of professionals with programs that target the nutrition needs of older individuals in the community. The extent to which older adults can maintain their independence (for example, through home-delivered meals) may depend on their ability to be linked with the services they need. Community nutrition professionals can function as a conduit to connect older adults with the services they need.

Special Dietary Needs of Older Adults

Thirst and Fluid Requirements

Renal mass, renal blood flow, and fluid excretion decrease with age.[55,56] The regulation of body water relies on thirst and an individual's response to that thirst. Thirst is reduced in elders in general, and specifically in those with an elevated serum sodium and osmolality. Illness compounds the problem, as the lack of thirst may lead to severe dehydration and reduced mental acuity.[57]

Dehydration among older adults expresses itself as a swollen tongue, constipation, electrolyte disturbance, nausea and vomiting, hypotension, mental confusion, sunken eyeballs, increased body temperature, and decreased urine output. Older adults who are immobile may decrease water and fluid intake so they do not need to ask for assistance with toileting functions.[57]

For normal hydration, eight 8-ounce glasses of water or fluid is needed each day. Common sources include plain water, milk, juice, carbonated beverages, soups, and hydrous fruits. Caffeine-containing beverages such as coffee and tea are not good water sources.

Care Alerts

The Clinton administration awarded grants totaling $450,000 to support educating communities and empowering families to improve nutrition and hydration in long-term care facilities. The grantees are the National Association of Area Agencies on Aging; the National Long Term Care Ombudsmen Resource Center; the National Center on Elder Abuse; and the National Policy and Resource Center on Nutrition and Aging.

This is a joint effort of the Administration on Aging (AOA) and the Health Care Financing Administration (HCFA). Although there are many contributing factors, a large part of unintended weight loss, dehydration, and abuse can be avoided when warning signs are identified early and the nursing home industry and the general public are better informed and aware.

The National Policy and Resource Center on Nutrition and Aging in Miami, Florida, has a demonstration project, Reducing Malnutrition and Dehydration in Nursing Homes, to use nutrition care alerts as warning signs and action steps for caregivers in nursing facilities (see Appendix 10–A). Focusing on early detection can prevent poor nutrition and involve caregivers at all levels. CNPs, mainly RDs, can increase awareness of the warning signs by conducting in-service programs focusing on the nutrition care alerts. Morbidity, mortality, and healthcare cost reductions are projected.[58]

Appetite and Satiety

Age has an inverse effect on the variety of foods eaten.[59,60] How this may occur is interesting. The change in palatability of a food once an individual begins to eat it is called sensory-specific satiety. This type of satiety is associated with a decreased intake of one food and a switch to another food during that ingestion period. The sensory-specific satiety mechanism promotes more variety and potentially a more well-balanced eating pattern.[61]

The mechanism has been shown to diminish among individuals as they age when comparing groups 12 to 15 years, 22 to 35 years, 45 to 60 years, and 65 to 82 years.[62] It is not known whether this is the result of a rather monotonous selection of foods, a lower calorie content of foods, denture problems, or lack of taste or seasoning of food. This area of research is relatively new but of interest to community nutrition professionals who plan and prepare meals and snacks for older adults.

Taste and Smell

Taste buds turn over constantly every 10.5 days; olfactory receptors in the nasal cavity have an average turnover time of 30 days.[63] Losses in taste and smell begin at about 60 years of age and may peak by age 70. Chemosensory losses include the following[63]:

- ageusia—absence of taste
- hypogeusia—diminished sensitivity of taste
- dysgeusia—distortion of normal taste
- anosmia—absence of smell
- hyposmia—diminished sensitivity of smell
- dysosmia—distortion of normal smell

The detection threshold for taste and smell varies with the molar conductivity values of the anions. The threshold for distinguishing odors among elders may be as much as 11 times higher than that of younger individuals. In addition, the ability to distinguish the odors of certain items varies. For example, the ability to distinguish the odor of breads, vegetables, and coffee declines greatly with age, but elders retain the ability to identify green bell pepper.[63]

Several medical conditions affect the sense of taste and smell (see Table 10–3). Many seniors take multiple medications every day, as depicted in Figure 10–1. Drugs such as local anesthetics, opiates (codeine, morphine), antihypertensive agents (diltiazem and nifedipine), and antimicrobial agents (allicin, streptomycin, tyrothricin) also influence the sense of smell. Certain types of drugs affect the sense of taste, including anesthetics (benzocaine, lidocaine), antihistamines (chlorpheniramine maleate), antirheumatics (allopurinol, colchicine, hydrocortisone, salicylates), drugs for Parkinson's disease (levodopa, baclofen), vasodilators (nitroglycerin patch), and amphetamines. As taste and smell sensitivities decrease, decreases in stimulation of salivary glands, gastric acid, and pancreatic secretions occur and increases in plasma insulin and pancreatic polypeptide occur. When the senses are stimulated by food, plasma-free fatty acids may decline and sympathetic nervous system activity and metabolic rate may increase. With a reduction of taste and smell, metabolic processes can be altered.[63]

TABLE 10–3   Medical Conditions That Affect the Senses of Taste and Smell

Condition	Effect on Taste	Effect on Smell
Nervous	Bell's palsy	Head trauma
	Damage to chorda tympani	Korsakoff's syndrome
	Familial dysautonomia	Multiple sclerosis
	Head trauma	Parkinson's disease
	Multiple sclerosis	Tumors and lesions
	Raeder's paratrigeminal syndrome	
Nutritional	Cancer	Chronic renal failure
	Chronic renal failure	Liver disease including
	Liver disease including cirrhosis	vitamin B_{12} deficiency
	Niacin (vitamin B_3) deficiency	Thermal burn
	Zinc deficiency	
Endocrine	Adrenal cortical insufficiency	Adrenal cortical insufficiency
	Congenital adrenal hyperplasia	Cushing's syndrome
	Pseudohypoparathyroidism	Hypothyroidism
	Panhypopituitarism	Diabetes mellitus
	Cushing's syndrome	Gonadal dysgenesis
	Cretinism	(Turner's syndrome)
	Hypothyroidism	Hypogonadism
	Diabetes mellitus	Primary amenorrhea
Local	Facial hypoplasia	Adenoid hypertrophy
	Glossitis and other oral disorders	Allergic rhinitis and atrophy
	Leprosy	Bronchial asthma
	Oral Crohn's disease	Leprosy
	Radiation therapy	Ozena
	Sjögren's syndrome	Sinusitis and polyposis
		Sjögren's syndrome
		Viral infections
		Acute viral hepatitis
		Influenza-like infections
Other	Hypertension	Familial (genetic)
	Influenza-like infections	Laryngectomy Olfactory
	Laryngectomy	sarcoidosis

Source: Adapted from: Schiffman S. Changes in taste and smell: drug interactions and food preferences. *Nutrition Reviews.* 1994;52(8 part II): S11-S14.

Potassium Loss

Many potent diuretics produce significant potassium losses. Potassium is the main ion inside body cells; it maintains fluid balance, electrolyte balance,

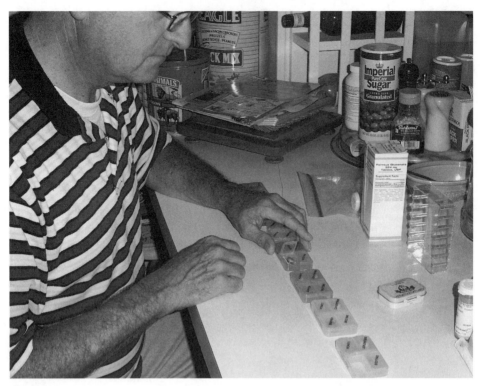

FIGURE 10-1   A Daily regimen of multiple medications frequently organizes the life of a senior with chronic disease. *Source:* Lew Carter.

and cell integrity. Potassium is essential to maintaining the heartbeat; a lack of potassium from fasting or severe diarrhea may cause heart failure. Dehydration is dangerous, because the loss of potassium from brain cells makes the victim unaware of the need for water.[64]

Most eating patterns do not provide enough potassium to compensate for the amount lost due to diuretics. Proper choice of foods can effectively replace potassium losses. Food that are high in potassium are bran cereals, cooked dried fruit such as apricots, peaches, prunes, bananas, baked or boiled potatoes, sweet potatoes, pumpkin, winter squash, stewed tomatoes, spinach, asparagus, cantaloupe, watermelon, lima beans, cooked dry beans, peas, lentils, and milk and yogurt (all types).

Dyslipidemia

Data based on a sample of 610 women and 387 men between 70 and 104 years suggest that elders do not incur an increased risk of heart attack, angina, or death from any cause if they have either low high-density lipoprotein (HDL) cholesterol or high total serum cholesterol levels. Baseline measures in 1990 showed 32% of women and 16% of men with cholesterol levels greater than 240 mg/dL versus 9% of women and 26% of men with low HDL levels. Women with total cholesterol levels greater than 240 mg% had the longest survival; women with 200 to 240 mg% had the lowest survival. There was no significant effect of total cholesterol or HDL on heart attacks or mortality rates for men or women.[65]

Hip Fractures

Hip fractures among women over 65 increased 40% between 1988 and 1996, with about a third suffering serious falls annually.[66] The Centers for Disease Control and Prevention attributes the increase to a growing number of people 85 and older. The United States had 31 million people 65 and over in 1990 and that number will double by 2040. Older adults are hospitalized for fall-related injuries 5 times more often than for other injuries. Women are nearly 3 times more likely than men to be hospitalized for falls.[66]

People are living longer as we reduce heart disease, stroke, and cancer, but seniors fall more frequently because they are generally more sedentary, have weaker muscles, poorer balance, and experience polypharmacy that can make them dizzy. In 1996, 340,000 people 65 and over were hospitalized with a broken hip and 80% were women. In 1988, the rate of hospitalization among women 65 and older was 972 per 100,000 compared to 1,356 per 100,000 in 1996.

More adults 65 and older die from fall-related injuries each year than from any other cause; 9,000 deaths occurred in 1997. One in three older adults require hospitalization for a fall annually, with a broken hip the most common and serious injury. Half of those who break a hip do not regain mobility or independence, resulting in admission to a nursing home or moving in with relatives. Hip fractures may initiate the beginning of the end as they may lead quickly to decline and death. Exercising to increase muscle strength and balance is a preventive strategy.

Info Line

CDC: www.cdc.gov/ncipc/olderadults.htm. National Resource Center for Safe Aging. Accessed January 9, 2007.

Constipation

The prevalence of constipation among older adults may be about 34%. Defined medically as defecation less than 3 times a week or every third day, constipation is a daily problem for many older adults. In a study of 211 frail elders receiving home care, 45% reported constipation as a problem and 11% felt it was a major problem. The major strategies to overcome constipation cited by 70 respondents were as follows: 4% changed bowel habits, 7% increased exercise, 34% changed what they ate, and 88% used medications. Of the 62 respondents who used medications, the types commonly used were as follows: 50% stool softeners, 24% bulk agents, 19% stimulants, 19% osmotics, 14% unknown, 10% combination laxatives, 8% cathartics, 2% lubricants, 10% enemas, and 2% suppositories.[67] These data suggest that public education about the role of fiber, especially the laxative effect of fresh fruit, is warranted.

Bereavement

Loneliness at mealtime may influence the amount and frequency of meal and snack consumption. For older adults who live alone, a question for those who may not meet their energy or nutrient needs is whether mealtime is viewed as a chore or a reminder of what meals used to be like.

Eating behaviors of 50 individuals over 60 years who were widowed within the previous 2 years were contrasted with eating behaviors of 50 married elders. Responses showed that 72% of the widowed elders felt that eating was a chore, and a favorite substitute for meals was low-nutrient-dense snacks; 84% experienced weight loss with an average of 7.6 pounds of body weight. The widowed group averaged 35% of total energy intake from fat, compared with 32% for the married respondents. Grief resolution showed a positive association with dietary components, which suggests that emotional and nutritional status may be mediated by the eating pattern.[68]

Oral Health

Dental caries, missing teeth, infections, mucosal lesions, and diseased gums make chewing difficult and decrease the variety and amount of food ingested. Inadequate oral health care, which increases weight loss and the onset of malnutrition, can be resolved with regular dental care.[10,57]

Alzheimer's Disease

Alzheimer's disease was identified in 1907 by Alois Alzheimer, who uncovered abnormal structures of amyloid plaques and neurofibrillary tangles in the brain of a woman. The disease affects 4 million Americans who are over 65 years of age and is among the top 5 causes of death among the elderly.[69-70] One in 10 people over 65 and nearly half of those over 85 have Alzheimer's disease. About 60% of the elderly in long-term care facilities have Alzheimer's disease.[69,71]

Alzheimer's disease costs the United States at least $100 billion a year, including $26 billion in workplace productivity lost because of caregiver duties. More than 7 out of 10 Alzheimer's disease patients live at home. Half of all people who live in nursing homes suffer from Alzheimer's disease or a related disorder. Alzheimer's patients live an average of 8 years and may live as long as 20 years after symptoms begin.[72]

Alzheimer's disease is slow and progressive. The cause is unknown.[71-75] The process involves degeneration of neurons in the hippocampus and cerebral cortex due to a 40–90% decline in choline acetyltransferase activity.[69-77] There is an association between the number of plaques and the degree of cell loss with the severity of dementia expressed as memory loss, decline in cognition, and distant-type behavior.[75,76]

There is no known cure for Alzheimer's disease, but drugs are used to treat symptoms of depression, agitation, or sleep disorders.[74] Symptoms occur for an average of 6 to 10 years, but the span from onset to death can be from 3 to 20 years. Respiratory diseases and bronchopneumonia are the major causes of death.[76,78]

Alzheimer's disease has 3 stages that are summarized in Table 10–4. [69,70,76,79] The need for nutritional support increases with each stage. During

TABLE 10–4   Major Stages of Alzheimer's Disease

Stage	Symptoms
1	Is still alert.
	Purchases and prepares own food; feeds self.
	Complains of memory loss.
	Has decreased vocational abilities.
	Is increasingly unable to think abstractly and make proper judgments.
	Displays mood and personality changes, irritability, hostility, and agitation.
2	Is completely unable to learn and recall information.
	Is disoriented with time and place; needs assistance for daily living.
	Can feed self, but needs direction and assistance at mealtime.
	Is at risk of falling.
	Shows signs of depression, agitation, hostility, uncooperativeness, and physical aggressiveness.
	Begins pacing needlessly.
3	Is severely impaired intellectually.
	Is completely disoriented.
	Requires total assistance.
	Cannot feed self; may refuse to chew and swallow food.
	May become incontinent and bedridden.
	Is at risk for malnutrition, infection, pneumonia, and pressure sores.
	Coma may occur.

Source: Huey E. *Nutritional Assessment of Patients With Alzheimer's Disease in Three Stages of the Disease* [master's thesis]. California State University Long Beach; 1995:2.

stage 1, individuals may need assistance shopping, storing, or cooking food. In stage 2, individuals often begin to pace, have chewing or swallowing problems, and need assistance feeding themselves. In stage 3, individuals may not recognize foods, forget to eat, or forget what to do with the food. A loss of muscle mass and body fat results from the reduced eating.[78-80] The need for home care increases, until 24-hour care is appropriate.

Limited nutritional data are available for Alzheimer's disease, because few studies exist and there is a lack of standard criteria used to evaluate nutritional status of patients. The RDAs evaluate food intake, but standards exist only for healthy adults up to 50 years of age.[25] Community nutrition and healthcare professionals must recognize this limitation when they are using the RDAs to evaluate eating patterns, because individuals with Alzheimer's often exceed age 65 and may have different nutritional needs. Huey reported below-normal hemoglobin and hematocrit levels for stage 2 patients; stage 3 patients had lower energy intakes than patients in stages 1 and 2, even when the stage 3 patients had nutritional supplements.[73]

Foods That May Protect Against Alzheimer's

A small but growing body of research suggests that diet might be linked to one's chances of developing Alzheimer's disease. Researchers from Erasmus

Medical Center in Rotterdam, the Netherlands, found that people who ate lots of vegetables and other foods containing vitamins E and C were less likely to develop Alzheimer's disease or vascular dementia, caused by hardening of the arteries.[72]

The dietary habits of nearly 8,000 men and women who were at least 55 years old and free of dementia were studied. The participants answered questions about their eating habits, were reexamined twice, the second time 6 years after enrolling. Of the participants, 146 had Alzheimer's and 29 had vascular dementia. A higher dietary intake of vegetables and vitamins E and C was associated with a lower risk of developing either type of dementia.

Researchers at Rush-Presbyterian-St. Luke's Medical Center, Chicago, supported the Dutch scientists' findings. In people 65 and older, they found, high vitamin E intake was associated with reduced decline in memory and other brain functions.

It may be premature to recommend eating vegetables and other foods high in vitamins E and C to protect against Alzheimer's, but antioxidants do protect against heart disease and some cancers and may have a role in Alzheimer's prevention. The same observation regards fish.

Framingham Heart Study participants were followed for almost a decade, observing who ended up with Alzheimer's disease and researchers compared the concentration of DHA in their blood to the DHA in the blood of people who did not develop dementia. Adults with the highest DHA levels ate 3 servings of fish a week and were only about half as likely to develop dementia by the time they were in their 80s as those with the lowest levels. One and a half to two weekly servings were associated with a reduced risk for dementia in later years. The mechanism is thought to be related to DHA.

While only 3–4% of fatty acids in the blood plasma are DHA, the proportion is closer to 40% in the brain. Regarding mechanism, DHA fatty acids are present in cell membranes, which surround each brain cell. When they contain DHA, it makes the membranes more fluid than they would be with other fatty acids, which might make it easier for messages to get from one brain cell to another, improving memory and cognition.[81]

A new observation regards the use of alcohol. Alcohol raises good HDL cholesterol, for some people, but their bad LDL cholesterol goes up by as much as 15–20% when HDL cholesterol may increase only a little.

The Human Genome Project mapped every gene in every human chromosomes. Twelve percent of the population carries a version of a gene on chromosome number 19, the ApoE gene, that makes the body handle alcohol and fat differently. That same gene mutation places people at higher risk for developing Alzheimer's disease. It makes obese men more prone to diabetes.

Of almost 3,000 people, the very overweight men with the gene variation averaged at least 10% more sugar in their blood and 15% more insulin than obese men without that gene. Their blood sugar levels registered them as having impaired glucose tolerance, a diabetes precursor.[81]

"The Dwindles" or Failure to Thrive

Failure to thrive is neither a normal part of aging nor the inevitable result of chronic disease. It is a consequence of a number of factors: normal aging;

malnutrition; and specific physical, psychological, and/or social determinants (see Figure 10–2). Medical nutrition therapy is the cornerstone of the treatment of elder adults with failure to thrive. Several factors enhance failure to thrive. Each may be relatively mild, but in combination with malnutrition and aging the synergy is lethal. Eleven factors that enhance failure to thrive and create a dwindling condition include the following[82]:

1. diseases (chronic obstructive lung disease, heart failure, cancer, infections, hyperthyroidism, hypothyroidism, or uncontrolled diabetes)
2. dementia
3. delirium
4. drinking alcohol
5. drug use
6. dysphagia
7. deficit of senses creating deafness and blindness
8. depression
9. desertion by family and friends
10. destitution and poverty
11. despair

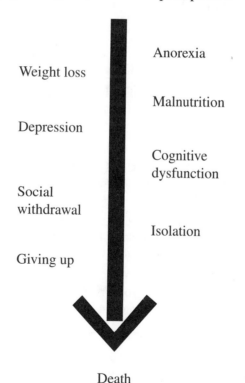

Normal changes of aging plus physical, psychological, and social precipitants

Anorexia

Weight loss

Malnutrition

Depression

Cognitive dysfunction

Social withdrawal

Isolation

Giving up

Death

FIGURE 10–2 The downward spiral of geriatric failure. *Source:* The "Dwindles" Failure to thrive in older patients. *Postgrad Med* 1993;94:199-212.

RDAs for Healthy Older Adults

Many nutritional surveys of elders report only a low or moderate prevalence of clear nutrient deficiency but show an increased risk for malnutrition and subclinical deficiencies. This has a cyclic effect: nutritional status influences the age-related rate of functional decline for body organs, influences body composition, and predisposes to chronic diseases.[83-85]

The nutritional needs of older adults vary due to the age range of this population. One notices this when contrasting 50- to 60-year-olds with 80- to 90-year-olds in terms of habits, activities, and abilities. Specific RDAs for each decade after 50 years of age are relevant.[86,87] Nutrient needs are related to observed body functions and changes that take place after a person passes 50 years of age. The rationale for variations in nutrient requirements for individuals over 50 years of age is based on the following needs and/or changes[87]:

- the need for vitamins B_6 and E to promote immune response
- reduced ability to absorb vitamin B_{12} and folic acid due to less hydrochloric acid produced
- the need for vitamin B_6 for glucose tolerance and normal cognitive function
- the need for vitamin B_6, B_{12}, and folate to protect against homocysteine
- decreased ability to convert vitamin D to an active form
- the need for vitamins C and E and beta-carotene to reduce risk for coronary heart disease, cancer, and cataracts
- marginal zinc deficiency leading to mental lethargy, delayed wound healing, and loss of taste
- vitamin-disease associations (e.g., folate with cervical dysplasia, and vitamin C with atrophic gastritis)

Older adults experience subclinical deficiencies that impact the body's ability to maintain good health. Dietary challenges include:

- Vitamin B_6—to keep the immune system functioning properly to reduce illness. Older adults need more than younger adults, yet 50–90% of older adults do not meet their daily needs.
- Vitamin D—to preserve bone density. Loss is accelerated with aging, increasing the risk of fractures, stooped posture, and osteoporosis.

A solution is eating more nutrient-dense foods: more fruits, vegetables, whole grains, low- and nonfat dairy foods, and lean meats; and fewer high-calorie, nutrient-poor snacks and desserts. The nutrient-dense foods contain the following nutrients[88]:

1. Calcium—Found in dairy products like milk and yogurt, canned salmon and sardines with bones, calcium-fortified orange juice, broccoli, kale, beans.
2. Folate—Obtained by eating beans, green vegetables, fortified grain foods—bread, cereal, pasta, and rice.
3. Riboflavin—Commonly found in milk, dark green vegetables, meat, whole-grain and enriched-grain foods.
4. Vitamin B_6—Available in baked potatoes with skin, bananas, chicken, beef, canned tuna, and whole-grain foods.

5. Vitamin B_{12}—Available in meat, fish, poultry, cheese, and fortified cereal products.
6. Vitamin D—Acquired by consuming milk (which comes fortified with the nutrient), some fortified cereals (check labels), fatty fish, including salmon, sardines, herring, and mackerel.

Adults over 70 years are vulnerable to compromised nutrient intake because as they age, energy needs decrease, and a decrease in food intake follows. Among adults over 70 years old surveyed in NHANES III, about 40% consumed less than two thirds of the RDA for energy (NHANES III 1988–1994). The Food Guide Pyramid categories should highlight specific selections with a high ratio of nutrients to energy (nutrient density) to ensure adequate nutrient intakes, and it should be narrowed to reflect lowered energy needs.[89]

Several organizations will need to modify their food pyramid for over-70 adults because a new design was presented in 2005. Any pyramid for the over-70 over adult must be based on the principles of the *2005 Dietary Guidelines for Americans.* Attention must be given to plenty of variety; patterns high in grain products, vegetables, and fruits; patterns low in saturated fatty acids and cholesterol; low to moderate use of sugar, salt, and alcohol; and physical activity in balance with energy intake. Flagging and using symbols for water and fiber are needed. An older person will be challenged to obtain adequate intakes of particular nutrients due to (1) reduced portion sizes, (2) reduced number of food servings being ingested, and (3) restrictions in food choices secondary to medical conditions (for example, hypertension and low-sodium foods). The nutrients that are of particular concern in the elderly are calcium, vitamin D, and vitamin B_{12}. Specific food guides for seniors are as follows:

- *Bread, cereal, and pasta group:* whole grain, enriched, or preferably fortified. The Food and Drug Administration (FDA) issued regulations that require enriched cereal grains to be fortified with folic acid at 140 µg/100 g of product. Although the purpose was to prevent birth defects, seniors may benefit by lowering blood homocysteine levels, potentially by reducing cardiovascular disease.
- *Vegetable group:* deeply colored, dark green, orange, or yellow fresh, frozen, or canned vegetables for vitamin C, folic acid, vitamin A (in the form of provitamin A carotenoids) and high dietary fiber, cruciferous vegetables, like turnips, kale, cabbage, and broccoli, with antioxidant phytochemicals such as indoles, flavones, and isothiocyanates.
- *Milk, yogurt, and cheese group:* low-fat dairy products, lactose-free foods, live culture fermented dairy products and lower fat cheeses, which are concentrated sources of protein, calcium, vitamin D (milk only), and riboflavin.
- *Meat, poultry, fish, dry beans, egg, and nuts group:* selection should be based on preference, availability, ease of preparation, chewability, and cost.
- *Fats and sugar:* fat intake should be kept at 30% or less of energy, saturated fat to 10% or less of energy, and cholesterol to 300 mg/d, which may not apply to the total over-70 population.[90] In certain situations, somewhat greater fat intake may be warranted (e.g., underweight individuals, diabetics with hypertriglyceridemia). Trans fatty acids found

predominantly in hydrogenated fats have a biological effect similar to saturated fat and should be limited.[91]

- *Fiber (grain, fruits, vegetables, meat-legumes groups):* help prevent constipation, diverticulosis and diverticulitis,[92] lower cholesterol, cardiovascular disease, and cancer levels.[93,94] Generally 20 g/d or more is needed to provide health benefits.[95]
- *Fluids:* needs are influenced by the amount of physical activity, the medications taken, renal function, and ambient temperature. Aging compromises homeostatic mechanisms, e.g., decreased thirst sensation. In addition, lack of fluid can be a major contributory factor in constipation. Elderly people should drink 2 quarts (about 2 liters) of fluid per day.[25] Alcohol, coffee, and tea should not be included in the total fluid intake due to their diuretic effect.
- *Supplements:* Calcium, vitamin D, and vitamin B_{12} supplementation are recommended.[96-100]

Even though the scientific data are not available to make definitive decisions and choose exact criteria, the United States has recognized the need to address uniqueness of the graying population and various requirements at different stages of elder life. Exhibit 10-2 details the RDAs for macronutrients and AIs for vitamins and minerals for adults 51 years old and older.

Older Americans Act of 1965

The Nutrition Program for Older Americans was mandated by the 1972 Title VII Amendment to the Older Americans Act of 1965. In the United States, nutrition services assist older Americans to live independently by promoting better health through improved nutrition and reduced isolation. In 1977, the US Congress approved funding of home-delivered meals under Title IIIC of the Older Americans Act. Title IIIC is a federal program coordinated with other supportive services.[101]

Nutrition services include the procurement, preparation, transport, and service of meals; nutrition education; and nutrition counseling to older persons at congregate sites or in their homes. Nutrition-related supportive services include outreach, transportation, and escort of older persons to nutrition sites, as well as food shopping assistance.

In most states, Title IIIC is administered through a department of aging or a nutrition section. Program goals are generally to maintain or improve the physical, psychological, or social well-being of elders by providing or securing appropriate nutrition services. Program objectives may include the following[101]:

- to give preference to elders in greatest economic or social need, with particular attention to low-income minority individuals
- to maintain or increase the number of meals served consistent with funding levels and inflation rates
- to serve meals that are nutritious, safe, of good quality, at the lowest reasonable cost
- to promote increased cost-effectiveness through improved program and food service management

Exhibit 10–2 Select Recommended Dietary Allowances*† and Adequate Intakes for Adults 51 Years Old and Older

Life Stage Group	Fat	Protein	CHO	Fiber	Vitamin A	Iron	Zinc	Iodine	Calcium	Folate
Group	(g)	(g)	(g)	(g)	(µg RE)‡S	(mg)	(mg)	(µg)	(mg)	(µg)
Females										
51–70	25–35	46	130	21	700	8	8	150	1,200	400
>70	25–35	46	130	21	700	8	8	150	1,200	400
Males										
51–70	25–35	56	130	30	900	8	11	150	1,200	400
>70	25–35	56	130	30	900	8	11	150	1,200	400

*The allowances, expressed as average daily intakes over time, are intended to provide for individual variations among most normal persons as they live in the United States under usual environmental stresses. Diets should be based on a variety of common foods in order to provide other nutrients for which human requirements have been less well defined. For more information, navigate to www.nap.edu.

†This table does not include nutrients for which dietary reference intakes (DRI) have recently been established (see *DRIs for Calcium, Phosphorus, Magnesium, Vitamin D, and Fluoride* [1997], *DRIs for Thiamin, Riboflavin, Niacin, Vitamin B₆, Folate, Vitamin B₁₂, Pantothenic Acid, Biotin, and Choline* [1998], and *DRIs for Vitamin E, Vitamin C, Selenium, and Carotenoids* [2000]). Note: AIs are bold in table above.

‡Retinol equivalents 1 retinol equivalent=1 µg retinal or 6 µg β-carotene.

Source: Adapted from: Monsen ER. Dietary reference intakes for the antioxidant nutrients: vitamin C, vitamin E, selenium, and carotenoids. *J Am Diet Assoc.* 2000;100:637–640.

- to promote or maintain high food safety and sanitation standards
- to promote or maintain coordination with other supportive services

To be eligible for congregate meals, a person must be either 60 years old or over, the spouse of any person aged 60 or over, or a disabled person under age 60 who resides in housing facilities occupied primarily by elderly persons who receive congregate nutrition services. To be eligible to receive a home-delivered meal, the above criteria apply, and a telephone interview or a home visit to the applicant is usually required. Verification of need for the service is determined through home assessment, and, if eligible, the recipient receives meal service within 1 week.

In most states, the following criteria must be met for individuals to be eligible to receive a home-delivered meal[101]:

- any person aged 60 or over
- the spouse of any person aged 60 or over
- any person aged 60 or over who is frail, homebound by reason of illness or incapacitating disability, or otherwise isolated
- a spouse of a recipient may receive a home-delivered meal if the agency concludes that it is in the best interest of the home-bound older person

The following individuals are also eligible to receive a congregate or home-delivered meal:

- a nonelderly, disabled person who resides with an elderly person who receives either home-delivered or congregate meals
- a volunteer of any age who provides essential services during program hours (may be offered a meal and the opportunity to contribute to the meal cost)
- a guest less than 60 years of age (may be offered a meal and shall pay a fee)
- nutrition service staff

Each congregate and home-delivered meal is planned to supply one third of the RDAs as established by the Food and Nutrition Board of the National Academy of Sciences-National Research Council (see Table 10–5).[25] When feasible and appropriate, the cultural and religious preferences and special dietary needs of eligible persons are considered.

In most communities, a local agency is set up to develop, implement, and monitor policies, procedures, and standards that comply with all applicable laws and regulations of the state and county, including health and fire safety inspections. The staff at an agency generally includes a nutrition services director. If the agency provides its own meal and delivery service, then it may employ its own project community nutrition professional, food service manager, and diet technician.

The community nutrition professional usually has a bachelor's degree in nutrition, dietetics, institutional food service management, or a closely related field from an accredited college or university. Postgraduate course work and/or a graduate degree is desirable in nutrition, dietetics, institutional food service management, public health nutrition, home economics with an emphasis in nutrition and food service management, or gerontology. A master's degree is encouraged but not mandatory. The community nutrition professional or nutritionist is generally required to be an RD with the American

TABLE 10–5 Minimum Menu Requirements for Congregate and Home-Delivered Meals, Title IIIC

Meal Component	Food Sources
Protein	A 3-ounce cooked edible portion of meat, fish, fowl, eggs, or cheese. Meat alternatives may be used only once per week and include cooked dried beans, peas, lentils, nuts, nut butter (peanut butter and others), or products made from these foods.
Vegetable/fruit	Two half-cup servings of vegetables or fruits or their juices.
Bread or alternate	One serving whole-grain or enriched bread, biscuits, muffins, rolls, sandwich buns, cornbread, or other hot breads. Bread alternates include enriched or whole-grain cereals, rice, spaghetti, macaroni, noodles, dumplings, pancakes, waffles, and tortillas.
Milk	Eight ounces of fortified skim or low-fat milk or buttermilk, or the calcium equivalent.
Margarine	One teaspoon of fortified margarine or butter.
Dessert/Coffee	Each meal shall contain 1 half-cup serving of a dessert such as fruit, pudding, gelatin, ice cream, ice milk, or sherbet. Cake, pie, cookies, and similar foods shall be limited to once per week. Coffee, tea, and decaffeinated beverages may be used, but shall not be counted as fulfilling any part of the meal pattern requirements.

Source: Adapted from Older Americans Act Title IIIC. US Congress; 1965.

Dietetic Association and have 3 years of professional experience in nutrition and dietetics, food service management, geriatric nutrition, or community nutrition. A minimum of 1 year of experience in food service management is often required. Completion of a 1-year dietetic internship may be substituted for 1 year of experience.

The job responsibilities of the professional generally include participating in developing policies, procedures, and standards; annually assessing each nutrition service provider on-site; and providing technical assistance to other agency personnel and nutrition service providers. The nutritionist provides nutrition education to participants in congregate and home-delivery meal programs and approves and certifies menus prior to use. He or she participates in needs assessments for applicants and the development of public service announcements for local radio, television, and newspaper.

The nutritionist regularly schedules on-site monitoring of nutrition service providers and evaluates how efficiently and effectively services are provided. He or she conducts problem solving, information sharing, and continuing education activities among service provider staff. The nutritionist reviews and approves nutrition-related contracts and monitors contracts for adherence, quality, and effectiveness.

The number of hours needed for nutrition consultation to perform all duties is usually determined by the administrator, but it may vary from 1 day per week to full-time. Often the nutritionist and all nutrition service contracts are selected through a competitive bid process. Providers who apply often furnish the appropriate congregate or home-delivered meals and a nutrition consultant or a food service manager.

Info Line

NUTRITION EDUCATION SERVICES FOR CONGREGATE AND
HOME-DELIVERED MEAL PARTICIPANTS

Nutrition education is generally required no less than once every
other month per fiscal year, and preferably monthly at each congregate site. The nutrition education for congregate sites is defined as
demonstrations, audiovisual presentations, lectures, or small group
discussions, which are planned, approved, and coordinated by a
qualified nutritionist. Home-delivered nutrition education occurs no
less than quarterly. Home-delivered education is usually an educational brochure, questionnaire, or fact sheet on nutrition. The Gerontological Nutrition Dietetic Practice Group provides camera-ready
nutrition education sheets as inserts in its monthly newsletter (see
Figure 10–3).[102]

  The purpose of nutrition education is to inform individuals
about available facts and information that will promote improved
food selection and eating habits. One nutrition education session
per year addresses the sources and prevention of food-borne illness.
The education may guide older persons in making sound food
choices and in obtaining the best food to meet nutritional needs for
the least money. Or the education can make older persons aware of
community-sponsored health programs that encourage and promote
sound nutritional habits and good health. Often the education assists
older persons with special diets.

  Nutrition education services are based on the particular needs of
congregate and homebound older persons. This is usually determined by an annual needs assessment and evaluation of the service.
All nutrition education activities are documented with signatures of
attendees, a copy of any handout material, and a description of the
verbal presentation or talk kept on file in the agency office.

Meal Service Requirements

The *Dietary Guidelines for Americans* are used throughout the United States
for Title IIIC menus.[95] Guidelines include increasing the consumption of complex carbohydrates and fiber and lowering intake of fat, sodium, and simple
sugars. Low-sodium meats, flavorings, and stocks are strongly encouraged, as
well as whole grains, meat alternates, and raw fruits and vegetables to increase the fiber content of menus. Low-fat salad dressings, cheeses, and
gravies made without drippings and fats are strongly recommended, as well
as baking, broiling, and steaming foods rather than frying them in fat.

  Detailed nutritional analyses must accompany the menus. The menus must
meet one third of the RDAs for males age 51 and above for these nutrients:
protein, thiamin, riboflavin, niacin, vitamin B_6, folacin, vitamin B_{12}, vitamin A,
vitamin C, vitamin D, calcium, iron, phosphorus, magnesium, zinc, and vitamin E (see Appendix 10–B for a nutritionally adequate meal pattern). The
menus must provide a protein source, vegetable and/or fruit, bread or bread alternate, and milk, and provide more than 500 kilocalories per meal.

30 Snacks for less than 1 gram of fat

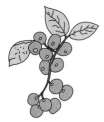

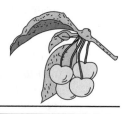

When you cut the fat out of your diet, there is still plenty of room for fun and tasty snacks. Try one of the following when you need a snack or a quick meal. Each contains less than 1 gram of fat.

- Two pretzel rods

- Fresh fruit chunks sprinkled with cinnamon

- Two rice cakes spread with fruit spread

- A small whole wheat pita stuffed with sliced tomatoes. cucumbers, sprouts, and a sauce of lemon juice and Dijon mustard

- A cinnamon-raisin bagel spread with apple butter

- A flour tortilla wrapped around vegetarian refried beans

- Eight ounces of Bloody Mary mix with a stalk of celery (and without the vodka)

- Popcorn sprinkled with salt and chili powder

- One cup of Wheat Chex sprinkled with Cajun seasoning mix and baked in an oven until crisp

- One half cup of applesauce sprinkled with nutmeg

- A juicy dill pickle

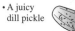

- A cup of pasta tossed with fresh tomatoes and basil

- A cup of beans cooked in sloppy joe sauce served on toast

- An English muffin spread with tomato sauce and mushrooms and baked until hot—to make a mini cheeseless pizza

- A frozen banana

- A cup of herb tea stirred with a cinnamon stick

- Four breadsticks

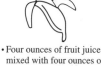

- Four ounces of fruit juice mixed with four ounces of club soda to make a fruit juice spritzer

- Six melba rounds dotted with strawberry jam

- One half cup of split pea soup with 4 nonfat crackers

- One Dole frozen fruit and juice bar

- Twenty frozen grapes

- Raw vegetables dipped in fat-free dressing

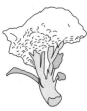

- One fresh ear of corn lightly sprinkled with salt

- A skewer of mushrooms grilled over the coals until lightly browned

- A steaming baked potato stuffed with hot vegetables

- Three ginger snaps

- One slice of toast sprinkled with cinnamon and sugar

- A homemade oat bran muffin spread with raspberry jam

- One fruit kabob– assorted melon balls and fruit chunks on a skewer

FIGURE 10–3 Nutrition education handout for older adults as prepared by the Gerontological Nutrition Dietetic Practice of the American Dietetic Association. Courtesy of the Physicians Committee for Responsible Medicine, Washington, DC.

All foods for congregate and home-delivered meals are packaged and transported in a manner that protects them from potential contamination including dust, insects, rodents, unclean equipment and utensils, and unnecessary handling. Hot food is maintained at or above 140°F, and cold food is maintained at or below 45°F throughout the meal service period or until delivered to the homebound participant.[101]

Systematic temperature checks of food are taken and recorded daily at several points; at the end of production, at delivery, at serving time for congregate sites, and at the point of packaging for home-delivered foods. Temperatures are taken no less than 1 time per week per route prior to handing the food to the recipient.

For food safety and reduced chance of food-borne illness, holding time between the completion of cooking and beginning of food service at the congregate site is not to exceed 2 hours. For home-delivered meals, the holding time between the completion of cooking and delivery of the last meal is not to exceed 2 hours. Frozen, home-delivered meals may exceed the 2-hour time limit when the food is maintained at 32°F or less and in a frozen state until delivery[101] (see Chapter 6 for more detail on food safety).

Effect of Home-Delivered Meals

Two important questions about the home-delivered meal programs in the United States have been posed recently: (1) Does the program serve those who are currently most needy? (2) Does the meal program reduce the need for higher levels of care?[103] Roe stated that the rationale for serving home-delivered meals has generally been based on nonnutritional criteria (e.g., a warm meal, contact with a deliverer, improved quality of life, alleviation of distress and food insecurity among the disabled) and that the indices of benefit are rarely quantitative.

Assessment of older adults' needs for food assistance have been based on anecdotal reports by elderly of the number of times they go without food, the type of discharge diet order from the hospital, living status, and advanced age.[104–106] The assessment method has been haphazard, and no generally accepted system of assessment has been defined.

A 1984 survey conducted by the Texas Department of Aging reported that dependence on a meal served by a community agency was higher among the homebound than among those who obtained meals at congregate sites. The need was greater in geographic areas of poverty and among minority groups.[107] However, another study showed that in geographic areas that contained a large minority population, programs were the least innovative and fewer meals were provided during the week.[108]

Studies have shown that meal recipients have fewer hospitalizations and a better meal quality; however, among minority groups, those who receive meals are more likely than nonminority elders to have several hospitalizations due to lack of management of their diabetes and hypertension.[109,110] Recommendations that have been made regarding home-delivered meals are as follows[103]:

- Make provisions for weekends and evenings.
- Focus on special diets (e.g., individuals with diabetes).
- Reduce the amount of fat in the meals.
- Ensure good sources of folate, since this is often lacking in the food prepared or selected by older adults.
- Conduct research to determine if the home meals program reduces hospital costs and institutionalization.
- Determine if meal program deficiencies are due to lack of innovation, lack of case management, or unequal access to health care.

Several variations of the Food Guide Pyramid have been developed for seniors. One variation promotes plant-based foods,[111] e.g.:

- The serving size of a plant protein choice is based on the protein equivalent of 1 serving of animal protein (3 ounces), or 11/2 cups.
- Serving sizes are listed for added fats, sweets, and snacks.
- Dairy foods are calculated using 2% milk as a worst-case scenario and lean meat at 55 calories per ounce.
- No more than 15% of calories are allowed from the fat group.
- Seniors can choose higher fat dairy products or animal proteins and still meet the 30% or fewer calories from fat recommendation.

Any elder-sensitive Food Guide Pyramid (FGP) can convey important concepts, but it may be less practical for elders on a limited income or at least a lower literacy. The Senior Nutrition Awareness Project (SNAP) of the University of Rhode Island and University of Connecticut is a 2-state USDA Family Nutrition Program. It combines staff, resources, and ideas to create effective nutrition education to seniors such as small group programs, mass media, a free hotline, and direct mail both to seniors and to providers. A practical, elder-friendly pyramid consisting of a large-print, 4-page foldout was designed. It can be used as part of face-to-face programming or as a single nutrition education piece.

Compared with the standard USDA FGP:

- Background symbols were removed to simplify the visual.
- Nutrient-dense, high-fiber, lower fat food choices were listed.
- The tool Foods to Choose More Often was used with the pyramid to illustrate nutrient density and words were used in place of symbols.
- A variety of beverages including water were used.
- The word *supplements* was replaced by the words *seniors may need more* to promote the idea that seniors should choose whole foods.
- A foldout addresses supplements.
- Plant proteins are included in the protein food group.
- Serving size of 1 plant protein is based on the protein equivalent of 3 ounces of animal protein.
- A serving of plant proteins is 1 1/2 cups.
- Serving sizes are given for added fats, sweets, and snacks.
- Dairy foods were calculated using 2% milk and lean meat at 55 calories per ounce.
- Higher fat milk products are recommended for those who may need to gain weight.

Another innovation has been Medicare's support of the Ornish diet. Medicare officials are paying up to 1,800 elderly Americans with severe heart disease to try the Ornish diet and lifestyle plan. The plan requires patients to become vegetarians, reduce fat intake to no more than 10% of total energy, exercise regularly, and practice stress management.

Conventional treatment for heart patients costs $16,000-$29,000/person. The Ornish plan averages $7,200. Medicare officials believe the Ornish plan will save a portion of the $6 billion/year spent on heart surgery for Medicare recipients alone. Patients' progress will be tracked for 4 years to determine efficacy.

Consistent reduction in blood lipids and hypertension and medication reduced by half have been reported. Success could lead HCFA to coverage of nutrition therapy for all Medicare beneficiaries. Recommendations from the Institute of Medicine's study, the Role of Nutrition in Maintaining Health in the Nation's Elderly: Evaluating Coverage of Nutrition Services for the Medicare Population, creates a healthcare environment posed for change, and this change may include the Ornish diet and lifestyle. [112]

Healthy Life for Seniors—A Choice or an Outcome?

Future cohorts of older people may be healthier and more independent well into their 80s and 90s. Fries suggests healthier lifestyles and better health care during youth and middle years will promote maximum life span in future years. Future cohorts may have fewer debilitating illnesses and may experience compressed morbidity—only a few years of major illness in very old age. Older adults of the future may die a natural death—death due to the natural wearing out of all organ systems by approximately age 100.[113] This change could significantly affect health services, employment, and leisure activities for future generations of elderly Americans. An increase in short-stay convalescent centers and home health services may occur.

In 1989, Verbrugge analyzed the National Health Interview Survey from 1958 to 1985 and reported that successive cohorts of middle-aged and older persons reported more morbidity in terms of short-term disability and days of restricted activity than previous cohorts. Morbidity rates increased over a 27-year interval for heart disease, cancer, diabetes, hypertension, and non–life-threatening diseases like arthritis. Mortality rates did not change.[114]

Earlier diagnosis and better secondary and tertiary prevention and clinical care with high-tech screening and treatment will promote survival from major illnesses. Recent cohorts of older adults experience more chronic conditions than previous cohorts, but gradual changes in health habits such as less smoking, less consumption of alcohol and saturated fats, increased exercise, and decreased loneliness—especially at mealtime (see Exhibit 10–3)—may improve the well-being of future elders.

Regarding marketing and communication, many messages and information about physical activity and exercise have been unclear, inconsistent, or confusing to older people. Marketing research is scarce, including older adult perceptions, beliefs, and concerns about physical activity and aging. Too few messages effectively communicate information about physical activity. The goal should be to address activities appropriate along the continuum of health and functional status from healthy to frail adults.[115]

Popular physical activities among senior adults are outlined in Table 10–6. Healthier lifestyles for people currently in their 20s and 30s will give them more years without illness and may result in fewer chronic health problems when they reach old age.[114]

Eating Better and Moving More

The Eating Better & Moving More concept from the Florida International University guidebook gives easy-to-use and inexpensive ways of implementing nutrition education and physical activity for older adults.[115] The guidebook outlines a 12-week program with topics including the Food Guide Pyramid;

Exhibit 10–3   Ideas to Combat Eating Alone Among Older Adults
Idea

- Plan meals as special events once or twice a week. Set the table, light candles, play music, or eat when a television show or sports event that you and your friends like is on.
- Invite friends over for meals, bring a part of the meal to a friend's house, or trade portions of planned leftovers for an early evening meal 2 or 3 nights a week.
- Eat out once a week or so. Many restaurants have lower prices and smaller portions at lunchtime for seniors. Some may offer reduced prices for older adults.
- Plan a daytime outing once a week with a friend. Go to lunch and visit a museum or attend an afternoon concert or theater performance.
- Visit or join a senior center for lunch; participate in meals offered by your local agency on aging.
- Form a gourmet club with others who eat alone.
- Participate in a church or community service club. Volunteer to participate in social functions.
- Choose a nonprofit health organization to support as a volunteer and give time during mealtime.

calcium and vitamin D and bone health; fruits and vegetables in the diet; fiber, portion sizes, and serving sizes; and health benefits of walking, drinking adequate fluids, and other types of physical activity.[116-117] Sample data collection forms are available at http://www.nutritionandaging.fiu.edu/ you_can.

A feasibility study of seniors at the Little Havana Activities and Nutrition Center (LHANC) congregate dining site in Miami-Dade County, Florida, measured:

- number of steps walked before and after activity classes
- flexibility and balance
- fruits, vegetables, dairy products, and fiber intake

Twenty Cuban-American women attendees consented to participate. The institutional review board at Florida International University approved the study and seniors were excluded if they were unable to do any physical activity due to functional or cognitive limitations. Data were recorded at weeks 1, 6, and 12. Physical activity questions from the modified Baecke validated questionnaire were used. Nutrition questions were adapted from the Performance Outcomes Measures Program (POMP), version 3 questionnaire. Flexibility and balance measures used a chair sit and reach technique and a functional reach test.

Participants wore digital step counters, had personalized step goals, and kept a weekly log of steps. Weekly didactic classes and biweekly 15–20 minute supervised group walks were held. After 12 weeks, 17 remained and had a significant improvement in steps walked, flexibility, balance, and self-reported increased numbers of shopping trips, and increased consumption of vegetables and alternate proteins such as tofu, soy, beans, and nuts.[118]

Crimmins studied National Health Interview Survey cohorts from 1969 to 1981 and reported greater limited activity for males up to age 74 and females

TABLE 10–6   Popular Exercises for Senior Adults With Benefits and Energy Expenditure

Exercise	Energy Expenditure	Benefits	Locations
Swimming	90 calories in 20 minutes	Increases heart rate; good source of exercise for people with arthritis or other joint problems; provides a daily dose of vitamin D if outdoors.	Local YMCA and colleges have pools for swimming classes and aqua aerobics.
Walking	148 calories in 20 minutes	Increases heart rate; burns calories; is a way to relax and socialize with friends; is a weight-bearing exercise, which is good for bone and muscle development; provides a daily dose of vitamin D from the sunlight.	An adult can walk just about anywhere. Some fun places to walk are the park, the school track, the shopping mall, or around the neighborhood.
Dancing	98 calories in 20 minutes	Is a weight-bearing exercise, is fun, and is a way to meet new friends and socialize.	Local colleges and YMCA often have dance classes.
Bowling	84 calories in 20 minutes	Is a way to socialize while having fun, a weight-bearing exercise, and a form of friendly competition with friends.	Local bowling lanes have leagues that an individual can join.

Source: Adapted from: Evans WJ. Exercise, nutrition and aging. *J Nutr.* 1992;122:796–801.

Info Line

The National Institutes of Health and the National Cancer Institute has an information service at 1 (800) 4-CANCER (1 (800) 422–6237). This service gives older adults information about various screening and treatment programs. Spanish-speaking staff are available. The mailing address is Office of Cancer Communications, National Cancer Institute, Building 31, Room 10A24, Bethesda, MD 20892.

up to age 72.[119] This contrasted with Palmore who studied 45- to 64-year-olds and reported no change in days of restricted activity but some decline in the number of days of bed disability.[120]

Schneider and Brody suggest that the average period of decreased livelihood will increase, since the number of very old people having multiple chronic illnesses will increase and some diseases will begin in old age.[121]

Rice and Feldman propose that there will be people who achieve advanced old age while still in very good health.[122] At the same time, another group of equally old people will experience extended morbidity.

The concept of *active* versus *dependent* life expectancy has arisen.[123] The end point of active life expectancy is defined as the loss of independence and the need to rely on others for most activities of family living.[123] Life expectancy has increased beyond 65 years, but about one fourth of those additional years will require dependent living.[124] A 65-year-old woman in 1990 had approximately 18.6 years of life remaining, with 12.6 years in active life expectancy and 6.0 years in dependency. A 65-year-old man could live 14.4 more years with 2.4 years in a dependent state. Some gerontologists suggest that a deficit in the active life expectancy of 1.0 to 2.5 years will occur for poor older adults compared with those who are not impoverished. Kane, Ouslander, and Abrass describe this as a growing bimodal distribution of older people, with one group healthier and free of disease and another, larger group of elders surviving diseases but living with compressed morbidity.[125] Many erroneous prejudices exist that form a barrier to the older adult's and society's enjoyment of elder life. This is called *ageism.*[126]

One important goal of health planners and practitioners is to approach a rectangular survival curve. Advances in medicine, public hygiene, and health have increased the percentage of people surviving into their 70s and 80s. Ideally all people would survive to a maximum life span and create a "rectangular curve" (see Chapter 1, Figure 1–4). Aging-related Web sites for support organizations are listed in Appendix 10–C.

"Exceptionally healthy aging" is a new phrase referring to a chronological process that is opposite of disease and reflects the following[127,128]:

1. exceptional longevity or health span as defined by absence of all components of a defined set of conditions
2. exceptionally favorable risk factor profiles
3. exceptionally slow rates of aging changes

This does not necessarily simply reflect absence of disease risk factors, but rather novel protective factors, or a combination of factors that may exist. It is reported that heritability of longevity in the general population is only about 30%. Assessment of the general environment interactions are needed. Please visit http//www.longevityconsortium.org/.

Guidelines to assist older adults to eat well and to remain independent prompting longevity are listed in Table 10–7.

Info Line

> Nutrition across the age spectrum includes the unique biological needs of seniors and is the focus of many professional organizations like the American Dietetic Association, which publishes position papers on relevant issues, e.g., Nutrition Across the Spectrum of Aging published in the *Journal of the American Dietetic Association* in 2005 and located in volume 105, issue 4, on pages 616–633.

TABLE 10–7   Guidelines to Help Older Independent Adults Eat Well

Problem	Solution
Can't shop	• Use local food store delivery service to bring groceries to residence. May be free or involve a small charge. • Seek church, synagogue, or local volunteer center help. • Seek family member or neighbor to shop, pay if necessary, or hire home health workers a few hours each week. Check yellow pages of the telephone book under Home Health Services.
Can't cook	• Purchase TV dinners, frozen entrees, vegetables, or deli meals. • Join congregate meal programs for seniors including meal delivery programs. • Explore relocating to a family member's home or senior residence.
Limited income	• Purchase high-quality, low-cost foods, such as split pea soup, canned beans. • Clip and use coupons for foods you like. • Purchase store-brand foods. • Explore local church or synagogue programs with free or low-cost meals. • Alternate days or weeks to eat at local senior programs. • Check eligibility for food stamps by calling county government reviewing blue pages of telephone book.

Source: Adapted from: Announcement: eating well for older people. *Nutr Today.* 2004;39(5):199.

Nutrition Screening Initiative

The broadest multidisciplinary effort ever initiated in the United States to encourage the incorporation of nutrition screening, assessment, and care of elders into a healthcare system is called the Nutrition Screening Initiative. The initiative responds to the 1988 surgeon general's Workshop on Health Promotion and Aging and the *Healthy People 2010* objectives for increased interdisciplinary collaboration assessing nutritional status and providing nutrition intervention.[129,130] Focusing on an initial 5-year period, the American Dietetic Association, the American Academy of Family Physicians, and the National Council on the Aging joined with 35 key health, aging, and medical organizations and professionals to form a coalition for the initiative.[131] If older persons are at risk of poor nutrition, screening can identify the problem(s) and possible primary, secondary, and tertiary interventions. The major risk factors of poor nutritional status are inappropriate food intake, poverty, social isolation, dependency/disability, acute/chronic diseases or conditions, chronic medication use, and advanced age (80 and above). Table 10–8 identifies major and minor indicators of poor nutritional status. The screening process can likewise build professional collaboration to expand programs on a community level.

Screening can be administered at 3 levels using instruments developed by the Nutrition Screening Initiative: the Determine Your Nutritional Health

TABLE 10–8   Major and Minor Indicators of Poor Nutritional Status of Older Adults

Major Indicators	Minor Indicators
Weight loss	Alcoholism
Under-/overweight	Cognitive impairment
Low serum albumin	Chronic renal insufficiency
Change in functional status	Multiple concurrent medications
Inappropriate food intake	Malabsorption syndromes
Mid-arm muscle circumference less than 10th percentile	Anorexia, nausea, dysphagia
	Change in bowel habit
Triceps skinfold less than 10th percentile or greater than 95th percentile	Fatigue, apathy, memory loss
	Poor oral/dental status, dehydration
Obesity	Poorly healing wounds
Nutrition-related disorders	Loss of subcutaneous fat and/or muscle mass
• Osteoporosis	Fluid retention
• Osteomalacia	Reduced iron, ascorbic acid, zinc
• Folate deficiency	
• B_{12} deficiency	

Source: Adapted from: *Report of Nutrition Screening I: Toward a Common View.* Washington, DC: Nutrition Screening Initiative; 1991:2.

checklist, Level I screen for seniors, and the Level II screen for seniors (see Exhibits 10–D1 through 10–D3 in Appendix 10–D). The checklist has two elements[132,133]:

1. a self-assessment using a series of statements to which elders respond
2. a mnemonic device (the word DETERMINE) that provides basic education on nutritional risk factors

The checklist is a public-awareness instrument. It can be administered by any level of health care professional or self-administered. By summing the checklist, older adults receive a nutritional score that ranges from no risk, to moderate risk, to high nutritional risk.

The Level I screen is a basic nutrition screen designed for social service and health professionals to identify older Americans who may need medical or nutritional attention. This instrument can identify individuals who may be good candidates for meal assistance such as home or congregate meal programs or nutrition therapy and education.[131]

The Level II screen provides more specific diagnostic information on nutritional status. It is designed for health and medical professionals to use with older adults who have a potentially serious medical or nutritional problem. This instrument contains a detailed history of weight change and laboratory and clinical indicators of protein and calorie malnutrition, obesity, and other disorders. Specific health and social service professionals are easily identified to save time and money and to reduce confusion. To promote monitoring of

Info Line

> For more information and to obtain materials, contact The Nutrition
> Screening Initiative, 2626 Pennsylvania Avenue NW, Suite 301,
> Washington, DC 20037. Telephone: (202) 625–1662.

nutritional status, a few of the items in the checklist can be repeated when
the Level I and Level II screens are administered.

The Nutrition Screening Initiative convened an intervention roundtable
to identify practical ways to prevent and to treat nutritionally related problems. Health care professionals who work with older adults in any of 6 key
areas (social services, oral health, mental health, medication use, nutrition
education and counseling, and nutrition support) can choose among a variety of interventions. A manual entitled *Implementing Nutrition Screening and
Intervention Strategies* provides a step-by-step process to develop and refine
programs for nutrition screening and intervention.[134] The programs can
evolve in community-based care, acute and long-term care, and outpatient
or ambulatory care settings. An algorithm that identifies the flow from the
checklist to interventions in different types of health care is provided in
Figure 10–4.[134]

The Nutrition Screening Initiative was used in addition to 14 demographic
questions to survey 11,891 older adults in a study in Indiana. Congregate meal
service was provided to 7,670 (65%) respondents, and home-delivered meals
served 4,223 (36%). Respondents were 70% female and 27% male, with missing data on 3% of the respondents; 85% were white and not of Hispanic origin, and 8% were African American.[135]

The residential location of respondents reflected 72% who lived independently in their home or apartment and 21% who lived in a retirement complex. Of the respondents, 38% resided in a town with a population of 10,000
to 50,000, 30% lived in a rural setting of less than 10,000 people, 6% lived
on a farm, 13% resided in a suburb or central city with more than 50,000
people, and 13% did not complete the information.

Of the respondents, 69% were 75 to 106 years old, and 31% were 60 to
74 years old. Over one half (55%) were widowed; 27% were married; and
60% lived alone. Thirty-two percent had completed high school; an additional 12% had completed some or all of college; and 17% had completed a
minimum of an eight-grade education. Of the respondents, 68% owned and
used a microwave oven. Fifty-seven percent stated that the noon meal received from the congregate or home delivery was their main meal of the day;
59% described the meal as well-balanced and healthy.

Responses from the Determine Your Nutritional Health checklist revealed
that 53% eat alone most of the time, and 52% take 3 or more different prescribed or over-the-counter drugs daily. Thirty-five percent state that they
have an illness or condition that makes them change the kind and/or amount
of food they eat. The compilation of responses to the checklist showed 37%
were at no nutritional risk, 30% were at moderate risk, and 33% were at high
nutritional risk.[135]

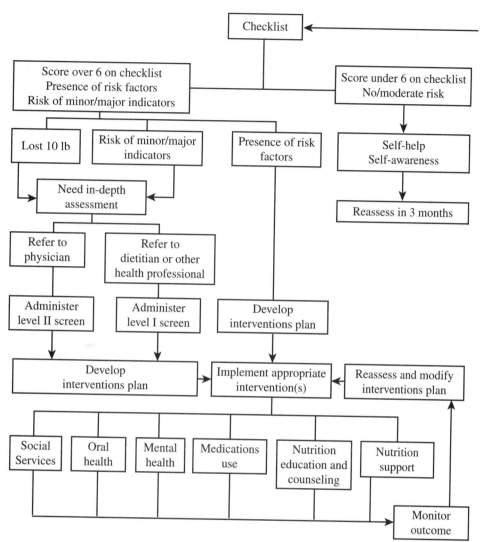

FIGURE 10–4 Flow of nutrition screening data from checklist to outcome. *Source:* Nutrition Screening Initiative. *Report of Nutrition Screening I: Toward a Common View.* Washington, DC: Nutrition Screening Initiative, 1991.

A similar assessment was conducted among Medicare beneficiaries 70 years and older in New England. A 14-item checklist provided information. Of the respondents, 24% were at high nutritional risk. Of these, 56% reported their health as fair or poor; 38% had dietary patterns with less than 75% of the RDAs for 3 or more nutrients.[136]

Two study groups of inner-city African-American seniors were compared against whites from New England. The 2 African-American groups included 115 public housing residents over 50 from North St. Louis and 115 public housing residents age over 50 from East St. Louis. The Nutritional Screening Initiative Checklist measured nutritional risk among the participants finding 48% of the North St. Louis sample and 66% of the East St. Louis sample scoring high on the checklist. They had a limited intake of fruits, vegetables, and milk; more dental problems; a lack of money for food; a high-fat eating pattern; and an inability to shop.[137]

Responses from 18,885 adults aged 20 or older from 1988 to 1994 in the National Health and Nutritional Examination Study III (NHANES III) showed 35% of African Americans with leisure time inactivity compared to 18% of other ethnic groups.[138] A major contributor to obesity, i.e., the intake of fatty foods, is also a behavior that places African Americans at risk. The NIH-sponsored study included cholesterol screening and education in New England and a pool of 9,803 participants, 562 of whom were African American.

Factors associated with high nutritional risk of older women have been identified as having an income equal to or below 125% of the federal poverty level, being African American, living alone, and being between 60 and 74 years of age.[139] African-American women who live alone and who are 60–74 years of age have exceptionally high levels of overall nutritional risk compared with other ethnic groups.[140] Of 196 participants in a study of type 2 diabetes, 51% of the men and women were African American. Over 75% had received diet and exercise counseling, but less than half were following dietary recommendations; 25% were not getting proper exercise.[141]

Only 6% of the participants in a Title IIIC Nutrition program achieved adequate energy and nutrient intakes within a 72-hour period; 41% had eating behaviors that placed them at risk for malnutrition. Non-Hispanic African-American adults were more likely to have lower intakes of calcium than other groups.[142]

Physicians Need More Nutrition Training

The Intersociety Professional Nutrition Education Consortium (IPNEC), a federally funded consortium founded in 1997, includes members of the American Society for Clinical Nutrition (ASCN), the American College of Nutrition, and the American Dietetic Association. The purpose is to create a physician-nutritionist specialty, along with the requisite curriculum to assure that nutrition education and information are provided to those in medical schools.

One area of training involves geriatrics. Fewer than 6% of medical school graduates now receive adequate nutrition training. The US Congress mandated better nutrition education in all US medical schools in 1990. Training as nutrition support physicians may yield physicians who not only incorporate sound dietary recommendations into daily practice but also specialize in the treatment of obesity or other chronic diseases and are skilled in the care of the aging population.

The American Academy of Family Physicians has been dedicated to the Nutrition Screening Initiative (NSI) for 10 years to improve an understanding of nutritional problems, nutrition therapy, and the role of RDs. Physician interest in nutrition may ensure high quality nutrition education and interventions to patients and identify how nonpharmacological interventions, like supplements and alternative medical therapies, may continue as clinically legitimate interventions.[143]

At the same time seniors are actively involved in seeking their continued vitality, quackery and fraud is common and frequently waged against seniors

(Table 10–9). Many seniors seek over-the-counter treatments for their ills. Few spend personal money for seek professional assistance for their nutritional well-being.

In December 2000, the US Congress approved legislation to provide America's senior citizens with access to medical nutrition therapy (MNT) to assist them in managing diabetes and kidney disease. The Medicare legislation also establishes RDs as Medicare providers. This action is a monumental achievement for the nation, for our seniors who rely on the Medicare program for their health care and for the dietetics profession. The elderly, who struggle with diabetes and kidney disease, will now be able to work with RDs to manage their disease and to prevent further complications through MNT. The American Dietetic Association worked for many years to establish the effectiveness of MNT in treating and controlling a number of diseases, including diabetes and kidney disease. Patients who receive these services require fewer hospitalizations and medications and have reduced incidence of complications. The legislation, sponsored by Representative Nancy Johnson (R-Conn) and Senators Jeff Bingaman (D-NM) and Larry Craig (R-Idaho), won wide bipartisan support as House and Senate members recognized the critical importance of providing this vital, basic service to the Medicare population. The new Medicare benefit was available January 1, 2002. The Health Care Financing Administration (HCFA) established regulations implementing medical nutrition therapy coverage. MNT is effective for patients with heart disease, stroke, high cholesterol, and other life-threatening conditions, and advocacy for MNT coverage in other areas will likely be sought.

TABLE 10–9   Fifteen Treatment Areas Included in Top Health Frauds Often Directed Toward Seniors

1. Relieve stress, tension, and anxiety
2. Rejuvenate skin/remove wrinkles
3. Relieve pain without medication
4. Prevent disease
5. Reduce cholesterol level
6. Increase strength
7. Reduce the risk of cancer
8. Stop smoking painlessly
9. Eliminate body poison
10. Slow down the aging process
11. Restore hair or promote growth
12. Enhance memory or intelligence
13. Remove cellulite
14. Improve sexual performance
15. Increase bust size

Source: FDA Backgrounder: Top Health Frauds. Washington, DC: Food and Drug Administration;1990:1–2.

Info Line

NUTRITION SCREENING INITIATIVE—OLDER AMERICAN'S PRAYER

The Nutrition Screening Initiative and the Nutrition Institute of Louisiana at Methodist Hospital are my advocates, I shall not starve;

They consider me at risk for poor nutrition status if I suddenly lie down in green pastures or alternative settings;

They screen me and intervene to assure that I receive appropriate foods and waters;

They restoreth my depleted nutrients, activity, independence and dignity;

They guideth me in straight dietary paths for the sake of prevention of illness, dependence and disability;

Yea, though I swim, jog or walk, even with assistive devices, through the valley of the shadow of ignorance and inadequate reimbursement, I will fear no evil, for they art with me;

Their component organizations, individuals and staff, they comfort me;

They preparest a table, meal or artificial nutrition support before me despite limited resources;

They have anointed my head and other parts of my body, with moderate amounts of unsaturated oils;

If my cup runneth over, they will adjust my calorie and fluid needs;

Surely goodness and mercy shall follow me all the days of my life because through their interventions, I will optimize my independence and execute a living will while I am still competent;

And I shall dwell in various environments, but preferably at home, enjoying a good quality of life, until my final residence when I shall dwell in the house of the Lord forever.

Source: Reprinted from Barrocas A. *Older American's Prayer.* New Orleans, La.1991 in memory of Bess Handmacher and the Nutrition Screening Initiative.

National Institutes of Health Research with Older Adults

Several research initiatives are directed specifically toward women in the later adult years but some target men and women.[144]

Postmenopausal Estrogen/Progestin Interventions

Postmenopausal estrogen/progestin interventions (PEPI) tested the effects of various postmenopausal estrogen-replacement therapies on risk factors for osteoporosis and selected cardiovascular risk factors (e.g., HDL cholesterol, systolic blood pressure, fibrinogen, and insulin). Women ages 45 to 64 from all ethnic groups and with or without uteruses were randomized to 1 of 5 treatment arms.[145]

Women's Health Trial: Feasibility Study in Minority Populations

The Women's Health Trial (WHT) evaluates the feasibility of recruiting 2,250 women 50 to 69 years old and of different socioeconomic status and minority groups to determine if they can reach and practice a modified fat-eating pattern. Eligibility required that women have an eating pattern of about 38% or more of total calories from fat at the beginning of the study. The aim is to reduce total fat to 20% of calories; reduce saturated fat and dietary cholesterol intakes; and increase intake of fruits, vegetables, and grains. Three clinical centers are involved: 1 enrolls at least 50% African-American women, 1 enrolls at least 50% Hispanic women, and 1 reflects the US female population in general.

Cardiovascular Health Study

The Cardiovascular Health Study of men and women 65 years and older determines the degree to which known risk factors predict coronary heart disease (CHD) and stroke among older adults.

Randomized Trial of Low-Dose Aspirin in Female Nurses (Women's Health Study)

The Women's Health Study began in 1991 to study 41,600 postmenopausal female nurses 45 years and older, who had no previous history of heart disease or contraindications to aspirin. The purpose is to evaluate the effect of low-dose aspirin and the antioxidants beta-carotene and vitamin E in the primary prevention of heart disease in postmenopausal women. Aspirin has been efficacious in preventing and reducing vascular disease in men, and data are emerging to show that the use of low-dose aspirin and antioxidants may reduce vascular risk among women.

Trial of Antioxidant Therapy of Cardiovascular Disease in Women

This trial studies the effects of antioxidant therapy (beta-carotene, vitamin C, or vitamin E) on the cardiovascular health of about 8,000 women 45 years and older who had a prior history of disease.

Systolic Hypertension in the Elderly Program

The Systolic Hypertension in the Elderly Program determines the effect of long-term use of antihypertensive therapy on isolated systolic hypertension. Approximately 4,736 men and women 60 years and over (57% women and 14% African-American men and women) compose the study sample. Results show a 36% decline in stroke, a 27% reduction in CHD, and a 32% reduction in all cardiovascular disease events with antihypertensive therapy.

Women's Health Initiative

The WHI study population is composed of approximately 160,000 postmenopausal women, ages 50 to 79. The collaborative study has 2 goals: to evaluate the effectiveness of specific, untested preventive approaches to cancer, heart disease, and osteopathic fractures; and to evaluate strategies at the community level to achieve healthful behaviors (see Chapter 9).

Senior Profile

To honor a distinguished nutrition researcher among the oldest old, Exhibit 10–4 describes the life and accomplishments of Elsie Widdowson.

Method Alert

A new area of training for CNPs involves using various assessment techniques such as telephones and computers to reach seniors. Jonnalagadda et al examined the accuracy of a computer-assisted, interactive, multiple-pass telephone interview technique for completing 24-hour dietary recalls. The

Exhibit 10–4   Elsie Widdowson, British Expert on Nutrition, Died at 93 Years of Age in Barrington, England

Elsie Widdowson (1906–2000), a nutritionist, used the discipline of wartime rationing to prescribe the healthiest diet in British history. The diet was an experimental plan for the government to promote for the citizens of Britain once its imports were impeded in World War II. She wrote it with her research partner of 60 years, Dr R.A. McCance. It was based on bread, cabbage, and potatoes, all of which were in relatively plentiful supply. Though aging British people are most apt to remember the numbing taste of such questionable delicacies as dried eggs, they say the lean, mean diet was the most nutritious the English ever forced down.

The team known as "Mac and Elsie" profoundly affected how the world assessed nutritional values, how it investigated dietary deficiencies, and how mammalian development was perceived. The 2 researchers would from time to time starve or overfeed volunteers of different age groups to study their metabolism. Their findings in the late 1930s on the body's need for salt became a key part of care for patients in diabetic comas and those with other ailments.

Working on her own at 80, Dr Widdowson chased seals on the Labrador ice floes to study their eating habits. A decade later, she published a paper on the physiology of the newborn bear.

Known for the twinkle in her eye, she kept generations of cats on her little farm; raised tomatoes, apples, and bees; and ate lots of butter and eggs, which she considered good for people. Her sense of humor is suggested by her final advice after many an academic lecture: "Take it with a grain of salt." She even gave the lie, or at least a whole new spin, to the old British maxim, "as different as chalk and cheese." To deal with the lack of calcium in people's diets due to cheese shortages during World War II, she and Dr McCance persuaded the government to add chalk to bread.

She obtained her doctorate from Imperial College in London studying the chemistry of the compounds produced in ripening and stored fruit. At Kings College in London doing postgraduate work, she found herself spending time in hospital kitchens. She met a young doctor, McCance, who was studying the chemical consequences of cooking food. She realized his analyses of the carbohydrates in fruit were incorrect and told him. He arranged a grant so she could work with him.

Their collaboration continued until his death in 1993. The initial step was to combine her research on fruits and vegetables and his on meat, then collect information on foods generally. The result was their 1940 book, *The Composition of Foods*, which is known as the dietitian's bible and is now about to be published in its sixth edition.

With the onset of rationing, the 2 made guinea pigs of themselves and other scientists, living on questionable treats like Woolton pie; it consisted of vegetables and bread crumbs and was named for Lord Woolton, the wartime minister of food, who fiercely promoted their very lean cuisine. To prove the diet's effectiveness, the scientists decamped to the Lake District for vigorous exercise. In 1 day, they walked 36 miles and climbed 7,000 feet, burning 4,700 calories. They were none the worse for it. The only serious worry was a lack of calcium, a problem handled by adding ground chalk to bread flour.

After the war, Dr Widdowson studied how to treat the gross starvation suffered by survivors of Nazi concentration camps and children in 2 German orphanages. She was amazed to find children who had been given extra bread, jam, and orange juice did worse than those who had not. Dr Widdowson explained the growth difference by the personality of the director who was very stern. Children and staff were in constant fear of her criticisms. Love was the healthiest food of all.

Source: Martin D. Elsie Widdowson, British expert on nutrition, dead at 93. *New York Times* Company. June 26, 2000.

goal was to estimate energy intakes among 78 men and women (22 to 67 years old) from the Dietary Effects on Lipoprotein and Thrombogenic Activity (DELTA) study.[146]

Three-day, multiple-pass, 24-hour recalls were obtained on randomly selected days first during a self-selected diet period, when participants prepared their own meals, then again when all meals were prepared by the study. During the dietary intervention, body weight was maintained and dietary intake was monitored. Using a t-test statistic, men and women underestimated energy intake by 11% and 13%, respectively, during the self-selected diet period. During the meal-provided period, men underestimated energy intake by 13%; women overestimated energy by 1.3%. This research suggests gender and eating condition influence perceived intake.[146]

Healthy People 2010 Actions

In the *Healthy People 2010* objectives, attention has been given to improving the quality of life and reducing any disparity in care among older adults of different ethnic groups (see Exhibit 10–5). *Healthy People 2010* physical activity objectives have been developed to serve as general framework for goals for increasing physical activity among adults 50 years and older and include[115]:

- reduce the proportion engaging in no leisure-time physical activity from 40 to 20%

Exhibit 10–5   DATA 2010: The Healthy People 2010 Database—November 2000: Objectives for Seniors

Objective Number	Objective	Baseline Year	Baseline	Target 2010
01–03b	Counseling about health behaviors—Diet and nutrition (adults aged 18 years and older)	UK	UK	UK
07–12	Older adult participation in community health promotion activities (age adjusted, persons aged 65 years and older)	1998	12	90
	American Indian or Alaska native	1998	UK	90
	Asian or Pacific Islander	1998	22	90
	Black or African American	1998	8	90
	White	1998	12	90
	Hispanic or Latino	1998	12	90
	Not Hispanic or Latino	1998	12	90
	Female	1998	13	90
	Male	1998	10	90
	Education level (persons aged 65 years and older)			
	Less than high school (persons aged 65 years and older)	1998	6	90
	High school graduate (persons aged 65 years and older)	1998	10	90
	At least some college	1998	20	90
	Poor	1998	8	90
	Near poor	1998	9	90

	Middle/high income	1998	16	90
	Persons with activity limitations	1995	10	90
	Persons without activity limitations	1995	12	90
	Sexual orientation	1998	UK	90
19–01	Healthy weight in adults (age adjusted, adults aged 20 years and older)	1988–94	42	60
	American Indian or Alaska native	1988–94	UK	60
	Asian or Pacific Islander	1988–94	UK	60
	Black or African American	1988–94	34	60
	White	1988–94	42	60
	Hispanic or Latino	1988–94	UK	60
	Mexican American	1988–94	30	60
	Not Hispanic or Latino	1988–94	43	60
	Female	1988–94	45	60
	Male	1988–94	38	60
	Lower income level (≤130% of poverty threshold)	1988–94	38	60
	Higher income level (≥130% of poverty threshold)	1988–94	43	60
	Persons with disabilities	1991–94	32	60
	Persons without disabilities	1991–94	41	60
	20 to 39 years	1988–94	51	60
	40 to 59 years	1988–94	36	60
	60 years and older	1988–94	36	60

Continued

Exhibit 10–5   DATA 2010: The Healthy People 2010 Database—November 2000: Objectives for Seniors

Persons with arthritis	1991–94	36	60
Persons without arthritis	1991–94	36	60
Persons with diabetes	1988–94	26	60
Persons without diabetes	1988–94	43	60
Persons with high blood pressure	1988–94	27	60
Persons without high blood pressure	1988–94	46	60
22–05 Flexibility—Adults (age adjusted, persons aged 18 years and older)	1998	30	43
American Indian or Alaska native	1998	26	43
Asian or Pacific Islander	1998	34	43
Black or African American	1998	26	43
White	1998	30	43
Hispanic or Latino	1998	22	43
Not Hispanic or Latino	1998	31	43
Female	1998	30	43
Male	1998	30	43
Less than high school (persons aged 25 years and older)	1998	16	43
High school graduate (persons aged 25 years and older)	1998	23	43

At least some college (persons aged 25 years and older)	1998	36	43
Poor	1998	21	43
Near poor	1998	24	43
Middle/high income	1998	34	43
Urban (metropolitan statistical area)	1998	32	43
Rural (nonmetropolitan statistical area)	1998	25	43
18 to 24 years	1998	36	43
25 to 44 years	1998	32	43
45 to 64 years	1998	28	43
65 to 74 years	1998	24	43
75 years and older	1998	22	43
Persons with arthritis symptoms	1998	UK	43
Persons without arthritis symptoms	1998	UK	43

UK = unknown

Source: Adapted from: US Department of Health and Human Services. DATA2010—the *Healthy People 2010* Database. *CDC Wonder.* Atlanta, Ga: Centers for Disease Control; November 2000.

- increase the proportion participating in moderate physical activity daily for at least 30 min/d from 15 to 30%
- increase the proportion engaging in vigorous physical activity that promotes the development and maintenance of cardiorespiratory system more than 3 d/wk for more than 20 minutes each from 23 to 30%
- increase the proportion performing physical activities that enhance and maintain muscular strength and endurance from 18 to 30% and flexibility from 30 to 43%
- increase the proportion of US schools providing access to physical activity spaces and facilities for all persons outside normal school hours
- increase the proportion of work sites offering employer-sponsored physical activity and fitness programs from 46 to 75%
- increase the proportion of trips walking rather than riding from 17 to 25%
- increase the proportion of biking rather than riding from 0.6 to 2%

Community nutrition professionals have several avenues to develop and to implement programs for senior adults. Action steps can mobilize community resources in several ways:

1. Organizations should identify strategies they already address and collaborate with other groups that focus their interests in those strategies.
2. Actions should involve those with a reasonable expectation of success.
3. Tactical planning can delineate specific actions to achieve strategies.
4. Financial planning to allocate money and people for coalition and collaborative efforts are instituted.
5. Health organizations and government agencies can exchange and disseminate best practices with workable systems.
6. Evaluation with measurable objectives is essential in all implementation steps.

This blueprint for adults supports an increase in physical activity and improves the health and well-being of all Americans. Success depends on developing and targeting resources and working collaboratively to move the evidence about the benefits of physical activity into national action.[115]

References

1. Riley MW, Riley J. Longevity and social structure: the potential of the added years. In: Pifer A, Bronte L, eds. *Our Aging Society: Paradox and Promise.* New York: WW Norton; 1986:53-77.
2. Perry D. The links of aging research to disease prevention. *Nutr Rev.* 1994;52(8):S48.
3. Lawton MP, Nahemow L. Ecology and the aging process. In: Eisdorfer C, Lawton MP, eds. *Psychology of Adult Development and Aging.* Washington, DC: American Psychological Association; 1973:619-674.
4. Hooyman NR, Kiyak HA. *Social Gerontology—A Multidisciplinary Perspective.* 3rd ed. Boston, Mass: Allyn & Bacon, Inc; 1993.
5. Social Security Administration, US Department of Health and Human Services. *Social Security Bulletin: Annual Statistical Supplement.* Washington, DC: US Government Printing Office; 1990.
6. American Association of Retired Persons. *A Profile of Older Americans 1990.* Washington, DC: American Association of Retired Persons; 1990.

7. Rosenwaike IA. A demographic portrait of the oldest old. *Milbank Memorial Fund Q: Health and Society.* 1985;63:187-205.

8. US Bureau of the Census. *Marital Status and Living Arrangements. Current Population Reports.* Washington, DC: US Dept of Commerce; March 1990. Series P-20, no. 1450.

9. Newman C. Older, healthier and wealthier. *Washington Post.* August 10, 2000:A3.

10. Sullivan DH, Martin WE, Flaxman N, et al. Oral health problems and involuntary weight loss in a population of frail elderly. *J Am Geriatr Soc.* 1993;41:725-731.

11. Wong ND, Wilson PWF, Kannel WB. Serum cholesterol as a prognostic factor after myocardial infarction: the Framingham Study. *Ann Intern Med.* 1991;115:687-698.

12. Evans WJ, Meredith CN. Exercise and nutrition in the elderly. In: Munro HN, Danford DE, eds. *Nutrition, Aging and the Elderly.* New York: Plenum Publishing Corporation; 1989:89.

13. Keller HH. Malnutrition in institutionalized elderly: how and why? *J Am Geriatr Soc.* 1993;41:1212-1218.

14. CDC. *Health, United States, 1999 Report.* Atlanta, Ga. Available at: http://www.cdc.gov/nchs. Accessed January 9, 2001.

15. Warner HR, Butler RN, Sprott RL, et al, eds. *Modern Biological Theories of Aging.* New York: Raven Press; 1987.

16. Schneider EL, Reed JD. Life extension. *N Engl J Med.* 1985;313:1159-1168.

17. Institute of Medicine. *Extending Life, Enhancing Life: A National Research Agenda on Aging.* Washington, DC: National Academy Press; 1992.

18. Finch CE. *Longevity, Senescence and the Genome.* Chicago: University of Chicago Press; 1991.

19. McCormick AM, Campisi J. Cellular aging and senescence. *Curr Opinion Cell Biol.* 1991;3:230-234.

20. Goldstein S. Replicative senescence: the human fibroblast comes of age. *Science.* 1990;249:1129-1133.

21. Hayflick L, Moorhead PS. The serial cultivation of human diploid cell strains. *Exp Cell Res.* 1961;25:585-621.

22. Harman D. The free radical theory of aging. In: Warner HR, Butler RN, Sprott RL, et al, eds. *Modern Biological Theories of Aging.* New York: Raven Press; 1987.

23. Shock NW, Greulich RG, Andres RA, et al. *Normal Human Aging: The Baltimore Longitudinal Study of Aging.* Washington, DC: US Government Printing Office; 1984.

24. National Institutes of Health. National Institute on Aging. *In Search of the Secrets of Aging.* Bethesda, Md: National Institutes of Health; May 1993:1-35. NIH publication No. 93-2756.

25. National Research Council, Commission on Life Sciences, Food and Nutrition Board. *Recommended Dietary Allowances.* 10th ed. Washington, DC: National Academy Press; 1989.

26. Soldo B, Agree E. America's elderly. *Popul Bull.* 1988;43:1-46.

27. US Department of Health and Human Services. *Health, US; 2004.* Atlanta, Ga: CDC, NCHS; November 2004. DHHS Publication No. 2005-0152.

28. Torres-Gil F. Hispanics: a special challenge. In: Pifer A, Bronte L, eds. *Our Aging Society.* New York: WW Norton; 1986.

29. Lopez-Aqueres W, Kemp B, Plopper M, et al. Health needs of the Hispanic elderly. *J Am Geriatr Soc.* 1984;32:191-198.

30. US Bureau of the Census. *Age, Sex, Race and Hispanic Origin Information from the 1990 Census.* Washington, DC: US Dept of Commerce; 1991.

31. Lacayo C. Hispanics. In: Palmore E, ed. *Handbook on the Aged in the United States.* Westport, Conn: Greenwood Press; 1984.

32. US Senate Special Committee on Aging. *Developments in Aging: 1989.* Vol. 1. Washington, DC: US Government Printing Office; 1990.

33. US Bureau of the Census. *State Population and Household Estimates With Age, Sex and Components of Change: 1981-1988.* Washington, DC: US Dept of Commerce; 1989. Current Population Reports. Special Studies Series P-25, no. 1044.

34. Longino CF, Biggar JC, Flynn CB, et al. *The Retirement Migration Project: A Final Report to the National Institute on Aging.* Coral Gables, Fla: University of Miami; 1984.

35. Rudman D, Feller AG. Protein-calorie undernutrition in the nursing home. *J Am Geriatr Soc.* 1989;37:173-178.

36. Baker H, Frank O, Thind IS, et al. Vitamin profiles in elderly persons living at home or in nursing homes, versus profile in healthy young subjects. *J Am Geriatr Soc.* 1979;27:444-450.

37. Abbasi AA, Rudman D. Undernutrition in the nursing home: prevalence, consequences, causes and prevention. *Nutr Rev.* 1994;52(4):119.

38. Stiedemann M, Jansen C, Harrill I. Nutritional status of elderly men and women. *J Am Diet Assoc.* 1978;73:132-139.

39. Phillips P. Grip strength, mental performance and nutritional status as indicators of mortality risk among female geriatric patients. *Age and Aging.* 1986;15:53-56.

40. Katz IR, Beaton-Wimmer P, Parmelle P, et al. Failure to thrive in the elderly: exploration of the concept and delineation of psychiatric components. *J Geriatr Psychiatry.* 1993;6:161-169.

41. Verdery RB, Goldberg AP. Hypercholesterolemia as a predictor of death: a prospective study of 224 nursing home residents. *J Gerontol.* 1991;46:M84-90.

42. Goldberg AF, Mattson DE, Rudman D. The relationship of growth to alveolar ridge atrophy in an older male nursing home population. *Special Care in Dentistry.* 1988;8:184-186.

43. Veis SI, Logemann JA. Swallowing disorders in persons with cerebrovascular accident. *Arch Phys Med Rehabil.* 1985;66:372-375.

44. Palmer ED. Dysphagia in parkinsonism. *JAMA.* 1974;229:1349.

45. Cheah KC, Beard OW. Psychiatric findings in the population of a geriatric evaluation unit: implications. *J Am Geriatr Soc.* 1980;28:153-156.

46. Rovner BW, Kafonek S, Filipp L, et al. Prevalence of mental illness in a community nursing home. *Am J Psychiat.* 1986;143:1446-1449.

47. Gallagher A. Leading the way... the dietitian's role as team leader in the interdisciplinary management of anorexia and unintentional weight loss in the elderly. USA: MultiMedia HealthCare. *Global Monitor,* PAR-04541; 2004:1-9.

48. Kamel HK. Underutilization of calcium and vitamin D supplements in an academic long-term care facility. *J Am Med Dir Assoc.* 2004;5(2):98-100.

49. Winograd CH, Brown EM. Aggressive oral refeeding in hospitalized patients. *Am J Clin Nutr.* 1990;52:967-968.

50. Morley JE, Kraenzle D. Causes of weight loss in a community nursing home. *J Am Geriatr Soc.* 1994;42(6):583-585.

51. Anthony P, Ireton-Jones CS. Dietitians in home care: a new challenge. *Support Line.* 1994;16(6):1-5.

52. Howard L, Heaphey L, Timchalk M. A review of the current national status of home parenteral and enteral nutrition from the provider and the consumer perspective. *J Parenteral and Enteral Nutr.* 1986;10:416-424.

53. Collopy B, Dubler N, Zuckerman C. The ethics of home care: autonomy and accommodation. *Hastings Center Report.* March/April 1990:20(2);1S-16S.

54. Regenstein M. Reimbursement for nutrition support. *Nutr in Clin Prac.* 1989;4:194-202.

55. Pfeil LA, Katz PR, Davis PJ. Water metabolism. In: Morley JE, Glick Z, Rubenstein LZ, eds. *Geriatric Nutrition.* New York: Raven Press; 1990:193-202.

56. Crowe MJ, Forsling ML, Rolls BJ, et al. Altered water excretion in healthy elderly men. *Age and Aging.* 1987;16:285-293.

57. Chernoff R. Thirst and fluid requirements. *Nutr Rev.* 1994;52(8, part II): S3-S5.

58. American Dietetic Association. *Nutrition Screening Initiatives.* Winter 1999; 28:2.

59. Fanelli MT, Stevenhagen KJ. Characterizing consumption patterns by food frequency methodologies: core foods and variety of foods in diets of older Americans. *J Am Diet Assoc.* 1985;85:1570-1576.

60. Brown EL. Factors influencing food choices and intake. *Geriatrics.* 1976;31:89-92.

61. Rolls B. Appetite and satiety in the elderly. *Nutr Rev.* 1994;52(8, part II): S9-S10.

62. Rolls B, McDermott T. Effects of age on sensory specific satiety. *Am J Clin Nutr.* 1991;54:988-996.

63. Schiffman S. Changes in taste and smell: drug interactions and food preferences. *Nutr Rev.* 1994;52(8, part II):S11-S14.

64. Hamilton EMN, Whitney EN, Sizer FS. *Nutrition Concepts and Controversies.* 5th ed. Whitney EN, Sizer FS, eds. New York: West Publishing Company; 1991.

65. Krumholz HM, Seeman TE, Merrill SS, et al. Lack of association between cholesterol and coronary heart disease mortality and morbidity and all-cause mortality in persons older than 70 years. *JAMA.* 1994;272:1335-1340.

66. Centers for Disease Control. National Resource Center for Sage Aging; 2000. Available at: http:/www.safeaging.org. Accessed January 9, 2007.

67. Wolfsen CR, Barker JC, Mitteness LS. Constipation in the daily lives of frail elderly. *Arch Fam Med.* 1993;2:853-858.

68. Rosenbloom CA, Whittington FJ. The effects of bereavement on eating behaviors and nutrient intakes in elderly widowed persons. *J Gerontol.* 1993;48:223S-229S.

69. Butler RN. Senile dementia of the Alzheimer type (SDAT). In: Abrams WB, Berkow B, eds. *The Merck Manual of Geriatrics.* Rahway, NJ: Merck Sharp & Dohme Research Laboratories; 1990:933-937.

70. Claggett SM. Nutritional factors relevant to Alzheimer's disease. *J Am Diet Assoc.* 1989;89:392-396.

71. National Institute on Aging. *Alzheimer's Disease Costs the Nation an Estimated 90 Billion Dollars per Year.* Washington, DC: US Dept of Health and Human Services; 1993. NIH pub no. 93-3409.

72. Alzheimer's Association. "Smart Pills" make headway. Rubin R. *USA Today.* July 7, 2004.

73. Huey E. *Nutritional Assessment of Patients With Alzheimer's Disease in Three Stages of the Disease* [master's thesis]. Long Beach, Calif: California State University Long Beach; 1995.

74. Katzman R. Medical progress—Alzheimer's disease. *N Engl J Med.* 1986;312:964-971.

75. McKhann G, Drachman D, Folstein M, et al. Clinical diagnosis of Alzheimer's disease: report of the NINCDS-ADRDA work group under the auspices of Department of Health and Human Services Task Force on Alzheimer's disease. *Neurology.* 1984;34:939-944.

76. Gray GE. Nutrition and dementia. *J Am Diet Assoc.* 1989;849:1795-1802.

77. Wolf-Klein GP, Silverston FA, Levy AP. Nutritional patterns and weight change in Alzheimer patients. *Int Psychogeriatrics.* 1992;4(10):103-118.

78. Breteler MB, Claus JJ, Duijn CM, et al. Epidemiology of Alzheimer's disease. *Epidemiol Rev.* 1992;14:59-82.

79. Litchford MD, Wakefield LM. Nutrient intakes and energy expenditures of residents with senile dementia of the Alzheimer's type. *J Am Diet Assoc.* 1987;87:211-213.

80. Singh S, Mulley GP, Losowsky MS. Why are Alzheimer patients thin? *Age and Aging.* 1988;17:21-28.

81. Tufts nutrition: translating the research for use at your table. *Tufts University Health & Nutrition Letter.* 2004; (suppl):3.

82. Egbert AM. "The Dwindles": failure to thrive in older patients. *Postgrad Med.* 1993;94:199-212.

83. Bendich A, Butterworth CE, eds. *Micronutrients in Health and in Disease Prevention.* New York: Marcel Dekker Inc; 1991.

84. Young VR. Amino acids and proteins in relation to the nutrition of elderly people. *Age and Aging.* 1990;19:S10-S24.

85. Committee on Diet and Health, Food and Nutrition Board, Commission on Life Sciences, National Research Council. *Diet and Health: Implications for Reducing Chronic Disease Risk.* Washington, DC: National Academy Press; 1989.

86. Blumberg JB. Considerations of the recommended dietary allowances for older adults. *Clin Appl Nutr.* 1991;1:18-19.

87. Blumberg J. Nutrient requirements of the healthy elderly—should there be specific RDAs? *Nutr Rev.* 1994;52(8, part II):S15-S18.

88. Growing older presents new nutrition challenges. *Tufts University Health & Nutrition Letter.* October 2003;21(8):1,8.

89. Russell R, Rasmussen H, Lichtenstein A. Modified food guide pyramid for people over seventy years of age. *J Nutr.* 1999;129:751-753.

90. Krauss RM, Deckelbaum RJ, Ernst N, et al. Dietary guidelines for healthy American adults. *Circulation.* 1996;9:1795-1800.

91. Lichtenstein AH. Trans fatty acids, plasma lipid levels, and the risk of developing cardiovascular disease. A statement for healthcare professionals from the American Heart Association. *Circulation.* 1997;9:2588-2590.

92. Brodribb JM. Dietary fiber in diverticular disease of the colon. In: Spiller GA, Kay RM, eds. *Medical Aspects of Dietary Fiber.* New York: Plenum Press; 1980:43-66.

93. Kromhout D, Bosschieter EN, de Lezenne C. Dietary fiber and 10-year mortality from coronary heart disease, cancer, and all causes: the Zutphen Study. *Lancet.* 1982;2:518-521.

94. Rimm EB, Ascherio A, Givanucci E, Spiegelman D, Stampfer MJ, Willett WC. Vegetable, fruit, and cereal fiber intake and risk of coronary heart disease among men. *JAMA.* 1996;275:447-451.

95. *Dietary Guidelines for Americans.* 5th ed. Washington, DC: US Dept of Agriculture and Dept of Health and Human Services; 2005.

96. Institute of Medicine. *Dietary Reference Intakes: Calcium, Phosphorus, Magnesium, Vitamin D, and Fluoride.* Washington, DC: National Academy Press; 1997.

97. Hurwitz A, Brady DA, Schaal ES, Samloff IM, Dedon J, Ruhl CE. Gastric acidity in older adults. *JAMA.* 1997;278:659-662.

98. Krasinski SD, Russel RM, Samloff IM, et al. Fundic atrophic gastritis in an elderly population. *J Am Geriatr Soc.* 1986;34:800-806.

99. Carmel R. In vitro studies of gastric juice in patients with food-cobalamin malabsorption. *Dig Dis Sci.* 1994;39:2516-2522.

100. Suter PM, Golner BB, Goldin BR, Morrow FD, Russel RM. Reversal of protein-bound vitamin B$_{12}$ malabsorption with antibiotics in atrophic gastritis. *Gastroenterology.* 1991;101:1039-1045.

101. Older Americans Act, Title IIIC USC (1965).

102. Gerontological Nutrition Dietetic Practice Group. 30 snacks for less than 1 gram of fat. Chicago, Ill: American Dietetic Association;1994.

103. Roe D. Development and current status of home-delivered meals program in the United States: are the right elderly served? *Nutr Rev.* 1994;52(1):30-33.

104. Food Research and Action Center. *A National Survey of Nutritional Risk Among the Elderly.* Washington, DC: Food Research and Action Center; 1987.

105. Bernard MA, Rombeau JL. Nutritional support for the elderly patient. *Nutrition, Aging and Health.* New York: Alan R Liss; 1989:229-258.

106. Lowe BF. Future directions for community-based long-term care research. *Milbank Q.* 1988;66:552-571.

107. Hunger and Nutrition Research Project. *Hunger Among the Elderly: Myth or Reality [final report].* Austin, TX: Texas Department of Aging; 1984.

108. Balsam AL, Rogers BL. *Service Innovations in the Elderly Nutrition Program. AARP Report.* Boston, Mass: Tufts University; July 1988.

109. Roe DA, HoSang G. *Supplemental Nutrition Assistance Program (SNAP)* [final report]. Albany, NY: New York State Department of Health: August 1988.

110. Roe DA. *Supplemental Nutrition Assistance Program (SNAP)* [final report]. Albany, NY. October 1989.

111. Nutritionists try out new food guide pyramid for seniors. *Gerontological Nutritionists Newsletter.* Winter 1999:1,9.

112. Medicare. *Nutrition Screening Initiatives.* Winter 1999;(28):1

113. Fries JF. Aging, natural death, and the compression of morbidity. *N Engl J Med.* 1980;303:130-135.

114. Verbrugge L. Recent, present and future health of American adults. *Ann Rev Public Health.* 1989;10:333-361.

115. The Robert Wood Johnson Foundation. *National Blueprint: Increasing Physical Activity Among Adults Age 50 and Older.* Princeton, NJ: RW Johnson Foundation; 2003:25.

116. Institute of Medicine. *Dietary Reference Intakes for Water, Potassium, Sodium, Chloride, and Sulfate.* Washington, DC: National Academy Press; 2004.

117. National Policy and Resource Center on Nutrition and Aging. *Eating Better and Moving More Guidebook.* Miami, FL: Miami-Florida International University; 2003.

118. Cuervo Leon J, Kirk-Sanchez NJ, Pan YL, Weddle DO, Wellman, NS. Helping older adults to eat better and move more. *Gerontological Nutritionists.* Summer 2004:14.

119. Crimmins EM. Evidence on the compression of morbidity. *Gerontologica Perspecta.* 1987;1:45-49.

120. Palmore EB. Trends in the health of the aged. *Gerontologist.* 1986;26:298-302.

121. Schneider EL, Brody JA. Aging, natural death, and the compression of morbidity: another view. *N Engl J Med.* 1983;309:854-856.

122. Rice DP, Feldman JJ. Living longer in the United States: demographic changes and health needs of the elderly. *Milbank Fund Memorial Q: Health and Society.* 1983;61:362-396.

123. Katz S, Branch LG, Granson MH, et al. Active life expectancy. *N Engl J Med.* 1983;309:1218-1224.

124. Manton KG, Stallard E. Cross-sectional estimates of active life expectancy for the US elderly and oldest-old populations. *J Gerontology.* 1991;46:S170-182.

125. Kane RL, Ouslander JG, Abrass IB. *Essentials of Clinical Geriatrics.* 2nd ed. New York: McGraw-Hill; 1989.

126. Butler RN. Ageism: another form of bigotry. *Gerontologist.* 1969;9:243-246.

127. Terry D, Wilcox M, McComick MA, et al. Cardiovascular advantages among the offspring centenarians *J Gerontol A Biol Sci Med Sci.* 2003;58(5):M425-M43;1.

128. Hadley E. *Epidemiologic Studies on Longevity and Healthy Aging.* Betheseda, Md: Geriatrics and Clinical Gerontology Program. National Institute on Aging 2002.

129. *Surgeon General's Workshop on Health Promotion and Aging.* Washington, DC: US Government Printing Office; 1988. No. 1988-201-875/83669.

130. US Department of Health and Human Services, Public Health Service. *Healthy People 2000. National Health Promotion and Disease Prevention Objectives.* Boston, Mass: Jones and Bartlett Publishers; 1992.

131. Nutrition Screening Initiative. *Report of Nutrition Screening I: Toward a Common View.* Washington, DC: Nutrition Screening Initiative; 1991.

132. Nutrition Screening Initiative. *Nutrition Screening Manual for Professionals Caring for Older Americans.* Washington, DC: Nutrition Screening Initiative; 1991.

133. Nutrition Screening Initiative. *Nutrition Interventions Manual for Professionals Caring for Older Americans.* Washington, DC: Greer, Margolis, Mitchell, Grunwald & Associates, Inc; 1992.

134. Nutrition Screening Initiative. *Implementing Nutrition Screening and Intervention Strategies.* Washington, DC: Nutrition Screening Initiative; 1993.

135. Eigenbrod J, Spangler AA. The Nutrition Screening Initiative Survey of elderly nutrition program participants in Indiana. Presented at: Indiana Dietetic Association annual meeting; November 1994; Nappanee, Ind.

136. Posner BM, Jette AM, Smith KW, et al. Nutrition and health risks in the elderly: the Nutrition Screening Initiative. *Am J Public Health.* 1993;83:972-978.

137. Gans KM, Burkholer GJ, Risica PM, Lasater TM. Baseline fat-related dietary behaviors of white, Hispanic, and black participants in a cholesterol screening and education project in New England. *J Am Diet Assoc.* June 2003;103(6):699-706.

138. Crespo CJ, Smit E, Andersen RE, Careter-Pokras O, Ainsworth BE. Race/ethnicity, social class and their relation to physical inactivity during leisure time: results from the third National Health and Nutrition Examination Survey, 1988-1994. *Am J Rev Med* 2001;18(1):46-53.

139. Sharkey JR, Schoenberg NE. Variations in nutritional risk among black and white women who receive home-delivered meals. *J Women Aging.* 2002;14(3-4):99-119.

140. Sharkey JR, Schoenberg NE. Prospective study of black-white differences in food insufficiency among homebound elders. *J Aging Health.* August 2005;17(4):507-527.

141. Cox RH, Carpenter JP, Bruce FA, Poole KP, Gaylord CK. Characteristics of low-income African American and Caucasian adults that are important in self-management of type 2 diabetes. *J Community Health*. April 2004;29(2):155-170.

142. Ervin RB, Kennedy-Stephenson J. Mineral intakes of elderly adult supplement and non-supplement users in the third national health and nutrition examination survey. *J Nutr*. November 2002;132(11):3422-3427.

143. Nutrition Screening Initiatives. *Study Says Physicians Need More Nutrition Training*. Winter 1999;(28):3,6.

144. National Institutes of Health. *Heart Memo*. Bethesda, Md: National Institutes of Health; 1994.

145. The Writing Group for the PEPI Trial. Effects of estrogen and estrogen/progestin regimens on heart disease risk factors in postmenopausal women. *JAMA*. 1995;273:199-208.

146. Jonnalagadda S, Mitchell D, Smiciklas-Wright H, et al. Accuracy of energy intake data estimated by a multiple-pass, 24-hour dietary recall technique. *J Am Diet Assoc*. 2000;100:303-308,311.

SECONDARY AND TERTIARY PREVENTION—MANAGING DISEASE AND AVOIDING COMPLICATIONS

CORONARY HEART DISEASE

Learning Objectives

- Discuss the epidemiology of cardiovascular heart disease in the United States.
- Define the role of nutrition in the etiology, prevention, and treatment of cardiovascular heart disease.
- Identify the *Healthy People 2010* objectives for cardiovascular heart disease.
- Describe how community nutritionists can be actively involved in primary, secondary, and tertiary care of coronary heart disease in the United States.
- List the major food components that increase or decrease coronary heart disease.

High Definition Nutrition

Arteriosclerosis–a group of diseases characterized by thickening and loss of elasticity of arterial walls.

Atherosclerosis–a common form of arteriosclerosis with plaques forming within the intima of medium and large arteries.

Dyslipidemia–abnormal blood lipids or fats; the most common form is hypercholesterolemia.

Endogenous–developing or originating within the organism.

Exogenous–developing or originating outside the organism.

Food synergy–an additive influence of foods and constituents, which, when eaten, have a beneficial effect on health.

Protein–any one of a group of complex organic nitrogenous compounds widely distributed in plants (i.e., vegetable protein) and animals (i.e., animal protein).

Thrombosis—the formation or presence of a blood clot within a blood vessel during life.

Vitamin A toxicity—intake of at least 100,000 IU of vitamin A per day for 10 years.

Vitamin D toxicity—chronic intake of at least 6,000 IU of vitamin D per day.

An Overview of Coronary Heart Disease

Coronary heart disease (CHD) is the result of atherosclerosis or hardening of arteries due to the development of lipid-laden, calcified plaques in the arterial wall. The integrity of the arteries and the flow of blood are reduced. If this occurs in the coronary arteries, a myocardial infarction or sudden death can result; strokes result from atherosclerosis in the cerebral arteries. CHD remains the number 1 cause of death in the United States among men and women; see Figure 11–1. About 1 million people have angina pectoris, and 1,250,000 experience a myocardial infarction (MI) each year.[1]

Heart disease deaths in the United States today exceed all cancers, accidents, and suicide. Cardiovascular disease (CVD) prevalence data from the NHANES survey (1999–2002) is outlined in Figure 11–2. Some data are collected from self-reports showing that the prevalence of myocardial infarction (MI) and electrocardiogram-defined MI were greater in men than in women but angina was reported higher in women than in men. In women, MI reports were higher in blacks than whites. In men, there was a higher prevalence among whites than blacks.[2]

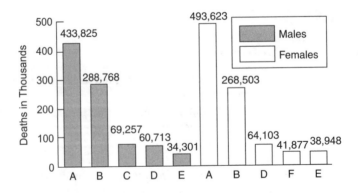

Leading causes of death for all males and females—
United States; 2002.

A Total CVD (preliminary)   D Chronic lower respiratory diseases
B Cancer   E Diabetes mellitus
C Accidents   F Alzheimer's disease

FIGURE 11–1   Leading Causes of Death
Source: CDG/NCHS

Prevalence of cardiovascular diseases in Americans age 20 and older by age and sex— NHANES; 1999–2002.
These data include CHD, CHF, stroke, and hypertension.

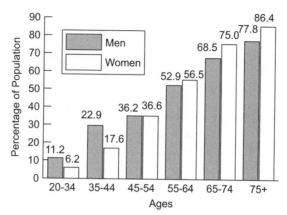

FIGURE 11–2 Prevalence of Cardiovascular Disease
Source: CDG/NCHS and NHLBI.

Incidence, Prevalence, and Mortality Rates of US Population for Cardiovascular Disease and Coronary Heart Disease

Almost 60,000,000 Americans have 1 or more forms of cardiovascular disease, which includes the following[3]:

Prevalence: High blood pressure 50,000,000; stroke 4,400,000; coronary heart disease 12,200,000 (myocardial infarction 7,700,000 and angina pectoris 6,300,000); rheumatic fever/heart disease 1,800,000; congenital cardiovascular defects 1,000,000; and congestive heart failure 4,600,000.[3]

Ethnicity: The estimated adjusted prevalence of CVD in adults for white men was 30%, for women 23.8%, for black men 40.5%, for black women 39.6%, for Mexican-American men 28.8%, and for Mexican-American women 26.6%.[3]

Age and gender: The highest estimated prevalence of CVD of the population is among those age 75 and older; 79.0% for women and 70.7% for men. The second highest prevalence of CVD is between the ages of 65–74; 65.2% for women and 65.2% for men.[3]

Mortality from CVD: Cardiovascular diseases claim over 1 million lives annually.

Ethnicity and gender: The death rates caused by CVD in 2002 were 428,461 white female deaths and 375,392 white male deaths.[4]

Coronary Heart Disease (CHD)

Prevalence: The estimated prevalence is 12,200,000 people alive today have a history of heart attack, angina pectoris, or both. It is estimated that 7,200,000 Americans age 20 and older have a history of myocardial infarction, that is 4.4 million men and 2.8 million women.[3]

Info Line

American Heart Association guidelines take a personal approach to preventing cardiovascular disease in women. Important statistics focus on CVD and women as follows[5]:

- CVD ranks first among all disease categories in hospital discharge for women.
- CVD, particularly coronary heart disease (CHD) and stroke, remains the leading cause of death of women in America and most developed countries, with over 5% of all female deaths in the United States occurring from CVD.
- CVD is a particularly important problem among minority women. The death rate due to CVD is higher in black women than in white women.
- One in 2.5 women who die do so of heart disease, stroke, and other cardiovascular disease compared with 1 in 30 who die of breast cancer.
- In 2001, CVD claimed the lives of 498,863 females; cancer claimed 266,693.
- Coronary heart disease claims the lives of 248,184 females annually compared with 41,394 lives from breast cancer and 65,632 from lung cancer.
- About 38% of women, compared with 25% of men, will die of a heart attack within 1 year.
- Of the approximately 4.8 million stroke survivors alive today, 56% are women.
- Misperceptions still exist that CVD is not a real problem for women.

Aggressive treatment for women should be linked to whether each woman has low, intermediate, or high risk of having a heart attack in the next 10 years, based on a standardized scoring method developed by the Framingham Heart Study. Low risk means a woman has < 10% chance of having a heart attack in the next 10 years, intermediate risk is a 10–20% chance, and high risk is > 20% chance.

Lifestyle interventions such as smoking cessation, regular physical activity, heart-healthy diet, and weight maintenance were given high priority in all women to reduce existing CVD and to prevent major risk factors from developing. The recommendation for a heart-healthy diet includes consistently eating a variety of fruits, vegetables, grains, low-fat or nonfat dairy products, fish, legumes, and sources of protein low in saturated fat, e.g., poultry, lean meats, and plant sources. Women should limit saturated fat intake to < 10% of calories, limit cholesterol intake to < 300 mg/d, and limit intake of trans fatty acids.[4]

The weight maintenance or reduction recommendation includes consistent balance of physical activity, caloric intake, and formal behavioral programs to maintain or achieve a BMI between 18.5 and 24.9 kg/m^2 and a waist circumference < 35 in. Omega-3 fatty acids supplementation may be an adjunct to food for high-risk women as well as folic acid supplementation, if a higher-than-normal level of homocysteine has been measured. A complete list of clinical recommendations is located at http://circ.ahajournals.org/cgi/content/full/109/5/672/TBL4?ck=nck.

Ethnicity, age, and gender: Among American adults age 20 and older the prevalence of CHD is 6.9% for white men; 5.4% for white women; 7.1% for black men; 9.0% for black women; 7.2% for Mexican-American men; and 6.8% for Mexican-American women. The prevalence for ages 35 to 44 is 2.2% for men and 4.0% for women. In the age group 45 to 54, it is 6.7% for men and 5.5% for women.[3]

Incidence: An estimated 11,000,000 Americans will have a new or recurrent coronary attack and more than 40% of these people will die.[3] The rate of new and recurrent CHD in nonblack men ages 65 to 74 is 23.0 per 1,000 population; for ages 75 to 84 it is 35.3; and for age 85 and older it is over 50. For nonblack women it is 9.8, 24.9, and over 25, respectively. For black men the rates are 16.3, 54.9, and 40.8; and for black women the rates are 13.3, 18.3, and 14.1, respectively. Among American Indians ages 65 to 74, the rates of new and recurrent heart attacks are 25.1 for men and 9.1 for women per 1,000.[4]

Mortality of CHD: Approximately 225,000 people a year die a sudden death from a coronary attack.[3]

Risk factors for CHD: A number of risk factors have been linked to the development of CHD and the rate of its development, including genetic predispostion, sex, age, elevated serum total cholesterol, cigarette smoking, elevated blood pressure, obesity, and physical inactivity. Hyperlipidemia is the major risk factor for CHD. Hyperlipidemia results from an overproduction of cholesterol, triglyceride, and very-low-density lipoprotein (VLDL) by the liver, and the defective removal of lipids and lipoproteins by the liver—that is, an altered removal of low-density lipoprotein (LDL), the chief transport modality for cholesterol, by the LDL receptor in the liver. A high-fat diet has a direct impact on serum total cholesterol level.[1]

Fifty-one percent of US adult men and 54% of adult women have blood cholesterol levels over 200 mg/dL. Among whites only, 17.8% of men and 19.9% of women have levels of 240 mg/dL or higher.[6] A concomitant concern is the increase in the number of adults exceeding a healthy body weight (body mass index of 25.0 kg/m^2 and greater noted for 69.4% of men and 57.2% of women. More than one half of blacks and Mexican-American women have excess body weight.[6]

Youth demonstrate CHD risk early in life. Estimates are that 36.5% of US youth aged 19 and under, or 27.7 million, have blood cholesterol levels of 170 mg/dL or higher. This includes 8.4 million white males, 9.2 million white females, 2.2 million black males, and 2.7 million black females.[3]

The pathophysiology of atherosclerosis is directly related to levels of total serum cholesterol, LDL, VLDL, and remnant particles; it is inversely associated with high-density lipoproteins (HDL).[2] High CHD rates occur among individuals who have elevated blood cholesterol levels (greater than 240 mg/dL or 6.21 mmol/L). However, many CHD cases are diagnosed in individuals who have a serum total cholesterol less than 240 mg/dL. The average cholesterol level for US adults is 210 mg/dL.[1]

Stabilization and reversibility of atherosclerotic coronary lesions have been demonstrated. During the past 30 years, several clinical trials have shown that not only can CHD be prevented, but that life expectancy can be increased. Important trials include the following:

1. The multicenter Lipid Research Coronary (LRC) Primary Prevention Trial—a randomized trial with middle-aged men assigned to cholestyramine or placebo; both groups followed a moderate, low-cholesterol diet.
2. The Cholesterol-Lowering Atherosclerosis Study—a randomized, placebo-controlled trial with drug and diet.
3. The Leiden Study—a noncontrol group trial of men with stable angina prescribed a low-cholesterol, high-polyunsaturated fat, vegetarian diet.
4. The Oslo Trial—a diet and smoking intervention of normotensive men with elevated cholesterol levels.
5. The Cardiff, Wales Trial—a test of a high-fish diet.
6. The Lifestyle Heart Trial in San Francisco—a less than 10% fat, high-fiber diet with stress management for men and women.
7. The Helsinki Heart Study—a double-blind, placebo-controlled trial of 2 mental hospital populations.

Thrombosis is the major complication of atherosclerosis. If it were not present, the atherosclerosis would be far less serious. Lifelong dietary habits can either promote or prevent thrombosis by affecting coagulation and platelets. Dietary fat and cholesterol serve as precursors for prostaglandins. Saturated fat and cholesterol suppress the LDL receptor, resulting in increased LDL levels. In addition, saturated fat is thrombogenic (tending to produce blood clots within blood vessels). Polyunsaturated vegetable oils contain omega-6 fatty acids, which lower plasma LDL levels; monounsaturated vegetable fats have less saturated fat and can lower LDL; and omega-3 fatty acids from fish decrease plasma LDL and VLDL and lower cholesterol and triglyceride levels.[5] Stearic acid is a saturated fatty acid and especially potent in raising the LDL level of blood.

After a fatty meal, particles and remnants circulate in the plasma. The stypven time, analogous to the prothrombin time or the time required to coagulate the blood, is greatly accelerated due to the fat; fibrinolysis is lessened. Levels of lipoprotein-a (Lp-a) increase, and Lp-a binds to fibrin and prevents plasmin from dissolving clots that occur naturally. Lp-a is high in cholesterol and may promote atherosclerosis. Fatty acids are also released when lipoprotein lipase acts on triglyceride-rich remnants after chylomicron breakdown. The released fatty acids also become atherogenic.[5]

Ketogenic, low-calorie diets (which convert protein residue to ketone bodies) may promote thrombosis in overweight coronary patients due to the resulting high plasma-free fatty acid levels and reduced prostacyclin concentrations. Obese hypertriglyceridemic patients have increased levels of activated factor VII, which is highly associated with thrombosis.

Saturated fatty acid (SFA) intake expressed as the percentage of total energy has repeatedly shown a strong correlation with CHD mortality rates across multiple countries.[7] When graphing the percentage of total energy from saturated fat against CHD, the slope is nearly 2½ times steeper than the slope of serum cholesterol and CHD. A study of Japanese migrants to Hawaii and San Francisco demonstrates the positive effect of dietary fat composition on CHD rates.[8] However, within a population, it has been difficult to observe and to document a significant effect of exogenous saturated fat intake on CHD. Various dietary components that influence plasma lipid and lipoprotein levels have been identified[9] (see Table 11–1).

A 10–20% reduction of plasma total cholesterol occurs in concert with dietary saturated fatty acids and cholesterol at ≤ 7% of energy and ≤ 200 mg per day, respectively. Increasing soluble fiber can accentuate the loss, with an additional reduction up to 10% in plasma total cholesterol.[9]

The current recommendation is that SFA should contribute less than 10% of total energy and less than 7% for the treatment of elevated plasma total cholesterol and LDL cholesterol levels. The US eating pattern contains about 13% of energy from SFA and about 7% of energy from omega-6 fatty acids.[6] The literature is extensive regarding the role of food composition and eating habits on lipid levels.

A 1970 study of about 12,000 men in 18 populations from 7 countries (Finland, Greece, Italy, Japan, the Netherlands, the United States, and Yugoslavia) opened our eyes to the food-lipid association. The percentage of energy from SFA was highly correlated with the 5-year CHD incidence rate and with serum cholesterol concentration. Among the groups, 80% of the serum cholesterol variability was explained by SFA intake.[7] When the Framingham Study[10] could not confirm these results, several reasons were given[11]:

- the homogeneity of the dietary pattern within a population
- a large intraindividual variation from day to day in the fat composition of food intake

TABLE 11–1 Major Dietary Components and Their Effect on Plasma Total Cholesterol and LDL Cholesterol

Effect	Component
Lowers total cholesterol and LDL cholesterol levels	Omega-6 fatty acids Monounsaturated fatty acids Soluble fiber Carbohydrate Vegetarianism Alcohol
Raises total cholesterol and LDL cholesterol levels	Saturated fatty acids Cholesterol Overweight/obesity Omega-3 fatty acids*

*Omega-3 fatty acids are hypotriglyceridemic and hypocholesterolemic. For individuals with hypertriglyceridemia, omega-3 fatty acids elevate LDL cholesterol levels.
Source: Adapted from: Kris-Etherton, Krummel D, Russel ME, et al. The effect of diet on plasma, lipids, lipoproteins, and coronary heart disease. *J Am Diet Assoc.* 1988;88:1373. Used with permission of the American Dietetic Association.

- genetic and metabolic heterogeneity within a population
- unrefined dietary assessment methods
- confounding variables

Diets with less saturated fat tend to lower the plasma total cholesterol[12-15] (see Table 11–2). SFAs are found in animal fat, coconut fat, and palm and palm kernel oils. Omega-5 fatty acids are hypocholesterolemic. They are found mainly in vegetable oils.

TABLE 11–2   Sources and Effect of Dietary Fatty Acids on Plasma Lipids

Fatty Acids	Common Sources	Major Effect on Plasma Lipids
Saturated		
C12:0 (lauric)	Coconut, palm kernel oil	Increases plasma total cholesterol
C14:0 (myristic)	Coconut	Increases plasma total cholesterol
C16:0 (palmitic)	Palm oil, beef	Increases plasma total cholesterol
C18:0 (stearic)	Cocoa butter, beef	Decreases plasma total cholesterol, has no effect, or raises it less than expected
Monounsaturated		
C18:1(oleic)	Oil, beef, olive oil, rapeseed	Decreases plasma total cholesterol*
Polyunsaturated		
Omega-6		
C18:2 (linoleic)	Corn oil, cottonseed oil, soybean oil, sunflower oil	Decreases plasma total cholesterol†,‡
Omega-3		
C20:5 (Eicosapentaenoic)	Atlantic and king mackerel	Decreases plasma total cholesterol§
C22:6 (Docosahexaenoic)	Atlantic and Pacific herring (sardines), lake trout, chinook salmon, albacore tuna, Atlantic and sockeye salmon, bluefish, pink and chum salmon, Atlantic halibut, coho salmon, marine lipids (cod liver oil and omega-3 fatty acid supplements)	Decreases plasma triglycerides, variable LDL cholesterol, and HDL cholesterol effects§

*Snook JT, Delany JP, Vivian VM. Effect of moderate to very low-fat defined formula diets on serum lipids in healthy subjects. *Lipids.* 1985;20:808.
†Bronsgeest-Schoute DC, Hautvast JGAJ, Hermus RJJ. Dependence of the effects of dietary cholesterol and experimental conditions on serum lipids in man. *Am J Clin Nutr.* 1979;32:283.
‡Grundy SM, Nix D, Whelon MF, et al. Comparison of three cholesterol-lowering diets in normolipemic men. *JAMA.* 1986;256:2351.
§Kuusi T, Ehnholm C, Huttunen J, et al. Concentration and composition of serum lipoproteins during a low-fat diet at two levels of polyunsaturated fat. *J Lipid Res.* 1985;26:360.
Source: Modified from Kris-Etherton, Krummel D, Russel ME, et al. The effect of diet on plasma, lipids, lipoproteins, and coronary heart disease. *J Am Diet Assoc.* 1988;88:1373.

The quantities of SFA, omega-6 fatty acids, and cholesterol are important determinants of blood lipid level. Two predictive equations were developed to determine the magnitude of change in plasma total cholesterol when there are changes in the fatty acid composition of an individual's eating pattern.[16,17] The effect of the quality and quantity of fat on blood cholesterol when exogenous cholesterol is modified is seen in the Keys[16] and Hegsted[17] predictive equations.[18] Keys's (Minnesota) equation is as follows:

$$\Delta \text{ CHOL} = 1.35 \ (2 \ \Delta S - \Delta P) + 1.52 \ \Delta Z$$

Hegsted's (Harvard) equation is as follows:

$$\Delta \text{ CHOL} = 2.16 \ \Delta S - 1.65 \ \Delta P + 0.0677 \ \Delta C - 0.53$$

Where g CHOL = estimated change in serum cholesterol in mg/dL
ΔS = change in percentage of daily calories from saturated fat
ΔP = change in percentage of daily calories from polyunsaturated fat
ΔZ = change in the square root of daily dietary cholesterol in mg/1,000 kcal
ΔC = change in dietary cholesterol in mg/day

Both equations predict a twofold plasma cholesterol-raising effect of SFA that is approximately twice the cholesterol-lowering effect of omega-6 fatty acids. The effect of dietary fat on serum cholesterol is a function of the expression $2S - P$, where S = saturated fat and P = polyunsaturated fat.[19] CHD research in Italy and Australia shows:

- Diet composition continues to relate to CHD risk factors. In Northern Italy, 352 adults, 46% females and 48% males (6% not reporting gender), reported their diets were high in protein (animal/vegetable ratio 1.7 in women and 1.4 in men) and high in fat and low in carbohydrates. The atherogenic potential of the diet, evaluated by the cholesterol/saturated fat index, was high in about 50% of the population. Thiamin and riboflavin intakes were lower than the Italian recommended allowances in more than 60% of the people tested, but vitamin A intake was adequate for 70%. A positive association among men and women 20 to 39 years old for energy, alcohol, total and saturated fats, and some blood lipids was noted. Among older people blood lipids were correlated with body mass index.[20]
- Dietary composition remains consistent. Over the last 4 decades there has been extensive research into the links between diet and coronary heart disease. Australia's National Heart Foundation's nutrition policy is partly based on extensive research linking diet and coronary heart disease with key points as follows[21]:
  1. A high intake of saturated fatty acids is strongly associated with elevated serum cholesterol and LDL -cholesterol levels and increased risk of coronary heart disease.
  2. The n-6 polyunsaturated fatty acids (principally linoleic acid) lower serum cholesterol levels when substituted for saturated fats and probably have an independent cholesterol-lowering effect.

3. The n-3 polyunsaturated fatty acids (fish oils) reduce serum triglyceride levels, decrease the tendency to thrombosis, and may further reduce coronary risk through other mechanisms.

4. Monounsaturated fatty acids reduce serum cholesterol levels when substituted for saturated fatty acids. It is not clear whether this is an independent effect or simply the result of displacement of saturates.

5. Trans fatty acids may increase serum cholesterol levels and can be reckoned to be equivalent to saturated fatty acids.

6. Total fat intake, independent of fatty acid type, is not strongly associated with coronary heart disease but may contribute to obesity. Associations between total fat intake and coronary heart disease are primarily mediated through the saturated fatty acid component.

7. Dietary cholesterol increases serum cholesterol levels in some people and may increase risk of coronary heart disease.

8. A high intake of alcohol increases blood pressure and serum triglyceride levels and increases mortality from cardiovascular disease. Light alcohol consumption reduces the risk of coronary heart disease.

9. The consumption of sugar is not associated with coronary heart disease.

10. High salt intake is related to hypertension especially in the subset of salt-sensitive people. Potassium intake may be inversely related to hypertension.

11. Abdominal obesity increases the risk of coronary heart disease probably by adversely influencing conventional risk factors.

12. A high intake of plant foods reduces the risk of coronary heart disease through several mechanisms, including lowering serum cholesterol and blood pressure levels.

Lipid Response to Dietary Change

Cocoa butter is composed of the SFA stearic acid (C18:0). In dietary manipulation studies, it has either decreased,[22] not affected,[23] or increased[16] plasma total cholesterol. When stearic acid replaces palmitic acid, it can lower cholesterol,[24] but different SFAs evoke different responses (e.g., stearic acid is hypocholesterolemic [lowers blood cholesterol] compared with palmitic acid but hypercholesterolemic [raises blood cholesterol] compared with linoleic acid). For this reason, healthcare providers must consider individual food selections when promoting a less than 10% SFA intake.

The extent of plasma lipid response is related to an individual's baseline plasma lipid level.[15,25-28] Cholesterol-lowering responses have ranged from +4% to −17%, with a mean level of −11%. LDL and plasma total cholesterol levels tend to decline when lipid-lowering foods are consumed; HDL levels have decreased in some studies.

In an Australian study of 163 men and 66 women, 16 to 80 years old, adipose tissue level of linoleic acid was positively associated with coronary artery disease (CAD) involvement. Platelet linoleic acid levels had a positive association with CAD; and by controlling for possible confounding factors, the platelet concentration of eicosapentaenoic acid (i.e., omega-3) had an inverse association with CAD for men, whereas the docosapentaenoic acid concentration had an inverse association with CAD for women.[29]

Speculation is that the linoleic acid increases the risk of new atherosclerotic lesions,[30-34] but further research is warranted. Saturated fatty acids consistently raise plasma total cholesterol, and omega-6 fatty acids lower it. Their effects differ, as saturated fatty acids are twice as powerful as omega-6 fatty acids. A 1% increase in the SFA intake increases plasma total cholesterol by 2.7 mg/dL. A 1% increase in omega-6 fatty acids results in a 1.4 mg/dL reduction in total cholesterol.[16]

Fish oil can lower plasma triglyceride, but intake must be about 90 to 120 grams for an effect. This amount is abnormally high for average individuals to consume. A realistic eating pattern would contain 2 to 3 fish meals a week as a healthy, preventive approach.[35] Studies of West Greenland Eskimos and white Danes show great contrast in eating and in health outcome.[36,37] Total fat intake was similar, but the Danes consumed about twice as much SFA and omega-6 fatty acids as the Eskimos. The age-adjusted mortality from myocardial infarction for Greenland Eskimos was about 10% of the mortality for Danes. For the Eskimos, plasma total cholesterol, triglycerides, LDL, and VLDL levels were lower, and HDL levels were higher. Eskimos consume about 5 to 10 g/day of omega-3 fatty acids by eating fish, seal, walrus, and whale.[36,37]

Omega-3 fatty acids reduce triglyceride levels and may lower cholesterol level.[38] The effect is dose related.[39] Fish oil may also serve other roles (for example, it may lessen the hypercholesterolemic effect of dietary cholesterol, reduce platelet aggregation and blood clotting, lessen inflammation, and reduce the viscosity of blood by improving the oxygen supply to tissues and narrowed vessels).[35,40,41]

Fish oil containing omega-3 fatty acids alters platelet function. Using the fish oil diet, a 14% decrease in platelet adhesiveness and a 4-minute increase in bleeding time has been observed.[42] These changes are due to prostaglandins, which are made from essential fatty acids.

A decreased production of thromboxane A2 and increased synthesis of prostacyclins are responsible for the antithrombic action of the omega-3 fatty acids. Fish oil stops the formation of the atherosclerotic plaque by reducing cellular growth factors and the adhesion of macrophages to the endothelium. Fish oils also promote the endothelial-derived relaxing factor and inhibit the synthesis of interleukin-1-alpha from monocytes. Recurrent stenosis after coronary angioplasty was less in patients who were given fish oil before the procedure.[42] Fish oil decreases blood viscosity, which is a thrombosis-inducing factor, and it reduces fat level in the blood after a fatty meal. The omega-3 fatty acids in fish and fish oil prevent 2 important aspects of CHD: the lipid-rich atherosclerotic plaque and thrombosis. Incorporating fish and fish oil into the low-cholesterol, low-saturated-fat diet is essential to achieve maximal beneficial effects.[42]

A daily intake of 90 to 120 grams of fish oil tends to create a positive lipid profile with lower plasma triglycerides and total cholesterol levels. A 30-71% lowering of plasma triglycerides using capsules in hypercholesterolemic and hypertriglyceridemic patients was reported. Patients took 20 1-gram capsules containing 0.18 grams eicosapentaenoic acid and 0.12 grams docosapentaenoic acid per capsule daily for 2 years.[42]

Strong warnings have been issued against the routine continuous use of fish oil supplements.[43] Concerns include safety, proper dosages, length of treatment, side effects, and the effects of long-term use. At a level of 30 to 40 mL codliver oil per day, risk of vitamin A and D toxicity can occur. Vitamin A toxicity is known to occur in some persons who ingest as little as 100,000 IU per day for about 10 years or 200,000 IU per day for 5 years. Other side effects include increased bleeding, alteration of impaired immune function,[44] and potential intake of environmental toxins. Individuals with normal plasma lipid levels should not use fish oil supplements since their role as a CHD preventive therapy is not clear.[8]

When monounsaturated fatty acids (MUFAs) such as those provided by olive and peanut oil are substituted for SFA, lower plasma total cholesterol and LDL cholesterol levels without lower HDL levels are reported.[12,45,46] A level of 12–15% of calories from MUFAs is recommended.[46] A 3-week eating pattern that was 38% of calories from fat, 10% from SFA, 25% from MUFA (mainly olive oil), and 4% from omega-6 fatty acids lowered plasma apolipoprotein by 7.4% more.[47] This suggests that an eating pattern with the fat mainly of MUFA may be one of the most effective lipid-lowering patterns.

Considering the various lipid responses to fatty acid composition of the eating pattern, current findings strongly suggest that healthcare providers use percentage of energy from SFA, MUFA, polyunsatured fatty acids (PUFA), and omega-6 fatty acids and not use a polyunsaturated to saturated fatty acid ratio when making eating pattern recommendations. This provides a more accurate description of the healthful amounts of the various fatty acids.[48] This approach allows individuals to learn about the various sources of fat and their effects, as well as how to apply this information to individual eating patterns.[48]

Salmon has been presented as one of several foods people should limit to reduce their risk of cancer but consume to reduce heart attacks. This controversy heightened when salmon raised on farms in the United States and Europe was reported to have higher levels of pollutants than salmon caught in the wild. Eating farmed salmon once a month was recommended.[49]

The US Food and Drug Administration (FDA) stated that consumers should not reduce their intake of farmed or wild salmon while Britain reminded people that the levels of pollutants reported in the study are within internationally recognized safety limits. Trace amounts of polychlorinated biphenyls (PCBs) were found in farm-raised salmon, but PCBs aren't proven human carcinogens. Contaminant levels in salmon have decreased 90% in the past 30 years, and long-term studies of factory workers exposed to high levels of PCBs show no increase in the incidence of cancer.

Concentrations of PCBs in farm-raised salmon were only 1.8% of the level FDA finds tolerable or an average of 36.6 ppb compared with 2,000 ppb in the FDA's guidelines. If a person eats 8 ounces of farmed salmon every week for 70 years, the PCBs would increase his cancer risk by 1 in 100,000, according to the Environmental Protection Agency. Salmon is a rich source of omega-3 fatty acids, which reduce heart attacks. Omega-3 in salmon assists brain development in utero and early life and may prevent Alzheimer's disease and breast cancer.[49]

A German chemical company, BASF, is participating in a new project designed to trace Norwegian farmed salmon throughout the entire production chain as part of a qualitative move to boost sales through improving consumer confidence. The tracing project, named Technology Development for Profitable Fishfarming (TELOP), is supported by the Norwegian government and monitored by independent research institutes and is designed to give a high degree of consumer protection by supplying detailed information about the way the salmon is treated at every stage of the production process.

BASF supplies vitamins and amino acids in the feed given to the salmon, as well as the carotenoid astaxanthin, which gives the famed fish its characteristic pink color. Users can trace the origin of any filet of salmon they buy to determine where the salmon was processed, the feed received, and any additives used. The process ensures transparency greater than that required by European Union legislation effective in January 2005.[50]

Preventing the release of polybrominated diphenyl ethers (PBDEs) into the environment removes contamination from water, air, and food matter, reducing a public health problem.[51]

- PBDEs are brominated organic compounds that persist and accumulate to a toxic level.
- PBDEs are used as flame retardants, comprising up to 30% of product weight, due to their ease of mixing into the product. This increases their ease of release into house dust and sewage sludge.
- North Americans' PBDE tissue levels are 20 times greater than Europeans, with US PBDE concentrations doubling within 4–6 years.
- Octa- and penta-PBDE were banned in Europe in 2004. North American companies voluntarily phased out their production of these by the end of 2004.
- Deca-PBDEs have a low bioaccumulation and transport potential because of their large molecular size. Whether they degradate to different PBDE congeners is being studied.
- PBDEs accumulated from air vapor and skin exposure from furniture have been recently identified as potentially significant sources of PBDEs.
- PBDE levels in food are measured in parts per billion; dust contaminants in indoor air are measured in parts per million.
- PBDE levels in food are not believed to be a food safety issue in commercially produced foods.
- Little is known about the toxicity of PBDEs. Developmental neurotoxicity and alterations to the thyroid are the critical effects. PBDEs have been shown to have dioxin-like toxicity, but are much less potent when compared to PCBs or dioxins/furans. PBDEs do not appear to be genotoxic, suggesting that these compounds are not DNA-reactive carcinogens. The toxicological potencies of the different individual constituents of the mixtures, known as congeners, have not been determined.
- Concentration of PBDEs in US and Canadian foods and the relative contribution of PBDEs in different food groups to total dietary intake is needed.
- PBDEs accumulate in fats, fish, and other fatty foods.

The Role of Total Fat

Even though fat composition has a major influence on blood lipids, total fat intake has influenced the CHD morbidity and mortality in 3 different populations.[52] Plasma lipids respond the same to a low-fat diet[12] and a high-fat diet[28] when saturated and polyunsaturated fat composition are the same.

The total amount of fat may be more influential than nutritionists once thought. A significant correlation between total fat intake and the percentage of body fat was reported for 155 moderately overweight, middle-aged men.[53] The hypothesis is that first, a high-fat diet may contribute to obesity; second, exogenous fat is stored in body fat more efficiently than carbohydrate; and third, the outcome is an increased CHD risk.[54] Studies show that women who follow a 15–20% fat-eating pattern consume 11% fewer calories than women who have 45–50% of their total calories from fat, and they experience a 15% energy surplus.[55]

The Role of Dietary Cholesterol

Exogenous cholesterol increases plasma total cholesterol and lipoprotein cholesterol levels. Cholesterol-rich chylomicron and VLDL remnants may be atherogenic and increase as cholesterol is ingested.[56] Total daily cholesterol intake should not exceed 300 mg/day. Plasma cholesterol response is greatest with changes in cholesterol intake below 500 mg/day.

The first report of a correlation between dietary cholesterol and plasma cholesterol levels ($r = 0.90$) involved a study of the Tarahumara Indians.[57] This Mexican population was unacculturated and inhabited the Sierra Madre Occidental Mountains. At the same time in US cross-sectional studies, a lack of association between cholesterol intakes and plasma cholesterol levels was consistently reported when intakes were between 200 and 1,500 mg per day.[58-59] Reasons given then and now for the lack of significant correlation are[56]:

- the large day-to-day variation in the plasma cholesterol level
- an inadequate number of 24-hour recalls to estimate dietary cholesterol accurately
- a similar or narrow range of dietary cholesterol intake
- inappropriate end points
- undefined independent variables affecting blood cholesterol

Two major studies, the Western Electric Study and the Lipid Research Clinics Coronary Primary Prevention Trial, reported a significant association between exogenous cholesterol change and changes in plasma total cholesterol.[60-61] Observations from the Western Electric Study involved a 25-year follow-up and reported a positive and independent association between dietary cholesterol and risk of CHD death.[61]

In other studies, participants were assigned to regimens that either added a specified number of eggs each day to their usual eating pattern or involved eating a prepared meal.[62] The dietary manipulations involved 1 or more of the following:

- varying amounts of dietary cholesterol
- different time periods for the experimental diet

- men only, women only, or men and women combined
- various ages of individuals
- different baseline blood cholesterol levels
- alteration of the quantity and quality of fat
- crossover and double-blind research designs
- various numbers of blood cholesterol samples due to -5% to $+10\%$ change in level[62] per day for an individual

Plasma cholesterol responds to dietary cholesterol. The response to cholesterol intake between 0 and 500 mg/day can be termed as linear or curvilinear.[56] Most individuals compensate for different exogenous cholesterol levels and show no serum cholesterol change. Other individuals are sensitive to changes in cholesterol intake.

In 1 study, 80% of the participants responded to dietary change and the response was predictable.[63] For 20%, the plasma response was either much higher or much lower than expected. It appears that about one half of individuals have a predictable or greater than anticipated cholesterol response; 16% have less than one half of the predicted response.[64]

The Role of Trans Fatty Acids and Vegetable Oils

Vegetable Oils

Health-conscious consumers have recently become concerned with trans fatty acids, which appear naturally in the fat of beef, butter, milk, and lamb.[65] Commercially prepared, partially hydrogenated margarines and solid cooking oils are also high in trans fatty acids.

Trans fatty acids are produced during the hydrogenation of vegetable oils. This process adds hydrogen to unsaturated fatty acids in the oil and modifies the fat by changing it from a liquid to a soft or solid state. Partially hydrogenated vegetable oils are used to replace naturally solid, saturate-rich fats, such as lard and beef tallow. They are used in margarines, baked foods, and in commercial frying, where vegetable oils cannot be used. Margarines made in the United States are composed of 0–30% trans fatty acids; stick margarines have more trans fatty acids than soft, tub margarines. The main sources of trans fatty acids in the US eating pattern are stick margarine, shortening, commercial frying fats, and high-fat baked goods.[65]

Clinical trial data show that at high levels, trans fatty acids resemble saturated fatty acids and raise serum LDL cholesterol and modestly lower HDL levels. Trans fatty acids do not reduce HDL cholesterol when ingested at current average levels. The US population currently consumes about 12–14% of total energy from saturated fatty acids, and about 2–4% from trans fatty acids. This is an average 8 to 13 grams of trans fatty acids per day.[65]

In the Netherlands, consumption of trans fatty acids is approximately twice that of US residents, yet no adverse effects on heart disease have been attributed to their ingestion. Dutch, US, and Australian researchers have shown that trans fatty acids have far more moderate effects on blood cholesterol levels than saturated fatty acids. A recent US Department of Agriculture (USDA) study involving healthy persons who consumed an average amount of trans fatty acids did not report a lower HDL level among the treatment group. Consuming twice the level of trans fatty acids reduced HDL levels by 2.8%.[65]

Mortality from CHD has declined in the United States during the past 20 years. At the same time, there has been a change from consuming highly saturated animal fats to eating more unsaturated vegetable oils and margarines, which contain no cholesterol but have the essential fatty acid, linoleic acid, and the antioxidant, vitamin E.[65]

Partially hydrogenated vegetable fats and oils can be used to replace saturated animal fats in foods, replace saturate-rich frying, and substitute for saturated baking fats. Totally liquid vegetable oils are often unsuitable for fried and baked products because they form oxidation products during frying and do not perform well in baked foods. Partially hydrogenated vegetable oils, which can be used in baked products, decrease the saturated fatty acid intake and maintain the quality of commercially baked goods.

Data from the Nurses' Health Study of 87,000 women were evaluated for the association of trans fatty acid content of foods on plasma LDL cholesterol. Dietary data were obtained from a semiquantitative food frequency with 61 foods. Women were followed for 8 years; within that time, 431 new cases of CHD were documented. During the analysis of the data, the age and the total energy intake of the women were controlled. A direct association appeared between trans fatty acid intake and CHD risk, and a relative risk of 1.50 resulted when comparing the highest with the lowest quintile of trans fatty acid intake. Multivitamin use; saturated and monounsaturated fat; linoleic acid; dietary cholesterol; fiber; and vitamins E, C, and A intakes did not enhance or dilute the association. By analyzing data only for women with a consistent margarine intake for 1 decade, a relative risk of 1.67 was noted. Further, a significant association was reported between higher risk for CHD and intakes of major food sources of trans fatty acids. This means that as intake of margarine, cookies, cake, and white bread increased, the risk of CHD increased.[66]

The plasma lipid modifying effects of feeding vegetable oil sterol esters (VOSE) in salad dressings were determined in 26 men and 27 women fed controlled, isocaloric diets for 6 weeks. Diets contained typical American foods that provided 33% of energy from fat with a PUFA:MUFA:SFA ratio of 1.3:1.4:1.0. to determine blood lipid effects of fat level and VOSE in salad dressings; 3.6 g VOSE/d (2.2 g sterol equivalent) was divided into 2 servings/d of either ranch dressing (8 g fat per serving), or Italian dressing (4 g fat per serving), added to the same basal diet, and compared in a parallel design. Within each type of dressing, diets having dressing without (control) and with VOSE (test) were fed for a 3-wk/diet and crossed over randomly. Control and test dressings had similar fat and fatty acid concentrations.[67]

The type of salad dressing or gender did not affect plasma LDL-C, HDL-C, or triglycerides (TG) ($p > 0.05$). With data for dressings and gender combined, switching from a self-selected baseline diet to the control diet with no VOSE resulted in reduction in LDL-C of 8.4% ($p < 0.0001$), HDL-C of 3.1% ($p = 0.009$), and triglycerides (TG) of 9.2% ($p < 0.0001$). Daily consumption of 3.6 g VOSE resulted in further decreases in LDLC of 9.7% ($p < 0.0001$), and in TG of 7.3% ($p = 0.005$). No further decrease in HDL-C was observed. Total plasma carotenoids, uncorrected for plasma lipids, decreased by 11.6% ($p < 0.0001$) with VOSE consumption compared to control consumption. Plasma carotenoids on all diets remained within normal ranges. Low-fat foods, e.g., reduced-fat salad dressings, appear effective carriers for VOSE and fit in a healthy eating pattern to lower blood cholesterol.[67]

To investigate the effect of different doses on cholesterol lowering, investigators compared 3 different levels of plant sterols (0.83, 1.61, 3.24 g/d) in a randomized, double-blind, placebo-controlled study. The spreads were butter, a commercially available spread, and 3 spreads fortified with different amounts of plant sterols. A hundred healthy volunteers with normal or mildly elevated cholesterol each consumed 4 spreads for a period of 3.5 weeks. Compared to the control spread intake, total cholesterol decreased by 0.26, 0.31, and 0.35 mmol/L, for daily consumption of 0.83, 1.61, and 3.24 g of plant sterols, respectively. LDL cholesterol decreases were 0.20, 0.26, and 0.30. Decreases in the LDL:HDL ratio were 0.13, 0.16, and 0.16 units, respectively. Cholesterol reductions between the different plant sterol doses were not statistically significant. Plasma vitamin K_1, vitamin D, lycopene, and alpha-tocopherol were not affected by plant sterol enriched spreads. Plasma (alpha + beta) carotene concentrations were decreased by about 11 and 19% with daily consumption of 0.83 and 3.24 g plant sterol spreads, respectively.[68]

The 3 low-dosage plant sterols had a significant cholesterol-lowering effect ranging from 4.9 to 6.8%, from 6.7 to 9.9%, and from 6.5 to 7.9%, for total, LDL cholesterol, and LDL:HDL cholesterol ratio, respectively. No dramatic effect was observed for lipid-soluble (pro) vitamins. Consumption of about 1.6 g of plant sterols per day appears to beneficially affect plasma cholesterol concentrations without seriously affecting plasma carotenoid concentrations.[68]

The Role of Carbohydrate

The complement of a low-fat eating pattern is a high-dietary-carbohydrate (CHO) pattern. An eating pattern with approximately 80% of calories from CHO (i.e., a very-high-CHO and very-low-fat diet), which is markedly different from the typical American eating pattern, decreases plasma total cholesterol, LDL, and HDL.[69,70] An eating pattern with 50–65% of calories from CHO has also significantly lowered plasma lipids.[71]

There is no clear consensus about the temporal response of plasma triglycerides to dietary CHO. An increased consumption of simple CHOs may create a greater plasma triglyceride response than that observed for complex CHOs.[72] Factors affecting the plasma lipid response to increased dietary CHOs include the following:

- the rate at which dietary CHO is increased
- the fiber content of the eating pattern
- the type of carbohydrate
- initial plasma lipid, lipoprotein, glucose, and insulin status of the individual

These issues need to be investigated in well-controlled experiments.

The Role of Fiber

Soluble fiber has a beneficial effect on plasma lipid levels by binding choles-terol and bile acids in the small intestine and carrying them into the colon for elimination. Plasma total cholesterol and LDL cholesterol are lowered, and HDL cholesterol is either unchanged or raised when soluble fiber is added to the eating pattern (see Table 11–3). Current recommendations are to increase dietary fiber intake to 20 to 25 g/day but not to exceed 40 to 50 g/day.[73] This includes oats, legumes, pectin, psyllium, and selected gums.

A long-term, longitudinal study of healthy, middle-aged men in Eng-land reported that energy and fiber consumption has a significant associa-tion with the incidence of CHD.[74] A lower incidence of CHD was noted for men who ate high-fiber cereals and abundant calories. Forty-five men who developed clinically significant heart disease consumed 6.7 grams dietary fiber per day from cereals, not fruits, vegetables, and nuts. The 292 men who developed clinical CHD during the study had an average daily fiber intake of 8.9 grams. In the Zutphen Study, CHD mortality was about 4 times higher for men in the lowest quintile of dietary fiber intake than for those in the highest quintile.[75]

Pectin and guar gum have each reduced plasma total cholesterol by 10% or more.[76–78] Ten grams per day of psyllium hydrophilic mucilloid has low-ered serum total cholesterol by 15% and LDL by 20% in hypercholesterolemic men.[79] Consuming 5 to 11 grams of soluble fiber for 6 weeks has demon-strated an additional 5.6 to 6.5 mg/dL lowering of plasma total cholesterol after the effect of a moderate cholesterol-lowering eating pattern.[80] The addi-tion of 1 cup of hot oat bran cereal and 5 oat bran muffins daily (47 grams dietary fiber) creates a significant plasma lipid response;[81] however, the study methods are questionable. In addition, the practicality of the regimen is a concern. Pectin is sticky, difficult to add to foods, and attaches to the oral mucosa for hours. A possible alternative is eating apples; the pectin in 2 to 8 apples a day can have a hypocholesterolemic effect.[82]

High fiber only from fruits and vegetables that provide 42 grams per day did not decrease plasma total cholesterol in 1 study,[83] whereas small amounts of legumes and especially beans effectively lower both plasma total choles-terol and triglycerides. When an eating pattern high in fiber from citrus pectin (28 grams) is ingested, a significant reduction in plasma total choles-terol by 13 mg/dL has been observed. Eating patterns very high in both CHO (72% of kcal) and fiber (74 grams per day) have lowered fasting plasma tryg-lycerides in hypertriglyceridemic individuals with diabetes.[84] Some dietary fibers bind bile acids, increase fecal bile acid, enhance steroid excretion, and decrease lipid and sterol absorption.[77]

In a double-blind, placebo-controlled trial with men and women 21 to 70 years old with primary hypercholesterolemia (i.e., total serum cholesterol greater than 220 mg/L), 37 followed a high-fat diet and 81 consumed a low-fat diet. Participants were randomly assigned to take either 5.1 grams of psyl-lium or a placebo 2 times daily. The total cholesterol levels of participants on psyllium and on either the low- or high-fat diet declined 10 to 15 mg/dL, and cholesterol values decreased by 11-13 mg/dL.[85] The importance of this trial is that it showed that psyllium has an independent effect and may be a substitute for drug therapy among primary hypercholesterolemic individuals.

TABLE 11-3 Plasma Lipid Change With Various Dietary Fibers

Type of Fiber	Hyperlipidemic Participant	Food	Dry Weight (g/day)	Total C	% Change LDL-C	% Change HDL-C	% Change Triglyceride
Soluble							
Pectin	No	Fruits	31	−13	NR	—	—
	No		40–50	−13	NR	NR	—
	Yes			−13	NR	NR	−13
Guar	No	Oats	20	−13	NR	—	—
	Yes		13	−13	−15	—	—
Legumes	Yes	Beans	115	−19	−24	−12	—
	Yes		140	−7	—	—	−25
Oats	Yes	Oatmeal	100	−13	−14	—	—
	Yes		100	−19	−23	−5	—
Insoluble							
Cellulose	No	Wheat	15	—	—	—	—
Lignin	No	Vegetables	12	—	—	—	—

NR = not reported.

Source: Adapted from: Kris-Etherton P, Krummel D, Russel ME, et al. The effect of diet on plasma, lipids, lipoproteins, and coronary heart disease. *J Am Diet Assoc.* 1988;88:1373. Used with permission of the American Dietetic Association.

Oats May Be a Protective Food

Meydani et al discovered that certain compounds called avenanthramides in oats hinder the ability of blood cells to stick to artery walls. The accumulation—called atherosclerosis, could block the blood vessel. Oats clean high-fiber content cholesterol that would otherwise circulate in the bloodstream from the digestive system. Apoproteins combine with non–water-soluble cholesterol to form low-density lipoprotein that accumulates in the body. High-density lipoproteins clean excess cholesterol from the liner by carrying them for elimination. Water-soluble fiber in oats may reduce LDL cholesterol circulating in blood due to avenanthramides in oats and the anti-inflammatory activity.[86]

Dietary Fiber, Weight Gain, and Cardiovascular Risk

Dietary fiber intake can predict serum insulin level, weight gain, and other risk factors for cardiovascular disease (CVD) more strongly than intake of total or saturated fat.[87] Two thousand nine hundred nine healthy black and white adults, 18 to 30 years old at baseline, participated in the Coronary Artery Risk Development in Young Adults (CARDIA) Study for 10 years. After controlling for potential confounding factors, dietary fiber intake assessed with a quantitative food frequency questionnaire was significantly inversely associated with values for body weight, waist:hip ratio, serum insulin, and weight gain during the 10-year follow-up period. Dietary fiber intake was inversely associated with blood pressure, serum triglyceride level, high-density lipoprotein cholesterol level, low-density lipoprotein cholesterol level, and serum fibrinogen level, but associations were lessened after adjustment for serum insulin level measured during fasting.[87]

The Role of Protein

Epidemiological studies have shown that animal protein in an eating pattern is positively correlated ($r = 0.78$) and the vegetable protein is negatively correlated ($r = -0.40$) with CHD mortality rates.[57] In human studies, when animal protein is replaced with soybean protein, there is either a small hypolipidemic effect or no effect.[88-90] Several studies conducted with hypercholesterolemic patients have reported that soy protein lowers serum total cholesterol more effectively than casein.[91]

The Role of Dietary Iron

An interesting hypothesis about the role of high iron status as a risk for heart disease is being explored. There are limited data to suggest that iron is a pro-oxidant and may have an etiological role in cardiovascular disease. The rationale is that oxidation of LDL contributes to arterial plaque formation and that oxidation has an immediate role in damaging tissue during and immediately following heart attack and stroke.[92-95]

The pros of this hypothesis are as follows:

- Iron protects premenopausal women due to loss of iron during menstrual bleeding.
- Postmenopausal estrogen therapy may cause intermittent bleeding, resulting in a lowering of body iron stores.
- Aspirin protects an individual because it causes gastrointestinal blood and iron loss.
- Coronary risk reduction may be linked to exercise because exercise increases runner's anemia.
- The low mortality from CHD in developing countries may be due to high rates of iron-deficiency anemia.

Epidemiologic studies that have supported the hypothesis include a cohort of 1,931 men in Finland with 51 experiencing a myocardial infarct during the 3-year follow-up period. If serum ferritin was equal to or greater than 200 micrograms/L, the men had 2.2 times increased risk of infarct. Exogenous iron intake had a positive association with the risk of infarct; a 5% increase in risk occurred for each 1 mg increase in iron intake.[96] Another study supporting this hypothesis was an 11-country study in which CHD mortality rates were associated with iron and serum cholesterol levels.[97]

The cons of this hypothesis are as follows:

- Hormones are primarily responsible for the changes in women with menopause.
- Exercise primarily influences cardiovascular fitness.
- Geographic differences in CHD are due to lifestyle differences (e.g., smoking, energy intake, and expenditure).
- Iron status cannot account for the trends in CHD mortality.

Studies that have not supported the iron and CHD hypothesis are as follows: (1) a US study of 45,720 men, for whom 880 were diagnosed with CHD in the 4-year follow-up period and no associations were noted between iron and CHD risk[98]; (2) a US study with 238 experimental and 238 control males, showing that men with high ferritin levels did not have a higher risk of infarct[99]; (3) a study of 171 older men and 406 older women reporting no significant difference in serum ferritin levels for those with and without coronary artery disease[100]; and (4) a US study with 1,827 white men and 2,410 white women for whom 489 had an infarct and 900 developed CHD in the 16-year follow-up period. For women only, serum iron was inversely linked to infarct, but total iron-binding capacity, transferrin saturation, and exogenous iron were not associated with infarct for men or women. Serum iron and transferrin saturation did have an inverse association with CHD for both men and woman.[101]

The Role of Coffee

The United States experienced a surge in coffee consumption during the 1990s. In 1989 there were about 200 specialty coffee outlets in the United States, compared to 4,500 in 1994. In addition, there are numerous opportunities to

Info Line

> *Cappuccino* is coffee made with espresso, a minimal amount of steamed milk, and a large foam cap made from a few ounces of milk. It is named because of the cap of foam on top, which resembles the hooded robe of the Capuchin friars or Roman Catholic monks. It provides 51–130 mg caffeine per serving. *Espresso*, derived from the same bean as coffee but brewed with less water, provides 30–57 mg caffeine per serving. *Latte*, a basic espresso with steamed milk and often a dollop of frothed milk on top, provides 51–130 mg caffeine per serving. *Mocha* is generally espresso with a small amount of steamed milk, 1 to 2 ounces of mocha or chocolate syrup, and sometimes a dollop of frothed milk. It provides 57–130 mg caffeine per serving.

request or purchase coffee in nearly every restaurant, fast food facility, gasoline station, bank, and grocery store. America's fondness for coffee includes espresso, latte, mocha, and cappuccino.[102]

Findings regarding coffee consumption and plasma lipid levels are not consistent.[9] Both an association and a causal relationship have been noted. The recommended range of intake varies from 1 to 2 cups per day to 9 or fewer cups per day.

In Norway, the Tromso Heart Study reported coffee consumption as a major determinant of total serum cholesterol level.[103] Coffee intake was correlated with total serum cholesterol level in the 14,667 men and women—even after adjustment for age, logarithm of body-mass index, leisure-time physical activity, cigarette smoking, and alcohol consumption.

Serum total cholesterol was 31 mg/dL higher in men who drank more than 9 cups per day compared with men who drank less than 1 cup per day. A corresponding increase of 26 mg/dL was noted for women. HDL cholesterol was higher in both men and women who drank 1 to 4 cups than for individuals who drank less than 1 cup per day. At 5 or more cups per day, HDL cholesterol was lower for women, but this was not true for men. In effect, each cup of coffee raised serum total cholesterol by 1.6 mg/dL in men and 1.3 mg/dL in women.[104]

In a prospective study of 1,130 medical students followed for 19 to 35 years, heavy coffee drinkers (5 or more cups per day) had 2 to 3 times greater risk for CHD, even after adjustment for age, smoking, blood pressure, and baseline serum cholesterol.[105] In 2 studies, abstinence from coffee for 4 to 5 weeks created a greater than 10% decrease in plasma total cholesterol.[106,107]

Haffner et al opened a new avenue of speculation by reporting that the regression coefficients in the multiple regression analyses were more significant when coffee rather than caffeine was the independent variable.[104] This implicates components in coffee other than caffeine. To provide conclusive data on the effects of coffee, decaffeinated coffee, and caffeine on plasma lipid levels, further clinical investigations are recommended.[108]

The Role of Alcohol

Epidemiological and clinical studies have reported a protective effect of moderate alcohol consumption (i.e., 7 to 14 ounces of alcohol per week) on the incidence of CHD, and an additional beneficial effect of alcohol on HDL cholesterol levels. Cross-sectional data of 4,855 male and female participants in the Lipid Research Clinics Program Prevalence Study showed a significant association between alcohol consumption and HDL cholesterol levels ($r = 0.21$ for men and 0.25 for women).[109] Men aged 50 to 69 years with the highest alcohol consumption (42 to 85 grams per day) had an HDL cholesterol level of 55 mg/dL, which reflected levels of young women; nondrinkers had 42 mg/dL level. In addition, alcohol consumption explained 4–6% of the total variance in HDL cholesterol.

A small amount of alcohol (i.e., 1 drink a day) may protect against CHD because it affects the subfractions HDL_2 and HDL_3 and may be an anticlotting factor. Three weeks of abstinence decreased total HDL and HDL_3. Both increased when alcohol intake resumed.[110] Other researchers have reported that about 9 grams of alcohol per day for a month can raise HDL cholesterol by 7%, primarily due to an increase in HDL_2.[111]

To reduce the impact of risk factors on CHD in the general population, in 2001 the American Heart Association (AHA) recommended a population-wide alcohol goal that consumption should not exceed 2 drinks (1 to 2 oz of ethanol) per day for men and 1 drink per day for women.[112] In addition, the beneficial effect of wine appears to be the same as that achieved by grape juice.[113]

Alcohol increases plasma triglyceride levels. It is associated with hypertension, alcoholic hepatitis, and cirrhosis. Certain cancers, fetal alcohol syndrome, psychosocial problems, and serious accidents are linked to habitual alcohol intake. Increasing alcohol intake to favorably change HDL cholesterol and hence lower CHD risk appears inappropriate. If one drinks, moderation of alcohol intake is recommended.[109]

Vegetarianism

A vegetarian diet that is low in total fat, SFA, and cholesterol and high in fiber has been shown to promote a favorable plasma lipoprotein profile. Plasma lipid and lipoprotein levels of 73 men and 43 women on a vegetarian eating pattern were lower when compared with omnivores (i.e., total cholesterol, 126 and 184; LDL cholesterol, 73 and 118; VLDL cholesterol, 12 and 17; and HDL cholesterol, 42 and 49).[114] The lower HDL cholesterol level among vegetarians is reflected in a lower HDL_2 cholesterol level.[115]

Further research is needed to identify the factor(s) creating plasma lipid variations between vegetarians and omnivores. Plasma total cholesterol, LDL cholesterol, and HDL cholesterol all decline when omnivores follow a vegetarian eating pattern (i.e., 13%, 15%, and 10%, respectively). Apolipoprotein A-1 removal rate is accelerated for vegetarians and persons who consume low-fat, high-CHO foods.[116,117] LDL production rate is lower for vegetarians.[117] A higher linoleic acid and lower arachidonic acid concentration in platelets is reported for vegans and lacto-ovovegetarians compared with omnivores.[118]

The Role of Folate

The folic acid-heart disease relationship surfaced in the literature in 1969, focusing on a rare genetic disorder, homocystinuria, that prematurely hardens arteries and promotes death by heart attack or stroke early in life. Homocysteine converts to methionine, requiring folic acid and vitamin B_{12}. High homocysteine levels due to impaired conversion damage arterial walls, and cholesterol plaque forms. Women with high homocysteine and low folate levels have double the risk of heart attack.[119] Women who have high levels of homocysteine have low levels of serum folate. Homocysteine elevations are reversible if folic acid intake is increased, but research has not shown that a decrease in serum homocysteine levels actually decreases morbidity and mortality of cardiovascular disease. Omenn et al calculate that 9% of male and 5.4% of female coronary artery deaths in the United States could be prevented by fortification of flour and cereal products using 350 mcg folic acid per 100 g food.[120,121]

The Role of Antioxidants

Antioxidants, including vitamin E, beta-carotene, and vitamin C, donate electrons to electron-seeking compounds. They stop oxidizing agents from breaking double bonds of fatty acids and prevent the alteration of DNA by electron-seeking substances. Data connecting antioxidants to a reduced risk of CHD are limited, but the Nurses' Health Study and the Health Professionals Follow-Up Study report a decreased risk of CHD for men and women with higher vitamin E intakes.

The Nurses' Health Study enrolled 87,000 women, 34 to 59 years old, in 1976 and followed them for 8 years. The sample reported 552 cases of documented CHD during the follow-up period. The relative risk of CHD for women with the highest vitamin E intake, 2.8 IU per day, was 0.66 (95% confidence interval (CI) of 0.50–0.87). Women with more than 2 years of vitamin E supplementation had a relative risk of 0.59 (95% CI of 0.38–0.91). Interestingly, dietary sources of vitamin E, multivitamin supplement users, and vitamin C intake were not linked to reduced risk.[122,123]

The Health Professionals Follow-Up Study analyzed the association of CHD risk and vitamin E intake. In 1986, 51,529 men 40 to 75 years old with no CHD were enrolled; the study reported 667 new CHD cases 4 years later. A significant trend of lower CHD risk with higher vitamin E intakes was noted ($p = 0.003$). Men who consumed 60 or more IU of vitamin E each day had a relative risk of 0.64, compared to men who ingested 7.5 IU a day. Men who took 100 IU of vitamin E per day had a relative risk of 0.63 (95% CI of 0.47–0.84).[124]

These 2 studies suggest that men and women who take vitamin E supplementation may have a lower CHD risk. However, the US Nutrition Labeling and Education Act (see Chapter 2) recommends an increased intake of fruits and vegetables rather than vitamin supplementation. The National Academy of Science's Food and Nutrition Board is considering revisions of the recommended dietary allowances to include potential supplementation for nutrients that demonstrate preventive effects on chronic diseases (see Chapter 2).

Vitamin K Protects Arteries

Vitamin K stops vascular calcification. It appears to activate a protein in artery walls that keeps calcified hardened sections of blood vessels from expanding and causing more damage. In a clinical trial, 450 people ages 60 to 80 had 500 micrograms of vitamin K or a placebo every day. Progression of vascular calcification via CT scans were measured. The theory was that those who take vitamin K supplements will develop less hardening of the arteries.[125]

Adults 60 and older average 120 micrograms of vitamin K daily. That may be sufficient for blood to clot properly, but insufficient for the nutrient to help bones retain their strength and for arteries to retain their suppleness.[125]

Traditional reliance on whole foods is being challenged in the scientific community, which seems reasonable. What does not appear reasonable is the decision by the free enterprise system to market megavitamin doses when research data are not consistent and have not reached a consensus.

Food Synergy

Food synergy is the additive influence of foods and constituents which, when eaten have a beneficial effect on health. The following 4 constituents were studied and provided examples of food synergy:

1. **Fish Oil.** Thirty-six postmenopausal women grouped by exogenous hormone use were randomized to take 8 capsules/d of either placebo oil (control) or n-3 fatty acid–enriched oil (supplement). The supplement provided 2.4 g eicosapentaenoic acid (EPA) plus 1.6 g docosahexaenoic acid (DHA) daily. Supplementation with n-3 fatty acids was associated with 26% lower serum triacylglycerol concentrations ($p < 0.0001$), a 28% lower overall ratio of serum triacylglycerol to HDL cholesterol ($p < 0.01$), and markedly greater EPA and DHA concentrations in serum phospholipids ($p < 0.05$). This shows a favorable influence with fish oil supplements.[126]

2. **Carotenoids.** In 1984, 73,286 female nurses completed a semiquantitative food-frequency questionnaire about carotenoid intake. During the 12 years of follow-up (803,590 person-years), 998 cases of MI were reported. A significant inverse association between the highest quintiles of intake of β-carotene and α-carotene and risk of MI was noted. No significant relation with smoking and intakes of lutein/zeaxanthin, lycopene, or β-cryptoxanthin was observed.[127]

3. **Chronic Disease Patterns.** Risk appears to be lower with consumption of whole-grain rather than refined-grain intake. Benefit is greatest when all edible parts of the grain are included (bran, germ, and endosperm). Phytochemicals in the fiber matrix may be responsible for the reduced risk.[128]

4. **The Chicago Heart Association Detection Project in Industry.** This study included 6,766 men and women, aged 36 to 64 years on various eating patterns. None had diabetes mellitus or myocardial infarction at baseline (1967–1973). After a 26-year follow-up questionnaire in 1996 when they were 65 years and older, the best health scores were noted for normal-weight individuals (BMI 18.5 to < 25.0). The

worst scores were reported for obese persons (BMI $\geq$ 30.0). A higher percentage of normal-weight persons reported excellent or very good health compared with overweight and obese persons; for example, for women, 46.8% versus 37.9% and 24.3%; and for men, 53.8% versus 49.1% and 36.5% ($p < 0.001$). This points to the effect of balanced food and physical activity to create a healthy body weight.[129]

The National Cholesterol Education Program

In 1984, the National Institutes of Health (NIH) Consensus Development Conference on Lowering Blood Cholesterol to Prevent Heart Disease recommended creating and implementing a national cholesterol education program. The National Cholesterol Education Program (NCEP) began in 1985 with the goal to reduce the prevalence of elevated blood cholesterol in the United States and contribute to the reduction of CHD morbidity and mortality. The NCEP has issued several reports, including the Adult Treatment Panel I, II, and III guidelines, the Population Strategies Panel report, and the report of the Panel on Blood Cholesterol Levels in Children and Adolescents.[130-134]

1988 Cholesterol Guidelines—Adult Treatment Panel I

With the first report of the Adult Treatment Panel (ATP I), an LDL cholesterol level of 160 mg/dL or higher placed an individual at high risk for CHD.[10] A level of 130 to 159 mg/dL was classified as a borderline value, with less than 130 mg/dL considered desirable. A triglyceride level greater than 250 mg/dL was considered elevated. Other major risk factors for CHD included male sex, cigarette smoking, hypertension, diabetes mellitus, family history of premature myocardial infarction or sudden death, an HDL cholesterol level below 35 mg/dL and confirmed by repeated measurement, history of occlusive peripheral vascular disease or cerebrovascular disease, and severe obesity (more than 30% above ideal body weight).[130] The goals of treatment were to reduce LDL below 160 mg/dL or below 130 mg/dL in the presence of CHD or 2 or more CHD risk factors.

The ATP I report stated that modification of diet and increased exercise level were the cornerstones of therapy of patients with dyslipidemia. In the step 1 diet, dietary fat was restricted to less than 30% of total energy. Dietary saturated fat was restricted to less than 10% of total energy, cholesterol to less than 300 mg/dL, and calories were restricted in overweight individuals. All individuals at risk were to be referred to a registered dietitian for an initial assessment of their present eating pattern, instruction, and follow-up.

If the minimal goals of therapy were not achieved by 3 months, the step 2 diet was to be adopted, which restricted saturated fats to less than 7% of total energy and cholesterol to less than 200 mg/day. Medical nutrition therapy was to continue for at least 6 months prior to considering medication, unless the patient had established CHD or pancreatitis. If medical nutrition therapy was not effective in reaching target LDL cholesterol values, or if CHD or pancreatitis was established, then drug therapy was to be considered as an adjunct to diet. At the time of ATP I, the use of severe dietary fat restriction rather than an increase in monounsaturated fat to lower LDL cholesterol levels was being evaluated. Currently, lowering saturated fat by replacing it with complex carbohydrates is preferred because this is less calorically dense and promotes weight loss.

1990 Expert Panel on Population Strategies for Blood Cholesterol Reduction

In 1990, epidemiological, clinical, and experimental evidence clearly demonstrated that the likelihood that a person will develop or die from CHD is directly related to the level of blood cholesterol.[1] Data from the 361,662 men screened for the Multiple Risk Factor Intervention Trial demonstrate a continuous association, with risk increasing as cholesterol increases.

In the 1990 report, approaches to lowering blood cholesterol were redefined. The average cholesterol level for the adult US population in 1990 was about 210 mg/dL. Approximately 55% of US adults had cholesterol levels at or above 200 mg/dL.[1] For these reasons, 2 kinds of strategies were recommended: (1) a patient-based strategy, which seeks to help those who have a high risk of CHD because of their high blood cholesterol level; and (2) a population-based strategy, which seeks to reach all Americans. The population approach promoted the adoption of eating patterns to lower the blood cholesterol level of individuals and to reduce the average cholesterol level throughout the population. If both approaches were used, the effect was thought to be synergistic.[1]

Figures 11–3 through 11–6 illustrate conceptually the anticipated effects of these two approaches, both separately and combined. The result was a reduction of 10% or more in the average blood cholesterol level of the US population leading to an approximate reduction of 20% or more in CHD and, consequently, to significant improvement in the health and quality of life of Americans.

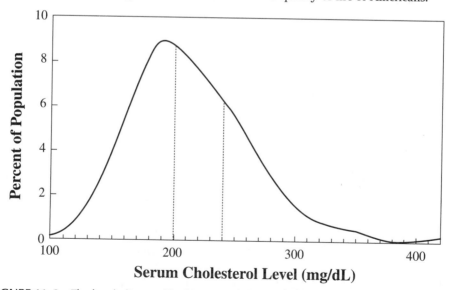

FIGURE 11–3   The borderline and high cutoff levels are shown as dotted lines to indicate the proportions of the population above or below 200 or 240 mg/dL.
Source: Reprinted from *Report of the Expert Panel on Population Strategies for Blood Cholesterol Reduction* by the National Cholesterol Education Program, p. 10, U. S. Department of Health and Human Services, Public Health Service, NIH Publication No., 90–3046, November 1990.

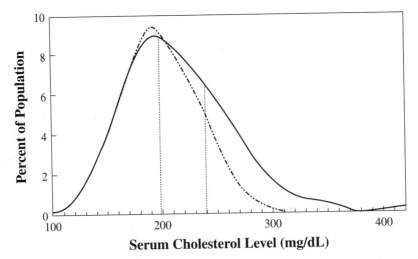

FIGURE 11–4   Expected shift in population distribution of serum cholesterol values with widespread application of Adult Treatment Panel guidelines. The dotted-dashed line represents an estimate of the effect of treating many people with elevated cholesterol levels. *Source: Report of the Expert Panel on Population Strategies for Blood Cholesterol Reduction* by the National Cholesterol Education Program, p. 10, U.S. Department of Health and Human Services, Public Health Service, NIH Publication No., 90–3046, November 1990.

The panel recommended the following average nutrient intakes for healthy Americans and complemented other national guidelines[131-133]:

- less than 10% of total calories from saturated fatty acids
- an average of 30% or less of total calories from all fat

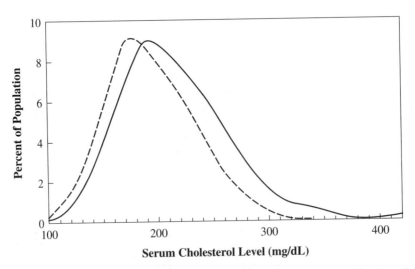

FIGURE 11–5   Expected shift in population distribution of serum cholesterol values if the recommendations of the Expert Panel on Population Strategies for Blood Cholesterol Reduction result in a 10% decrease in blood cholesterol of Americans. The dashed line shows the effect of the recommendations. *Source: Report of the Expert Panel on Population Strategies for Blood Cholesterol Reduction* by the National Cholesterol Education Program, p. 10, U.S. Department of Health and Human Services, Public Health Service, NIH Publication No. 90-3046, November 1990.

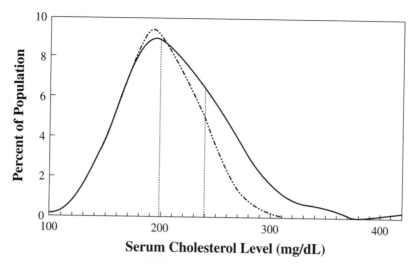

FIGURE 11-6 Anticipated combined effects of the recommendations of the Adult Treatment Panel (dotted-dashed line) and the Expert Panel on Population Strategies for Blood Cholesterol Reduction (dashed line).
Source: Report of the Expert Panel on Population Strategies for Blood Cholesterol Reduction by the National, Cholesterol Education Program, p. 10, U.S. Department of Health and Human Services, Public Health Service, NIH Publication No., 90–3046, November 1990.

- dietary energy levels needed to reach or maintain a desirable body weight
- less than 300 mg of cholesterol per day

The panel recommended that healthy Americans select, prepare, and consume foods that contain lower amounts of saturated fatty acids, total fat, and cholesterol to lower blood cholesterol levels. In addition, eating patterns were suggested to be compatible with cultural and ethnic considerations and with personal preferences for good food as follows[1]:

- Eat a greater quantity and variety of fruits, vegetables, breads, cereals, and legumes.
- Consume more low-fat dairy products, such as skim or low-fat milk and skim or low-fat milk products, in place of high-fat milk products.
- Eat moderate amounts (e.g., about 6 ounces per day, cooked) of trimmed, lean red meat, poultry without skin, or fish, in place of foods high in saturated fatty acids.
- Eat egg yolks only in moderation. Egg whites do not contain cholesterol, and they can be eaten often.
- Use oils, margarines, and shortenings with vegetable oils that contain primarily unsaturated fatty acids instead of saturated or partially hydrogenated fatty acids.
- Read food labels. Choose foods with lower amounts or proportions of fat and/or saturated fatty acids.
- Choose prepared baked goods that have been made with unsaturated vegetable oils and, at most, small amounts of egg yolk.
- Choose convenience foods guided by low saturated fatty acid, total fat, and cholesterol content and cost.

- When preparing foods, keep use of fats to a minimum, use smaller amounts of ingredients high in saturated fatty acids, and use low-fat alternatives.
- In restaurants and fast-food outlets, select menu items that are low in saturated fatty acids, total fat, and cholesterol, as well as cooked foods that are baked, boiled, or broiled without fat.
- Recognize that no single food or supplement (e.g., fish oil supplements or dietary fiber) is the answer to achieving a desirable blood cholesterol level, and that a habitual pattern of eating that is consistently low in saturated fatty acids, total fat, and cholesterol is recommended.

1993 Cholesterol Guidelines—Adult Treatment Panel II

The National Cholesterol Education Program (NCEP) issued the Second Report of the Expert Panel on Detection, Evaluation, and Treatment of High Blood Cholesterol in Adults (ATP II) 5 years after the first report.[134] ATP II classified blood cholesterol levels for adults as desirable, borderline, and high and focused on the clinical approach to lowering cholesterol, making new recommendations in 3 important areas: cholesterol-lowering treatment in relation to CHD risk status, including age; HDL cholesterol; and an expanded approach to medical nutrition therapy.[117]

The ATP II report listed the ages at which a patient's risk of CHD is strong enough to warrant more aggressive treatment. These ages are 45 years and older for men and 55 years and older for women. Women who have undergone premature menopause and receive no estrogen-replacement therapy would need more aggressive treatment at an earlier age.

Positive risk factors for CHD were identified as family history of CHD at an early age, smoking cigarettes, hypertension, a low HDL cholesterol (below 35 mg/dL), and diabetes. A high HDL cholesterol (60 mg/dL or greater) is considered a negative risk factor, because it lowers the risk for CHD. The risk of CHD increases with age and the report recommended lowering high blood cholesterol among both healthy elderly persons and postmenopausal women. Treatment would rely primarily on dietary therapy. The report recommends that drug therapy not be used with these patients unless CHD risk is high.

The ATP II report noted that clinical trials had not yet answered the question of whether lowering high blood cholesterol with drugs also reduced total mortality. Reliance was placed on dietary therapy, until large clinical trials provided an answer about total mortality.[134]

The report concluded that prevention and treatment of high blood cholesterol can be cost effective if diet is used as the mainstay of therapy and drugs are reserved for high-risk patients. Prevention of CHD through lowering cholesterol could substantially reduce the country's annual cost from CHD in medical treatments and lost wages—a cost currently between $50 billion and $100 billion.

Additional NCEP Activities

Additional activities for NCEP include the following:

- to combine clinical and public health strategies to help reduce blood cholesterol levels among high-risk individuals and the general population

- to disseminate the NCEP reports and patient education brochures widely to more than 41 organizations representing a diverse group of health professionals from the public and private sectors
- to encourage all health professionals to use the ATP II guidelines to identify and to target coronary patients and others at high risk of CHD for aggressive therapy. (Many of these individuals are not receiving cholesterol-lowering treatment, and they will account for nearly half of all future heart attacks.)[134]

The Adult Treatment Panel III (ATP III) Report of the National Cholesterol Education Program is an evidence-based set of guidelines on cholesterol management.[135] Therapeutic lifestyle changes (TLC) remain a centerpiece for clinical management, but cholesterol-lowering therapy is warranted for high-risk patients (see Table 11–4) to lower low-density lipoprotein cholesterol (LDL-C) to < 100 mg/dL. Older persons can benefit from therapeutic lowering of LDL-C and a high-risk patient with high triglycerides or low high-density lipoproteins cholesterol (HDL-C) should be given a fibrate or nicotinic acid with an LDL-lowering drug. For moderately high-risk persons (2+ risk factors and 10-year risk 10-20%), the recommended LDL-C goal is < 130 mg/dL. A person at high risk or moderately high risk with obesity, physical inactivity, elevated triglycerides, low HDL-C, or metabolic syndrome should have TLC to modify these factors regardless of LDL-C level. Lower-risk individuals should still attend to a healthy lifestyle and low LDL cholesterol levels[135,136] (see Table 11–5).

TABLE 11–4   ATP III LDL-C Goals and Cutpoints for TLC and Drug Therapy in Different Risk Categories and Proposed Modifications Based on Recent Clinical Trial Evidence

Risk Category	LDL-C Goal	Initiate TLC	Consider Drug Therapy
High risk			
CHD 10-year risk > 20%	< 100 mg/dL	≥ 100 mg/dL	≥ 100 mg/dL
			(< 100 mg/dL consider drug options)
Moderately high risk > 2 risk factors and 10-year risk 10–20%	< 130 mg/dL	≥ 130 mg/dL	≥ 130 mg/dL
			(100–129 mg/dL consider drug options)
Moderate risk > 2 risk factors and 10-year risk < 10%	< 130 mg/dL	≥ 130 mg/dL	≥ 160 mg/dL
Lower risk			
0-1 risk factor	< 160 mg/dL	≥ 160 mg/dL	≥ 190 mg/dL
			(160–189 mg/dL and LDL drug optional)

Source: National Cholesterol Education Program (NCEP) Expert Panel on Direction, Evaluation, and Treatment of High Blood Cholesterol in Adults (Adult Treatment Panel III). *Circulation.* 2004;110:227–239.

TABLE 11–5 Recommendations for Modifications to Enhance the ATP III Treatment Design for LDL-C

Recommendation

1. Therapeutic lifestyle changes (TLC) to reduce CVD risks

2. For high-risk individuals, LDL-C goal is < 100 mg/dL
   - However, LDL-C goal of < 70 mg/dL is optional especially for individuals at very high risk
   - If LDL-C goal of ≥ 100 mg/dL, TLC and drug therapy
   - If baseline LDL-C is < 100 mg/dL, TLC and optional drug therapy
   - If low LDL-C and high triglycerides, combined fibrate or nicotinic acid with drug; if triglycerides are ≥ 200 mg/dL, goal becomes < 130 mg/dL

3. For moderately high-risk individuals, base therapy on LDL-C level as outlined above

4. For high risk or moderately high risk with lifestyle-related risk factors, TLC regardless of LDL-C level

5. If LDL-lowering drug therapy used, intensity level needed to achieve a 30–40% reduction in LDL-C levels

6. For low risk, TLC and monitor risk level

Source: National Cholesterol Education Program (NCEP) Expert Panel on Direction, Evaluation, and Treatment of High Blood Cholesterol in Adults (Adult Treatment Panel III). *Circulation.* 2004;110:227–239.

Lowering Cholesterol Levels

Data from the third NHANES survey show that the average blood cholesterol levels in the United States dropped significantly from 1976 to 1988.[137] There has been a substantial reduction in the proportion of adults with high blood cholesterol.

Between the NHANES II (1976–1980) and the first phase of the NHANES III (1988–1991), the average cholesterol level among adults ages 20 to 74 declined from 213 to 205 mg/dL. Mean cholesterol levels decreased in men and women, in African Americans and whites, and in all age groups.

This significant 12-year drop in cholesterol levels is part of a trend that has occurred over the past 46 years. This drop has coincided with declining blood pressure levels and smoking rates and a 54% decrease in mortality from CHD.[137] Decreases in high blood cholesterol, smoking, and high blood pressure have made a major contribution to the decline in CHD deaths. Lifestyle improvements and better diagnosis and treatment of CHD have also contributed.

The decline in overall cholesterol levels occurred because of declining LDL levels. The mean LDL level dropped from 136 to 128 mg/dL. The decline in LDL levels may be due to changes in the consumption of saturated fat and dietary cholesterol, use of lipid-lowering drugs, hormone use, or changes in the prevalence of other factors such as obesity or physical activity.[137]

The decline in average cholesterol levels is accompanied by a shift in distribution of cholesterol values among the entire population. The proportion of the population with high blood cholesterol levels, 240 mg/dL and above, dropped from 26 to 20%. The proportion with borderline-high total cholesterol levels, 200 to 239 mg/dL, has not changed significantly (from 30 to 31%). There has been a substantial increase from 44 to 49% in the proportion of the population with desirable cholesterol levels below 200 mg/dL. There has also been a decline in the proportion of the population who need dietary therapy (from 36 to 29%).[137]

It appears that public health programs designed to reduce serum cholesterol levels are proving successful. Combined public health and clinical strategies recommended by the NCEP and many cooperating organizations have made a substantial contribution to the decline in cholesterol levels as a whole and to the decline in the percentage of individuals with especially high levels.

The NCEP recommends 2 strategies for lowering the cholesterol levels of Americans. One is a clinical strategy, which detects and treats individuals at high risk of coronary heart disease. The second is a public health strategy, which attempts to shift the cholesterol levels of the entire population to a lower range through dietary changes.[134]

Applying the ATP definitions of treatment to the NHANES III data, the percentage of adults over age 20 who would be candidates for dietary therapy is estimated to be 29%. This is a decline from 36% derived by the application of the ATP definitions to the NHANES II.

There is a greater emphasis on physical activity and weight loss in combination with medical nutrition therapy as the secondary prevention approach for high blood cholesterol. Patients with existing CHD require aggressive therapy to lower their cholesterol levels. About 32% of men and 27% of women are candidates for dietary therapy. Of 52 million adults (29%) who would require dietary therapy, 11 million people already have CHD.[138]

Drug therapy is reserved for patients at high risk for coronary heart disease and only after unsuccessful dietary therapy. In contrast to the 29% of adults who would require medical nutrition therapy, the analysis of the NHANES III data indicates that about 7% of all adults, or 12.7 million Americans, might require cholesterol-lowering drug treatment. Of those patients who are candidates for drug therapy, about 4 million would be patients with CHD.

The national goal to reduce the mean serum cholesterol level of US adults to below 200 mg/dL appears to be attainable. Another *Healthy People 2010* objective, to reduce the prevalence of high blood cholesterol to no more than 20% of adults, essentially has been achieved. However, 52 million US adults still need medical nutrition therapy as a secondary prevention for high blood cholesterol. There remains a huge challenge.[134]

Some clinicians have found that to lower LDL levels by more than 15% effectively, medications must include 1 of the following: bile acid-binding resins (cholestyramine and colestipol), nicotinic acid, and the hydroxy methyl glutanyl coenzyme A (HMG CoA) reductase inhibitors (lovastatin, pravastatin, and simvastatin).[10] In asymptomatic patients over 45 years of age, resins may be preferred. If the individual is unwilling or unable to take resins, or target values are not achieved, then nicotinic acid could be used. If the individual is unwilling or unable to take nicotinic acid or target values are not achieved, then an HMG CoA reductase inhibitor can be used. Combinations of resins and nicotinic acid, or resins and an HMG CoA reductase inhibitor are also very effective if target values cannot be achieved with a single agent.

In individuals with established heart disease, an HMG CoA reductase inhibitor is the drug of choice because of compliance issues.

For individuals with combined elevations of LDL and triglyceride, nicotinic acid is preferred. If nicotinic acid is contraindicated if the individual is unwilling or unable to take this agent, or if target values are not achieved, then an HMG CoA reductase inhibitor can be used. Combinations of bile acid-binding resin and nicotinic acid, resin and gemfibrozil, or resin and an HMG CoA reductase inhibitor can also be used. If heart disease is diagnosed, then an HMG CoA reductase inhibitor is preferred and compliance is usually good.

Individuals with severe hypertriglyceridemia (greater than 1,000 mg/dL) are treated with diet, exercise, and weight reduction. If diabetes is present, glucose control is important. If triglyceride levels remain greater than 1,000 mg/dL, then gemfibrozil can be prescribed to lower triglyceride levels to less than 500 mg/dL and to reduce the risk of recurrent pancreatitis. Other medications that can be used include fish-oil capsules and, in nondiabetic participants, nicotinic acid.

Drug therapy is not recommended for the treatment of HDL deficiency, moderate hypertriglyceridemia in combination with HDL deficiency, or hypertriglyceridemia alone. Modifying lifestyle, as previously mentioned, and attempting to correct secondary causes are important. While prospective studies support the view that raising HDL cholesterol levels is beneficial in reducing CHD, no prospective primary or secondary trial has been conducted with individuals who have HDL deficiency.[10,11] Individuals with CAD frequently have decreased HDL cholesterol levels.[130] For isolated hypertriglyceridemia, even less information is available. Elevated triglyceride levels have not been clearly shown to be a risk factor for CAD, nor has lowering triglyceride levels clearly been shown to reduce CAD risk.

For individuals with established CHD, efforts should be made to optimize the lipid profile, specifically to lower LDL levels to below 100 mg/dL, lower triglyceride levels to below 200 mg/dL, and increase HDL levels to above 40 mg/dL. These goals are often difficult to achieve without combination drug therapy. Medications that can be used include HMG CoA reductase inhibitors, gemfibrozil, or nicotinic acid. The combinations of nicotinic acid and resins, HMG CoA reductase inhibitors and resins, or gemfibrozil and resins, can be used. Some combinations are not well tolerated. The combination of HMG CoA reductase inhibitor and gemfibrozil is currently not recommended because of the potential for myositis. For individuals without CHD but with 2 or more CHD risk factors, especially when decreased HDL levels are present, the goal is to lower LDL levels to below 130 mg/dL, to raise HDL levels to above 40 mg/dL, and to keep triglyceride levels below 200 mg/dL, using both medical nutrition and drug therapy. For other patients, efforts should be made to keep the LDL level below 160 mg/dL with medical nutrition therapy and, if necessary, with the addition of pharmacologic therapy.[130]

Results from a 12-year follow-up of 316,099 men who were 35 to 57 years of age when screened for participation in the Multiple Risk Factor Intervention Trial give detailed and precise determination of associations of serum cholesterol, blood pressure, and cigarette smoking to risk of death from CHD.[139] A strong incremental association with coronary death was observed for serum total cholesterol at levels above 180 mg/dL. At high levels, a 10 mg/dL lower level of serum cholesterol was associated with 10% lower risk of coronary death. Strong incremental associations with coronary death were observed for cigarette smoking, systolic blood pressure at levels above 110 mm Hg, and diastolic pressure at levels above 70 mm Hg. The age-adjusted coronary death rate for a nonsmoker with systolic blood pressure below 118 mm Hg and serum cholesterol below 182 mg/dL was 3.1 deaths per 10,000 person-years. In contrast, the corresponding rate for a smoker with systolic blood pressure of at least 142 mm Hg and serum cholesterol of at least 245 mg/dL was 20 times higher, or 62.6 deaths per 10,000 person-years. These results support the inference that the great majority of coronary deaths in middle-aged men could be prevented if cigarette smoking were eliminated and if blood pressure and serum cholesterol were maintained at optimal levels by hygienic means from youth through adulthood.

Prevention of CHD

Can a lifelong low-fat eating pattern exert beneficial effects on CHD rates beyond an influence on blood cholesterol? New approaches to cholesterol reduction are needed, and a few are outlined in the following sections.

Work-Site Intervention

In Ohio, 80 upper-management male employees participated in a company-sponsored, comprehensive physical exam. The 70 participants who had a triglyceride level above 5.17 mmol/L (mg% cholesterol) were invited to participate in a nutrition education program. The study was nonrandomized, with 33 men in the intervention and 37 in the control group. All participants completed 3-day dietary records before and after the nutrition education program. The intervention included a year-long program of individualized instruction, group sessions, and telephone follow-up. Participants in the intervention group decreased their intakes of energy, cholesterol, and percentage of energy from total fat and protein. Carbohydrate and dietary fiber intakes increased. Significant decreases in plasma total cholesterol (from 6.15 ± 0.17 mmol/L to 5.43 ± 0.16 mmol/L), triglycerides (from 1.68 ± 0.87 mmol/L to 1.49 ± 0.67 mmol/L), body weight (from 86 ± 2.3 kg to 81 ± 1.6 kg), and body fat (from 24% ± 3.5% to 21% ± 3.5%) were observed for the intervention group. This work-site intervention suggests that primary prevention programs can decrease risk factors associated with coronary heart disease.[140]

Parent-Child Tutorial Program

During a nutrition education intervention pilot study, 44 children from 4 to 10 years of age were identified as having plasma LDL cholesterol levels between the 90th and 99th percentiles. They were randomized to either a parent-child tutorial program or a usual-care setting. The tutorial program was home-based and included a picture book and an audiotaped story complemented by activities and a guide for parents. Knowledge of health-promoting foods, food records, and biochemical measures were obtained at baseline, 3-month, and 6-month observation points. At the 6-month follow-up, significant increases in knowledge were reported, cholesterol intake increased for the control children but decreased for the treatment children, and both groups experienced a 10% decline in the average LDL cholesterol levels.[141]

Lifestyle Heart Trial

The Lifestyle Heart Trial was conducted in San Francisco with 41 middle-aged men randomized to either an 8% fat, vegetarian eating regimen or a control group. Stress management, moderate aerobic exercise, and smoking cessation were included in the experimental arm. Annual coronary angiograms demonstrated regression of coronary lesions in the experimental group and progression among the control subjects. Changes in total cholesterol and LDL cholesterol levels from baseline to 1 year for treatment and control groups were: experimental—225 to 171 mg/dL total cholesterol and 151 to 95 mg/dL LDL; control—244 to 231 mg/dL total cholesterol and 167 to 157 LDL.[142]

Garlic Consumption

Several alternative therapies have emerged in the CHD prevention arena. One approach has been the use of garlic for reducing total serum cholesterol when it is above 200 mg/dL. When combining data from 5 studies, a statistically significant treatment effect was noted. The mean difference in cholesterol change for the treatment compared to the placebo group was a decrease of 23 mg/dL. It appears that individuals with a total serum cholesterol over 200 mg/dL can lower their blood cholesterol by 9% by consuming one half to 1 clove of garlic per day for 4 to 6 months.[143]

Data from 13 studies with about 800 people found that garlic created a 4% decline in cholesterol levels, whereas a 5% reduction occurred from dietary changes alone or 17% from statin drugs.[144]

Modified Eating Behavior

Research on the role of dietary factors in the etiology of CHD has prompted the American Heart Association, the National Cholesterol Education Program, and others to recommend changes from the current American diet to a diet lower in saturated fats and cholesterol. Changing people's eating habits, however, is not an easy task and involves more than making dietary prescriptions. Inducing a person to change eating behavior is not simply determined by what is good for him or her but is affected by a variety of psychological factors.[145]

It has been suggested that lowering plasma cholesterol by either dietary change or medication may result in elevated levels of depression and/or aggressive hostility, one component of Type A behavior.[146] Accordingly, depression could increase the likelihood for suicide, and aggressive hostility could elevate the risk of dying from other violent episodes. If this hypothesis is correct, one should expect increases in depression and aggressive hostility among those who change their diet to reduce plasma cholesterol levels.

Contrary to the above hypothesis, data gathered from the Family Heart Study indicate that those who improved their diet and reduced their plasma cholesterol levels showed reductions in depression and aggressive hostility.[145] These results are consistent with predictions derived from the psychological theory of self-efficacy.[147]

Intervention studies have verified the importance of modified eating behavior in reducing coronary risk. Interventions to reduce coronary risk may be most beneficial for Type A, coronary-prone individuals, especially after they are convinced that their own behavior can influence their health status. Participation in cholesterol-lowering programs is not associated with reduced psychological well-being. Improvements in diet appear to be associated with reductions in depression and aggressive hostility, as well as with lowered plasma cholesterol levels. Overall, psychological factors are powerful predictors of health outcomes and appear to be influenced by health behaviors.

Physical Activity

Sesso et al[148] followed 12,516 middle-aged and older men (mean age 57.7 years, range 39 to 88 years) from 1977 through 1993. Physical activity was assessed as blocks walked, flights climbed, and participation in sports or recreational activities. They found that total physical activity and vigorous activities showed the strongest reductions in CHD risk. Moderate and light activities, which may be less precisely measured, showed nonsignificant inverse associations.[148]

The Effects of Serum Total Cholesterol Reduction on Mortality from Noncardiovascular Causes

At a time when high serum total cholesterol has been shown to have a positive association with cardiovascular disease, cancer, and all-cause mortality, some researchers have questioned lowering serum cholesterol.[149-152] Some data suggest that a low serum cholesterol may increase mortality from noncardiovascular causes.

The Multiple Risk Factor Intervention Trial (MRFIT) observed an excess number of deaths among men with low serum cholesterol levels.[153] Men with a serum total cholesterol below 160 mg/dL had a 6% higher death rate from lung cancer, suicide, chronic obstructive lung disease, hepatic cirrhosis, alcohol dependence, liver cancer, lymphatic and hematopoietic cancers, or hypertension-induced intracerebral hemorrhage.[139] Of consideration is whether these diseases contributed to a lowered serum total cholesterol, rather than the low cholesterol inducing the diseases and mortality. Community-based intervention studies such as MRFIT, the OSLO, World Health Organization, and European Collaborative trials used strategies to change eating behavior and reported fewer CHD events and lower CHD mortality and all-cause mortality.[139,154,155]

Is the US eating pattern healthy? The preferred eating pattern is one that contains a wide variety of foods. Kant and colleagues analyzed the relation between dietary variety and all-cause mortality using the NHANES I Epidemiologic Follow-Up Study, 1982 to 1987, database. The study sample included 4,160 men and 6,264 women between 25 and 74 years of age at baseline in 1971 to 1975. Total intake of 5 major food groups was assessed by assigning the presence of the food group in a 24-hour recall a score of 1 and following with an additional 1 for each of the different 5 food groups consumed.[137]

The results showed that 25% of the participants had a food group score of less than 4; about 5% had a score below 3. Fruit, dairy, and vegetable groups were the food groups most frequently missed by the study participants.

More men than women had a lower score. Income and education both had a positive association with the score. For women, body mass index was inversely associated with the score. Compared with women, men who smoked had lower scores.

For both men and women, there was an inverse association between the age-adjusted risk of all-cause mortality and the food group score. When potential confounders were controlled, the relative risk for men consuming 2 or fewer food groups was 1.5; the relative risk for women was 1.4.[137] This data analysis suggests that a food group analysis can be linked with total mortality and, specifically, lack of variety accompanies increased risk of death.

Several concerns have been raised about these data. First, use of one 24-hour food record limits the representativeness of individual intake. The large sample size might minimize this effect. Second, accuracy of the amount of food reported as eaten and the consistent assignment of what constitutes a serving in any one of the 5 food groups is assumed, but not known. Third, changes in eating behaviors for health promotion in the general population between 1971 and 1975 were probably much less than the changes individuals made in the 1980s. The extent of dietary behavioral change in this cohort during the latency period was not known. Fourth, it is not known whether an improvement in food quality (i.e., eating patterns that have balance, variety, or moderation) can lower all-cause mortality including CHD deaths.

The Current Challange

Powerful medical nutrition and drug therapies are now available to achieve both intensive plasma lipid lowering and an antithrombotic effect. Both are important for the management of every individual at risk or with overt CHD. Not only is an improved understanding of the atherosclerotic process needed, but also it is necessary to understand to the role of healthy eating on longer life among low- versus high-risk individuals. The Lipid Research Clinic Trial demonstrated that, for every 1% lowering of the plasma cholesterol concentration, there was a 2% reduction in CHD events. The challenge continues to be to implement therapies to lower plasma cholesterol levels in the US population.

How Low (Fat) Should You Go to Reduce Risk of Cardiovascular Disease?

The American Heart Association (AHA) claims that eating a low-fat diet can reduce some risk factors associated with heart disease and stroke, but reducing fat in the diet to very low levels may not provide any additional benefit. The AHA states that data are insufficient to recommend very low-fat diets as a strategy to reduce blood levels of total cholesterol, and in particular the bad cholesterol, LDL. Very low-fat diets cannot be recommended to reduce body weight or the risk of death from heart disease on a population-wide basis.[119]

Very low-fat diets are defined as $\leq$ 15% of total calories from dietary fats. This contrasts with the 30% of total calories consumed daily to come from fat, with no more than 10% from saturated fats currently recommended. Very low-fat diets may be associated with reduced risks for cardiovascular disease, but there remain numerous unanswered questions that make population-wide recommendations of such diets premature since very low-fat diets may increase triglycerides and decrease good cholesterol, or HDL, levels without yielding additional decreases in LDL levels.

Increased consumption of fruits, vegetables, and whole grains and increased physical activity levels and weight loss raise HDL cholesterol and lower LDL cholesterol in some individuals. Very low-fat diets provide enough nutrients, such as vitamins and minerals. Individuals eating a very low-fat diet appear to make up at least some, if not all, of the calories that would have been consumed as fat with simple and/or complex carbohydrates. Groups at high risks when eating very low-fat diets are young children, pregnant women, the elderly, and individuals with insulin-dependent diabetes mellitus or elevated blood levels of triglycerides.[119]

The AHA step 1 diet is reduced in total and saturated fat and sets a general guideline for the US population. Reductions in saturated fat intake to no more than 7% of total calories characterizes the AHA step 2 diet and is recommended for individuals at an increased risk of CHD.[119]

NCEP Recommendations for Health Partners

The National Cholesterol Education Program endorses the following recommendations:

- Health professionals should both practice and advocate recommended eating patterns. They should ensure that education of future health professionals includes appropriate nutrition education. Health professionals should work with industry, government, volunteer groups, and healthcare agencies to facilitate adoption of the recommended eating patterns.[1]
- The food industry, food and animal scientists, and food technologists should increase efforts to design, modify, prepare, promote, label, and distribute good-tasting, safe foods that are lower in saturated fatty acids, total fat, and cholesterol.
- Government agencies should provide consistent, coordinated nutrition statements and policies emphasizing low saturated-fatty acid, low-fat, and low-cholesterol eating patterns; expand and standardize food labeling requirements to identify clearly the content of saturated fatty acids, total fat, cholesterol, and total calories; and take other steps to improve the consumer comprehension necessary to achieve the recommended eating patterns.
- Education at all levels should incorporate curricula that emphasize the background, benefits, and methods of achieving eating patterns that are lower in saturated fatty acids, total fat, and cholesterol. This recommendation includes elementary through high schools, vocational programs (especially in culinary arts), colleges, universities, and health professional schools.
- Measurement of blood cholesterol, followed by appropriate education and counseling, is best initiated in the healthcare setting; but in specific circumstances and especially for selected segments of hard-to-reach population groups, public screening for blood cholesterol, when carried out with high-quality standards, is appropriate.

Info Line

> The American Heart Association (AHA) is a national volunteer health organization whose mission is to reduce death and disability from cardiovascular disease and stroke. AHA recommendations, if implemented, will promote adoption of eating patterns that will help most Americans lower their levels of blood cholesterol and their risk of CHD. Affiliates are organized by city and county throughout the United States. Professional subunits focus on cardiovascular education and research topics (e.g., epidemiology, high blood pressure, and arteriosclerosis). The national office is located at 7272 Greenville Avenue, Dallas, TX 75231–4596.

- Research and surveillance must be ongoing to develop new information concerning diet, blood lipids, and CHD; the development of better databases concerning food composition, food consumption patterns, illness rates, food product development, and nutrition education and communication is critical.

The Extent of CHD in Europe

The British Heart Foundation published an article outlining the extent of coronary heart disease in Europe indicating that the highest mortality rate of CHD was in Ireland with 246 deaths per 100,000 35- to 74-year-olds.[156] The presence of tobacco growers and the agricultural policy in Europe continues to subsidize tobacco growers, and only 4% of the budget is spent on fresh produce.[156] The country with the third highest death rate and the lowest rate of coronary artery bypass operations is the United Kingdom.[156]

In May 1999, the first report from the Monitoring Trends and Determinants in Cardiovascular Disease Study (MONICA) showed mortality decreasing. For example, Spain's mortality rate of coronary heart disease is 76 men per 100,000.[157] However, in 1995, the mortality rate appeared to decrease in Spain; the rate for men ages 35 to 74 was 125 per 100,000 according to the World Health Organization (WHO).[158] The trend in mortality rates across most of western Europe has decreased annually for men ages 35 to 64 as follows: France –5.7%; Sweden –3.8%; Italy –3.4%. However, in the East the rates have increased at an alarming rate and are substantially higher for the Czech Republic (+1.3%), Russia (+2.0%), and Poland (+2.2%).[157] The rates for these eastern countries are 266, 285, and 378 per 100,000, respectively.[157] The WHO reported in 1995 that for women ages 35 to 74, the mortality rates in Russia, Romania, and Hungary are 255, 176, and 169 per 100,000 population, respectively.[158]

The European Society of Cardiology (ESC) is an organization of executive scientific committees and working groups that "share the responsibility of counteracting the rapidly increasing prevalence of cardiovascular disease in the non-industrialized world and must find reasons for this prevalence and be active in the prevention."[159] The ESC is now trying to focus its mission on underdeveloped countries across Africa and Southeast Asia. In 1990, 1.8 million men and 1.7 million women in the developing world died from coronary disease and by 2020 those figures will likely reach 4.2 million and 3.5 million, respectively.[160]

The American Heart Association has been concerned with the international issues of cardiovascular heart disease; although the United States has had substantial success in the battle against the tobacco industry, other nations should target the tobacco companies as a key force in reducing the risk of cardiovascular disease.[161] The smoking cessation initiative, published in the *European Heart Journal* by the World Heart Federation, provides an overview of the burden of cardiovascular disease in developing nations.[162] The project gathered data from risk-factor surveys of heart disease and stroke, prevention programs, medical training facilities, and government programs[150] in developing countries and countries in economic transition (e.g., central and eastern Europe).[157]

In summary, the mortality rates of eastern Europe are alarming aside from the rates in Ireland. An increased focus of prevention and treatment of CHD is needed on a global scale by the World Health Organization, American Heart Association, European Society of Cardiology, and other organizations to address the future epidemic of heart disease in underdeveloped countries.

Dietary Fat and Cholestrol Assessment Instruments

Several dietary fat and cholesterol assessment instruments are available. A few are described next:

- Fat/Cholesterol Avoidance Scale—a 7-item, self-administered scale allows individuals to report their food selection and preparation practices. Scores can be used to assess and/or group individuals into those with heart-healthy versus unhealthy eating.[163,164]
- A Cholesterol-Saturated Fat Index (CSI)—calculated as follows:

$$CSI = (1.01 \times g \text{ saturated fat}) + (0.05 \times mg \text{ cholesterol})$$

A low CSI indicates low saturated fat and/or cholesterol content or hypocholesterolemic and low atherogenic potential, respectively. For example, a typical 2,000 kcal American eating pattern with 40% fat, 14% or 31 g saturated fat, and 400 mg cholesterol, has a CSI of 51.[165]
- The Block Fat Screen—a self-administered frequency tool that requires about 4 minutes. Foods are based on a medium portion and reflect high fat content. An average fat intake can be calculated to categorize individuals as low- or high-fat consumers.[166]
- The New American Eating Pattern—an approach to eating that involves a gradual modification of current habits through careful, programmed changes in high-fat, high-cholesterol, low-complex carbohydrate, and high-salt diet. The program is people friendly and based on beneficial experiences of 233 families. Changes in eating pattern are directed by 3 phases and self-assessment to gauge achievement of goals.[167]
- The Eating Pattern Assessment Tool—a self-administered instrument divided into 2 sections (1 that assesses intake of food characterized by high fat and cholesterol and another that contains lower-fat food

groupings as an alternate). The instrument is designed to assess overall fat and cholesterol intake and the frequency of such intakes and to educate people about fat-containing foods with educational messages.[168]

Method Alert

Household Activity Scale

Some women try to do housework immediately after they've had a heart attack even if they are told to go home and rest. It has been suggested that if a woman does fewer household chores, then she must be feeling very poor, and this might be due to a coronary condition. Women are generally committed to their housework, and because they are more inclined to ignore or downplay any symptoms compared with men, they do not believe they are at risk of CHD even though it's the number 1 killer of women.

Kimble Household Activities Scale

The Kimble Household Activities Scale lists 14 tasks that people do to take care of their homes (Table 11–6).[169] Depending on what women can or cannot

TABLE 11–6   Kimble Household Activity Scale

Household Activity	Perform Without Difficulty 1	Perform, but Slower Than Previously 2	No Longer Attempt 3	Never Have Performed 4
Cooking				
Washing dishes by hand				
Loading the dishwasher				
Scrubbing pots and pans				
Carrying baskets of laundry				
Loading/unloading washer and dryer				
Carrying 10-lb bags of groceries into house				
Unpacking groceries and placing on shelves				
Vacuuming				
Sweeping the floor				
Mopping the floor				
Scrubbing the floor on hands and knees				
Changing bed linens				
Moving furniture				

Source: Adapted from: Kimble A. For women only: 14 questions that could reveal hidden heart disease. *Tufts University Health and Nutrition Letter.* 2002;17(12):4-5.

perform, the severity of disease can be assessed. Women with CHD can answer the questions every 6 months to monitor cardiac symptoms, medication change, or change in treatment.

This list of chores reflects what people do to take care of their homes. If chest pain and discomfort, shortness of breath, or other symptoms of heart disease occur, then people might change or stop these activities. An individual evaluates his/her ability to perform these household activities as follows: (1) without difficulty; (2) not as easily because symptoms may be related to heart disease; (3) no longer attempted because symptoms occur; and (4) never have performed the activities because a spouse or someone else has always done them.

In summary, the more activities one can no longer do or cannot do as easily as once before, then the greater likelihood a physician's evaluation is needed to rule out other causes. Reassessment at 6-month intervals is suggested, especially for women who may not be aware that certain lifestyle habits can affect them as negatively as the lifestyles affect men.[169]

Healthy People 2010 Objectives

Reducing dietary fat, increasing complex carbohydrate and fiber-containing foods, lowering obesity, and monitoring blood cholesterol levels are the focus of *Healthy People 2010* objectives to lower CHD deaths. Community nutrition professionals can integrate numerous community-based and high-risk approaches into their programs to address the number 1 cause of death in the United States[163] (see Exhibits 11–1 and 11–2).

Exhibit 11–1 DATA2010: The *Healthy People 2010* Database—November 2000, Focus Area: 12—Cardiovascular

Objective Number	Objective	Baseline Year	Baseline	Target
12–01	Reduce coronary heart disease deaths to no more than 166 per 100,000 people. (Age-adjusted baseline: 208 per 100,000 in 1998)			
	All	1998	126	166
	American Indian	1998	126	166
	Blacks	1998	252	166
	Asian-Pacific Islander	1998	123	166
	Hispanic	1998	145	166
	White	1998	206	166
12–13	Mean total blood cholesterol levels—mean number in mg/d: (age adjusted, adults aged 20 years and older).			
	American Indian or Alaska native	1988–1997	UK	199
	Asian or Pacific Islander	1988–1997	UK	199

continued

Exhibit 11-1   continued

Black or African American	1988–1997	204	199
White	1988–1997	206	199
Hispanic or Latino	1988–1997	UK	199
Not Hispanic or Latino	1988–1997	206	199
Female	1988–1997	207	199
Male	1988–1997	204	199
Poor	1988–1997	205	199
Near poor	1988–1997	204	199
Middle/high income	1988–1997	206	199

12-14   High blood cholesterol levels (age adjusted, adults aged 20 years and older).

American Indian or Alaska native	1988–1994	UK	17
Asian or Pacific Islander	1988–1994	UK	17
Black or African American	1988–1994	21	17
White	1988–1994	21	17
Hispanic or Latino	1988–1994	UK	17
Not Hispanic or Latino	1988–1994	UK	17
Female	1988–1994	22	17
Male	1988–1994	19	17
Less than high school education	1988–1994	22	17
High school graduate	1988–1994	22	17
At least some college education	1988–1994	19	17

12-15   Blood cholesterol screening—adults screened within preceding 5 years (age adjusted, persons aged 18 years and older).

American Indian or Alaska native	1998	58	80
Asian or Pacific Islander	1998	68	80
Black or African American	1998	67	80
White	1998	67	80
Hispanic or Latino	1998	59	80
Not Hispanic or Latino	1998	68	80
Female	1998	70	80
Male	1998	64	80
Less than high school education	1998	58	80
High school graduate	1998	69	80
At least some college education	1998	78	80
Rural	1998	63	80
Persons with activity limitations	1998	72	80
Persons without activity limitations	1998	66	80

UK = unknown

Source: Adapted from: US Department of Health and Human Services. DATA 2010–the *Healthy People 2010* Database. *CDC Wonder.* Atlanta, Ga: Centers for Disease Control; November 2000.

Exhibit 11–2 Model Nutrition Objective for Risk Reduction

By 20___, the chronic disease risk factor ___*___ among [*target population*] will be reduced from _____% to _____ %.

*Obesity; hypertension; elevated serum cholesterol; poor physical fitness; excess intake of dietary fat, cholesterol, sodium, alcohol, and sugar; inadequate intake of dietary fiber, fruits and vegetables, and calcium.

Source: Adapted from: *Model State Nutrition Objectives.* Washington, DC: The Association of State and Territorial Public Health Nutrition Directors; 1988.

References

1. National Cholesterol Education Program. *Report of the Expert Panel on Population Strategies for Blood Cholesterol Reduction.* Bethesda, Md: US Dept of Health and Human Services; 1990. NIH publication 90-3046.
2. Ford ES, Giles WH, Croft JB. Prevalence of nonfatal coronary heart disease among American adults. *Am Heart J.* March 2000;139(3):371-377.
3. *National Health and Nutrition Examination Survey III (NHANES II), 1988–1994.* CDC/NCHS and the American Heart Association; 1999. Available at: www.americanheart.org/statistics03cardio.html. Accessed January 10, 2006.
4. American Heart Association. American Heart Association Guidelines. *Circulation.* 2004;109:672-693.
5. Berg Sloan C, Ternus M. American Heart Association's new guidelines take a personal approach to preventing cardiovascular disease in women. *Networking News.* 2005;27(1):1,4.
6. Ford ES, Mokded AH, Giles WH, et al. Serum total cholestrol concentrations and awareness, treatment, and control of hyper-cholesterol among US adults. *Circulation.* 2003;107:2185-2189.
7. Keys A. Coronary heart disease in seven countries. *Circulation.* 1970;41:1.
8. McGee D, Reed D, Yano K, et al. Ten-year incidence of coronary heart disease in the Honolulu Heart Program: relationship to nutrient intake. *Am J Epidemiol.* 1984;119:667-676.
9. Kris-Etherton PM, Krummel D, Russel ME, et al. The effect of diet on plasma, lipids, lipoproteins, and coronary heart disease. *J Am Diet Assoc.* 1988;88:1373.
10. Castelli WP, Garrison RJ, Wilson PWF, et al. Incidence of coronary heart disease and lipoprotein cholesterol levels: the Framingham Study. *JAMA.* 1986;256:2835.
11. Samuel P, McNamara DJ, Shapiro J. The role of diet in the etiology and treatment of atherosclerosis. *Ann Rev Med.* 1983;34:179.
12. Grundy SM. Comparison of monounsaturated fatty acids and carbohydrates for lowering plasma cholesterol. *N Engl J Med.* 1986;314:745.
13. Mensink RP, Katan MB. Effect of monounsaturated fatty acids versus complex carbohydrates on high density lipoproteins in healthy men and women. *Lancet.* 1987;1:122.
14. Weisweiler P, Janetschek P, Schwandt P. Influence of polyunsaturated fats and fat restriction on serum lipoproteins in humans. *Metabolism.* 1985;34:83.
15. Schwandt P, Janetschek P, Weisweiler P. High density lipoproteins unaffected by dietary fat modification. *Atherosclerosis.* 1982;44:9.

16. Keys A, Anderson JT, Grande F. Serum cholesterol response to changes in the diet. IV. Particular saturated fatty acids in the diet. *Metabolism.* 1965;14:776.

17. Hegsted DM, McGandy RB, Meyers ML, et al. Quantitative effects of dietary fat on serum cholesterol in man. *Am J Clin Nutr.* 1965;17:281.

18. Bronsgeest-Schoute DC, Hautvast JGAJ, Hermus RJJ. Dependence of the effects of dietary cholesterol and experimental conditions on serum lipids in man. *Am J Clin Nutr.* 1979;32:2183.

19. Anderson JT, Grande F, Keys A. Cholesterol-lowering diets. *J Am Diet Assoc.* 1973;62:133.

20. Porrini M, Simonetti P, Testolin G, Roggi C, Laddomada M, Tenconi M. Relation between diet composition and coronary heart disease risk factors. *J Epidemiol Community Health.* June 1991;45(2):148-151.

21. Shrapnel W, Calvert G, Nestel P, Truswell A. Diet and coronary heart disease: the National Heart Foundation of Australia. *Med J Aust.* May 4, 1992;156(suppl):S9-S16.

22. Connor WE, Witiak DT, Stone DB, et al. Cholesterol balance and fecal neutral steroid and bile acid excretion in normal men fed dietary fats of different fatty acid composition. *J Clin Invest.* 1969;48:1363-1375.

23. Grande F, Anderson JT, Keys A. Comparison of effects of palmitic and stearic acids in the diet on serum cholesterol in man. *Am J Clin Nutr.* 1970;23:1184.

24. Bonanome A, Grundy SM. Effect of dietary stearic acid on plasma cholesterol and lipoprotein levels. *N Engl J Med.* 1988;318:1244.

25. Snook JT, DeLany JP, Vivian VM. Effect of moderate to very low fat defined formula diets on serum lipids in healthy subjects. *Lipids.* 1985;20:808.

26. Grundy SM, Nix D, Whelan MF, et al. Comparison of three cholesterol-lowering diets in normolipemic men. *JAMA.* 1986;256:2351.

27. Kuusi T, Ehnholm C, Huttunen J, et al. Concentration and composition of serum lipoproteins during a low-fat diet at two levels of polyunsaturated fat. *J Lipid Res.* 1985;26:360.

28. Weisweiler P, Drosner M, Janetschek P, et al. Changes in very low and low density lipoproteins with dietary fat modifications. *Atherosclerosis.* 1983;49:325.

29. Hodgson JM, Wahlquist MR, Boxall JA, et al. Can linoleic acid contribute to coronary artery disease? *Am J Clin Nutr.* 1993;58:228-234.

30. Logan RL, Thomson M, Riemersma RA, et al. Risk factors for ischaemic heart-disease in normal men aged 40—Edinburgh-Stockholm Study. *Lancet.* 1978;1:949-954.

31. Riemersma RA, Wood DA, Butler S, et al. Linoleic acid content in adipose tissue and coronary heart disease. *Br Med J.* 1986;292: 1423-1427.

32. Wood DA, Riemersma RA, Butler S, et al. Adipose tissue and platelet fatty acids and coronary heart disease in Scottish men. *Lancet.* 1984;2:117-121.

33. Wood DA, Riemersma RA, Butler S. Linoleic and eicosapentaenoic acids in adipose tissue and platelets and risk of coronary heart disease. *Lancet.* 1987;1:177-183.

34. Blankenhorn DH, Johnson RL, Mack WJ. The influence of diet on the appearance of new lesions in human coronary arteries. *JAMA.* 1990;263:1646-1652.

35. National Dairy Council. Nutrition and health effects of unsaturated fatty acids. *Dairy Council Dig.* 1988;59:1.

36. Dyerberg J. Linolenate-derived polyunsaturated fatty acids and prevention of atherosclerosis. *Nutr Rev.* 1986;44:125.
37. Bang HO, Dyerberg J, Hjorne N. The composition of food consumed by Greenland Eskimos. *Acta Med Scand.* 1976;200:69.
38. Herold PM, Kinsella JE. Fish oil consumption and decreased risk of cardiovascular disease: a comparison of findings from animal and human feeding trials. *Am J Clin Nutr.* 1986;43:566.
39. Simons LA, Hichie JB, Balasubramaniam S. On the effects of dietary omega-3 fatty acids (MaxEPA) on plasma lipids and lipoproteins in patients with hyperlipidemia. *Atherosclerosis.* 1985;54:75.
40. Nestel PJ. Fish oil attenuates the cholesterol induced rise in lipoprotein cholesterol. *Am J Clin Nutr.* 1986;43:752.
41. Leaf A, Weber PC. Cardiovascular effects of omega-3 fatty acids. *N Engl J Med.* 1988;318:549.
42. Saynor R, Verel D, Gillott T. The long-term effect of dietary supplementation with fish lipid concentrate on serum lipids, bleeding time, platelets and angina. *Atherosclerosis.* 1984;50:3.
43. Omega-3 fatty acids: eat fish, or fish oils? *CNI Weekly.* 1987;17:6.
44. Simopoulos AP, Salem N, Purslane. A terrestrial source of omega-3 fatty acids. *N Engl J Med.* 1986;315:833.
45. Mattson FH, Grundy SM. Comparison of effects of dietary saturated, monounsaturated, and polyunsaturated fatty acids on plasma lipids and lipoproteins in man. *J Lipid Res.* 1985;26:194.
46. Grundy SM, Bonanome A. Workshop on monounsaturated fatty acids. *Arteriosclerosis.* 1987;7:644.
47. Baggio G, Pagan A, Muraca M, et al. Olive oil-enriched diet: effect on serum lipoprotein levels and biliary cholesterol saturation. *Am J Clin Nutr.* 1988;47:960.
48. Nichaman MZ, Hamm P. Low-fat, high-carbohydrate diets and plasma cholesterol. *Am J Clin Nutr.* 1987;45:1155.
49. Santene C. Eat your salmon. *Wall Street Journal.* February 11, 2004.
50. Nutia USA. Tracing salmon from farm to fork. May 27, 2004. NOVIS. Frederiksterg, Denmark.
51. Editorial. *Salmon of the Americas. PCDE Facts.* Newark, NJ; *Salmon of the Americas.* 2004.
52. Gordon T, Kagan A, Garcia-Palmieri M, et al. Diet and its relation to coronary heart disease and death in three populations. *Circulation.* 1981;63:500.
53. Dreon DM, Frey-Hewitt B, Ellsworth N, et al. Dietary fat: carbohydrate ratio and obesity in middle-aged men. *Am J Clin Nutr.* 1988;47:995.
54. Acheson KJ, Flatt JP, Jequier E. Glycogen synthesis versus lipogenesis after a 500 g carbohydrate meal in man. *Metabolism.* 1982;31:1234.
55. Lissner L, Levitsky DA, Stupp BJ, et al. Dietary fat and the regulation of energy intake in human subjects. *Am J Clin Nutr.* 1987;46:886.
56. Grundy SM, Barrett-Connor E, Rudel LL, et al. Workshop on the impact of dietary cholesterol on plasma lipoproteins and atherogenesis. *Arteriosclerosis.* 1988;8:95.
57. Connor WE, Cerqueira MT, Connor R, et al. The plasma lipids, lipoproteins, and diet of the Tarahumara Indians of Mexico. *Am J Clin Nutr.* 1978;31:1131.
58. *The Framingham Study—An Epidemiological Investigation of Cardiovascular Diseases. Sec. 24. The Framingham Diet Study.* Washington, DC: US Dept of Health, Education and Welfare; 1970.
59. Gordon T, Fisher M, Ernst N, et al. Relation of diet to LDL cholesterol, VLDL cholesterol, and plasma total cholesterol and triglycerides in white

adults: the Lipid Research Clinics Prevalence Study. *Arteriosclerosis.* 1982;2:502.

60. Shekelle RB, Shryock AM, Paul O. Diet, serum cholesterol, and death from coronary heart disease: the Western Electric Study. *N Engl J Med.* 1981;304:65.

61. Gordon DJ, Salz KM, Roggenkamp KJ, et al. Dietary determinants of plasma cholesterol change in the recruitment phase of the Lipid Research Clinics Coronary Primary Prevention Trial. *Arteriosclerosis.* 1982;2:537.

62. Hegsted DM, Nicolosi RJ. Individual variation in serum cholesterol levels. *Proc Natl Acad Sci USA.* 1987;84:6259.

63. Jacobs DR, Anderson JT, Hannan P, et al. Variability in individual serum cholesterol response to change in diet. *Arteriosclerosis.* 1983;3:349.

64. Katan MB, Beynen AC, De Vries JHM. Existence of constant hypo- and hyper-responders to dietary cholesterol in man. *Am J Epidemiol.* 1986;123:221.

65. Food and Nutrition Science Alliance: the American Dietetic Association (ADA), American Institute of Nutrition (AIN), American Society for Clinical Nutrition, Inc. (ASCN), Institute of Food Technologists (IFT). *Statement on Trans Fatty Acids.* Chicago, Ill: Food and Nutrition Science Alliance; 1994.

66. Willett WC, Stampfer MJ, Manson JE, et al. Intake of trans fatty acids and risk of coronary heart disease among women. *Lancet.* 1993;341:581–585.

67. Judd J, Baer D, Clevidence B, Chen S, Meijer G. Effect of dietary sterol esters in salad dressings on blood lipids, lipoproteins and carotenoids. Baltimore, Md: Beltsville Human Nutrition Research Center, ARS, USDA, Beltsville MD and Lipton; 2000.

68. Hendriks HJ, Weststrate JA, van Vliet T, Meijer GW. Spreads enriched with three different levels of vegetable oil sterols and the degree of cholesterol lowering in normocholesterolaemic and mildly hypercholesterolaemic subjects. *Eur J Clin Nutr.* 1999;53:319–327.

69. Keys A, Fidanza F, Scardi V, et al. Studies on serum cholesterol and other characteristics of clinically healthy men in Naples. *Arch Intern Med.* 1954;93:328.

70. Keys A, Kimura N, Bronte-Stewart B, et al. Lessons from serum cholesterol studies in Japan, Hawaii, and Los Angeles. *Ann Intern Med.* 1958;48:83.

71. Hallfrisch J, West S, Fisher C, et al. Modification of the United States' diet to effect changes in blood lipids and lipoprotein distribution. *Atherosclerosis.* 1985;57:179.

72. Glinsmann WH, Irausquin H, Park YK. Evaluation of health aspects of sugar contained in carbohydrate sweeteners: report of Sugars Task Force, 1986. *J Nutr.* 1986;116(suppl):55.

73. Floch MH, Maryniuk MD, Bryant C, et al. Practical aspects of implementing increased dietary fiber intake. *Nutr Today.* 1986;21:27.

74. Morris JN, Marr JW, Clayton DG. Diet and heart: a postscript. *Br Med J.* 1977;2:1307–1314.

75. Kromhout D, Bosschieter EB, DeLezenne Coulander C. Dietary fibre and 10-year mortality from coronary heart disease, cancer, and all causes: the Zutphen Study. *Lancet.* 1982;1:518.

76. Jenkins DJA, Reynolds D, Leeds AR, et al. Hypocholesterolemic action of dietary fiber unrelated to fecal bulking effect. *Am J Clin Nutr.* 1979;32:2430.

77. Miettinen TA, Tarpila S. Effects of pectin on serum cholesterol, fecal bile acids, and bilary lipids in normolipidemic and hyperlipidemic individuals. *Clin Chim Acta.* 1977;70:471.

78. Jenkins DJA, Reynolds D, Slavin B, et al. Dietary fiber and blood lipids: treatment of hypercholesterolemia with guar crisp bread. *Am J Clin Nutr.* 1980;33:575.

79. Anderson JW, Zettwoch N, Feldman T, et al. Cholesterol-lowering effects of psyllium hydrophilic mucilloid for hypercholesterolemic men. *Arch Intern Med.* 1988;148:292.

80. Van Horn LV, Liu K, Parker D, et al. Serum lipid response to oat product intake with a fat-modified diet. *J Am Diet Assoc.* 1986;86:759.

81. Anderson JW, Story L, Sieling B, et al. Hypocholesterolemic effects of oat-bran or bran intake for hypercholesterolemic men. *Am J Clin Nutr.* 1984;40:1146.

82. Truswell AS. Effects of different types of dietary fiber on plasma lipids. In: Heaton KW, ed. *Dietary Fiber: Current Developments of Importance to Health.* London, England: Libbey and Co; 1978.

83. Stasse-Wolthuis M, Albers HFF, Van Jeveren JGC, et al. Influence of dietary fiber from vegetables and fruits, bran or citrus pectin on serum lipids, fecal lipids and caloric function. *Am J Clin Nutr.* 1980;33:1745.

84. Anderson JW, Chen WL. Plant fiber, carbohydrate and lipid metabolism. *Am J Clin Nutr.* 1979;32:346.

85. Sprecher DL, Harris BV, Goldberg AC, et al. Efficacy of psyllium in reducing serum cholesterol levels in hypercholesterolemic patients on high or low-fat diets. *Ann Intern Med.* 1993;119:545-554.

86. Bliss RM. Oats may keep arteries out of sticky situations. *Ag Res.* June 2004;52(6):7.

87. Ludwig DS, Pereira MA, Kroenke CH, et al. Dietary fiber, weight gain, and cardiovascular disease factors in young adults. *JAMA.* 1999;282:1539-1546.

88. Van Raaij JM, Katan MB, Hautvast JG, et al. Effects of casein versus soy protein diets on serum cholesterol and lipoproteins in young healthy volunteers. *Am J Clin Nutr.* 1981;34:1261.

89. Carroll KK, Giovannetti PM, Huff MW, et al. Hypocholesterolemic effect of substituting soybean protein for animal protein in the diet of healthy young women. *Am J Clin Nutr.* 1978;31:1312.

90. Sacks FM, Breslow JL, Wood PG, et al. Lack of an effect of dairy protein (casein) and soy protein on plasma cholesterol of strict vegetarians: an experiment and a critical review. *J Lipid Res.* 1983;24:1012.

91. Carroll KK. Hypercholesterolemia and atherosclerosis: effects of dietary protein. *Fed Proc.* 1982;41:2792.

92. Langseth L. Is high iron status a risk for heart disease? *Food and Nutr News.* 1994;66(3):17-19.

93. Steinberg D, Parthasarthy S, Carew TE, et al. Beyond cholesterol: modifications of low-density lipoprotein that increase its atherogenicity. *N Engl J Med.* 1989;320:915-924.

94. Luc G, Fruchart JC. Oxidation of lipoproteins and atherosclerosis. *Am J Clin Nutr.* 1991;53:206S-209S.

95. Goldhaber JI, Weiss JN. Oxygen free radicals and cardiac reperfusion abnormalities. *Hypertension.* 1992;20:118-127.

96. Salonen JT, Nyyssonen K, Korpela H, et al. High stored iron levels are associated with excess risk of myocardial infarction in eastern Finnish men. *Circulation.* 1992;86:803-811.

97. Lauffer RB. Iron stores and the international variation in mortality from coronary artery disease. *Med Hypothesis.* 1991;35:96-102.

98. Rimm EB, Ascherio A, Stampfer MJ, et al. Dietary iron intake and risk of coronary disease among men. *Circulation.* 1994;89(3):969-974.

99. Stampfer MJ, Grodstein F, Rosenberg I, et al. A prospective study of plasma ferritin and risk of myocardial infarction in US physicians. *Circulation.* 1993;87:688.

100. Aronow WS. Serum ferritin is not a risk factor for coronary artery disease in men and women aged ≥ 62 years. *Am J Cardiol.* 1993;72:347-348.

101. Cooper RS, Liao Y. Iron stores and coronary heart disease: negative findings in the NHANES I Epidemiologic Follow-Up Study. *Circulation.* 1993;87:686.

102. Specialty Coffee Association of America. *The Specialty Coffee Chronicle.* May/June 2004.

103. Thelle DS, Arnesen E, Forde OH. The Tromso Heart Study. *N Engl J Med.* 1983;308:1454.

104. Haffner SM, Knapp JA, Stern MP, et al. Coffee consumption, diet and lipids. *Am J Epidemiol.* 1985;122:1.

105. Lacroix AZ, Mead LA, Liang KY, et al. Coffee consumption and the incidence of coronary heart disease. *N Engl J Med.* 1986;315:977.

106. Forde OH, Knutsen SF, Arnesen E, et al. The Tromso Heart Study: coffee consumption and serum lipid concentrations in men with hypercholesterolemia: a randomized intervention study. *Br Med J.* 1985;290:893.

107. Arnesen E, Forde OH, Thelle DS. Coffee and serum cholesterol. *Br Med J.* 1984;288:1960.

108. Leonard-Green TK, Watson RR. Caffeine and health risk [author's reply to letter]. *J Am Diet Assoc.* 1988;88:370.

109. Ernst N, Fisher M, Smith W, et al. The association of plasma high density lipoprotein cholesterol with dietary intake and alcohol consumption: the Lipid Research Clinics Program Prevalence Study. *Circulation.* 1980;62(suppl IV):41.

110. Haskell WL, Camargo C, Williams PT, et al. The effect of cessation and resumption of moderate alcohol intake on high-density-lipoprotein subfractions. *N Engl J Med.* 1984;310:805.

111. Burr ML, Fehily AM, Butland BK, et al. Alcohol and high-density-lipoprotein cholesterol: a randomized controlled trial. *Br J Nutr.* 1986;56:81.

112. Krauss R, Eckel R, Howard B, et al. AHA dietary guidelines, revision 2000: a statement for healthcare professionals from the nutrition committee of the American Heart Association. *Circulation.* 2000;102:2284-2311.

113. Miyagi Y, Miwa K, Inoue H. Inhibition of human low-density lipoprotein oxidation by flavonoids in red wine and grape juice. *Am J Cardiol.* 1997;80:1627-1631.

114. Gear JS, Mann JI, Thorogood M, et al. Biochemical and hematological variables in vegetarians. *Br Med J.* 1980;280:1415.

115. Lock DR, Varhol A, Grimes S, et al. Apo A-I/Apo A-II ratios in plasma of vegetarians. *Metabolism.* 1983;32:1142.

116. Nestel PJ, Billington T, Smith B. Low density and high density lipoprotein kinetics and sterol balance in vegetarians. *Metabolism.* 1981;30:941.

117. Blum CB, Levy RI, Eisenberg S, et al. High density lipoprotein metabolism in man. *J Clin Invest.* 1977;60:795.

118. Fisher M, Levine P, Weiner B, et al. The effect of vegetarian diets on plasma lipids and platelet levels. *Arch Intern Med.* 1986;146:1193.

119. Malinow MR, Bostom AG, Krauss RM. Homocyst(e)ine, diet, and cardiovascular diseases—a statement for healthcare professionals from the nutrition committee, American Heart Association. *Circulation.* 1999;99:178-182.

120. Omenn GS, Beresford SA, Motulsky AG. Preventing coronary heart disease: B vitamins and homocysteine. *Circulation.* February 10, 1998;97(5):421-424.

121. McLaughlin R. Neural tube defects. *Digest.* 1998;1,3.

122. Dugan L. Antioxidants in the prevention of coronary heart disease. *Scan Pulse.* 1994;13(3):1-2.

123. Stampfer MJ, Hennekens CH, Manson JE, et al. Vitamin E consumption and the risk of coronary disease in women. *N Engl J Med.* 1993;328:1444-1449.

124. Rimm EB, Stampfer MJ, Ascherio A, et al. Vitamin E consumption and the risk of coronary disease in men. *N Engl J Med.* 1993;328: 1450-1456.

125. Tufts nutrition: translating the research for use at your table. *Health & Nutrition Letter.* February 2004; (suppl):4.

126. Stark K, Park E, Maines V, Holub B. Effect of a fish-oil concentrate on serum lipids in postmenopausal women receiving and not receiving hormone replacement therapy in a placebo-controlled, double-blind trial. *Am J Clin Nutr.* 2000;72:389-394.

127. Osganian S, Stampfer M, Rimm E, Spiegelman D, Manson J, Willett W. Dietary carotenoids and risk of coronary artery disease in women. *Am J Clin Nutr.* 2003;77:1390-1399.

128. Jacobs DR Jr, Steffen L. Nutrients, foods, and dietary patterns as exposures in research: a framework for food synergy. *Am J Clin Nutr.* 2003;78:508S-513S.

129. The Chicago Heart Association. Body mass index in middle age and health-related quality of life in older age: the Chicago Heart Association detection project in industry study. *Arch Intern Med.* 2003;163(20):2448-2455.

130. Shaefer EJ. Hyperlipoproteinemia. In: Rakel RD, ed. *Conn's Current Therapy 1991.* Philadelphia, Pa: WB Saunders; 1991:515-522.

131. National Research Council. *Diet and Health: Implications for Reducing Chronic Disease Risk.* Washington, DC: National Academy Press; 1989.

132. American Heart Association. *Dietary Treatment of Hypercholesterolemia. A Handbook for Counselors.* Dallas, Tex: American Heart Association; 1988.

133. US Department of Agriculture/US Department of Health and Human Services. *Nutrition and Your Health: Dietary Guidelines for Americans.* 2nd ed. Washington, DC: US Government Printing Office; 1985. HG-232.

134. National Cholesterol Education Program. Second report of the Expert Panel on Detection, Evaluation, and Treatment of High Blood Cholesterol in Adults: summary report. *JAMA.* 1993;269(23):3015-3023.

135. National Cholesterol Education Program (NCEP) Expert Panel on Direction, Evaluation, and Treatment of High Blood Cholesterol in Adults (Adult Treatment Panel III). Implications of recent clinical trials for NCEP ATP III Guidelines. *Circulation.* 2004;110:227-239.

136. Grundy SM, Cleeman JI, Merz NB, et al. Implications of recent clinical trials for the national cholesterol education program adult treatment panel III guidelines. *Circulation.* 2004;110:227-239.

137. Kant AK, Schatzkin A, Harris TB, et al. Dietary diversity and subsequent mortality in the first National Health and Nutrition Examination Survey Epidemiologic Follow-Up Study. *Am J Clin Nutr.* 1993;57:434-440.

138. *Healthy People 2000: National Health Promotion and Disease Prevention Objectives.* Washington, DC: US Dept of Health and Human Services; 1991. DHHS (PHS) publication 91-50212.

139. Neaton JD, Wentworth D. Serum cholesterol, blood pressure cigarette smoking, and death from coronary heart disease. *Arch Intern Med.* 1992;152:56-64.

140. Baer JT. Improved plasma cholesterol levels in men after a nutrition education program at the worksite. *J Am Diet Assoc.* 1993;93:658-663.

141. Stallings VA, Cortner JA, Shannon BM, et al. Preliminary report of a home-based education program for dietary treatment of hypercholesterolemia in children. *Am J Health Promot.* 1993;8:106-108.

142. Ornish D, Brown SE, Scherwitz LW, et al. Can lifestyle changes reverse coronary heart disease? *Lancet.* 1990;336:129-133.

143. Warshafsky S, Kamer RS, Sivak SL. Effect of garlic on total serum cholesterol: a meta-analysis. *Ann Intern Med.* 1993;119:599-605.

144. O'Neil J. Garlic to cut cholesterol? Don't bother. *New York Times.* September 26, 2000:D8.

145. Weidner G, Connor SL, Hollis JF, et al. Improvements in hostility and depression in relation to dietary change and cholesterol-lowering: the Family Heart Study. *Ann Intern Med.* 1992;117:820-823.

146. Muldoon MF, Manuch SB, Matthews KA. Lowering cholesterol concentrations and mortality: a quantitative review of primary prevention trials. *Br Med J.* 1990;301:309-314.

147. Bandura A. *Social Foundations of Thought and Action: A Social Cognitive Theory.* Englewoood Cliffs, NJ: Prentice Hall; 1986.

148. Sesso H, Paffenbarger R, Lee I. Physical activity and coronary heart disease in men: the Harvard Alumni Health Study. *Circulation.* 2000;102:975-980.

149. WHO Expert Committee on the Prevention of Coronary Heart Disease. *Prevention of Coronary Heart Disease.* Geneva, Switzerland: World Health Organization; 1982. Technical report series no. 678.

150. Klag MJ, Ford DE, Mead LA, et al. Serum cholesterol in young men and subsequent cardiovascular disease. *N Engl J Med.* 1993;328:313-318.

151. Stamler J. Established major coronary risk factors. In: Marmot M, Elliott P, eds. *Coronary Heart Disease Epidemiology: From Aetiology to Public Health.* New York: Oxford University Press; 1992:35-66.

152. Stamler J, Stamler R, Brown WV, et al. Serum cholesterol: doing the right thing. *Circulation.* 1993;88:1954-1960.

153. Hulley SB, Walsh JMB, Newman TB. Health policy on blood cholesterol: time to change directions. *Circulation.* 1992;86(3):1026-1029.

154. Holme I, Hjermann I, Helgeland A, et al. The Oslo Study: diet and anti-smoking advice. *Prev Med.* 1985;14:279.

155. World Health Organization European Collaborative Group. European Collaborative Trial of Multifactorial Prevention of Coronary Heart Disease: final report. *Lancet.* 1986;1:869-872.

156. Bradbury J. Europe needs to reduce heart disease [News]. *Lancet.* February 19, 2000;355 (9204).

157. Horton R. Future of European cardiology: continentally isolated or globally integrated? [Commentary]. *Lancet.* 1999;354(918F):791-792.

158. American Heart Association. *World Health Statistics Annual.* Geneva, Switzerland: World Health Organization; 2006.

159. Tunstall-Pedoe H, Kuulasmaa K, Mahonen M, Tolonen H, Ruokokoski E, Amouyel P. Contribution of trends in survival and coronary event rates to changes in coronary heart disease mortality: 10-year results from 37 WHO MONICA project populations. *Lancet.* 1999;353:1547-1557.

160. Institute of Medicine. *Control of Cardiovascular Disease in Developing Countries.* Washington, DC: National Academy Press; 1998.

161. Fuster V. Epidemic of cardiovascular disease and stroke: the three main challenges. *Circulation.* 1999;99:1132-1137.

162. Chockalingam A, Balaguer-Vintro I. Impending global pandemic of cardiovascular disease. Geneva, Switzerland: World Heart Federation, 1999.

163. Knapp JA, Hazuda HP, Haffner SM, et al. A saturated fat/cholesterol avoidance scale: sex and ethnic differences in a biethnic population. *J Am Diet Assoc.* 1988;2:172-177.

164. Frank GC, Zive M, Nelson J, et al. Fat and cholesterol avoidance among Mexican American and Anglo preschool children and parents. *J Am Diet Assoc.* 1991;8:954-961.

165. Connor SL, Artaud-Wild SM, Classick-Kohn CJ, et al. The cholesterol/saturated-fat index: an indication of the hypercholesterolemic and atherogenic potential of food. *Lancet.* 1986;1:1229-1232.

166. Block G, Clifford C, Naughton MD, et al. A brief dietary screen for high fat intake. *J Nutr Ed.* 1989;21(5):199-207.

167. Connor SL, Connor WE. *The New American Diet.* New York: Simon & Schuster; 1986.

168. Peters JR, Quiter ES, Brekke ML, et al. The eating pattern assessment tool: a simple instrument for assessing dietary fat and cholesterol intake. *J Am Diet Assoc.* 1994;94(9):1008-1022.

169. Kaufman M. *Nutrition in Public Health—A Handbook for Developing Programs and Services.* Gaithersburg, Md: Aspen Publishers, Inc; 1990:570.

CANCER

Learning Objectives

- Discuss the epidemiology of cancer in the United States.
- Define the role of nutrition in the etiology, prevention, and treatment of cancer.
- Identify the *Healthy People 2010* objectives for cancer.
- Describe how community nutritionists can be actively involved in a cancer control network in the United States.
- List the major food sources or food components and how they protect the body and reduce cancer risk.
- Identify the basic elements of a healthy eating pattern for primary and secondary prevention of cancer.

High Definition Nutrition

Antioxidants—vitamins C and E and beta-carotene, which neutralize free radicals and other reactive chemicals and terminate harmful chemical reactions.

Apoptosis—programmed cell death.

Carcinogenesis—the process of promoting cancer.

Chemoprevention—treatment with anticancer drugs. Systemic chemotherapy is injected into the bloodstream or taken by mouth and circulated throughout the body. Less often, chemotherapy is applied locally—to the skin or into the bladder.

Conjugated linoleic acid—a natural component in animal food, especially dairy products, which has a cancer-preventing effect.

Hormone replacement therapy—treatment with hormones or with drugs that interfere with hormone production or hormone action, or the surgical removal of hormone-producing glands. Hormone therapy may kill cancer cells or slow their growth.

Lignin—a phenol similar in structure to estrogen that is hypothesized to decrease estrogen exposure and cancer risk.

Malignant—cancerous; a growth with a tendency to invade and destroy nearby tissue and spread to other parts of the body.

Meta-analysis—aggregate analysis of similar studies to determine consistency of results.

Phytoestrogens—plant estrogens that may prevent binding of endogenous estrogens to the estrogen receptor.

SEER—the National Cancer Institute's surveillance, epidemiology, and end results data registry that tracks cancer incidence, patient survival, and mortality.

Stages of cancer:

- In-situ—neoplasms that fulfill all microscopic criteria for malignancy except invasion.
- Localized—neoplasms that appear entirely confined to the organ of origin.
- Regional—neoplasms that have spread by direct extension to immediately adjacent organs and/or have metastasized to regional lymph nodes and appear to have spread no further.
- Distant or remote—Neoplasms that have spread beyond the immediate adjacent organs or tissue by direct extension and/or have either developed secondary or metastatic tumors, metastasized to distant lymph nodes, or have been determined to be systemic in origin (leukemia, multiple myeloma, etc.).

Tumor—an abnormal mass of tissue that may be either benign or malignant.

Tumor latency—average time to develop a first tumor.

An Overview of Cancer

The epidemiology of cancer shows that cancer is not an inevitable outcome of aging. Cancer is related to metabolic stresses linked to individual lifestyles. Variables that define lifestyle are tobacco and alcohol use, food intake, leisure time activity, occupational and environmental exposure, family cohesion, and personality.[1]

Epidemiologic and experimental studies have yielded data to answer many questions about cancer incidence and the role of eating patterns. Epidemiologic data come from ecologic correlations, cohort studies, case-control studies, and metabolic epidemiologic studies. Experimental studies, likewise, give strong support for a diet-cancer link. Data from metabolic studies focus largely on the colon cancer and bile acid metabolite association, breast and estrogen relation, and prostate and androgen association.

A key element in cancer epidemiology is the role of nutrition. Nutrition is thought to affect many different cancers because it appears to be a cofactor to chemical carcinogenesis.[1] Biomarkers may be very important in nutritional carcinogenesis, because tests of a cancer-to-diet hypothesis in homogeneous populations are inconclusive. Some researchers believe that nutritional carcinogenesis may best be studied by comparing the food intakes of diverse populations and by focusing more on biomarkers. If research uses specific biomarkers, the pathogenesis of a cancer may be clarified, and then further exploration with preventive strategies may be possible.[1]

Incidence

Cancer incidence increases with age, and most cases affect adults at the middle of their adult life or older. For children aged 1 through 14, cancer causes more deaths in the United States than any other disease. More than 8 million US residents living today have a history of cancer. Of these, 5 million were diagnosed more than 5 years ago; those who have no evidence of the disease and are still living are considered cured. Their life expectancy is the same as a person who was never diagnosed with cancer.[2-4]

Each year, about 1,400,000 new cancer cases are diagnosed. In a given year, about 564,000 individuals will die of cancer—which is more than 1,500 people per day. A startling 25% of all deaths in the United States are from cancer, and the increase in cancer mortality has been steady during the past half century. Lung cancer accounts for the greatest increase in cancer mortality; removing lung cancer deaths from cancer mortality would create a decline of 14% for the period from 1950 to 1990.[2]

In 2004, approximately 1,368,030 Americans developed cancer, and 563,700 Americans died of the disease. Figure 12–1 shows the 2005 estimated numbers for US cancer cases and deaths. Figure 12–2 outlines incidence rates per 100,000 US residents separately for males and females.

Long-term survival from cancer has increased for each decade since 1900. Fewer than 20% of individuals diagnosed with cancer in 1930 survived 5 years. This contrasts with 62% for all cancers combined currently. The 5-year survival rate is commonly used to measure the success of early detection, treatment, and follow-up.[2]

Psychosocial and behavioral research demonstrate that lifestyle and environmental factors influence an individual's general health and chances of developing cancer, and also that lifestyle influences an individual's ability to cope with cancer and cancer treatment. Behavioral modification can assist with the management of cancer side effects (e.g., pain, nausea, and vomiting), as well the ability to handle stress during treatment and recovery.[2]

Several cancers are linked to eating behavior risk factors:

- Colon and rectum cancer are linked to high-fat and/or low-fiber food intake.
- Breast cancer is linked to variations in fat intake.
- Prostate cancer may be linked to dietary fat.

Info Line

Forty-nine percent of men in Los Angeles 40 years and older did not have a prostate exam in the past 2 years. Among uninsured men in this group, 71% did not have a prostate exam in the past 2 years. The percentage of men 40 years and older who did not have a prostate exam in the past 2 years was highest among Asians (64%), followed by Latinos (59%), African Americans (48%), and whites (42%).
Source: LA Health Profiles. Los Angeles, Calif: Los Angeles County Department of Health Services; 1999:33.

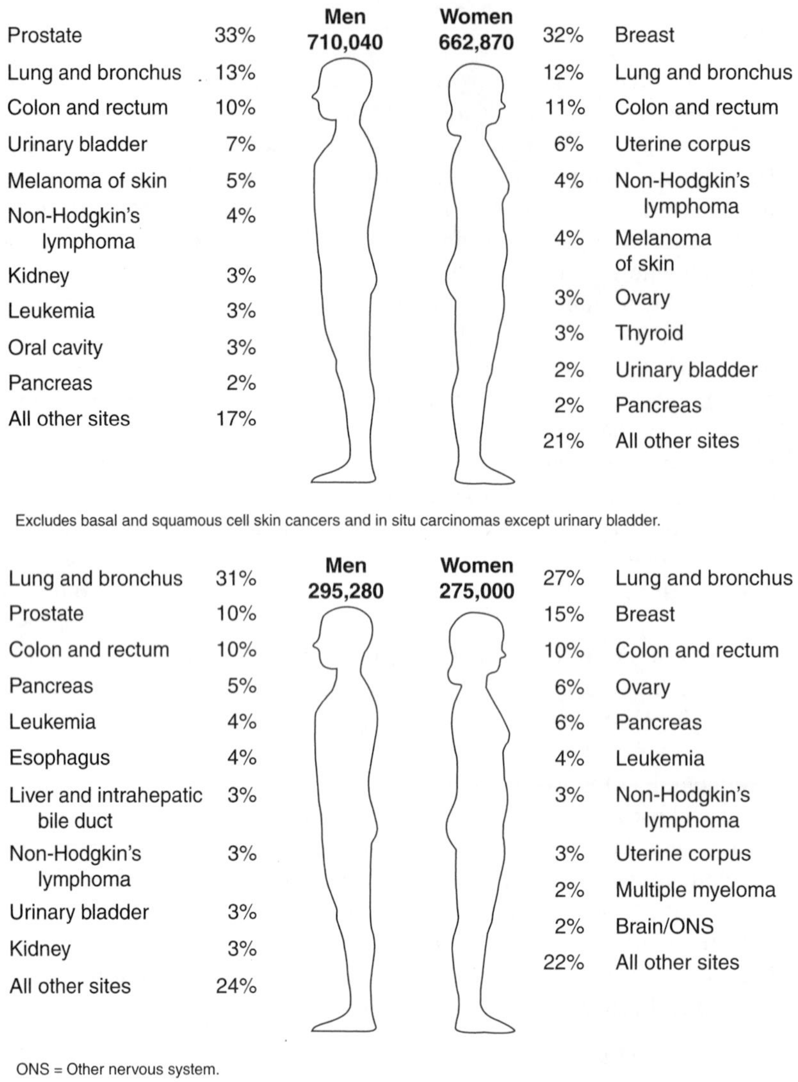

Prostate	33%	**Men** **710,040**	**Women** **662,870**	32%	Breast
Lung and bronchus	13%			12%	Lung and bronchus
Colon and rectum	10%			11%	Colon and rectum
Urinary bladder	7%			6%	Uterine corpus
Melanoma of skin	5%			4%	Non-Hodgkin's lymphoma
Non-Hodgkin's lymphoma	4%			4%	Melanoma of skin
Kidney	3%			3%	Ovary
Leukemia	3%			3%	Thyroid
Oral cavity	3%			2%	Urinary bladder
Pancreas	2%			2%	Pancreas
All other sites	17%			21%	All other sites

Excludes basal and squamous cell skin cancers and in situ carcinomas except urinary bladder.

Lung and bronchus	31%	**Men** **295,280**	**Women** **275,000**	27%	Lung and bronchus
Prostate	10%			15%	Breast
Colon and rectum	10%			10%	Colon and rectum
Pancreas	5%			6%	Ovary
Leukemia	4%			6%	Pancreas
Esophagus	4%			4%	Leukemia
Liver and intrahepatic bile duct	3%			3%	Non-Hodgkin's lymphoma
Non-Hodgkin's lymphoma	3%			3%	Uterine corpus
Urinary bladder	3%			2%	Multiple myeloma
Kidney	3%			2%	Brain/ONS
All other sites	24%			22%	All other sites

ONS = Other nervous system.

FIGURE 12–1   2005 estimated US cancer cases and deaths

- Pancreatic cancer is linked to high fat intake.
- Oral cancer is linked to excess use of chewing tobacco and alcohol-containing mouthwash before and after eating.

Ethnic Differences

Cancer incidence rates are higher for African-American men than for white men—689 versus 557 per 100,000. Mortality is higher for African-American men and women than for white adults. A comparison of the rates for various ethnic groups is given in Figure 12–3.

African Americans have significantly higher incidence and mortality rates for most cancers. Their survival rate compared to whites is lower, which

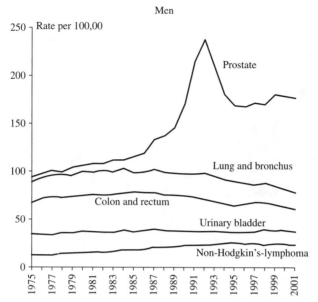

*Age-adjusted to the 2000 US standard population.

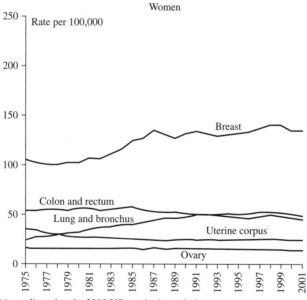

*Age-adjusted to the 2000 US standard population.

FIGURE 12–2 Cancer incidence rates for men and women, United States, 1975-2001

may be in part due to late diagnosis (see Table 12–1). Many of these cancer sites have screening tests available, which strengthens the argument for early detection and timely treatment. Hispanics and Native Americans also have lifestyle and cultural differences that influence participation in screening and prevention activities. Values and belief systems and socioeconomic factors including access to care are important influential factors in overall diagnosis and survival.[2]

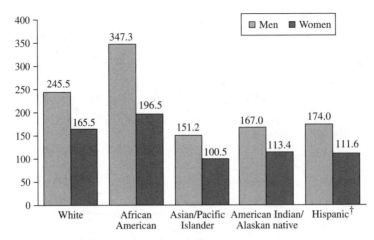

*Per 100,000, age-adjusted to the 2000 US standard population.
†Hispanic is not mutually exclusive from whites, African Americans, Asian/Pacific
Islanders, and American Indians.

FIGURE 12–3 Cancer death rates* by race and ethnicity, United States, 1997-2001

TABLE 12–1 Cancer Survival (%) by Site and Race, 1995-2000*

Site	White	African American	Difference
All sites	66	55	11
Breast (female)	89	75	14
Colon	64	54	10
Esophagus	16	9	7
Leukemia	48	39	9
Non-Hodgkin's lymphoma	60	51	9
Oral cavity	61	39	22
Prostate	100	96	4
Rectum	65	55	10
Urinary bladder	83	62	21
Uterine cervix	74	66	8
Uterine corpus	86	63	23

*5-year relative survival rates based on cancer patients diagnosed from 1995 to 2000 and followed
through 2001.
Source: Surveillance, Epidemiology, and End Results Program, 1975-2001. Bethesda, Md: Division
of Cancer Control and Population Sciences, National Cancer Instiute; 2004.

Lifetime probabilities of developing various cancers are given in Table 12–2.
Probabilities reflect the average experience of people in the United States and
do not take into account individual behavior and risk factors. Colon cancer is
more likely for men than stomach cancer, but each is linked to eating behavior. For women, the lifetime probability of breast cancer is 1 in 7 compared
to a 1 in 81 probability for pancreas cancer, but alcohol and eating behavior
may link to each.[2]

TABLE 12–2   Lifetime Probability of Developing Cancer, by Site, Men and Women, United States, 1999-2001

Site (Men)	Risk
All sites	1 in 2
Prostate	1 in 6
Lung and bronchus	1 in 13
Colon and rectum	1 in 17
Urinary bladder	1 in 28
Non-Hodgkin's lymphoma	1 in 46
Melanoma	1 in 53
Kidney	1 in 67
Leukemia	1 in 68
Oral cavity	1 in 73
Stomach	1 in 81
Site (Women)	**Risk**
All sites	1 in 3
Breast	1 in 7
Lung and bronchus	1 in 18
Colon and rectum	1 in 18
Uterine corpus	1 in 38
Non-Hodgkin's lymphoma	1 in 56
Ovary	1 in 68
Melanoma	1 in 78
Pancreas	1 in 81
Urinary bladder	1 in 88
Urinary cervix	1 in 130

Source: DevCan, *Version 5.2: Probability of Developing or Dying of Cancer Software.* Statistical Research and Applications Branch, NCI; 2004. Available at: http://srab.cancer.gov/devcan. Accessed September 2006.

Genetics

Studies of twins make it possible to estimate the overall contribution of inherited genes to the development of malignant diseases.[5] Data on 44,788 pairs of twins listed in the Swedish, Danish, and Finnish twin registries were combined to assess the risks of cancer at 28 anatomical sites for the twins of persons with cancer. Statistical modeling was used to estimate the relative importance of heritable and environmental factors in causing cancer at 11 of those sites. At least one cancer occurred in 10,803 persons among 9,512 pairs of twins. An increased risk was found among the twins of affected persons for stomach, colorectal, lung, breast, and prostate cancer. Statistically significant effects of heritable factors were observed for prostate cancer (42% of the risk may be explained by heritable factors; 95% confidence interval,

29-50%), colorectal cancer (35%; 95% confidence interval, 10-48%), and breast cancer (27%; 95% confidence interval, 4-41%).

Inherited genetic factors make a minor contribution to susceptibility to most types of neoplasms. This finding indicates that the environment has the principal role in causing sporadic cancer. The relatively large effect of heritability in cancer at a few sites (such as prostate and colorectal cancer) suggests the importance of our knowledge about the genetics of cancer.[5]

Japanese researchers identified a messenger gene that plays a role in the death of cancerous cells. When a cell's DNA becomes damaged, a tumor-suppressing gene, p53, instructs the cell to destroy itself. If p53 becomes mutated, damaged cells survive, which can lead to cancer. It appears that the tumor suppressor gene does not communicate directly with the cell's suicide mechanism, but activates other genes to act as the bearer of bad news. How to know which genes are messengers has been unclear.

A gene called Noxa may be one of the messengers involved in the suicide of damaged cells. When p53 activates Noxa, Noxa triggers cell suicide. When the researchers blocked the activation of Noxa, damaged cells did not commit suicide, but continued to thrive.[6]

Monitoring

The best end point for cancer intervention should be reduction in the incidence of cancer.[1] Surveillance, epidemiology, and end results (SEER) data registries show changes in incidence and mortality for specific cancers and changes in trends. SEER is the major component of the National Cancer Institute's system for tracking cancer incidence, patient survival, and mortality. The SEER program currently collects and publishes cancer incidence and survival data from 14 population-based cancer registries and 3 supplemental registries covering approximately 26% of the US population. Information on more than 3 million in situ and invasive cancer cases is included in the SEER database, and approximately 170,000 new cases are added each year within the SEER coverage areas. National surveillance and monitoring must continue to acknowledge the successful reduction of any cancers that appear preventable.[3,4] The Web site is www.seer.cancer.gov.

The Cancer Intervention and Surveillance Modeling Network (CISNET) is a consortium of NCI-sponsored investigators whose focus is to use modeling to improve our understanding of the impact of cancer control interventions, e.g., prevention and screening treatment on population trends in incidence and mortality. These models are also used to project future trends and to help determine optimal cancer control strategies.[3,4]

Cancer Control Objectives

The National Cancer Institute (NCI) has established goals for the nation to significantly reduce the US cancer mortality rate. A reduction in the mortality rate is possible through full and rapid application of existing knowledge of cancer prevention, screening and detection, and state-of-the-art treatment methods. Reducing cancer mortality depends on a reduction in smoking, the adoption of prudent eating pattern and screening measures, and accelerated and widespread application of gains in state-of-the-art cancer treatment methods.[4]

The 2005 National Cancer Institute goals and budget of $112.12 million is allocated as follows:

- *Strengthening cancer prevention:* Tobacco control, energy balance research, prevention vaccines and drugs, and translation of research into improved outcomes and public policy ($75 million)
- *Developing and improving early detection options:* Biospecimen repositories, lung screening image library, biomarkers and molecular imaging for precancerous lesions, evaluation, and monitoring ($16.5 million)
- *Predicting cancer risk and treatment success:* Risk prediction markers and models, intervention and surveillance modeling, markers of risk in high-risk populations, and endoscopic imaging ($18.75 million)
- *Management and support:* ($1.87 million)

A set of specific cancer control objectives has been chosen to help guide the nation's cancer control program toward this overall goal. Linked to the objectives is a set of cancer control indicators that NCI uses to measure progress toward achievement of the objectives (see Table 12–3). These objectives can be adjusted to reflect specific regional cancer rates and cancer control problems. They can direct the development of and serve as objectives for regional cancer control efforts across the United States.[4]

Much of cancer incidence can be prevented through changes in smoking and diet. The scientific evidence for smoking as a cancer cause has been recognized for over 20 years. The evidence for diet has emerged over the past decade and has progressed to the extent that recommendations for dietary change are widespread.[4]

Smoking

About 30% of all cancer deaths (over 130,000 deaths per year) are related to smoking. Approximately 54 million Americans—about 1 in every 3 adults—smoke cigarettes daily, and those who smoke 2 or more packs daily have lung cancer mortality rates 20 times higher than nonsmokers. Since 1953, lung cancer rates have increased 172% among men and 256% among women (see Figure 12–4). Lung cancer exceeds breast cancer as the leading cause of cancer death among women in all states in the United States. Cigarette smoking is further associated with cancers of the larynx, head and neck, esophagus, bladder, kidney, pancreas, and stomach. These facts are tempered, however, by the knowledge that cancer risk returns to near normal within 10 years after stopping smoking for all smoking-induced cancers, except for lung cancer, which requires about 15 years for risk to return to normal.[4]

Progress has been made in reducing the percentage of adult smokers since the 1964 surgeon general's report on smoking and health. Smoking prevalence rates for high school students are listed in Figure 12–5. These figures present both a promise—that declines are possible—and a challenge—to reinforce and accelerate the decline into a consistent trend in smoking reduction, and to stop smoking and other tobacco use among our nation's youth.[4] An additional challenge is to provide strategies to assist individuals

TABLE 12–3 Cancer Surveillance Indicators

Indicator	Measure	Source
Mortality	Deaths per 100,000 persons	National Center for Health Statistics mortality data
Incidence	Cases per 100,000 persons	SEER*; other population-based registries
Survival	Relative survival by cancer site	SEER; other registries, either population- or hospital-based
Smoking	Percentage of adults and children who smoke; time since quitting	National Health Interview Survey; Current Population Survey
Diet	Percent obesity; percent fat and fiber in the diet	National Health and Nutrition Examination Survey; US Department of Agriculture Survey
Occupation	Percent exposed; percent screened in workplace	National Health Interview Survey; Current Population Survey; other population surveys
Screening	Percentage of eligible persons screened	National Health Interview Survey; Current Population Survey; other population surveys
Treatment	Distribution by cancer stage of diagnosis; percentage of cancer patients treated via multidisciplinary approaches; cancer patient survival	SEER; population-based, hospital-based, or cancer center-based registry; Medicare data system; directory of medical specialties
Knowledge, attitudes, and beliefs	Percentage of population/ethnic groups with particular knowledge and beliefs about cancer	Supplement to National Health Interview Survey; independent population surveys
Costs	Indirect/direct	Medicare data system; National Medical Care Utilization and Expenditure Survey; surveys of medical insurance

*SEER: Surveillance, Epidemiology, and End Results Program.
Source: Data from the American Cancer Society; Cancer Facts: Figures, 2004. pp. 1-44.

who stop smoking from gaining weight. Smoking and chewing tobacco are habits some individuals use to curb their appetite and to maintain their body weight.[7]

Smoking cigarettes appears more closely tied to colon cancer than previously known. More than 1,900 people with precancerous polyps, known as adenomas, or colon cancer answered questionnaires about smoking habits. Higher rates of both cancer types were noted among people who smoked cigarettes.[8]

Upper body fat and body weight at age 30 are as important to survival of breast cancer patients as they are to the risk of developing the disease. Women who continue to gain weight over their adult years and whose body fat is predominantly in the upper body in a manlike or android distribution

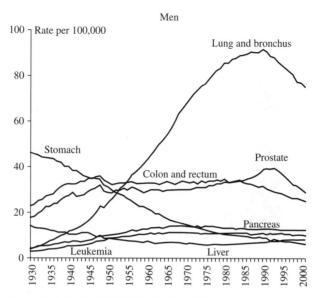

*Age-adjusted to the 2000 US standard population.

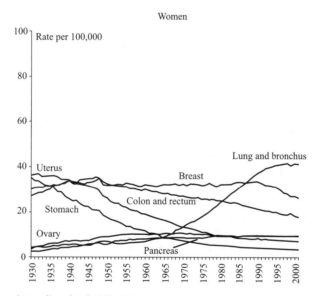

*Age-adjusted to the 2000 US standard population.

FIGURE 12–4   Cancer death rates for men and women, United States, 1930-2001

of fat not only have a greater risk of developing breast cancer but also a greater risk of dying from the cancer.[9]

Kumar et al analyzed the effects of obesity and body fat composition in 166 women with breast cancer, of whom 83 died during the 10-year follow-up period.[10] Upper body fat distribution was a significant indicator for decreased survival after controlling for the stage of the disease itself. Body weight and percentage of body fat at diagnosis did not have a significant influence on survival, the investigators observed.

Weight gained by age 30 or during the third decade of life is probably more important as it signifies adult weight gain that is predominantly in the abdomen.

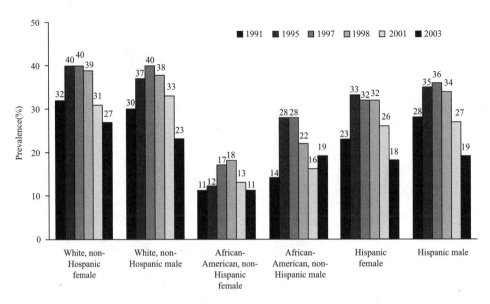

* Smoked cigarettes on one or more of the 30 days preceding the survey.

FIGURE 12–5   Current cigarette smoking prevalence (%) by gender and race/ethnicity, high school students, United States 1991-2003

Although weight gain in later years may be significant, body fat distribution, particularly increases in the abdomen when an individual is in his or her 30s, is a high risk factor in hormonal cancers in women and in diabetes and hypertension for men and women. The ratio of waist fat to the fat fold in the thigh is a good indicator of whether a person's body fat distribution is predominantly android (masculine, upper body) or gynoid (female, lower body) distribution.

Upper body fat and weight gain in adulthood can be modified by changes in lifestyle such as diet and exercise and offer the greatest means for preventing recurrence and death. Recommendations from the American Institute of Cancer Research are that adult weight gain must not exceed 11 pounds or it should be taken seriously.

No evidence exists that certain types of exercise will eliminate fat or help spot reduce in specific areas of the body, but if a person is overweight and attempts to reduce by exercise and a healthy diet, a significant reduction of upper body fat will occur.[9]

Dietary Components

Doll and Peto conducted an extensive review of cancer causes and estimated that 35% of cancer deaths may be related to dietary components, with the possible range of effect being 10-70%. A midrange estimate of 35% would mean that about 150,000 lives could be saved annually through dietary changes. These estimates cannot be considered definitive. Research to test the effectiveness of dietary interventions to reduce cancer incidence and mortality for particular cancer sites is currently under way. Even the most conservative estimates represent a potentially significant impact on cancer mortality.[11]

Certain changes in eating behavior are prudent because they will reduce cancer incidence. Limiting the consumption of fat to 30% of total calories and eating fruits, vegetables, and whole-grain cereal products daily will lower the risk of cancer.[12] The NCI concurs and recommends a diet low in fat and high in fiber-rich foods.

The NCI estimates that a minimum of one third of the number of people dying in 2006 from cancer could be saved in the year 2010 based on modification of dietary factors. Current clinical trials show positive results of reducing the incidence of cancer by changing eating patterns or using chemopreventive agents. Current research in chemoprevention, diet, and nutrition supports estimates that 35% of all cancers could possibly be prevented by modifying diet and nutrition.[4] Table 12–4 lists the American Cancer Institute nutritional and physical activity guidelines.

Advances in Cancer Screening and Treatment

Community nutrition professionals may find that primary and secondary prevention of all cancers must involve a more aggressive approach toward eating behavior. Likewise, understanding the screening and detection approaches recommended for several major cancers, even if there is no known dietary link, equips professionals with skills to communicate more effectively with their clients.[4]

Screening

Statistics indicate that, for most cancers, detection and treatment of early-stage disease provides a much greater chance of patient survival than detection and treatment at later stages of the disease. Consequently, cancer mortality for

TABLE 12–4 Diet and Health Guidelines for Cancer Prevention

1. Eat a variety of healthful foods, with an emphasis on plant sources.
   - Eat 5 or more servings of a variety of vegetables and fruits each day.
   - Choose whole grains in preference to processed (refined) grains and sugars.
   - Limit consumption of red meats, especially those high in fat and processed.
   - Choose foods that help maintain a healthful weight.
2. Adopt a physically active lifestyle.
   - Adults: Engage in at least moderate activity for 30 minutes or more on 5 or more days of the week.

     o 45 minutes or more of moderate to vigorous activity on 5 or more days per week may further enhance reductions in the risk of breast cancer and colon cancer.
   - Children and adolescents: Engage in at least 60 minutes per day of moderate to vigorous physical activity at least 5 days per week.
3. Maintain a healthful weight throughout life.
   - Balance caloric intake with physical activity.
   - Lose weight if you are currently overweight or obese.
4. If you drink alcoholic beverages, limit consumption.

Source: Adapted from: American Cancer Society. *The Complete Grade—Nutrition and Physical Activity.* Atlanta, Ga: American Cancer Society; October 2006.

breast, colorectal, and prostate cancers can be greatly reduced through aggressive screening (see Exhibit 12–1).

Breast cancer accounts for about 18% of all cancer deaths among women, and recent data show that the age-adjusted incidence and mortality from breast cancer in women has not changed during the past decade. Results from a long-term clinical study of over 60,000 women enrolled in the Health Insurance

Exhibit 12–1   Screening Guidelines for the Early Detection of Various Cancers

---

Breast Cancer

- Yearly mammograms are recommended starting at age 40 and continuing for as long as a woman is in good health.
- A clinical breast exam should be part of a periodic health exam, about every 3 years for women in their 20s and 30s, and every year for women 40 and older.
- Women should know how their breasts normally feel and report any breast changes promptly to their healthcare providers. Breast self-exam is an option for women starting in their 20s.
- Women at increased risk (e.g., family history, genetic tendency, past breast cancer) should talk with their doctors about the benefits and limitations of starting mammography screening earlier, having additional tests (i.e., breast ultrasound and MRI), or having more frequent exams.

Colorectal Cancer

- Beginning at age 50, men and women should follow one of the following examination schedules:
  - A fecal occult blood test (FOBT) every year.
  - A flexible sigmoidoscopy (FSIG) every 5 years.
  - Annual fecal occult blood test and flexible sigmoidoscopy every 5 years.*
  - A double-contrast barium enema every 5 years.
  - A colonoscopy every 10 years.

Combined testing is preferred over either annual FOBT, or FSIG every 5 years alone.

*People who are at moderate or high risk for colorectal cancer should talk with a doctor about a different testing schedule.

Prostate Cancer

- The prostate-specific antigen (PSA) test and the digital rectal examination (DRE) should be offered annually, beginning at age 50, to men who have a life expectancy of at least 10 more years.
- Men at high risk (African-American men and men with a strong family history of one or more first-degree relatives diagnosed with prostate cancer at an early age) should begin testing at age 45.
- For men at average risk and high risk, information should be provided about what is known and what is uncertain about the benefits and limitations of early detection and treatment of prostate cancer so that they can make an informed decision about testing.

Source: American Cancer Society. American Cancer Society Guidelines for the early detection of cancer. Available at: https//www.cancer.org/doc_root/PED/PED_2.asp. Accessed January 11, 2007.

Plan of New York show that breast cancer mortality is reduced 30% in women over age 50 who are screened for breast cancer by mammography and physical examination.[13] A study from Sweden duplicates the 30% mortality reduction found in the Health Insurance Plan study.[14] The fact that breast cancer mortality for women over 50 has not decreased indicates that women may not be taking advantage of screening. An American Cancer Society survey reports that only 15% of women over 50 reported receiving an annual mammogram.

Cervical cancer screening has long been known to be effective. Use of the Papanicolaou (Pap) smear can reduce the risk of mortality from invasive cervical cancer by as much as 75%.[15] This fact, coupled with current screening figures, yields the estimate that use of the Pap smear for screening could reduce mortality from cervical cancer in the United States by at least 25%. Surveys indicate that, at most, 79% of women aged 20 to 39 and 57% of women aged 40 to 70 for whom the risk of cervical cancer is great follow recommended guidelines on screening for cervical cancer.

Treatment

Data from NCI's SEER program indicate that the likelihood of surviving cancer for at least 5 years from the point of detection, compared with the survival of the general population, is over 49% for cases diagnosed in 1976 through 1981, compared to 48% for cases diagnosed in 1973 through 1975, and an estimated 38% for cases diagnosed in 1960 to 1963.[3] If lung cancer is removed from the most recent figure, the chances of surviving cancer for at least 5 years, which for most cancer sites indicates a cure, is 56%. The figures show a steady gain in survival rates, and for some cancers the gains have been dramatic. In 1960, only 40% of patients survived Hodgkin's disease for more than 5 years; the latest SEER figures show the rate to be 74%, an increase attributable to improvements in radiation and chemotherapy.

Survival from testicular cancer has increased from 76% in 1973-1975 to 87% among patients diagnosed between 1977 and 1981, because of significant advances in treatment. For women, NIH Cancer Center development panel concluded that mortality from breast cancer can be reduced through adjuvant postsurgical therapies. These include chemotherapy in premenopausal women and hormonal or tamoxifen therapy in postmenopausal women. Both treatments are recommended for women with positive lymph node involvement and treatments are recommended for postmenopausal women with positive estrogen receptors.[4]

The increased survival rate for many specific sites is small, but a steady trend toward an overall increase in cancer survival during past decades is apparent. Analysis of data from the NCI SEER program indicates the rate of increase in the overall cancer survival rate is about 0.5% annually. The primary reasons for this steady improvement are gains in treatment efficacy and/or earlier detection. For other sites, such as prostate cancer, the increased survival is not fully understood. These improved survival rates may be influenced strongly by the increased detection of asymptomatic disease that might otherwise have remained undiagnosed or by improved attention to eating and exercise patterns. Another avenue for medical nutrition therapy for nutrition professionals is tertiary prevention, such as assisting cancer patients during treatments and helping to reduce symptoms. Table 12-5 outlines nutrition-related problems and recommended treatments that comprise the majority of tertiary treatment.[16]

TABLE 12–5 Managing Cancer Symptoms—Common Nutritional Problems and Recommended Medical Nutrition Therapy

Nutrition-Related Problems	Recommended Treatment
Stomatitis/esophagitis	Eat foods at room temperature or cold foods.
	Eat soft, moist, and tender foods.
	Use a straw for liquids.
	Avoid mouth irritants (citrus, spicy, salty, or rough foods).
	Practice good oral hygiene.
	Use oral anesthetics.
	Use nutritional supplements.
Anorexia	Relax at mealtime.
	Stay active.
	Eat nutrient-dense foods.
	When hungry, eat small, frequent meals and snacks.
	Vary eating places.
	Use nutritional supplements consistently but sparingly.
Nausea	Keep lips moistened.
	Use sugarless hard candies, gum, and popsicles.
	Moisten foods with gravies.
	Avoid nutrient-dense foods like margarine, juices.
	Try saliva substitutes.
	Avoid fluids with meals.
	Eat small, but frequent meals slowly.
	Eat bland, dry foods.
	Avoid fried, spicy-hot, very sweet, and very tart foods.
	Drink plenty of fluids.
	Avoid foods with strong odors.
	Eat foods at room temperature or cooler.
	Avoid favorite spicy or high-fat foods to prevent nausea.
Constipation	Drink plenty of fluids.
	Include high-fiber foods such as raw fresh fruits and vegetables, bran, whole grains, and legumes.
	Keep active.
	Try a hot beverage a half hour before usual time for a bowel movement.
	Only use medication per doctor's order.
Weight gain	Do *NOT* go on a diet. Evaluate cause of weight gain.
	Use behavior modification techniques.
	Avoid high-fat, high-sugar foods in excess.
	Keep active.
Dysphagia	Eat finely chopped foods.
	Swallow food and follow with a fluid.

Source: Adapted from: National Cancer Institute. *Eating Tips: Tips and Recipes for Better Cancer Treatment.* Bethesda, Md: NIH; 1994.

Dissemination and application of existing state-of-the-art cancer therapy can significantly increase national cancer survival rates. When current survival figures from the SEER program are compared with estimated survival from state-of-the-art treatments, the differences in survival translate into a 15% reduction in the cancer mortality rate. In addition to the gains in survival reasonably expected with aggressive application of state-of-the-art cancer treatment, further advances in research are confirmed. If trends in improved survival are also taken into account and estimated through the year 2010, then the reduction in mortality from increased application of state-of-the-art treatment could reach 25%.

Patterns of Cancer Occurence

The prospect of surviving cancer is not the same for all Americans. Survival rates can potentially be improved through application of state-of-the-art primary, secondary, and tertiary treatment. Survival differences have been observed for different ethnic groups and, most importantly, for different socioeconomic groups. Patients with lower socioeconomic status (SES) characteristics have lower survival rates for the cancer sites studied to date. If differences in survival by SES are related to access to the healthcare system early in the disease or access to state-of-the-art treatment, then the potential for mortality reduction would be even greater than it is now projected.[4]

Estimates of survival by race show that blacks have a lower chance of surviving cancer. Five-year analyses show that much of the difference can be explained by socioeconomic status. On the whole, both black and white Americans with low incomes have a poorer prognosis from cancer than those whose incomes are above the median.[17] A challenge facing the healthcare community is to develop systems that enable professionals to practice state-of-the-art technology and allow patients to have access to state-of-the-art treatment and screening. With the current proposals for healthcare reform, neither condition is ensured.

Other evidence of differential survival among population groups has been demonstrated over the past 20 years. For example, Mormons and Seventh Day Adventists have cancer death rates far below the general population. Mortality from colorectal cancer among California Mormons is only 70% and 78% of the general white population for men and women, respectively. Their incidence of cancers of the lung; larynx; tongue, gums, and mouth; esophagus; and bladder is 55% lower than for the US population.[18]

In addition, there are geographic differences in cancer mortality rates adjusted for age and sex differences. For example, 22 states exceed the US incidence rate for colorectal cancer of 53.1 per 100,000. Twenty-three states exceed the US incidence rate for prostate cancer of 161.2 per 100,000. The US mortality rate for colorectal cancer was 19.6 per 100,000, and the *Healthy People 2010* objective is 13.9 per 100,000. No state has met the 2010 objective. Twenty-seven states have met the 2010 prostate cancer goal of 28.8 deaths per 100,000.[3]

As noted earlier, many US ethnic minorities have a worse cancer experience than US whites. The exceptions to this are certain segments of the US Asian population, who have better overall cancer survival rates and better survival rates for certain cancer sites than whites. Addressing the cancer prevention and treatment needs of minorities is critical to achieve a 50% lower cancer mortality by the year 2010. Ethnic-specific cancer incidence, mortality excess, and poorer survival experience require aggressive and long-term catch-up efforts to achieve the overall goal.

The most extensive cancer data available on US minorities are for blacks. Blacks have greater age-adjusted incidence and mortality rates from many cancers and lower survival rates than whites for all but brain, ovary, and stomach cancer. Blacks experience high rates of smoking-related cancers. Many of these cancers (lung, esophagus, and pancreatic cancers) have high fatality rates in all population groups. This suggests the need to control these illnesses through primary prevention rather than through treatment—the intervention being the prevention and cessation of tobacco use. Cancers with poorer survival for blacks compared to whites include some cancers with lower incidence in blacks (bladder and uterus cancer). The cancer survival differences between blacks and whites are not completely understood. Socioeconomic factors influence the survival differences, and there is a greater proportion of blacks than whites at low socioeconomic levels.[19]

Socioeconomic status is associated with a variety of factors, including host factors—immune and nutritional status/function—that influence cancer development and response to treatment. Furthermore, unequal distribution of health facilities and trained health personnel may result in poor access to cancer screening, detection, and treatment among certain segments of the population. Socioeconomic status also affects educational attainment and, thus, occupation. Occupation may affect exposure rates to occupational carcinogens. For example, studies of cancer risk in the steel and rubber industries show that black employees work in the most hazardous work sites, including those with toxic/carcinogen exposures.[20]

A possible factor in surviving cancer is an individual's general health status. Low-income persons tend to have poorer health and a shorter life expectancy than affluent persons. Therefore, community nutrition efforts aimed at improving general health status address improved cancer survival.[20]

Strength of the Cancer Control Network

The ability to effect a reduction in cancer mortality depends in part on the existence and application of a number of resources, including the following: (1) the means to provide information on prevention, screening, and treatment to the public and to healthcare professionals, including community nutrition professionals; (2) a system of providing patients access to state-of-the-art cancer prevention and treatment; (3) a mechanism for maintaining continued research progress and for fostering new research; and (4) a cancer control network with organizational and personnel capabilities for a variety of cancer interventions.

A network of cancer research centers has been developed, although some of the areas of the country remain underserved. Programs are being developed and evaluated to increase the pace of clinical research and to bring the benefits of clinical research to communities (e.g., the Community Clinical Oncology Program and the Cooperative Group Treatment Outreach Program). Physician Data Query, a computerized information system on cancer treatment, has been introduced and is available to clinicians through the National Library of Medicine or through commercial information systems. The capability to monitor progress in cancer control has been increased through the expansion of the SEER program. The Cancer Information System maintains a nationwide, toll-free telephone network for immediate answers to cancer-related questions from cancer patients, their families, the general public, and health professionals.

Actions and coordination of multiple actions are necessary to decrease cancer mortality before the year 2010. The overall goal is to reduce the projected cancer mortality rate by 50%. Predictions are that a 7-10% reduction in cancer mortality rate can be realized if dietary fat is lowered to less than 25% of total calories and dietary fiber is increased to 20 to 30 grams per day. A concerted effort with specific action plans at the local, state, and professional levels have been recommended as follows[4]:

- *National Cancer Institute*—to guide and support basic and applied research in screening, diagnosis, treatment, and public education; to provide information and technical assistance to other agencies and organizations interested in conducting cancer control activities; and to conduct public and professional education programs.
- *Other federal agencies*—to sponsor appropriate research and data collection; to publicize information nationally; to offer technical assistance to program planners; and to promote appropriate regulatory measures.
- *State agencies*—to integrate cancer control techniques into state health-care delivery and health promotion programs; to develop survey and surveillance capabilities; to collaborate on an interstate basis in forming coalitions and implementing programs; to coordinate program planning among various state agencies (e.g., agriculture, environmental protection, health, aging); and to develop policies that promote cancer prevention.
- *Local government*—to promote primary prevention through health education in schools; to develop local health promotion programs and coalitions; to provide technical assistance to community organizations that are planning health promotion programs; to cooperate with state and federal agencies to provide survey data or capability; and to offer screening programs through local health clinics.
- *Private industry*—to offer health promotion and work-site wellness programs and screening programs to employees; to collaborate with employee groups to promote work-site health promotion programs; to monitor employee use of measures to prevent exposure to carcinogens in the workplace; to offer on-site food options consistent with cancer prevention; and to develop insurance policies that reward risk-avoidance behavior.
- *Professional organizations*—to incorporate cancer control knowledge into basic training curricula and continuing education; to increase the number of questions about cancer prevention and control on licensure examinations; to include more articles in journals about cancer control and the role of the health professional; to counsel patients about prevention steps they can take for themselves; and to provide assistance to other organizations and agencies developing cancer control programs.
- *Volunteer organizations*—to increase offerings of health education and screening programs at the community level; to form coalitions for cancer control; and to collaborate with federal agencies in disseminating health information and materials nationally.

• *The media*—to increase coverage about cancer causes, prevention, and control, especially about tobacco and dietary components; to communicate more closely with scientists and health professionals; and to enhance their understanding of research methods and implications for technology transfer.

Info Line

> The American Cancer Society is the nationwide, community-based volunteer health organization dedicated to eliminating cancer as a major health problem by preventing cancer, saving lives from cancer, and diminishing suffering from cancer through research, education, and services. Affiliates are set up at the local and regional levels and listed in the white pages of the telephone book.
>
> Annually, March 15-April 15 is National Cancer Control Month. Contact the American Cancer Society, 1599 Clifton Road NE, Atlanta, GA 30329-4251; (800) ACS-2345.

Surveillance Actions

An NCI surveillance working group formulated a set of actions to track the progress of cancer control and included indicators that measure progress toward specific health and eating behavior objectives (i.e., percent fat, fiber, and obesity). The actions are as follows:

• Identify sources of baseline information for indicators.
• Establish cooperative working arrangements for data collection.
• Monitor and report annually on changes in the indicators.
• Detail progress toward the objectives every 5 years (2010 and 2015).

Update on the Etiology and Treatment of Cancer-Associated Anorexia and Cachexia

One half of cancer patients experience weight loss at some point in their treatment, with even a higher percentage in the terminal phases of their disease. Patients not only suffer from anorexia, a decreased desire for food intake, but also from cachexia—the involuntary weight loss and wasting syndrome that is common to many chronic diseases. Cachexia is actually the cause of death in up to 20% of cancer patients and is, at least, present in up to 80% of cancer patients at the time of their death. The weight loss is disproportionate to the degree of anorexia and food intake and, unlike other starvation syndromes, more prominently involves the loss of skeletal muscle in addition to adipose tissue. A major problem is the inability to correct the problem solely with refeeding. A cardinal feature of the depression that so often accompanies the diagnosis of cancer is loss of appetite.

There is also increasing evidence for a central role for proteolytically generated peptides derived from tumors in producing cancer cachexia. The activation of proinflammatory cytokines has been strongly implicated in cancer cachexia. Tumor necrosis factor, TNF, originally called cachexin, caused a wasting syndrome in tumor-bearing laboratory animals.[21] Cytokines act upon multiple sites, creating a complex biological cascade.[22-23]

An altered metabolism has been noted in cancer patients with cachexia. Competition for nutrients between the host and the tumor, called "the parasitic nature of tumors," is an additional problem.[24] This points to the inefficiency of anaerobic metabolism, which is a feature of many tumors. Hypoxic tumor cells require 40 times the amount of glucose to provide the equivalent energy provided under aerobic conditions.

Cancer patients have a well-described insulin resistance when a high TNF level is present. The insulin resistance results in reduced glycogen synthesis in skeletal muscle and a lack of inhibition of gluconeogenesis in the liver.[22,25] Corticosteroids are well known to increase appetite in cancer patients.[26] Megesterol acetate (MA) and dexamethasone can stimulate appetite but promote gastric irritation.[27]

Cyclooxygenase-2 (COX-2) inhibitors may be more attractive drugs in avoiding these side effects, such as seen with non-steriodal anti-inflammatory drugs (NSAIDs), but their clinical usefulness in reversing cachexia is limited to laboratory and animal experiments.[28] The most successful agent in stimulating appetite has been MA.[29,30] N-3 polyunsaturated fatty acids eicosapentaenoic acid (EPA) may regulate cytokines as demonstrated in 2 studies of pancreatic cancer patients treated with EPA. Some researchers showed that there was a significant fall in peripheral blood mononuclear cell (PBMC) IL-6 and PIF production in association with weight gain in cachectic pancreatic cancer patients who received 2 g of EPA supplementation per day, but this result could not be confirmed in a larger randomized clinical trial. [31]

Dietary Modification—Breast and Colon Cancer Incidence

Breast Cancer

For US women, breast cancer has the highest incidence and, after lung cancer, the second highest mortality. Approximately 1 of every 9 women will develop breast cancer during her life. Breast cancer incidence has increased about 2% per year since the early 1970s, but mortality rates have declined over the past 10 years.

International correlation studies show a linear relationship between breast cancer and total dietary fat availability and fat consumption. Studies of individuals who migrated from areas with diets low in animal fat and protein to areas with a more typical western diet show higher cancer rates among the migrants when compared with incidence in the country of origin (e.g., migration from Japan to Hawaii and from Italy to Australia). International correlation studies also show a strong positive association of per capita fat consumption with breast cancer incidence and mortality rates. Breast cancer is more common in countries with high average consumption of total and saturated fat, protein (particularly animal protein), and total calories. For example, breast cancer incidence is more than 5 times higher in the United States than in Japan.[3,13,32]

Persons migrating from areas with low rates of fat consumption to areas with high rates acquire the higher cancer rates of their adopted country; for example, Japanese migrants to Hawaii and Italian migrants to Australia experience higher rates of breast cancer, suggesting that environmental factors are important. Although consistent evidence from animal studies supports a positive association between increased dietary fat intake and increased risk of breast cancer, analytical epidemiologic studies of individuals including both case-control and cohort studies have produced inconsistent results. This may be partly due to the known difficulty of quantifying individual dietary intake.

Except for dietary fat, few nutritional factors in adult life have been associated with breast cancer. Extensive data from animal models, international correlations, and case-control studies support the hypothesis that a high-fat diet promotes the development of breast cancer in postmenopausal women.[33] Avoiding adult weight gain and maintaining a healthy body weight may decrease breast cancer risk and mortality.[34] Research with 127 breast cancer cases and 242 matched controls concluded that higher serum n-6 polyunsaturated fatty acids (PUFA) linoleic acid and lower monounsaturated fatty acids (MUFA) levels predicted less breast cancer.[35]

Recurrence of breast cancer and mortality among 385 postmenopausal women in remission for breast cancer was studied. Antioxidant supplement users compared with nonusers were less likely to have a breast cancer recurrence or breast cancer-related death (OR = 0.54, 95% confidence intervals (CI) = 0.27 − 1.04). Vitamin E supplements showed a modest protective effect when used for more than 3 years (OR = 0.33, 95% CI = 0.10 − 1.07). Prior vitamins C or E from diet, supplements, or both showed no relationship with risk. Risks of recurrence and disease-related mortality were reduced when vitamin C and vitamin E supplements were used for more than 3 years.[36]

Culturally diverse women 40 to 60 years of age were interviewed about their food perceptions. The women included 29 breast cancer survivors and 32 women with no breast cancer. Three different perspectives on healthful eating were identified: (1) traditional, with regular meals of meat, potatoes, and vegetables and no specific claims about the diet-breast cancer relationship; (2) mainstream, with increasing vegetables and fruits and decreasing fat intake to improve health, reduce cardiovascular disease risk, and, possibly, reduce breast cancer risk; and (3) alternative, with belief in toxins, carcinogens, and protective factors in food that affect cancer risk.[37]

None of the overall perspectives were related to participants' breast cancer status, but they were related to what participants thought.

Colorectal Cancer

Colorectal cancer is the third leading cause of cancer deaths in US women, and the incidence is second only to that of breast cancer. Approximately 78,500 new cases were diagnosed in 1991, and approximately 31,000 deaths from colorectal cancer occurred.

Colon Cancer in the United States

Approximately 145,000 new cases of colorectal cancer will be diagnosed in the year 2005.[3] The estimated prevalence of colorectal cancer in the United States as of 1998 was 862,000 (400,000 males and 462,000 females).[38]

In the year 2005 that colon and rectum cancer accounted for approximately 10% of all new cases of cancer in males, and 11% of all new cases of cancer in females. Colon and rectum cancer will continue to account for 10% of deaths related to cancer in males, and 10% in females.[39] Colon cancer is ranked third in number of deaths from cancer behind lung/bronchus and prostate for males and lung/bronchus and breast for females. Estimated new cases of colon cancer for the year 2005 were 48,290 for males and 56,660 for females. Estimated new cases of rectum cancer were 23,530 for males and 16,810 for females.[39] Newer validated data are not available.

When colorectal cancer is diagnosed at a localized stage, death rates are low; only about 10% of patients will die within 5 years. The various stages of cancer progression can be demonstrated with colorectal cancer. With progression to a regional stage, 35% of patients will die within 5 years. With progression into advanced stages (spreading to distant sites), death rates are high; about 92% will die within 5 years. An estimated 56,300 Americans died of colorectal cancer in 2005.[3]

African Americans are more likely than whites to be diagnosed with colorectal cancer at a more advanced stage and are therefore more likely to die from the cancer. The incidence of cases from 1992-1998 was highest for blacks, followed by whites, Asian/Pacific Islanders, Hispanics, and American Indians. The incidence rates per 100,000 population for these ethnic groups were 50.1, 42.9, 38.2, 28.4, and 28.6, respectively. The mortality rates follow a similar pattern. The mortality rates per 100,000 population were 22.8, 16.8, 10.7, 10.2, and 10.3, respectively.[3]

Risk for colon cancer generally increases with age. People 50 years of age or older account for 90% of all cases of colorectal cancer.[40] The 1- and 5-year survival rates for patients with colon and rectum cancer are 81% and 61%, respectively, for all races combined. If the cancer is detected early, the 5-year survival rate is 90%.[39]

Colon Cancer Worldwide

An estimated 876,000 new cases of colorectal cancer occurred worldwide in 1996; 445,000 occurred in males and 431,000 in females.[39] The incidence of colon and rectal cancer is higher in developed countries than in developing countries. The lifetime probability of developing colorectal cancer in developed countries is 4.6% in men and 3.2% in women. The highest incidences are in Australia/New Zealand, North America, and northern and western Europe. In Australia/New Zealand, incidence rates are 45.81 per 100,000 population for males and 34.78 per 100,000 population for females. Moderately high incidence rates are seen in southern and eastern Europe. Incidence rates are low in Africa and Asia, with the exception of Japan, where the incidence is on the rise. In Miyagi, Japan, the rate among males increased from 19.7 per 100,000 in 1978-1981 to 41.5 per 100,000 in 1988-1992, and the rate among females rose from 16.8 per 100,000 to 24.8 per 100,000. In middle Africa the incidence of colon and rectal cancer for males and females is 2.26 and 3.36 per 100,000 population, respectively. Incidence rates in India and Thailand are around 10 per 100,000 population per year.[39]

Survival at 5 years is 41% for males, 42% for females as reported by European and Indian cancer registries and slightly lower in China and developing countries (32% for males and 38% for females). The lowest estimated survival is in eastern Europe (30%).[39] World age-standardized incidence rates are lowest, around 10 per 100,000 per year in Africa, India, Thailand, and in some Chinese populations.[38]

The World Health Organization statistics for colon and rectum cancer show high mortality rates in Hungary and low mortality rates in Kyrgyzstan and Portugal. Colon cancer mortality in 1998 in Hungary was 29.3 per 100,000 population for males and 28.4 per 100,000 for females. In Kyrgyzstan colon cancer mortality in 1998 was 1.8 per 100,000 population in males and 2.6 per 100,000 population for females. Rectum cancer mortality in 1998 in Hungary was 18.3 per 100,000 population for males and 11.8 per 100,000 for females. In Portugal, rectum cancer mortality was 9.3 per 100,000 population for males and 5.5 per 100,000 population for females. High mortality rates are observed in Austria and the Czech Republic, and low mortality rates are reported in Bulgaria, Romania, and the Ukraine.[41]

Epidemiologic and animal studies conducted over the past few decades have established a strong link between dietary factors and colorectal cancer. Various dietary constituents have been implicated, including fat, excess calories, and reduced dietary fiber.[3,13,32]

Calcium may protect the colon by reducing the abnormal growth of cells that can develop into colon polyps and cancer. A major clinical study influenced gastroenterology practice, as people who took 1,200 mg of calcium daily for at least 9 months reduced their risk of colon polyp recurrence.[42,43] Essential activities for colon health include maintaining a high-fiber, low-fat diet, exercising regularly, and having routine check-ups. Men and women 50 years and older should consume 1,200 mg calcium daily, compared with 1,000 mg for younger adults, to help maintain strong bones and a healthy colon.[44]

In observational studies, the link between dietary fat and colorectal cancer is inconsistent. The large Nurses' Health Study showed a positive correlation between total fat intake and colon cancer risk. High intake of fruits and vegetables has been consistently related to lower risk of colon cancer, whereas the consumption of cereal grain products has been either unrelated or associated with lower risk of colon cancer. The majority of analytic epidemiological studies that have had reasonable capability assessing dietary fiber have generally shown a protective effect of fiber. A worksheet to aid individuals in evaluating their fiber intake is presented in Table 12–6.[20,32] Later in this chapter, fiber research studies are discussed.

Due to the high animal protein intake in the United States, when fat is reduced in the diet, protein is usually decreased. When phenylalanine and tyrosine were restricted in the diets of animals with melanomas, prostate cancer, and breast cancer, tumor invasion stopped and apoptosis was promoted. Fed a specially formulated food, laboratory mice implanted with melanoma cells lost some weight but thrived on the low-protein diet, which also inhibited metastasis. The amino acid-restricted diet had a major effect on containing the malignant melanoma. Blood levels of these 2 amino acids declined by 30 to 40%.[45]

To test the effect in humans, students ate a low-protein diet, along with a commercially available protein supplement, and no harmful effects were observed. The greatest challenge to making such a nutritionally based treatment available to people is the reluctance of physicians to test it in clinical trials. Some physicians question if nutrition has any role in cancer prevention or treatment. Most clinical trials are not set up to test adjuvant therapy, like a restricted amino acid diet. Researchers look for a silver bullet and targeting drug therapies. Often this involves a signaling molecule, and with the heterogeneic nature of cancer cells, multiple therapies are required.[45,46]

Eating a variety of plant foods amid a low-protein eating pattern provides many different phytochemicals to prevent disease. The low incidence of colon cancer among native Africans is related to a diet low in animal fat and

TABLE 12–6 How to Rate Your Fiber Intake

Food	Serving Size	Usual Number of Servings per Day	Grams of Fiber per Serving	Fiber Intake
Beans: pinto, red, lima, navy, black-eyed	$1/2$ cup	_____	3	_____
Broccoli	1 cup	_____	3	_____
Brown rice	$3/4$ cup	_____	3	_____
Carrots	$3/4$ cup	_____	2	_____
Green peas	$1/2$ cup	_____	4	_____
Lentils	$1/2$ cup	_____	8	_____
Pears	1 small	_____	3	_____
Strawberries/blueberries	1 cup	_____	3-4	_____
Wheat bran cereals	1 cup	_____	5-10	_____
Wheat bran muffins and breads	1 muffin/slice	_____	2	_____
		Your average daily fiber intake		_____

Rating (count the number of servings of food you ate):
- 2 or fewer—try adding a few more. It's easy!
- 3-5—You're on your way to better health!
- 6 or more servings—you're doing fine. Keep it up!

Source: Adapted from: National Center for Nutrition and Dietetics. *Nutrition Fact Sheet: Focus on Fiber.* Chicago Ill: American Dietetic Association; 1994. Used with permission.

protein.[47] A diet high in animal fat and protein may suppress healthful bacteria in the colon and promotes the growth of damaging microbes, producing polyps and promoting cancer. About 400 species of bacteria live in the human colon, but it has not been known until recently how microbes interact with different dietary components. Four types of colonic bacteria are[47]:

1. Methanogenic bacteria, which break down dietary carbohydrates to produce short-chain fatty acids (SCFAs) for the integrity of the lining of the colon and production of methane gas, a sign of a healthy colon. Methanogenic bacteria were found in the colons of 82% of native Africans, but only 45% of white South Africans who eat a different, typically western diet.
2. Sulfur-reducing bacteria, a by-product of high animal protein intake, suppress methanogenic bacteria, reducing the production of SCFAs. Sulfur-reducing bacteria damage colon cells.
3. Seven-alpha hydroxylating bacteria convert bile acids from high-fat foods into substances toxic to the colon's lining. This bacteria may be much more common in the colons of westerners, regardless of race, than of native Africans.[48]
4. *Lactobacilli* microbes produce lactic acid and suppress the growth of harmful colonic bacteria. *Lactobacilli* are common in the colons of Africans, but rare in Westerners, regardless of race, unless consumed in probiotics and prebiotics. Probiotics include yogurt, kefir (fermented milk drink), tempeh (cake made of fermented, cooked soybeans), miso (fermented soybean paste), and sauerkraut. Prebiotics include whole

grains, like barley and oatmeal; legumes; vegetables and fruits like onions, dark leafy greens, berries, and bananas; flaxseed; and foods containing inulin, like yogurts and nondairy frozen desserts.

A comparison of intakes of these foods and levels of the 4 types of colonic bacteria are being studied among 20 African Americans, 20 white Americans, and 20 healthy adult native Africans. The study will further our knowledge of how to eat to protect the colon.[49]

An additional area of interest regards the foods that may promote healthy bacterial growth. One way to promote the growth or metabolic activity of beneficial bacteria is to eat probiotic and prebiotic foods. Probiotic foods like yogurt contain bacteria, while prebiotic foods provide nutrients that healthy bacteria use for fuel. Yogurt with live bacterial cultures can alleviate acute diarrhea in children and adults. In a recent randomized controlled study of adult hospital patients, live culture yogurt decreased the incidence and duration of diarrhea brought on by antibiotics. There is a possible role for probiotic bacteria in diminishing inflammatory bowel diseases, irritable bowel syndrome, colitis, lactose intolerance, urinary tract infections, high blood cholesterol and high blood pressure, and enhancing the immune system.[50]

Lactic acid bacteria generate acid and lower sugar. Lactic acid tends to inhibit the growth of less acid-tolerant organisms like *E. coli* and the *Clostridium* species, which are harmful. They can pass through the intestine in large numbers to exert their influence. Probiotics are available in supplements, but foods contain a variety of nutrients with synergistic effects, which may improve the effects of probiotics. A regular intake maintains the beneficial effect.[50]

Estrogen, Isoflavones, Lycopene, and Fiber

Exposure to estrogens is associated with increased risk of estrogen-dependent cancers such as cancers of the breast, endometrium, and prostate.[28] Scientific data suggest that diet may influence risk of estrogen-dependent cancers by altering estrogen exposure. Obesity may increase estrogen levels, and vegetarian diets may decrease estrogen levels. The mechanisms by which diet influences estrogen levels relate to estrogen synthesis and metabolism. Estrogens originate in the ovary, adipose and muscle tissue, and liver. Estradiol produced in the ovary is the primary circulating estrogen in premenopausal women. Estrone, produced mainly in adipose and muscle tissue, is the primary estrogen in postmenopausal women. Higher levels of estrone-sulfate and 16-hydroxylated estrogens were noted in breast cancer patients than in control subjects.[51]

Factors that alter the levels of sex hormone-binding globulin (SHBG) may influence estrogen availability, and factors that influence enterohepatic circulation of estrogens may affect estrogen excretion and alter plasma levels. Plant estrogens (phytoestrogens) may prevent binding of endogenous estrogens to the estrogen receptor.[51]

Weight reduction, anorexia nervosa, and starvation lower estrogen levels and increase SHBG. Vegetarian diets are associated with a low incidence of cancers of the breast, endometrium, and prostate.[52] Vegetarian diets reduce estrogen exposure by (1) decreasing enterohepatic circulation of plasma estrogen with concomitant increases in fecal estrogens and decreased plasma and urinary estrogens; (2) decreasing estradiol availability by increasing SHBG;

(3) decreasing hepatic estrogen sulfation with subsequent decreased plasma estrone-sulfate levels[53]; and (4) altering estrogen metabolism.[52]

Isoflavone Phytoestrogens

One of the most important classes of dietary compounds known to influence estrogen exposure is the phytoestrogens, plant compounds that possess weak estrogenic activity (see Figure 12–6).[53-55] Phytoestrogens inhibit estrogen synthesis, blocking the actions of potent estrogens, interfering with estrogen receptor replenishment, and increasing SHBG synthesis.

Phytoestrogens include isoflavones, and daidzein and genistein are the 2 most common ones. Phytoestrogens have been shown to act as antiestrogens (see Table 12–7). They bind to the estrogen receptor and prevent more potent compounds from binding and exerting their effects. They contain phytochemicals that are known or believed to block specific pathways that lead to the development of breast cancer (see Figure 12–7).[56]

Soybeans and other legumes are the primary food sources of daidzein and genistein in humans[57] and may be a contributing factor for low incidence of

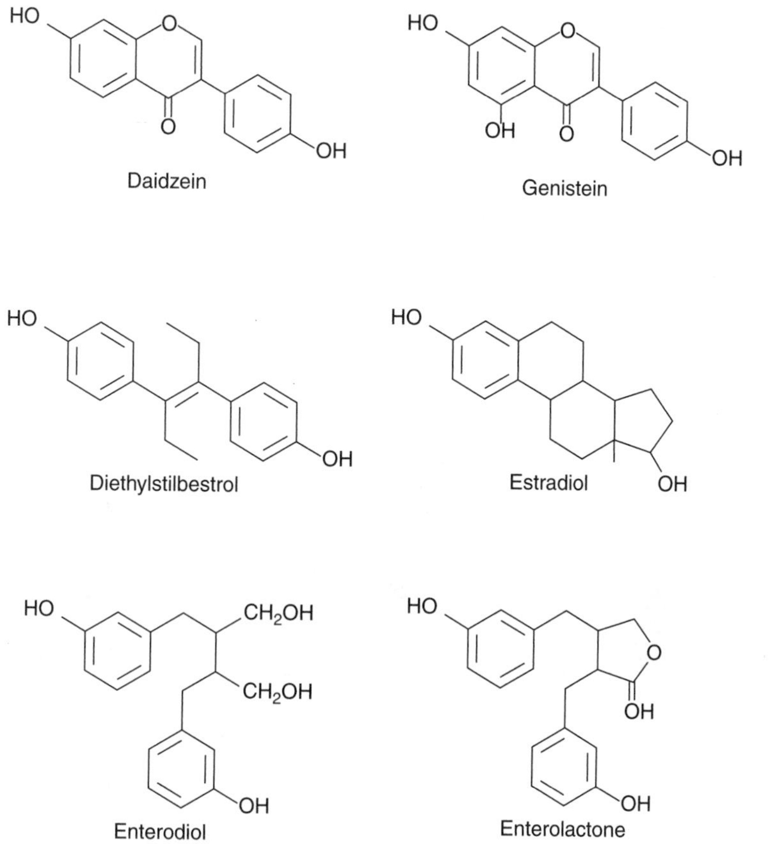

Daidzein

Genistein

Diethylstilbestrol

Estradiol

Enterodiol

Enterolactone

FIGURE 12–6 Comparison of the structures of selected isoflavone phytoestrogens (daidzein and genistein), lignins (enterodiol and enterolactone), and estrogens (diethylstilbestrol and estradiol).
Source: Reprinted from Kurzer MS. Diet, estrogen and cancer. *Contemporary Nutr.* 1992;17(7):1-2.

Table 12–7   14 Major Plant Phytochemicals With Cancer-Protective Properties

	1	2	3	4	5	6	7	8	9	10	11	12	13	14
Garlic	*						*	*		*				
Green tea			*	*		*				*				
Soybeans		*	*		*	*		*	*	*				
Cereal grains		*	*	*	*	*		*		*				
Cruciferous	*		*	*	*	*	*	*		*	*	*		
Umbelliferous			*		*	*	*	*		*			*	*
Citrus			*	*	*	*	*	*		*				
Solanaceous			*	*	*	*	*	*		*				
Cucurbitaceous			*		*	*	*	*		*				
Licorice root			*			*		*		*				
Flaxseed			*			*			*	*				

Key: 1 = sulfides; 2 = phytates; 3 = flavonoids; 4 = glucarates; 5 = carotenoids; 6 = coumarins; 7 = monoterpenes; 8 = triterpenes; 9 = lignins; 10 = phenolic acids; 11 = indoles; 12 = isothiocyanates; 13 = phthalides; 14 = polyacetylenes.
Source: Reprinted from Caragay AB. Cancer preventive foods and ingredients. *Food Technology.* April 1992; 46(4):65-68. Used with permission of the Institute of Food Technologists.

breast and prostate cancer in Japanese women and men.[58] Dietary soy has been shown to be inversely associated with breast cancer risk in Singapore.[59] Animal studies have shown that dietary soy decreases mammary tumor development in rats[60] and reduces precancerous changes in a prostatic cancer model for mice.[61]

Soy foods are important sources of several phytochemicals including isoflavones, phenolic acids, and saponins, which have beneficial effects. When incorporating soyfoods into the eating pattern, one will eat less saturated fat

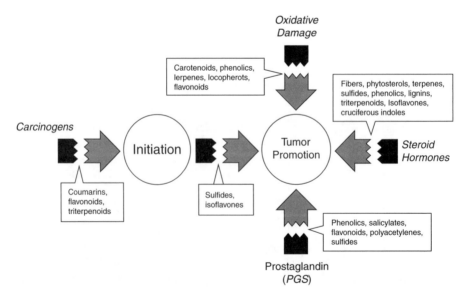

FIGURE 12–7   Potential role of dietary phytochemicals in breast cancer progression. Certain phytochemicals are known or believed to block specific pathways that lead to the development of breast cancer.
Source: Reprinted from Caragay AB. Cancer preventive foods and ingredients. *Food Technology.* April 1992;46:65-68. Used with permission of the Institute of Food Technologists.

and cholesterol and more fiber (in the case of soybeans, tempeh and textured vegetable protein). The process of eating soy foods helps establish a new diversified eating pattern, whereas taking pills minimizes food behavior change and relies on supplements.

Why increase soy food intake?

- Flavonoid intake is shown as inversely associated with heart disease mortality and the incidence of heart attack.[62] Flavonoids extend the activity of vitamin C, which acts as an antioxidant, and not only protect LDL cholesterol from oxidation, but also inhibit blood clot formation and cause an anti-inflammatory and antitumor action. Genistein and daidzein are antioxidants influencing the atherosclerotic process. Genistein intake may decrease thrombosis and inhibit the growth of both human breast and prostate cancer cells in vitro.
- Anderson et al confirmed that soy protein significantly reduces total and LDL cholesterol levels and triglycerides without lowering HDL cholesterol levels.[63]
- Although hormone replacement therapy (HRT) is a common treatment for the prevention and treatment of cardiovascular disease and osteoporosis in postmenopausal women, some women prefer not to take HRT. Soy products containing isoflavones are a viable alternative because soybeans are one of the richest sources of phytoestrogens, i.e., isoflavones, especially if they contain most or all of the bean, such as in soy milk, sprouts, flour, and tofu with 1–3 mg isoflavones per gram soy protein.[64]
- Genistein, the major isoflavone in soy, binds to estrogen receptors. Additionally, genistein and daidzein have estrogenic action, which is positive for bone health. Sixty-six postmenopausal, hypercholesterolemic women experienced a lower serum cholesterol level and improved bone mineral density by consuming soy.[65] An exact daily intake of soy has not been established, even though beneficial effects have been reported.[66]

Soy and Prostate Cancer Reduction

The anticancer effects of soy are by no means limited to breast cancer.[67] Breast cancer and prostate cancer mortality rates in Asian countries are extremely low in comparison to western countries where 4-5 times more men die of prostate cancer.[68,69] The difference in prostate cancer incidence between these 2 countries is not large, but Japanese men rarely die from it. Soy food consumption may contribute by delaying the clinical appearance of prostate tumors by a few years. Incidence rates show $< \frac{1}{4}$ of prostate cancer diagnoses each year are in men under 65[68] and one half of breast cancer diagnoses occur in women under 65.[70]

The primary isoflavone in soybeans, genistein, inhibits the growth of both hormone-dependent and hormone-independent prostate cancer cells.[71] Genistein inhibits the metastatic activity of prostate cancer cells independent of its effect on cell growth.[72] In dose-dependent studies, genistein inhibited the incorporation of 3HTHY (a measure of tissue growth) by 44-88% in cultured benign prostate hypertrophy tissue and prostate cancer tissue.[69,73]

A human study has shown that isoflavones may be twice as concentrated in the prostatic fluid compared to blood levels.[74] One week prior to surgery, a man consumed daily 160 mg of phytoestrogens (from red clover). The prostate cancer tissue showed significant apoptosis (programmed cell death).[75]

Severson et al conducted a prospective study with 7,999 men in Hawaii and followed them for 18-21 years. Tofu consumption was associated but not significantly associated with a markedly reduced risk of prostate cancer (< 1/wk vs > 5/wk; age-adjusted relative risk = 0.35; $p < 0.054$).[76]

The effects on prostate tumor development of an eating pattern consisting of a soy protein isolate with a low isoflavone content[77] versus one with a higher isoflavone content produced no difference in final tumor outcome. A 27% increase in tumor latency in the high isoflavone group was observed primarily when isoflavones were fed prior to the administration of the carcinogen.

Isoflavones are weak estrogens. The potential mechanism of action to inhibit prostate cancer is by signal transduction. Genistein inhibits protein tyrosine kinase activity, and tumor inhibition has been associated with a decrease in protein phosphorylation.[73] Testosterone, or its active metabolite, dihydrotestosterone, may play a role in prostate cancer. Very preliminary findings from a short-term study in men found that soy consumption may decrease levels of a metabolite of testosterone.[73,78]

Studies on Soy and Prostate Health

Soy protein is being tested clinically in human trials as an adjuvant therapy for treatment of prostate cancer as follows[79,80]:

- Men diagnosed as having prostate cancer, with a prostate specific antigen (PSA) greater than 4 and not under treatment were randomized to lifestyle changes, vegan diet, exercise, and stress management. Participants met 1 hour/week at a church for blood pressure and weight measurement and education. They received 1 year of group support, group dinners, and cooking and tasting demonstrations. Participants kept written records of stress management, exercise, and diet. Dietary goals included 50-100 mg isoflavones/day.
- A National Cancer Institute (NCI) Phase III randomized study monitors the effect of a diet low in fat and high in soy, fruits, vegetables, green tea, vitamin E, and fiber on PSA levels in prostate cancer patients. One hundred fifty-four patients are stratified by treatment (prostatectomy vs radiotherapy) and PSA level (less than 5 mg/mL vs 5 or greater mg/mL). For diet intervention, participants meet weekly for 8 weeks, then every 2 weeks for 2 months, then monthly for 14 months. Control patients follow NCI nutrition guidelines with counseling and monitoring every 2 months for 18 months.
- One hundred men with prostate cancer are being followed postprostatectomy and eating a 20% fat diet that is high in fiber (25-35 g) with 40 grams soy isolate containing 40 mg genistein, 200 mcg selenium, and lycopene in the form of tomato products.
- Prostate cancer patients at a University of Texas research project are counseled on a special daily diet that includes:
  - less than 20% calories from fat
  - at least 5 fruits/vegetables per day
  - 25-30 grams of fiber
  - 800 IU vitamin E

- 500 mg vitamin C
- 40-60 grams of soy protein as powder and whole soy foods

Follow-up involves telephone calls, educational handouts, and access to an extensive list of soy foods in the US soy foods directory.

Lignins

Lignins are heterocyclic phenols similar in structure to estrogens and isoflavones that are hypothesized to decrease estrogen exposure and cancer risk. Lignins are abundant in seeds, especially flaxseed, in the form of a glycoside[81] that is converted into mammalian lignins—enterolactone and enterodiol—and excreted in the urine. Enterolactone, the most important animal lignin, may have antiestrogenic properties. Postmenopausal women with breast cancer, as compared with omnivorous and vegetarian control subjects, excrete lower amounts of urinary lignins. Enterolactone and enterodiol are excreted in significantly lower amounts in urine of nonvegetarians as compared to vegetarians.[82]

Enterolactone and other lignin metabolites have been shown to inhibit in vitro estrogen synthesis.[83] They also have been shown to bind to the estrogen receptor[84] and to inhibit estradiol-stimulated breast cancer cell growth in vitro.[85]

Flaxseed is the most concentrated food source of lignin precursors.[81] When expressed per 100 grams net weight, flaxseed consumption results in an average hundred-fold greater total lignin production than consumption of other oil seeds, cereals, and legumes. Fruit and vegetable consumption results in very low lignin production. These foods, however, may contribute significantly to lignin production when consumed in amounts greater than normally consumed.[81,55]

The link between a high-fiber eating pattern and health promotion has been suggested for many years.[86] Burkitt's report in 1969 heightened the interest.[87] Some researchers report that specific foods high in dietary fiber—such as fruits, vegetables, and grains—protect against degenerative disease.[86,88,89] Approximately 45% of total dietary fiber intake in the United States is from fruits and vegetables; grains provide 25% of fiber.[90] All other foods provide the remaining 30%.

Adlercreutz has suggested that phytoestrogens or lignins, not dietary fiber, protect against western diseases. The link connecting colon and breast cancer to diet in epidemiologic studies is that certain populations consume small amounts of specific fiber-rich foods, especially grain, that contain lignins, which are precursors to mammalian lignins. Phytoestrogens and lignins are thought to be anticarcinogenic, antiproliferative, and antihormonal. Thus, a diet high in fiber increases fecal bulk and is speculated to influence estrogen metabolism in a favorable direction, giving protection against both colon and breast cancer. Since lignins are associated with high-fiber foods—such as grains, certain berries, and seeds—it is difficult to distinguish the protective properties of phytoestrogens or lignins from dietary fiber.[84,91,92]

Prostate Cancer

Most cases of prostate cancer occur in men older than 50, and more than 70% of these cases are in men over 65. For reasons that are still unknown, African-American men are more likely than white men to develop prostate cancer and are more than twice as likely to die from it. Having 1 or more close relatives with prostate cancer also increases a man's risk of developing this disease, as does eating a diet high in animal fat. Prostate cancer can usually be found in its early stages by having a PSA blood test and a digital rectal exam (DRE).[93]

Large Bowel Cancer and Fiber

Correlation studies that compare national colorectal cancer incidence or mortality rates with estimates of national dietary fiber consumption suggest that fiber intake may protect against colon cancer.[94] Case-control studies[94,95] support the protective role of dietary fiber in colorectal cancer. A recent case-control study in Argentina reports that dietary fiber is highly protective against colon cancer.[96]

Different fiber sources were associated with varying risks of colon and rectal cancer in a western New York population.[97] Patients with pathologically confirmed, single, primary cancers of the colon and rectum, as well as age-, sex-, and neighborhood-matched control subjects were interviewed regarding usual quantity and frequency of consumption of foods. For colon cancer, risk decreased with intake of grain fiber for both females and males and with intake of fruit/vegetable fiber for males only. For rectal cancer, fruit/vegetable fiber intake was associated with decreased risk, whereas grain fiber was not. This study suggests that different fibers have different protective effects on cancer risk, which may also vary by gender.[97]

Health Benefits of Wheat Bran

A study by McBurney et al[98] involved 567 individuals who completed a 3-year treatment with or without wheat bran fiber to decrease recurrence of colorectal adenomas. At least 1 adenoma was diagnosed in 338 participants in the high-fiber group (47%) and in 229 participants in the low-fiber group (51%); relative risk (RR) was 0.88, or not different from control (95% confidence interval 0.70 to 1.11; $p = 0.28$). Recurrence rates for males versus females were not different. Fewer recurrent adenomas occurred in the high-fiber group (50.0) compared to the low-fiber group ($p < 0.05$) but not in male participants who underwent a 1-year follow-up colonoscopy. There were no treatment effects on adenoma size or histology although a higher proportion of participants with 3 or more recurrent adenomas was found in the high- versus. low-fiber treatments ($p < 0.03$).[98]

Lack of effect may have resulted from:

- an inadequate follow-up time
- increases in total dietary fiber and cereal fiber among the high-fiber relative to the low-fiber participants
- beneficial effects only experienced among individuals with lower baseline intake
- treating people with wheat bran fiber who have preexisting adenomas may not be useful
- wheat bran fiber may have protective effects only in the prevention of new adenomas or in slowing the progression of large adenomas to carcinomas

Key messages for the community about the health benefits of fiber are found in Appendix 12-A.

A prospective study of colon cancer risk among women reports no association between dietary fiber intake and colon cancer.[99] Low intake of fiber from fruits may contribute to colon cancer risk, but not statistically independent of meat intake. Colon cancer risk reduction has been reported in a prospective study where individuals had a more frequent consumption of vegetables and high-fiber grains.[100] Human observational studies and animal experiments suggest that calcium may decrease the risk of colorectal cancer, possibly because increased formation of the calcium salt of bile acids decreases promotion of cancer. The vitamin D and calcium supplementation trial in the Women's Health Initiative will answer questions regarding the effect of supplementation on colorectal cancer (see Chapter 9).

Breast Cancer and Fiber

Fat and fiber content of one's eating pattern are generally inversely related, and it is difficult to separate their independent effects. International comparisons show an inverse correlation between breast cancer death rates and consumption of fiber-rich foods.[97] An exception is Finland, where intake of both fat and fiber is high and the breast cancer mortality rate is low. Data suggest that the high level of fiber in the rural Finnish diet can modify the breast cancer risk associated with a high-fat diet.[101]

A meta-analysis of 12 case-control studies of dietary factors and risk of breast cancer found that high dietary fiber intake was associated with a reduced breast cancer risk.[102] Graham et al found that the risk of breast cancer was lowest in those who reported the highest intakes of dietary fiber.[103] Willett et al found no indication of a protective effect of fiber consumption on breast cancer incidence in a prospective cohort of 89,494 women who were 34 to 59 years of age and were followed for 8 years in the Nurses' Health Study.[104] These authors suggest that the relationship between dietary fiber and breast cancer risk warrants further research since they could not exclude the possibility that specific fractions of dietary fiber may protect against breast cancer.

Dietary fiber increases intestinal transit rate and bulk and thereby dilutes intestinal constituents that may promote carcinogenesis.[88,94,105] Lampe et al found that different dietary fibers have different effects on bowel function and that these differences vary between men and women.[106,107] Kashtan et al studied colonic fermentation and markers of colorectal cancer risk in patients with polyps.[108] They found no significant differences between oat bran, a more fermentable fiber, and wheat bran, a less fermentable fiber, on putative risk factors for colon cancer.

Lipkin and colleagues suggest that proliferation rates of epithelial cells that line colorectal mucosa crypts are related to risk of colorectal cancer, with proliferation rates highest in colon cancer patients and lowest in noncancer patients.[109,110] Intermediate rates occur for patients with familiar polyposis. DeCosse et al found that a daily dietary supplement of 22.5 grams of wheat bran fiber significantly reduced the number of adenomatous polyps in the low sigmoid colon and rectum of patients with familial polyposis.[111] Alberts et al studied the effects of wheat bran fiber on rectal epithelial cell proliferation in patients with resection for colorectal cancers. They found that the wheat bran fiber supplement inhibited DNA synthesis and rectal mucosa cell proliferation in this high-risk group, suggesting that fiber could be used as a chemopreventive agent for colorectal cancer.[112]

Few studies have examined the effects of dietary fiber on hormone metabolism while holding fat content of the eating pattern constant. Rose et al found that when wheat bran was added to the usual eating pattern of premenopausal women, it significantly reduced serum estrogen concentrations, while neither corn bran nor oat bran had the same effect.[113] High-fiber intakes may diminish the extent to which unconjugated estrogens undergo intestinal absorption. Dietary fiber intake was increased from about 15 grams per day to 30 grams per day in this study, an increase similar to that recommended by the National Cancer Institute. Rose believes an increase in dietary fiber intake to about 30 grams per day can favorably modify breast cancer risk by reducing circulating estrogens.[114]

Lycopene

Antioxidants like lycopene, are internal bodyguards that protect human cells from free radicals. These radicals are highly reactive oxidized molecules that disturb the body's cell membranes and attack the internal genetic material. The degenerative effect is called "oxidative stress." It is suspected to be a main culprit of heart disease, cancer, and aging. Free radicals promote arterial blockages, joint deterioration, and nervous system degradation.

In November 1998, researchers at the University of Toronto reported that regular consumption of a variety of processed tomato products, like ketchup, tomato juice, and tomato sauce, significantly raises the blood levels of lycopene in the human body. A flood of scientific research on lycopene, including supplements, has occurred.

Consumers who eat tomato products every day increased from 17.5% in December 1998 to 20.9% in April 1998. About 50% of consumers eat tomato products 2 to 5 times weekly; 16.5% have a tomato intake of only once per week and 5.6% are occasional eaters.

About 84% of consumers prefer fresh tomatoes over processed. Eating tomatoes in general is good, however, heat processing of tomatoes increases lycopene levels 5 times.[115]

Wine Antioxidant Kills Cancer

Resveratrol helps control atherosclerosis, heart disease, arthritis, and autoimmune disorders. It appears that resveratrol starves cancer cells by stopping the action of a key protein, nuclear factor-kappa B (NF-kB), responsible for cell survival. Physiologically relevant doses of resveratrol were used in research studies and produced dramatic effects. Human cancer cells treated with resveratrol died due to a compound called tumor necrosis factor alpha (TNF α). Resveratrol initiates a reaction in the NF-kB molecule that causes cancer cells to self-destruct in a process called apoptosis.

The total amount of resveratrol in 1 glass of wine drunk 3 or 4 times a week is the right amount to block the protein from feeding cancer cells. Resveratrol is an antioxidant found in a number of plants, including grape skins, raspberries, mulberries, and peanuts. In nature it fights fungus during the rainy season.[116]

Info Line

The Cancer Research Foundation of America is a national nonprofit
health organization whose mission is the prevention of cancer
through scientific research and education. Founded in 1985 by
Carolyn Aldige, the organization's commitment is fueled by the fact
that certain cancers are preventable through lifestyle and health policy changes, yet more than 550,000 Americans die from the disease
annually. Since its inception, the foundation has supported research,
education, and early detection programs in excess of $28 million.

Animal Studies

Cohen et al reported that rats fed a diet supplemented with wheat bran developed significantly fewer mammary tumors than rats on diets not supplemented
with wheat bran.[117] Boffa et al found that fiber-free and 20% high-fiber diets
were associated with hyperproliferation, a risk factor for colon cancer. They
suggest that moderate amounts of fiber, 5% and 10% in their animal model,
may have protective effects on cell proliferation, differentiation, and carcinogenesis, while fiber-free diets and diets supplemented with too much fiber have
the potential to promote colon carcinogenesis.[118] Increasing current intake of
dietary fiber to 20 to 35 grams per day from a variety of food sources, including vegetables, legumes, and grains, appears prudent and necessary.[119]

Safety of Saccharin

The National Toxicology Program's ninth report on carcinogens, released in
May 2001 removed saccharin from the list of substances previously listed as
a carcinogen in people. Reviewers believe that our understanding has
advanced, which allows us to now make finer distinctions about research.
These distinctions indicate that the rat bladder tumors shown from earlier
research activated mechanisms not relevant to humans. Thus, saccharin is
now considered safe for human consumption.

Conjugated Linoleic Acids

A recent area of investigation has been the role of conjugated linoleic acid
(CLA) in the inhibition of uncontrolled cell growth or neoplasia.[120] Linoleic
fatty acid is essential for tumor growth.[121] However, it can be modified to
yield protective properties. When linoleic acid is heated, the double bonds
migrate from the cis 9 and 12 positions to the cis or trans 9 and 11 or 10 and
12 positions. The biologically active form appears to be the 9-cis, 11-trans
isomer.[122]

In 1991, Ip et al demonstrated that a test diet with 1.0% or 1.5% CLA reduced tumor incidence by 42% and 50%, and it reduced tumor multiplicity
by 56% and 59%, respectively.[123] In related research, a daily 0.5-gram dose

of CLA for 22 weeks not only lowered plasma total and LDL cholesterol by 13% and 17%, respectively, but it also reduced the severity of atherosclerosis in rabbits.[124,125]

CLA is found naturally in animal foods, especially dairy products. The proposed cancer-preventing effect occurs at a level slightly above the estimated daily US consumption.[126] The concern is to balance an intake that provides protection with one that does not exceed the 30% total fat intake.

Phytosterols

Phytosterols may function as anticancer agents with β-sitosterol shown to inhibit cell proliferation of human colon cancer.[127-131] The mechanism may be twofold, i.e., promoting the sphingomyelin cycle and increasing apoptosis via an increase in ceramide. Ceramide-based enzymes may inhibit cell growth and stimulate apoptosis.[131-132]

Several Asian societies have lower incidence rates of colon, prostate, and breast cancers compared to western societies. The Asian cultures consume about 4 times the amount of phytosterols.[131] Peanuts are a good source of phytosterols with 153 mg sitosterol (SIT) per 100 g of refined peanut oil compared to pure olive oil having 117 mg SIT/100 g. Peanuts and peanut butter average 61-134 mg SIT/100 g and peanut flour averages 44-48 mg SIT/100 g. In common servings, 1.2 oz of roasted peanuts, 1.3 oz of peanut butter, and 1 oz of peanut oil each provide about 50 mg of SIT. [131]

Genetically Modified Organisms (GMOs)

About one fourth of the US cropland contains genetically modified crops comprising 35% of all corn, 55% of all soybeans, and nearly 50% of all cotton. Fifty genetically engineered or biotech (bt) plants are approved by USDA[133]: soybeans, corn, canola, flax, papaya, potatoes, sugar beet, tomatoes, yellow squash, radicchio, cotton, and dairy products (see Table 12–8).

Labeling is not required and yet many consumers may not be able to define the process. The term "genetically modified" describes a laboratory

Table 12–8

Biotech or Genetically Modified Products Available in Grocery Stores After 2000

Corn, soybeans, and potatoes that require fewer applications of herbicides/pesticides.

Tomatoes that soften slower and remain on the vine longer, resulting in enhanced flavor and color.

Soybeans that are lower in saturated fats and higher in oleic acid.

Virus-resistant papayas.

Peppers that are modified to be sweeter and firmer.

Oils, such as soybean and canola oils, developed to contain more stearate, which makes margarine and shortenings more healthful.

Peas grown to remain sweeter and produce higher crop yields.

Source: Adapted from: Future foods or frankenfoods? The controversy over GMOs. *Supermarket Savvy*. March/April 2000.

technique used by scientists to change the DNA of microorganisms, plants, and animals. Bt applications began in 1800 BC when yeast was used to leaven bread and ferment wine. About 4,000 years later, it was used to breed plants through deliberate cross-pollination.

When plants are cross-bred, all genes are mixed, producing random combinations. With advanced molecular technology, specific genes can be transmitted from one organism to any other allowing transfer among all living organisms. A virus gene in potatoes can be transferred to corn to protect against disease. A cow can be injected with a bovine growth hormone that is produced by genetically engineered bacteria.[133]

One third of consumers surveyed by the International Food Information Council (IFIC) were aware that bts are available in the supermarket. Two out of three support the use of biotechnology, but some fear and concern remains among one third of consumers.[134] Go to http://ificinfo.org for more information.

Benefits

- Bt reduces crop losses and increases yields by reducing the need for chemical pesticides. This is essential because food production must increase to feed the global population of 9 billion people by 2050.
- Bt crops can adapt to severe environments like drought, soil with high salt content, and temperature extremes.
- Bt results in increased plant tolerance to environmentally safe herbicides that discourage weeds but leave plants unaffected.
- Bt causes functional qualities of foods such as reduced allergenicity or toxicity, delayed ripening, increased starch content or prolonged shelf life, and nutritional characteristics, e.g., altered protein or fat content or higher phytochemical content.

Safety

Consumer Reports concluded that there is no evidence that bt foods on the market are unsafe to eat, but that vigilance is warranted; a potential for increased natural toxins or decreased nutrients in some foods, even production of new allergens exists.[134] Europe has required labeling of bt foods since September 1998. The FDA requires special labeling when a food is produced under certain conditions, e.g., when biotechnology introduces an allergen that substantially changes the food's nutritional content, e.g., vitamins or fat.

Further, the US House and Senate are discussing a required labeling of genetically modified foods sold to consumers.[133] The future holds bt oatmeal and breads that lower cholesterol and oranges having multivitamin content. To avoid bt, consumers should buy organic foods. The certifying organizations for producers of organic foods prohibit the use of bt ingredients.

The Need for a Controlled Trial of a Low-Fat Eating Pattern

Many different types of epidemiologic studies have addressed the hypothesis that dietary intakes of fat, grains, fruits, and vegetables are related to the incidence of breast and colorectal cancers. Animal experiments are important for demonstrating plausible biological mechanisms and for confirming or explaining the results of epidemiological studies, but the results cannot on their own be extrapolated to humans. If a marker for disease exists, then clinical metabolic studies may be performed to test the effect of dietary modifications on the marker. No such marker currently exists for breast or colorectal cancer.

Studies correlating international data on incidence of disease with food disappearance data and migrant studies provide useful evidence for these hypotheses. However, this information is not entirely reliable, because the studies do not link dietary habits with disease incidence at the individual level. They also cannot adequately control for confounding factors that may influence the disease rate.

Case-control studies overcome some of these problems but suffer from possible biases in the selection of case and control subjects, differential recall of dietary intake by case and control subjects, and nondifferential error in the measurement of dietary intake. Prospective cohort studies avoid selection and recall biases but still rely upon food questionnaires that are known to involve substantial measurement error. These problems are compounded by the narrow range of intakes of the populations typically entering a case-control or cohort study.

The role of antioxidant vitamins C and E and beta-carotene in cancer prevention is of considerable interest. These nutrients neutralize free radicals and other reactive chemicals and terminate the harmful chemical reactions. Beta-carotene, the most common plant source of vitamin A, is a food colorant. The rich yellow, orange, and red pigment of fruits and vegetables is due to its presence. However, beta-carotene has another unique property. Beta-carotene, vitamin C, and vitamin E all assist the body to resist unstable chemicals that damage cells.

More than 100 population-based studies showed a strong association between lowered risk of chronic diseases (e.g., heart disease and cancer) and the high daily intake of antioxidant vitamins. Such studies are still being conducted. However, health authorities in the United States have become proactive and recommend a minimum of 5 fruits and vegetables a day and the use of whole-grain products as a means of achieving the RDAs for the antioxidants.[135] Good food sources of vitamin C, vitamin E, and beta-carotene are outlined in Table 12–9.[136] Americans average about 1.5 mg of beta-carotene per day, which is only 25-30% of the RDA.[137-138] Figure 12–8 shows the trends in 5 A Day intakes among adults.

The United Nations' Food and Agriculture Organization (FAO) launched a campaign to increase consumption of fruits and vegetables worldwide. Researchers determined that inadequate fruit and vegetable consumption was one of the top 10 causes of death annually among the world's population. Noncommunicable diseases (NCD) such as diabetes, obesity, heart disease, and some forms of cancer represent 45% of global disease overall and are responsible for 60% of deaths annually. FAO statistics project that the fiber, vitamins, minerals, and antioxidants in fruits and vegetables could help prevent some of those diabetes cases, as well as 31% of heart disease cases and 11% of strokes. The WHO International Agency for Research on Cancer estimates that the percentage of cancers that are preventable through increased fruit and vegetable intake ranges from 5 to 12% for

TABLE 12–9   Food Sources of Vitamin C, Vitamin E, and Beta-Carotene

Nutrient	Good Food Sources
Vitamin C	Vegetables such as asparagus, broccoli, brussels sprouts, cauliflower, cabbage, green peppers, kale, snow peas, and sweet potatoes Fruits such as cantaloupes, grapefruits, honeydew melons, oranges, tangerines, and strawberries
Vitamin E	Almonds, hazelnuts Peanut butter Salad/vegetable oils Sunflower seeds Wheat germ
Beta-carotene	Dark, green leafy vegetables such as collard greens, kale, mustard greens, peppers, spinach, turnip greens, and Swiss chard Yellow-orange vegetables such as carrots, pumpkins, sweet potatoes, and winter squash Yellow-orange fruits such as apricots, cantaloupes, mangoes, papayas, and peaches

Source: Adapted from: *Food Sources of Vitamin C, E, and Beta Carotene.* American Cancer Society brochure; Atlanta, Ga.

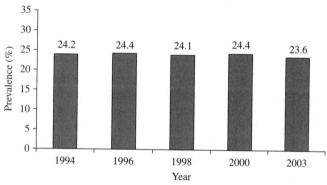

Note: Data from participating states and the District of Columbia were aggregated to represent the United States.

FIGURE 12–8   Trends in consumption of five or more recommended vegetable and fruit servings for cancer prevention, adults 18 and older. United States, 1994-2003

all cancers, and from 20 to 30% for upper gastrointestinal tract cancers.

The FAO said it will work with the 5 A Day marketing partnerships launched in several countries, including the United States, that help support farmers by promoting fruit and vegetable consumption. Farmers will also be given education in farming techniques that will increase production of fruits and vegetables to meet what the FAO hopes is an increased demand for them without compromising food safety.[139] The United Nations FAO Web site is at www.fao.org/english/newsroom/focus/2003/fruitveg1.htm.

Behavior Change

A culturally diverse convenience sample of 30 women aged 40 to 60 years diagnosed with breast cancer 6 months to 15 years previously were studied to explore dietary changes. Women had many different beliefs about diet's role in breast cancer and in their own cancer diagnosis. Dietary actions were not always consistent with reported beliefs. The factors that did seem to influence dietary changes were family support, employment, financial status, culture, and other health concerns. Taking dietary supplements may be a common, but temporary response to a diagnosis. Women should explore cancer prevention through healthy eating and seek professionals to help them evaluate benefits of dietary options.[140]

Cancer prevention efforts have generally been in the form of recommendations regarding overall health and nutrition. Studies reveal that there is a weak association between nutrition knowledge and beliefs and dietary behavior. The objective of 1 study was to determine if people who have more knowledge of cancer-prevention behaviors do in fact follow them. [139]

Data were obtained from the 1992 National Health Interview Survey, Cancer Epidemiology Supplement. Respondents answered a series of questions regarding the relationship between diet and disease and completed a food frequency questionnaire to estimate daily fruit and vegetable intake. As knowledge levels increase, diets come closer to the dietary recommendations. Perceived barriers to eating a healthful diet were examined. The investigators concluded that individuals who perceived barriers to eating a healthful diet did not in fact achieve their dietary recommendations. Barriers include ease of eating a healthful diet, perceived taste of the foods, social support, and education level.

Telephone interviews of a population-based sample of 126 breast, 114 prostate, and 116 colorectal cancer patients were conducted to investigate the prevalence and predictors of changes in diet, physical activity, and dietary supplement use among cancer patients. About 66.3% of patients reported making lifestyle changes; 40% made 1 or more dietary changes, 21% added new physical activity, and 48% began supplement use. Women were more than twice as likely as men to take a new supplement ($p < 0.01$). Adults 60 and older were significantly less likely to make dietary changes (odds ratio = 0.39 and 0.54, for those 60 and older and those under 60, respectively) or to take new supplements (odds ratio = 0.42 and 0.69, respectively). Patients receiving 3 or more treatments for their cancer were more likely to make dietary changes (odds ratio = 3.0). Patients diagnosed 24 months before the interview were just as likely to make lifestyle changes as those diagnosed less than a year before the interview. A major predictor of starting a new supplement was a stronger desire for personal control or a strong internal locus of control (for trend $p < 0.05$ for both). Cancer survivors are likely to modify their lifestyle and they represent individuals who could benefit from counseling on diet and physical activity.[141]

Future diet and health-related programs should educate people about the importance of good nutrition. CNPs must address perceived barriers to change and conduct general and focused nutrition education for cancer prevention.[139]

Even though multiple strategies have been used to encourage behavior change, none have proven more successful than others. Motivational interviewing is a new strategy taking a different approach. It allows people to recognize and then act on problems currently existing or those occurring in the future. The individual becomes responsible for the change in his or her behavior. Techniques involve persuasion and support to increase intrinsic motivation.[142]

Five principles form the foundation of motivational interviewing. CNPs who wish to apply the principles should learn to:

1. *Express empathy*—Seek to understand the client's feelings without judgment.
2. *Accept discrepancy*—Encourage clients to voice their perceptions and the discrepancies that may exist between where they are and where they want to be.
3. *Avoid argumentation*—Minimize defensiveness.
4. *Roll with resistance*—Allow perceptions to shift.
5. *Support self-efficacy*—Encourage clients to believe that they can complete tasks successfully.

Behavioral research suggests that these techniques can empower a person to change, especially when CNPs treat individuals with respect and encourage them as the change process begins.[142]

Work-Site Intervention

Major preventive efforts have taken the form of organized intervention at the job site. The many benefits include having the support of management for employee wellness; using the physical environment for instruction including exercise rooms, cafeterias, walking areas, and meeting rooms; scheduling classes conveniently before, during, and after work; using the group dynamics of the employees to form classes and to develop healthy competition if needed.

The Treatwell Intervention

Primary prevention efforts involving work-site interventions often include separate treatment and control groups.[143,144] In the Treatwell intervention in Massachusetts, 1,762 employees represented 8 control and 5 intervention companies. Eligibility criteria for participation were:

- company size (200-2,000 employees)
- presence of a cafeteria with a kitchen in which to implement the cafeteria-based intervention
- an annual employee turnover rate of less than 25%
- fewer than 25% of employees working rotating shifts, part-time, or off-site
- company stability, defined as having no plans for geographic relocation or major layoffs during the intervention period

The purpose of the intervention was to reduce fat consumption and increase consumption of fiber in the eating patterns of the intervention group using food-focused messages (see Table 12-10). The secondary effect of the dietary changes on other nutrients was evaluated. Each participant completed a health-habits questionnaire before and after the 15-month intervention.

TABLE 12–10   Eating Pattern Messages Linked to Food Items in the Treatwell Food Frequency Questionnaire (FFQ)

Message	FFQ Items*
Trim fat	
• Choose fish	• Fish
• Choose skinned turkey or chicken.	• Ratio of chicken and turkey without skin to chicken and turkey with skin
• Choose lean red meat.	• Red meat • Hamburger fat score
–Keep to 6 oz or less (cooked) a day.	• Unable to quantify
• Choose low-fat dairy products. –skim, 1%, or 2% milk	• Ratio of skim and low-fat to whole milk
–low-fat yogurt, cheese, and ice milk	• Unable to quantify
• Use half the amount of fat or oil you normally use. –in cooking or baking –as spreads	 • Fats and oils added in cooking • Margarine and butter
Add fiber	
• Eat at least one serving of a high-fiber cereal every day.	• Proportion of cold cereal eaters who consumed low- and high-fiber cereals at baseline and at follow-up
• Eat at least one serving of fruit per meal and for snacks.	• All fruit
• Eat at least one serving of vegetables at lunch and dinner.	• All vegetables
• Eat at least one of these foods at each meal: –whole-grain bread –rice or pasta –potato –dried beans, peas, or lentils	 • Dark and whole-grain bread • Rice and pasta • Potatoes, mashed or baked • Beans or lentils, dried

*Food items derived from the FFQ that are related to the eating pattern messages, or derivations based on one or more FFQ responses.
Source: Reprinted from Hunt MK, Hebert JR. Impact of worksite cancer prevention program on eating patterns of workers. *J Soc Nutr Education.* 1993;25(5):236-243. Used with permission of the Society for Nutrition Education.

In addition, the nutrient and energy intakes were determined from the Willett semiquantitative food frequency questionnaire.[145]

Participants in the intervention group decreased their use of margarine and butter as spreads ($p < 0.01$) and increased their intake of vegetables ($p < 0.02$) significantly more than did workers in control companies. The greatest change in nutrient content occurred for nontargeted dietary components. Specifically, significantly greater increases were observed for vitamin A and beta-carotene. Marginally significant increases were noted for vitamin B_6, moderate decreases were seen for saturated and monounsaturated fats, and small increases were noted for polyunsaturated fats.[143] This observation is important because analysis of the total nutrient intake beyond the targeted nutrients is warranted. Healthy eating refers to the total composition of an eating pattern, not just the fat or sodium content.

Of equal importance is the choice of research instruments when trying to assess nutrient composition in a large study group. The Willett food frequency questionnaire is useful when ranking individuals into percentiles of intake and to identify outliers for specific dietary components. Frequencies in general should not be used to estimate the mean nutrient intake of an individual or a group.

Women's Intervention Nutrition Study

The purpose of the Women's Intervention Nutrition Study (WINS) was to evaluate the feasibility of integrating dietary fat intake reduction into adjuvant treatment strategies for postmenopausal women with breast cancer by determining the degree of adherence to such a dietary program.[146] WINS was a step-by-step, individualized approach to reduce total fat intake and fat components (see Table 12–11). It was based on behavioral and social learning theory about dietary behavioral change (see Table 12–12).[147,148]

The primary end point was group dietary fat intake using 4-day food records and unannounced 24-hour telephone recalls. Fasting blood for lipid analysis was obtained at baseline and at 3, 6, 12, 18, and 24 months.

TABLE 12–11 Changes in Eating Pattern Composition From Baseline to 6 Months for Treatment and Control Participants; WINS Study

| | Daily Intake by Dietary Group | | | |
| | Intervention (96 Subjects) | | Control (100 Subjects) | |
Nutrient	Baseline	6 Months	Baseline	6 Months
Total energy, kcal	1,755 ± 447	1,466 ± 395	1,731 ± 395	1,544 ± 369
Protein, g	73 ± 20	70 ± 19	75 ± 18	68 ± 16
Carbohydrate, g	218 ± 65	223 ± 72	212 ± 57	195 ± 57
Fiber, g	17.4 ± 5.7	18.4 ± 6.7	16.9 ± 6.2	16.6 ± 6.4
Fat total, g	66 ± 23	33 ± 14*	66 ± 20	56 ± 20
Calories	11.3 ± 4.5	6.8 ± 3.0*	11.4 ± 4.2	10.2 ± 4.3
From total fat, %	33.4 ± 6.0	20.5 ± 6.2*	34.3 ± 5.6	32.1 ± 7.3
From monounsaturated fats, %	12.3 ± 4.1	7.6 ± 4.1*	11.7 ± 3.5	12.4 ± 5.1
From polyunsaturated fats, %	6.6 ± 2.8	4.6 ± 2.7*	6.7 ± 2.9	6.7 ± 3.1
Linoleic acid (c18:2)	12.8 ± 6.1	6.4 ± 3.4*	12.1 ± 4.7	10.7 ± 5.1

Note: Values are mean ± SD.
*Difference from baseline to 6 months is for intervention versus control group ($p < 0.001$).
Source: Reprinted from Buzzard IM, Asp EH, Chlebowski RT, et al. Diet intervention methods to reduce fat intake: nutrient and food group composition of self-selected low-fat diets. *J Am Diet Assoc.* 1990;90:42-49. Used with permission of the American Dietetic Association.

TABLE 12–12   **The Women's Intervention Nutrition Study Dietary Intervention Protocol for Low-Fat Eating**

Step	Content
1	Teaching basic concepts about low-fat and high-fat foods, recipe modification, and food preparation methods via 4 biweekly visits, 8 monthly visits, and 2 bimonthly visits
2	Establishing an individualized, daily fat-gram goal (initially, 20% energy as fat, then 15% energy as fat); monitoring with a food diary and the following tools: • fat-gram counter • brand-name guide • keeping score booklet
3	Setting individual long- and short-term goals for eating behaviors

Source: Data from Buzzard IM, Asp EH, Chlebowski RT, et al. Diet intervention methods to reduce fat intake: nutrient and food group composition of self-selected low-fat diets. *J Am Diet Assoc.* 1990;90:42-49. Used with permission of the American Dietetic Association.

Anthropometric data collection included body weight, height, and waist and hip circumference taken at baseline and at 3-month intervals.

Changes in mean intake of energy, total fat, and percentage of energy from fat calculated from 4-day food record data show total fat and percent energy derived from fat significantly different between the 2 dietary groups ($p < 0.001$). The percentage of energy from fat determined 3 months' postrandomization was lower (19.5% versus 22.2% when the target was 15%).[146]

The low-fat eating plan in the dietary intervention group did not involve changes in total energy intake. This group had reduced body weights compared with the weights seen in the dietary control group at all observation points. The body weight difference was 3.26 kg 18 months after randomization (1.46 ± 5.01 kg weight loss versus 1.80 ± 6.34 kg weight gain, for intervention and control group patients, respectively, $p < 0.001$).[146]

This study demonstrated that significant dietary fat intake reduction can be achieved during breast cancer treatment and maintained for at least 2 years by patients in a multicenter study. Feasibility of the fat modification was established. A definitive trial is now needed to test the hypothesis that a program of dietary fat intake reduction that complements systemic adjuvant therapy can reduce disease recurrence and increase survival duration of postmenopausal women with localized breast cancer.[146]

This fat intake reduction program could be broadly implemented by registered dietitians at the hospital and community levels. The approximate cost of instruction for the low-fat eating plan is projected to be about $375 to $400. This is based on current professional charges for 5 hours of a registered dietitian's service and reflects the percentage of effort required in the WINS. Costs associated with breast cancer management, including costs for local therapy to the diseased breast, are approximately $10,000. Tamoxifen for 5 years plus chemotherapy would cost $15,000. A program for dietary fat intake reduction costing $375 represents less than a 2% increase in the $25,000 cost associated with current management of early-stage breast cancer.[149]

The Women's Health Initiative

The randomized, controlled clinical trial component of the Women's Health Initiative (WHI) enrolled 68,135 postmenopausal women 50 to 79 years of age at 40 clinical centers. This trial had 3 interventions, and women can enroll in 1 or more of the intervention components. The first will evaluate the effect of a low-fat dietary pattern on prevention of breast and colon cancer and coronary heart disease. The second will examine the effect of hormonal-replacement therapy on prevention of coronary heart disease and osteoporotic fractures. The third will evaluate the effect of calcium and vitamin D supplementation on prevention of osteoporotic fractures and colon cancer (see Chapter 9).[150]

The WHI Community Prevention Study of strategies to enhance adoption of healthful behaviors will evaluate how the many behaviors of proven value to women's health can be widely adopted. This aspect of WHI will mobilize community resources to enhance adoption of these behaviors through education, removal of barriers, and improvement of social supports. The behaviors to be targeted are derived from the national goals described in *Healthy People 2010*. Special emphasis will be focused on minorities, the medically underserved, and socioeconomically disadvantaged populations, as these groups have received too little attention and have lagged in adoption of preventive behaviors.[150]

Method Alert

In clinical trials and community-based interventions that focus on cancer, many of the instruments previously used in cardiovascular research are adopted.

The Willett Semi-Quantitative Food Frequency questionnaire is a dietary assessment instrument based on the principle that the average eating pattern over weeks, months, or years is preferred to a recall or record of foods eaten for a short period of time (e.g., 1 to 7 days). It consists of a food list of about 60 to 100 foods and a 5- to 7-item frequency response component. It can be either self-administered or administered in a 1-to-1 interview. Foods included are eaten fairly often by a majority of individuals, provide nutrients or dietary components of interest (e.g., vitamin C or cholesterol), or allow the investigator to discriminate or rank individuals on intake. Guidelines for development of a food frequency questionnaire and testing the reproducibility and validity of the instrument are available.[151]

Healthy People 2010 Actions

Several Healthy People *2010* objectives are directed toward cancer risk reduction using dietary behavior modification (see Exhibit 12-2). Dietary fat, fiber, complex carbohydrate, and total energy intakes are the major focus. Community nutrition professionals can blend these objectives with national cancer control objectives to direct their programs and to target high-risk subgroups in the population (see Exhibit 12-3).

Exhibit 12–2   DATA2010: The *Healthy People 2010* Database—November 2000.
Focus area: 03-Cancer

Objective Number	Objective	Baseline Year	Baseline	Target 2010
03-01	Overall cancer deaths (age-adjusted rate per 100,000 persons of all ages)	1998	202.4	160
	American Indian or Alaska native	1998	129.3	160
	Asian or Pacific Islander	1998	124.2	160
	Black or African American	1998	255.1	160
	White	1998	199.3	160
	Hispanic or Latino	1998	123.7	160
	Not Hispanic or Latino	1998	206.6	160
	Female	1998	169.2	160
	Male	1998	252.4	160
	Education level (persons aged 65 years and older)			
	Less than high school	1998	137.8	90
	High school graduate	1998	139.7	90
	At least some college	1998	79.6	90
03-03	Reduce the breast cancer death rate	1998	28	22
03-05	Reduce the colorectal cancer death rate	1998	21	14
03-07	Reduce the prostate cancer death rate	1998	32	29

Source: Adapted from: US Department of Health and Human Services. DATA2010—the *Healthy People 2010* database. *CDC Wonder.* Atlanta, Ga: Centers for Disease Control, November 2000.

Exhibit 12–3   Model Nutrition Objective for Reduced Risk Reduction

By 20____, the chronic disease risk factor _____*_____ among [*target population*] will be reduced from _____% to _____%.

*Obesity; hypertension; elevated serum cholesterol; poor physical fitness; excess intake of dietary fat, cholesterol, sodium, alcohol, or sugar; inadequate intake of dietary fiber, fruits and vegetables, or calcium.
Source: Adapted from: *Model State Nutrition Objectives.* Washington, DC: The Association of State and Territorial Public Health Nutrition Directors; 1988.

References

1. Wynder EL. Metabolic epidemiology and the causes of cancer. Presented at UCLA extension conference, Nutritional Medicine in Medical Practice; January 22-23, 1993; Santa Monica, Calif.
2. American Cancer Society. *Cancer Facts and Figures*. Atlanta, Ga: American Cancer Society; 2005.
3. Ries LAG, Eisner MP, Kosary CL, et al, eds. *SEER Cancer Statistics Review, 1975-2002*. Bethesda, Md: National Cancer Institute. Available at: http://seer.cancer.gov/csr/1975_2002/. Accessed January 10, 2000.
4. National Cancer Institute. *Cancer Control Objectives for the Nation*. Bethesda, Md: National Cancer Institute; 1993.
5. Lichtenstein P, Niels H, Verkasalo K, et al. Environmental and heritable factors in the causation of cancer—analyses of cohorts of twins from Sweden, Denmark, and Finland. *N Engl J Med*. 2000;343:78-85.
6. Oda E, Ohki R, Murasawa H, et al. Noxa, a BH3-Only Member of the Bd-2 Family and Candidate Mediator of p53-Induced Apoptosis. *Science*. 2000;288:1053-1057.
7. Ogden J, Fox P. Examination of the use of smoking for weight control in restrained and unrestrained eaters. *Int J Eating Disorders*. 1994;16:177-185.
8. Hayes R. Smoking, colon cancer link called stronger. *OC Register*. April 5, 2000.
9. Warsorich MJ, Cunningham J. Diet, individual responsiveness and career prevention. *J Nutr*. July 2003;133:24005-24035.
10. Kumar NB. Android obesity at diagnosis and breast carcinoma survival. Evaluation of the effects of anthropometric variables at diagnosis, including body composition and body fat distribution and weight gain during life span, and survival from breast carcinoma. *Cancer*. 2000;88:2751-2757.
11. Doll R, Peto R. The causes of cancer: quantitative estimates of available risks of cancer in the United States today. *J Natl Cancer Inst*. 1981;66:1191-1308.
12. National Research Council. *Diet and Health: Implications for Reducing Chronic Disease Risk*. Washington, DC: National Academy Press; 1989.
13. Shapiro S, Venet W, Strax P, et al. *Periodic Screening for Breast Cancer. The Health Insurance Plan Project and Its Sequelae, 1963-1986*. Baltimore, Md: Johns Hopkins University Press; 1988.
14. Tabar L, Faqerberg CJ, Gad A, et al. Reduction in mortality from breast cancer after mass screening with mammography: randomized trial from the breast cancer screening working group of the Swedish National Board of Health and Welfare. *Lancet*. 1985;1(8433):829-832.
15. Stenkvist B, Bergshrome R, Eklund G, et al. Papanicolaou smear screening and cervical cancer: what can you expect? *JAMA*. 1984;252:1423-1426.
16. National Cancer Institute. *Eating Tips: Tips and Recipes for Better Cancer Treatment*. Bethesda, Md: National institutes of Health; 1994.
17. Pollack ES. Tracking cancer trends: incidence and survival. *Hospital Practice*. 1984;19(8):99-102, 105-108, 111-112.
18. Mills PK, Beeson WL, Phillips RL, et al. Cohort study of diet, lifestyle, and prostate cancer in Adventist men. *Cancer*. 1989;64:598-604.
19. Hunter CP, Redmond CK, Chen VW, et al. Breast cancer: factors associated with stage at diagnosis in black and white women, black/white cancer survival study group. *J Natl Cancer Inst*. 1993;85:1129-1137.

20. Public Health Service. *Occupational Hazard Rates Among Black Employees*. Bethesda, Md: US Dept of Health and Human Services; 1985.

21. Cerami A, Ikeda Y, Le Trang N, et al. Weight loss associated with an endotoxin-induced mediator from peritoneal macrophages: the role of cachectin (tumor necrosis factor). *Immunol Lett*. 1985;11(3-4):173-177.

22. Tisdale MJ. Cancer anorexia and cachexia. *Nutrition*. 2001;17:438-442.

23. Argiles JM, Lopez-Soriano FJ. The role of cytokines in cancer cachexia. *Med Res Rev*. 1999;19:112-248.

24. van Halteren HK, Bongaerts GP, Wagener DJ. Cancer cachexia: what is known about its etiology and what should be the current treatment approach? *Anticancer Res*. 2003;23:5111-5115.

25. von Haeling S, Genth-Zotz S, Anker SD, Volk HD. Cachexia: a therapeutic approach beyond cytokine antagonism. *Int J Cardiol*. 2002;85:173-183.

26. Moertel CG, Schutt AJ, Reitemeier RJ, Hahn RG. Corticosteroid therapy of preterminal gastrointestinal cancer. *Cancer*. 1974;33:1607-1609.

27. Loprinzi CL, Kugler JW, Sloan JA, et al. Randomized comparison of megestrol acetate versus dexamethasone versus fluoxymesterone for the treatment of cancer anorexia/cachexia. *J Clin Oncol*. 1999;17:3299-3306.

28. McMillan DC, Wigmore SJ, Fearon KC, et al. A prospective randomized study of megestrol acetate and ibuprofen in gastrointestinal cancer patients with weight loss. *Br J Cancer*. 1999;79:495-500.

29. Loprinzi CL, Ellison NM, Schaid DJ, et al. Controlled trial of megestrol acetate for the treatment of cancer anorexia and cachexia. *J Natl Cancer Inst*. 1992;82:1127-1132.

30. Yeh SS, Hafner A, Schuster MW, et al. Relationship between body composition and cytokines in cachectic patients with chronic obstructive pulmonary disease. *J Am Geriatr Soc*. 2003;51(6):890-891.

31. Jatoi A, Rowland K, Loprinzi CL, et al. An eicosapentaenoic acid supplement versus megestrol acetate versus both for patients with cancer-associated wasting: a North Central Cancer Treatment Group and National Cancer Institute of Canada collaborative effort. *J Clin Onocol*. 2004;22(12):2469-2476.

32. National Center for Nutrition and Dietetics. *Nutrition Fact Sheet: Focus on Fiber*. Chicago, Ill: American Dietetic Association; 1994.

33. Blackburn GL, Copeland T, Khaodhiar L, Buckley RB. Diet and breast cancer. *J Womens Health*. March 2003;12(2):183-192.

34. Barnett JB. The relationship between obesity and breast cancer risk and mortality. *Nutr Rev*. February 2003;61(2):73-76.

35. Rissanen H, Knekt P, Järvinen R, Salminen I, Hakulinen T. Serum fatty acids and breast cancer incidence. *Nutr Cancer*. 2003;45(2):168-175.

36. Fleischauer AT, Simonsen N, Arab L. Antioxidant supplements and risk of breast cancer recurrence and breast cancer-related mortality among postmenopausal women. *Nutr Cancer*. 2003;46(1):15-22.

37. Chapman GE, Beagan B. Women's perspectives on nutrition, health, and breast cancer. *J Nutr Educ Behav*. May-June 2003;35(3):135-141.

38. Janne P, Mayer R. Chemoprevention of colorectal cancer. *N Engl J Med*. 2000;342(26):1960-1968.

39. Winawer S. *Colorectal Cancer: The Importance of Prevention and Early Detection*. Atlanta, Ga: Centers for Disease Control and Prevention; 2000. Available at: www.cdc.gov/cancer/colorectal/. Accessed January 10, 2007.

40. National Cancer Institute. *SEER Cancer Statistics Review, 1973-1996*. Bethesda, Md: National Cancer Institute; 1999.

41. National Cancer Institute. *Surveillance, Epidemiology, and End Results Program 1973-1996*. Washington, DC: Division of Cancer Control and Population Sciences, National Cancer Institute; 1999.

42. Bond JH. Polyp guideline: diagnosis, treatment, and surveillance for patients with colorectal polyps. *Am J Gastroenterol.* 2000;95:3053-3063.

43. Baron JA, Beach M, Mandel JS, et al. Calcium supplements for the prevention of colorectal adenoma. *N Engl J Med.* 1999;340:101-107.

44. Wyeth. *Calcium for Colon Protection* [brochure 6087-69]. Madison, NJ: Wyeth Consumer Healthcare; 2002.

45. Fu YM, Yu ZX, Li YQ, et al. Specific amino acids dependency regulates invasiveness and viability of androgen-independent prostate cancer cells. *Nutr Cancer.* 2003;45:60-73.

46. American Institute of Cancer Research. Do amino acids build cancer? *Science Now.* 2004;9:3.

47. O'Keefe SJD. Differences in diet and colonic bacterial metabolism that might account for the low risk of colon cancer in native Africans. *Gastroenterology.* 2004;126(4):M2097.

48. O'Keefe SJD, Kidd M, Espitalier-Noel G, et al. The rarity of colon cancer in Africans is associated with low animal product consumption not fiber. *Am J Gastroenterol.* 1999;94:1373-1380.

49. A gut reaction. *AICR Science Now.* 2004;9:1-2.

50. Choices and changes—yogurt: a wonder food? *AICR Science Now.* 2004;9:2.

51. Kurzer MS. Diet, estrogen and cancer. *Contemporary Nutr.* 1992;17(7):1-2.

52. Adlercreutz H. Western diet and western diseases: some hormonal and biochemical mechanisms and associations. *Scan J Clin Lab Invest.* 1990;50(suppl):3-23.

53. Woods MN, Gorbach SL, Longcope C, et al. Low-fat, high-fiber diet and serum estrone sulfate in premenopausal women. *Am J Clin Nutr.* 1989;49:1179-1183.

54. Setchell KDR, Adlercreutz H. Mammalian lignins and phyto-oestrogens: Recent studies on their formation, metabolism and biological role in health and disease. In: Rowland IR, ed. *Role of the Gut Flora in Toxicity and Cancer.* London, England: Academic Press; 1988:316-345.

55. Messina M, Barnes S. The role of soy products in reducing risk of cancer. *J Natl Cancer Inst.* 1991;83:541-547.

56. Caragay AB. Cancer preventive foods and ingredients. *Food Technol.* April 1992;46(4):65-68.

57. Gustafson DR, Kurzer MS. Flavonoid inhibition of aromatase enzyme activity (AA) in human adipose stromal cells (ASC). *Fed Proc.* 1991;5(5):A931.

58. Adlercreutz H, Honjo H, Higashi A, et al. Urinary excretion of lignins and isoflavonoid phytoestrogens in Japanese men and women consuming a traditional Japanese diet. *Am J Clin Nutr.* 1991;54:1093-1100.

59. Lee HP, Gourley L, Duffy SW, et al. Dietary effects on breast-cancer risk in Singapore. *Lancet.* 1991;337:1197-2000.

60. Messina M, Messina VJ. Increasing use of soyfoods and their potential role in cancer prevention. *J Am Diet Assoc.* 1991;91:836-840.

61. Makela S, Pylkkanen L, Santti R, et al. Role of plant estrogen and estrogen-related altered growth of the mouse prostate. In: *Effects of Food on the Immune and Hormonal Systems.* Schwerzenbach, Switzerland: Swiss Federal Institute of Technology and University of Zurich; 1991:135-139.

62. Hertog MGL, Feskens EJM, Hollman PCH, et al. Dietary antioxidant flavonoids and risk of coronary heart disease. *Lancet.* 1993;342:1007-1011.

63. Anderson JW, Johnstone BM, Cook-Newell ME. Meta-analysis of the effects of soy protein intake on serum lipids. *N Eng J Med.* 1995;333:276-282.

64. Hesseltine CW, Wang HL. Fermented soybean food products. In: Smith AK, Circle SJ, eds. *Soybeans: Chemistry and Technology.* Westport, Conn: AVI Press; 1992.

65. Erdman JW, Potter S. Soy and bone health. *Soy Connection.* 1997;5(2):1,4.

66. Samour P, Coffield E. Behavior modification in changing to diets containing soy. *Soy Connection.* 1998;6(3)1-2.

67. Messina M, Persle V, Setchell K et al. Soy intake and cancer risk: a review of the in vitro and in vivo data. *Nutr Cancer.* 1994;21:113-31.

68. American Cancer Society. *Cancer Facts and Figures.* Atlanta, Ga: American Cancer Society; 1998.

69. Messina M. Soy shows promise in slowing prostate cancer rate of growth. *Connection.* 1998;6(4):1,3.

70. American Cancer Society. *Breast Cancer Facts and Figures.* Atlanta, Ga: American Cancer Society; 1996.

71. Peterson G, Barnes S. Genistein and biochanin A inhibit the growth of human prostate cells but not epidermal growth factor receptor tyrosine autophosphorylation. *Prostate.* 1993;22(4):335-345.

72. Santibanez JF, Navarro A, Martinez J. Genistein inhibits proliferation and in vitro invasive potential of prostatic cancer cell lines. *Anticancer Res.* March-April 1997;17(2A):1199-1204.

73. Geller J, Sionit L, Partido C, et al. Genistein inhibits the growth of human-patient BPH and prostate cancer in histoculture. *Prostate.* February 1, 1998;34(2):75-79.

74. Morton MS, Matos-Ferreira A, Abranches-Monteiro L, et al. Measurement and metabolism of isoflavonoids and lignins in the human male. *Cancer Letters.* March 19, 1997;114(1-2):145-151.

75. Stephens FO. Phytoestrogens and prostate cancer: possible preventive role. *Med J Aust.* August 9, 1997;167(3):138-140.

76. Severson RK, Nomaura AM, Grove JS, Stemmermann GN. A prospective study of demographics, diet, and prostate cancer in men of Japanese ancestry in Hawaii. *Cancer Res.* April 1, 1989;49(7):1857-1860.

77. Pollard M, Luckert PH. Influence of isoflavones in soy protein isolates on development of induced prostate-related cancers in L-W rats. *Nutr Cancer.* 1997;28(1):41-45.

78. *Am Assoc Cancer Res.* 1996;37:270. Abstract 1841.

79. Yip I, William A, Heber D. Nutritional approaches to the prevention of prostate cancer progression. *Adv Exp Med Biol.* 1996;399;173-181.

80. Patterson A. Studies on soy and prostate health. *Connection.* 1998;6(4):1,4.

81. Thompson LU, Robb P, Serraino M, et al. Mammalian lignin production from various foods. *Nutr Cancer.* 1991;16:43-52.

82. Adlercreutz H, Heikkinen R, Woods M, et al. Excretion of the lignins enterolactone and enterodiol and of equol in omnivorous and vegetarian postmenopausal women and in women with breast cancer. *Lancet.* 1982;1:1295-1299.

83. Adlercreutz H, Bannwart C, Wahala K, et al. Inhibition of human aromatase by mammal lignins and isoflavonoid phytoestrogens. *J Steroid Biochem Molec Biol.* 1993;44:147-153.

84. Adlercreutz H, Mousavi Y, Clark J, et al. Dietary phytoestrogens and cancer: in vitro and in vivo studies. *J Steroid Biochem Molec Biol.* 1992;41:331-337.

85. Mousavi Y, Adlercreutz H. Enterolactone and estradiol inhibit each other's proliferative effect on MCF-7 breast cancer cells in culture. *J Steroid Biochem Molec Biol.* 1992;41:615-619.

86. Potter JD. Reconciling the epidemiology, physiology, and molecular biology of colon cancer. *JAMA*. 1992;268:157-177.

87. Burkitt DP, Walker AR, Painter NS. Effects of dietary fiber on stools and the transit times, and its role in the causation of disease. *Lancet*. 1972;2(792):1408-1412.

88. Klurfeld DM. Dietary fiber-mediated mechanisms in carcinogenesis. *Cancer Res*. 1992;5:2055S-2059S.

89. Block G, Patterson B, Subar A. Fruit, vegetables, and cancer prevention: a review of the epidemiological evidence. *Nutr Cancer*. 1992;18:1-29.

90. Block G, Lanza E. Dietary fiber sources in the United States by demographic group. *J Natl Cancer Inst*. 1987;79:83-91.

91. Thompson LU. *Contemporary Nutrition*. Minneapolis, Minn: General Mills Inc; 1992.

92. Slavin JL. Dietary fiber and cancer update. *Contemporary Nutr*. 1992;17(8):1-2.

93. American Cancer Society, Inc. *Cancer Facts for Men*. Atlanta, Ga: American Cancer Society; 2002. Publication no. 2008.

94. Bingham SA. Mechanisms and experimental and epidemiological evidence relating dietary fiber (nonstarch polysaccharides) and starch to protection against large bowel cancer. *Proc Nutr Soc*. 1990;49:153-171.

95. Willett W. The search for the causes of breast and colon cancer. *Nature*. 1989;338:389-394.

96. Iscovich JM, Abbe KA, Castelleto R, et al. Colon cancer in Argentina: II. Risk from fiber, fat, and nutrients. *Int J Cancer*. 1992;51:858-861.

97. Freudenheim JF, Graham S, Horvath PJ, et al. Risks associated with source of fiber and fiber components in cancer of the colon and rectum. *Cancer Res*. 1990;50:3295-3300.

98. Massimino SP, McBorney MI, Field CJ, et al. Fermentable fiber increases GLP-1 secretion and improves glucose homeostasis despite increased intestinal glucose transport capacity in healthy dogs. *J Ntr*. 1998;128:1786-1793.

99. Willett WC, Stampfer MJ, Colditz GA, et al. Relation of meat, fat, and fiber intake to the risk of colon cancer in a prospective study among women. *N Engl J Med*. 1990;33:1664-1672.

100. Thun MJ, Calle EE, Namboodini MM, et al. Risk factors for fatal colon cancer in a large prospective study. *J Natl Cancer Inst*. 1992;84: 1491-1500.

101. Rose DP. Dietary fiber, phytoestrogens, and breast cancer. *Nutrition*. 1992;8:47-51.

102. Howe GR, Hirohata T, Hislop TG, et al. Dietary factors and risk of breast cancer: combined analysis of 12 case-control studies. *J Natl Cancer Inst*. 1990;82:561-569.

103. Graham S, Hellmann R, Marshall J, et al. Nutritional epidemiology of postmenopausal breast cancer in western New York. *Am J Epidemiol*. 1991;134:552-566.

104. Willett WC, Hunter DJ, Stampfer MJ, et al. Dietary fat and fiber in relation to risk of breast cancer: an 8-year follow-up. *JAMA*. 1992;268:2037-2044.

105. Eastwood MA. The physiological effect of dietary fiber: an update. *Annual Rev Nutr*. 1992;12:19-35.

106. Lampe JW, Fredstrom SB, Slavin JL, et al. Sex differences in colonic function: a randomized trial. *Gut*. 1993;34:531-536.

107. Lampe JW, Slavin JL, Melcher EA, et al. Effects of cereal and vegetable fiber feeding on potential risk factors for colon cancer. *Cancer Epid Biomarkers Prevention*. 1992;1:207-211.

108. Kashtan H, Stern HS, Jenkins DJ, et al. Colonic fermentation and markers of colorectal-cancer risk. *Am J Clin Nutr.* 1992;55: 723-728.

109. Lipkin M, Enker WE, Winawer SJ. Tritiated-thymidine labeling of rectal epithelial cells in "non-prep" biopsies of individuals at increased risk for colonic neoplasia. *Cancer Lett.* 1987;37:153-161.

110. Terpstra OT, van Blankenstein M, Dees J, et al. Abnormal pattern of cell proliferation in the entire colonic mucosa of patients with colon adenoma or cancer. *Gastroenterology.* 1987;92:704-708.

111. DeCosse JJ, Miller HH, Lesser ML. Effect of wheat fiber and vitamins C and E on rectal polyps in patients with familiar adenomatous polyposis. *J Natl Cancer Inst.* 1989;81:1290-1297.

112. Alberts DS, Einspahr J, Rees-McGee S, et al. Effects of dietary wheat bran fiber on rectal epithelial cell proliferation in patients with resection for colorectal cancers. *J Natl Cancer Inst.* 1990;8: 1280-1285.

113. Rose DP, Goldman M, Connolly JM, et al. High fiber diet reduces serum estrogen concentration in premenopausal women. *Am J Clin Nutr.* 1991;54:520-525.

114. Rose DP. Plasma estrogens, diet, and breast cancer. *Nutrition.* 1990;7:139-140.

115. Lessons in lycopene [news release]. Pittsburgh, Pa: HJ Heinz Company; April 28, 1999.

116. Mayo M, et al. *J Euro Molecular Biology Organization (EMBO).* Available at: www.foodnavigator.com/news. Accessed. May 27, 2004.

117. Cohen LA, Kendall ME, Zang E, et al. Modulation of N-nitromethylurea-induced mammary tumor promotion by dietary fiber and fat. *J Natl Cancer Inst.* 1991;83:496-501.

118. Boffa LC, Lupton JR, Mariani MR, et al. Modulation of colonic epithelial cell proliferation, histone acetylation, and luminal short chain fatty acids by variation of dietary fiber (wheat bran) in rats. *Cancer Res.* 1992;52:5906-5912.

119. Pilch SM. *Physiological Effects and Health Consequences of Dietary Fiber.* Bethesda, Md: Life Sciences Research Office, Federation of American Societies for Experimental Biology; 1987:149-157.

120. Ha YL, Grimm NK, Pariza MW. Anticarcinogens from fried ground beef: heat altered derivatives of linoleic acid. *Carcinogenesis.* 1987;8:1881-1887.

121. Ip C, Carter CA, Ip MM. Requirement of essential fatty acid for mammary tumorigenesis in the rat. *Cancer Res.* 1985;45:1997-2001.

122. Kritchevsky D. Diet and cancer, conjugated linoleic acid in food: scientists study its role as inhibitor of cancer-causing substances. *Food Nutr News.* 1994;66(3):22-23.

123. Ip C, Chin SF, Scimeca JA, et al. Mammary cancer prevention by conjugated dienoic derivative of linoleic acid. *Cancer Res.* 1991;51: 6118-6124.

124. Lee KN, Kritchevsky D, Pariza MW. Conjugated linoleic acid and atherosclerosis in rabbits. *Atherosclerosis.* 1994;108(1):19-25.

125. Nicolosi RJ, Courtemanche KV, Laitinen L, et al. Effect of feeding diets enriched in conjugated linoleic acid on lipoproteins and aortic atherogenesis in hamsters. *Circulation.* 1993;88(suppl):2458.

126. Ip C, Singh M, Thompson HJ, et al. Conjugated linoleic acid suppresses mammary carcinogenesis and proliferation activity of the mammary gland in the rat. *Cancer Res.* 1994;54:1212-1215.

127. Raicht RF, Cohen BI, Fazzini EP, Sarwal AN, Takahashi M. Protective effect of plant sterols against chemically induced colon tumors in rats. *Cancer Res.* February 1980;40(2):403-405.

128. Awad AB, Garcia MD, Fink CS. Effect of dietary phytosterols on rat tissue lipids. *Nutr Cancer.* 1997;29(3):212-216.

129. Rao AV, Agarwal S. Role of antioxidant lycopene in cancer and heart disease. *J Am Coll Nutr.* October 2000;19(5):563-569.

130. Awad AB, Chen YC, Fink CS, Hennessey T. Beta-sitosterol inhibits HT-29 human colon cancer cell growth and alters membrane lipids. *Anticancer Res.* September-October 1996;16(5A):2797-2804.

131. Awad AB, Fink CS. Phytosterols as anticancer dietary components: evidence and mechanism of action. *J Nutr.* september 2000;130(9): 2127-2130.

132. Hannun YA. Functions of ceramide in coordinating cellular responses to stress. *Science.* December 13, 1996;274(5294):1855-1859.

133. Future foods or frankenfoods? The controversy over GMOs. *Supermarket Savvy.* March/April 2000. Available at: www.Supermarketsavvy.com. Accessed January 11, 2007.

134. US Consumer Attitudes Toward Food Biotechnology. Wirthlin Group Quorom Surveys. 1999.

135. National Cancer Institute. *5-A-Day Initiative.* Bethesda, Md: National Cancer Institute; 1992.

136. American Cancer Society. *Food Sources of Vitamin C, E, and Beta Carotene.* Public information brochure. Atlanta, Ga: American Cancer Society; date unknown.

137. Human Nutrition Information Service. *Nationwide Food Consumption Survey: Continuing Survey of Food Intakes by Individuals. Women 19-50 Years and Children 1-5 Years, 1 Day, 1985.* Washington, DC: US Dept of Agriculture; 1985:102.

138. Patterson BH, Block G, Rosenberger WF, et al. Fruit and vegetables in the American diet: data from the NHANES II survey. *Am J Public Health.* 1990;80:1443-1449.

139. United States Department of Agriculture. UN launches campaign to encourage fruit, vegetable consumption. *Nutr Week.* 2003;33(22):3.

140. Beagan B, Chapman G. Eating after breast cancer: influences on women's actions. *J Nutr Educ Behav.* 2004:36:181-188.

141. Patterson R, Neuhouser M, Henderson M, Schwartz S, Standish L, Bowen D. Changes in diet, physical activity, and supplement use among adults diagnosed with cancer. *J Am Diet Assoc.* 2003;103: 323-328.

142. Miller WR, Rollnick S. Preparing people to change addictive behavior. *Motivational Interviewing.* New York, NY: The Gulford Press.

143. Hunt MK, Hebert JR, Sorensen G, et al. Impact of worksite cancer prevention program on eating patterns of workers. *J Soc Nutr Ed.* 1993;25:236-243.

144. Hebert JR, Harris DR, Sorensen G, et al. A work-site nutrition intervention: its effects on the consumption of cancer-related nutrients. *Am J Public Health.* 1993;83:391-394.

145. Willett WC, Reynolds RD, Cottnell-Hoehner S, et al. Validation of a semi-quantitative food frequency questionnaire: comparison with a 1-year diet record. *J Am Diet Assoc.* 1987;87:43-47.

146. Chlebowski RT, Blackburn GL, Buzzard IM, et al. Adherence to a dietary fat intake reduction program in post menopausal women receiving therapy for early breast cancer. *J Clin Oncology.* 1993;11:2072-2080.

147. Buzzard IM, Asp EH, Chlebowski RT, et al. Diet intervention methods to reduce fat intake: nutrient and food group composition of self-selected low-fat diets. *J Am Diet Assoc.* 1990;90:42-49.

148. Chlebowski RT, Nixon DW, Blackburn GL, et al. A breast cancer nutrition adjuvant study (NAS): protocol design and initial patient adherence. *Breast Cancer Res Treat.* 1987;10:21-29.

149. Eddy DM. Screening for breast cancer. *Ann Intern Med.* 1989;111: 389-399.

150. National Institutes of Health. *Women's Health Initiative.* Bethesda, Md: National Heart Lung and Blood Institute; 1994.

151. Willett W. *Nutritional Epidemiology.* New York: Oxford University Press; 1990:69-126.

DIABETES MELLITUS

Learning Objectives

- Identify the warning signs of insulin-dependent and non–insulin-dependent diabetes mellitus.
- Compare prevalence of diabetes mellitus among different ethnic groups.
- Identify risk factors for developing diabetes and its complications.
- Identify how medical nutrition therapy can reduce cardiovascular disease risks and other complications.

High Definition Nutrition

Blood glucose monitoring—a way of testing how much glucose (sugar) is in the blood. A drop taken from the fingertip is placed on a specially coated testing strip that changes color according to how much glucose is in the blood. A person can tell if the level of glucose is low, high, or normal in 1 of 2 ways: first, by comparing the color on the end of the strip to a color chart that is printed on the side of the test strip container, and second, by inserting the strip into a small meter which reads the strip and shows the level of blood glucose in a digital window display. Blood testing is more accurate than urine testing in monitoring glucose levels because it shows what the current level of glucose is, rather than a prior level.

Capsaicin—a topical ointment made from chili peppers used to relieve the pain of peripheral neuropathy.

Certified diabetes educator (CDE)—a healthcare team professional who is qualified by the American Association of Diabetes Educators to teach people with diabetes how to manage their condition.

Complications—both insulin-dependent and non–insulin-dependent diabetes may precipitate tissue-damaging complications. Microvascular complications affect small blood vessels in 3 organ systems: retinopathy (the eyes), nephropathy (the kidneys), and neuropathy (the nerves).

Dawn phenomenon—a sudden rise in blood glucose levels in the early morning hours for people with insulin-dependent diabetes and (rarely) in people with non–insulin-dependent diabetes. Unlike the Somogyi effect, it is not a result of an insulin reaction, and it may warrant blood glucose monitoring during the night and adjustments in evening snacks or insulin dosages.

Diabetes Control and Complications Trial (DCCT)—a 10-year study (1983-1993) funded by the National Institute of Diabetes and Digestive and Kidney Diseases (NIDDK) to assess the effects of intensive therapy on the long-term complications of diabetes. The study proved that intensive management of insulin-dependent diabetes prevents or slows the development of the eye, kidney, and nerve damage caused by diabetes.

Diabetologist—a physician who treats people with diabetes mellitus.

Gestational diabetes mellitus (GDM)—a type of diabetes mellitus that can occur when a woman is pregnant generally in the second half of the pregnancy when glucose (sugar) in the blood is higher than normal. When the pregnancy ends, the levels return to normal in about 95% of all cases.

Glycemic index (GI)—the area under the postprandial glucose curve for a particular food. It is expressed as a percentage of the response compared to a reference food such as white bread when the carbohydrate content is the same for both foods. The index is not popular and not widely used by medical professionals, but the public is sensitized to the concept.

HbA1c or glycated hemoglobin—describes glucose control over a 3-month period by measuring the amount of glucose that becomes incorporated into hemoglobin. Hemoglobin is the blood protein molecule that transports oxygen to body tissues. A high percentage of HbA1c indicates poor control, whereas a low percentage (< 6%) indicates good control.

Insulin-dependent diabetes mellitus—also known as IDDM or type 1 diabetes, commonly develops in people under 30 years of age. Insulin is required; without insulin, life-threatening diabetic ketoacidosis called diabetic coma occurs. IDDM accounts for 5-10% of all cases of diabetes.

Macrovascular disease—a disease of the large blood vessels that sometimes occurs when a person has had diabetes for a long time. Fat and blood clots build up in the large blood vessels and stick to the vessel walls. Three kinds of macrovascular disease are coronary disease, cerebrovascular disease, and peripheral vascular disease.

Microvascular complications—disease of the smallest blood vessels that sometimes occurs when a person has had diabetes for a long time. The walls of the vessels become abnormally thick but weak, and therefore they bleed, leak protein, and slow the flow of blood through the body. Then some cells, for example, the ones in the center of the eye, may not get enough blood and may be damaged.

Non–insulin-dependent diabetes mellitus—also known as NIDDM or type 2 diabetes, it is the most common form of diabetes (90-95% of all cases). It generally begins in middle age but can occur earlier or later. Individuals are instructed to follow a modified eating and exercise pattern and are placed on oral hypoglycemic drugs (e.g., biguanides or sulfonylureas); many receive insulin.

Oral hypoglycemic agents—pills or capsules that people whose pancreas still makes some insulin take to lower the level of glucose (sugar) in the blood by causing the cells in the pancreas to release more insulin.

Sorbitol—a sugar alcohol that the body uses slowly, is a sweetener in diet foods, and is called a nutritive sweetener with 4 calories in every gram. Sorbitol is produced by the body and in excess can cause cellular damage. Diabetic retinopathy and neuropathy may be related to too much sorbitol in the cells of the eyes and nerves.

Tight control—a phrase that indicates blood glucose levels equal to a standard.

Xylitol—a sweetener found in plants, a substitute for sugar and called a nutritive sweetener providing calories like sugar.

Overview of Diabetes Mellitus

Diabetes mellitus affects 18 million Americans, nearly 1 in every 20 people, creating about 1 million new cases each year. The frightening fact is that only about 50% of diabetes cases are thought to be diagnosed. Early detection is the challenge and over 5 million people do not know they have the disease. Distinct differences are noted for the incidence of diabetes among ethnic groups (see Table 13–1).

Diabetes is neither a mild disease nor a curable disease. Insulin is crucial to the daily survival of over a million people, but it is not a cure. People with diabetes are at risk for serious health complications.[1,2]

In the last decade diabetes increased 38% among Hispanics, 29% among whites, and 25% among blacks. Researchers state that the association between

TABLE 13–1   Diabetes Among Persons 20 Years of Age and Over by Sex, Age, Race, and Hispanic Origin: United States, 1999-2000 as Percentage of the US Population

Sex, Age, Race, and Hispanic Orgin	Physician-Diagnosed Diabetes[*] %	Undiagnosed Diabetes[†] %
20 years and over, age adjusted		
Both sexes	6.1	2.5
Male	6.6	2.7
Female	5.7	2.3
Not Hispanic or Latino:		
White	4.8	2.6
Black or African American	11.7	3.0
Mexican	9.6	2.4
Age Group		
20-39 years	1.4	0.8
40-59 years	5.8	3.3
60 years and older	15.0	4.2

[*]Diagnosed diabetes excludes women who reported diabetes only during pregnancy.
[†]Undiagnosed diabetes is defined as a fasting blood glucose of at least 126 mg/dL.
Source: Centers for Disease Control and Prevention, National Center for Health Statistics, National Health and Nutrition Examination Survey. Prevalence of diabetes and impaired fasting glucose in adults—United States, 1999-2000. *MMWR.* 2003;52(35). Available at: www.cdc.gov/mmwr/preview/mmwrhtml/mm5235al.htm. Accessed January 17, 2007.

obesity and the risk of diabetes is as strong as the association between smoking and the risk of lung cancer.[3] Annual healthcare costs associated with diabetes totaled $132 billion in 2002. The largest increase in diabetes, i.e., 70%, occurred in people ages 30 to 39 with college educations. Associated factors are being busy, more time on the computer and commuting to their jobs, spending less time being physically active, and eating in fast food establishments. The thrifty gene theory purports that humankind lived through feast or famine by storing fat so it could be available during a famine. Diabetes is increasing globally to epidemic proportions in industrialized and developing nations. In Arabic countries, 15% of the population has diabetes, and in India, 10% of the people have diabetes.[2]

The complications are macrovascular and/or microvascular. Macrovascular complications are due to atherosclerosis of large blood vessels. The result is reduced blood flow to tissues. Complications include angina, heart attacks, strokes, and amputations. Smoking, high blood pressure, and abnormal blood lipid levels are additional risk factors, with complications including heart disease, stroke, kidney disease, blindness, nerve damage, and severe infection leading to gangrene and foot and leg amputations. Microvascular complications lead to visual loss, kidney failure, and multiple neurological symptoms. Some patients experience pain, burning, and loss of sensation in their lower limbs as a neurological complication and may resort to topical treatment with capsaicin to relieve pain.[1]

People with diabetes are 2 to 4 times more likely than others to develop heart disease and are more likely to die from heart attacks than people who don't have the disease. The ADA guidelines recommend the use of drugs called statins for people with diabetes over the age of 40 who have a total cholesterol level that is greater than or equal to 135 mg/dL. The primary goal continues to be an LDL < 100 mg/dL. People with diabetes and overt cardiovascular disease who are at very high risk for further events should be treated using a high dose of a statin, and, in these high-risk patients, an LDL cholesterol of < 70 mg/dL is the goal.[4]

An individual with diabetes cannot uptake glucose from the blood into energy for cellular use. High levels of glucose in the blood and urine result. Individuals with diabetes have a genetic tendency to develop the disease, but the environment also has an impact.

In normal metabolism, glucose is absorbed from the digestive tract, transported by the blood to the body's cells, and assisted by insulin to enter the cells. The cells either use the glucose for immediate energy or store it. Insulin is a hormone produced by the pancreas. Individuals with diabetes may lack sufficient insulin, have a defect in insulin function, or have decreased receptors on cells. Body cells are then unable to use the glucose, which increases in the blood and spills into the urine. To prevent complications, blood glucose levels must be kept near a normal range.[1] Professionals such as Certified Diabetes Educators and Diabetologists focus on treatment and prevention of further complications.

There are 2 main types of diabetes with distinctly different warning signs (see Table 13–2). Insulin-dependent diabetes mellitus, type 1, occurs most often in children and young adults and requires treatment with insulin injections that is coordinated with dietary and physical activity habits. This form of diabetes was previously called juvenile-onset diabetes. Approximately 5% of all

TABLE 13–2   The Warning Signs of Diabetes

IDDM	NIDDM
Rapid onset	Gradual onset
Frequent urination	Any of the insulin-dependent symptoms
Excessive thirst	Unrecognized symptoms
Extreme hunger	Recurring or hard-to-heal skin, gum, or bladder infections
Dramatic weight loss	Fatigue
Irritability	Blurred vision
Weakness and fatigue	Tingling or numbness in hands or feet
Nausea and vomiting	Itching

Source: Adapted from: *Who We Are, What We Do.* Alexandria, Va: American Diabetes Association; 1988:1. Used with permission of the American Diabetes Association.

cases are type 1. Non–insulin-dependent diabetes mellitus, or type 2 diabetes, occurs most often in adults over 40, especially the obese. This type has previously been called adult-onset diabetes. The adults most at risk for diabetes are those who are overweight; over 40; have a family history of diabetes; or are of black, Hispanic, or Native American descent.[1] Approximately 95% of all diabetes cases are type 2. The most important public health goal is early detection.

Type 1 diabetes may result from a genetically transmitted autoimmune process that destroys insulin-producing beta cells of the pancreas,[5] but not all carriers develop the disease. In some individuals, the process interacts with the early consumption of cow's milk.[6-10] The preferred food during the first year of life is breast milk. When breastfeeding is discontinued, iron-fortified infant formula rather than cow's milk is the best substitute throughout the first year of life.[5]

The American Diabetes Association Position Statement in 2002 based its recommendations for treatment and prevention on evidence-based research.[11] Glucose control with diet, physical activity, and medication are primary goals to maintain quality of life and to slow the progression to further complications.

Diabetes, in fact, is sometimes considered an accelerated model of aging. Not only do its complications mimic the physiologic changes that can accompany old age, but its victims have shorter-than-average life expectancies. It is recommended that a diabetes mellitus diagnosis be confirmed on a subsequent day by 1 of the following[12]:

1. Symptoms of diabetes plus casual plasma glucose concentration ≥ 200 mg/dL (11.1 mmol/L). Casual is defined as any time of day without regard to time since last meal. The classic symptoms of diabetes include polyuria, polydipsia, and unexplained weight loss.
2. Fasting postprandial glucose (FPG) ≥ 126 mg/dL (7.0 mmol/L). Fasting is defined as no caloric intake for at least 8 h.
3. Two-hour postload glucose ≥ 200 mg/dL (11.1 mmol/L) during an oral glucose tolerance test (OGTT). The test should be performed as described by WHO, using a glucose load containing the equivalent of 75 g anhydrous glucose dissolved in water.

In the absence of unequivocal hyperglycemia, these criteria should be confirmed by repeat testing on a different day. The third measure (OGTT) is not recommended for routine clinical use.

Recommended Eating Pattern for Patients with Type 2 Diabetes

Type 2 diabetes is a heterogeneous disorder demonstrated by insulin resistance and abnormalities in insulin secretion.[13,14] A clear genetic susceptibility exists, but environmental factors play a major role. Diet, physical fitness, and obesity affect insulin resistance.[13,15-17] Obesity is a major predisposing factor and is found in approximately 80% of people who develop type 2 diabetes.[18]

Medical nutrition therapy goals for type 2 diabetes patients are[11]:

1. Attain and maintain optimal metabolic outcomes including:
   - Blood glucose levels in the normal range or as close to normal as is possible to prevent or reduce the risk for complications of diabetes.
   - A lipid and lipoprotein profile that reduces the risk for macrovascular disease.
   - Blood pressure levels that reduce the risk for vascular disease.
2. Prevent and treat the chronic complications of diabetes. Modify nutrient intake and lifestyle as appropriate for the prevention and treatment of obesity, dyslipidemia, cardiovascular disease, hypertension, and nephropathy.
3. Improve health through healthy food choices and physical activity.
4. Address individual nutritional needs, taking into consideration personal, ethnic, and cultural preferences and lifestyle while respecting the individual's wishes and willingness to change.

Specific goals for select groups are[11]:

1. Youth with type 1 diabetes, to provide adequate energy to ensure normal growth and development; integrate insulin regimens into usual eating and physical activity habits.
2. Youth with type 2 diabetes, to facilitate changes in eating and physical activity habits that reduce insulin resistance and improve metabolic status.
3. Pregnancy and lactation, to provide adequate energy and nutrients needed for optimal outcomes.
4. Older adults, to provide for the nutritional and psychosocial needs of an aging individual.
5. Persons treated with insulin or insulin secretagogues, to provide self-management education for treatment (and prevention) of hypoglycemia, acute illnesses, and exercise-related blood glucose problems.
6. Persons at risk for diabetes, to decrease risk by encouraging physical activity and promoting food choices that facilitate moderate weight loss or at least prevent weight gain.

Referral to the ADA diet and use of the term *ADA diet* are discouraged.[19] Since 1994, the ADA has not endorsed any single meal plan or specified percentages of macronutrients. Current nutrition recommendations advise individualization based on treatment goals, physiologic parameters, and medication usage.

Due to the complexity of eating patterns, a registered dietitian (RD), knowledgeable and skilled in MNT, should serve as the team member who provides medical nutrition therapy (MNT). The RD is responsible for integrating information about the patient's clinical condition, eating, and lifestyle habits and for establishing treatment goals in order to determine a realistic plan for nutrition therapy.[19]

The rationale is to reduce microvascular complication (i.e., neuropathy, nephropathy, and retinopathy) and to retard the atherosclerotic macrovascular disease. The development of microvascular complications is linked to lack of glycemic control,[12] whereas atherosclerosis is associated with risk factors of diabetes (e.g., obesity, dyslipidemia, hyperinsulinemia, hypertension, platelet dysfunction, and other metabolic abnormalities unique to diabetes).[1]

Physical activity, oral hypoglycemic agents (e.g., metformin, a biguanide), and eating behavior are the focus to prevent macrovascular complications. This is important, because deaths from cardiovascular disease occur 2 to 3 times more often in diabetics compared to nondiabetics and represent the major cause of death in patients with diabetes.[12]

Biochemical indicators of diabetes control are outlined in Table 13-3. Hypertriglyceridemia and hypercholesterolemia are more common among individuals with diabetes than in the general population. They are major risk factors for coronary heart disease (CHD) in persons with diabetes.[20] At any level of serum cholesterol, mortality from CHD is 3 to 5 times greater among persons with diabetes compared to persons who are not diabetic.[21]

An optimal eating pattern is moderate in protein (15-20%) and moderate in carbohydrate and fat (60-70% of energy from carbohydrates and monounsaturated fat). Saturated fat intake kept at < 10% is recommended.[11]

Info Line

All oral hypoglycemic agents belong to a class of drugs known as sulfonylureas. Each type of pill is sold under 2 names: one is the generic name as listed by the Food and Drug Administration; the other is the trade name given by the manufacturer. Six types of these pills are for sale in the United States. Four are known as first-generation drugs and have been in use for some time. They are:

Generic Name	Trade Name
tolbutamide	Orinase
acetohexamide	Dymelor
tolazamide	Tolinase
chloropropamide	Diabinese

These two recent drugs are the second generation and are stronger with fewer side effects:

Generic Name	Trade Name
glipizide	Glucotrol
glyburide	Diabeta, Micronose

TABLE 13–3   Summary of Recommendations From the American Diabetes Association for Biochemical Indices and Values for Adults With Diabetes

Glycemic control	
A1c	< 7.0%[*]
Preprandial capillary plasma glucose	90-130 mg/dL (5.0-7.2 mmol/L)
Peak postprandial capillary plasma glucose[+]	< 180 mg/dL (< 10.0 mmol/L)
Blood pressure	< 130/80 mm Hg
Lipids[‡]	
LDL	< 100 mg/dL (< 2.6 mmol/L)
Triglycerides	< 150 mg/dL (< 1.7 mmol/L)
HDL	> 40 mg/dL (> 1.1 mmol/L)[§]

[*]Referenced to a nondiabetic range of 4.0-6.0% using a DCCT-based assay.
[+]Postprandial glucose measurements should be made 1-2 h after the beginning of the meal, generally peak levels in patients with diabetes.
[‡]Current NCEP/ATP III guidelines suggest that in patients with triglycerides ≥ 200 mg/dL, the non-HDL cholesterol (total cholesterol minus HDL) be used. The goal is ≤ 130 mg/dL (31).
[§]For women, it has been suggested that the HDL goal be increased by 10 mg/dL.
Source: American Diabetes Association, Inc. Position statement—diagnosis and classification of diabetes mellitus. *Diabetes Care.* 2005;28:S37-S42.

There is no restriction in mono- or disaccharides if total energy intake promotes a reasonable body weight. This type of eating pattern demonstrates that glycemic control can occur with a varied eating pattern. If serum cholesterol levels are elevated, individuals should have eating patterns low in both total and saturated fat.[21,22] The American Diabetes Association recommends increasing the fiber content of foods to prevent colorectal cancer and views the general alcohol recommendation of no more than 2 drinks a day for men and no more than 1 alcoholic beverage a day for women as acceptable. The key is to customize the eating pattern for acceptance and glycemic control.

Blood sugar may vary in its response to different foods, but the glycemic index (GI) is not used widely. High carbohydrate diets may adversely effect glycemic control, raise very-low-density lipoprotein (VLDL) and triglyceride levels, and reduce high-density lipoprotein (HDL) cholesterol levels. Foods with low GI values produce low postprandial glycemic levels. Most grain products, breads, and cereals have a high GI, but data do not show a clear benefit of low versus high glycemic index diets.[11]

Legumes including beans, peas, and lentils; pastas; whole grains like oats, barley, and corn; and raw fruits have a low GI. Total and soluble dietary fiber content of food and the form of starch granules influence the GI. White pasta and some legumes are either less accessible or inhibit the activity of digestive enzymes. Resistant starch-containing foods are thought to modify postprandial glycemic response but reports of long-term studies are not available.[11]

Liu et al examined the association between intake of whole versus refined grain and the risk of type 2 diabetes mellitus. Using a food frequency questionnaire for repeated dietary assessments, they prospectively evaluated the relation between whole-grain intake and the risk of diabetes mellitus among

75,521 women, 38 to 63 years old. No previous diagnosis of diabetes or cardiovascular disease existed. During the 10-year follow-up, 1,879 cases of diabetes mellitus were diagnosed. The highest and lowest quintiles of intake were compared and the age and energy-adjusted relative risks were 0.62 (95% confidence interval [CI] = 0.53, 0.71, P trend < 0.0001) for whole grain, 1.31 (95% CI = 1.12, 1.53, P trend = 0.0003) for refined grain, and 1.57 (95% CI = 1.36, 1.82, P trend < 0.0001) for the ratio of refined- to whole-grain intake. The observations were strongest for women with a body mass index > 25 and were not entirely explained by dietary fiber, magnesium, and vitamin E.[20]

Sugar replacers or polyols are sugar-free sweetening ingredients used in the same amount as sugar, but not adding as many kcals. Foods with sugar replacers are labeled "sugar-free" or "no sugar added" and may be packaged with the FDA health claim, "does not promote tooth decay," if noncariogenic. These foods include hard candies, chocolate, baked goods, chewing gum, jams, fruit spreads, sugar-free breath mints, cough drops, and throat lozenges. Nonnutritive intense sweeteners may be combined with sugar replacers to increase product sweetness.

Saccharin, aspartame, acesulfame K, neotame, and sucralose are currently approved for use as sugar substitutes or nonnutritive sweeteners in the United States by the Food and Drug Administration (FDA). See Exhibit 13–1.

The FDA establishes an acceptable daily intake (ADI) of all food additives including nonnutritive sweeteners. The ADI is the amount that can be safely consumed daily over an individual's lifetime without adverse effects. The level includes a hundredfold safety factor. Actual intake by persons with diabetes for all nonnutritive sweeteners is well below the ADI.[23] A 2-week aspartame intake consumption for individuals with diabetes is 2-4 mg/kg body weight (BW) daily. The ADI is 50 mg/kg BW in the United States and 40 mg/kg BW in Europe.[24]

Monounsaturated fat may not increase and may even lower low-density lipoprotein (LDL) cholesterol levels.[25-27] LDL cholesterol levels may not change, VLDL and triglyceride levels may decline, and HDL cholesterol levels may increase when more than 50% of the food energy is from fat and about 35% is from carbohydrate compared to a 60% or higher carbohydrate eating pattern. Other studies have shown that if high-carbohydrate diets are primarily refined

Info Line

Individuals with diabetes may use a variety of food products sweetened with artificial sweeteners or sugar alcohols like sorbitol and xylitol.

Web sites about sweeteners:

www.splenda.com, www.sweetone.com, www.neotame.com, www.nutrasweet.com, www.sweetnlow.com, www.natrataste.com, and www.caloriecontrol.org.

Telephone contacts:

Sweet'N Low Helpline: 1 (800) 221-1763, The Nutrasweet Center: 1 (800) 323-5316, Sweet One Hotline: 1 (800) 544-8610, NatraTaste: 1 (800) 828-7211, and Splenda: 1 (800) 777-5363.

Exhibit 13–1   Approved Nonnutritive Sweeteners in the United States

Nonnutritive Sweetener	Information
Saccharin	• oldest nonnutritive sweetener in the US food supply
	• widely used for 100 years
	• 300 to 400 times sweeter than sucrose
	• well absorbed and nonaccumulative in body tissue
	• metallic, bitter aftertaste, frequently used with a buffer, such as dextrose, to eliminate aftertaste
	• only sweetener available in the United States during World Wars I and II and use increased because of sugar rationing
	• in 1977, a ban on saccharin was proposed, based on research showing saccharin caused malignant tumors in second-generation male rats and intensive review of the research occurred
	• pregnant women are advised to limit use
	• sold as Sweet 'N Low, Sugar Twin, and Sweet Magic
Aspartame	• a dipeptide containing phenylalanine and aspartic acid, approved by FDA in 1981 as a tabletop sweetener
	• on June 27, 1996, approved as a general purpose sweetener
	• 200 times sweeter than sucrose
	• nonnutritive, with a sweet, clean, and bitterless taste
	• not heat stable, but may be added to products after cooking
	• > 100 million individuals around the world use products containing aspartame
	• acceptable daily intake (ADI) is 50 mg/kg BW in adults; the estimated daily intake of aspartame in children is 8 to 17 mg/kg body weight (BW) in children 2 to 5 years; 40 mg/kg BW in European adults
	• safe during pregnancy and lactation
	• persons with phenylketonuria (PKU) must restrict intake
	• in 1999, the FDA's Center for Food Safety and Applied Nutrition received requests for information regarding an e-mail alleging that breakdown products of aspartame, i.e., methanol and formate, caused systemic lupus, multiple sclerosis, seizures, and brain tumors; none of these allegations was proved valid
	• US consumption increased from 8.4 million pounds in 1986 to 17.5 million pounds in 1992; sold as Equal, Nutrasweet, SweetMate, and NatraTaste

Exhibit 13–1   continued

Acesulfame potassium	• also known as acesulfame K, or Ace-K, was approved by FDA in 1988
	• a derivative of acetoacetic acid, is 200 times sweeter than sucrose
	• safety determined using multigenerational rat studies
	• is safe for pregnant women
	• intakes in children average 3 to 9 mg/kg BW, which is less than the ADI
	• sold as Sweet One and Swiss Sweet
Sucralose	• the only nonnutritive sweetener made from sucrose
	• approved by FDA on April 1, 1998
	• received the broadest initial approval FDA ever granted to a food additive
	• approved as a general purpose sweetener
	• no warning labeling required
	• tastes like sugar with no aftertaste
	• contains no calories
	• does not promote tooth decay
	• approximately 600 times sweeter than sugar
	• so stable, it is not broken down in the body
	• passes through the body unchanged quickly after it is ingested
	• sold as Splenda

Source: Cicinelli-Timm DJ. Nonnutritive sweeteners in the US. *DCE Newsflash: Diabetes Care and Education.* 2000;21:10-14.

and also high in dietary fiber, then adverse effects on glycemic control, VLDL, and triglycerides may not occur.[28,29]

Weight loss lowers insulin resistance and improves glucose use.[30] The Prospective Diabetes Study in the United Kingdom evaluated the response of 3,044 new non–insulin-dependent diabetes mellitus (NIDDM) patients to dietary modification. Overweight or obese patients followed a 3-month, low-calorie diet that had 30% of calories from fat. Of the patients, 16% with a 13% reduction in body weight experienced a near normal fasting plasma glucose due to the weight loss.[31]

Twenty urban, free-living, obese native Hawaiians received a high-fiber, 7% fat, and 78% carbohydrate diet. They could eat when and as much as they wanted. An automatic decline in energy intake of about 1,000 kcal per day occurred 3 months later. In addition, a significant mean weight loss of 17 pounds with a range of 4.4 to 33 pounds was observed. Fasting serum glucose declined from 160 mg/dL to 122 mg/dL. Hypoglycemia was common for several women, warranting a change in medications. Significantly lower fasting serum triglycerides, total cholesterol, LDL cholesterol, and systolic and diastolic blood pressures were also reported.[32]

Ten overweight NIDDM patients living in Derby, Western Australia, were returned to a 7-week hunter-gatherer existence. All experienced a reduction in dietary fat from 40% of calories to 13% of calories. Physical activity increased, and an average weight loss of 17.6 pounds occurred. Fasting plasma glucose concentrations declined from 207 mg/dL to 118 mg/dL, and a significant reduction in fasting plasma insulin and triglycerides occurred.[33]

One can identify the optimal carbohydrate-containing foods for persons with diabetes by using the postprandial glycemic effect of foods. In one 12-week crossover study, high- and low-GI diets were compared. Glycemic control improved for individuals on the low-GI diet compared with those on the high-GI diet. The low-GI diet produced a lower 8-hour plasma glucose profile, less glycosuria, and a significantly lower glycosylated hemoglobin level (i.e., 7.0 ± 0.3% versus 7.9 ± 0.5%).[34]

Alpha-lipoic acid (ALA) is the component of interest. Patients with diabetes have been found to have elevated levels of free radicals in their bodies. ALA is unique among known antioxidants because of its combination water and fat solubility. By scavenging free radicals in both water- and fat-based tissues, and by recycling other important antioxidants including vitamins C and E and glutathione, ALA is proving effective in preventing cataracts, treating diabetic neuropathy, and controlling blood sugar levels. Although high doses of ALA are needed to achieve these effects, only minor side effects have been documented. It has been estimated that as many as 15% of US endocrinologists already prescribe ALA to their patients with diabetes.

Vitamin B_{12} has also shown promise in treating diabetic neuropathy. In 1 double-blind, placebo-controlled study, 50 patients with diabetic neuropathy were treated with either 1,500 mg (divided into 3 daily doses) of methylocobalamin or placebo over a 4-month period. Somatic and autonomic symptoms of neuropathy were significantly improved in those receiving the vitamin B_{12}. Additional research is needed to further evaluate the role of vitamin B_{12} in diabetic neuropathy.

Because many conventional diabetes drugs have serious side effects or lose effectiveness when used long term, the search for safe and effective alternatives has spread worldwide. Numerous herbal and other natural remedies that have been used historically are now being examined scientifically.[35]

- Preliminary studies have shown the extract of the maitake mushroom to be effective in controlling blood glucose levels and reducing insulin resistance. Clinical trials are currently in progress to determine the usefulness of maitake mushrooms in diabetes treatment.
- The leaves of *Gymnema sylvestre*, a bush that grows in western India, have been shown to be effective in the treatment of types 1 and 2 diabetes. Clinical trials confirmed the ability of *Gymnema* to induce insulin production in the pancreas, leading to decreased blood glucose, glycosylated hemoglobin, and glycosylated plasma protein levels.
- *Momordica charantia*, known as bitter melon, also native to India, has been found to have hypoglycemic effects in patients with type 2 diabetes.

Extracts of *M charantia* contain a mixture of β-sitosterol and several other active polypeptides.

- Fenugreek seed, a seasoning believed to promote digestion, has been shown to have both hypoglycemic and hypolipidemic effects. Proteins in the seeds have been shown to stimulate insulin production, while the defatted fiber-rich sections of the seeds help delay gastric emptying, thereby slowing glucose absorption. Gels in the fenugreek fiber inhibit cholesterol absorption from the small intestine and bile acid reabsorption from the large intestine.

- A few studies have found the ginsenosides and eleuthorosides in ginseng root to have a hypoglycemic effect. It has been speculated that ginseng may cause an elevation in mood, which improves self-care, leading to improved glucose control. American ginseng may reduce blood sugar levels up to 20% in people with and without diabetes.

A few studies have compared eating pattern with meal frequency. Smaller, frequent meals can reduce postprandial insulin secretion and enhance peripheral tissue insulin sensitivity. A 1-day evaluation among 11 NIDDM patients showed that nibblers who consumed food with hourly snacks had significant reductions in mean blood glucose, serum insulin, and C-peptide concentration during a 9.5-hour study period when compared with those who ate 3 meals and 1 snack.[36] This suggests that eating over a longer period (grazing) and consuming foods that are slowly absorbed (foods high in soluble fiber) or that have a low GI can be beneficial.

The Diabetes Control and Complications Trial

Secondary and tertiary prevention in the form of nutrition counseling that leads to self-management may lower additional medical cost for individuals with diabetes.

The Diabetes Control and Complications Trial was a multicenter, randomized clinical trial designed to compare intensive with conventional diabetes therapy and the effects on the development and progression of the early vascular and neurologic complications of insulin-dependent diabetes mellitus (IDDM).[37] A total of 1,441 patients 13 to 39 years old were recruited at 29 centers from 1983 through 1989. In June 1993, after an average follow-up of 6.5 years (range 3 to 9 years), the independent data monitoring committee determined that the study results warranted terminating the trial.[38]

Conventional therapy for 143 patients consisted of 1 or 2 daily injections of insulin that contained mixed, intermediate, and rapid-acting insulins; daily self-monitoring of urine or blood glucose; and extensive education about a tailored eating pattern and exercise.[39] The goals of conventional therapy included the absence of symptoms attributable to glycosuria or hyperglycemia; the absence of ketonuria; the maintenance of normal growth, development, and reasonable body weight; and freedom from severe or frequent hypoglycemia.

Intensive therapy for 77 patients included the administration of insulin 3 or more times daily by injection or an external pump. The pump dosage was adjusted according to the results of self-monitoring of blood glucose performed at least 4 times per day, dietary intake (see Table 13–4), and anticipated exercise. The goals of the intensive therapy were as follows:

- preprandial blood glucose concentrations between 70 and 120 mg per deciliter (i.e., 3.9 to 6.7 mmol per liter)
- postprandial concentrations of less than 180 mg per deciliter (i.e., 10 mmol per liter)
- a weekly 3 AM measurement of greater than 65 mg per deciliter (i.e., 3.6 mmol per liter)
- HbA1c (glycated hemoglobin) monthly measurement within the normal range (e.g., less than 6.05%)[37]

Adherence and effectiveness were reflected in the substantial difference over time between the HbA1c values of the intensive therapy group and those of the conventional therapy group. A statistically significant difference in the average HbA1c value was maintained after baseline between the intensive therapy and conventional therapy groups in both cohorts ($p < 0.001$).

After 5 years, the cumulative incidence of retinopathy in the intensive therapy group was approximately 50% less than in the conventional therapy group. After an average of 6 years of follow-up, retinopathy developed in 23 patients in the intensive therapy group and 91 patients in the conventional therapy group. Intensive therapy lowered the adjusted mean risk of retinopathy by 76%, with a 95% confidence interval of 62-85%. During the study period, intensive therapy reduced the average risk of retinopathy progression

TABLE 13–4 Dietary Guidelines Used in the Diabetes Control and Complications Trial

Dietary Component	Guideline
Energy	To achieve and maintain 90-120% of reasonable body weight and/or provide for normal growth and development.
Carbohydrate	50% of total daily energy intake; 45-55% is the acceptable range. Simple sugars should contribute no more than 25% of energy from carbohydrate.
Fat	30% of total energy intake with upper acceptable limit of 35%.
Cholesterol	Intake of no more than 600 mg/day. Amended in July 1988 to be consistent with the National Cholesterol Education Program Step 1 guidelines (i.e., intake of cholesterol < 300 mg/day; total fat < 30% of total energy; saturated fatty acids < 10% of total energy; polyunsaturated fatty acids up to 10% of total energy; monounsaturated fatty acids 10-15% of total energy).
Polyunsaturated to saturated fat ratio	One is desirable; 0.8 is the acceptable lower limit.
Fiber	Encouraged without use of pharmacologic fiber supplements.
Alcohol	In moderation.
Protein	10-25% of total daily energy intake but no less than 0.8 g/kg for adults, 0.84 g/kg for persons aged 15 to 18 years, and 1.0 g/kg for persons aged 11 to 14 years.

Source: Adapted from: DCCT. Nutrition interventions for intensive therapy in the Diabetes Control and Complications Trial. *J Am Diet Assoc.* 1993;93(7):768-772. Used with permission of the American Dietetic Association.

by 54% (95% confidence interval of 39-66%). Intensive therapy reduced hypercholesterolemia by 34%, defined as a serum concentration of low-density lipoprotein cholesterol greater than 160 mg per deciliter or 4.14 mmol per liter (95% confidence interval of 7-54%, $p = 0.02$). When all major cardiovascular and peripheral vascular events were combined, intensive therapy reduced the risk of macrovascular disease by 41%. This was 0.5 events per 100 patient-years, from 0.8 events (95% confidence interval of 10% to 68%).[37]

The incidence of severe hypoglycemia, including multiple episodes in some patients, was approximately 3 times higher in the intensive therapy group than in the conventional therapy group ($p < 0.001$). In the intensive therapy group, there were 62 hypoglycemic episodes per 100 patient-years in which assistance was required, as compared with 19 such episodes per 100 patient-years in the conventional therapy group. This included 16 and 5 episodes of coma or seizure per 100 patient-years in the respective groups.

There were no deaths, myocardial infarctions, or strokes definitely attributable to hypoglycemia, and no significant differences between groups with regard to the number of major accidents requiring hospitalization (20 in the intensive therapy group and 22 in the conventional therapy group). There were 2 fatal motor vehicle accidents, 1 in each group, in which hypoglycemia may have had a causative role. In addition, a person not involved in the trial was killed in a motor vehicle accident involving a car driven by a patient in the intensive therapy group who was probably hypoglycemic. There were 54 brief hospitalizations to treat severe hypoglycemia in 40 patients in the intensive therapy group, as compared with 36 hospitalizations in 27 patients in the conventional therapy group. This includes 7 and 4 hospitalizations, respectively, to treat hypoglycemia-related injuries.

Weight gain was a problem for individuals who received intensive therapy. There was a 33% increase in the mean adjusted risk of becoming overweight (defined as a body weight more than 120% above the ideal). There were 12.7 cases of excess weight per 100 patient-years in the intensive therapy group, versus 9.3 in the conventional therapy group. At 5 years, patients who received intensive therapy had gained a mean of 4.6 kg more than patients who received conventional therapy.

The final recommendations from the study were as follows[40,41]:

- Most individuals with IDDM should be treated with closely monitored intensive regimens, with the goal of maintaining their glycemic status as close to the normal range as safely possible.
- Due to the risk of hypoglycemia, intensive therapy should be implemented with caution, especially in patients with repeated severe hypoglycemia or those unaware of hypoglycemia.
- The risk-benefit ratio with intensive therapy may be less favorable in children under 13 years of age and in patients with advanced complications, such as end-stage renal disease or cardiovascular or cerebrovascular disease.
- Individuals with proliferative or severe nonproliferative retinopathy may be at high risk for accelerated retinopathy after the start of intensive therapy and should be followed closely by their ophthalmologists.

The Diabetes Control and Complications Trial did not include individuals with type 2 diabetes. Hyperglycemia is associated with the presence or progression of complications in both types 1 and 2.[42,43] The main conclusions of this trial emphasize the benefits of reducing glycemia in IDDM. However, these conclusions are applicable to individuals with NIDDM. Care should be taken to address age, capabilities, and coexisting diseases when defining the preferred management. Healthcare professionals should be cautious about the use of therapies other than medical nutrition therapy that are aimed at achieving euglycemia in patients with NIDDM.[37,43]

The Diabetes Prevention Trial-Type 1, sponsored by the National Institute of Diabetes and Digestive and Kidney Diseases (NIDDK), is nationwide in the United States and in Canada. The purpose is to evaluate the onset of diabetes among high-risk people. Information is available at (800) HALT-DM1 or http://www.niddk.nih.gov.

Comorbidities in Diabetes

People with diabetes are an important and growing subset of the hypertensive population. Of diabetic complications, 30-75% can be attributed to hypertension. The control of hypertension is essential to reduce the likelihood of stroke and coronary heart disease. By controlling hypertension, one can slow the progression of renal failure and potential onset of heart disease.

Hypertension (HTN) (blood pressure $\geq$ 140/90 mm Hg) is a common comorbidity of diabetes, affecting the majority of people with diabetes, depending on type of diabetes, age, obesity, and ethnicity. HTN is also a major risk factor for cardiovascular (CVD) and microvascular complications such as retinopathy and nephropathy. In type 1 diabetes, HTN is often the result of underlying nephropathy. In type 2 diabetes, HTN may be present as part of the metabolic syndrome (i.e., obesity, hyperglycemia, and dyslipidemia) that is accompanied by high rates of CVD.

Randomized clinical trials have demonstrated the benefit (reduction of CHD events, stroke, and nephropathy) of lowering blood pressure to < 130 mm Hg systolic and < 80 mm Hg diastolic in individuals with diabetes.[44-47] Epidemiologic analyses show that blood pressure > 115/75 mm Hg is associated with increased cardiovascular event rates and mortality in individuals with diabetes.[44,48,49] Therefore, a target blood pressure goal of < 130/80 mmHg is reasonable if it can be safely achieved.

Although there are no well-controlled studies of diet and exercise in the treatment of HTN in individuals with diabetes, reducing sodium intake and body weight (when indicated); increasing consumption of fruits, vegetables, and low-fat dairy products; avoiding excessive alcohol consumption; and increasing activity levels have been shown to be effective in reducing blood pressure in nondiabetic individuals.[50] These nonpharmacological strategies may also positively affect glycemia and lipid control. Their effects on cardiovascular events have not been well measured.

Elevated blood pressure can be reduced with weight loss of 4 to 8 kg minimum, limiting sodium intake to 2,400 mg per day, limiting alcohol intake to no more than 2 drinks a day, increasing exercise from none or once to 3 to 4 times a week, and stopping smoking if applicable. Alternate approaches include an increase in potassium, calcium, and fish oil, with a decrease in total fat and caffeine intakes. An acute 5 to 15 mm Hg increase in blood pressure is noted 15 minutes after ingestion of 250 mg of caffeine. These alternate approaches to reducing blood pressure vary in effect among individuals, and they remain the focus of continued research.[51]

Elevated levels of insulin may make people prone to blood clots.[52] Individuals with type 2 diabetes are resistant to insulin and experience elevated insulin levels. About 75% of people with the most common type of diabetes die of heart attacks or strokes. This has been previously assigned to high blood pressure and low levels of HDL cholesterol.

Of about 3,000 participants in the Framingham Offspring Study, both diabetics and nondiabetics had both elevated insulin levels and levels of PAI-1 antigen, a chemical that stops the blood's ability to dissolve clots. Insulin resistance reduces the blood's ability to dissolve clots. Exercise increases the effectiveness of insulin and improves the dissolution of blood clots, possibly lowering the risk of cardiovascular disease.[11] Exhibit 13-2 provides guidelines for the management of comorbidities with diabetes mellitus.

Exhibit 13-2   Management of Comorbidities With Diabetes Mellitus

---

Hypertension
- The optimal BP goal for patients with diabetes is unknown. In general, the goal of therapy is to reduce BP to ≤ 140/90, in a gradual, stepwise fashion to avoid hypotension. A further reduction to ≤ 130/85 is reasonable if tolerated; control of HTN can decrease nephropathy, cerebrovascular disease, and coronary artery disease.
- Optimize lifestyle modifications (diet, exercise, weight management).
- Angiotensin converting enzyme inhibitors (ACEIs) and low-dose diuretics or α-blockers.
- Calcium channel blockers use in diabetics is controversial and might increase risk of vascular events.

Hyperlipidemia
- The most common presentation is normal LDL-C (although the LDL-C is small, dense, and atherogenic), low HDL-C, and high TG. Abnormalities resolve as diabetic control improves.
- The recommended LDL-C goal is ≤ 130 mg/dL (3.35 mmol/L) in patients without CAD and ≤ 100 mg/dL (2.6 mmol/L) in patients with CAD.
- Diet and lifestyle changes first; drug therapy second.
- If medication is indicated to meet LDL-C target goal, an HMGCoA reductase inhibitor (lovastatin or simvastatin) is recommended. A 25-45% decrease in LDL-C is anticipated when using these agents. Triglycerides usually fall about 5-15%.
- Fibrates such as gemfibrozil or fenofibrate may be considered in patients where a very high triglyceride, e.g, ≥ 500 mg/dL, is the primary lipid abnormality.
- Niacin can decrease LDL-C and triglycerides by approximately 20% and 40%, respectively; however, it can cause glucose intolerance, so it should be tried with caution.

---

continued

Exhibit 13-2   continued

- Bile acid resins may cause hypertriglyceridemia.
- Annual screening for dyslipidemia is recommended.

Diabetic Neuropathy
- Sixty percent of patients will develop neuropathy after 25 years of DM.
- There are several different types of diabetic neuropathy, the most common being distal polyneuropathy with burning, shooting, or stabbing pain in the feet and lower extremities.
- Good glycemic control, warm baths, pressure garments that decrease the movement of hair follicles, and analgesics like acetaminophen or aspirin help to relieve symptoms.
- If the above measures do not control pain, low-dose tricyclic antidepressants may be tried. Commonly, amitriptyline, imipramine, or nortriptyline 25 mg at bedtime is given with the dose gradually increased to a maximum of 150 mg if needed. Monitor patients for side effects such as confusion, orthostatic hypotension, and urinary retention.
- Patients with localized burning, hyperesthetic, or stabbing pain can be treated topically with 0.025% and 0.075% capsaicin cream, applied 3-4 times/day for 3-4 weeks.

Diabetic Nephropathy
- Defined as ≥ 300 mg of urine albumin in a 24-hour period, retinopathy, and no other identifiable cause of renal disease.
- Optimal control of hypertension, glucose levels, and the use of ACEIs.
- Screening for microalbuminuria for type 2 diabetics should be done at the time of diagnosis and annually thereafter.

Cardiovascular Disease
- Control contributing risk factors.
- Aspirin therapy:
  o Enteric-coated 81-325 mg/day if no aspirin allergy, bleeding tendency, or anticoagulant therapy.

Note: For women of childbearing age, discuss contraception and emphasis of diabetes control before conception and during pregnancy.
Source: American Diabetes Association, Inc. Position statement—diagnosis and classification of diabetes mellitus. *Diabetes Care*. 2005;28:S37-S42.

Diabetes and Disordered Eating

Diabetes may predispose some individuals to aberrant eating patterns. Several physiologic and psychodynamic risk factors are identified, and stages of progression to disordered eating have been described[53] (see Exhibit 13-3). An acute concern for individuals with diabetes who have a disordered eating pattern is ketoacidosis, which results from severe hypoglycemia or hyperglycemia.[54]

The hypoglycemia condition results from food restrictions, delayed meals or snacks, purging to vomit food, frequent use of laxatives or enemas, and excess insulin to hide overeating or binging. Hyperglycemia may be acute or can span several hours. It is strengthened by lack of judgment during the stressful period around a binge, inappropriate management of insulin and

Exhibit 13–3   Stages of Progression to Disordered Eating

Abnormal Eating
- May or may not eat in response to dysphoria.
- Deliberately cheats.
- Overeats at meals frequently.

Compulsive Eating
- Loses concept of normal eating.
- Binges at mealtimes.
- Hoards food.
- Has feelings of being denied food that others are allowed.

Addictive Eating
- Manipulates to obtain food.
- Denies eating.
- Feels guilty about eating.
- Anxious about not having enough food.

Eating Disorder
- Obsessed with weight and food.
- Has a body-image distortion.
- Binges at meal or nonmeal times.
- Starves.
- Purges to relieve guilt or anxiety or to maintain weight, including skipping insulin.
- Uses food as weapon.

Source: Adapted from: Davidow DN, Turner M. Complications of coexisting diabetes mellitus and eating disorders in IDDM. *On the Cutting Edge.* 1994;15(6):9. Used with permission of the American Dietetic Association.

Info Line

The National Digestive Diseases Information Clearinghouse (NDDIC) is a service of the National Institute of Diabetes and Digestive and Kidney Diseases (NIDDK), one of the National Institutes of Health (NIH), under the US Department of Health and Human Services. Established in 1980, the clearinghouse provides information about digestive diseases to people with these conditions and to their families, healthcare professionals, and the public. NDDIC responds to inquiries; develops, reviews, and distributes publications; and works closely with professional and patient organizations and government agencies to coordinate resources about digestive diseases. Its Web site is at www.niddk.nih.gov.

The Diabetes Care and Education Dietetic Practice Group of the American Dietetic Association Web site is at www.dce.org. Features include *Recipe of the Month,* where diabetic recipes with nutrient analysis are posted, and *Diabetes Newswires,* where daily newswires are scanned for articles on diabetes and nutrition and are posted.

TABLE 13–5   Problems That Cause Overeating Among Individuals With Diabetes

Situation	Description
Negative emotions	Individual is tempted to overeat to cope with stress and negative emotions.
Resisting temptation	Food, food cues, or cravings are temptations to eat inappropriate foods.
Eating out	Eating at restaurants makes adherence difficult.
Feeling deprived	Individual is tempted to give up trying because of feelings of deprivation.
Time pressure	Time pressure makes eating right or treating reactions very difficult.
Temptation to relapse	Individual considers giving up and no longer trying to eat right.
Planning	Hectic life makes planning what and when to eat difficult.
Competing priorities	Responsibilities and obligations get in the way of eating right.
Social events	Parties, holidays, and socializing are temptations to overeat and make poor food choices.
Family support	Family's behaviors are less than supportive.
Food refusal	People offer inappropriate foods, and it is difficult to refuse without hurting their feelings.
Friends' support	Friends' behaviors are less than supportive.

Source: Adapted from: Schlundt DG. Emotional eating. *On the Cutting Edge.* 1994;15-19. Used with permission of the American Dietetic Association.

other medications, and lack of attention to self-care.[55,56] A cluster analysis compiling data from 26 adults with diabetes (12 insulin-dependent and 14 non-insulin-dependent adults) identified everyday problem situations that cause overeating (see Table 13–5).[56]

Rapid weight gain from fluid retention or insulin edema and efficient use of food energy frequently occur when blood glucose returns to a normal range. The success in glucose control complicates the management of disordered eating, as the individual may be very anxious about the weight gain and react with a purge or binge.[57] A successful strategy has been flexible insulin administration, which involves allowing the individual to administer an amount of insulin consistent with the amount of food energy consumed. Adjustments are made for premeal blood glucose, exercise plans, and any potential stressors that may occur. Individuals given this liberalization of management should be able to deal honestly with themselves and the amount of food they eat. Individuals with unsuccessful management of eating and diabetes may require counseling with a psychotherapist to curb the binging behavior and regulate their blood glucose levels while taking care of their personal needs.[57]

Management Strategies

All people do not follow similar eating patterns, nor do they eat at the same times or places each day. Tastes, cultural differences, and economics influence the eating patterns of individuals with diabetes as much as they influence people without diabetes. The goal of secondary prevention approaches to diabetes is to help individuals develop self-management skills and the approaches may vary.[11] Meal planning alternatives need flexibility and ease of understanding.

Medical nutrition therapy was central to the intensive intervention in the Diabetes Control and Complications Trial (DCCT). Post-DCCT recommendations emphasize goals, not rules or regulation; practical and achievable recommendations; and customized or tailored plans. Benefits for the DCCT intensive-therapy group included neuropathy reduced by 60%; microalbuminuria decreased by 39% for people with no renal disease at baseline, and severe albuminuria slowed by over 54%; retinopathy reduced by 76% in primary prevention and by 54% in secondary prevention groups compared with conventional-therapy groups. The current medical nutrition therapy for diabetes involves the following[22]:

Type 1

- If receiving conventional therapy, maintain a consistent timing and amount of food, match insulin with food preferences, disregard fractionated calories using snacks, but synchronize food with insulin.
- Monitor blood glucose and adjust short-acting insulin in relation to the amount of food eaten to create a tight control of blood glucose.
- If multiple injections or the insulin pump is used, integrate insulin with lifestyle (e.g., adjust premeal insulin doses to exercise and food alterations).
- Strive for consistency and optimal blood glucose level.
- Alter dietary composition (i.e., fat, carbohydrate, and protein), based on other risk factors and biochemical measures.
- Recognize that sucrose and fructose have no significant advantage or disadvantage and can be a part of the overall pattern.
- Monitor blood glucose during the night for the dawn phenomenon.

Type 2

- Strive for moderate weight loss of 10 to 20 pounds minimum, with the goal to achieve a reasonable body weight.
- Space smaller meals and snacks throughout the day to attenuate post-meal hypoglycemia due to impaired insulin secretion.
- Develop an exercise program that can be followed.
- Use a weight-control eating pattern that has either a reduced-calorie (eating 500 fewer kcal/day) or very low-calorie pattern (< 800 total kcal/day).
- Dietary composition applies as outlined for type 1.
- Maintain an intense, ongoing program with contact at 1- or 2-week intervals.

The landmark DCCT evaluated the lifetime risk for diabetes mellitus in the United States since 1 in 3 people born in the United States will develop diabetes, and it may reduce his or her life by 10 or more years.[58]

Ten key challenges for the diabetes community to address over the next few decades are[59]:

1. continuing the improvements in diabetes care
2. recognizing and addressing the complexities of diabetes management
3. improving the system of care
4. broadening the definition of the medical/healthcare office
5. addressing the dual impact of the diabetes epidemic

6. recognizing and dealing with nonhealth forces on diabetes prevention and control
7. taking special opportunities for health professionals
8. empowering patients for more than good self-care
9. achieving a balance between individuality and community
10. accepting and embracing globalization

Targeted community screening for kidney disease in a high-risk population can identify individuals with chronic kidney disease, increase awareness of the disease, and improve health-seeking behavior.[60]

Additional Strategies

Conducting counseling sessions with individuals with diabetes requires baseline data, an instruction plan with user-friendly materials, and a follow-up strategy. After the initial 1 or 2 visits, a strategy to ensure adherence for a new lifestyle is warranted. It cannot be overemphasized that newly diagnosed individuals with diabetes as well as veterans of the disease need continuous booster sessions. Reinforcement of their positive efforts and realignment of misconceptions and unhealthy practices are essential to maintain control. Exhibit 13–4 delineates adherence techniques for healthcare providers.

The Transtheoretical Model and Type 2 Diabetes Mellitus

The Transtheoretical Model[61-63] has been applied in the past 20 years in research on health behavior change[64,65] because programs based on it may increase the effectiveness of interventions and help people make change that lasts.[65-68]

The basic premise of the model is that behavior change is a dynamic process—when people change a behavior, they move through a virtually

Exhibit 13–4   Techniques for Encouraging Adherence

- Involve the individual and the primary decision maker as a vital part of the team.
- Establish a supportive working relationship by being nonjudgmental, positive, and helpful.
- Use appropriate language for the individual's understanding.
- Address the individual's concerns.
- Meet his/her expectations.
- Enlist the family and include them in the education process.
- Individualize the medical nutrition therapy to the individual's lifestyle.
- Give feedback on progress: blood glucose, glycosylated hemoglobin, lipid levels, weight.
- Use contingency plans.
- Use relapse prevention therapy.
- Use role-playing scenarios for decision making.
- Schedule frequent follow-up.
- Reward adherence to medical regimens.

Source: Adapted from: Powers MA, ed. *Nutrition Guide for Professionals: Diabetes Education and Meal Planning.* Alexandria, Va: American Diabetes Association and the American Dietetic Association; 1988:9. Used with permission.

universal series of 5 sequential and predictable stages of change. To facilitate forward movement through the stages, health professionals can use methods (called change processes) that are appropriate (or matched) to the client's stage (see Table 13–6). Health professionals can guide clients to reevaluate their views about the pros and cons of behavior change (decisional balance) and help them develop the confidence needed to adopt a new way of eating and resist temptations to continue or revert to old behavior patterns (self-efficacy).[66]

Info Line

The American Diabetes Association is a nonprofit organization of professionals and volunteers who are concerned with diabetes and its complications. A central theme of diabetes care is to know the causes and strategies to manage high and low blood sugar levels. Spanish and English versions of materials are often available. The association extends to more than 70 countries with over 800 affiliates.

The American Diabetes Association funds meritorious research, publishes the latest scientific findings, and provides services to people with diabetes, their families, healthcare professionals, and the public. *Diabetes Forecast* is a monthly publication of the American Diabetes Association for the public. It translates research data into layperson's terms and highlights events in the lives of individuals living with diabetes.

The American Diabetes Association may be the central resource for diabetes education in a community. The strength of any nonprofit organization depends on the size and enthusiasm of its volunteer force. Family members often become avid volunteers and, in the process, learn how to assist their own family members better. In Los Angeles, the Latino Outreach Programs of the American Diabetes Association provide volunteer opportunities targeted to high-risk groups. For example, volunteers can sign up to assist with the following:

- Program planning committee—to develop educational activities for patients with diabetes and their families, and publicly represent the American Diabetes Association through participation in community events, health fairs, and media interviews.
- Patient education—to organize and implement monthly patient education programs and seminars.
- Support groups—to facilitate bilingual Latino support groups.
- Youth programs—to organize educational and social programs for Latino children with diabetes and maintain an active youth registry.
- Unidos Contra la Diabetes Health Fair—to plan and implement the annual public education and screening fair, including identification of sponsors, exhibitors, product donations, screening providers, event promotion, and event day logistics.
- Unidos Contra la Diabetes, Una Noche de Honor fundraising committee—to participate in the annual testimonial dinner including identifying honorees and soliciting sponsors and auction item donations.

For more information, contact the American Diabetes Association, Customer Service Department, 1660 Duke Street, Alexandria, VA 22314. Telephone (800) 232-3472 or (703) 549-1500.

TABLE 13–6 Common Change Processes for Each Stage of Behavioral Change Based on the Transtheoretical Model and Applicable to Diabetes Mellitus

		Stage		
Precontemplation	**Contemplation**	**Preparation**	**Action**	**Maintenance**
Consciousness raising	————————>			
Social liberation				
	Emotional arousal ————>			
	Self-reevaluation ————>			
		Commitment		
			Countering ——————>	
			Environmental control ——>	
			Rewards ——————>	
			Helping relationships ——>	

Source: Adapted from: Byrd-Bredbenner C, Finckenor M. Putting the transtheoretical model into practice with type 2 diabetes mellitus patients. *Top Clin Nutr.* 2000;15(3):44-58.

Special Issues in Managing Diabetes

During Childhood and Adolescence

The initial classification of diabetes is usually based on the clinical picture at intake. Children with immune-mediated type 1 diabetes are not overweight but have recent weight loss, polyuria, and polydipsia. As the US population becomes increasingly overweight, however, the percentage of children with immune-mediated type 1 diabetes who are obese is increasing with 24% overweight at the time of diagnosis. Children with immune-mediated diabetes usually have a short duration of symptoms and frequently have ketosis; 30-40% have ketoacidosis at intake.[69] After metabolic stabilization, children have brief diminished insulin requirements called the honeymoon period, then required insulin for survival and are at continual risk for ketoacidosis. Of children with immune-mediated type 1 diabetes, 5% have a first- or second-degree relative with the same disease.[69]

Conversely, most children with type 2 diabetes are overweight or obese at diagnosis and have glycosuria without ketonuria, absent or mild polyuria and polydipsia, and little or no weight loss. About 33% have ketonuria at diagnosis and 5-25% of patients who are subsequently classified as having type 2 diabetes have ketoacidosis at presentation. These patients may have ketoacidosis without any associated stress, other illness, or infection. Children with type 2 diabetes usually have a family history of type 2 diabetes, and those of non-European ancestry (Americans of African, Hispanic, Asian, and American Indian descent) are disproportionately represented.[70]

Type 2 diabetes mellitus among American Indian/Alaska native youth is an alarming new morbidity that, without intervention, will lead to significant increased morbidity and mortality during adulthood. Healthcare professionals must address multiple medical and psychosocial concerns within the context of a medical home with the goal of coordinating comprehensive services from healthcare professionals and the community. Healthcare professionals who care for families affected by type 2 diabetes mellitus face the challenge of motivating people to adopt significant behavioral changes. Several interventions have proved effective in preventing diabetes complications among adults, and evaluation of these interventions in children with type 2 diabetes mellitus is urgently needed.[71]

As with adults, a multidisciplinary team approach is recommended (e.g., a physician, a registered dietitian who may be a community nutrition professional, a nurse, and a behavioral specialist trained in pediatric diabetes). A complete nutrition assessment forms the foundation of the eating pattern. It should include the following[11]:

- Probable reasons for poor weight gain or linear growth should be assessed. Usually these are due to poor glycemic control, inadequate insulin, and overrestriction of food energy. Excessive weight gain may be caused by excessive energy intake, overtreatment of hypoglycemia, overinsulinization, or low activity level.
- The role of parents and caregivers and extent of previous nutrition education should be assessed. Prior food likes and dislikes, lifestyle, and family economics should be determined.
- A 24-hour recall or food record to reveal a typical day can be computerized to determine total energy, macro- and micronutrient intake, and

TABLE 13–7   Plasma Blood Glucose and A1c Goals for Type 1 Diabetes by Age of Child

Values by Age (years)	Plasma Blood Glucose Goal Range (mg/dL)		A1c (%)	Rationale
	Before Meals	Bedtime/ Overnight		
Toddlers and preschoolers (< 6)	100-180	110-200	≤ 8.5 (but ≥ 7.5%)	• High risk and vulnerable to hypoglycemia
School age (6-12)	90-180	100-180	< 8%	• Risks of hypoglycemia and relatively low risk of complications prior to puberty
Adolescents and young adults (13-19)	90-130	90-150	< 7.5%*	• Risk of hypoglycemia • Developmental and psychological issues

*A lower goal (< 7.0%) is reasonable if it can be achieved without excessive hypoglycemia.
Source: American Diabetes Association, Inc. Position statement—diagnosis and classification of diabetes mellitus. *Diabetes Care.* 2005;28:S37-S42.

meal and snack distribution. The child's total eating environment can be reviewed to acquire an accurate picture of the usual eating routine and food sources, including school routine, weekday routine, relationships with siblings and friends, and factors that influence food choices such as self-care skills.

Plasma blood glucose and A1c goals for children with type 1 diabetes are outlined in Table 13–7.

Due to the increased diagnosis of type 2 diabetes among children, an emergency plan to treat hypoglycemia has been developed for schools as a quick response. The school nurse usually coordinates care, but all personnel responsible for students with diabetes should be involved.[72]

When symptoms of hypoglycemia are observed for a child, school personnel should give a quick-acting sugar product equivalent to 15 grams of carbohydrate. This may include 3 or 4 glucose tablets, 3 teaspoons (or three fourths of a tube) of glucose gel, 4 ounces of juice, or 6 ounces (half a can) of nondiet soda. The child's blood glucose level should be checked 10 to 15 minutes later and repeated if blood glucose level is not within student's target range.[72]

Appendix 13–A outlines a quick reference emergency plan for a student with either hyperglycemia or hypoglycemia.

During Adult and Older Adult Years

Fung et al assessed the associations between major dietary patterns and risk of type 2 diabetes in adult women. Dietary information was collected 4 times between 1984 and 1994 from 69,554 women 38 to 63 years old. None had a history of diabetes, cardiovascular disease, or cancer in 1984. Factor analysis identified 2 major dietary patterns: prudent and western. The prudent pattern included higher intakes of fruits, vegetables, legumes, fish, poultry, and whole grains, while the western pattern included higher intakes of red and processed meats, sweets and desserts, french fries, and refined grains. In 14 years of follow-up, 2,699 incident cases of type 2 diabetes occurred. After adjusting for potential confounders, a relative risk for diabetes of 1.49 (95% confidence interval [CI], 1.26-1.76, P for trend, < 0.001) was found when comparing the highest to lowest quintiles of the western pattern. Positive associations were also observed between type 2 diabetes and red meat and other processed meats. The relative risk for diabetes for every 1-serving increase in intake is 1.26 (95% CI, 1.21-1.42) for red meat, 1.38 (95% CI, 1.23-1.56) for total processed meats, 1.73 (95% CI, 1.39-2.16) for bacon, 1.49 (95% CI, 1.04-2.11) for hot dogs, and 1.43 (95% CI, 1.22-1.69) for processed meats.[73]

Approximately one half of US individuals with type 2 diabetes are over 65 years old. The major reason for glucose intolerance observed among older adults is insulin resistance. Medications to treat comorbidity and polypharmacy in general may complicate diabetes therapy among senior adults. Medications that may increase hyperglycemia include diuretics, glucocorticoids, nicotinic acid, lithium, and other antidepressants. Medications that enhance hypoglycemia are beta-blockers, monoamine oxidase inhibitors, phenylbutazone, large doses of aspirin, and cimetidine. Seniors are at a greater risk from acute illnesses and complications of chronic illnesses. Their recovery from physiologic insults of fractures and acute illness is also slower and impaired when they have diabetes.[21,74] Specific concerns for seniors include the following:

- acute hyperglycemia and dehydration, which can lead to a hyperglycemic hyperosmolar nonketotic syndrome (a very high blood glucose without ketones—i.e., 400 to 2,800 mg/dL); mortality rate is 20% to 40% of patients
- hypoglycemia
- persistent hyperglycemia, which has deleterious effects on the body's defense against infection

During Illness

When illness occurs, glucose levels may rise but individuals must still take insulin. Appetite often wanes, which restricts food intake. To avoid hypoglycemia, carbohydrates should be replaced during illness. At least 50 grams of carbohydrate should be eaten every 3 to 4 hours (e.g., 2.5 cups of carbonated beverages, three fourths cup of sherbet, and 3 to 5 slices of toast). Eight to twelve ounces of liquid should be consumed every hour. Salty foods and beverages are advised if vomiting and diarrhea have occurred to replace electrolytes.

During Pregnancy

The goal of medical nutrition therapy is to reduce the incidence of birth defects and risk of macrosomia, which can cause a complicated delivery and high-risk nursery care.[75,76] Birth defects are marked by abnormal glucose tolerance during pregnancy. Without monitoring and control, the elevated blood glucose can lead to fetal or infant sickness and potentially death.[77] Infants born to women with gestational diabetes often exceed average birth weights (e.g., over 10 pounds at birth) and may experience increased risk of obesity and impaired glucose tolerance later in life.

Five nonrandomized studies compared rates of major congenital problems among infants whose mothers participated in preconception diabetes care programs or intensive diabetes management after they were already pregnant. The preconception care programs were multidisciplinary and involved diabetes self-management with diet, insulin, and testing glucose levels. More than 80% of the moms achieved normal A1c concentrations before they became pregnant. In all 5 studies, the incidence of major congenital malformations in women who participated in preconception care (range 1.0-1.7% of infants) was much lower than the incidence in women who did not participate (range 1.4-10.9% of infants).[78-82] It is not known for sure if the lower congenital problems were due to improved diabetes care, but it appears that malformations can be reduced or prevented by careful management of diabetes before pregnancy.

Recommendations for the management of pregnant women who have diabetes are as follows[11]:

- A1c levels should be normal or as close to normal as possible (< 1% above the upper limits of normal) in an individual patient before conception is attempted.
- All women with diabetes and child-bearing potential should be educated about the need for good glucose control before pregnancy. They should participate in family planning.
- Women with diabetes who are contemplating pregnancy should be evaluated and, if indicated, treated for diabetic retinopathy, nephropathy, neuropathy, and CVD.
- Among the drugs commonly used in the treatment of patients with diabetes, statins should be discontinued before conception. ACE inhibitors in the first trimester may give maternal benefit that can outweigh fetal risk, but later in the pregnancy they should generally be discontinued. Use of metformin and acarbose before and during pregnancy should be reviewed for the individual woman.

After delivery, gestational diabetes mellitus (GDM) disappears in 90% of the mothers.[83] Table 13-8 outlines ways to identify women with gestational diabetes.

When Postexercise, Late-Onset Hypoglycemia Occurs

Hypoglycemia can occur 6 to 15 hours after strenuous exercise. This is different from the more immediate type of hypoglycemia that occurs 1 to 2 hours after exercise. Postexercise, late-onset (PEL) hypoglycemia can result in stupor, coma, and/or seizures. This can be the result of vigorous swimming for 3 hours or starting a 3 mile/day running program. In a 2-year prospective case study of 300 persons with IDDM, 48 (16%) had PEL hypoglycemia. Frequent

TABLE 13-8 Methods to Identify Women With Gestational Diabetes

Method 1—Screening and a 3-Hour 100-Gram OGTT	Method 2—2-Hour, 75-gram OGTT
• All pregnant women screened at 24-28 weeks gestation, or earlier if risk factors present. Women who present for their first prenatal visit later than 28 weeks are screened at that first visit, any time of the day. Fasting is not required.	• Test no later than 24-48 weeks; earlier if risk factors present.
• Administer a 50-gram glucose load followed by a 1-hour plasma glucose: Negative if < 140 mg/dL Positive if ≥ 140 mg/dL	• 75-gram 2-hour oral glucose tolerance test is done after an overnight fast for at least 8 hours but not more than 14 hours and after at least 3 days of unrestricted diet and physical activity.
• Values ≥ 140 mg/dL but ≤ 190 mg/dL require follow-up with a 3-hour 100-gram oral GTT.	
• If the blood glucose screening value is ≥ 191 mg/dL, a fasting blood glucose should be checked. An elevated screening value and fasting value ≥ 95 mg/dL would provide 2 abnormal values; treatment for gestational diabetes is recommended. A 3-hour GTT is not required and if administered may result in an unnecessary blood glucose elevation.	
• The 3-hour 100-gram GTT is done after an overnight fast for 8 hours, but not more than14 hours and after 3 days of unrestricted diet and physical activity.	• Abnormal values with 2 values equaled or exceeded to diagnose GD:
• Abnormal 3-hour 100-gram GTT with 2 out of 4 values must be equaled or exceeded to diagnose GD:	Fasting glucose level ≥ 95 mg/dL 1-hour glucose level ≥ 180 mg/dL 2-hour glucose level ≥ 155 mg/dL
Fasting glucose level ≥ 95 mg/dL 1-hour glucose level ≥ 180 mg/dL 2-hour glucose level ≥ 155 mg/dL 3-hour glucose level ≥ 140 mg/dL	

Source: Adapted from: Carpenter MW, Coustan DR. Criteria for screening tests of gestational diabetes. *Amer J Ob Gyn.* 1992;144:768.

monitoring of blood sugar in the evening and overnight is recommended. Food should be added if the person is weak, exhausted, or hungry. Insulin should be reduced.[84,85]

Legislation and a Global Approach

In 2000, Medicare Part B coverage for MNT of diabetes mellitus and kidney disease was approved by the US Congress. The Medicare legislation establishes registered dietitians as Medicare providers. The benefit became available January 1, 2002.

A call to Congress by the American Diabetes Association in May of 2004, in Washington, DC, involved more than 400 diabetes care and prevention advocates from every state in the United States. Visually, the red shirts and the 8,000 phone calls strengthened the same message to Capitol Hill. Requests included:

- cosponsoring the Diabetes Prevention and Treatment Act, which authorizes money for preventing diabetes and its complications
- supporting within the budget an additional $10 million for the division of diabetes at the Centers for Disease Control and Prevention, in the next budget
- increasing the National Institutes of Health budget by 10% to further lead diabetes research[86]

"Sharing global perspectives—building our common ground" was the theme of the XIV International Congress of Dietetics (ICD), in Chicago, on May 28-31, 2004. Dietetics professionals from 34 countries addressed the global scope of dietetics practice with 5 broad topics:

1. building healthy communities
2. food security
3. issues in the dietetics profession
4. food administration management
5. nutrition strategies for new epidemics

MNT for diabetes remained a priority topic for attendees, especially since estimates of worldwide diabetes cases predict an increase from 171 million in 2000 to 366 million in 2030.[87]

The American Cancer Society, American Diabetes Association, and American Heart Association joined forces in June 2004 to prevent chronic degenerative diseases. Their joint recommendations for Americans included: have blood pressure monitored every 2 years, body mass index (BMI) measured at regular health visits, blood cholesterol levels checked every 5 years starting at age 30, and a blood glucose (sugar) test every 5 years starting at age 45 years. Learn more at http://www.everydaychoices.com.

A Case for Primary Prevention of Diabetes

Can we slow or alter the conversion from a normal glucose tolerance to an impaired glucose tolerance? Longitudinal studies that track this process have not been conducted previously, but there is a growing body of data that points to the role of dietary composition on the incidence of diabetes. The intakes of vegetable fat, potassium, calcium, and magnesium were shown to be inversely associated with the 6-year incidence of self-reported diabetes of 84,360 US nurses.[88] Male Seventh-Day Adventists who had higher meat intake also had an increased death rate due to diabetes.[89] Two short-term studies reported that fish and legume intake were inversely associated and intake of pastries was positively associated with the 4-year risk of glucose intolerance.[90] A high-fat intake among individuals with impaired glucose tolerance was significantly associated with the 2-year risk of developing NIDDM.[91]

Data from the 30-year follow-up of men in the Seven Countries Study showed that of the 338 men available, 21% had an impaired glucose tolerance. These men had a higher proportion of simple sugars in their eating pattern compared with men with normal glucose tolerance, as well as a higher body mass index. For those with newly diagnosed diabetes, current fat intake and previous intakes of fat, saturated and monounsaturated fatty acids, and cholesterol were higher than intakes of men with no diabetes. Multiple regression analysis identified total fat and saturated fatty acids as independently and positively associated with 2-hour plasma glucose level; the analysis revealed that higher intakes of vitamin C, fish, potatoes, vegetables, and legumes were associated with reduced 2-hour plasma glucose levels.[92]

The authors of this study hypothesized that the role of dietary factors may differ at different stages of diabetes development. This difference is related to the 2-stage process in the development of NIDDM.[93] If the 2-step model of NIDDM development is real and food components aid in the process, then individuals should be able to slow or alter the conversion of glucose tolerance to intolerance with dietary modification. Thus, primary prevention may become a reality.

The Pima Indians: Pathfinders for Health

History paints a colorful portrait of the American Indians who live today in the Gila River Indian Community. Their ancestors were among the first people to set foot in the Americas 30,000 years ago. They have lived in the Sonoron Desert near the Gila River in what is now southern Arizona for at least 2,000 years.

Called the Pima Indians by exploring Spaniards who first encountered them in the 1600s, these early Americans called themselves "O'Odham," the river people, and those with whom they intermarried, "Tohono O'Odham," the desert people.

Archaeological finds suggest that the Pima Indians descended from the Hohokam, "those who have gone," a prehistoric people who originated in Mexico. Strong runners, the Pima Indians were also master weavers and farmers who could make the desert bloom. Once trusted scouts for the US Cavalry, the Pima Indians are pathfinders for health, helping scientists from the National Institute of Diabetes and Digestive and Kidney Diseases (NIDDK), a part of the National Institutes of Health (NIH), learn the secrets of diabetes, obesity, and their complications.[94]

Migrating from Mexico, the people settled the land up to where the Gila River and the Salt River meet, in what is now Arizona. They established a sophisticated system of irrigation that made the desert fertile with wheat, beans, squash, and cotton. The women of the community made exquisite baskets so intricately woven that they were watertight. They were also a generous people. They sheltered the Pee Posh (or Maricopa Indians) who fled attack by hostile tribes, and who also became part of the Gila River community. Anyone who followed the Gila River, the main southern route to the Pacific, encountered these peaceful and productive traders who gave hospitality to travelers for hundreds of years. "Bread is to eat, not to sell. Take what you want," they told Kit Carson in 1846.

Today, the Pima Indians of the Gila River Indian Community are still an agricultural people, nurturing orchards of orange trees, pistachios, and olives. They are still giving, too. Eleven thousand strong, the members of the Gila River Indian Reservation have participated in 30 years of research helping people avoid diabetes challenges to their eyes, hearts, and kidneys, and understanding how and why people gain weight and what can be done to prevent it.[94]

Diabetes Around the World: Singapore

The prevalence of diabetes in Singapore is as follows[95]:

- GDM: 8.6% of pregnancies
- Type 2 diabetes: 9% of adult population, noted in the 1998 National Health Survey
- Type 1 diabetes: 3.5 per 100,000 children aged 0 to 12 yrs

Ethnic or cultural food practices can help or hinder diabetes management. The high prevalence of saturated fats in cooking (coconut milk, palm oil, animal fat) makes it difficult for patients to control saturated fat intake. Most Singaporeans believe that healthier foods are not tasty. Standards of care or practice guidelines used for diabetes care and education include frequency of blood glucose monitoring: type 1, 1-2 days a week, 7 times per day; type 2, monthly to every 3 months (random or fasting); and GDM, 1-2 days a week, several times per day.[95] Targets of glycemic control are outlined in Table 13–9.

TABLE 13–9   Glycemic Control Targets for Diabetic Patients in Singapore

Age Group (yrs)	Pre-Meal* Blood Glucose Levels (mmol/L)	HbA1c (%)
< 6	5-12	7–9
6-12	4-10	6–8
> 13	4-8	6–8
GDM adult	< 5.5	6.5–7
	6.7[†]	6.5–7
	6.1-8	6.5–7
	7.1-10[†]	6.5–7

*To convert mmol/L glucose to mg/dL multiply mmol/L by 18.0
[†]2 h postmeal
Source: Ong C. Diabetes care and education around the world: Singapore. *Diabetes Care and Education Newsletter.* 2000;21:7-8.

Exhibit 13–5   DATA2010: The Healthy People 2010 Database–November 2000. Focus Area: 05-Diabetes

Objective number	Objective	Baseline Year	Baseline	Target
04-07	Kidney failure due to diabetes (rate per million, persons of all ages)	1996	113	78
	American Indian or Alaska native	1996	482	78
	Asian or Pacific Islander	1996	156	78
	Black or African American	1996	329	78
	White	1996	79	78
	Hispanic or Latino	1996	UK	78
	Not Hispanic or Latino	1996	UK	78
	Female	1996	103	78
	Male	1996	112	78
	Under 20 years	1996	0	78
	20 to 44 years	1996	35	78
	45 to 64 years	1996	276	78
	65 to 74 years	1996	514	78
	75 years and older	1996	263	78
05-01	Diabetes education (age adjusted, persons aged 18 years and older)	1998	45	60
	American Indian or Alaska native	1998	UK	60
	Asian or Pacific Islander	1998	UK	60

continued

Exhibit 13–5   continued

Objective number	Objective	Baseline Year	Baseline	Target
	Black or African American	1998	45	60
	White	1998	46	60
	Hispanic or Latino	1998	34	60
	Not Hispanic or Latino	1998	47	60
	Female	1998	49	60
	Male	1998	42	60
	Less than high school (persons aged 25 years and older)	1998	26	60
	High school graduate (persons aged 25 years and older)	1998	43	60
	At least some college (persons aged 25 years and older)	1998	56	60
	Under 18 years (not age adjusted)	1998	UK	60
	18 to 44 years (not age adjusted)	1998	48	60
	45 to 64 years (not age adjusted)	1998	47	60
	65 to 74 years (not age adjusted)	1998	40	60
	75 years and older (not age adjusted)	1998	27	60
05-02	New cases of diabetes (rate per 1,000, persons of all ages)	1994–1996	3.5	2.5
	American Indian or Alaska native	1994–1996	UK	2.5

Asian or Pacific Islander	1994-1996	UK	2.5
Black or African American	1994-1996	5.7	2.5
White	1994-1996	3.2	2.5
Hispanic or Latino	1994-1996	5.7	2.5
Not Hispanic or Latino	1994-1996	3.3	2.5
Female	1994-1996	3.9	2.5
Male	1994-1996	3.1	2.5
Less than high school (persons aged 25 years and older)	1994-1996	6.9	2.5
High school graduate (persons aged 25 years and older)	1994-1996	4.5	2.5
At least some college (persons aged 25 years and older)	1994-1996	4.3	2.5
Under 18 years (not age adjusted)	1994-1996	UK	2.5
18 to 44 years (not age adjusted)	1994-1996	2.0	2.5
45 to 64 years (not age adjusted)	1994-1996	6.9	2.5
65 to 74 years (not age adjusted)	1994-1996	9.3	2.5
75 years and older (not age adjusted)	1994-1996	9.4	2.5
05-03 Overall cases of diagnosed diabetes (age adjusted rate per 1,000, persons of all ages)	1997	40	25
American Indian or Alaska native	1997	UK	25
Asian or Pacific Islander	1997	UK	25
Black or African American	1997	74	25

continued

Exhibit 13–5   continued

Objective number	Objective	Baseline Year	Baseline	Target
	White	1997	36	25
	Hispanic or Latino	1997	61	25
	Not Hispanic or Latino	1997	38	25
	Female	1997	40	25
	Male	1997	39	25
	Less than high school (persons aged 25 years and older)	1997	95	25
	High school graduate (persons aged 25 years and older)	1997	58	25
	At least some college (persons aged 25 years and older)	1997	44	25
	Under 18 years (not age adjusted)	1997	UK	25
	18 to 44 years (not age adjusted)	1997	16	25
	45 to 64 years (not age adjusted)	1997	76	25
	65 to 74 years (not age adjusted)	1997	143	25
	75 years and older (not age adjusted)	1997	117	25
05-05	Diabetes deaths (age adjusted rate per 100,000, persons of all ages)	1997	75	45
	American Indian or Alaska native	1997	107	45

	Asian or Pacific Islander	1997	62	45
	Black or African American	1997	130	45
	White	1997	70	45
	Hispanic or Latino	1997	86	45
	Not Hispanic or Latino	1997	74	45
	Female	1997	67	45
	Male	1997	87	45
	Under 45 years	1997	3	45
	45 to 64 years	1997	64	45
	65 to 74	1997	281	45
05-07	Cardiovascular disease deaths in persons with diabetes (age adjusted rate per 100,000, persons of all ages)	1997	343	309
	American Indian or Alaska native	1997	93	309
	Asian or Pacific Islander	1997	223	309
	Black or African American	1997	283	309
	White	1997	359	309
	Hispanic or Latino	1997	270	309
	Not Hispanic or Latino	1997	351	309
	Female	1997	339	309
	Male	1997	363	309
	Less than high school	1997	145	309

continued

Exhibit 13–5 continued

Objective number	Objective	Baseline Year	Baseline	Target
	High school graduate	1997	247	309
	At least some college	1997	125	309
	Under 45 years (not age adjusted)	1997	38	309
	45 to 64 years (not age adjusted)	1997	306	309
	65 to 74 years (not age adjusted)	1997	850	309
	75 years and older (not age adjusted)	1997	3,222	309
05-12	Annual glycosylated hemoglobin measurement: in persons with diabetes	1998	24	50
	American Indian or Alaska native	1998	29	50
	Asian or Pacific Islander	1998	48	50
	Black or African American	1998	21	50
	White	1998	25	50
	Hispanic or Latino	1998	22	50
	Not Hispanic or Latino	1998	25	50
	Female	1998	24	50
	Male	1998	25	50
	18 to 44 years (not age adjusted)	1998	29	50
	45 to 64 years (not age adjusted)	1998	23	50
	65 to 74 years (not age adjusted)	1998	13	50
	75 years and older (not age adjusted)	1998	11	50

05-17	Self-blood-glucose-monitoring—in persons with diabetes—at least once daily	1998	42	60
	American Indian or Alaska native	1998	53	60
	Asian or Pacific Islander	1998	30	60
	Black or African American	1998	40	60
	White	1998	43	60
	Hispanic or Latino	1998	36	60
	Not Hispanic or Latino	1998	43	60
	Female	1998	43	60
	Male	1998	41	60
	18 to 44 years (not age adjusted)	1998	43	60
	45 to 64 years (not age adjusted)	1998	41	60
	65 to 74 years (not age adjusted)	1998	44	60
	75 years and older (not age adjusted)	1998	38	60

UK = unknown
Source: Adapted from: US Department of Health and Human Services. DATA2010—the *Healthy People 2010* database. *CDC Wonder.* Atlanta, Ga: Centers for Disease Control; November 2000.

Materials are available in English, Amharic, Cambodian, Oromo, Somali, Spanish, Tigrean, and Vietnamese. Topics include a class flyer, sick-day management, exercise, meal planning, and meal portions on a multicultural diabetes Web site. A Web site on multicultural diabetes classes can be found at http://ethnomed.org/ethnomed/patient_ed/diabetes/diabetes_index.html.

Healthy People 2010 Actions

Several HP 2010 objectives address diabetes mellitus, risk factors of diabetes mellitus, or eating behaviors to improve overall health of Americans predisposed to or diagnosed with diabetes mellitus (see Exhibit 13–5). Targets are defined for blacks, Native Americans, and Hispanics. Kaufman has outlined a model nutrition objective for risk reduction.[96] Community nutrition professionals can use this blueprint to develop diabetes self-management programs (see Exhibit 13–6).

Exhibit 13–6   Model Nutrition Objective for Risk Reduction

By 20____, the chronic disease risk factor ____*____ among [*target population*] will be reduced from _____% to _____%.

*Obesity; hypertension; elevated serum cholesterol; poor physical fitness; excess intake of dietary fat, cholesterol, sodium, alcohol, and sugar; inadequate intake of dietary fiber, fruits and vegetables, and calcium.

Source: Adapted from: *Model State Nutrition Objectives.* Johnstown, Pa: The Association of State and Territorial Public Health Nutrition Directors; 1988.

References

1. *American Diabetes Association: Who We Are, What We Do.* Alexandria, Va: American Diabetes Association; 2005.
2. Sherman N. Too fat + too lazy = diabetes. *HealthScout Reporter.* August 24, 2000.
3. Glasgow RE, Haire-Joshu D. Diabetes and smoking: why you should kick butts. *Diabetes Forecast.* September 2000.
4. *American Diabetes Association: Clinical Practice Recommendations 2005.* Alexandria, Va: American Diabetes Association; January 25, 2005;1:(51)1-79.
5. Shead NF. Cow's milk, diabetes, and infant feeding. *Nutr Rev.* 1991; 51(3):79-81.
6. Savilahti E, Akerblom HK, Tainio V-M, et al. Children with newly diagnosed insulin-dependent diabetes mellitus have increased levels of cow's milk antibodies. *Diabetes Res.* 1988;7:137-140.
7. Yokota A, Yamaguchi Y, Ueda Y, et al. Comparison of islet cell antibodies, islet cell surface antibodies, and anti-bovine serum albumin antibodies in type 1 diabetes. *Diabetes Res Clin Pract.* 1990;9:211-217.
8. Scott FW. Cow milk and insulin-dependent diabetes mellitus: is there a relationship? *Am J Clin Nutr.* 1990;51:489-491.
9. Martin JM, Trink B, Daneman D, et al. Milk proteins in the etiology of insulin-dependent diabetes mellitus. *Ann Intern Med.* 1991;23:447-452.

10. American Academy of Pediatrics, Committee on Nutrition. Statement on cholesterol. *Pediatrics.* 1992;90:469-473.

11. American Diabetes Association. Position statement: evidence-based nutrition principles and recommendations for the treatment and prevention of diabetes and related complications. *JAMA.* 2002;102(1):109-118.

12. American Diabetes Association. Position statement–diagnosis and classification of diabetes mellitus. *Diabetes Care.* 2005;28:S37-S42.

13. DeFronzo RA, Ferrannini E. Insulin resistance: a multifaceted syndrome responsible for NIDDM, obesity, hypertension, dyslipidemia and atherosclerotic cardiovascular disease. *Diabetes Care.* 1991;14:173-194.

14. Ward WK, Beard JC, Halter JB, et al. Pathophysiology of insulin secretion in non–insulin-dependent diabetes mellitus. *Diabetes Care.* 1984;7: 491-502.

15. Lovejob J, DiGirolamo M. Habitual dietary intake and insulin sensitivity in lean and obese adults. *Am J Clin Nutr.* 1992;55:1174-1179.

16. Helmrich SP, Ragland DR, Leung RW, et al. Physical activity and reduced occurrence of non–insulin-dependent diabetes mellitus. *N Engl J Med.* 1991;325:147-152.

17. Toeller M, Greis FA, Dannehl K. Natural history of glucose intolerance in obesity: a ten-year observation. *Int J Obesity.* 1982;6:145-149.

18. Anderson JW. Nutrition management of diabetes mellitus. In: Shils ME, Young VR, eds. *Modern Nutrition in Health and Disease.* 7th ed. New York: Lea and Febiger; 1988:840-872.

19. American Diabetes Association. Diabetes nutrition recommendations for health care institutions [position statement]. *Diabetes Care.* 2004;27 (suppl 1):S55-S57.

20. Liu S, Manson J, Stampfer M, et al. A prospective study of whole-grain intake and risk of type 2 diabetes mellitus in US women. *Am J Public Health.* 2000;90:1409-1415.

21. Bierman EL. Atherogenesis in diabetes. *Arteriosclerosis Thrombosis.* 1992;12:647-656.

22. American Diabetes Association and the Diabetes Care and Education Practice Group of the American Dietetic Association. *Maximizing the Role of Nutrition in Diabetes Management.* Alexandria, Va: American Diabetes Association; 1994.

23. Powers MA, Warshaw H. Low-calorie sweeteners and fat replacers: the ingredients, use in foods, and diabetes management. In: Powers MA, ed. *Handbook of Diabetes Medical Nutrition Therapy.* Gaithersburg, Md: Aspen Publishers, Inc; 1996.

24. Holler HJ, Pastors JP. *Diabetes Medical Nutrition Therapy.* Chicago, Ill: American Dietetic Association; 1997.

25. Garg A, Bonanome A, Grundy SM, et al. Comparison of a high-carbohydrate, sucrose-containing diet in patients with non–insulin-dependent diabetes mellitus. *N Engl J Med.* 1988;319:829-834.

26. Garg A, Grundy SM, Unger RH. Comparison of effects of high and low carbohydrate diets on plasma lipoproteins and insulin sensitivity in patients with mild NIDDM. *Diabetes.* 1992;41:1278-1285.

27. Grundy SM. Comparison of monounsaturated fatty acids and carbohydrates for lowering plasma cholesterol. *N Engl J Med.* 1986; 314:745-748.

28. Simpson HCR, Lousley S, Gelkie M, et al. A high carbohydrate leguminous fiber diet improves all aspects of diabetic control. *Lancet.* 1981;1:1-5.

29. Howard BV, Abbott WGH, Swinburn BA. Evaluation of metabolic effects of substitution of complex carbohydrates for saturated fat in individuals with obesity and NIDDM. *Diabetes Care.* 1991;14:786-795.

30. Ravusine E, Bogardus C, Schwartz RS, et al. Thermic effect of infused glucose and insulin in man: decreased response with increased insulin resistance in obesity and NIDDM. *J Clin Invest.* 1993;72:893-902.

31. UKPDS Group. UK Prospective Diabetes Study 7: response of fasting plasma glucose to diet therapy in newly presenting type II diabetic patients. *Metabolism.* 1990;39:905-912.

32. Shintani TT. Obesity and cardiovascular risk intervention through the ad libitum feeding of traditional Hawaiian diet. *Am J Clin Nutr.* 1991;153:1647S-1651S.

33. O'Dea K. Marked improvement in carbohydrate and lipid metabolism in diabetic Australian aborigines after temporary reversion to traditional lifestyle. *Diabetes.* 1984;33:596-603.

34. Brand JC, Colaqiuri S, Crossman S, et al. Low-glycemic index foods improve long-term glycemic control in NIDDM. *Diabetes Care.* 1991;14:95-101.

35. Fragakis AS. *Popular Dietary Supplements.* 2nd ed. Chicago, Ill: American Dietetic Association; 2002.

36. Jenkins DJA, Ocana A, Jenkins AL, et al. Metabolic advantages of spreading the nutrient load: effects of increased meal frequency in non–insulin-dependent diabetes. *Am J Clin Nutr.* 1992;55:461-467.

37. Diabetes Control and Complications Trial Research Group. The effect of intensive treatment of diabetes on the development and progression of long-term complications in insulin-dependent diabetes mellitus. *N Engl J Med.* 1993;329:977-986.

38. Siebert C, Clark DM Jr. Operational and policy considerations of data monitoring in clinical trials: the Diabetes Control and Complications Trial experience. *Diabetes Care.* 1993;14:30-44.

39. Diabetes Control and Complications Trial Research Group. *DCCT Manual of Operations.* Springfield, Va: US Dept of Commerce; 1993. National Technical Information Service publication 93-183382.

40. Lawson PM, Champion MC, Canny C, et al. Continuous subcutaneous insulin infusion does not prevent progression of proliferative and preproliferative retinopathy. *Br J Ophthalmol.* 1982;66:762-766.

41. Klein R, Klein BE, Moss SE, et al. The Wisconsin epidemiologic study of diabetic retinopathy. III. Prevalence and risk of diabetic retinopathy when age at diagnosis is 30 or more years. *Arch Ophthalmol.* 1984;102:527-532.

42. Nathan DM, Singer DE, Godine JE, et al. Retinopathy in older type II diabetics: association with glucose control. *Diabetes.* 1986;35:797-801.

43. American Diabetes Association. Implications of the diabetes control and complications trial. *Diabetes Care.* 1993;16:1517-1520.

44. Chobanian AV, Bakris GL, Black HR, et al. The seventh report of the Joint National Committee on Prevention, Detection, Evaluation, and Treatment of High Blood Pressure: the JNCN 7 report. *JAMA.* 2003;289:2560-2572.

45. UK Prospective Diabetes Study Group. Tight blood pressure control and risk of macrovascular and microvascular complications in type 2 diabetes: UKPDS 38. *BMJ.* 1998;317:703-713.

46. Hansson L, Zanchetti A, Carruthers SG, et al. Effects of intensive blood-pressure lowering and low-dose aspirin in patients with hypertension: principal results of the Hypertension Optimal Treatment (HOT) randomised trial: the HOT Study Group. *Lancet.* 1998;351:1755-1762.

47. Adler AI, Stratton IM, Neil HA, et al. Association of systolic blood pressure with macrovascular and microvascular complications of type 2 diabetes (UKPDS 36): prospective observational study. *BMJ.* 2000;321:412-419.

48. Lewington S, Clarke R, Qizilbash N, Peto R, Collins R. Age-specific relevance of usual blood pressure to vascular mortality: a meta-analysis of individual data for one million adults in 61 prospective studies. *Lancet.* 2002;360:1903-1913.

49. Stamler J, Vaccaro O, Neaton JD, Wentworth D. Diabetes, other risk factors, and 12-yr cardiovascular mortality for men screened in the Multiple Risk Factor Intervention Trial. *Diabetes Care.* 1993;16:434-444.

50. Sacks FM, Svetkey LP, Vollmer WM, et al. Effects on blood pressure of reduced dietary sodium and the Dietary Approaches to Stop Hypertension (DASH) diet: the DASH-Sodium Collaborative Research Group. *N Engl J Med.* 2001;344:3-10.

51. National High Blood Pressure Education Working Group. Report on hypertension in diabetes. *Hypertention.* 1994;23:145-158.

52. Heart Protection Study Collaborative Group: MRC/BHF Heart Protection Study of cholesterol-lowering with simvastatin in 5963 people with diabetes: a randomised placebo-controlled trial. *Lancet.* 2003;361:2005-2016.

53. Davidow DN, Turner M. Complications of coexisting diabetes mellitus and eating disorders in IDDM. *On the Cutting Edge.* 1994;15(6):8-10.

54. Marcus MD, Wing RR, Jawad A, et al. Eating disorders symptomatology in a registry-based sample of women with insulin-dependent diabetes mellitus. *Int J Eating Disorders.* 1992;12:425-430.

55. King NL. Overview of eating disorders in diabetes management. *On the Cutting Edge.* 1994;15(6):5-7.

56. Schlundt DG, Pichert JW, Rea MR. Situational obstacles to adherence for adolescents with diabetes. *Diabetes Ed.* 1994;20:207-211.

57. Bossetti BM. Compulsive overeating, obesity and diabetes. *On the Cutting Edge.* 1994;15(6):12-14.

58. Riddle M. Diabetes: too big and too bad to ignore any longer. *Clin Diabetes.* 2004;22:90-91.

59. Vinicor F. The future of diabetes: what is there besides new medicines? *Clin Diabetes.* 2004;22:94-96.

60. National Kidney Foundation. Kidney Early Evaluation Program (KEEP). *Diabetes Educator.* 2004;30:196-209.

61. Boyle RG, O'Connor PJ, Pronk NP, Tan A. Stages of change for physical activity, diet, and smoking among HMO members with chronic conditions. *Am J Health Promo.* 1998;12:170-175.

62. Campbell MK, Symons M, Demark-Wahnefried W, et al. Stages of change and psychosocial correlates of fruit and vegetable consumption among rural African-American church members. *Am J Health Promo.* 1998;12:185-191.

63. Nitzke S, Auld G, McNulty J, et al. Stages of change for reducing fat and increasing fiber among dietitians and adults with a diet-related chronic disease. *J Am Diet Assoc.* 1999;99:728-731.

64. Prochaska JO, Velicer WF. The transtheoretical model of health behavior change. *Am J Health Promo.* 1997;12:38-48.

65. Greene GW, Rossi SR. Stages of change for reducing dietary fat intake over 18 months. *J Am Diet Assoc.* 1998;98:529-534.

66. Byrd-Bredbenner C, Finckenor M. Putting the transtheoretical model into practice with type 2 diabetes mellitus patients. *Top Clin Nutr.* 2000;15(3):44-58.

67. Marcus BH, Simkin LR. The transtheoretical model: application to exercise behavior. *Med Sci Sports Exerc.* 1994;26:1400-1404.

68. Mhurchu CN, Margetts BM, Speller VM. Applying the stages-of-change model to dietary change. *Nutr Rev.* 1997;55:10-16.

69. American Diabetes Association. Type 2 diabetes in children and adolescents. *Diabetes Care.* 2003;23(3):381-382.

70. American Diabetes Association. *Medical Management of Type 1 Diabetes.* 3rd ed. Alexandria, Va: American Diabetes Association; 1998:246.

71. Gahagan S, Silverstein J, and the Committee on Native American Child Health and Section on Endocrinology. Prevention and treatment of type 2 diabetes mellitus in children, with special emphasis on American Indian and Alaska native children. *Pediatrics.* 2003;112(4):343.

72. USDHHS. *Helping the Student with Diabetes Succeed.* Washington, DC: US Dept of Health and Human Services; 2003:13-19.

73. Fung TT, Schulze M, Manson JE, Willet WC, Hu FB. Dietary patterns, meat intake, and the risk of type 2 diabetes in women. *Arch Intern Med.* 2004;164:2235-2240.

74. Avioli LV. Significance of osteoporosis: a growing international health care problem. *Calcif Tissue Int.* 1991;49:S5-S7.

75. Kitzmiller JL, Gavin LA, Gin GD, Jovanovic-Peterson L, Main EK, Zigrang WD. Preconception care of diabetes: glycemic control prevents congenital anomalies. *JAMA.* 1991;265:731-736.

76. Jovanovic-Peterson L, Peterson CM, Reed GF, et al. Maternal postprandial glucose levels and infant birth weight: the Diabetes in Early Pregnancy study. *Am J Obstet Gynecol.* 1991;164:103-111.

77. Sizer FS, Whitney EN. *Nutrition Concepts and Controversies.* 8th ed. Belmont, Calif: Wadsworth Thomson Learning; 2000.

78. Miller E, Hare JW, Cloherty JP, Dunn PJ, et al. Elevated maternal hemoglobin Alc in early pregnancy and major congenital anomalies in infants of diabetic mothers. *N Engl J Med.* 1981 304:1331–4.

79. Goldman JA, Dicker D, Feldberg D, Yeshaya A, Samuel N, Karp M. Pregnancy outcome in patients with insulin-dependent diabetes mellitus with preconceptional diabetic control: a comparative study. *Am J Obstet Gynecol.* 1986;155:293-297.

80. Rosenn B, Miodovnik M, Combs CA, Khoury J, Siddiqi TA. Pre-conception management of insulin-dependent diabetes: improvement of pregnancy outcome. *Obstet Gynecol.* 1991;77:846-849.

81. Tchobroutsky C, Vray MM, Altman JJ. Risk/benefit ratio of changing late obstetrical strategies in the management of insulin-dependent diabetic pregnancies: a comparison between 1971-1977 and 1978-1985 periods in 389 pregnancies. *Diabetes Metab.* 1991;17:287-294.

82. Willhoite MB, Bennert HW Jr, Palomaki GE, et al. The impact of preconception counseling on pregnancy outcomes: the experience of the Maine Diabetes in Pregnancy Program. *Diabetes Care.* 1993;16:450-455.

83. Green OC, Winter RJ, Depp R, et al. Fuel-mediated teratogenesis: prospective correlations between anthropometric development in childhood and antepartum maternal metabolism. *Clin Res.* 1987;35:657A.

84. Barnard RJ, Ugianskis EJ, Martin DA, et al. Role of diet and exercise in the management of hyperinsulinemia and associated atherosclerotic risk factors. *Am J Cardiol.* 1992;69:440-444.

85. Goodyear LJ, Smith RJ. Post exercise late onset hypoglycemia. In: Kahn CK, Weir GL, eds. *Joslin's Diabetes Mellitus.* Philadelphia, Pa: Lea and Febiger; 1994:451-507.

86. Krauss B. Two groups are better than one for congressional matters. *Newsflash.* 2004;25(5):12.

87. Geil P. It's a small world after all! The 2004 International Congress of Dietetics. *Newsflash.* 2004;25(5):13.

88. Colditz GA, Manson JE, Stampfer MJ, et al. Diet and risk of clinical diabetes in women. *Am J Clin Nutr.* 1992;55:1018-1023.

89. Snowdon DA, Philips RL. Does a vegetarian diet reduce the occurrence of diabetes? *Am J Public Health.* 1985;75:507-512.

90. Feskens EJM, Bowles CH, Kromhout D. Inverse association between fish intake and risk of glucose intolerance in normoglycemic elderly men and women. *Diabetes Care.* 1991;14:935-941.

91. Marshall JA, Hoag S, Shetterly S, et al. Dietary fat predicts conversion from impaired glucose tolerance to NIDDM: the San Luis Valley Diabetes Study. *Diabetes Care.* 1994;17:50-56.

92. Feskens E, Virtanen SM, Rasanen L, et al. Dietary factors determining diabetes and impaired glucose tolerance. *Diabetes Care.* 1995;18: 1104-1112.

93. Saad MF, Knowler WC, Pettitt DJ, et al. A two-step model for the development of non–insulin-dependent diabetes. *Am J Med.* 1991;90: 229-235.

94. National Institute of Diabetes and Digestive and Kidney Diseases. The Pima Indians. *Pathfinders for Health.* May 2002:1-2.

95. Ong C. Diabetes care and education around the world: Singapore. *DCE DPG Newsletter,* Winter, 2004. 7-8.

96. Kaufman M. *Nutrition in Public Health—A Handbook for Developing Programs and Services.* Gaithersburg, Md: Aspen Publishers, Inc; 1990:570.

CHAPTER FOURTEEN

HYPERTENSION

Learning Objectives

- Identify the incidence and prevalence of hypertension in the United States.
- List and define the magnitude of influence of dietary components and lifestyle behaviors on blood pressure level.
- Describe major clinical trials and primary prevention studies that use eating behavior change as an intervention.

High Definition Nutrition

Blood pressure–the force that flowing blood exerts against artery walls.
Diastolic blood pressure–blood pressure occurring when the heart relaxes between contractions.
Systolic blood pressure–blood pressure occurring when the heart contracts.

Prevalence

High blood pressure (HBP) is defined as systolic pressure of 140 mm Hg or higher, or diastolic pressure of 90 mm Hg of higher; taking antihypertensive medicine; and/or being told at least twice by a physician or other health professional that you have high blood pressure (Figure 14–1). Prehypertension is systolic pressure of 120-139 mm Hg, or diastolic pressure of 80-89 mm Hg, and both not taking antihypertensive medication, or not being told on 2 occasions by a doctor or other health professional that you have hypertension. Nearly 1 in 3 adults has HBP. About 28% of American adults age 18 and older, or about 59 million people, have prehypertension.[1]

Overall, 39% of all US adults are normotensive, 31% are prehypertensive, and 29% are hypertensive. The age-adjusted prevalence of prehypertension is

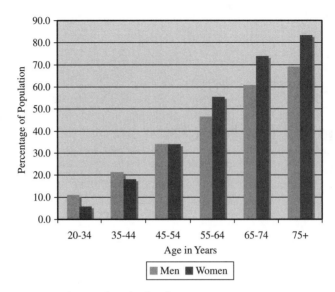

FIGURE 14–1   Prevalence of High Blood Pressure in Americans.
Source: CDC/NCHS and NHLBI

greater in men (39%) than in women (23.1%). African Americans aged 20 to 39 years have a higher prevalence of prehypertension (37.4%) than whites (32.2%) and Mexican Americans (30.9%), but their prevalence is lower at older ages because of a higher prevalence of hypertension earlier in life.[2]

Of those with HBP, 30% do not know why they have it; 34% are on medication and have it controlled; 25% are on medication but do not have their HBP under control; and 11% are not on medication. A higher percentage of men than women have HBP until age 55. After that a much higher percentage of women have HBP than men do. HBP is 2-3 times more common in women taking oral contraceptives, especially in obese and older women, than in women not taking them.[1]

About half of people who have a first heart attack and two thirds who have a first stroke have blood pressure higher than 160/95 mm Hg.[3] People with systolic blood pressure of 160 mm Hg or higher have a relative risk for stroke about 4 times greater than for those with normal blood pressure (BP).[4] The prevalence of HBP among blacks and whites in the southeastern United States is greater and death rates from stroke are higher than among those in other regions. Hypertension precedes the development of congestive heart failure (CHF) in 91% of cases. HBP is associated with a 2-3 times higher risk for developing CHF.[5]

Race/Ethnicity and HBP

The prevalence of hypertension among ethnic groups varies but blacks in the United States have the highest blood pressure for any ethnic group in the world. Compared with whites, blacks develop HBP earlier in life and their average blood pressures are much higher. As a result, compared with whites, blacks have 1.3 times greater rate of nonfatal stroke, a 1.8 times greater rate of fatal stroke, a 1.5 times greater rate of heart disease death, and a 4.2 times greater rate of end-stage kidney disease.[1,2] Within the African-American community, rates of hypertension vary substantially.[6]

- Those with the highest rates are more likely to be middle-aged or older, less educated, overweight, or obese, physically inactive, and to have diabetes.
- Those with the lowest rates are more likely to be younger, but also overweight or obese.
- Those with uncontrolled HBP who are not on antihypertensive medication tend to be male, younger, and have infrequent contact with a physician.

The awareness, treatment, and control of HBP among those in the Cardiovascular Health Study (CHS) age 65 and older improved during the 1990s. The percentages who were aware of and treated for HBP were higher among blacks than among whites. Prevalences with HBP under control were similar. For both groups combined, the control of blood pressure (BP) to lower than 140/90 mm Hg increased from 37% in 1990 to 49% in 1999. Improved control was achieved by an increase in antihypertensive medications per person and by increasing the proportion of the CHS population treated for hypertension from 34.5% to 51.1%.[7]

A study of children and adolescents from 1988-1994 and 1999-2000, among ages 8 to 17 showed that among non-Hispanic blacks, mean systolic BP levels increased 1.6 mm Hg among girls and 2.9 mm Hg among boys, when compared with non-Hispanic whites. Among Mexican Americans, girls' systolic BP increased 1.0 mm Hg and boys' systolic BP increased 2.7 mm Hg when compared with non-Hispanic whites.[8]

Mortality

HBP was listed as a primary or contributing cause of death in about 261,000 of 2,443,387 US deaths in 2002.[1]

- From 1992 to 2002, the age-adjusted death rate from HBP increased 26.8%, and the actual number of deaths rose 56.6%.
- The 2002 overall death rate from HBP was 17.1%. Death rates were 14.4% for white males, 49.6% for black males, 13.7% for white females, and 40.5% for black females.
- As many as 30% of all deaths in hypertensive black men and 30% of all deaths in hypertensive black women may be due to HBP.

Cost

In 2005 the estimated direct and indirect cost of high blood pressure was $59.7 billion.[9]

Historic Perspectives in Salt and Blood Pressure

"Mankind can live without gold but not without salt."—Cassiodorus, a Roman official and historian, AD 490-583.

"Season all your grain offerings with salt. Do not leave the salt of the covenant of your God out of your grain offerings: add salt to all your offerings."–Moses's proclamation to the people of Israel (Leviticus 2:13).[10]

An historic review shows Roman Catholics using salt as a sign of purity and for baptizing babies. Salt's importance to humankind also involves a complex set of integrated systems regulating sodium balance. The control systems in animals and humans have a wide range with set points and there is flexibility in the amount creating minimal risk versus extreme risk when either too little or too much sodium intake is ingested.

Interest in the regulation of salt intake was stimulated by Richter's pioneering studies during the 1930s, which showed increased salt appetite in adrenalectomized rats.[11] Stimulation of central angiotensin receptors results in sodium retention and increased sodium intake,[12] whereas their blockade reduces sodium appetite.[13]

When sodium intake is 10 times greater than normal it does not raise blood pressure in spontaneously hypertensive rats or borderline hypertensive rats unless a certain level of social stress is present. When sodium intake is quickly lowered by 50-100% in animals and humans, neural and hormonal actions occur to maintain homeostasis. Long-term reduction in sodium intake may be associated with reduced sympathetic and neurohumoral adjustments.

Low sodium intake did not affect young people's responses to upright tilting, but older adults could not compensate to tilting, suggesting impaired baroreceptor reflexes.[14] Endocrine changes occur for both high- or low-sodium diets[15-18]; plasma rennin and angiotensin concentrations are inversely related to dietary sodium.[19-21]

In humans, psychologic stress may induce sodium and fluid retention as reported for male college students 18 to 22 years old experiencing 1 hour of competitive tasks.[22] Those retaining sodium, fluid, or both during stress had reduced glomerular filtration rates, increased reabsorption of sodium, or both. Most men with sodium retention had a hypertensive parent, suggesting a genetic relation.

Increased blood pressure in population studies and sodium appetite may result from increased psychosocial stress.[23,24] Data from Central Africa show that with a low (2 g/d) salt intake, blood pressure rose with age in a social system where traditional ways were changing and psychosocial stress was high.[25] Timio et al measured blood pressure in a group of nuns who consumed < 12 g salt/d; their average blood pressure of 127 mm Hg at 58 years was the same as that recorded at age 38 y.[26] In the control group of women living in the city, blood pressure increased from 127 to 167 mm Hg during the same period. Psychosocial stress was not assessed but higher stress in the city women could evoke this response.

Sodium handling appears to be determined by both genetic and environmental influences.[27] Some individuals may be salt sensitive only under stressful conditions. Salt sensitivity when hypertension exists is associated with renal, hemodynamic, and metabolic disturbances that may increase the risk of cardiovascular and renal morbidity.[28] Low-salt diets lowered blood pressure in 30-60% adults with essential hypertension[28-31] and in 25-40% of normotensives.[29,32] Potential physiologic or genetic markers of salt-sensitive individuals to predict who may best benefit from salt reduction include calcium metabolism,[33-35] plasma rennin concentrations,[29,36,37] sympathetic nervous system (SNS) function,[30-32,38-40] haptoglobin phenotypes,[41] abnormal renal and adrenal responses to angiotensin II,[42] natriuretic hormone alternations,[33-43] different types of salts,[44-47] abnormal renal acid-base regulation,[48] and renal retention of sodium.[36,37,49]

Essential hypertension is a multifactorial condition affecting 62 million adults. Blood pressure regulation is the result of cardiac output and peripheral vascular resistance, which are both influenced by sympathetic outflow and hormones such as angiotensin, insulin, noradrenaline, prostaglandins, kinins, and atrial natriuretic factor. Stress; extracellular and intracellular cations of sodium, potassium, calcium, and magnesium; and various food components including cations, fats, and alcohol influence cardiac output and peripheral vascular resistance.[50]

Increased energy intake may increase insulin secretion and sympathetic outflow. High energy intakes often accompany high sodium intake, fluid retention, and alteration of intracellular electrolytes. Low sodium intakes may increase angiotensin and noradrenaline and also cause calcium retention.[50]

Three major nutritional factors are associated with hypertension. These are obesity, high alcohol intake, and high sodium intake.

Obesity

Epidemiologic studies show an association between obesity and hypertension in a wide variety of socioeconomic, racial, and ethnic groups.[51-54] A strong correlation exists between body weight and blood pressure and between increases in body weight and subsequent development of hypertension.[51,53]

Intervention studies show that weight reduction may reduce arterial pressure in overweight, hypertensive patients. A drop in pressure may occur with caloric restriction only, even without reduction in sodium intake and before ideal body weight is achieved. Weight reduction in obese individuals can reduce cardiovascular risk factors, such as hyperlipidemia and glucose intolerance. Obesity is the strongest risk factor for hypertension. Approximately 50% of women and 39% of men with high blood pressure are overweight. The data are strong and consistent as briefly discussed next.

Many studies have reported a stepwise increase in blood pressure as body weight concomitantly increases. Individuals who are overweight or obese have an increased prevalence and incidence of hypertension compared to individuals who are not overweight or obese.[55,56] In general, an individual who is overweight is at 2 to 6 times higher risk of developing hypertension.[53,57]

Since excess weight is common among minority populations, certain groups (i.e., African Americans, Hispanics, Native Americans, and Asian/ Pacific Islanders) are at a higher risk of hypertension. The National Health and Nutrition Examination Survey IV cutoff points for obesity are body mass index (BMI) greater or equal to 30.0 for men and women and greater than or equal to 25.0 for men and women for overweight. Using these cutoff points, the prevalence of excess weight ranges from less than 20% in younger white men to greater than 60% in older African-American women[58,59] (see Chapter 15).

With the documented increasing body weight of US youths and adults, the population in general is at a greater risk. Approximately 20-30% of hypertension prevalence has been influenced by this trend toward increasing body weight. [52,53]

The estimated prevalence of high blood pressure for US women ages 20 and older varies by ethnicity. See Figure 14–2. Blacks (45% women and 42% men) develop high blood pressure at an earlier age, and experience a more severe form at any decade of life. One outcome is a 5-times greater rate of end-stage kidney disease for blacks when compared to whites.[60] Surveys estimate that 2.2 million Americans 15 years and older have costly disabilities from high blood pressure. For Mexican Americans, 28.7% of women and 27.8% of men have hypertension compared to 16.7% of Asians and 21.2% of American Indians or Alaskan natives.[1]

An inverse relationship between fish intake and risk of stroke has been reported.[61-64] Fish may inhibit platelet aggregation[65] or lower blood viscosity[66]; it may also suppress formation of leukotrienes and reduce plasma fibrinogen,[67] blood pressure levels,[68] and insulin resistance.[69] Average food supply per capita for omega-3 fatty acids (eicosapentaenoic acid and docosahexaenoic acid) for residents in the United States is 0.1 to 0.2 g/d[70] and lower than that of Danish whites (0.8 g/d) and Greenland Eskimos (10.5 g/d)[71] minimizing risk of hemorrhagic stroke as noted among Greenland Eskimos.[72]

The association between fish and omega-3 polyunsaturated fatty acid intake and risk of strokes in women was examined. A cohort of 79,839 women aged 34 to 59 years in the Nurses' Health Study were followed up for 14 years. To be eligible, women had to be free from prior diagnosed cardiovascular disease, cancer, and history of diabetes and hypercholesterolemia, and they had to complete a food frequency questionnaire including questions about consumption of fish and other frequently eaten foods.[73]

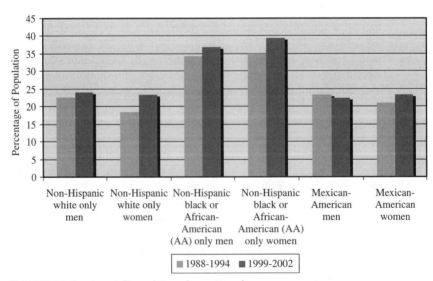

FIGURE 14–2   Age-Adjusted Prevalence Trends.
Source: CDC/NCHS.

Relative risk of stroke compared by category of fish intake and quintile of omega-3 polyunsaturated fatty acid intake was examined for the 574 strokes that occurred. Compared with women who ate fish less than once per month, those with higher intake of fish had a lower risk of total stroke; the multivariate relative risks (RRs), adjusted for age, smoking, and other cardiovascular risk factors, were 0.93 (95% confidence interval [CI] 0.65-1.34) for fish consumption 1 to 3 times per month, 0.78 (95% CI, 0.55-1.12) for once per week, 0.73 (95% CI, 0.47-1.14) for 2 to 4 times per week, and 0.48 (95% CI, 0.21-1.06) for 5 or more times per week (*p* for trend = 0.06).[73]

A prospective cohort of 75,521 US women 38 to 63 years old without previous diagnosis of diabetes mellitus, coronary heart disease, stroke, or other CVDs completed detailed food frequency questionnaires (FFQs) in 1984, 1986, 1990, and 1994. In this 12-year follow-up of the Nurses' Health Study, a higher intake of whole-grain foods was associated with a lower risk of ischemic stroke.[74]

An interesting finding by British researchers was that tall men had a reduced risk of stroke compared with their shorter peers. Fetal growth, early life socioenvironmental circumstances, infection, and nutrition in childhood can influence both a man's height and his risk for stroke.[75] McCarron et al measured the height of over 4,800 British men, 45-59 years old; 287 had suffered at least 1 stroke. Men without a history of stroke were slightly taller than those who had suffered a stroke. The average height of the stroke-free men was 171.7 centimeters (67.6 inches) versus 170.3 centimeters (67.0 inches) in those who had strokes. After adjusting for age, blood pressure, weight, smoking, social class, and other risk factors, height was associated with ischemic strokes caused by a blood clot, but not by hemorrhagic strokes of uncontrolled bleeding in the brain.[75,76]

The Seven Countries Study[77] demonstrated a direct relation of systolic and diastolic blood pressures within 16 communities to coronary death rates. These data showed a doubling in risk for every increment of 10 mm Hg in the population's median systolic blood pressure. Within individuals, further evidence of a direct relation of increasing systolic and diastolic blood pressure levels with the subsequent incidence of coronary heart disease (CHD) mortality over 11.6 years of follow-up is documented in men initially free of CHD screened for the Multiple Risk Factor Intervention Trial.[78] The pooling of results from 9 prospective observational studies including 418,343 persons initially free of CHD shows the increase in risk for CHD mortality to begin at levels of diastolic blood pressure between 73 and 78 mm Hg and to increase more than fivefold between levels of 73 and 105 mm Hg.[79]

Even with the disease burden attributable to hypertension, the level of awareness, treatment, and control of this condition is considered a national tragedy. US blood pressure control rates fall well below the 55% goal for the year 2010. In selected populations, the challenge is even greater.

Large subgroups of the general population are reported to be most sensitive to the blood pressure effects of changes in dietary salt intake. They include African Americans, the elderly, diabetics, the obese, those with renal impairment, and the vast majority of hypertensives.[80] In addition to a direct effect on blood pressure, sodium restriction augments the response to other antihypertensives and reduces potassium loss in patients on diuretics.[81]

Alcohol

A classic study of alcohol intake among the French military found that those who consumed 3 liters or more of wine per day had increased chance of being hypertensive.[82] This finding spurred researchers to explore the alcohol and blood pressure hypothesis. Almost all of the 30 or more cross-sectional studies to date have shown a small but significant elevation in blood pressure among individuals who consume 3 or more drinks per day (i.e., 40 grams of ethanol) compared with nondrinkers. The relationship has persisted after controlling for potentially confounding factors including body mass index, cigarette smoking, and age.[83]

About 5-7% of the prevalence of hypertension is assigned to the ingestion of 3 or more alcoholic drinks per day, which has been noted as a threshold. The prevalence is 2 times greater in the 6-or-more-drinks group than in the 2-or-fewer group.[84,85]

Intervention studies demonstrate a short-term pressor effect of alcohol consumption, short-term drops in blood pressure from abstinence or less than 1 drink per day in heavy drinkers, and normalization of blood pressure in former heavy drinkers who stop drinking.[86] It appears that excess alcohol intake may lead to elevated blood pressure, poor adherence to antihypertensive therapy, and, occasionally, refractory hypertension.[86-88]

Sodium

The average person consumes about 3,000 mg per day of sodium.[89,90] Differences in salt intake are largely explained by the amount of processed food eaten, which can provide as much as 75-85% of the sodium consumed in Western countries.[91,92] The National Research Council recommends that Americans consume no more than 2,400 mg of sodium per day. Intake varies throughout the world and is much lower in less developed countries, e.g., 25 mg per day, while intake in northern China exceeds 6,000 mg per day. The human body accommodates different intakes by producing the hormone aldosterone, which, in turn, conserves sodium. If sodium levels are high, aldosterone levels drop, allowing more sodium to be excreted.

An important finding is that blood pressure at all levels correlates with heart disease risk, which means that even slightly elevated pressure that is not defined as hypertension can increase risk.[93] Research suggests that about 25% of people with normal blood pressure and 50% with hypertension respond to changes in sodium intake.[94] Sodium is strongly associated with increased risk for cardiovascular disease for overweight people.[95] Excess sodium can cause significant damage to the heart, brain, kidneys, and arteries, independent of its effects on blood pressure.[96,97]

When one excretes sodium, she or he excretes calcium. A study of postmenopausal women reported 500 mg of sodium caused a loss of about 10 mg of calcium.[98] An average sodium intake of 3,000 mg per day, which is typical in the United States, could cause an average daily loss of 60 mg of calcium. With reduced absorption as one ages, an increase in dietary requirements to 500 mg of calcium may be needed to offset bone calcium loss. One epidemiological study reported an association between high urinary sodium excretion reflecting high sodium intake and increased loss of bone from the hip.[90,99]

Cross-sectional studies show a weak but significant relationship between salt intake and prevalence of hypertension. This weak observation may be due to the lack of standardized blood pressure measurements and sodium intake estimates based upon dietary recall. Primitive, unacculturated societies with sodium intake of less than 50 to 80 mEq/day of sodium have no hypertension and no increase of blood pressure with age. Confounding variables include exercise, lean body mass, societal stress, and potassium intake.[100-102]

Population studies in western countries have not demonstrated a correlation between habitual salt intake and blood pressure, but the range of sodium intake is limited in western societies.[103] Intervention studies demonstrate a modest reduction of blood pressure (8 mm Hg systolic and 4 mm Hg diastolic) with sodium intake of less than 100 mEq/day. Sodium restriction may decrease the amount of diuretic and other antihypertensive drugs needed.[101]

The Intersalt Study involved over 10,000 adults from 52 countries. Researchers collected 24-hour urine samples and anthropometric measures. Major observations were as follows[104-106]:

- A change of 100 mEq per day in sodium excretion was associated with a change in systolic blood pressure of 2.2 mm Hg.
- A reduction of 100 mEq of sodium intake per day could lower the rise in systolic blood pressure for adults 25 to 55 years old by 9 mm Hg.
- Diastolic blood pressure could be lowered by 4.5 mm Hg.
- BMI and alcohol intake were predisposing factors for blood pressure elevation.

Research suggests that there is probably a subset of salt-sensitive individuals in whom sodium intake is an important determinant of blood pressure.[107,108] High sodium intake may limit the effectiveness of some antihypertensive drugs. Therefore, sodium restriction to 70 to 100 mEq per day (4 to 5 grams of salt) is recommended for all hypertensive patients.[109]

Potassium, Calcium, Magnesium, Fat, and Fiber

Studies suggest but do not confirm the following[104,105,110-113]:

- Reduced potassium intake may be associated with high blood pressure.
- High potassium intake (greater than 80 mEq or 3 to 4 g/day) has a modest blood pressure-lowering effect.
- Increased intake of calcium may lower blood pressure in some individuals.
- A within-person or intraindividual relationship exists between dietary magnesium and blood pressure.
- Low intake of saturated fat and high intake of polyunsaturated fat, particularly from fish and fiber, are associated with lower arterial pressure.

Potassium

Potassium supplementation can lower blood pressure. For over 50 years, various mechanisms have been proposed (e.g., a direct natriuretic effect, suppression of the renin-angiotensin and sympathetic nervous systems, baroreceptor function improvement, and less peripheral vascular resistance).[114,115] The first controlled trial to test the effect of potassium supplementation occurred in 1980; this was followed by almost 2 dozen randomized, controlled trials with crossover designs among normotensive individuals. In addition, clinical trials among hypertensive individuals that demonstrate an overall lowering in both systolic and diastolic blood pressure have been conducted. Potassium's effect on lowering blood pressure may be more powerful among subgroups (e.g., African Americans).

Multicountry studies identify an inverse association between blood pressure and serum, urine, and total body levels and dietary intake of potassium.[105,116] After adjusting for age, sex, body mass index, alcohol intake, and urinary sodium excretion in addition to correcting for a regression to the mean phenomenon, the Intersalt Study reported a 2.7 mm Hg reduction in systolic blood pressure for a 60 mmol/24-hour higher excretion of urinary potassium.[105]

The ratio of urinary sodium to potassium is a more powerful factor than the level of potassium alone. The Intersalt Study predicted that a reduction of the sodium-to-potassium ratio of 3.1 to 1.0 was associated with a 3.4 mm Hg decrease in the average level of systolic blood pressure.[104] Other studies suggest that a lower intake of dietary potassium among African Americans may be related to the higher prevalence of hypertension in this subgroup.[117]

The evidence about potassium as a beneficial dietary component and the use of potassium supplementation is still developing. Increased potassium intake is recommended as a general preventive approach, primarily for individuals who have normal renal function and who are not taking drugs known to raise serum potassium levels.[109] The drugs could be potassium-sparing diuretics and angiotensin-converting enzyme inhibitors.

Calcium

Increased intake of calcium has been reported to lower blood pressure in some individuals.[118] Some studies suggest that a direct relationship exists between serum calcium concentration and blood pressure.[119] The calcium-blood pressure hypothesis is fueled by many observational studies reporting an inverse association between calcium intake and either blood pressure level or the prevalence and incidence of hypertension.[113,120-126] The results show a favorable role of calcium and blood pressure for African Americans and women in general, but less influence on white men. Cross-sectional studies have involved samples in Europe, East Asia, South Africa, the Caribbean, and North America, and prospective studies (e.g., the Nurses' Health Study) in the United States.[113,120-122,124,125,127-130] In the Nurses' Health Study, a significantly lower relative risk of 0.78 for hypertension was associated with dietary calcium intake of 800 mg/day compared with an intake of 400 mg/day.[125] Maternal calcium intake was found to be inversely associated with blood pressure of infants before 1 year of age.[131]

In more than 25 randomized, clinical trials, most used calcium tablets rather than calcium-rich foods as the intervention. In trials using dietary calcium sources, reductions in both systolic and diastolic blood pressure are noted. However, pooled analysis of trials with normotensive participants suggests an average blood pressure change of 0.99 systolic and −0.54 diastolic (95% confidence interval of −2.20, +0.22 and −1.31, +0.23). The pooling of 23 trials with hypertensive participants suggests an average of −1.48 for systolic (2.40, −0.56) and −0.29 for diastolic pressure (−0.88, +0.30).[126,132-135]

One concern about calcium supplementation is that the risk for developing renal calculi may increase with increased calcium intake. Because the design of many of the calcium supplementation studies and trials did not control for extraneous variables such as sodium intake, other electrolytes, alcohol intake, and exercise, the hypothesis still needs to be tested.

Magnesium

Data regarding magnesium, zinc, and lead are too meager to justify any recommendations. In phase 1 of the Trials of Hypertension Prevention Study, oral supplementation with magnesium resulted in a small lowering of both systolic and diastolic blood pressure (−0.2 and −0.1 mm Hg, respectively). Gastrointestinal upsets were observed among the intervention group, which were deemed unacceptable side effects when the influence of the supplement on blood pressure appears small.[112,136-138]

Fat and Fiber

Contradictory studies suggest that low saturated fat and high polyunsaturated fat intakes are associated with lower arterial blood pressure. Increased intake of vegetable proteins and complex carbohydrates as observed among vegetarians in industrialized countries show lower blood pressure levels.[139] Dietary fiber in the form of wheat, wheat bran, pectin, and oat bran have been studied for their hypotensive influence. Results are neither strong nor consistent but warrant further exploration.

The large Multiple Risk Factor Intervention Trial (see Chapter 11) with 12,000 participants showed an independent association between systolic blood pressure and saturated fat, exogenous cholesterol per 1,000 kcal, and complex carbohydrate. This observation was not confirmed in studies involving more than 138,000 nurses and healthy male professionals.[140-142]

Observation studies suggest that eating large amounts of fish rich in polyunsaturated omega-3 fatty acids lower rates of coronary artery disease and may lower serum triglycerides, but their role in hypertension control is not known.[140,142-144] Evidence is still inadequate to recommend specific dietary changes in fat for hypertension control, even though these changes could potentially lower blood cholesterol and reduce coronary artery disease risk. Further research and exploration of hypotheses linking dietary fat composition amid individuals with different body mass indices and baseline blood pressure levels are needed.

The Effect of Healthy Eating

Healthy eating can improve the efficacy of some pharmacologic agents. Nutritional approaches can be effective as definitive intervention alone but also as adjuncts to pharmacologic therapy. An experimental trial called Trials of Hypertension Prevention was conducted by a collaborative research group. The trial, which involved nonpharmacologic interventions to lower blood pressure, included 2,182 persons with high normal diastolic blood pressure of 80 to 89 mm Hg. Randomization assignment was one of 3 lifestyles (weight reduction, sodium reduction, and stress management) and 4 nutritional supplementation groups (calcium, magnesium, potassium, and fish oil). After 6 months, significant decreases in diastolic and systolic blood pressure were noted for the weight reduction and sodium reduction intervention groups. Even with high compliance, neither stress management intervention nor nutritional supplements significantly lowered blood pressure.[112]

The multiple-step intervention program included a sodium-light lifestyle intervention (see Exhibit 14–1). Eight group meetings and two 1-on-1 meetings were held in the first 3 months. These sessions were followed by less intensive counseling. Positive support was given throughout the study.

Exhibit 14–1   Sodium-Light Lifestyle Intervention Approach in Phase I of the Trials of Hypertension Prevention

- Intervention objective: To reduce the group average 24-hour urinary sodium excretion to a mean of 80 mmol (1,800 mg)
- Nutrition counseling objective: To reduce the individual's 24-hour sodium intake to 60 mmol (1,400 mg) without changing other nutrient intakes
- Contact pattern
  –Eight group and two individual counseling sessions over a 3-month period
  –Periodic group meetings and individual telephone or in-person contacts throughout follow-up
- Program content
  –Sodium content of foods
  –Food shopping, label reading, recipe modification, restaurant selections
  –Sodium-specific dietary behavior problem solving
  –Food tasting
  –Take-home packages of low-sodium foods and product samples
  –Local shopping guide for sodium-reduced products
  –Peer support and family involvement
  –Field trips (e.g., to restaurants, supermarkets)
  –Motivational activities
- Adherence monitoring/enhancement
  –Food diaries
  –Attendance
  –Overnight (8-hour) urinary sodium excretion

Source: Reprinted from Kumanyika SK. Feasibility and efficacy of sodium reduction in the trials of hypertension prevention, phase I. *Hypertension.* 1993;22:502-512. Used with permission of the American Heart Association.

A total of 327 individuals were assigned to active intervention; 417 were assigned to the control group. An average weight loss of 8.5 pounds and reduction of 2.9 mm Hg and 2.3 mm Hg systolic and diastolic blood pressure, respectively, were reported after 18 months of intervention. The weight loss alone was associated with a 51% reduction in the incidence of hypertension.[112,145]

The 5-year Primary Prevention of Hypertension Trial used a multifactorial intervention with reductions of total energy, sodium, and alcohol intake, and increased physical activity for normotensive individuals. An average 5.9 pounds of weight loss and a reduction of 1.3 mm Hg systolic and 1.2 mm Hg diastolic blood pressure occurred. Individuals involved in the intervention had a 50% lower 5-year incidence of hypertension than those who received the usual care.[146]

A third major trial, Hypertension Prevention Trial, demonstrated that energy reduction alone could lower blood pressure and the incidence of hypertension. An average reduction in systolic blood pressure and diastolic blood pressure of 2.4 mm Hg and 1.8 mm Hg, respectively, was experienced by participants who only reduced their total energy intake.[147]

To determine the effect on blood pressure of 2 multicomponent/behaviorial interventions, participants averaging 50 years of age were randomized to 1 of 3 intervention groups. The participants were hypertensive and not taking antihypertensive drugs.

Treatment groups were:

A. *Advice only group.* A registered dietitian (RD) discussed nonpharmocological factors that affect blood pressure such as weight, sodium intake, physical activity, and the DASH diet, and printed materials were provided for the 273 members.
B. *Established group.* Goals established for this group of 268 included weight loss of at least 15 lb at 6 months for those with BMI of at least 25, moderate intensity physical activity, daily intake of no more than 100 mEq of Na, and daily intake of 1 oz or less of alcohol for men and $^1/_2$ oz for women.
C. *Established plus DASH diet group.* These 269 individuals had the same goals as the established group, but they also received instruction and counseling on the DASH diet. Participant goals were designed to accomplish the DASH diet and increase consumption of fruits and vegetables (9-12 servings per day) and low-fat dairy products (2-3 servings/day) and reduce intake of saturated fat (less than 7% of total energy) and total fat intake (less than 25% of total energy intake).

During the initial 6 months, 18 face-to-face intervention contacts were made. Participants kept food diaries, recorded physical activity, and monitored calorie and sodium intake. The established plus DASH diet group monitored intake of fruits, vegetables, dairy, and fat intakes.

Blood pressure; weight and height; 24-hour urine collections for Na, K, P, and urea nitrogen; treadmill tests; waist circumference; 24-hour dietary recalls; and physical activity recall were obtained. Results showed the smallest blood pressure reduction in the advice only group while the greatest blood pressure reduction was in the established plus DASH diet group. In this group, 77% of individuals with stage 1 hypertension at baseline had a systolic BP < 140 and diastolic BP < 90 at 6 months.[148]

Appel et al enrolled 459 adults, 22 years of age or older, who were not taking antihypertensive medication in a study. Average systolic blood pressures were 160 mm Hg and diastolic blood pressures ranged from 80 to 95 mm Hg. The major exclusions were uncontrolled diabetes mellitus (DM), hyperlipidemia, chronic illness, renal insufficiency, and an alcoholic beverage intake of more than 14 drinks per week.

A control diet low in fruits, vegetables, and dairy products with a fat content typical of the average diet in the United States was eaten for 3 weeks. Afterward, these participants were randomly assigned for 8 weeks to either the control diet, high in fruits and vegetables, or a combination diet, which was rich in fruits and vegetables and low-fat dairy products while being low in saturated and total fat intake. Sodium intake and body weight were maintained.

At each of 3 screening visits, trained staff members measured the participants' standard blood pressure twice with a 5-minute resting period between measures. During the run-in phase, 2 blood pressures were measured on each of 4 separate days, a 24-hour urine sample was collected, and a questionnaire on symptoms was completed. The intervention phase was 8 weeks of assigned diets. Once each week during the first 6 weeks, blood pressure was measured. During the last 2 weeks, 2 blood pressure measures were obtained on each of 5 separate days, as were a 24-hour urine sample, a description of symptoms, and a physical activity recall questionnaire.

At baseline, the mean systolic and diastolic blood pressures were 131 ± 10.8 mm Hg and 84.7 ± 4.7 mm Hg, respectively. The combination diet lowered systolic and diastolic BP by 5.5 and 3.0 mm Hg more than the control diet. The fruit and vegetable diet reduced systolic blood pressure by 2.8 mm Hg more and diastolic BP by 1.1 mm Hg more than the control diet. For participants with hypertension, the combination diet reduced BP by 11.4 and 5.5 mm Hg, systolic and diastolic, respectively, than those on the control diet. For adults without hypertension, the reduction was 3.5 mm Hg and 2.1 mm Hg, respectively.[149]

Sacks et al randomly assigned 412 participants to either a control diet typical of US foods or the DASH diet. In the assigned diet, participants ate foods with high, intermediate, and low levels of sodium for 30 consecutive days in random order. The 3 sodium levels were high, 150 mmol per/day with a calorie intake of 2,100 Kcal; intermediate, 100 mmol per day; and low, 50 mmol/day, the level hypothesized to lower blood pressure. The daily sodium intake was proportionate to the total calorie requirements of participants.

The DASH diet compared to the control diet resulted in significantly lower systolic blood pressure at every sodium level and in a significantly lower diastolic blood pressure at the high and intermediate sodium levels. It had a larger effect on both systolic and diastolic blood pressure at high sodium levels than it did at low ones. Compared with the high-sodium control diet, the low-sodium DASH diet produced greater reductions in systolic and diastolic blood pressures than either the DASH diet alone or a reduction in sodium alone. The reduction of sodium intake below 100 mmol per day and the DASH diet both lower blood pressure substantially.[150]

The Effect of Hypertension Control

The number of Americans who receive medication for high blood pressure has increased significantly over the last 20 years. In 1991, 73% of hypertensives took drugs. The number of hypertensive individuals whose blood pressure was controlled was about 75%.[151-155] Awareness of high blood pressure has improved in the last 30 years, but with 60 million Americans with high blood pressure, treatment and control are challenging.

African-American men are at high risk for high blood pressure, but NHANES III data show a 60% increase in the number of black men whose high blood pressure is under control. African Americans with blood pressure above 140/90 mm Hg have higher rates of awareness, treatment, and control of the high blood pressure than other ethnic groups. However, for hypertensive individuals with blood pressure above 160/95 mm Hg, the rate of treatment and control among blacks is less than among individuals of all other ethnic groups with hypertension.[151]

About 50% of US adults 50 years old and older do not know their BP, which increases their risk for undetected and untreated hypertension. Awareness and action plans are urgently needed. Of 1,500 Americans 50 years of age and older surveyed, 69% had not discussed the physical consequences of high BP with a doctor or nurse in the past 12 months, 27% knew the importance of systolic BP as the indicator of high BP, but 46% incorrectly believed that stress is a cause of high BP. The National Council on Aging estimates that one third, or about 30 million Americans affected by high BP are unaware that they have hypertension and only 27% are treated to the recommended goal of 140/90 mm Hg.[153]

Adults 40 to 59 years old appear to be the most aware (73%) and have their blood pressure controlled (66%) compared to younger adults 18 to 39 years old (52% aware and 52% controlled). A reported 44% of adults over 60 years old are controlled and treated for their high blood pressure. Among ethnic groups, Mexican Americans have the lowest percentage aware (58%) and controlled (44%) compared to non-Hispanic whites (70% aware and 56% controlled). Non-Hispanic blacks have the highest awareness at 74%, but only a reported 45% is treated and controlled.[154]

To guide practitioners, the 7th NIH Joint National Committee on Detection, Evaluation, and Treatment of High Blood Pressure established guidelines for the treatment of elevated blood pressure. The guidelines are based on a classification system (see Table 14–1). Depending on the severity of an individual's high blood pressure, the committee recommends a certain course of action. The recommended treatment begins with changing the patient's lifestyle (i.e., reducing weight, increasing exercise, and limiting salt and alcohol intake). If this course of action does not work, the committee recommends medication.[151]

A corresponding report by the working group of the National High Blood Pressure Education Program calls for continuation of the national education program. The campaign educates the general public about high blood pressure, targets high-risk groups such as African-American men, and educates healthcare providers.[152]

TABLE 14-1   Classification and Management of Blood Pressure for Adults

Blood Pressure Classifications	SPB* mm Hg	DBP* mm Hg	Lifestyle Modification	Initial Drug Therapy With No Compelling Indication	Initial Drug Therapy With a Compelling Indication
Normal	< 120	and < 80	Encourage	No antihypertensive drug indicated.	Drug(s) for compelling indications.[†]
Prehypertension	120-139	or 80-89	Yes		
Stage 1 hypertension	140-159	or 90-99	Yes	Thiazide-type diuretics for most. May consider ACEI, ARB, BB, CCB, or combination.	Drug(s) for the compelling indications.[†] Other antihypertensive drugs (diuretics, ACEI, ARB, BB, CCB) as needed.
Stage 2 hypertension	≥ 160	or ≥ 100	Yes	Two-drug combination for most[‡] (usually thiazide-type diuretic and ACEI or ARB or BB or CCB).	

DBP = diastolic blood pressure; SBP = systolic blood pressure.
Drug abbreviations: ACEI, angiotensin converting enzyme inhibitor; ARB, angiotensin receptor blocker; BB, beta-blocker; CCB, calcium channel blocker.
* Treatment determined by highest BP category.
† Treat patient with chronic kidney disease or diabetes to BP goal of < 130/80 mmHg.
‡ Initial combined therapy should be used cautiously in those at risk for orthostatic hypotension.

Source: US Department of Health and Human Services. *The Seventh Report of the Joint National Committee on the Prevention, Detection, Evaluation, and Treatment of High Blood Pressure. National High Blood Pressure Education Program.* Washington, DC: National Institutes of Health, NHLBI; December 2003. NIH Publication No 03-5233.

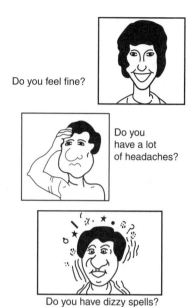

With high blood pressure, you could

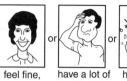

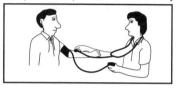

FIGURE 14–3 Strike Out Stroke health education materials developed for low-literacy adults in North Carolina. The materials emphasize the symptoms one can experience and the need to have blood pressure checked frequently.
Source: Reprinted from *Info Memo: Easy-to-Read Materials.* Bethesda, Md: Four Stroke Belt Projects, National High Blood Pressure Prevention and Control Program, National Heart, Lung, and Blood Institute; 1993:17.

Because about 80% of a person's daily sodium intake is from processed foods, the working group specifically solicits the following[152]:

- food manufacturers to reduce sodium in their products
- supermarkets to label shelves to direct customers to low-sodium foods
- food service operators to label foods and provide salt substitutes

Preventing strokes means lowering blood pressure or controlling hypertension. The United States has experienced a 37% drop in age-adjusted death rates from stroke or cerebrovascular disease from 1979 to 1992. Among non-Hispanic whites age 20 and older, 2.3% of men and 2.6% of women have had a stroke. The estimated stroke incidence is 277,000 for white males and 312,000 for white females. In 2002, 52,959 white males and 86,760 white females died of stroke. Further, stroke is the third major cause of death in the United States.[9]

Four states with a high incidence of high blood pressure and stroke developed easy-to-read health education materials to explain risk factors for strokes.[155] North Carolina developed materials for low-literacy clients by using focus groups to respond to fourth- and seventh-grade level materials (see Figure 14–3). The focus group participants emphasized the need for simple, direct materials that clearly showed which foods to control and demonstrated the specific ethnic groups being targeted.

Recent Research Regarding Strokes

Stroke in Young Adults: A Retrospective Analysis

Recent data suggest that stroke in young adults is more frequent than previously reported. To explore clinical and discharge characteristics of young adults with stroke, a retrospective chart review was completed for all adults, 18 to 45 years of age, hospitalized in 1992 with a diagnosis of stroke. The group consisted of 37 patients with an average age of 36 years. The 16 men and 21 women represented 8.4% of that hospital's 441 patients with stroke treated in 1992. A total of 25 (67.6%) had ischemic strokes (37.8% cerebral infarction and 29.8% transient ischemic attacks), and[156] 12 (32.5%) had hemorrhagic strokes (18.9% subarachnoid and 13.4% intracerebral hemorrhage). The distribution of cerebral infarction/transient ischemic attack subtypes included 16% atherothromboembolic, 32% cardiogenic, 4% lacunar, 16% other causes, and 32% of undetermined cause. Hemorrhagic stroke subtypes included 25% hypertensive, 41.6% aneurysmal, 16.7% other vascular anomalies and 16.7% of undetermined cause. Among those who survived, 88% were discharged directly home, and 12% required rehabilitation. During the acute phase, 11% of the population died. These data suggest that strokes in young adults (1) are more frequent than previously recognized, (2) have multiple etiologic and pathologic factors, and (3) in many cases, are treatable. In general, these patients have a good prognosis.[156]

Diabetes Mellitus as a Risk Factor for Stroke

To evaluate the relative potency of diabetes mellitus as a risk factor for stroke, the relative frequency of stroke symptoms was compared among cohorts with and without diabetes. Stroke symptoms were classified as atherothrombotic cerebral infarctions, transient ischemic attacks, reversible ischemic neurologic deficits, and multi-infarct dementia. The groups were compared according to the occurrence of these symptoms, and both cross-sectional and longitudinal designs were used to study 293 consecutive patients.[157] Hypertension, heart disease, and stroke symptoms and signs were more frequent among diabetics than among age-matched nondiabetics. Among diabetics, strokes occurred at an earlier age and were more common among men. Regression analyses assigned diabetes second to hypertension as a risk factor for stroke, followed by heart disease and smoking. Diabetes associated with hypertension or hyperlipidemia added significantly to stroke risk. Initially, cerebral blood flow values and cognitive test scores were equivalent among diabetics and nondiabetics; after 3 years, cognition became significantly impaired among diabetics, despite better maintenance of cerebral blood flow among treated diabetics compared with nondiabetics. Diabetes acts to compound risk for stroke not only by promoting cerebral atherogenesis but also by aggravating other risk factors including hypertension, heart disease, and hyperlipidemia.[157]

The Causes of Stroke in the Young

In a group of 75 patients under the age of 45 years with stroke, ischemic cerebral infarction was diagnosed in 60 patients and primary intracerebral hemorrhage in 15. Trauma was found to be the commonest identifiable predisposing factor to cerebral infarction, being present in 13 cases (22%). Migraine was the second most commonly identified predisposing factor while atheroma and hypertension were infrequent. Such a high frequency of preceding trauma has not previously been described, perhaps because it is not generally appreciated that the delay between the traumatic event and subsequent stroke may be considerable. The diagnostic management of young stroke patients is considered with particular reference to the indications for specialized cardiac and neuroradiological investigations.[158]

Intake of fruit and vegetables (f/v), especially cruciferous and green leafy vegetables, and citrus fruit and juice, is inversely associated with risk of ischemic stroke.[159] Between 1980 and 1994, 75,596 women, 34 to 59 years old, participated in the Nurses' Health Study; and 38,683 men, 40 to 75 years old, participated in the Health Professionals' Follow-Up Study, from 1986 to 1994.

Adjusting for standard cardiovascular risk factors, adults with f/v in the highest quintile (median = 9.2 servings/day for men and 10.2 servings/day for women) versus the lowest quintile (median = 2.6 servings/day for men and 2.9 servings/day for women) had a 0.59 relative risk for ischemic stroke. A 1-serving/day incremental increase in f/v produced a 6% decrease in risk of ischemic stroke. Protective effect of total f/v against ischemic stroke was greatest for cruciferous vegetables, green leafy vegetables, and citrus fruit and juice.[159]

High-Risk Subgroups

Hypertension Among Older Adults

Hypertension occurs in approximately 60% of non-Hispanic whites, 71% of non-Hispanic blacks, and 61% of Mexican Americans 60 years or older.[151] Systolic hypertension is a known, independent risk factor for coronary heart disease, stroke, and cardiovascular disease. The prevalence of isolated systolic hypertension—defined as systolic blood pressure of 140 mm Hg or greater with diastolic blood pressure less than 90 mm Hg—increases after age 60. The sudden onset of hypertension in older patients suggests the presence of secondary hypertension.

Treating hypertension in older patients is recommended.[160] The Systolic Hypertension in Elder People Study (SHEP) assigned individuals to treatment with a low-dose diuretic, chlorthalidone. If warranted, atenolol or reserpine was added. Individuals who received treatment were compared to those on a placebo who had baseline average systolic blood pressure of 160 mm Hg or greater and diastolic blood pressure greater than 90 mm Hg. The results after an average of 4.5 years clearly favored active treatment. There were 36% fewer fatal and nonfatal strokes and 27% fewer fatal and nonfatal myocardial infarctions in actively treated versus placebo-treated participants. Benefit occurred in all age, race, sex, and blood pressure subgroups. Data from other clinical trials indicate that older patients who have diastolic blood pressure of 90 mm Hg or greater can also benefit from active antihypertensive therapy.

The working group on hypertension in the elderly has issued a report to guide clinicians in their care of elderly, hypertensive patients.[161] The report states that the absolute risk of cardiovascular disease is greater among the elderly but that the benefits of control are also greater. Secondary intervention for elderly hypertensives first addresses lifestyle, focusing on weight control, increased physical activity, and reduction in alcohol and sodium intake. Antihypertensive drug therapy is the second approach, with diuretics and beta-blockers commonly prescribed if lifestyle modification alone does not reduce blood pressure levels.[161]

Hypertension Among Individuals with Diabetes Mellitus

Patients with both hypertension and diabetes mellitus are at high risk for cardiovascular complications. The control of hypertension and dyslipidemia and cessation of cigarette smoking can reduce the risk. The blood pressure goal for high-risk individuals is 130/85 mm Hg or less. Lifestyle changes that can improve health outcome include weight reduction among obese individuals with insulin resistance.[162]

Hypertension During Pregnancy

Hypertension during pregnancy can create life-threatening outcomes for both mother and fetus. Four diagnostic categories are as follows[163]:

- chronic hypertension
- preeclampsia-eclampsia
- chronic hypertension with superimposed preeclampsia
- transient hypertension

The criteria for diagnosing hypertension in pregnancy are systolic pressure increases of 30 mm Hg or greater and diastolic pressure increases of 15 mm Hg or greater, compared with the mother's average blood pressure before 20 weeks of gestation. If prior blood pressure is not known, 140/90 mm Hg or above is considered abnormal. Chronic hypertension is defined as high blood pressure observed before pregnancy or diagnosed before the 20th week of gestation.

A pregnancy-specific condition called preeclampsia is characterized by an increased blood pressure accompanied by proteinuria, edema, or both. The contemporary phrase is pregnancy-induced hypertension. Occasionally, abnormalities of coagulation and liver function can occur. Preeclampsia may progress rapidly to a convulsive phase called eclampsia. Medical nutrition therapy (e.g., moderate sodium restriction) given along with drug therapy may be effective in reducing complications.[163]

Hypertension During Childhood and Adolescence

Studies of a biracial population of children 5 to 14 years old in 2 communities in Louisiana (the Franklinton and Bogalusa Heart Studies) indicated that height and weight, not age, were the strongest determinants of blood pressure in growing children. Taking 9 blood pressures per child in a rigorous, randomized design, registered nurses recorded the resting blood pressures of the children in an unhurried, relaxed atmosphere. Stepwise multiple regression analyses were used to determine variables accounting for the variability of blood pressure. These variables included mood score, community, and previous attendance at an examination. Height accounted for 32% of the variability in systolic blood pressure, and body mass index explained an additional 5-6% of the variability. Other analysis demonstrated a 2.7 mm Hg higher systolic and 1.1 mm Hg higher diastolic blood pressure for black children compared to white children. These data provide supportive evidence that hypertension originates during youth. The exact mechanisms that contribute to the early onset need delineation so primary prevention activities can be developed and implemented.[164]

Dietary Sodium in Children and Adolescents

Secular changes in the typical North American eating pattern of both children and adults show a progressive increase in sodium.[165] An increase in processed foods amid a decrease in natural foods low in sodium and high in potassium have increased sodium intake and changed the sodium-to-potassium ratio. Processed foods add sodium to food intake, and family eating styles have an increased use of modular, deli, and restaurant take-out meals. These selections influence preferences and choices of children.[166]

Simons-Morton et al analyzed children's intake of foods high in fat and sodium and reported that 9- to 11-year-old children had only a few foods accounting for most selections, with selections fairly consistent from day to day. The frequently eaten foods were nutrient poor and either high in fat or sodium.[166]

Average sodium intakes of children and youth exceed their need. Surveys report an average daily sodium intake of youth as > 3.5 g (> 130 mmol), consistency over different regions and ethnic groups, a consistently higher intake of sodium than expected or needed, and sodium-potassium ratios generally > 1.0.[167] In an adolescent urban population in Philadelphia, sodium intake averaged ≈406 mg/MJ (1.7 mg/kcal), or 3.8 g sodium/day, and Sinaiko et al reported for 13-year-old children in Minneapolis a baseline average sodium excretion of 140-160 mmol/24 hours.[168]

Short children may be at risk for high blood pressure in old age. Adults who were short as children may be more likely to have high blood pressure in early old age, putting them at increased risk for heart disease and other chronic illnesses. Data from about 150 men who were 5 to 8 years old in 1937 and 1939 were compared when they were in their 60s in 1997 and 1998. Early growth reflected the development of the stress response system, which also controlled blood pressure. Chronic stress can influence growth and inhibit the production of growth hormone. Chronic stress results in a less effective stress response system and makes children more vulnerable to stress and more likely to suffer from high blood pressure as adults. Prior research showed an association between family conflict and slowed growth. These observations may explain why some shorter adults are at greater risk for heart disease.[169]

Systolic blood pressure (SBP) was highest in those men who were short as children and lowest in men who were tall as children. Average systolic pressure was about 168 in the shortest men and 151 in the tallest. A systolic blood pressure reading above 140 is considered high. Associations remained regardless of smoking status, social class, height, weight, and diet as adults, as well as their health and SES as a child. No association was noted between adult height and blood pressure. Diastolic blood pressure (DBP) was not affected by height and tends to be less responsive to stress.[169]

The Seventh Report of the Joint National Committee (JNC) on Prevention, Detection, Evaluation, and Treatment of High Blood Pressure classifies blood pressure into stages based on both systolic (SBP) and diastolic (DBP) blood pressure levels. When a disparity exists between SBP and DBP stages, patients are classified into the higher stage (they are "up-staged").[170]

Hypertension Classifications

Lloyd-Jones et al evaluated the effect of disparate levels of SBP and DBP on blood pressure staging and eligibility for therapy. They examined 4,962 Framingham Heart Study participants between 1990 and 1995 and determined each individual's blood pressure stage based on SBP alone, DBP alone, or both. After excluding the 1,306 subjects who were on antihypertensive therapy 3,656 adults (mean age 58 ± 13 years; 55% women) were eligible. In this sample, 64.6% had congruent stages of SBP and DBP, 31.6% were up-staged on the basis of SBP, and 3.8% on the basis of DBP; thus, SBP alone correctly classified JNC-VI stage in 96% (64.6% + 31.6%) of the adults.

For adults > 60 years of age, SBP alone correctly classified 99%; in those 60 years old, SBP alone correctly classified 95%. Of the 1,488 adults with high-normal blood pressure or hypertension, 13.0% had congruent elevations of SBP and DBP, 77.7% were increased by one stage based on SBP, and 9.3% were up-staged on the basis of DBP; SBP alone correctly classified 91%, whereas DBP alone correctly classified only 22%. SBP elevation in relation to DBP is common in middle-aged and older persons. SBP appears to play a greater role in the determination of blood pressure stage and eligibility for therapy. Given these results, combined with evidence from hypertension treatment trials, Lloyd-Jones et al recommended that future guidelines might consider a greater role for SBP than for DBP in determining the presence of hypertension, risk of cardiovascular events, eligibility for therapy, and benefits of treatment.[171]

Treatment strategies have generally focused on lowering a patient's diastolic pressure, because diastolic pressure accurately predicted heart disease and stroke risk in younger patients. This practice excludes the elderly, who not only tend to have higher systolic pressures and lower diastolic pressures but who also have the least controlled blood pressures of all age groups. Franklin et al found that for adults 50 and older,[172] high pulse pressure was linked to mortality, and, when systolic pressure was considered, diastolic pressure showed a negative association.[172] Systolic blood pressure, unlike diastolic blood pressure, increases dramatically with age. Inadequate control of systolic hypertension contributes to an increase in deaths and hospitalizations for heart failure. A major criterion for diagnosis, staging, and managing hypertension in middle-aged and older Americans is systolic blood pressure.[173]

Info Line

A normal blood pressure for most adults is less than 120/80, and high blood pressure medicine is recommended if blood pressure is at or over 140/90. Take Action for Healthy BP is a program from Novartis. Information on the program is available at 1-888-BPHELP3 or www.HealthyBPhelp.com.

Community Programs for Blood Pressure Control

Modification of nonpharmacologic or lifestyle factors as primary prevention could potentially reduce the prevalence of hypertension nationally by at least 30% and could reduce the need for antihypertensive drugs in those who are hypertensive.[50]

A primary prevention approach can be complemented by special attempts to lower blood pressure among individuals at high risk of developing hypertension. A high-risk approach targets persons with a high normal blood pressure, a family history of hypertension, and one or more lifestyle factors that predispose them as they age to increases in blood pressure.[112] Achievement of the intervention goals may be constrained by a number of societal barriers. These barriers include a lack of acceptable low-sodium food substitutes and the absence of a national campaign to foster adoption of healthy habits.[174]

Community programs may be an important strategy for primary prevention of hypertension. The Joint National Committee on Detection, Evaluation and Treatment of High Blood Pressure suggests that communities consider the following[151,174]:

- detection, education, and referral for other cardiovascular risk factors
- various strategies to improve adherence:
  1. public, patient, and professional education activities
  2. culturally sensitive approaches
  3. informative food labeling
  4. heart-healthy menus in restaurants
  5. safe trails for walking and biking
- multiple channels for outreach:
  1. healthcare settings
  2. schools
  3. work sites
  4. churches and community centers
  5. supermarkets and pharmacies
- media promotion
- second-order prevention efforts directed toward individuals with normal risk factor levels who need education and support to maintain preventive behaviors (i.e., weight control, exercise, and good nutrition)

Modest activities can expand to become comprehensive programs. Coordination with clinicians and other healthcare providers may increase support of the community program. Advisory boards or community high blood pressure councils facilitate cooperation with professional agencies, local health departments, voluntary health agencies, hospitals, industry, and other interest groups. Community advisory boards or councils can identify community problems and local resources, set priorities, list practical solutions to problems, and formulate methods of evaluating program effectiveness.[175-178] In addition, community involvement fosters a sense of ownership. Ownership strengthens the community's acceptance of responsibility for its health problems and potential solutions.

The JNC-VII report contains the latest guidelines as follows[170]:

- In persons older than 50 years, systolic blood pressure greater than 140 mm Hg is a much more important cardiovascular disease (CVD) risk factor than diastolic blood pressure.
- The risk of CVD beginning at 115/75 mm Hg doubles with each increment of 20/10 mm Hg; individuals who are normotensive at age 55 have a 90% lifetime risk for developing hypertension.
- Individuals with a systolic blood pressure of 120-139 mm Hg or a diastolic blood pressure of 80-89 mm Hg should be considered as prehypertensive and require health-promoting lifestyle modifications to prevent CVD.
- Thiazide-type diuretics should be used in drug treatment for most patients with uncomplicated hypertension, either alone or combined with drugs from other classes. Certain high-risk conditions are compelling indications for the initial use of other antihypertensive drug classes (angiotensin converting enzyme inhibitors, angiotensin receptor blockers, beta-blockers, calcium channel blockers).
- Most patients with hypertension will require 2 or more antihypertensive medications to achieve goal blood pressure (< 140/90 mm Hg, or 130/80 mm Hg for patients with diabetes or chronic kidney disease).
- If blood pressure is more than 20/10 mm Hg above goal blood pressure, consideration should be given to initiating therapy with 2 agents, 1 of which usually should be a thiazide-type diuretic.
- The most effective therapy prescribed by the most careful clinician will control hypertension only if patients are motivated. Motivation improves when patients have positive experiences with, and trust in, the clinician. Empathy builds trust and is a potent motivator; however, the responsible physician's judgment remains paramount.

Convenient reference guides are available, such as pocket-sized cards that serve as a handy classification reference during physical examinations. Information on the macronutrients and micronutrients found in foods and as recommended in the DASH diet are also available.[179-180] See Table 14-2. Other diet intervention tools include:

- *DASH diet screener*—A self-administered diet screener to evaluate achieving the DASH eating pattern. One can score his or her diet and receive tips for improvement.
- *DASH diet and meal plan*—A sheet presents the DASH diet basics and a day's worth of food choices.
- *Blood pressure record sheet*—A monthly record allows a permanent list of a patient's blood pressure measurements.

For more information go to http://www.nhlbi.nih.gov to review JNC-VII.

Method Alert

Observational studies can explore the possible determinants of health problems but cannot directly assess the effects of interventions, whereas randomized, controlled trials can answer key questions concerning causes and benefits of intervention.[181]

TABLE 14–2 Outline of the DASH Eating Plan

The DASH eating plan shown below is based on 2,000 calories a day. The number of daily servings in a food group may vary from those listed depending on energy (caloric) needs. Use this table to help plan menus or to shop for groceries.

Food Group	Daily Servings (except as noted)	Serving Size Examples	Food Examples	Importance
Grains and grain products	7-8	1 slice bread 1 cup dry cereal* 1/2 cup cooked rice, pasta, or cereal	Whole wheat bread, English muffin, pita bread, bagel, cereals, grits, oatmeal, crackers, unsalted pretzels, and popcorn	Major sources of energy and fiber
Vegetables	4-5	1 cup raw, leafy vegetable 1/2 cup cooked vegetable 6 oz vegetable juice	Tomatoes, potatoes, carrots, green peas, squash, broccoli, turnip greens, collards, kale, spinach, artichokes, green beans, lima beans, sweet potatoes	Rich sources of potassium, magnesium, and fiber
Fruits	4-5	6 oz fruit juice 1 medium fruit 1/4 cup dried fruit 1/2 cup fresh, frozen, or canned fruit	Apricots, bananas, dates, grapes, oranges, orange juice, grapefruit, grapefruit juice, mangoes, melons, peaches, pineapples, prunes, raisins, strawberries, tangerines	Important sources of potassium, magnesium, and fiber
Low-fat or fat-free dairy foods	2-3	8 oz milk 1 cup yogurt 1 1/2 oz cheese	Fat-free (skim) or low-fat (1%) milk, fat-free or low-fat buttermilk, fat-free or low-fat regular or frozen yogurt, low-fat and fat-free cheese	Major sources of calcium and protein
Meats, poultry, and fish	2 or less	3 oz cooked meats, poultry, or fish	Select only lean; trim away visible fats; broil, roast, or boil, instead of frying; remove skin from poultry	Rich sources of protein and magnesium

continued

TABLE 14-2   continued

Food Group	Daily Servings (except as noted)	Serving Size Examples	Food Examples	Importance
Nuts, seeds, and dry beans	4-5 per week	1/3 cup or 1 1/2 oz nuts 2 tbsp or 1/2 oz seeds 1/2 cup cooked dry beans	Almonds, filberts, mixed nuts, peanuts, walnuts, sunflower seeds, kidney beans, lentils, and peas	Rich sources of energy, magnesium, potassium, protein, and fiber
Fats and oils[†]	2-3	1 tsp soft margarine 1 tbsp low-fat mayonnaise 2 tbsp light salad dressing 1 tsp vegetable oil	Soft margarine, low-fat mayonnaise, light salad dressing, vegetable oil (such as olive, corn, canola, or safflower)	Besides fats added to foods, remember to choose foods that contain less fats
Sweets	5 per week	1 tbsp sugar 1 tbsp jelly or jam 1/2 oz jelly beans 8 oz lemonade	Maple syrup, sugar, jelly, jam, fruit-flavored gelatin, jelly beans, hard candy, fruit punch, sorbet, ices	Sweets should be low in fat

*Serving sizes for dry cereals vary between $1/2$-$1^{1}/4$ cups. Check the food's nutrition label.
[†]Fat content changes serving counts for fats and oils: For example, 1 tbsp of regular salad dressing equals 1 serving; 1 tbsp of a low-fat dressing equals 1/2 serving; 1 tbsp of a fat-free dressing equals 0 servings.
Source: National Institutes of Health, National Heart, Lung, and Blood Institute. *National High Blood Pressure Education Program.* Bethesda, Md: NIH; 2003. NIH publication No 03-4082.

Quantitative questions about nutrition challenge scientists because of the difficulty and expense to determine the effects of single nutrients amid many nutrients and their interactions. No simple, definitive research method provides the answer. A combination of current scientific methods may be insufficient to measure effect. Current scientific techniques provide some power for determining if individual dietary factors can harm healthy people or whether modification of factors reduce the potential harm. Examples of questions to ask to help make this determination include[181]:

1. Does excessive dietary sodium cause more harm than good?
2. Does lowering the daily consumption below a certain amount shift the balance from harm to good?[182]

Three essential parts to any public policy decision regarding dietary intake must include:

1. evidence
2. circumstances including resources and priorities
3. preferences and values about reasonable and appropriate recommendations and actions

Austin Bradford Hill, one of the fathers of modern medical epidemiology, proposed diagnostic tests for establishing causation and his recommendations remain standard.[183,184] They are outlined next.

Is There Evidence From Experiments in Humans?

The strongest, least biased evidence about whether a substance causes harm comes from randomized, controlled trials in which some individuals receive a harmful dose and others do not. The participants are then followed closely to determine any relation between the adverse outcomes of interest and the treatment groups. For example, randomized, controlled trials (RCT) exist in which people are given various amounts of salt and biochemical agents and blood pressure outcomes are measured.

Is the Association Strong?

Traditional study designs provide information on strength of association. Freedom from bias is the issue and is strongest for randomized, controlled trials, followed by nonrandomized trials, observational studies with cohorts, case comparisons, and finally, surveys.

Cohort studies: People initially free of the outcome of interest, e.g., hypertension, are assessed for their exposure to the causative agent, e.g., they consume their usual daily intake of salt and are then followed to determine the outcome rate. Variables potentially related to risk are measured at baseline and adjusted to determine the independent effect of the exposure. In a randomized, controlled trial, the baseline level of exposure may be due to some unmeasured factor, e.g., a causative agent.

Case-control studies: Case subjects with an outcome of interest, e.g., hypertension, are assessed for prior exposure to the factor of interest and the same factor is assessed for a control group. A common problem is that there are many sources of bias that can influence the observations.[185]

Survey: This involves a simultaneous assessment of both exposure and outcome of interest. A toxic effect can be overlooked if individuals with an adverse effect are not well enough to be surveyed or have reduced exposure as a result of the outcome and appear unaffected.

Is the Association Consistent Across Studies?

A causal association is likely when repeated studies yield similar conclusions among different investigators.

Is the Temporal Relation Correct?

An exposure that is a cause must precede an outcome. Experiments and cohort studies meet the temporal requirement.

Is There a Dose-Response Gradient?

When larger exposures yield higher risk, a causal relation exists.

Does the Association Make Epidemiologic Sense?

People in countries with high dietary salt intake have a higher prevalence of hypertension compared with those with lower salt intake. Exposure and outcome vary, making findings difficult to interpret.

Does the Association Make Biological Sense?

The biological soundness of the mechanism and cell response are the basis of scientific acceptance.

A scale to evaluate research evidence, Figure 14–4, shows the contribution from observational studies, including cohort studies, case-control studies, and surveys versus true experiments. The Canadian Task Force on the Periodic Health Examination has another system of codes for study types, as shown in Table 14–3.[186]

When incorporating scientific evidence into policy, one must consider:

- *circumstances* such as effect, feasibility, cost, and alternative demands on resources
- *values* including society's current ethical standards, preferences, and the vested interests of key stakeholders.

Strategic actions are necessary when establishing a nutrition or dietary policy. When vested interests request data review for establishment of a policy, if after review there is no cause for concern or health risk, then the policy action can be suspended. If the review is inconclusive, then a systematic review should be scheduled. If public debates occur, specific evidence and detail should be presented.

Observational Studies Focusing on Dietary Salt Intake

Observational studies lead to hypotheses for further testing such as RCTs. Rigorous interventional studies with salt and blood pressure have been conducted

Diagnostic Test in Descending Order of Strength of Association	Consistent With Causation*	Neutral or Inconclusive	Opposes Causation
Randomized, controlled trial in humans	+ + + +	- - -	- - - -
↓			
RCT	+ + + +	- - -	- - - -
↓			
Cohort study	+ + +	- -	- - -
↓			
Case-control study	+	- -	- - -
↓			
Surveys	+	-	-
↓			
Consistency	+ + +	- -	- - -
↓			
Temporality	+ +	- -	- - - -
↓			
Gradient	+ +	-	- -
↓			
Epidemiologic sense	+ +	-	- -
↓			
Biological sense	+	0	-

* +, Causation supported; 0, causal association not affected; -, causation rejected.

FIGURE 14–4 Flow chart to evaluate importance of diagnostic.
Source: Adapted from: Haynes R. Nature and role of observational studies in public health policy concerning the effects of dietary salt intake on blood pressure. *Am J Clin Nutr.* 1997;65(suppl):622S-625S; and from Goldbloom R, Battista RN, Haggerty J. The periodic health examination: 1. Introduction. *Can Med Assoc J.* 1989;141:205-207.

and these supersede prior observational studies, forming the foundation for any policy about salt and hypertension. The policy might address the merit of low sodium as a preventive approach or contain advice for nonhypertensives. If studies demonstrate no effect on blood pressure, then the policy debate can stop. Larger studies might be needed to demonstrate a sustained, clinical effect on health.

TABLE 14–3   Gradations of Contributions From Research Studies

Code	Level	Study Type
1	High	randomized, controlled trials
2-1	Medium	nonrandomized, controlled trials
2-2		cohort studies or case-control studies
2-3		comparisons between times or places with or without intervention (surveys)
3	Low	opinions of authorities, based on clinical experience, descriptive studies, or reports of expert committees

Source: Adapted from: Haynes R. Nature and role of observational studies in public health policy concerning the effects of dietary salt intake on blood pressure. *Am J Clin Nutr.* 1997;65(suppl):622S-625S; and from Goldbloom R, Battista RN, Haggerty J. The periodic health examination: 1. Introduction. *Can Med Assoc J.* 1989;141:205-207.

HEALTHY PEOPLE 2010 ACTIONS

Healthy People 2010 objectives for lifestyle changes to address high blood pressure prevention and control are presented in Exhibit 14–2. The composition of eating patterns (i.e., fat, complex carbohydrate, fiber, and sodium intake) is the primary focus. Attaining an appropriate body weight and controlling blood pressure are listed as objectives for individuals from adolescence throughout the adult years. An important action is to increase to 90% the proportion of men and women who take direct responsibility for their blood pressure control. Black men and white men are specific high-risk groups targeted by this objective. Community nutrition professionals can direct their program planning toward the lifestyle changes that include eating behavior and support blood pressure prevention and control (see Exhibit 14–3).

Exhibit 14–2   DATA2010: The *Healthy People 2010* Database—November 2000

Objective Number	Objective	Baseline Year	Baseline	Target 2010
12-08	Knowledge of early warning symptoms of stroke	UK	UK	UK
12-09	High blood pressure (age adjusted, adults aged 20 years and older)	1988-1994	28	16
	American Indian or Alaska native	1988-1994	UK	16
	Asian or Pacific Islander	1988-1994	UK	16
	Black or African American	1988-1994	40	16
	White	1988-1994	27	16
	Hispanic or Latino	1988-1994	UK	16
	Not Hispanic or Latino	1988-1994	28	16
	Female	1988-1994	26	16
	Male	1988-1994	30	16
	Poor	1988-1994	32	16
	Near poor	1988-1994	30	16
	Middle/high income	1988-1994	27	16
	Persons with disabilities	1991-1994	32	16

Exhibit 14–2   continued

	Persons without disabilities	1991-1994	27	16
	Persons with diabetes	1988-1994	UK	16
	Persons without diabetes	1988-1994	UK	16
12-10	High blood pressure control (age adjusted, adults aged 18 years and older)	1988-1994	18	50
	American Indian or Alaska native	1988-1994	UK	50
	Asian or Pacific Islander	1988-1994	UK	50
	Black or African American	1988-1994	19	50
	White	1988-1994	18	50
	Hispanic or Latino	1988-1994	UK	50
	Mexican American	1988-1994	13	50
	Not Hispanic or Latino	1988-1994	UK	50
	Female	1988-1994	28	50
	Male	1988-1994	13	50
	Poor	1988-1994	25	50
	Near poor	1988-1994	20	50
	Middle/high income	1988-1994	16	50
	Persons with disabilities (aged 20 years and older)	1991-1994	24	50
	Persons without disabilities (aged 20 years and older)	1991-1994	16	50
	Persons with diabetes	1988-1994	UK	50
	Persons without diabetes	1988-1994	UK	50
12-11	Action to help control blood pressure (age adjusted, adults aged 18 years and older)	1998	82	95
	American Indian or Alaska native	1998	UK	95
	Asian or Pacific Islander	1998	76	95
	Black or African American	1998	86	95
	White	1998	80	95
	Hispanic or Latino	1998	74	95
	Not Hispanic or Latino	1998	83	95
	Female	1998	83	95
	Male	1998	80	95
	Poor	1988	80	95
	Near poor	1988	79	95
	Middle/high income	1988	81	95
	Urban (metropolitan statistical area)	1988	83	95
	Rural (nonmetropolitan statistical area)	1988	80	95
	Persons with activity limitations	1994	84	95
	Persons without activity limitations	1994	76	95
	Persons with diabetes	1998	UK	95
	Persons without diabetes	1998	UK	95
12-2	Blood pressure monitoring—persons who know whether their blood pressure is high or low (age adjusted, adults aged 18 years and older)	1998	50	95
	American Indian or Alaska native	1998	89	95
	Asian or Pacific Islander	1998	86	95

continued

Exhibit 14–2 continued

Black or African American	1998	92	95
White	1998	90	95
Hispanic or Latino	1998	84	95
Not Hispanic or Latino	1998	91	95
Female	1998	92	95
Male	1998	87	95
Less than high school (persons aged 25 years and older)	1998	84	95
High school graduate (persons aged 25 years and older)	1998	90	95
At least some college (persons aged 25 years and older)	1998	93	95
Persons with activity limitations	1994	90	95
Persons without activity limitations	1994	84	95

UK = unknown

Source: Adapted from: US Department of Health and Human Services. DATA2010–the *Healthy People 2010* database. *CDC Wonder.* Atlanta, Ga: Centers for Disease Control; November 2000.

Exhibit 14–3   Model Nutrition Objective for Risk Reduction

By 20____, the chronic disease risk factor * among [*target population*] will be reduced from _____ % to _____%.

*Obesity; hypertension; elevated serum cholesterol; poor physical fitness; excess intake of dietary fat, cholesterol, sodium, alcohol, and sugar; inadequate intake of dietary fiber, fruits, vegetables, and calcium.

Source: Adapted from: *Model State Nutrition Objectives.* Johnstown, Pa: The Association of State and Territorial Public Health Nutrition Directors; 1988.

References

1. Fields LE, Burt VL, Cutler JA, et al. The burden of adult hypertension in the United States 1999 to 2000: a rising tide. *Hypertension* 2004;44: 398-404.
2. Greenlund K, Croft J, Mensah G. Prevalence of heart disease and stroke risk factors in persons with prehypertension in the United States, 1999-2000. *Arch Intern Med.* 2004;164:2113-2118.
3. Hurst W. *The Heart, Arteries and Veins.* 10th ed. New York: McGraw-Hill; 2002.
4. MacMahon S, Rodgers A. The epidemiological association between blood pressure and stroke: implications for primary and secondary prevention. *Hypertens Res.* 1994;17(suppl. 1):S23-S32.
5. Levy D, Larson M, Vasan R, Kannel W, Ho K. The progression from hypertension to congestive heart failure. *JAMA.* 1996;275:1557-1562.

6. Collins R, Winkleby M. African American women and men at high and low risk for hypertension: a signal detection analysis of NHANES III, 1988-1994. *Prev Med.* 2002;35:303-312.

7. Psaty B, Manolio T, Smith N, et al. Time trends in high blood pressure control and the use of antihypertensive medications in older adults: the Cardiovascular Health Study. *Arch Intern Med.* 2002;162:2325-2332.

8. Muntner P, He J, Cutler J, Wildman R, Whelton P. Trends in blood pressure among children and adolescents. *JAMA.* 2004;291:2107-2113.

9. *Heart Disease and Stroke Statistics—2005 Update.* Dallas, Tex: American Heart Association; 2005.

10. Batterson M, Boddie WW, eds. *Salt: The Mysterious Necessity.* Midland, Mich: Dow Chemical Co; 1972.

11. Richter CP. Increased salt appetite in adrenalectomized rats. *Am J Physiol.* 1936;115:155-161.

12. Phillips MI. Central effects of angiotensin II on hypertension and sodium intake. In: Fregly MJ, Kare MR, eds. *The Role of Salt in Cardiovascular Hypertension.* New York: Academic Press; 1982:127-145.

13. Buggy J, Jonklaas J. Sodium appetite decreased by central angiotension blockade. *Physiol Behav.* 1984;32:749-753.

14. Shannon RP, Wei JY, Rosa RM, Epstein FH, Rowe JW. The effect of age and sodium depletion on cardiovascular response to orthostasis. *Hypertension.* 1986;8:438-443.

15. Freeman RH, Davis JO. Factors controlling rennin secretion and metabolism. In: Genest J, Kuchel O, eds. *Hypertension.* New York: McGraw-Hill; 1983:225-250.

16. Williams GH, Dluhy RG. Control of aldosterone secretion. In: Genest J, Kuchel O, eds. *Hypertension.* New York: McGraw-Hill; 1983:320-337.

17. Kuchel O. The autonomic nervous system and blood pressure regulation in human hypertension. In: Genest J, Kuchel O, eds. *Hypertension.* New York: McGraw-Hill; 1983:140-160.

18. DeWardener HE, MacGregor W. The natriuretic hormone and its possible relationships to hypertension. In: Genest J, Kuchel O, eds. *Hypertension.* New York: McGraw-Hill; 1983:89-94.

19. Denton DA, Coghlan JP, Fei DT, et al. Stress, ACTH, salt intake and high blood pressure. *Clin Exp Hypertens.* 1984;A6:403-415.

20. Sybertz EJ, Salvin CS, Morgan RM. Influence of angiotensin converting enzyme inhibition with captopril on blood pressure and adrenergic function in normal and sodium restricted rats. *Clin Exp Hypertens.* 1981;A3:105-107.

21. Volpe M, Lembo G, Morganti A, Condorelli M, Trimarco B. Contribution of the rennin-angiotensin system and of the sympathetic nervous system to blood pressure homeostasis during chronic restriction of sodium intake. *Am J Hypertens.* 1988;1:353-358.

22. Light KC, Koepke JP, Obrist PA, Wilis PW. Psychological stress induces sodium and fluid retention in men at high risk for hypertension. *Science.* 1983;220:429-431.

23. Denton D. *The Hunger of Salt.* Heidelberg, Germany: Springer-Verlag; 1982.

24. Waldron J, Nowotarski M, Freimer M, Henry JP, Post N, Witten C. Cross-cultural variation in blood pressure: a quantitative analysis of the relationships of blood pressure to cultural characteristics; salt consumption and body weight. *Soc Sci Med.* 1982;16:419-430.

25. Simmons D, Barbour G, Congleton J, et al. Blood pressure and salt intake in Malawi: an urban rural study. *J Epidemiol Commun Health.* 1986;40:188-192.

26. Timio M, Verdecchia P, Ronconi M, Gentili S, Francucci B, Bichiasao E. Blood pressure changes over 20 years in nuns in a secluded order. *J Hypertens.* 1985;3:S387-S388.

27. Oparil S, Chen Y-F, Yand R-H, et al. The neuronal basis of salt sensitivity. In: Rettig R, Ganten D, Luft FC, eds. *Salt and Hypertension.* Berlin, Germany: Springer Verlag, 1989:83-96.

28. Campese VM. Salt sensitivity in hypertension: renal and cardiovascular implications. *Hypertension.* 1994;23:531-550.

29. Weinberger MH, Miller JZ, Luft FC, et al. Definitions and characteristics of sodium sensitivity and blood pressure resistance. *Hypertension.* 1986;8(suppl II):127-134.

30. Takeshita A, Imaizumi T, Ashihara T, Nakamura M. Characteristics of responses to salt loading and deprivation in hypertensive subjects. *Circ Res.* 1982;51:457-464.

31. Koolen MI, van Brummelen PV. Adrenergic activity and peripheral hemodynamics in relation to sodium sensitivity in patients with essential hypertension. *Hypertension.* 1984;6:820-825.

32. Skrabal F, Herholz H, Neumayer M. Salt sensitivity in humans is linked to enhanced sympathetic responsiveness and to enhanced proximal tubular reabsorption. *Hypertension.* 1984;6:152-158.

33. Oshima T, Matsuura H, Kido K, et al. Factors determining sodium chloride sensitivity of patients with essential hypertension: evaluation of multivariate analysis. *J Hypertens.* 1989;7:223-227.

34. Resnick LM, Laragh JH, Sealey JE, Alderman MH. Divalent cations in essential hypertension: relations between serum ionized calcium, magnesium, and plasma rennin activity. *N Engl J Med.* 1983;309:888-891.

35. McCarron DA, Rankin LI, Bennett WM, et al. Urinary calcium excretion at extremes of sodium intake in normal man. *Am J Nephrol.* 1981;1:84-90.

36. Kawaskai T, Delea CS, Bartter FC, Smith H. The effect of high sodium and low-sodium intakes on blood pressure and other related variables in human subjects with idiopathic hypertension. *Am J Med.* 1978;64:193-198.

37. Fujita T, Henry WL, Bartter FC, et al. Factors influencing blood pressure in salt-sensitive patients with hypertension. *Am J Med.* 1980;69:334-344.

38. Morgan T, Creed R, Hopper J. Factors that determine the response of people with mild hypertension to a reduced sodium intake. *Clin Exp Hypertens A.* 1986;A8:941-962.

39. Campese VM, Myers MR, DeQuattro V. Neurogenic factors in low rennin essential hypertension. *Am J Med.* 1980;69:83-91.

40. Dichtchekenian V, Sequeira DMC, Andriollo A, et al. Salt sensitivity in human essential hypertension: effect of rennin-angiotensin and sympathetic nervous system blockade. *Clin Exp Hypertens A.* 1989; AI(suppl 1):379-387.

41. Weinberger MH, Miller JZ, Fineberg NS, et al. Association of haptoglobin with sodium sensitivity and resistance of blood pressure. *Hypertension.* 1987;10:443-446.

42. Hollenberg NK, Chenitz WR, Adams DF, Williams GH. Reciprocal influence of salt intake on adrenal glomerulosa and renal vascular responses to angiotensin II in normal man. *J Clin Invest.* 1974;54:34-42.

43. Ashida T, Kuramochi M, Jojima S, et al. Effect of dietary sodium on the Na-K-ATPase inhibitor in patients with essential hypertension. *Am J Hypertens.* 1989;2:560-562.

44. Kotchen TA, Luke RG, Oh CE, Galla JH, Whitescarver S. Effect of chloride on rennin and blood pressure responses to sodium chloride. *Ann Intern Med.* 1983;98:817-822.

45. Kurtz TW, Al-Bander HA, Morris RC Jr. "Salt-sensitive" essential hypertension in man: is the sodium ion alone important? *N Engl J Med.* 1987; 317:1043-1048.

46. Luft FC, Zemel MB, Sowers JA, et al. Sodium bicarbonate and sodium chloride: effects on blood pressure and electrolyte homeostasis in normal and hypertensive man. *J Hypertens.* 1990;8:633-670.

47. Shore AC, Markandu ND, MacGregor GA. A randomized crossover study to compare the blood pressure response to sodium loading with and without chloride in patients with essential hypertension. *J Hypertens.* 1988;6:613-617.

48. Sharma AM, Krobben A, Schattenfroh S, Cetto C, Distler A. Salt sensitivity in humans is associated with abnormal acid-base regulation. *Hypertension.* 1990;16:407-413.

49. Dustan HP, Bravo EM, Tarazi RC. Volume-dependent essential and steroid hypertension. *Am J Cardiol.* 1973;31:606-615.

50. Maxwell MH. *Nutritional Medicine in Medical Practice.* Los Angeles, Calif: UCLA Extension; January 22-23, 1993.

51. Stamler J. Epidemiologic findings on body mass and blood pressure in adults. *Ann Epidemiol.* 1991;1(4):347-362.

52. Chiang BN, Perlman LV, Epstein FH. Overweight and hypertension: a review. *Circulation.* 1969;39:403-421.

53. MacMahon S, Cutler J, Brittain E, et al. Obesity and hypertension: epidemiological and clinical issues. *Eur Heart J.* 1987;8:57-70.

54. Fortmann SP, Haskell WL, Vranizan K, et al. The association of blood pressure and dietary alcohol: differences by age, sex, and estrogen use. *Am J Epidemiol.* 1983;118:497-507.

55. Van Itallie TB. Health implications of overweight and obesity in the United States. *Ann Intern Med.* 1985;103:983-988.

56. Kannel WB, Gordon T. Evaluation of cardiovascular risk in the elderly: the Framingham Study. *Bull NY Acad Med.* 1978;54:573-591.

57. National Institutes of Health Consensus Development Panel on the Health Implications of Obesity. Health implications of obesity: National Institutes of Health Consensus Development. *Ann Intern Med.* 1985;103:981-1077.

58. Shaper AG. Communities without hypertension. In: Shaper AG, Hutt MSR, Fejfar Z, eds. *Cardiovascular Disease in the Tropics.* London, England: British Medical Association; 1974:77-83.

59. Beilin LJ. The fifth George Pickering memorial lecture. Epitaph to essential hypertension—a preventable disorder of known aetiology? [editorial review]. *J Hypertension.* 1988;6:85-94.

60. American Heart Association. *Heart Facts.* Dallas, Tex: American Heart Association; 1998.

61. Kori SO, Feskens EJM, Kromhout D. Fish consumption and risk of strokes: the Zutphen Study. *Stroke.* 1994;25:328-332.

62. Gillum RF, Mussolino ME, Madans JH. The relationship between fish consumption and stroke incidences the NHANES I Epidemiologic Follow-Up Study. *Arch Intern Med.* 1996;156:537-542.

63. Marris MC, Manson JE, Rosner B, Buring JE, Willett WC, Hennekens CH. Fish consumption and cardiovascular disease in the Physicians' Health Study: a prospective study. *Am J Epidemiol.* 1995;142:166-175.

64. Orentia AJ, Daviglus ML, Dyer AR, Shekelle RB, Starnler J. Fish consumption and stroke in men; 30-year findings of the Chicago Western Electric study. *Stroke.* 1996;27:204-209.

65. Dyerberg J, Bang HO, Stoffersen E, Moneada S, Vane JR. Eicosopentaenoic acid and prevention of thrombosis and atherosclerosis. *Lancet.* 1978;2:117-119.

66. Tetrano T, Hirai A, Hamazald T, et al. Effect of oral administration of highly purified eicosapentaenoic acid on platelet function, blood viscosity and red cell deformability in healthy human subjects. *Atherosclerosis.* 1983;46:321-331.

67. Hostmark AT, Bjerkedal T, Klenulf P, Flaten H, Ulahagen K. Fish oil and plasma fibrinogen. *BMJ.* 1988;297:180-181.

68. Knapp HR, FitzGerald GA. The antihypertensive effects of fish oil: a controlled study of polyunsaturated fatty acid supplements in essential hypertension. *N Engl J Med.* 1989;320:1037-1043.

69. Starlien LH, Kraegen EW, Chisholm DJ, Ford GL, Bruce DG, Pascoe WS. Fish oil prevents insulin resistance induced by high-fat feeding in rats. *Science.* 1987;237:885-888.

70. Raper NR, Cronin PJ, Exler J. Omega-3 fatty acid content of the US food supply. *J Am Coll Nutr.* 1991;11:304-308.

71. Bang HO, Dyerberg J, Sinclair HM. The composition of the Eskimo food in Greenland. *Am J Clin Nutr.* 1980;33:2657-2661.

72. Kromann N, Gregg A. Epidemiological studies in the Upemavik district, Greenland: incidence of some chronic diseases, 1950-1974. *Acta Med Scand.* 1980;208:401-406.

73. Iso H, Rexrode KM, Stampfer MJ, et al. Intake of fish and omega-3 fatty acids and risk of stroke in women. *JAMA.* 2001;285:304-312.

74. Liu S, Manson J, Stampler M, et al. Whole grain consumption and risk of ischemic stroke in women. *JAMA.* September 27, 2000;284:12.

75. McCarron P. Adult height is inversely associated with ischemic stroke. The Caerphilly and Speedwell Collaborative Studies. *J Epidemiol Community Health.* 2000;54:239-240.

76. Reuters Health. *Short men and stroke risk.* London: England: Reuters Limited; March 10, 2000.

77. Keys A. Seven countries: a multivariate analysis of death and coronary heart disease. Cambridge, Mass: Harvard University Press; 1980.

78. Stamler J, Stamler R, Neaton JD. Blood pressure, systolic and diastolic, and cardiovascular risks: US population data. *Arch Intern Med.* 1993;153:598-615.

79. McMahon S, Peto R, Cutler J, et al. Blood pressure, stroke, and coronary heart disease: part 1. Prolonged differences in blood pressure: prospective observational studies corrected for the regression dilution bias. *Lancet.* 1990;335:765-774.

80. Weinberger MH. Salt sensitivity of blood pressure in humans. *Hypertension.* 1996;27:481-490.

81. Joint National Committee on Prevention, Detection, Evaluation, and Treatment of High Blood Pressure. The sixth report of the joint national committee on prevention, detection, evaluation, and treatment of high blood pressure. *Arch Intern Med.* 1997;157:2413-2446.

82. Lian C. L'Alcoolisme cuse d'hypertension arterielle. *Br Acad Med.* 1915;74:525-528.

83. Criqui MH, Meban I, Wallace RB, et al. Multivariate correlates of adult blood pressures in nine North American populations: the Lipid Research Clinics Prevalence Study. *Prev Med.* 1982;11:391-402.

84. Friedman GD, Klatsky AL, Siegelaub AB. Alcohol, tobacco, and hypertension. *Hypertension.* 1982;4(suppl III):III-143-III-150.

85. MacMahon SW, Blacket RB, Macdonald GJ, et al. Obesity, alcohol consumption and blood pressure in Australian men and women: the National Heart Foundation of Australia Risk Factor Prevalence Study. *J Hypertension.* 1984;2:85-91.

86. Potter JF, Beevers DG. Pressor effect of alcohol in hypertension. *Lancet.* 1984;1:119-122.

87. Gordon T, Doyle JT. Alcohol consumption and its relationship to smoking, weight, blood pressure and blood lipids: the Albany Study. *Arch Intern Med.* 1986;146:262-265.

88. Puddey IB, Beilin LJ, Vandongen R, et al. Evidence for a direct effect of alcohol consumption on blood pressure in normotensive men: a randomized controlled trial. *Hypertension.* 1985;7:707-713.

89. Engstrom A, Tobelmann RC, Albertson AM. Sodium intake trends and food choices. *Am J Clin Nutr.* 1997;65(suppl):704.

90. Sodium and health. *Loma Linda University Vegetarian Nutrition and Health Letter.* February 2000;2(2):1-3.

91. Mattes RD, Donnelly D. Relative contributions of dietary sodium sources. *J Am Coll Nutr.* 1991;10:383.

92. James WP, Ralph A, Sanchez-Castillo CP. The dominance of salt in manufactured food in the sodium intake of affluent societies. *Lancet.* February 1987;21:426-429.

93. Stamler J. The INTERSALT Study: background, methods, findings, and implications. *Am J Clin Nutr.* 1997;65(suppl):624-626.

94. Messerli FH, Schmieder RE, Weir MR. Salt: a perpetrator of hypertensive target organ disease? *Arch Intern Med.* 1997;157:2449-2452.

95. He J, Ogden LG, Vupputuri S, Bazzano LA, Loria C, Whelton PK. Dietary sodium intake and subsequent risk of cardiovascular disease in overweight adults. *JAMA.* 1999;282:2027-2034.

96. Yu HC, Burrell LM, Black MJ, et al. Salt induces myocardial and renal fibrosis in normotensive and hypertensive rats. *Circulation.* 1998;98(23):2621-2628.

97. Sullivan JM, Ratts TE, Schoeneberger AA, Samaha JK, Palmer ET. The effect of diet on echocardiographic left ventricular dimensions in normal man. *Am J Clin Nutr.* 1979;32(12):2410-2415.

98. Nordin BE, Polley KJ. Metabolic consequences of the menopause: a cross-sectional, longitudinal and intervention study on 557 normal postmenopausal women. *Calcified Tissue Int.* 1987;41:S1-S59.

99. Devine A, Criddle RA, Dick IM, Kerr DA, Prince RL. A longtitudinal study of the effect of sodium and calcium intakes on regional bone density in postmenopausal women. *Am J Clin Nutr.* 1995;62(4):740-745.

100. Dahl LK. Salt and hypertension. *Am J Clin Nutr.* 1972;25:231-244.

101. Law MR, Frost CD, Wald NJ. By how much does dietary salt reduction lower blood pressure? I. Analysis of observational data among populations. *Br Med J.* 1991;302:811-815.

102. Fregly MS, Fregly MJ. The estimates of sodium intake by man. In: Fregly MJ, Kare MR, eds. *The Role of Salt in Cardiovascular Hypertension.* New York, Academic Press; 1982:3-15.

103. Watt GCM, Foy CJW. Dietary sodium and arterial pressure: problems of studies within a single population. *J Epidemiol Community Health.* 1982;36:197-201.

104. Stamler R. Implications of the Intersalt study. *Hypertension.* 1991; 17(suppl I):I-16-I-20.

105. Intersalt Cooperative Research Group. Intersalt: an international study of electrolyte excretion and blood pressure; results for 24 hour urinary sodium and potassium excretion. *Br Med J.* 1988;297:319-328.

106. Intersalt Cooperative Research Group. Sodium, potassium, body mass, alcohol and blood pressure: the Intersalt Study. *J Hypertension.* 1988;6(suppl 4):584S-586S.

107. Muntzel M, Drueke T. A comprehensive review of the salt and blood pressure relationship. *Am J Hypertension.* 1992;5:1S-42S.

108. Grobbee DE, Hofman A. Does sodium restriction lower blood pressure? *Br Med J.* 1986;293:27-29.

109. Subcommittee on Nonpharmacological Therapy of the 1984 Joint National Committee on Detection, Evaluation, and Treatment of High Blood Pressure. Nonpharmacological approaches to the control of high blood pressure. *Hypertension.* 1986;8:444-467.

110. Witteman JCM, Willett WC, Stampfer MJ, et al. A prospective study of nutritional factors and hypertension among US women. *Circulation.* 1989;80:1320-1327.

111. Ascherio A, Rimm EB, Giovanucci EL, et al. A prospective study of nutritional factors and hypertension among US men. *Circulation.* 1992;86:1475-1484.

112. The Trials of Hypertension Prevention Collaborative Research Group. The effects of nonpharmacologic interventions on blood pressure of persons with high normal levels: results of the Trials of Hypertension Prevention, Phase I. *JAMA.* 1992;267:1213-1220.

113. He J, Tell GS, Tang Y-C, et al. Relation of electrolytes to blood pressure in men: the Yi People Study. *Hypertension.* 1991;17:378-385.

114. Treasure J, Ploth D. Role of dietary potassium in the treatment of hypertension. *Hypertension.* 1983;5:864-872.

115. Tannen RL. Effects of potassium on blood pressure control. *Ann Intern Med.* 1983;98:773-780.

116. Whelton PK, Klag MJ. Potassium in the homeostasis and reduction of blood pressure. *Clin Nutr.* 1987;6:76-82.

117. Langford HG. Can black/white differences in blood pressure and hypertensive mortality in the US be explained by differences in potassium intake? In: Whelton PK, Whelton A, Walker WG, eds. *Potassium in Cardiovascular and Renal Medicine—Arrythmias, Myocardial Infarction, and Hypertension.* New York: Marcel Dekker; 1986:397-400.

118. Medical Research Council Working Party. Medical Research Council trial of treatment of hypertension in older adults: principal results. *Br Med J.* 1992;304:405-412.

119. Dahlof B, Linholm LH, Hansson L, et al. Morbidity and mortality in the Swedish Trial in Old Patients with Hypertension (STOP-Hypertension). *Lancet.* 1991;338:1281-1285.

120. Kromhout D, Bosschieter EB, Coulander C de L. Potassium, calcium, alcohol intake and blood pressure: the Zutphen Study. *Am J Clin Nutr.* 1985;41:1299-1304.

121. Ackley S, Barrett-Connor E, Suarez L. Dairy products, calcium, and blood pressure. *Am J Clin Nutr.* 1983;38:457-461.

122. Connor SL, Connor WE, Henry H, et al. The effects of familial relationships, age, body weight, and diet on blood pressure and the 24 hour urinary excretion of sodium, potassium, and creatinine in men, women, and children of randomly selected families. *Circulation.* 1984;70:76-85.

123. Gruchow HW, Sobocincki KA, Barboriak JJ. Alcohol, nutrient intake, and hypertension in US adults. *JAMA.* 1985;253:1567-1570.

124. Joffres MR, Reed DM, Yano K. Relationship of magnesium intake and other dietary factors to blood pressure: the Honolulu Heart Study. *Am J Clin Nutr.* 1987;45:469-475.

125. Witteman JCM, Willett WC, Stampfer MJ, et al. A prospective study of nutritional factors and hypertension among US women. *Circulation.* 1989;80:1320-1327.

126. Belizan JM, Villar J, Pineda O, et al. Reduction of blood pressure with calcium supplementation in young adults. *JAMA.* 1983;249:1161-1165.

127. Elliott P, Fehily AM, Sweetnam PM, et al. Diet, alcohol, body mass, and social factors in relation to blood pressure: the Caerphilly Heart Study. *J Epidemiol Community Health.* 1987;41:37-43.

128. Feinleib M, Lenfant C, Miller SA. Hypertension and calcium. *Science.* 1984;226:384-386.

129. Garcia-Palmieri MR, Costas R Jr, Cruz-Vidal M, et al. Milk consumption, calcium intake, and decreased hypertension in Puerto Rico: Puerto Rico Heart Health Program Study. *Hypertension.* 1984;6:322-328.

130. Hung J-S, Huang T-T, Wu DL, et al. The impact of dietary sodium, potassium, and calcium on blood pressure. *J Formosan Med Assoc.* 1990;89:17-22.

131. McGarvey ST, Zinner SH, Willett WC, et al. Maternal prenatal dietary potassium, calcium, magnesium, and infant blood pressure. *Hypertension.* 1991;17:218-224.

132. Bierenbaum ML, Wolf E, Bisgeier G, et al. Dietary calcium: a method of lowering blood pressure. *Am J Hypertension.* 1988;1:149S-152S.

133. Grobbee DE, Hofman A. Effect of calcium supplementation on diastolic blood pressure in young people with mild hypertension. *Lancet.* 1986;2:703-706.

134. Johnson NE, Smith EL, Freudenheim JL. Effects on blood pressure of calcium supplementation of women. *Am J Clin Nutr.* 1985;42:12-17.

135. Lyle RM, Melby CL, Hyner GC, et al. Blood pressure and metabolic effects of calcium supplementation in normotensive white and black men. *JAMA.* 1987;257:1772-1776.

136. Mascioli S, Grimm R Jr, Launer C, et al. Sodium chloride raises blood pressure in normotensive subjects: the study of sodium and blood pressure. *Hypertension.* 1991;17(suppl I):I-21-I-26.

137. Whelton PK, Klag MJ. Magnesium and blood pressure: review of the epidemiologic and clinical trial experience. *Am J Cardiol.* 1989;63:26G-30G.

138. Henderson DG, Schierup J, Schodt T. Effect of magnesium supplementation on blood pressure and electrolyte concentrations in hypertensive patients receiving long term diuretic treatment. *Br Med J.* 1986;293:664-665.

139. Sacks FM, Kass EH. Low blood pressure in vegetarians: effects of specific foods and nutrients. *Am J Clin Nutr.* 1988;48:795-800.

140. Brussard JH, van Raaij JMA, Stasse-Wolthuis M, et al. Blood pressure and diet in normotensive volunteers: absence of an effect of dietary fiber, protein, or fat. *Am J Clin Nutr.* 1981;34:2023-2029.

141. Swain JF, Rouse IL, Curley CB, et al. Comparison of the effects of oat bran and low-fiber wheat on serum lipoprotein levels and blood pressure. *N Engl J Med.* 1990;322:147-152.

142. Mensink RP, Janssen M-C, Katan MB. Effect on blood pressure of two diets differing in total fat but not in saturated and polyunsaturated fatty acids in healthy volunteers. *Am J Clin Nutr.* 1988;47:976-980.

143. Sacks FM, Rouse IL, Stampfer MJ, et al. Effect of dietary fat and carbohydrate on blood pressure of mildly hypertensive patients. *Hypertension.* 1987;10:452-460.

144. Sacks FM, Stampfer MF, Munoz A, et al. Effect of linoleic and oleic acids on blood pressure, blood viscosity, and erythrocyte cation transport. *J Am Coll Nutr.* 1987;6:179-185.

145. Kumanyika SK. Feasibility and efficacy of sodium reduction in the trials of hypertension prevention, phase I. *Hypertension.* 1993;22:502-512.

146. Stamler R, Stamler J, Gosch FC, et al. Primary prevention of hypertension by nutritional-hygienic means: final report of a randomized, controlled trial. *JAMA.* 1989;262:1801-1807.

147. Hypertension Prevention Trial Research Group. The Hypertension Prevention Trial: three-year effects of dietary changes on blood pressure. *Arch Intern Med.* 1990;150:153-162.

148. Writing group of the Premier Collaborative Research Group. Effects of comprehensive lifestyle modification on blood pressure control. *JAMA.* 2003;289:2083-2093.

149. Appel L. A clinical trial of the effects of dietary patterns on blood pressure. *N Engl J Med.* 1997;336:1117-1124.

150. Sacks FM, Svetkey LP, Vollmer WM, et al. Effects on blood pressure of reduced dietary sodium and the dietary approaches to stop hypertension (DASH) diet. *N Eng J Med.* 2001;344:3-10.

151. National Heart, Lung, and Blood Institute. *The Fifth Report of the Joint National Committee on Detection, Evaluation, and Treatment of High Blood Pressure.* Bethesda, Md: National Institutes of Health; January 1993. NIH publication 93-1088.

152. Working Group on Health Education and High Blood Pressure Control, National High Blood Pressure Education Program. *The Physician's Guide: Improving Adherence Among Hypertensive Patients.* Bethesda, Md: US Dept of Health and Human Services, National Heart, Lung, and Blood Institute; March 1987.

153. Reuters Health. March 10, 2000. Available at www.reutershealth.com. Accessed January 22, 2007.

154. Trends in prevalence, awareness, treatment and control of hypertension in the United States, 1988-2000. *JAMA.* 2003;290:199-206.

155. National High Blood Pressure Prevention and Control Program. Easy-to-read materials produced by four stroke belt projects. *Info memo.* Bethesda, Md: National Heart, Lung, and Blood Institute; 1993.

156. Banet GA. Stroke in young adults: a retrospective analysis. *J Vasc Nurs.* 1994;12(4):101-105.

157. Mortel K, Meyer J, Sims P, McClintic K. Diabetes mellitus as a risk for stroke. *South Med J.* 1990;83(8):904-911.

158. Hilton-Jones D, Warlow C. The causes of stroke in the young. *J Neurol.* 1985;232(3):137-143.

159. Joshipura KJ, Ascherio A, Manson JE, et al. Fruit and vegetable intake in relation to risk of ischemic stroke. *JAMA.* 1999;282:1233-1239.

160. SHEP Cooperative Research Group. Prevention of stroke by antihypertensive drug treatment in older persons with isolated systolic hypertension. *JAMA.* 1991;265:3255-3264.

161. National High Blood Pressure Education Program Coordinating Committee. *Statement on Hypertension in the Elderly—Final Report.* Bethesda, Md: National Institutes of Health; 1980.

162. Epstein M, Sowers JR. Diabetes mellitus and hypertension. *Hypertension.* 1992;19:403-418.

163. National High Blood Pressure Education Program Working Group on High Blood Pressure in Pregnancy. Working group report on high blood pressure in pregnancy. *Am J Obstet Gynecol.* 1990;163:1689-1712.

164. National High Blood Pressure Education Program. *Working Group Report on Primary Prevention of Hypertension.* Bethesda, Md: National Institutes of Health; May 1993. NIH publication 93-2669.

165. Falkner B, Michel S. Blood pressure response to sodium in children and adolescents. *Am J Clin Nutr.* 1997;65(suppl):618S-621S.

166. Simons-Morton BG, Baranowski T, Parcel GS, O'Hara NM, Mattleson RC. Children's frequency of consumption of foods high in fat and sodium. *Am J Prev Med.* 1990;6:218-227.

167. Frank GC, Webber LS, Nicklas TA, Berenson GS. Sodium, potassium, calcium, magnesium, and phosphorous intakes of infants and children: Bogalusa Heart Study. *J Am Diet Assoc.* 1988;88:801-807.

168. Sinaiko AR, Gomez-Marin O, Prineas RJ. Effect of low sodium diet or potassium supplementation on adolescent blood pressure. *Hypertension.* 1993;21:989-994.

169. Montgomery S, Berney L, Blane D. Prepubertal stature and blood pressure in early old age. *Arch Dis Child.* 2000;82:358-363.

170. US Department of Health and Human Services. *The Seventh Report of the Joint National Committee on the Prevention, Detection, Evaluation, and Treatment of High Blood Pressure. National High Blood Pressure Education Program.* National Institute of Health, NHLBI; December 2003. NIH Publication No 03-5233.

171. Lloyd-Jones DM, Evans JC, Larson MG, O'Donnell CJ, Levy D. Differential impact of systolic and diastolic blood pressure–level on JNC-VI staging. *Hypertension.* 1999;34:3.

172. Franklin SS, Khan SA, Wong ND, Larson MG, Levy D. Is pulse pressure useful in predicting risk for coronary heart disease? The Framingham Heart Study. *Circulation.* 1999;100(4):354-360.

173. *Heart Memo.* Dallas, Tex: American Heart Association; Spring 2000:8.

174. Lefebvre RC, Lasater TM, Carleton RA, et al. Theory and delivery of health programming in the community: the Pawtucket Heart Health Program. *Prev Med.* 1987;16:80-95.

175. Mittelmark MB, Leupker RV, Jacobs DR, et al. Community-wide prevention of cardiovascular disease: education strategies of the Minnesota Heart Health Program. *Prev Med.* 1986;15:1-17.

176. Levine DM, Bone L. The impact of a planned health education approach on the control of hypertension in a high risk population. *J Hum Hypertension.* 1990;4:317-321.

177. Farquhar JW, Fortmann SP, Flora JA, et al. Effects of community wide education on cardiovascular disease risk factors: the Stanford Five-City Project. *JAMA.* 1990;264:359-365.

178. National High Blood Pressure Education Program. *Measuring Progress in High Blood Pressure Control: An Evaluation Handbook.* Bethesda, Md: US Dept of Health and Human Services, National Heart, Lung, and Blood Institute; April 1986. NIH publication 86-2647.

179. Sacks FM, Rosner B, Kass EH. Blood pressure in vegetarians. *Am J Epidemiol.* 1974;100(5):390-398.

180. Appee LJ, Moore TJ, Obarzanek E, et al. A clinical trial of effects of dietary patterns on blood pressure. DASH C Research Group. *N Engl J Med.* 1997;1336:1117-1124.

181. Haynes R. Nature and role of observational studies in public health policy concerning the effects of dietary salt intake on blood pressure. *Am J Clin Nutr.* 1997;65(suppl):622S-625S.

182. Lomas J. Making clinical policy explicit: legislative policy-making and lessons for developing practice guidelines. *Int J Technol Assess Health Care.* 1993;9:11-25.

183. Hill AB. *Principles of Medical Statistics.* 9th ed. London, England: *Lancet,* 1971.

184. Department of Clinical Epidemiology and Biostatistics, McMaster University Health Sciences Centre. How to read journals: IV. to determine etiology or causation. *Can Med Assoc J.* 1981;124:985-990.

185. Sackett DL. Bias in analytic research. *J Chronic Dis.* 1979;32:51-63.

186. Goldbloom R, Battista RN, Haggerty J. The periodic health examination: 1. introduction. *Can Med Assoc J.* 1989;141:205-207.

OBESITY

Learning Objectives

- Discuss the epidemiology of obesity in the United States.
- Define the role of eating behavior in the etiology, prevention, and treatment of obesity.
- Discuss voluntary methods practiced by individuals for weight loss and control.
- Identify the *Healthy People 2010* objectives for obesity.
- Describe how community nutritionists can be actively involved in the primary, secondary, and tertiary care of obesity in the United States.

High Definition Nutrition

Body mass index (BMI)—weight/height^2 calculated as kg/m^2.

Qualitative obesity—an abnormally high proportion of body fat.

Quantitative obesity—for adults, BMI > 30.

Overweight—for children, a body mass index (BMI) at or above the sex- and age-specific 95th percentile BMI cut point from the 2000 CDC growth charts; for adults, a BMI from 25 to 29.9.

Providers—includes any individual or organization involved in providing weight loss services or products to the public, e.g., physicians, clinical psychologists, dietitians, nutritionists, commercial programs, and products or publications marketed for weight loss or weight maintenance.

Stigma—any attribute that deeply discredits its possessor.

An Overview of Obesity

In 2005, over 100 million US adults were considered overweight or obese. One objective for *Healthy People 2010* is to reduce the prevalence of obesity among adults to less than 15%. When contrasted with data from 1994, the NHANES 1999-2002 data for adults 20 years old and older showed an alarming increase in the proportion who had become obese in the United States. The estimated age-adjusted obesity prevalence increased from 23% in 1994 to about 30% in 2002. In addition, the prevalence of overweight increased from 56% of the adult population to 65%.[1,2] See Figure 15–1. Women exceed men in prevalence of obesity at any year of assessment (see Figure 15–2). One third of women are obese compared to 28% of men.

Obesity-related health problems in the United States are complex, serious, and difficult to manage.[3] A National Institutes of Health (NIH) Consensus Development Conference Panel on Obesity concluded that a body mass index (BMI)—weight in kg/height in meters squared—greater than 26.9 in women and 27.2 in men indicates increased risk for many common diseases, including heart disease, certain cancers, stroke, diabetes mellitus, and atherosclerosis.[3,4] The cost of these diseases approaches $300 billion for health care alone.[5,6] Estimated annual healthcare cost due to obesity in the year 2000 in the United States was approximately $70 billion and over $33 billion per year was spent on weight control products and services. Prevention and treatment are paramount issues.[7]

A BMI of greater than 35 kg/m² is associated with a twofold increase in total mortality and a multifold increase in morbidity, yet a 10-20% weight loss can forestall or eliminate most obesity-related disease.[8] In addition, a definite reduction in healthcare costs as a result of improved cardiac function,

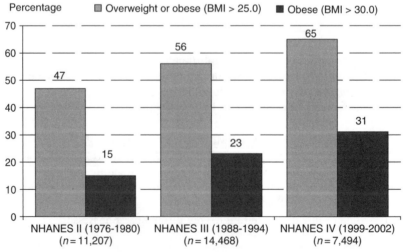

* Age-adjusted by the direct method to the year 2000 US Bureau of the Census
  estimates using the age groups 20 to 39, 40 to 59, and 60 to 74 years.

FIGURE 15–1   Age-Adjusted obesity prevalence
Source: CDC.

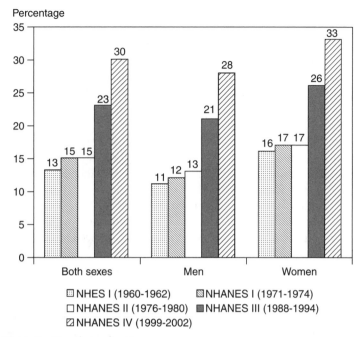

FIGURE 15–2 Trends in obesity.
Source: National Health Examination Survey 1960-1962, National Health and
Nutrition Examination Survey, 1971-1974, 1976-1980, 1988-1994, 1999-2002,
National Center for Health Statistics, Centers for Disease Control and Prevention,
2002, 2004.

improved lipid profiles, and improved glucose tolerance and the associated
decreased need for medication can be realized with weight loss.[9-11]

Overweight is defined for adults as a BMI of 25 to 29.9 kg/m^2 and obesity
as a BMI of $\geq$ 30 kg/m^2. Overweight and obesity are not mutually exclusive.
Obese persons are also overweight. A BMI of 30 is about 30 lb overweight and
equivalent to 221 lb in a 6'0" person. Overweight and obesity are especially
evident in some minority groups, those with lower incomes, and those with
less education.

Research has contributed to the understanding and management of body
weight from 3 major domains[12]:

1. *descriptive*—identification of characteristics of individuals with obesity
2. *theoretical*—explanation of various theories of human behavior to life
   situations
3. *experimental*—evaluation of the effectiveness of various nutrition education approaches

In the early 1980s, several researchers proposed a system of classification of levels of obesity, beginning with a standardization manual for data
collection,[13] but the attempt has continued to be challenging. Obesity can be
defined in terms of amount or distribution of body fat, mortality, or morbidity. Even skills such as the ability to possess eating restraint have been used
to characterize or to differentiate individuals with obesity.[14-16]

Due to the multifactorial nature of obesity, there is no consensus of what
is precisely a healthy level of body fatness, but many believe that a healthy

or good body weight range is one that is associated with the most favorable mortality experience.[17,18] Even with obesity being defined many different ways, the most common definitions are qualitative obesity and quantitative obesity.

Contributions from the theoretical or explanatory domain have evolved over the years. Most contemporary theories about obesity stem from response to the psychodynamic theory, even though the theory is limited to unique situations.[19,20] Other theories that have been tested in obesity research include behavioral theory involving antecedents and consequences or internal and external hunger cues.[21,22] Social learning theory, later termed *social cognitive theory*, explains behavior as the interplay of cognition, personal factors, and environmental factors.[23,24] The theory was expanded to focus on self-efficacy, and a scale with scores explaining a significant portion of the eating behavior of weight control participants has been tested.[25-27]

Self-efficacy has been shown to be associated with adherence, and nutrition education approaches teach individuals to become aware of their defeating thoughts and feelings and substitute negative thoughts with positive ones.[28] Two other theories that have been the basis of intervention programs include (1) the Health Belief Model, which incorporates an individual's perception of the seriousness of obesity with his or her ability to address and to change the problem[29,30]; and (2) the Theory of Reasoned Action, which assumes that humans' behavior can be predicted from their attitude, evaluation, and perception of others toward their behavior.[31]

Data from experimental studies have involved numerous therapeutic approaches that range from increasing the awareness of individuals about the energy content of foods to multifaceted strategies employing exercise, cognition, and skill development. Skill training as an indirect approach to empower individuals before working on changing behaviors has been recommended. Developing social support, buffering the effect of stress, uncovering the factors that bring on disinhibition, and setting up sequential stages of change have been explored.[16,32,33] Factors that appear to predict intention and dropout in weight-loss programs have been identified as demographic, type of program, personal variables, and environmental and attitudinal variables.[34]

The reasons for excess weight are multiple and mirror the characteristics of individuals who are more successful with their weight management. Those who are more successful with maintaining weight loss have achieved higher self-efficacy scores that reflect their taking responsibility for their efforts, defining a fitness or exercise program, developing a lifestyle using multiple resources, and participating in several programs to meet their needs. Reality checks about obesity can be administered and reviewed by community healthcare professionals to plan and to direct programs for individuals with obesity (see Exhibit 15–1).[35]

Gender and Ethnic Differences

Prevalence of obesity among ethnic groups is presented in Table 15–1. A greater percentage of minority groups and female minorities is obese. Black adult women display the highest prevalence among all groups for both obesity and severe obesity. Black men and white women have the lowest rates.[36]

Exhibit 15-1   Reality Checks for Healthcare Professionals—Obesity in the
United States

- One of every two Americans—about 100 million people—is overweight, and
  obesity-related health problems are complex, serious, and difficult to manage.
- A greater percentage of minority groups and female minorities is obese.
- Weight gain is an important indicator of obesity in the United States.
- Individuals at the extremes of body weight and BMI warrant special concern.
- Body fat placement influences health risk.
- There is a link between obesity and coronary heart disease risk factors.
- The incidence of non–insulin-dependent diabetes mellitus increases with rising
  BMI, and there is no evidence of a threshold.
- Mortality from all types of cancer increases with increasing weight among
  women and men.
- Most epidemiological studies report that excess body weight and excess BMI
  increases mortality.
- Depression appears to be a significant factor causing weight change among
  adults.
- Obesity can begin early in life; when it begins, it represents a cause for concern.
- One third of women and one fourth of men try to lose or control their weight.
- There is no single, effective strategy for weight loss.
- There are definite attitudinal and behavioral barriers to weight loss.
- Eating and exercise changes reinforced by behavior modification are the
  most common and preferred combined therapy.
- Professionals have a responsibility to assist overweight and obese individuals
  to lose weight.

Source: Author created

TABLE 15–1   Obesity Among Adults 20 to 74 Years of Age by Sex, Race, and
Hispanic Origin: United States, 1999-2000

Age, Race, and Hispanic Origin	Obese Percentage
All races and origins	31.1
Men	28.1
Women	34.0
White only, not Hispanic or Latino	30.0
Men	28.7
Women	31.3
Black or African American only, not Hispanic or Latino	39.6
Men	27.9
Women	49.6
Mexican	33.7
Men	29.0
Women	38.9

Note: Data are for the civilian noninstitutionalized population.
Source: Centers for Disease Control and Prevention, National Center for Health Statistics,
National Health Examination Survey and National Health and Nutrition Examination
Survey. *Health, United States, 2004.* Atlanta, Ga: Centers for Disease Control; 2,004.

The prevalence of obesity reaches 50% for Native-American, African-American, and Hispanic women in the United States. For Hispanic subgroups in the United States, prevalence of obesity has been reported for the 1982-1984 period using national data. With obesity defined as BMI at or above the 85th percentile and morbid obesity defined as BMI at or above the 95th percentile, the rates for obesity are 39%, 37%, and 34% for Mexican-American, Puerto Rican, and Cuban American women, respectively. For women, morbid obesity was noted for 16%, 14%, and 8% of Mexican Americans, Puerto Ricans, and Cuban Americans, respectively. For men, obesity was noted for 30%, 29%, and 25% of Mexican Americans, Cuban Americans, and Puerto Ricans, and morbid obesity was noted for 10%, 11%, and 8%, respectively.[36,37]

Data can be analyzed by education and income levels. Education can be stratified into 3 groups (0 to 8 years, 9 to 12 years, and over 12 years) and then subclassified by age (20 to 44 years and 45 to 74 years). For younger men and women, the majority who were obese had 9 or more years of education. For individuals 45 to 74 years old, especially Hispanics, a higher percentage of those who were obese were less educated. For individuals below the poverty level, prevalence of obesity was highest for black, Mexican-American, and Puerto Rican groups. Nearly one fourth of overweight Mexican-American and Puerto Rican males had incomes below the poverty level; almost one half of obese Puerto Rican women and one third of black and Mexican-American obese women were below the poverty level.[36,37] A sample of 936 Mexican Americans and 398 Anglo Americans from 3 culturally and socially distinct San Antonio neighborhoods reported a significantly greater prevalence of non–insulin-dependent diabetes mellitus among Mexican Americans compared with Anglo Americans at all 3 levels of body fatness.[38]

Five-year weight change was assessed in 4,207 young adults initially 18 to 30 years old at a CARDIA baseline exam (1985-1986). Weight gain was significantly ($p < 0.0001$) greater in black versus white men (13.2 versus 9.1 lb) and in black versus white women (13.2 versus 7.4 lb). Baseline weight and year-5 weight in all race and gender groups were strongly associated. This suggests a high degree of tracking of adiposity during young adulthood. Greater weight gain was noted for those with high school or less education versus college graduates among black women (14.4 versus 10.0 lb, $p < 0.05$), white women (10.2 versus 5.2 lb, $p < 0.0001$) and white men (10.2 versus 7.8 lb, $p < 0.001$). Significantly greater weight gain was observed in 18- to 24-year-old versus older 25- to 30-year-old men. No age-related difference was seen in women. Racial differences in weight gain remained after adjustment for age and level of education. The data indicate that young adults are at high risk of weight gain, weight gain was greatest among African Americans and among less educated participants, and primary prevention of adult obesity is warranted.[39]

Generally, the largest average increase in BMI over the past 10 years has occurred for black women compared with white women. Less education, lower income, and marrying during follow-up appeared a more important potential causal factor for both men and women gaining weight.[40-41]

Weight Among Parous Women—The SPAWN Study

Pregnancy is a vulnerability factor for some women to become overweight. Many studies suggest that weight gain associated with pregnancy averages

0.5 to 3.8 kg during 2.5 years of follow-up, and 73% of patients in an obesity clinic identified pregnancy as an important trigger for marked weight retention. Most retained more than 10 kg after each pregnancy. The SPAWN followed 2,342 women who delivered children in 1984-1985 in Stockholm and who completed 563 questionnaires about eating behavior and exercise after 15 years. Those women who became overweight had a higher prepregnant BMI (22.3+/-1.5 vs 20.5+/-1.6 kg/m^2, $p < 0.001$), gained more weight during pregnancy (16.3+/-4.3 vs 13.6+/-3.7 kg, $p < 0.001$), and had retained more at 1 year follow-up. The women who became overweight had a steeper weight trajectory, gaining more from 1 year follow-up to 15 years follow-up (11.1+/-6.5 vs 4.5+/-6.5 kg, $p < 0.001$), with a higher BMI at 15 years follow-up of 27.5+/-2.6 vs 22.5+/-2.3 5 kg/m^2 ($p < 0.001$). Differences between those who became overweight and those who did not was not explained by age, number of children, and various socioeconomic factors. Features of pregnancy that differed between the 2 groups were breastfeeding and smoking cessation. Women who became overweight had lower lactation scores than women who remained normal weight. More women who became overweight stopped smoking during pregnancy.[42]

In a cross-sectional, random-digit dialing telephone survey (Behavioral Risk Factor Surveillance System) of free-living adults (aged ≥ conducted between 1991 and 1998, BMI was calculated using self-reported weight and height. Prevalence of obesity, BMI ≥ 30, increased from 12.0% in 1991 to 17.9% in 1998, in all states, in both sexes, across all age, ethnic, and educational levels, and regardless of smoking status. Between 1991 and 1998, the largest increase occurred for 18 to 29 years, +69.9%, those with some college education and those who had completed college, +67.5% and +62.9%, respectively, and Hispanics, +80.0%. Increases in prevalence were +31.9% in the mid-Atlantic region, +67.2% in the south Atlantic region and by state, from +11.3% in Delaware to +101.8% in Georgia.[43] In fact, among the top 10 overweight US cities, 3 are in the South, and all have high percentages of African Americans; see Table 15-2.

TABLE 15–2   Top 10 Overweight Cities With the Highest Rates of Obesity for Adults 20 to 74, 33 largest US metro areas

Rank	Metro	Percentage Obese
1	New Orleans, La	37.6
2	Norfolk, Va	33.9
3	San Antonio, Tex	33.0
4	Kansas City, Mo	31.7
5	Cleveland, Ohio	31.5
6	Detroit, Mich	31.0
7	Columbus, Ohio	30.8
8	Cincinnati, Ohio	30.7
9	Pittsburgh, Pa	30.0
10	Houston, Tex	29.2

Note: Average for 33 largest metro areas is 28.8%.
Source: Adapted from: Doitch S. America weighs in. *Am Demographics.* Ithaca, NY. June 1997; 19(6):38-43.

Obesity and Food Insecurity

A study in the Netherlands found interesting associations between obesity and food deficit early in life. Men conceived during the Dutch famine, 1944-1945, had higher rates of obesity at age 19 years than men conceived before or after the famine. Ravelli et al found that women, not men, conceived during the famine had higher BMI and waist circumference at age 50 years than those conceived before or after the famine. Seven hundred forty-one infants born at term between November 1943 and February 1947 in Amsterdam were weighed at age 50 years and classified by exposure to famine and birth. Mean BMI of women exposed to famine in early gestation was a significant 7.4% higher than nonexposed women. In men, BMI was not significantly affected by exposure to famine during any stage of gestation.[44]

Food Insecurity and Risk of Obesity Among California Women

Food insecurity or the limited or uncertain availability of nutritionally adequate and safe foods may be associated with disordered eating and a poor diet. To evaluate if this increases risk for obesity and health problems, telephone interviews were conducted with 8,169 California women with BMI $\geq$ 30. Food insecurity was evaluated with 4 questions from the US Household Food Security module. Logistic regression was used to examine the association between food insecurity and obesity, controlling for income, race/ethnicity, education, country of birth, general health status, and walking. Food insecurity without hunger affected 13.9% of the population, and food insecurity with hunger, 4.3%. Almost one fifth (18.8%) of the population was obese. Obesity was more prevalent in food insecure (31.0%) than in food secure women (16.2%). Food insecurity without hunger was associated with increased risk of obesity in whites (OR = 1.36) and others (OR = 1.47). Food insecurity with hunger was associated with increased risk of obesity for Asians, blacks, and Hispanics (OR = 2.81) but not for non-Hispanic whites (OR = 0.82).[45]

Fat Placement, Stress, and Alcohol

Skinfold thickness on the trunk and extremities, circumference measures of the abdomen and hips and its ratio, and nuclear magnetic resonance imaging are ways to evaluate fat distribution.[46] Men have more abdominal fat or android fat; women have more gluteal fat and hip circumferences, called gynoid fat. Major complications of obesity (cardiovascular disease, diabetes mellitus, hypertension, and hyperlipidemia) are associated with increased abdominal fat.[47] This is true for men with a waist:hip ratio (WHR) greater than 0.95 and for women with WHR greater than 0.80.[48]

The age at which an individual becomes obese is important in relation to health risk. The risk for a comparable degree of obesity seems to be greater among individuals who became obese before age 40 than for those who became obese after age 40.[49] In addition, longitudinal studies show that weight gain accompanies a greater risk of cardiovascular disease than an unchanging level of obesity.[50]

Most premenopausal women store their fat around the hips. For women, stress and fat are linked at the waist according to Yale University researchers who found that women who are more upset by stressful circumstances and have a harder time adjusting to them are more likely to be fat around the middle. Stress causes the body to release a hormone called cortisol that causes fat storage centrally. Thirty women with abdominal fat who were not otherwise overweight and 29 women with extra weight in their hips but not elsewhere were compared on responses to stress.[51]

Women with abdominal fat reported feeling more threatened by stressful tasks, performed worse on the tasks, and consistently secreted more cortisol. The women were less able to adjust to the tasks even as they became familiar, meaning that their cortisol levels remained high on the second and third days of the experiment. Cortisol fell in the comparison group, whereas women with abdominal fat described themselves as having more negative moods and higher levels of life stress. Greater life stress or psychological vulnerability to stress may explain enhanced cortisol reactivity leading to accumulation of greater abdominal fat. Cortisol levels can be lowered by adequate sleep, exercise, and relaxation.[51]

Moderate Alcohol, Dietary Fat, and Abdominal Obesity in Women

In a study with 334 female twins (57.7+/-6.7 y) moderate alcohol consumers (12-17.9 g/d) had less total body fat (20.6+/-5.6 vs 24.8 +/-8.4 kg, $p = 0.03$) and central abdominal fat (CAF) (1.2+/-0.6 vs 1.6+/-0.7 kg, $p = 0.03$) than abstainers. In multiple regression, alcohol consumption remained independently associated with body fat distribution. Gene-environment interaction analysis indicated that this association was limited to women at high genetic risk of CAF. Among women at low genetic risk of CAF with polyunsaturated fat intakes in the highest tertile, about 50% had less CAF than women with intakes in the lowest tertile (0.9+/-0.4 vs 1.6+/-0.4 kg, $p = 0.0007$), an association absent in women with high genetic risk. Genetic risk modulates relationships between dietary factors and adiposity. Lower abdominal fat may mediate associations between dietary intake and type 2 diabetes risk.[52]

Data from 649 women in the the Postmenopausal Health Disparities Study in Oklahoma between 1994 and 1999 included 226 (34.9%) American Indians, 21 (3.2%) Asians, 78 (12.0%) blacks, 54 (8.3%) Hispanics, and 270 (41.6%) whites. Significant predictors for BMI were neuroendocrine factors, menopausal weight gain, smoking, mean fitness including difficulty performing physical activities, fat as percentage of total calories, moderate drinking, and being Asian or black.[53]

Development of Obesity

At a basic level, excess body fat can only occur when energy ingested exceeds energy requirements or when fat intake exceeds fat oxidation. This can occur due to behavioral causes (i.e., high intake of fat or of total energy or low levels of physical activity) or metabolic causes (i.e., low maintenance energy requirement or high energy efficiency).

Obesity Viewed as a Metabolic Problem

Obesity could be considered to be a metabolic problem in someone with an abnormally low rate of essential energy expenditure and an abnormally high food efficiency. However, based on current knowledge, a low rate of essential energy expenditure estimated by resting metabolic rate (RMR) is not a major cause of obesity.

Determinants of RMR are reasonably well understood, with 80-90% of the between-subject variation in RMR being explained by fat-free mass, body-fat mass, age, and gender. Some researchers have suggested a familial component to RMR. When these variables are considered, RMR is not substantially different between lean and obese individuals.[54]

Food efficiency can be approximated by the thermic effect of food (TEF), which consists of the costs of digestion, absorption, and metabolism of ingested food. Precise determinants of TEF and whether a low TEF is a factor in obesity development are controversial. Any existing between-subject differences in TEF are likely to be small and not of major importance in obesity development. No general abnormalities in essential energy expenditure or in food efficiency that would explain development of obesity have been identified. Based on current knowledge, the development of obesity cannot be solely blamed on metabolic causes.[55]

Systematic lean-obese metabolic differences are not identified, but small individual differences in essential energy expenditure or in food efficiency could influence the development of obesity under specific nutrition and environmental conditions. For example, individuals whose measured RMR is lower than their predicted RMR have been observed to have a higher incidence of weight gain over time than individuals whose measured RMR is higher than predicted RMR.[54] During overfeeding, individual differences are seen both in the amount of weight gained and in the composition of weight gain.[56] These differences could result from small individual differences in metabolism.

Obesity Viewed as a Behavioral Problem

Great difficulty occurs when researchers try to avoid classifying obesity as a problem in food intake. Regardless of energy expenditure, weight gain will not occur if energy intake is matched to energy expenditure. Individuals who practice an eating behavior with excess energy or fat intake may be at risk for positive energy and fat balance and ultimate gain in body fat. Similarly, individuals who reduce physical activity may be at risk of positive energy and fat balance if intake is not also adjusted downward.

Dietary composition is a factor in obesity development. High-fat foods promote fat storage by increasing total energy intake without any immediate increase in fat oxidation. Maintenance of a consistent body composition requires that, on average over time, the fuel mixture ingested equals the fuel mixture burned. Acute changes in protein and carbohydrate intake produce rapid changes in their oxidation. Fat oxidation is not acutely affected by changes in fat intake.[57]

Excess dietary energy from fat is stored as body fat more efficiently than excess energy from carbohydrate or protein. Even with the average percentage of calories from fat declining, individuals may be consuming more total energy and exercising less. They are in effect consuming more fat and expending fewer fat calories. The hypothesis that body fat is related to food composition and lifestyle and not total energy intake has become a popular research topic. Body fat may be closely related to the amount of fat in the foods consumed, as 97% of food energy from fat is available for immediate storage as body fat. Premeasures and postmeasures of social characteristics and weight-related attitudes and behaviors and body mass indices were examined for 304 Mexican-American women, 19 to 50 years old, living in Starr County, Texas. Path analysis revealed that women with higher socioeconomic characteristic scores had less frequent meals and ate less calorically dense foods. Dietary behaviors (e.g., frequency of meals and snacks, use of high- and low-caloric foods, and eating restraint) explained 17.4% of the variance in weight change.[58]

In another study, 3-day dietary records that included a 1-day recall were compared for 23 lean men, 17 lean women, 23 obese men, and 15 obese women. No differences were observed in total energy intake or energy intake relative to lean body mass between lean and obese participants. The obese men and women ate significantly more fat and less total carbohydrate than lean men and women; they consumed a similar amount of total sugar, but the obese men and women consumed a significantly greater percentage of added sugar.[59]

Several studies have reported similar results but some data suggest that obese individuals prefer a higher fat-to-sugar ratio in their food than normal-weight individuals. The high-fat foods may be selected due to taste, and for many high-fat foods, sugar is a complementary ingredient. Lean individuals may consume a substantial amount of sugar in the form of fruits and vegetables but naturally less fat. In other words, the source of the dietary sugar (added versus natural), not the actual amount, and the amount of dietary fat, not the source, appear more important than total energy, fat, and sugar.[60]

An additional consideration is dietary fiber intake. Fiber reduces intestinal transit time and increases postprandial satisfaction and the rate of glucose absorption. Whole grains, fruits, vegetables, and legumes are rich, natural sources of sugar and fiber. The fiber may influence the absorption rate of the natural sugars among lean individuals and retard fat deposition. This action is not present in the obese, as their dietary patterns are low in fiber and high in sugar and fat.[61]

Obesity Viewed as a Problem With the Interaction of Behavior and Metabolism

Obesity is not solely a metabolic or a behavioral problem. Whether a person becomes obese under a given set of nutritional circumstances is determined by an interaction between the behavioral and metabolic responses. These processes determine how much and what type of energy enters the system and the disposition of that energy within the body. Whether body weight and body composition remain the same, increase, or decrease over time depends on how closely metabolism matches behavior, so that energy intake equals energy expenditure and nutrient intake equals nutrient oxidation.

Treatment of Obesity to Produce Negative Energy Balance

Reducing body weight requires a negative energy balance. This is usually accomplished by calorie restriction. Since daily energy expenditure declines as body mass is lost, the amount of body energy lost will be less than the amount of negative energy balance produced. A common problem in obesity treatment is not producing weight loss but maintaining the reduced body weight. Poor success in maintaining weight reduction has led to the hypothesis that after weight reduction, the previously obese person has an abnormally high energy efficiency, virtually ensuring that weight regain will occur even if extremely low intake is maintained. An examination of the metabolic state after weight reduction may explain the ease of weight gain without the need to hypothesize an altered energy efficiency. Resting metabolic rate declines with weight reduction, since it is related to body mass. The majority of data suggest that the determinants of RMR after weight loss are the same as before. The thermal effect of food (described as a percentage of ingested energy) does not appear to change with weight reduction.[62]

A reduced body mass would lead to a decline in the energy cost of physical activity. Unless the amount of physical activity is increased, energy expenditure during activity may be reduced. Thus, total energy expenditure declines with weight loss, but the decline appears to be appropriate for the loss of body mass.

The composition of fuel burned is also altered by weight loss. The daily rate of fat oxidation seems to be proportional to the body fat mass, and since proportionally more body fat is lost compared to body stores of protein or carbohydrate, fat oxidation may decline to a greater extent than protein or carbohydrate oxidation. Thus, the weight-reduced individual is left with a lower rate of energy expenditure than before weight loss, and with a smaller proportion of this energy expenditure coming from fat than before. This situation favors weight regain, but not because of an abnormally high energy efficiency.[63]

Basically, if weight loss is to be maintained without exercise, sedentary individuals may have to consume 30-40% fewer calories than the average daily amount required for their weight. On the other hand, physically active individuals who expend about 200 extra calories per day in physical activity are able to maintain weight loss with a caloric consumption equal to the amount required for their weight.

Strategies to Avoid Weight Regain

Avoiding weight regain involves recognizing that altered body weight and body composition are associated with altered energy requirements, and altering behavior appropriately. Unless permanent changes in behavior are made to ensure that energy and nutrient balance are maintained, weight regain will occur. If the individual who was obese and is now reduced in weight reverts to pre–weight-loss behavior, weight regain will likely occur.

The importance of permanent changes in behavior for weight maintenance is illustrated by data showing that weight maintenance increases with length of behavioral therapy. The problem is that once a target weight is reached, the individual stops behavior therapy and begins to revert to previous behavior. Important strategies for avoiding a regain in body weight include a reduction in dietary fat (to meet the lower rates of fat oxidation) and an increase in physical activity. Physical activity is particularly important since it increases fat oxidation as well as total energy expenditure.[64]

Obesity cannot be blamed solely on overeating or on a low metabolism. Obesity develops when energy intake exceeds energy expenditure, and this can result from an increased energy intake or a decreased amount of exercise. Individual differences in behavior and metabolism can explain why some people maintain a higher body fat content than others. Obesity treatment involves creating negative energy balance, and differences in metabolism explain differences in weight loss. There is no convincing evidence that the reduced-obese person has an abnormal metabolic state. Because energy requirements are altered by a loss of body weight, weight regain will occur unless permanent changes are made in behavior to meet the altered energy requirements.

A comprehensive approach to weight loss and weight loss maintenance seems appropriate. Recommended components are as follows[65]:

- behavioral therapy
- cognitive intervention
- social support
- nutrition education

Behavioral therapy involves reducing caloric intake via stimulus control (e.g., reducing environmental food cues and the response to external cues). It involves modification of eating behaviors such as placing utensils on the table between bites, pausing during meals, and planning regularly scheduled meals. Behavior therapy also includes contingency management or providing positive feedback for healthful behavior and self-monitoring with effective problem solving.[66] Behavioral techniques that focus on fat intake reduction and increased energy expenditure should be emphasized.

Cognitive interventions involve restructuring the way an individual thinks and may include self-instructional training and relapse prevention techniques. A 6-month behavior, self-monitoring program was tested with 35 obese men and women and showed an average loss of 8 kg of body weight, 6 kg of fat, and 4% of body fat. No change was noted among the control group. The self-administered program included a workbook with simple self-evaluations of fat, carbohydrate, sugar, and water intake. The program emphasized exercise and making changes at home.[59]

Social support can be the common thread that continues after behavioral training if a spouse or significant other supports the weight loss. The significant other can assist with realistic weight goals, provide motivation, and assist with positive self-attitudes.[67] Nutrition education in the form of teaching individuals how to read labels, plan healthy meals, calculate energy intake and output, and modify recipes for less fat are important ways to assist individuals with how to create a new lifestyle rather than follow a diet at repeated intervals.

Theories of Obesity Development

Some researchers believe that obesity develops due to a pathological condition characterized by a defect in the regulation of body weight or body fat content. An alternative view is that an individual's body fat content is not regulated directly but is the consequence or the result of many other regulated metabolic processes. The body fat content can be considered as a settling point. This represents the body fat content present at the point where the other metabolic processes reach equilibrium so that energy and nutrient balance are achieved. Accordingly, obesity would not be a pathological condition, and no specific metabolic defect would be noted. This still raises important questions, such as why some individuals have such a high body fat content when the systems reach equilibrium and whether the settling point can be altered by changing behavior or metabolism.

The Link Between Obesity and Chronic Disease

In epidemiologic studies, the association between obesity and hypertension has been reported for a broad range of socioeconomic, racial, and ethnic groups. The Framingham Study found that relative body weight, body weight change, and skinfold thickness were related to blood pressure levels and to the subsequent development of hypertension. Weight gain and loss were associated with increased and decreased blood pressure, respectively.[68]

The Community Hypertension Evaluation Clinic screened about 1 million Americans. Individuals classifying themselves as overweight had rates of hypertension twice as high as individuals classifying themselves as normal weight. From the Intersalt Study, BMI was positively associated with systolic blood pressure and diastolic blood pressure. A 10-kg difference in body weight was associated with a 3 mm Hg diastolic and a 2.2 mm Hg systolic blood pressure difference. In NHANES I, BMI had the strongest relationship to blood pressure of all the nutritional variables. Upper-body obesity (android) correlated best with blood pressure.[69,70]

Several intervention trials observe that moderate weight reduction lowers blood pressure in normotensive and hypertensive individuals and that blood pressure reduction may not relate to salt intake. Blood pressure reduction does correlate with weight loss and, if weight is regained, blood pressure increases. Sodium restriction and weight loss are additive. Weight reduction reduces other cardiovascular risk factors of hyperlipidemia and glucose intolerance.[68]

Overweight individuals are more likely to have higher acidic urine, measured by a lower urinary pH. This places them at an increased risk of uric acid kidney stones. Type 2 diabetics are more likely to develop uric acid kidney stones compared with the general population, suggesting that insulin resistance in the kidneys leads to more acidic urine and uric acid stone formation. In addition to its effect on glucose metabolism, excess insulin in the kidneys may influence urinary acid excretion. This leads to abnormally acidic urine, which precipitates and results in uric acid stones. The hypothesis that urinary pH and body weight are inversely related was evaluated in 4,883 patients with kidney stones. Patients with more acidic urine had higher body weights, after controlling for the effects of age and patient factors that could affect urinary pH. These findings suggest that insulin resistance may be one of the important causes of gout and uric acid kidney stones.[71]

Obesity increases the risk of developing non–insulin-dependent diabetes, cardiovascular disease, and several other chronic diseases (see Chapters 11, 13, 14, and 16). Despite its prevalence and known association with other diseases, its treatment remains largely unsuccessful, in part because of an incomplete understanding of its etiology.

The Link Between Obesity and Lipoprotein Profile

Obesity, whether indicated by relative weight or by body mass index, has been positively associated with a more atherogenic lipoprotein profile. This is true for total cholesterol, low-density lipoprotein (LDL) cholesterol, and triglycerides. A negative correlation is noted with high-density lipoprotein (HDL) cholesterol. These associations have been reported for both adults and children. Framingham Study data predict that for each percentage increase in relative weight, a 1.1 mg/dL increase in serum cholesterol is expected.[72-73]

The cardiovascular disease cost attributed to obesity can be estimated. About 27% of cardiovascular disease, excluding hypertension, is diagnosed among men and women with BMI $\geq$ 29 kg/m^2. Among the obese, 70% of cardiovascular disease is attributed to obesity. This projects 19% of the total cardiovascular disease due to obesity or healthcare costs of $22.2 billion.[6]

Android obesity or excess fat deposits located predominantly in the upper body as opposed to gynoid or lower-body obesity is observed in individuals with carbohydrate and lipid abnormalities.[74] More recently, the relative contribution of body fatness to serum triglyceride, LDL cholesterol, and HDL cholesterol levels was insignificant compared to the effects of a central- or upper-fat pattern.[75]

Using the Gothenburg Study sample, the ratio of waist:hip circumference was associated most strongly with the incidence of ischemic heart disease, and waist:hip circumference was independently associated with the incidence of myocardial infarction.[76] In the Honolulu Heart Study cohort of 7,692 men, risk of coronary events had a positive association with subscapular skinfold thickness. This was independent of BMI.[77] Men in the highest tertile for subscapular skinfold thickness had more than twice the incidence of coronary heart disease during the 12-year follow-up compared with men in the lowest tertile. Abdominal skinfold was significantly and negatively correlated with the serum HDL cholesterol concentration (r = -0.16) in a different cohort of 421 healthy men over 18 years old.[78]

As early as 1914, relative mortality of insured men with large abdominal girths was greater than the already high mortality found in comparably overweight men with smaller waistlines.[79] Data from an adult, prospective cohort demonstrated that an elevated waist:hip ratio (WHR) in men and women was associated with an increased risk of developing coronary heart disease, stroke, and type 2 diabetes mellitus.[80,81] Upper body obesity was a more sensitive predictor of cardiovascular disease and diabetes than a high BMI (kg/m^2) was. This meant that overweight men and women with a low WHR exhibited a reduced risk of developing these comorbidities.

Waist circumference is easy to acquire, is strongly related to health risks, is not influenced by height, and is a convenient tool for self-diagnosis. Waistline may be a better predictor of health risk than BMI. Several cohort studies report 18% of the men and 24% of the women have a waist circumference ≥ 88 cm or 34.6 inches. Among these individuals, poor health and unsatisfactory quality of life was noted in 20%.[82]

However, the goal is to reduce body weight and to improve the lipoprotein profile. A 5-10% drop in plasma total cholesterol and LDL cholesterol levels has been reported for individuals on calorie-restricted weight-loss diets.[83] Some studies report unchanged posttreatment plasma total cholesterol and LDL-cholesterol levels with weight loss, and a few researchers have observed changes after 6 months of follow-up. Reductions in body weight due to exercise training have led to reductions in plasma total cholesterol and LDL cholesterol levels to the extent of 13 and 11 mg/dL, respectively.[84]

HDL level response varies with weight loss. HDL levels increased approximately 21% in obese patients (123 to 209% of ideal body weight) who lost a significant amount of weight.[85] A 15.6% increase in HDL levels was reported for 6 previously sedentary obese men who lost about 5.7 pounds following a moderate exercise and calorie-restricted regimen.[86] A 5% increase in HDL levels was reported for participants who lost weight by exercise training.[84]

Obesity and Diabetes

The incidence of type 2 diabetes mellitus increases with rising BMI, and there is no evidence of a threshold. Costs include the following[6]:

- routine care for uncomplicated diabetes
- morbidity and mortality from complications (e.g., diabetic ketoacidosis, diabetic coma, diabetic retinopathy, and diabetic neuropathy)
- excess prevalence of other disease conditions including visual, renal, and skin disorders

Data from the Nurses' Health Study show that 61% of non–insulin-dependent diabetes mellitus (NIDDM) cases were diagnosed among women 30 to 64 years old with BMI 29 kg/m^2 or greater, and 94% of NIDDM cases were attributed to obesity. Using 1986 population expenditures of $11.6 billion as the direct costs of healthcare expenditures and $8.2 billion as forgone productivity or indirect costs, and then applying the Nurses' Health Study data, 57% (0.61 × 0.94 = 0.57) of the costs of NIDDM are attributed to obesity. This equates to $11.3 billion.[6] Additional costs would be added for managing 40% of the costs attributed to morbid obesity.

Preventing Type 2 Diabetes With Weight Loss and Exercise

Modest changes in diet and physical activity can reduce the risk of type 2 diabetes. Nearly 9% of American women have diabetes, and women are particularly vulnerable to the risk of diabetes-related cardiovascular disease. The NIH Diabetes Prevention Program found that participants who lost at least 7% of their body weight and who completed at least 150 minutes of physical activity each week reduced their risk of developing type 2 diabetes by 58%.[87]

Reversing the Tide of Metabolic Syndrome

One in three Americans have a metabolic syndrome, which is characterized by central obesity, hypertension, and insulin resistance. Half of those diagnosed with metabolic syndrome have a family history of this syndrome. Several mechanisms influence the metabolic syndrome signs, symptoms, and the strategies for successful treatment.[88]

Obesity and Cancer

Mortality from all types of cancer increases with increasing weight among women and for men above desirable weight. Mortality ratios are higher for colon and prostate cancer among obese men, and for breast, endometrial, cervical, ovarian, and gall bladder cancer among obese women.[89] Using a 1986 total estimated cost of cancer in the United States of $75.1 billion and the cost due to cancers attributed in part to obesity, it is estimated that the combined contribution of obesity-promoted colon and breast cancer alone is 2.5% or $1.9 billion.[6]

Cancer epidemiology and clinical experiments have provided data that show an indirect link of obesity to reduced immunocompetence. Overall cancer death rate and the risk of certain types of cancer (i.e., cancer of the endometrium, colon, prostate, and breast) are elevated in obesity. Depressed immune function was noted for 28 obese children and adolescents attending a weight loss clinic. The impairment in immune function was associated with clinical and subclinical deficiencies of zinc and/or iron, which were more common in the obese versus the control group and reversed following appropriate supplementation therapy.[89-91]

Other researchers have observed at least a 50% reduction in the number of monocytes that matured into macrophages among obese individuals. Impaired monocyte maturation has been reported in association with certain kinds of cancers.[92] An additional finding has been the lower amount of a macrophage factor or cytokine that concentrates macrophages at an area of infection among obese, nonhyperglycemic individuals compared to normal weight controls.[93]

Obesity and Foods and Beverages

From 1971 to 2000, the prevalence of obesity in the United States increased from 14.5% to 30.9%.[94] Unhealthy diets and sedentary behaviors have been identified as the primary causes of deaths attributable to obesity.[95] Evaluating trends in dietary intake is an important step in understanding the factors that contribute to the increase in obesity. To assess trends in intake of energy (i.e., kilocalories [kcals]), protein, carbohydrate, total fat, and saturated fat from 1971 to 2000, the CDC analyzed data from 4 National Health and Nutrition Examination Surveys (NHANES): NHANES I (conducted from 1971 to 1974), NHANES II (1976-1980), NHANES III (1988-1994), and NHANES IV (1999-2000). This report summarizes the results of that analysis, which indicate that from 1971 to 2000, mean energy intake in kcals increased, mean percentage of kcals from carbohydrate increased, and mean percentage of kcals from total fat and saturated fat decreased.

From 1971 to 2000, a statistically significant increase in average energy intake occurred. For men, average energy intake increased from 2,450 kcals to 2,618 kcals ($p < 0.01$), and for women, from 1,542 kcals to 1,877 kcals ($p < 0.01$). For men, the percentage of kcals from carbohydrate increased between 1971-1974 and 1999-2000, from 42.4% to 49.0% ($p < 0.01$), and for women, from 45.4% to 51.6% ($p < 0.01$). The percentage of kcals from total fat decreased from 36.9% to 32.8% ($p < 0.01$) for men and from 36.1% to 32.8% ($p < 0.01$) for women. In addition, the percentage of kcals from saturated fat decreased from 13.5% to 10.9% ($p < 0.01$) for men and from 13.0% to 11.0% ($p < 0.01$) for women. A slight decrease was observed in the percentage of kcals from protein, from 16.5% to 15.5% ($p < 0.01$) for men and from 16.9% to 15.1% ($p < 0.01$) for women.

The decrease in the percentage of kcals from fat from 1971 to 1991 is attributed to an increase in total kcals consumed; absolute fat intake in grams increased.[96] USDA food consumption survey data from 1989-1991 and 1994-1996 indicated that the increased energy intake was caused primarily by higher carbohydrate intake.[97] Data from NHANES for 1971-2000 indicate similar trends. The increase in energy intake is attributable primarily to an increase in carbohydrate intake, with a 62.4-gram increase among women ($p < 0.01$) and a 67.7-gram increase among men ($p < 0.01$). Total fat intake in grams increased among women by 6.5 g ($p < 0.01$) and decreased among men by 5.3 g ($p < 0.01$).

A review of 8 years of patient data on 1,550 Mexican Americans and non-Hispanic white adults found that people who drink diet soft drinks were more likely to become overweight. For each diet soft drink drunk per day, participants were 65% more likely to become overweight during the next 7 to 8 years, and 41% more likely to become obese. Drinking sodas of any kind appeared to increase the risk of weight gain. Of 622 study participants who were of normal weight at the beginning of the study, about a third became overweight or obese.[98] Drinking any soda—regular or diet—was linked to a higher risk of becoming overweight. Regular soft drinks had very little connection with serious weight gain, but diet drinks did.

Parker and Folsom examined the association of voluntary vs involuntary weight loss with incidence of cancer in 21,707 older women from 1993 to 2000. Postmenopausal women initially free of cancer completed a questionnaire about intentional and unintentional weight loss episodes of ≥ 20 pounds during adulthood. Women who ever experienced intentional weight loss ≥ 20 pounds but no unintentional weight loss had incidence rates lower by 11% for any cancer (relative risk RR = 0.89, 95% CI: 0.79-1.00), by 19% for breast cancer (RR = 0.81, 95% CI: 0.66-1.00), by 9% for colon cancer (RR = 0.91, 95% CI: 0.66-1.24), by 4% for endometrial cancer (RR = 0.96, 95% CI: 0.61-1.52), and by 14% for all obesity-related cancer (RR = 0.86, 95% CI: 0.74-1.01) after adjusting for age, body mass index, waist:hip ratio, physical activity, education, marital status, smoking status, pack-years of cigarettes, current estrogen use, alcohol use, parity, and multivitamin use. Women who experienced intentional weight loss episodes of ≥ 20 pounds and were not currently overweight had an incidence of cancer similar to nonoverweight women who never lost weight.[99]

Obesity has a complicated relationship to both breast cancer risk and the clinical behavior of the established disease. In postmenopausal women, particularly the elderly, various measures of obesity are positively associated with risk. Before menopause, increased body weight is inversely related to breast cancer risk and related to estrogenic activity. Obesity has also been related to advanced disease at diagnosis and with a poor prognosis in both premenopausal and postmenopausal breast cancer. Breast cancer in African-American women, considering its relationship to obesity, exhibits some important differences from those described in white women, and the high prevalence of obesity in African-American women may contribute to the relatively poor prognosis compared with white American women. As it relates to expression of an aggressive tumor phenotype, insulin, insulin-like growth factor-I, leptin, and their relationship to angiogenesis and transcriptional factors are important.[100]

Although increased consumption of dietary fiber and grain products is widely recommended to maintain healthy body weight, little is known about the relation of whole grains to body weight and long-term weight changes. Liu et al examined the associations between the intakes of dietary fiber and whole- or refined-grain products and weight gain from 1984 to 1996 among 74,091 US female nurses, aged 38 to 63 years with no cardiovascular disease, cancer, and diabetes at baseline. They were followed for their dietary habits using validated food-frequency questionnaires and multiple models adjusted for covariates. Women who consumed more whole grains consistently weighed less than did women who consumed fewer whole grains; p for trend < 0.0001. Over 12 years, those with the highest increase in dietary fiber gained an average of 1.52 kg less than women with the smallest increase in dietary fiber; p for trend < 0.0001. Women in the highest quintile of dietary fiber intake had a 49% lower risk of major weight gain than women in the highest quintile (OR = 0.51; 95% CI: 0.39, 0.67; $p < 0.0001$). Weight gain was inversely associated with the intake of high-fiber, whole-grain foods but positively related to the intake of refined-grain foods, which indicated the importance of distinguishing whole-grain products from refined-grain products to aid in weight control.[101]

The inverse relationship between calcium intake and body weight in 564 women was evaluated for rate of weight gain. At the 25th percentile of calcium intakes, 15% of young women were overweight, but only 4% were overweight at calcium intakes at currently recommended levels. Obesity prevalence in this cohort fell from 1.4 to 0.2% across the same difference in calcium intakes. At midlife, women at the 25th percentile of intakes gained 0.42 kg/y. This gain declined to -0.011 kg/y when the recommended calcium intake was achieved. Calcium intake explains only a small fraction of the variability in weight or weight gain, but shifting the mean downward by increasing calcium intake might reduce the prevalence of overweight and obesity by perhaps as much as 60-80%.[102]

Body Weight and Mortality

New weight standards reflect results of several population-based studies that compared body weight to mortality. Body mass index (BMI) is the criterion recommended for defining a desirable weight index. It indicates relative fatness and has a minimal correlation to height. Using BMI, most epidemiological studies report that excess body weight increases mortality and that BMI is influenced by fat patterning, gender, and age. Similar increases in mortality are seen for individuals with a low BMI. For these individuals, lifestyle factors appear most important. Carefully measured weight and height are the easiest and most useful determinants of nutritional status and important predictors of mortality for the general population.

Ideal, desirable, or healthy body weights are defined as those associated with the lowest mortality. For over 50 years, reference weights developed by the Metropolitan Life Insurance Company have been popular. Their use is limited, however, because they underrepresent the lower socioeconomic class, minorities, and the elderly. They use arbitrary definitions of body frame size and refer to populations rather than individuals. They fail to remove early mortality from the overall analysis.[103]

Gender-specific height-weight tables are not used either. Instead, standards use the BMI (kg/m^2) to define a desirable weight index. BMI is not independent of stature (i.e., it declines as height increases). BMI is an acceptable surrogate for assessing percentage of body fat in most epidemiological studies. BMI below or above the recommended range is associated with worsened health and increased mortality. This weight and mortality association influences predicting hospitalization and healthcare expenditures, setting premiums for health insurance, strengthening preventive medicine, and establishing healthcare policy goals for the nation.

A curvilinear relationship between BMI and mortality was reported after review of 40 studies. BMI greater than 35 kg/m^2 has been associated with both a twofold increase in total mortality and a multifold increase in morbidity. This is due to diabetes, cerebrovascular and cardiovascular disease, and certain cancers that are more prevalent.[104]

Potential Errors in Data Collection

Potential errors in how weight data are collected reduce the ability to identify optimal weights for longevity. For example, survival analyses often reflect either a single body weight or a reported weight at 1 point in time. Individuals at various ages may comprise the sample. Reporting may be inaccurate, the weight scale may not be calibrated, garment weight may vary for different individuals, and individuals may have just eaten or not eaten prior to measurement. Change in body weight due to aging may not be considered during follow-up.

Body weight is determined by a complex interaction of behavioral, cultural, socioeconomic, psychological, physiological, and genetic factors. Each factor may independently influence longevity. Body weight may be a surrogate for another variable, which may have a positive or negative impact on mortality (e.g., leisure time activity, functional capacity, or the quantity and composition of the eating pattern).

Body weight and BMI provide only a snapshot view of an individual's fitness and are not sensitive to moderate changes in illness or aging. Men and women with the same BMI may look vastly different and have different body fatness and leanness. Likewise, body fat may accompany aging, but individuals may not see a change in BMI as they age. Morbidity is rarely reported as an outcome variable. If it were reported as an outcome variable, there might be a shift of optional weight ranges.

Data From Other Studies

Using evidence-based criteria, one can assess the magnitude of research in obesity. Exhibit 15–2 lists such evidenced-based criteria to evaluate research in obesity. A prospective 8-year study of obesity and coronary heart disease (CHD), the Nurses' Health Study, was conducted with 115,886 women, 30 to 55 years of age and 98% white.[105] In data analysis, adjustment was made for age and smoking. One important result was that relative weight had a strong positive association with the occurrence of fatal and nonfatal CHD. Obese women with a BMI greater than 29 kg/m² had a relative risk of 3.5 for fatal CHD compared to women with a BMI greater than 21 but less than 29 kg/m². When intermediate risk factors were controlled, the relative risk was under 2.0.

A 15-year follow-up study of 2,731 black females, 40 to 79 years old, who were members of the Kaiser Foundation Health Plan between 1966 and

Exhibit 15–2   Sources of Research Findings in Obesity

Evidence Category	Sources and Extent of Evidence	Definition
A	Randomized, controlled trials (RCTs). Rich body of data.	End points from well-designed RCTs (or trials that depart only minimally from randomization) that provide a consistent pattern of findings in the population for which the recommendation is made. Large numbers of studies with many participants are required.
B	Randomized, controlled trials. Limited body of data.	End points from intervention studies that include only a limited number of RCTs, post-hoc or subgroup analysis of RCTs, or meta-analysis of RCTs. Category is relevant when few randomized trials exist, sample size is small, and the trial results are inconsistent, or the trials involve samples other than the target population recommendation.
C	Nonrandomized trials. Observational studies.	Outcomes of uncontrolled or nonrandomized trials or observational studies.
D	Panel. Consensus. Judgment.	Synthesis of evidence from experimental research reported in the literature and/or derived from the consensus of panel members. Used only when compelling clinical literature was insufficient.

Source: NIH Clinical Guidelines on the Identification, Evaluation, and Treatment of Overweight and Obesity in Adults. Obesity Education Initiative. Bethesda, Md: National Institutes of Health; June 1998.

1973 presented a different picture.[106] Smoking, antecedent illness, education, and alcohol use were considered intermediate risk factors and controlled in the analysis. The resulting relative risk of death for women with a BMI greater than 25.8 was 1.00, compared to the lowest-mortality group with a BMI range of 23.5-25.8. A lack of association between BMI and mortality among black women has been reported in 2 smaller studies.[107,108]

BMI does not account for differences in body composition (e.g., fat distribution at various body sites). Increased central or visceral fat is a predictor of non–insulin-dependent diabetes mellitus, breast cancer, cardiovascular disease, and overall mortality.[47] BMI is an independent predictor of relative weight. The ratio of waist:hip circumference indicates body fat distribution. Beginning in the mid-1980s, several longitudinal studies of middle-aged adults reported an association between body fat distribution, increased risk for cardiovascular disease, and all-cause mortality.[76]

After a 12-year follow-up, the unadjusted odds ratio for the incidence of CHD for Swedish adults 54 years old was 3.2 for men compared to women. The ratio decreased to 3.1 after BMI and other cardiovascular risk factors were controlled. When waist:hip ratio was controlled, the odds ratio declined to 1.1 and eliminated the sex differences. This suggests that waist:hip ratio may be a marker of genetic, hormonal, or lifestyle factors closely related to CHD risk. Thereby, failing to control for body-fat pattern confounds any analysis of the association between excess body weight and mortality.[109]

Harris et al analyzed Framingham Study data of 1,723 nonsmoking men and women, 65 years old between 1957 and 1981.[110] Individuals in the upper 30% body weight range (BMI > 28.5 kg/m²) had a relative risk of mortality of 1.6 and 1.9, respectively, in contrast to those in the reference BMI range of 23.0 to 25.2 kg/m² for men and 24.1 to 26.1 kg/m² for women. The Framingham Study strengthened the observation that health risks of excess weight occur for individuals over the age of 65. However, BMI may become less associated with mortality as aging progresses.[111]

The National Institutes of Health recommends treatment of overweight only when patients have 2 or more risk factors or a high waist circumference. The focus should be on altering dietary and physical activity patterns to prevent weight gain and to produce moderate weight loss. Treatment should focus on producing substantial weight loss over a prolonged period; however, comorbities affect treatment options.[112]

Evidenced-based research exists showing that weight loss in overweight and obese individuals achieves increases in high-density lipoprotein (HDL) cholesterol and the following potential lowering:

- risk factors for type 2 diabetes and cardiovascular disease (CVD)
- blood pressure in both overweight hypertensive and nonhypertensive individuals
- serum trigylcerides
- total serum cholesterol and low-density lipoprotein (LDL) cholesterol
- blood glucose levels in overweight and obese persons with and without diabetes
- blood glucose levels and HbAlc in some individuals with type 2 diabetes

Mortality and Being Underweight

The association of mortality and relative weight is *J*- or *U*-shaped[89,113] (see Figure 15–3). Excess mortality occurs at very low and very high BMI. The nadir of the curve generally occurs at a BMI between 19.0 and 27.0 kg/m². It appears that healthy individuals below a desirable relative weight are at risk. A systematic overestimation of the influence of being underweight on mortality occurs if there is a failure to control for cigarette smoking or failure to account for subclinical disease precipitating an early mortality.[114]

The 14-year American Cancer Society prospective study of mortality involving 750,000 individuals confirmed that mortality among smokers in the lowest weight category was almost twice that of nonsmokers in the same category.[115] Mortality ratios of lean but heavy smokers (more than 20 cigarettes per day) were similar to ratios for individuals in the highest weight index. Cigarette smoking confounds mortality data among the underweight group, since the excess mortality of lean smokers is mainly caused by lung cancer

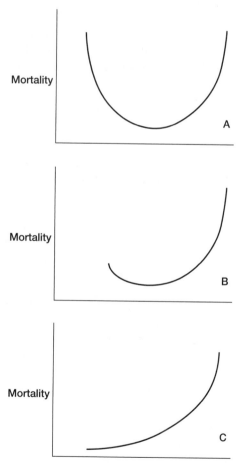

FIGURE 15–3 Schematic representation of the BMI-mortality relationship. Epidemiological studies suggest a *U*-shaped (A), *J*-shaped (B), or direct (C) association. *Source:* Adapted from: Kushner RF. *V Nutr Rev.* 1993;51(5):129.

and other diseases of the respiratory system. Failure to eliminate early mortality from the analysis due to clinical or subclinical illness can erroneously increase estimates of mortality due to lower weights.[89,115]

Smoking duration and intensity affect body leanness. Self-reported smoking data were collected from 12,000 adult men and women in NHANES II. As duration increased, BMI decreased for both men and women.[116] BMI of frequent male smokers was significantly greater than that of average smokers, whereas the data on women showed that there was no difference in weights among women having either average or high smoking rates. The Cancer Prevention Study I reported that cigarette smokers may have a higher waist:hip ratio than nonsmokers. This is independent of BMI and may increase mortality risk.[117]

Between 1977 and 1988, 11,703 men in good health were followed for all-cause, cardiovascular disease, and cancer mortality. Weight was reported but not measured. Five weight-change categories were defined. During the 11 years, 1,441 men died—including 345 from heart disease and 459 from cancer. Lowest all-cause mortality occurred for men who kept their weight within 1 kg of their baseline weight during the 11 years. In comparison, RR for death was the highest for men who lost more than 5 kg (RR = 1.57) or gained 5 kg (RR = 1.36); for CHD, the RRs were 1.75 and 2.01 for these weight-change categories. The higher RR for total mortality remained when cigarette smoking, physical activity, and initial BMI (< 25 versus > 25 kg/m^2) were controlled. Curiously, weight change did not predict cancer mortality, but this may be due to the overall low rate of cigarette smoking of 17.5%.[118]

NHANES I mortality data for 2,140 men and 2,550 women, age 45 to 71 years, was reviewed. Baseline data were collected in NHANES I (1971-1974), and the cohort was followed through 1987. All-cause, cardiovascular disease, and noncardiovascular disease mortality rates were evaluated, considering percent maximum weight loss and BMI. Percent maximum weight loss was calculated by subtracting measured weight from reported highest weight and expressed as a percentage. After adjusting for age, race, smoking, parity, and preexisting illness, the lowest death rate occurred for individuals with BMI less than 26 kg/m^2 and a loss of less than 5% of their maximum weight. A weight loss of more than 15% of maximum weight was associated with higher relative mortality for both men and women, irrespective of maximum BMI. The highest all-cause (RR = 2.8), cardiovascular disease (RR = 3.3), and noncardiovascular disease mortality (RR = 2.3) occurred for women with BMI greater than 29 and with weight loss greater than 15%.[119]

A 4-year follow-up of 10,529 Multiple Risk Factor Intervention Trial (MRFIT) men was conducted. The men were 35 to 57 years of age and free of cancer.[120] Weight change mirrored a 6- to 7-year time period and was expressed as both the intraindividual standard deviation (ISD) of weight and the type of weight change (e.g., no change, loss, gain, or weight cycling). Results were as follows:

- Men with a stable weight had the lowest adjusted risk of mortality.
- The highest relative risk for all-cause and cardiovascular disease mortality occurred in the highest ISD quartile.
- The average weight change was 1.4 kg.
- Adjusted relative risk of mortality was higher for individuals with sustained weight loss, not sustained weight gain.

- Relative risk for all-cause and cardiovascular mortality was dependent on baseline BMI.
- Men with a baseline BMI less than 28.8 kg/m² had a positive association between ISD of weight and mortality.

The trend emerging from various studies is that a sizable weight loss or gain is associated with higher relative rates of mortality. The causes of the changes in weight are not known. Data from 1,794 NHANES I participants identified depression as a significant factor causing weight change for about 27% of younger adults and 24% of older adults.[121] Voluntary weight loss was reported in 21,673 telephone interviews for approximately 25% of men and 40% of women attempting weight loss.[122]

Psychological Aspects of Obesity

Contempt for obesity appears widespread. This is becoming more common among multiethnic groups of youth.[123] Obese individuals are often subjected to intense prejudice that crosses age, sex, race, and socioeconomic strata. The prejudice and stigma appear to begin in childhood.[124] Six-year-old children describe silhouettes of an obese child as ugly, dirty, lazy, and stupid, among other adjectives.[125] When children are shown pictures of handicapped individuals missing limbs along with obese children, the obese children are chosen as the least likeable.[126-127] Interestingly, obese individuals also demonstrate a similar prejudice. Several systematic studies have reported that severely obese individuals do not demonstrate unusual levels of psychopathology using standard measures.[128]

Disparities are noted in acceptance rates for obese and nonobese individuals into universities and private colleges; employment rates by the armed forces, police, fire departments, and airlines; and salary levels.[129] Estimates are that each pound of fat incurs about $1,000 less per year for executives.[130]

As many as 78% of severely obese individuals undergoing surgery reported that they had always or usually been treated disrespectfully by medical professionals due to their weight.[131] A survey of 77 physicians documented their description of obese patients as ugly, awkward, and weak-willed.[132] Negative attitudes of medical professionals toward obese individuals may in part be based on unsuccessful attempts at treatment.[124] These data should alert professionals to the importance of their personal attitudes and expressions during contact with obese individuals.

Pediatricians in North Carolina were queried to determine their skill in managing obese patients and their willingness to advocate for policy changes. Only 12% of the 356 pediatricians reported high self-efficacy in obesity management. The main barrier to success with patients was identified as availability of fast food and soft drinks. Most felt that better counseling tools, including kits of materials, would be helpful and would allow them to participate in advocacy.[133] However, nearly one half of the overweight pediatricians did not identify themselves as overweight, which was more common for men than women. In addition, the self-classified thin pediatricians had nearly 6 times the odds (OR = 5.69) of reporting more counseling difficulty as a result of their weight than average weight pediatricians, and self-identified overweight pediatricians reported nearly 4 times as great counseling difficulty as average weight physicians (OR = 3.84).[134]

The first publicized case in which obesity was considered a disability was a 1985 decision regarding the New York handicapped employment law, *McDermott v Xerox Corporation*. After a medical exam, a tentative employment offer for McDermott—a 5-foot, 6-inch female who weighed 249 pounds—was terminated. The court upheld the state commission's finding of discrimination.[135] Similar court decisions were seen in *Gimello v Agency Rent-A-Car Systems*, where obesity was considered a disability under New Jersey law, and in *Cassisata v Community Foods* (1992), where the California Court of Appeals found that an employer had discriminated against a 305-pound female applicant due to her weight.[136]

In August 2005, a woman filed a lawsuit for false claims that drinking 3 cups of milk a day would help her lose weight and, in fact, she gained weight.[137] The lawsuit was dismissed but nutrition and obesity may take center stage in courts and grocery stores during the next decade.

Childhood Obesity

Over the past 40 years, there has been an increase in the percentage of overweight children and adolescents. Current estimates are that 16% of US children and adolescents are overweight using the BMI at or above the sex- and age-specific 95th percentile BMI cut point (see Figure 15–4). Anthropometric reference data (height, weight, and BMI) are detailed in Chapters 7 and 8.

Over 10% of preschool children between the ages of 2 and 5 are overweight, up from 7% in 1994. Among preschool children, 8.6% of non-Hispanic

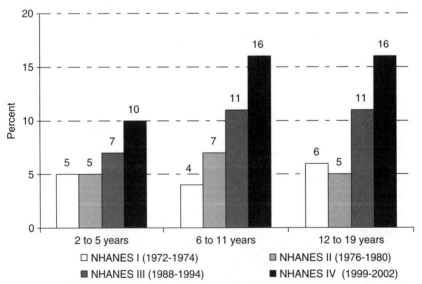

*Overweight is defined as being at or above the 95th percentile for body mass index by age and sex based on reference data.

FIGURE 15–4 Trends in Overweight US, 1971-2002. National Health and Nutrition Examination Survey, 1971-1974, 1976-1980, 1988-1994, 1999-2002, National Center for Health Statistics, Centers for Disease Control and Prevention, 2002, 2004.

whites are overweight. For children ages 6 to 11, 13.5% of non-Hispanic whites are overweight. Among adolescents ages 12 to 19, 13.7% of non-Hispanic whites are overweight, and 31% of children and teens ages 6 to 19 are considered at risk of becoming overweight (BMI from the 85th to the 95th percentile). Among non-Hispanic white children ages 6 to 11, 14.0% of boys and 13.1% of girls are overweight or obese using the 95th percentile of BMI values by age and sex on the CDC 2000 growth chart.[138]

Hispanic Health and Nutrition Examination Survey data indicate that Mexican-American boys and girls are shorter and relatively heavier than non-Hispanic white children. The excess weight appears to be related to fat of the upper trunk and not to lean body mass.[139]

The heights and weights of 1,670 elementary children in 3 central Harlem, New York, schools were measured and compared with the National Center for Health Statistics standards. The median weight- and height-for-age of these children exceeded the standard by 1.4 cm and 2.2 kg for boys and 2.7 cm and 2.8 kg for girls. For boys, the height-age was advanced by about 0.24 years, and for girls it was advanced by 0.47 years. For both boys and girls, about 14% were above the 95th percentile in weight-for-height.[140]

An obese child may embody more than 1 of the 6 major factors that contribute to obesity[141]:

1. genetic factors
2. lifestyle factors
3. emotional overeating
4. indulgence
5. neglect
6. medical factors

Obesity initiates a chain reaction for many children. It is generally complicated by the additional daily stress of problems with peers, social isolation, psychological distress, including low body esteem and self-esteem, physical limitations, illness, and lack of body skills to enhance participation in dance and sports.

In a case-control study of 100 obese participants and 100 age- and sex-matched, always-slender control subjects, subjects were queried about prior sexual abuse and depression. Sexual and nonsexual abuse in infancy, childhood, or adolescence was reported by 25% (sexual) and 29% (nonsexual) of the obese patients, compared with 6% and 14% of the always-slender group. Obesity was described frequently as a sexually protective device by overweight participants who also reported overeating to cope with emotional disturbances.[142]

Obesity in childhood carries a 70% risk of persistence into adulthood, when chronic disease expression occurs. An obese child often experiences adolescence earlier than his or her peers. This creates a shorter period for bone growth and a potentially shorter stature. Acute illnesses may surface (e.g., hyperinsulinemia, elevated serum lipids, and pulmonary and orthopedic problems).

Judgment of body size, attractiveness, and self-concept were compared for 19 diet-intervention mother-daughter pairs and 18 control pairs. Both mothers and daughters ranked large figures as less attractive than thin ones. Daughters wanted to be thinner than they perceived themselves to be; mothers tended to see their daughters as just right. Daughters' self-concept was inversely related to their age, and their own and their mothers' size.[143] Lower self-esteem was noted for girls with large body sizes and girls whose mothers had large body sizes. Control-group mothers with high BMI measures had lower levels of self-esteem; their daughters identified body size as an important factor in feelings of self-worth.[143]

Attempts to treat childhood obesity during the 1970s consisted of approaches that emphasized dieting, exercise, and behavioral change. Success was limited. Family-based strategies that emerged in the 1980s have been credited with sustained weight loss and a broader base for successful skill development. When the whole family addresses both the problems and the positive aspects of the child's life, each member can reorient attitudes and behaviors.

A decline in physical activity and an increase in television watching and sedentary activities such as video games may contribute to the increased prevalence of obesity among US youths. An International Food Information Council survey reported that 53% of 6- to 9-year-olds play outside after school and on weekends, but 80% report watching television.[144] Data from the National Health Examination Surveys show that the prevalence of obesity increased by 2% for each additional hour of television viewed, after controlling for numerous social and family variables. A reduction in resting metabolic rates may be the promoting factor. Resting metabolic rate declined by 12% for normal-weight girls, 8 to 12 years old, watching 25 minutes of nonviolent television programs; it declined by 16% for obese girls.[145-146]

Using the BMI graphs, parents and pediatricians can more accurately gauge whether children are overweight. This is a better way to track a child's physical development and alert parents and doctors if they should intervene with diet and exercise.

Info Line

How to Calculate a Child's BMI

- divide the child's weight (in pounds) by his or her height (in inches)
- divide the result again by the child's height
- multiply the result by 703
- using a BMI graph, plot where a child's age and BMI
  intersect to find the percentile

If the BMI places a child in the 85th to 95th percentile, he or she is considered at risk for being overweight. Those in the 95th percentile or higher are overweight.

Example:

A 10-year-old boy who weighs 120 pounds and is 5 feet tall has a BMI of 23, which would place him above the 95th percentile for his age and classify him as overweight. A 12-year-old girl weighing 125 pounds and being 5 feet, 4 inches would have a BMI of 21 and rank just above the 75th percentile for her age. In contrast to the BMIs for adults, BMI charts for children take into account gender and age, which is the reason that a BMI of 23 could be considered overweight for a 10-year-old boy but would be considered healthy for an adult.

If children are overweight by age 8, they are likely to become overweight adults. More than half of US adults are overweight or obese, placing them at increased risk for many health problems, including heart disease, diabetes, high blood pressure, and stroke. Between 11 and 15% of American children are believed to be overweight, and another 25% are believed to be at risk for becoming overweight. BMI takes into account body weight and height to calculate total body fat and is now widely used for adults age 20 and older.

Children whose BMI places them in the 85th to 95th percentile for their gender and age are considered at risk for being overweight and need to be monitored carefully. Depending on their family history, these children may need to be regularly tested for unsafe blood pressure and cholesterol levels. The 85th to 95th percentile equates to adults with a BMI of 25 to 29.9.

Youth with a BMI at the 95th percentile for their age are considered overweight, which is roughly equivalent to a BMI of 30 or more for adults. For these children, in addition to losing weight, blood pressure, blood cholesterol, and blood sugar should be measured to detect hypertension, unsafe cholesterol levels, and the early signs of diabetes. Type 2 diabetes, once seen only in adults, is a growing problem for children and teenagers. One benefit of the charts is the ability to track a child's weight up to age 20.

A family-based treatment of childhood obesity used parents as agents of change and compared it with the conventional approach, in which the children served as the agents of change. Sixty obese children aged 6 to 11 years were randomly allocated to the experimental or control group. Anthropometric, biochemical, sociodemographic, and family eating and activity habits questionnaires were completed. A clinical dietitian conducted 14 sessions for parents in the experimental group and 30 sessions for the children in the control group. The dropout rate of 9 was 9 times greater in the control group than in the experimental group, which had 1 dropout. Mean percentile weight reduction was significantly higher ($p < 0.03$) in children in the experimental group (14.6%) compared to the control group (8.1%). Treatment of childhood obesity with parents as the exclusive agents of change was superior to the conventional approach.[147]

Successful approaches to treat childhood obesity involve skill development and an interdisciplinary team of highly skilled health professionals who work with various aspects of the problem. A biopsychosocial assessment identifies the medical and psychosocial seriousness of the obesity. Intervention tackles the obese child's symptoms and factors that create the excess weight gain. The intervention may include marital, substance abuse, or individual counseling for family members.

Action and commitment at the national level to address the problem of childhood obesity in the United States has been sought. An improvement in the access to care for families with obese children is one direction. Mellin drafted 8 specific recommendations and submitted them to then-President Clinton, political leaders, and nutritional professionals to improve the overall well-being of children and to improve the availability, accessibility, and effectiveness of child obesity services. The recommendations were[141]:

1. Create a cabinet-level position on the child and family. This effort is needed to create a national agenda on childhood obesity and support legislation and policies.

2. Provide more economic and social support for low-income children. Support could be in the form of recreational areas; family-oriented programs; low-fat supplemental foods; and increases in fruits, vegetables, and grains.

3. Implement a national plan for high-quality after-school care and day care. Enhance after-school care so parents and children want to participate.

4. Mandate health-promoting environments in public schools. Endorse comprehensive school health that is reflected in required physical activity, healthy meals, nutrition education, and self- and body esteem.

5. Create an advisory committee on children and nutrition. With the commitment of a national advisory group, childhood obesity and hunger issues would remain priorities until solutions were found.

6. Extend coverage by health insurers to family-based, child-obesity services. Most obese children are denied a safe and effective medical care setting. Medical coverage for services is almost nonexistent, and costs of medical care when obesity is compounded with other chronic diseases is exceptionally high.

7. Designate increased funding for training. A shortage of healthcare providers for obese children and families escalates the need for training, ranging from undergraduate courses, to university fellowships, to professional education.

8. Designate increased research funding for the prevention and treatment of childhood obesity. Expand research support to address the handicapped, multiethnic groups, and practical approaches for working with young children and families.

Advocacy and Policy in Obesity Treatment and Prevention

To slow the rapid increase of obesity in the United States, strategies must include advocacy and creating public policies that improve healthcare delivery, research, education, and environmental changes to support healthy lifestyles.[148] In 2002, President Bush, then-Secretary of Health and Human Services Tommy Thompson, and US Surgeon General Richard Carmona focused on disease prevention encouraging the public to increase physical activity, select healthy foods more often, and avoid risky behaviors such as smoking. A national summit on prevention was held in Baltimore, Md, in 2003. Over 1,000 community leaders, policy makers, health officials, and others discussed multiple lifestyle strategies. Secretary Thompson initiated Steps to a Healthier US.[149]

In May 2004, the steps program set in place a plan to:

1. prevent diabetes among populations with prediabetes
2. increase rates of diagnosis
3. reduce complications of diabetes
4. prevent and reduce overweight and obesity
5. reduce the complications of asthma

Programs planned include the following:

1. promoting healthy choices away from home
2. encouraging labels on restaurant menus

3. establishing walking programs
4. helping local organizations to establish health-promoting programs and environments
5. establishing community-based education for all health programs in convenient locations
6. teaching providers preventive standards
7. enhancing systems to call individuals with chronic diseases for routine exams
8. using information technology to reach and teach about chronic diseases
9. training community workers
10. conducting media-awareness campaigns

Important legislation for obesity treatment and prevention includes Senate Bill 1172, the Improved Nutrition and Physical Activity (IMPACT) Act.[150] Components include:

1. training grants for healthcare professionals
2. grants to increase physical activity and improve nutrition
3. data collection regarding energy expenditure of children and analysis of data in the National Health and Nutrition Examination Survey (NHANES)
4. evaluation of food supplement and nutrition programs of the Department of Agriculture
5. a series of reports on obesity research and national campaigns to change children's behaviors and reduce obesity

Congresswomen Mary Bono, R-Calif, and Kay Granger, R-Tex, introduced a companion bill (HR 5412) to the IMPACT Act in the House of Representatives. Rep. Michael Castle, R-Del, introduced legislation aimed at reducing and preventing obesity among children with the Obesity Prevention Act, HF 2227. This act provides federal funding for physical fitness and nutrition.[150] Specific components include:

1. creating 20 demonstration programs for children and youth
2. developing a pilot program for 100 local school districts
3. establishing a national commission to coordinate activities among federal agencies
4. creating the President's Health and Fitness Awards and issuing them to schools
5. including nutrition and health education programs as allowable activities in after-school programs

Community Partnerships to Increase Health

Hearts n' Parks

In the summer of 1999, North Carolina communities hosted the Hearts n' Parks Y2K pilot program. Community parks and recreation departments integrated heart-healthy behaviors into new or existing community activities. The goal of the statewide pilot program is to increase the number of children and adults who engage in regular moderate-intensity physical activity and who follow a heart-healthy eating plan. Community partnerships include the

NHLBI's Cardiovascular Health Promotion Program (CHPP), the National Recreation and Park Association (NRPA), North Carolina State University, and Southern Connecticut State University.

Activities held at the 12 pilot sites include:

- The Roanoke Rapids Parks and Recreation Department taught nutrition basics to 4- to 6-year-old children at the FLIP (Fun for Little Interested People) camp. Arts and crafts involved children and aquacise involved seniors.
- The Albemarle Parks and Recreation Department put healthy snacks and health-related material into the children's summer day camp program. For adults, a local hospital collaborated for a walk about program, which combined walks, health education, and free blood pressure and blood glucose screenings.
- The Garner Parks and Recreation Department focused on fitness and food labels during a summer day camp for children. Keep the Beat . . . Circle Yourself in Health focused on seniors keeping journals and receiving prizes for healthier lifestyles.
- The Smithfield Parks and Recreation Department, a county health department, and a fitness center provided a 6-week senior exercise program that offered blood pressure, cholesterol, and body-composition screening.[151]

Centers for Obesity Research and Education

Physicians and other health workers were trained in managing obese patients through 8 centers in 7 states. Monthly workshops feature interactive hands-on activities and give participants practical information and tools for immediate use with patients. The Centers for Obesity Research and Education (CORE) curriculum treats obesity as a chronic disease, requiring ongoing treatment. Its developers have targeted the following goals: (1) to provide timely, relevant education and training about obesity and its management to primary care physicians and other healthcare professionals in communities; (2) to be an educational and informational resource in the field of obesity, nationally and in individual communities; and (3) to raise public awareness about the problem of obesity and the risk of excess weight, including options for prevention and management in fostering health improvement.

Program Sites:

- Mayo Clinic, Rochester, Minn
- Minnesota Obesity Research Center, Minneapolis, Minn
- New England Center for Health Education, Boston, Mass
- Northwestern Memorial Wellness Institute, Chicago, Ill
- Pennington Biomedical Research Center, Baton Rouge, La
- St. Luke's-Roosevelt Medical Center, New York, NY
- UCLA Center for Human Nutrition, Los Angeles, Calif
- University of Colorado Health Sciences Center, Denver, Colo

The *Obesity Management Journal* is published quarterly to provide insight and recommendations for the healthcare field to address obesity and weight management based on CORE findings.

Voluntary Weight Loss

The NIH Nutrition Coordinating Committee and the Office of Medical Applications of Research convened experts in obesity, nutrition, metabolism, epidemiology, biostatistics, behavior, and exercise physiology. Data on diet, exercise, behavior modification, and drug treatment in adults were presented. Surgery, liposuction, medical devices, the economics and ethics of weight-loss practices, and regulatory issues were not covered. This state-of-the-art information from the panel demonstrates the magnitude of the weight-loss challenge in the United States.[18]

Data from 4 national surveys of health practices indicate that 33-40% of adult women and 20-24% of men currently attempt weight loss; 28% of each group strive to maintain weight. For those trying weight loss, their efforts averaged 6.4 months for women and 5.8 months for men. Women averaged 2.5 attempts to lose weight in the past 2 years, compared to 2.0 attempts for men. Weight-loss efforts are not restricted to persons with high BMI.[18]

Fewer younger people try to lose weight compared with older persons. Weight-loss attempts increase with higher education, family income, and BMI. A higher percentage of Hispanic men attempt weight loss compared to all ethnic groups; the lowest percentage occurs for African-American men. A higher proportion of African-American and Hispanic women are overweight than are white women, but a similar percentage of all groups try weight-loss regimens.

Forty-four percent of female high school students and 15% of male students reported that they were trying to lose weight; 26% of female and 15% of male students were tying to keep from gaining weight.[18] Americans attempt weight loss for several reasons:

- to improve their self-image
- to reduce the risk of weight-related health problems
- to improve their perception of their health
- to increase societal acceptance of their weight

Concerns about future and current health, fitness, and appearance are the most important reasons that individuals try to lose weight. Individuals with higher BMI voice health concerns as an issue. Appearance and fitness are identified more frequently for individuals with a lower BMI. Appearance rather than fitness is more important to women. Weight loss after smoking cessation or pregnancy is also a priority.

Strategies for Weight Loss

Prevalence of Attempts

Serdula et al analyzed data on 107,804 adults, aged ≥ 18 years from the 1996 Behavioral Risk Factor Surveillance System random-digit telephone survey in 49 states. Respondents reported their current weight, goal weight, current weight loss or weight maintenance attempts, and strategies used to control weight. The prevalence of attempting to lose and maintaining weight was

28.8% and 35.1% for men and 43.6% and 34.4% for women. Common strategies were to eat less fat but not less energy for 34.9% of men and 40.0% of women and a combination of eating less energy and engaging in ≥ 150 minutes of leisure-time physical activity per week for 21.5% of men and 19.4% of women.[152]

Other researchers report that women try to lose weight by eating fewer calories (84%) and increasing physical activity (60-63%). Men also try to lose weight by eating fewer calories (76-78%) and increasing physical activity (60-62%). Race, education, income, and age influence which methods are used most often. Surveys of adults report that more than 80% of men and women who try to lose weight blend eating and exercise regimens. Popular methods used by adults include vitamins or meal replacements, over-the-counter products, weight-loss programs, and diet supplements. An individual's BMI influences the method she or he chooses.[18]

Students who attempted weight loss reported that for the week immediately prior to the survey, they used exercise (51% of females and 30% of males), skipped meals (49% and 18%, for females and males, respectively), used diet pills (4% and 2%), and practiced self-induced vomiting (3% and 1%). The general methods chosen include exercise (80% of females and 44% of males), diet pills (21% and 5%), and vomiting (14% and 4%).[18]

Do Healthcare Professionals Advise Obese Clients to Lose Weight?

The National Institutes of Health recommends that healthcare professionals advise obese patients to lose weight. Galuska et al obtained data from the Behavioral Risk Factor Surveillance System random-digit telephone survey and found 12,835 obese adults aged ≥ 18 years old with body mass index ≥ 30 based on self-reported height and weight had visited a physician for a routine check-up during the previous 12 months. Only 42% reported that they had been advised to lose weight. The advice was most often given to women, middle-aged adults, adults with high levels of education, and those with diabetes mellitus. Adults who reported receiving advice to lose weight were significantly more likely to attempt weight loss than those not receiving advice to lose weight (OR = 2.79).[153]

Success of Various Methods for Weight Loss and Control

Few scientific studies evaluate the effectiveness and safety of weight-loss methods. Participants lose weight, but after completing a program, they tend to regain the weight with time. Some weight-loss strategies may be harmful. Individuals should examine the scientific data on effectiveness and safety of the weight-loss program before adopting it. Over $30 billion is spent each year in the United States on weight-loss efforts. The proportion of persons who complete programs, how much weight they lose, and their success in maintaining the weight loss are not generally reported in peer-reviewed literature.[18]

Success rates are influenced by initial weight, the length of treatment, the magnitude of weight loss desired, and the motivation for wanting to lose weight. Effectiveness of unsupervised efforts to lose weight is suspect, because limited data exist on the personal strategies, individual compliance, and follow-up.[18]

An adjustable stomach band has been developed to treat severe obesity. With the Lap-Band system, surgeons position a plastic band, about the size of a wristwatch band, around the top of the stomach to section off a smaller portion. The idea is that when food fills the smaller stomach pouch, a patient should feel full after eating fewer calories and lose weight. The lap band can be adjusted without surgery through a port placed just under the skin in the upper abdominal muscles. It is believed that the band is less invasive and causes fewer complications than stapling or bypasses used to reduce stomach size. The band may replace all alternative procedures.[154]

Dietary Change

Most individuals try to lose weight by changing their eating pattern. They may reduce total calories; alter the percentage of calories from fat, protein, and carbohydrate; or use protein or fat substitutes. The effectiveness of these methods is unknown, because data are only available for programs following individuals about 5 years. Acute weight loss may be greater than 10% of initial body weight, but individuals may regain two thirds of the weight within 1 year. Some individuals maintain their weight loss for a few weeks to a few months; dropout rates may be higher than 80%.[18]

Frequently, individuals employ either a caloric restriction of 1,000-1,500 calories per day, which equals about 12 to 15 kcal/kg body weight, or 800 or fewer calories per day, which is approximately 6 to 10 kcal/kg body weight. Adverse side effects and excessive loss of lean body mass are reported for either level. Very-low-calorie diets produce more weight loss than low-calorie diets, but participants often return to preprogram weight within 5 years. Modifying the proportion of calories from macronutrients has a much smaller effect on weight loss than caloric restriction.

Very-low-calorie diets are generally provided as 1 part of a comprehensive program. Weight loss may average 1.5 to 2.5 kg/week, with a total loss of about 20 kg after 3 to 4 months on the regimen. To preserve lean body mass, foods with protein of a high biological value are needed at the minimum of 1 g per kg of ideal body weight per day. The diet can cause serious complications, with the most common complication being cholelithiasis.[155]

The Diet Fad of the 21st Century—High-Protein, Low-Carbohydrate Diets: Do They Work?

Successful dieting is a result of controlled calorie intake, but maintaining weight loss for a 6- to 9-month period becomes the challenge. Lifestyle changes that can be permanent and contribute to weight loss maintenance are preferred. The ideal macronutrient composition of a successful weight-loss diet remains controversial, leading one to search for a composition that can be maintained.[156]

A thorough review of popular weight-loss diets included studies on the effect of low-carbohydrate diets, but low carbohydrates had no metabolic advantage for a greater weight loss. Moderate fat diets, which include 20-30% of energy from fat, have often been compared for effectiveness with very-low-fat diets having 10-19% energy from fat. Low-fat diets coupled with caloric reduction have generally produced a greater weight loss than lower-fat diets alone, and they appear to be nutritionally balanced. The low- and very-low-fat diets are often too extreme and adherence for 6 to 9 months or more is unrealistic. Table 15–3 reviews several popular diets.[157]

The low-carbohydrate diets seem to be the meal plans earning the most popularity and creating the most controversy. See Table 15–4. Authors of the diet plans gaining the most attention have appeared on television shows including *Today*, *Good Morning America*, and *ABC World News Tonight*, as well as in newspapers and periodicals such as *USA Today*, *Time*, and *Newsweek*.[158] The more popular low-carbohydrate diets and their premises are[158]:

- *Carbohydrate Addict's Lifespan Program*. This plan claims that a dieter can break cravings for fat-causing carbohydrates by limiting intake of carbohydrate-containing foods. Of daily meals, 2 are composed of

TABLE 15–3   Comparison of Energy Composition of Diets Used for Weight loss

Type of Diet	Total Energy	Fat g (% of kcal)	CHO g (% of kcal)	Protein g (% of kcal)
High-fat, low carbohydrate	1,450	97	36	108
Percent energy		60	10	30
• Dr. Atkins' Diet Revolution				
• Protein Power				
• The Carbohydrate Addict's Diet				
• Dr. Berenstein's Diabetes Solution				
• Life Without Bread				
Moderate-fat, balanced-nutrient reduction	1,450	40	218	54
Percent energy		25	60	15
• USDA Food Guide Pyramid				
• DASH diet				
• National Cholesterol Education Program Step I and Step II diets				
• Weight Watchers				
• Jenny Craig				
• Nutri-Systems				
Low- and very-low-fat	1,450	16-24	235-271	54-72
Percent energy		10-15	65-75	15-20
• Ornish diet				
• Pritikin diet				

Source: Adapted from: Champagne CM. Diets for weight loss: low carbohydrates or low fat? *On the Cutting Edge.* 2004;25(6):17-19.

TABLE 15–4 A Comparison of Popular Protein Diets

Book	Dr. Atkins' New Diet Revolution by Robert C. Atkins, MD © 1992	Enter the Zone by Barry Sears, PhD © 1995	Protein Power by Michael R. Eades, MD and Mary Dan Eades, MD © 1996	Sugar Busters by Leighton Steward, Morrison C. Bethea, MD, Samuel S. Andrews, MD, and Luis A. Balart, MD © 1995
Author's background	Author Robert Atkins was a medical doctor and self-proclaimed nutrition pharmacologist.	Author Barry Sears has a PhD in biochemistry and no formal training in the area of nutrition.	Authors Michael and Mary Eades are medical doctors with no formal nutrition background.	The Authors are a CEO and 3 medical doctors.
Spin-off books	Dr. Atkins' New Diet Cookbook (1995), Dr. Atkins' New Carbohydrate Gram Counter (1997), and Dr. Atkins' Quick & Easy New Diet Cookbook (1997)	Mastering the Zone: The Next Step in Achieving Superhealth and Permanent Weight Loss (1996), Zone Perfect Meals in Minutes: 150 Fast and Simple Healthy Recipes (1997), Zone Food Blocks: The Quick & Easy, Mix & Match Counter for Staying in the Zone (1998), and Anti-Aging Zone (1998)	The Low-Carb Cookbook: The Complete Guide to the Healthy Low-Carbohydrate Lifestyles—With Over 250 Delicious Recipes (1997), The Protein Power Lifeplan (2000), and The Protein Power Lifeplan Carbohydrate Counter (2000)	Sugar Busters! Shopper's Guide (1999)
Book philosophy	Eating too many carbohydrates causes obesity and a variety of other health problems. Author believes ketosis leads to decreased hunger and results in a metabolic advantage.	Eating the right combination of foods leads to a metabolic state (lower insulin levels and desirable eicosanoid levels) in which the body works at peak performance, leading to decreased hunger, weight loss, and increased energy.	Eating carbohydrates releases insulin, which, if released in large quantities, can cause health problems such as heart disease, high blood pressure, elevated cholesterol levels, and diabetes and contributes to weight gain.	Sugar is toxic to the body, causing the body to release insulin, a hormone that promotes fat storage; obesity results from this insulin overload.

continued

TABLE 15–4   continued

Book	*Dr. Atkin New Diet Revolution* by Robert C. Atkins, MD © 1992	*Enter the Zone* by Barry Sears, PhD © 1995	*Protein Power* by Michael R. Eades, MD and Mary Dan Eades, MD © 1996	*Sugar Busters* by Leighton Steward, Morrison C. Bethea, MD, Samuel S. Andrews, MD, and Luis A. Balart MD © 1995
Diet composition	- Meat, fish, poultry, shellfish, eggs, cheese, and low-carbohydrate vegetables. - Butter and vegetable oils are allowed.	- 40% carbohydrates, 30% protein (based on lean body mass), 30% fat. - Meals or snacks with a 40/30/30 distribution. - Monounsaturated fatty acids. - Low-glycemic index foods. - Alcohol in moderation.	- 15-35% carbohydrate, 30-45% protein (based on lean body mass), 30-50% fat. - Monounsaturated fats. - 25 grams of fiber/day. - Meals and snacks are needed to avoid getting hungry. - 8 glasses of water/day.	- Protein and fat. No firm guidelines as to recommended percentages of macronutrient intakes. - Low-glycemic index carbohydrates (high-fiber vegetables, fruits, and whole grains, lean meats). - Olive and canola oils in moderation. - Alcohol in moderation. - 3 meals/day.
Diet specifics	- Carbohydrates—especially breads, pasta, most fruits and vegetables, milk, and yogurt. - Induction diet, during the first 2 weeks limits carbohydrate to 20 grams/day. - The next phase, ongoing weight-loss diet, limits	- Carbohydrates, specifically pasta, bread, breakfast sandwiches, carrots, and some type of fruit (e.g., bananas). - Saturated fat and arachidonic acid.	- Carbohydrates (says carbohydrates are not needed in the diet). - In phase I, intervention limits carbohydrates to 30 grams/day. Suggests following this intervention until loss of significant amounts of weight and/or	- Potatoes, white rice, corn, carrots, beets, white bread, all refined white products (e.g., cookies, cake, etc.). - Fruits 30 minutes before a meal or 2 hours after

a meal to avoid indigestion.

reduction or elimination of any prescribed medications for hypertension, diabetes, etc.
- In phase II intervention, carbohydrates are limited to 55 grams/day.
- In maintenance phase, one can increase daily carbohydrate by 10-gram increments until grams of carbohydrate equal grams of protein. If continuing to lose weight, one can increase carbohydrate until it exceeds protein by 30%.
- Allowed to subtract fiber grams from carbohydrate to allow a little higher carbohydrate intake in both interventions.
- Need to count carbohydrate grams from alcohol.

carbohydrates to 0-60 grams/day.
- The third phase, premaintenance, allows a gradual increase of carbohydrates over 2 months.
- The final phase, maintenance diet, limits carbohydrate to 25-90 grams/day.

1,000 calories, 71 g protein (28%), 114 g carbohydrate (46%), 28 g fat (25%), 7 g saturated fat, 16 g fiber. Low in some vitamins and minerals.

1,475 calories, 110 g protein (30%), 47 g carbohydrate (13%), 86 g fat (52%), 32 g saturated fat, 14 g fiber. Low in some vitamins and minerals.

1,340 calories, 111g protein (33%), 117 g carbohydrate (34%), 50 g fat (33%), 14 g saturated fat, 17 g fiber. Low in some vitamins and minerals.

Nutrient analysis of menu using The Food Processor nutrition and fitness software, version 7.20. Salem, Ore: ESHA Research; 1998.

Induction menu (1st 2 weeks) 1,400 calories, 125 g protein (36%), 28 g carbohydrate (8%), 83 g fat (53%), 29 g saturated fat, 5 g fiber
Ongoing weight-loss menu 1,840 calories, 161 g protein (35%), 33 g carbohydrate (7%),

continued

TABLE 15–4   continued

Book	Dr. Atkin New Diet Revolution by Robert C. Atkins, MD © 1992	Enter the Zone by Barry Sears, PhD © 1995	Protein Power by Michael R. Eades, MD and Mary Dan Eades, MD © 1996	Sugar Busters by Leighton Steward, Morrison C. Bethea, MD, Samuel S. Andrews, MD, and Luis A. Balart MD © 1995
	118 g fat (58%), 39 g saturated fat, 6 g fiber **Maintenance menu** 1,800 calories, 110 g protein (24%), 128 g carbohydrate (31%), 80 g fat (40%), 31 g saturated fat, 20 g fiber. Remaining percentage of calories from alcohol. Low in some vitamins and minerals.			
Supplements recommended	Take a basic supplement (created by Dr. Atkin's company) formulated for dieters (6 pills/day), chromium picolinate (300 mcg/day), essential oils (3–6/day), and carnitine, coenzyme Q10, and pyridoxine alpha-ketoglutarate if they help. Extensive recommendation for persons with heart disease and/or diabetes (more than 10 different supplements/day).	200 IU vitamin E.	A vitamin and mineral supplement; encourages 1,000 mg vitamin C, 200 mcg chromium, and 90 mg potassium.	None.

Practicality for everyday living	- Extreme limitations in food choices. - Not practical for eating out in restaurants or social situations. - If weight loss slows down, and more weight loss is desired, recommends a fat fast, which is pure fat. Eat 900 calories fat/day.	- Rigid rules. Users must calculate protein requirements based upon several tables and charts. Must also calculate the amount of protein and fat to eat when eating carbohydrates. (Eat 7 grams protein for every 9 grams carbohydrate and include ~ 2.5 grams fat). - Meals should be no more than 500 calories and snacks less than 100 calories. - Menu not appealing, lots of egg whites, nuts, olives, and peanut butter, and large portions of fruits and vegetables. - Never go more than 5 hours without eating. - Need to be in the zone before, during, and after exercise to get the most benefits. Encourages eating a zone-favorable snack 30 minutes before exercise.	- Not practical to think that carbohydrates are not needed. - Each meal must contain a serving of lean protein along with no more than the maximum amount of carbohydrate per meal recommended based on their intervention level (must check a chart to see protein equivalency).	- Must eliminate potatoes, corn, white rice, bread from refined flour, beets, carrots, and of course refined sugar, corn syrup, molasses, honey, sugared colas, and beers. - Drink alcohol with protein so it's not harmful. - Eat multiple meals/day to decrease insulin secretion. - Drink fluids between meals. - No larger meals after 8 PM to prevent increased cholesterol production.
Image presented regarding foods and eating behavior	- Indicates that diet is a way of life but plays on dieting mentality. Uses words like "indulge," "right foods," "lose more weight and fat than any other diet," and "eat as much as you want of permitted foods." - Suggests mini-binges are normal as long as you limit the time period of the binge.	- Treats food as if it were a drug. "You must eat food in a controlled fashion and in the proper portions—as if it were an intravenous drip." - Refers to food as good or bad.	Suggest that nutritional vacations are common and gives recovery guidelines (which involve restricting food for 1 week following vacation).	Uses typical diet terminology like "should" and capitalize on the fear factor—developing chronic diseases from sugar and refined starches.

continued

TABLE 15–4 continued

Book	*Dr. Atkin New Diet Revolution* by Robert C. Atkins, MD © 1992	*Enter the Zone* by Barry Sears, PhD © 1995	*Protein Power* by Michael R. Eades, MD and Mary Dan Eades, MD © 1996	*Sugar Busters* by Leighton Steward, Morrison C. Bethea, MD, Samuel S. Andrews, MD, and Luis A. Balart MD © 1995
Scientific evidence about health claims	Success documented through testimonial anecdotes. No scientifically validated studies published.	The theories of this book have not been validated scientifically, only supported by testimonials. Fat recommendation is supported by research.	The authors claim success through testimonial anecdotes and book sales. No scientifically validated studies published.	The book lists about 20 references throughout, many of them unknown textbooks and journals. No data published on their specific diet, only supported by testimonials and anecdotal claims.
Weight loss and maintenance	Loss but mostly water weight. A decreased carbohydrate diet causes liver and muscle glycogen depletion, which causes a large loss of water. It also leads to increased sodium excretion, which means more water loss. As body adjusts to water deficit, the weight loss slows or ceases.	Loss because of caloric reduction. Therefore, if followed carefully, this diet should result in weight control. However, the diet is not a realistic eating approach that can easily be followed for a lifetime.	No calorie guidelines are provided, but the menus do promote caloric restriction, which will result in weight loss.	Probably no loss unless you were eating a high-sugar diet beforehand.
Adjustments for persons with diabetes or heart disease?	- Yes, dedicates an entire chapter to hypoglycemia and the perils of diabetes. (Claims a low-carbohydrate diet is heart-protective. In fact, suggests a	- Yes, the author gives information on a study he conducted on 15 patients that demonstrates how effective the Zone diet is for people with type 2 diabetes.	- Yes, claims excess insulin is the cause of type 2 diabetes, elevated blood pressure, and heart disease. - Suggests their diet lowers blood glucose levels and	- Yes, the authors dedicated an entire chapter to these topics. - Claim use of refined sugar either directly or indirectly causes

high-saturated fat, low carbohydrate diet does not have a negative effect on lipids). - Has a fat-restricted diet for fat-sensitive individuals.	- Indicates too much insulin production, triggered by low-fat, high-carbohydrate diets, is the primary culprit for causing heart disease. - Suggests hyperinsulinemia is the best predictor of future heart attack and that hypercholesterolemia, hypertension, and hyperinsulinemia result from high-carbohydrate diets.	repairs pancreatic damage and restores tissues to normal levels. - Ketosis is encouraged for people with type 2 diabetes; indicates fat loss. - Claims strict adherence to a low-carbohydrate diet is the cornerstone of all diabetes therapy and is important in maintaining tight blood glucose control.	diabetes or speeds the onset. - Lists dietary sugar as an independent risk factor for cardiovascular disease. - Claims diets low in refined sugar and processed grain products keep blood glucose levels lower so there is less organ damage.
Lifestyle changes encouraged Exercise.	Exercise and smoking cessation.	Resistance training (no specific amount) and aerobic exercise.	Smoking cessation and aerobic exercise 4 times/week for 20 minutes.
Negative health implications Low-carbohydrate, high-protein diets such as these can result in ketosis (symptoms could include fatigue, nausea, weakness, and irritability), electrolyte loss, dehydration, exacerbate kidney disease and gout, and calcium depletion (contributing to osteoporosis). If the diets are high in saturated fat, they may increase a person's risk for colonary heart disease, high cholesterol levels, and other health problems. Diets may also contribute to vitamin and mineral inadequacies.			

Source: Adapted from: Boucher J. News you can use: the high-protein, low carbohydrate diet craze [news flash]. *Diabetes Care and Education Dietetic Practice Group.* 1999;20:26-30.

high-protein foods with very little carbohydrate; the third meal can include high-carbohydrate foods only if balanced with more high-protein foods.

- *Dr. Atkins' New Diet Revolution.* Dr. Atkins asserted that dieters can eat as much energy from fat and protein as desired so long as carbohydrates are severely restricted. The diet is composed of 4 phases; phase 1 allows approximately 4 g carbohydrate per day, and phase 4 allows no more than 40 to 60 g carbohydrate per day.
- *Sugar Busters!* On this plan, foods to avoid are classified according to glycemic index, because—according to the authors of this diet—sugar, not fat, is what causes extra weight and foods that cause surges in insulin increase the likelihood that energy will be stored as fat.
- *The Zone.* This plan is based on the ideal that every meal and snack must be 40% carbohydrate, 30% protein, and 30% fat for maximum burn of energy. The author of this diet claims that most people are insulin resistant, so the body produces too much insulin when a person eats carbohydrate foods, causing the body to store too much energy as fat.

A comparison of these 4 diets with a sample dinner and food restrictions are listed in Table 15–5.

Adjunct Therapy

Weight loss achieved in conjunction with exercise and energy restriction is preferred. Exercise has an independent effect on weight loss. It increases HDL cholesterol and lean body mass. Exercise can offset postprogram weight gain and provide a 4- to 7-pound weight loss in addition to the loss from caloric restriction.[18]

TABLE 15–5   A Comparison of 4 Popular Diets With a Sample Dinner

Diet	Sample Dinner	Some Food Restrictions
Atkins	Bacon cheeseburger (no bun, no fries), small salad.	High-sugar foods, breads, pasta, cereal, starchy vegetables, caffeine.
Carbohydrate Addict's Lifespan Program	Eat anything as a reward for following diet, but meal must be finished within 1 hour.	No fruit or fruit juices, potatoes, rice, pasta, sweets, or snack foods at any time except during reward meal; all other meals must be low-carbohydrate.
Zone	Lean-beef chili with nonfat cheese, onions, mushrooms, bell peppers, beans, tomatoes.	Pasta, breads, grains, starches, rice, beans, cantaloupe, honeydew melon, watermelon.
Sugar Busters	Grilled pork, brown rice, steamed green beans (fresh), water.	Refined sugar products, cookies, cake, pies, ice cream, potatoes, white bread, rice, carrots, most alcoholic drinks, watermelon, corn, bananas, all pasta (except whole wheat).

Source: Adapted from: Stein K. High-protein, low-carbohydrate diets: do they work? *J Am Diet Assoc.* 2000;100(7):760-761.

Behavior modification is a technique used for modifying eating and physical activity habits. It focuses on the following components:

- making small, consistent changes
- identifying adverse eating or lifestyle behaviors
- setting specific behavioral goals
- modifying determinants of the behavior(s) to be changed
- reinforcing desirable behavior
- participating in group or individual sessions with professionals or peer therapists
- participating in 16- to 18-week programs that result in a weight loss of 1 to 1.5 pounds per week

About one third of the weight that is lost in behavior modification programs is regained within 1 year. Most is regained within 5 years; however, a few participants maintain their weight loss. Investigational drugs have produced weight loss, but their prolonged use may slow weight loss and create a weight plateau. Phenylpropanolamine, an over-the-counter FDA-approved appetite suppressant, has produced weight loss. Long-term benefit is not well documented, and potential misuse is possible.[18]

Leptin is a peptide hormone in adipose tissue thought to signal the central nervous system about body fat stores and control appetite. A subset of 492 adults was selected from a larger cohort of young African-American and white adults. Cross-sectionally, leptin concentration was associated positively with body mass index, negatively with physical activity level, and was higher in women than men. The variables explained 72% of the variance in serum leptin. Leptin change correlated highly Pearson Product Moment correlations (r) ($r = 0.62$) with weight change over 8 years. The study suggests that adiposity determines leptin levels but leptin deficiency does not promote obesity in the general population.[159]

Moderate Physical Activity, Serum Leptin, and Appetite Satiety

Physical activity and snack intake may influence appetite sensations and subsequent food intake in obese women. Ten obese women, mean 50.0 +/- 8.5 y; mean BMI 37.2 +/- 6.5 kg/m^2 were randomized to 3 trials: moderate physical activity (20 min brisk walking), snack (58.5 g chocolate-based), and control (sitting, TV watching). Appetite and satiety were assessed by visual analogue scales, serum leptin, blood glucose, and plasma free fatty acids. A buffet-style dinner was provided immediately after the trials. The moderate physical activity and snack intake both produced lower appetite and higher satiety and fullness perceptions, compared to control, following the intervention. No significant differences were found in subsequent food intake. Serum leptin concentrations did not differ between trials and were not associated with appetite or satiety sensations at any time during the control or the snack trials. Leptin was correlated following moderate physical activity (prospective food consumption $r = -0.83$, $p = 0.003$; hunger $r = -0.79$, $p = 0.007$; desire to eat $r = -0.69$, $p = 0.02$; satiety $r = 0.71$, $p = 0.02$; fullness $r = 0.66$, $p = 0.04$). These associations were not influenced by BMI or fat mass.[160]

Moderate physical activity and snack intake acutely suppress the appetite of obese women. Associations between circulating leptin and appetite-satiety ratings suggest leptin involvement in short-term appetite regulation in response to physical activity-induced factors.

Dietary change and exercise, reinforced by behavior modification, is the most common combined therapy. A greater short-term weight loss occurs when diet and exercise are combined than when either is attempted alone. Behavior modification, including choices people make when eating out, may extend the period of time before weight is regained if participant contact is continuous. According to research commissioned by the National Restaurant Association (NRA), an overwhelming number of Americans oppose government-mandated portion sizes on high-fat foods served in restaurants and potential fat taxes on foods high in fat. Public-health advocates and some legislators have promoted both ideas. Consumers responding to the NRA poll indicate otherwise, i.e., 84% would oppose a law or regulation limiting restaurant portion sizes of food known to be high in fat, and 91% of respondents would oppose additional taxes on high-fat restaurant foods.[161]

Weight-Loss Enablers and Barriers

Success appears linked to therapies that promote practical dietary behaviors and to therapies or counselors who assist individuals with high-risk emotional and social situations. Success is also linked to behavioral strategies that employ self-monitoring of progress and encourage stress reduction. Barriers to weight loss include the following[18]:

- reduced self-efficacy
- inability to lose weight early in the program, causing individuals to stop their dietary and exercise changes
- lack of social or professional support
- deeply rooted social or psychological problems (e.g., depression)
- cultural norms and mores

Weight-loss information that should, at a minimum, be voluntarily provided to prospective patients/clients of weight loss programs includes the following:

Staff qualifications and program components–This includes a description of the program content and goals and pertinent information about weight management training, experience, certification, and education of the customer service personnel where the service, including distribution of products, is being provided, and which is appropriate to the program. The disclosure should include wording that encourages prospective patients/clients to ask additional questions about qualifications of the provider and should not be deceptive or misleading.

Risks associated with overweight and obesity–This includes information showing that obesity and overweight are associated with increased risk of heart disease, diabetes, some forms of cancer, gallbladder diseases, osteoarthritis, stroke, and sleep apnea, among other illnesses, and that moderate amounts of weight loss (5-10% of total weight) can reduce many of the risks.

Risks associated with the provider's product or program–This includes information about the risks associated with any drugs, devices, dietary supplements, or exercise plans that are provided in the course of the program or treatment and indicate:

1. that consultation with a medical professional is advisable for people who are under treatment for specific medical conditions or taking prescribed medications.
2. that unless medically indicated, weight loss after the first 2 or 3 weeks of dieting should not exceed a rate of 3 pounds or approximately 1-1.5% of body weight per week. More rapid weight loss may cause an increased risk of developing gallbladder disease, risk that is believed to be higher that the risk of developing gallbladder disease as a result of staying overweight/obese. People who are considered medically appropriate for more rapid weight loss should have their progress monitored by a physician.
3. that very-low-calorie diets (< 800 kcal per day) are designed to promote rapid weight loss in people whose obesity has resulted in, or has put them at medical risk of developing, serious health complications. Rapid weight loss may also be associated with some medical problems. This program provides medical supervision to minimize risks associated with rapid weight loss.
4. that people undergoing weight loss can experience physical changes in the body (dizziness, interruptions in the menstrual cycle, and hair loss, for example) that may indicate more serious conditions. People noticing such changes should be advised to talk immediately to their primary care physician.

Program costs—This includes information about:

- total program costs, including all fixed costs (administrative fees, entry fees, renewal fees, as appropriate)
- periodic costs such as weekly attendance fees or mandatory food purchases (except for food purchases at the option of the provider as either average approximate costs or a high/low range of costs per scheduled payment unit or per week)
- optional costs (such as fees charged for reentering the program or for any optional maintenance program)
- discretionary costs (medical tests, for example). Providers should also identify, clearly and prominently, any nonrefundable costs. If practical, providers should disclose total approximate program costs averaged across all dieters.

Outcome information—This would allow people to make informed choices among weight-loss products and services. Providers are encouraged to:

- collect data, e.g., how much weight consumers of a particular product or program have lost and how long they kept off all or part of their weight loss.
- disclose weight-loss and maintenance information to prospective clients/patients before they enroll.
- give a realistic statement suggesting that people who lose weight are likely to find it difficult to keep the weight off.

- explain that individuals can improve their chances of weight-loss maintenance by adopting a lifelong commitment that includes increased frequent and regular physical activity of at least moderate intensity, healthy eating in accordance with the *Dietary Guidelines for Americans,* emphasizing a reduction in total calories, a lower fat consumption, and increase in vegetables, fruits, and whole grains.
- provide information about the health benefits of modest weight loss equaling 5-10% of body weight or about 10-20 pounds.

These guidelines should remain in the program/procedures policy or staff manuals. Program description should include information about any required or optional products, e.g., drugs, devices, dietary supplements, herbal products, food substitutes, food. Failure to disclose information about the risks of obesity and the benefits of weight loss will not be considered inconsistent with the guidelines. Partnership for Healthy Weight Management has resolved to pursue means to develop research and to encourage the development of consumer education materials that provide guidance on outcome information and how consumers can use it.

It is worth noting that fresh fruits and vegetables (f/v) help people avoid excess calories and prevent chronic disease. Including f/v in meals is associated with income. Families having incomes less than 130% of the national poverty index eat f/v 20% less frequently than families with incomes at or above 350% of the poverty index. The rate is 70% less when potatoes are not included. Four situations seem to predict less fresh produce among low-income families.[162-168] They include:

1. Grocery stores in low-income areas are less likely to sell f/v compared to stores catering to higher income families.
2. Healthy foods, especially f/v, cost more than empty-calories foods.
3. F/v have increased in price more than any other food the past 25 years.
4. Social skills and managing a household are challenging for low-income individuals with few nutrition skills.

Health messages focusing on the problems individuals face can influence successful behavioral change, but this has not been consistent.[169-170] For example, success has been noted for reducing fat intake.

Message *targeting* became popular in the 1990s to focus on marketing brand and services.[171] Marketing by targeting occurs when sponsors of products, services, or causes direct messages from a population to a target group. This process cultivates change while being efficient in the process. Message tailoring customizes messages, thereby appealing to each individual while reaching a much larger population.[172]

Benefits and Risks of Weight Loss

Observational studies of persons who report weight loss and data from clinical trials document the association of weight loss to health. A reduction in the incidence and severity of non–insulin-dependent diabetes mellitus and hypertension in overweight persons is an immediate benefit. Diet and exercise-evoked weight loss can prevent the onset of hypertension and diabetes mellitus. Improved glycemic control and elimination of oral agents may occur for persons with diabetes. Randomized trial data indicate that weight loss among hypertensive patients accompanies significant declines in blood pressure and a decline in continued drug therapy. A positive effect on lipid and lipoprotein levels is also observed. What is not clear is whether short-term improvements confer permanent health benefits.[18]

For morbidly obese individuals, weight loss improves functional status, reduces work absenteeism, lessens pain, and increases social interaction. The prevalence and severity of sleep apnea can be markedly reduced by weight loss.[18] Very-low-calorie diets and fasting regimens can produce short-term adverse response (e.g., periodic fatigue, hair loss, and dizziness). Gallstones and acute gallbladder disease, cardiac arrhythmia, and death have been reported. Diets with high-quality protein, minerals, and electrolytes have offset serious, life-threatening complications. The effect of weight-loss programs on binge eating and bulimia needs further study. Many alternatives for weight loss are available to the public (see Exhibit 15–3). For further information about the adverse effects of weight loss, see F. Berg's *Health Risks of Weight Loss.*[173]

Exhibit 15–3   Popular Weight-Loss Programs

Do-It Yourself Programs

- *Overeaters Anonymous:* Nonprofit international organization that provides volunteer support groups patterned after the 12-step Alcoholics Anonymous program. Physical, emotional, and spiritual recovery aspects of compulsive overeating are addressed.
- *TOPS (Take Off Pounds Sensibly):* Nonprofit support organization of more than 300,000 members who meet weekly in groups. Does not prescribe or endorse particular eating or exercise regimen. Mandatory weigh-in at weekly meeting.

Nonclinical Programs

- *Diet Center:* Focuses on achieving healthy body composition through diet and personalized exercise recommendations under the name "Exclusively You Weight Management Program." A minimum 1,200 calorie diet is based on regular supermarket food. Diet Center prepackaged cuisine is optional. Clients are encouraged to visit center daily for weigh-in.
- *Jenny Craig:* Personal weight management menu based on Jenny Craig's cuisine with additional store-bought foods. Diet ranges from 1,000 to 2,600 kcal.

- *Nutri/System:* Menu plans based on Nutri/System's prepared meals with additional store-bought foods. Clients receive individual calorie levels ranging from 1,000 to 2,200 kcal/day. Multivitamin-mineral supplement available for clients.
- *Weight Watchers:* Emphasis on portion control and healthy lifestyle habits. Dieters choose from regular supermarket food, Weight Watchers Personal Cuisine (available in select markets to members only), or both. Reducing phase: Women average 1,250 kcal daily, men, 1,600 daily.

Clinical Programs

- *Health Management Resources (HMR):* Medically supervised, very-low-calorie diet (VLCD) or fortified, high-protein, liquid meal replacements (520 to 800 kcal daily) or a low-calorie option consisting of liquid supplements and prepackaged HMR entrees (800 to 1,300 kcal daily).
- *Medifast:* Medifast is a physician-supervised, very-low-calorie diet program of fortified meal replacements containing 450-500 kcal/day. Life Styles, The Medifast Program of Patient Support, prepares patients to maintain their goal weight after

continued

Exhibit 15–3   continued

completing the VLCD. Medifast also provides a low-calorie diet of approximately 860 kcal/day for those not indicated for the VLCD.

- *New Direction:* This system includes a medically supervised VLCD program of fortified meal replacements with 600-840 kcal/day, or programs with 1,000-1,500 kcal/day using regular foods, fortified bars, and beverage.
- *Optifast:* Medically supervised program of fortified liquid meal replacements and/or fortified food-bars, eventually including more regular foods. Dieters assigned an 800-, 950-, or 1,200-kcal plan.
- *Physicians in a Multidisciplinary Program:* Multidisciplinary programs

are similar to Health Management Resources, New Direction, and Optifast. The approach is food-based and weight-loss oriented but is a modified form of the 2. The multidisciplinary approach seeks coordination of services, the availability of individual and/or group counseling, and comprehensive health care.

- *Private Practice RDs:* Highly personalized approach to weight loss and maintenance. Exercise is encouraged as part of a safe, sensible weight-control plan. Clients identify barriers to their weight loss and maintenance and receive education about healthy lifestyles.

Source: Adapted from: Ward E. Programs for and approaches to treating obesity. *Environmental Nutrition.* 1994;1. Used with permission of Environmental Nutrition, Inc.

As discussed earlier, epidemiologic studies suggest that weight loss is associated with increased mortality, and yet the reason for weight loss may not be known (e.g., weight loss could be intentional by a healthy individual or it could be associated with illness and psychosocial distress). People who stop smoking gain weight and complicate the data. Weight cycling affects energy metabolism and may result in a faster regain of weight. Data about the long-term, negative effects of weight cycling on psychological and physical health are needed. Weight-reducing drugs appear safe in controlled studies, but these studies are short term. They involve older, more stable individuals who are not likely to abuse the drugs. Studies with adolescents and young adults are needed to evaluate the use of weight-reducing drugs among youths. Another alternative has been the use of diet preparations for jump-start weight loss, but they can be abused. Several chemical components are being used for weight loss.

Use of Diet Preparation

Several chemical components have been or are being used for weight loss (see Table 15–6).

Ephedrine or Ma Huang—Ephedrine, or ephedra, is a botanical, used in traditional Chinese medicine for centuries, a stimulant chemically similar to amphetamines affecting the central nervous system and heart. The plant provides ephedrine alkaloids of ephedrine and pseudoephedrine. When these products are "chemically synthesized and used in products," they fall under the Food, Drug, and Cosmetic Act regulations as a drug.[174]

Phenylpropanolamine (PPA)—The FDA has banned PPA, which has amphetamine-like properties suppressing appetite and causing short-term weight loss. The side effects include: acute hypertension (high blood pressure),

TABLE 15–6 Ingredients of Common OTC Diet Pills and Their Effects

Common Ingredients	Reported Effects	Possible Adverse Effects
Caffeine (including black and green tea leaves)	Stimulates central nervous system	Insomnia, restlessness, agitation, irritability; long-term use can result in anxiety, hallucinations, severe depression, or physical and psychological dependence.
Chitosan	Inhibits fat absorption	Persons with shellfish allergies should not consume. Flatulence and constipation.
Chromium polynicotinate	Controls blood sugar, high cholesterol, enhances athletic performance, weight loss	Hypoglycemia, kidney toxicity, cognitive and personality disorder.
DHEA	Slows aging, promotes weight loss, stimulates immunity, treats lupus and multiple sclerosis, increases strength and muscle mass, energy, sexual dysfunction, improves mood	Acne, voice deepening, excessive hair growth, menstrual irregularities, insulin resistance, hypertension, liver problems, etc. There are numerous drug interactions and negative side effects.
Garcinia cambogia	Hydroxycitric acid interferes with fat generation or deposition, suppresses appetite	Headache, upper respiratory tract symptoms, gastrointestinal symptoms.
Ginseng	Stimulates body during times of fatigue and stress	Not to be taken with other stimulants or antidepressant/ antipsychotic drugs, during pregnancy; and for individuals with diabetes, heart disease.
Guarana	High-powered stimulant	Disturbs sleep and causes agitation. Serious negative interactions with at least 22 drugs and supplements, including oral contraceptives.
Gymnema sylvestre leaf extract	Metabolic control, laxative, stimulant, diuretic	Lowers insulin and hypoglycemic drug levels, affects diabetics and hypoglycemics. Decreases iron absorption.
Hoodia gordonii cactus	Reduces hunger pains and feelings of hunger, appetite suppressant	No human studies have been released stating effectiveness or safety.
L-carnitine	Treats metabolism disorders, congestive heart failure, chronic fatigue syndrome, etc.	Gastrointestinal problems, tingling/numbness, headache, anemia, weakness, possible seizures, and serious side effects when taken with some supplements and many prescription drugs.

continued

TABLE 15–6   continued

Common Ingredients	Reported Effects	Possible Adverse Effects
Magnolia bark	Anti-stress, anti-anxiety, stimulant, induces sweating, digestive problems	Can cause drowsiness at high doses.
Passion flower	Reduces anxiety, aids in sleep	Liver and pancreatic toxicity. Increases bleeding when taken with other anticoagulant herbs or drugs, interaction with MAO inhibitors, and sedatives.
Piper nigum (pepper)	Antiflatulent, diuretic, induces sweating, increases gastric secretions, possible lipolysis	Increases absorption of drugs and other substances.

Source: Adapted from: Burkey H. The use and abuse of diet pills. *JHRC.* Spring 2005:9-15.

severe headaches, intracranial hemorrhages, seizures, and deaths due to strokes. PPA has been used in 106 over-the-counter (OTC) products, including many cough/cold medicines.[175] All products containing PPA were reformulated or eliminated due to the health and safety concerns for the public.[176-177]

Stimulants and Abusive Properties—Stimulants, analgesics, and tranquilizers are the most abused OTC products. Anxiety, hallucinations, severe depression, or physical and psychological dependence are some of the long-term effects of stimulant abuse. About 2% of hospital admissions are due to OTC medication adverse reactions and abuse by people taking the OTC diet pills/stimulants to lose weight, such as individuals with eating disorders, athletes, addicts, adolescents, students, and employees in odd-hours-jobs.[178-179]

Laxatives and Diuretics—Laxatives create elimination of the body wastes through bowel movements and include stimulants, bulk-forming, softening, lubricant, and osmotic forms. Abuse causes dehydration, dependency, cramping, severe diarrhea, malnutrition, electrolyte imbalance, fluid retention, rectal bleeding, permanent damage to the colon, cardiac arrhythmias, and kidney failure.[180]

Methods Alert

Treatments Recognized as Effective

Nutrition therapy including low-calorie and lower-fat diets; altering physical activity patterns; behavior therapy techniques; pharmacotherapy; surgery; and combinations of these are effective options. Therapy is a 2-step process involving assessment and treatment. Assessment determines the degree of overweight and overall risk. Treatment involves both reducing excess body weight and initiating control measures for existing risk factors.

Assessment

- BMI describes relative weight-for-height and is significantly correlated with total body fat content. It assesses overweight and obesity and can be used to monitor changes in body weight to determine efficacy of weight-loss therapy.

* Waist circumference is positively correlated with abdominal fat content. Excess fat in the abdomen in relation to total body fat is an independent predictor of risk factors and morbidity. A waist circumference of > 40 inches in men (102 cm) and > 35 inches in women (88 cm) with a BMI of 25 to 34.9 kg/m² places one at an increased risk for other health problems.

In 1997, the Food and Drug Administration (FDA) requested the voluntary withdrawal from the market of dexfenfluramine and fenfluramine due to a reported association between valvular heart disease and the use of dexfenfluramine or fenfluramine alone or combined with phentermine. Sibutramine is approved by FDA for long-term use. It has limited but definite effects on weight loss and can facilitate weight loss maintenance. FDA approved orlistat in 1999.

Risk Status

Risk status can define comorbidities, e.g., established coronary heart disease (CHD), type 2 diabetes, and sleep apnea; gynecological abnormalities; osteoarthritis; gallstones; and stress incontinence. These conditions place individuals at very high risk for disease complications and mortality. Additional cardiovascular risk factors include cigarette smoking, hypertension (systolic blood pressure ≥ 140 mm Hg or diastolic blood pressure ≥ 90 mm Hg, or the patient is taking antihypertensive agents), high-risk LDL cholesterol (≥ 160 mg/dL), low HDL cholesterol (< 35 mg/dL), impaired fasting glucose (fasting plasma glucose of 110 to 125 mg/dL), family history of premature CHD (definite myocardial infarction or sudden death at or before 55 years of age in father or other male first-degree relative, or at or before 65 years of age in mother or other female first-degree relative), and age (men ≥ 45 years and women ≥ 55 years or postmenopausal). High absolute risk means 3 risk factors exist requiring clinical management to reduce risk.

Physical inactivity and high serum triglycerides (> 200 mg/dL) add incremental absolute risk.

Patient Motivation

Assessment includes evaluating reasons and motivation for weight reduction; weight loss history and success; family, friends, and work-site support; one's understanding of the causes of obesity and how obesity contributes to several diseases; attitude toward physical activity; capacity to engage in physical activity; time availability for weight-loss intervention; and financial capability. Empowering patients by presenting new treatment plans provides hope for future weight loss.

Nutrition Therapy

General goals of weight loss and management are:

* at a minimum, to prevent further weight gain
* to reduce body weight
* to maintain a lower body weight over the long term

According to the National Cholesterol Education Program, when managing patients with hyperlipidemia, dietary modification including weight management are essential first steps, and RDs have the key responsibility to facilitate dietary and physical activity behavior changes. Twenty-three dyslipidemic males 50 to 70 years old in a lipid research trial requiring frequent dietary intervention with an RD were compared with 23 patients in another trial not requiring dietary intervention with an RD. Weight gain of ≥ 3 lb occurred in 43% of the non-RD group versus no weight increase in the RD-treated group ($p < 0.01$). Weight stabilization, i.e., gaining or losing ≤ 2 lb, occurred in twice as many men, or 61%, in the RD-treated group versus 30% in the other group ($p < 0.05$). Overall, compared with the non-RD treated group, the RD-treated group experienced a 57% additional health benefit and strengthened their rapport with an RD through medical nutrition therapy.[181]

Goals of Weight Loss and Management

The initial goal of weight loss is to reduce body weight by approximately 10% from baseline. A reasonable timeline is 6 months of therapy. For overweight patients with BMIs 27 to 35, a decrease of 300 to 500 kcal/day will result in weight losses of about 1/2 to 1 lb/week and 10% weight loss in 6 months. If BMIs are > 35, food energy deficits of up to 500 to 1,000 kcal/day will lead to weight losses of about 1 to 2 lb/week and a 10% weight loss in 6 months. Weight loss at the rate of 1 to 2 lb/week (calorie deficit of 500 to 1,000 kcal/day) commonly occurs for up to 6 months. After 6 months, the rate of weight loss usually declines and weight plateaus because of a lesser energy expenditure at the lower weight.

Lost weight may be regained unless a weight maintenance program with dietary therapy, physical activity, and behavior therapy is continued indefinitely. After 6 months of weight loss, maintenance efforts should be initiated. If more weight loss is needed, sequenced attempts should occur matched with eating and physical activity programs. If one is unable to lower weight, then prevention of further weight gain is important.

Special Treatment Groups

- Smokers: Cigarette smoking is a major risk factor for cardiopulmonary disease. Smoking and obesity have a synergistic effect on CVR, but concern for weight gain when one quits is a challenge.
- Older adults: Age alone should not deter treatment for obesity in senior men and women. Research shows similar cardiovascular risk improvement in older and younger adults.
- Diverse patient population: Tailored but standardized obesity treatment can address needs of diverse patient groups. The effect is not well documented, but research reports that attention to specific needs of the diverse population when setting expectations for weight loss may be beneficial.[112]

Healthy People 2010 Actions

Obesity is a fertile area for community nutrition professionals to apply group counseling skills for individuals at all ages. HP2010 objectives that focus on obesity address prevalence of the disorder, nutritionally balanced eating patterns with fat replaced by complex carbohydrate, and high-risk ethnic groups (see Exhibit 15–4). A model nutrition objective to reduce risk reduction for obesity is presented in Exhibit 15–5.[182]

Exhibit 15–4 *Healthy People 2010* Objectives for Reduction of Obesity

Objective Number	Objective	1988-97 Baseline for 20-Year-Olds and Older	2010 Target
19-01	Increase healthy weight to a prevalence of 60% among people aged 20 and older (Baseline: 42% for people aged 20 through 74 in 1988-94.)		
	Healthy weight prevalence among groups		
	Women	45	60
	Men	38	60
	Adults, 20 years and older		60
	20-39	51	60
	40-69	36	60
	60 and older	36	60
	Low income	38	60
	Black	34	60
	Hispanic-Mexican	30	60
	American Indians/Alaska natives	UK	60
	People with high blood pressure	27	60
	People with diabetes	26	60
	People with arthritis	43	60
19-03a	Overweight or obesity in children and adolescents		
	Children (children aged 6-11 years)	11	5
	American Indian or Alaska native	UK	5
	Asian or Pacific Islander	UK	5
	Black or African American	15	5
	White	15	5
	Hispanic or Latino	17	5

continued

Exhibit 15–4   continued

	Not Hispanic or Latino	11	5
	Female	11	5
	Male	12	5
	Lower income level (≤ 130% of poverty threshold)	11	5
	Higher income level (≥ 130% of poverty threshold)	11	5
	Persons with disabilities	UK	5
	Persons without disabilities	13	5
19-03b	Overweight or obesity in children and adolescents		
	Adolescents (aged 12-19 years)	11	5
	American Indian or Alaska native	UK	5
	Asian or Pacific Islander	UK	5
	Black or African American	13	5
	White	11	5
	Hispanic or Latino	14	5
	Not Hispanic or Latino	10	5
	Female	10	5
	Male	10	5
	Lower income level (≤ 130% of poverty threshold)	16	5
	Higher income level (> 130% of poverty threshold)	8	5
	Persons with disabilities	UK	5
	Persons without disabilities	11	5

UK = unknown
Source: Adapted from: US Department of Health and Human Services. DATA2010–the *Healthy People 2010* database. *CDC Wonder.* Atlanta, Ga: Centers for Disease Control; November 2000.

Exhibit 15–5   Model Nutrition Objective for Risk Reduction

By 20____, the chronic disease risk factor _____*_____ among [*target population*] will be reduced from _____% to _____%.

*Obesity; hypertension; elevated serum cholesterol; poor physical fitness; excess intake of dietary fat, cholesterol, sodium, alcohol, and sugar; inadequate intake of dietary fiber, fruits and vegetables, and calcium.

Source: Adapted from: *Model State Nutrition Objectives.* Johnstown, Pa: The Association of State and Territorial Public Health Nutrition Directors; 1988.

References

1. Flegal KM, Carroll MD, Ogden CL, Johnson CL. Prevalence and trends in obesity among US adults, 1999-2000. *JAMA*. 2002;288:1723-1727.
2. Hedley AA, Ogden CL, Johnson CL, Carroll MD, Curtin LR, Flegal KM. Overweight and obesity among US children, adolescents, and adults, 1999-2002. *JAMA*. 291:2847-2850.
3. US Department of Health and Human Services. *The Surgeon General's Report on Nutrition and Health*. Washington, DC: US Government Printing Office; 1988.
4. National Institutes of Health Consensus Development Conference Panel. Health implications of obesity. *Ann Intern Med*. 1985;103:1073.
5. Berg F. Obesity costs reach $39.3 billion. *Obes Health*. 1991;5:95.
6. Colditz GA. Economic costs of obesity. *Am J Clin Nutr*. 1992;55:503S-507S.
7. Obesity and our nation: What are the answers? [news release] Chicago, Ill: ADA; September 28, 2000.
8. Kanders BS, Blackburn GL. Reducing primary risk factors by therapeutic weight loss. In: Wadden TA, Van Itallie TB, eds. *Treatment of the Seriously Obese Patient*. New York: Guilford Press; 1992.
9. Benotti PN, Bistrian B, Benotti JR, et al. Heart disease and hypertension in severe obesity: the benefits of weight reduction. *Am J Clin Nutr*. 1992;55(suppl):586S-590S.
10. Gleysteen JJ. Results of surgery: long-term effects on hyperlipidemia. *Am J Clin Nutr*. 1992;55(suppl):591S-593S.
11. Pories WJ, MacDonald KG Jr, Morgan EJ, et al. Surgical treatment of obesity and its effect on diabetes: 10-year follow-up. *Am J Clin Nutr*. 1992;55(suppl):582S-585S.
12. Parham ES. Nutrition education research in weight management among adults. *J Nutr Ed*. 1993;25:258-267.
13. Schlundt DG, Taylor D, Hill JO, et al. A behavioral taxonomy of obese female participants in a weight-loss program. *Am J Clin Nutr*. 1991;53:1151-1158.
14. Herman CP, Mack D. Restrained and unrestrained eating. *J Personality*. 1975;43:647-660.
15. Stunkard AJ, Messick S. The three-factor eating questionnaire to measure dietary restraint, disinhibition, and hunger. *J Psychosomatic Res*. 1985;29:71-83.
16. Herman CP, Polivy J. A boundary model for the regulation of eating. In: Stunkard AJ, Stellar E, eds. *Eating and Its Disorders*. New York: Raven Press; 1984:141-156.
17. Bray GA, ed. *Obesity in Perspective*. Bethesda, Md: National Institutes of Health; 1978. DHEW publication 75-708. Fogarty International Series on Preventive Medicine. Vol 2, part 1.
18. National Institutes of Health. Technology Assessment Panel Statement. Methods for voluntary weight loss and control. *Nutr Rev*. 1992;50:340-345.
19. McReynolds WT. Toward a psychology of obesity: review of research on the role of personality and level of adjustment. *Int J Eating Disorders*. 1982;2:37-57.
20. Stuart RB, Davis B. *Slim Chance in a Fat World: Behavioral Control of Obesity*. Champaign, Ill: Research Press; 1972.
21. Brownell KD, Kramer FM. Behavioral management of obesity. *Med Clin North Am*. 1989;73:185-201.

22. Schachter S. Obesity and eating. *Science.* 1968;161:751-756.
23. Bandura A. *Social Learning Theory.* Englewood Cliffs, NJ: Prentice Hall; 1977.
24. Bandura A. *Social Foundations of Thought and Action: A Social Cognitive Theory.* Englewood Cliffs, NJ: Prentice Hall; 1986.
25. Bandura A. Self-efficacy: toward a unifying theory of behavior change. *Psychol Rev.* 1977;84:191-215.
26. Glynn SM, Ruderman AJ. The development and validation of an eating self-efficacy scale. *Cognitive Ther Res.* 1986;10:403-420.
27. Shannon B, Bagby R, Wang MQ, et al. Self-efficacy: a contributor to the explanation of eating behavior. *Health Ed Res.* 1990;5:395-407.
28. Bennett GA. An evaluation of self-instructional training in the treatment of obesity. *Addictive Behav.* 1986;11:125-134.
29. Sobal J, Stunkard AJ. Socioeconomic status and obesity: a review of the literature. *Psych Bull.* 1989;105:260-275.
30. Allon N. The stigma of overweight in everyday life. In: Wolman BJ, ed. *Psychological Aspects of Obesity.* New York: Van Nostrand Reinhold Co; 1981:130-174.
31. Ajzen I, Fishbein M. *Understanding Attitudes and Predicting Social Behavior.* Englewood Cliffs, NJ: Prentice Hall; 1980:278.
32. Thoits PA. Social support as coping assistance. *J Consul Clin Psychol.* 1987;54:416-423.
33. LaPorte DJ, Stunkard AJ. Predicting attrition and adherence to a very low calorie diet: a prospective investigation of the eating inventory. *Int J Obesity.* 1990;14:197-206.
34. Pratt CA. A conceptual model for studying attrition in weight-reduction programs. *J Nutr Ed.* 1990;22:177-182.
35. Kayman S, Bruvold W, Stern JS. Maintenance and relapse after weight loss in women: behavioral aspects. *Am J Clin Nutr.* 1990;52:800-807.
36. Kuczmarski RJ. Prevalence of overweight and weight gain in the United States. *Am J Clin Nutr.* 1992;55:495S.
37. Nielsen SJ, Siega-Riz AM, Popkin BM. Trends in energy intake in US between 1977 and 1996: similar shifts seen across age groups. *Obes Res.* 2002;10:370-378.
38. Stern MP, Gaskill SP, Hazuda HP, et al. Does obesity explain prevalence of diabetes among Mexican Americans? *Diabetologia.* 1983;24:272-277.
39. Pereira MA, Jacobs DR Jr, Van Horn L, et al. Dairy consumption, obesity, and the insulin resistance syndrome in young adults: the CARDIA Study. *JAMA.* 2002;287:2081-2089.
40. Kahn HS, Williamson DF, Stevens JA. Race and weight change in US women: the roles of socioeconomic and marital status. *Am J Public Health.* 1991;81:319-323.
41. Kahn HS, Williamson DF. The contributions of income, education and changing marital status to weight change among US men. *Int J Obes.* 1990;14:1057-1068.
42. Linné Y, Dye L, Barkeling B, Rössner S. Weight development over time in parous women: the SPAWN study–15 years follow-up. *Int J Obes Relat Metab Disord.* December 2003;27(12):1516-1522.
43. Mokdad AH, Serdulla MK, Dietz WH, Bownan BA, Marks JS, Koplan JP. The spread of the obesity epidemic in the United States, 1991-1998. *JAMA.* October 6, 1999;282:1519-1522.
44. Ravelli ACJ, van der Meulen JHP, Osmond C, Barker DJP, Bleker OP. Obesity at the age of 50 y in men and women exposed to famine prenatally. *Am J Clin Nutr.* 1999;70:811-816.

45. Adams EJ, Grummer-Strawn L, Chavez G. Food insecurity is associated with increased risk of obesity in California women. *J Nutr.* April 2003;133(4):1070-1074.

46. Lukaski HD. Methods for the assessment of human body composition: traditional and new. *Am J Clin Nutr.* 1987;46:537-556.

47. Bouchard C, Bray GA, Hubbard VS. Basic and clinical aspects of regional fat distribution. *Am J Clin Nutr.* 1990;52:946-950.

48. Bray GA. Pathophysiology of obesity. *Am J Clin Nutr.* 1992;55:488S-494S.

49. Bray GA. *The Obese Patient: Major Problems in Internal Medicine.* Vol. 9. Philadelphia, Pa: WB Saunders; 1976.

50. National Research Council. *Diet and Health: Implications for Reducing Chronic Disease Risk.* Washington, DC: National Academy Press; 1989.

51. O'Neil J. Vital signs–patterns: stress and fat linked at the waist. *New York Times.* September 28, 2000:D8.

52. Greenfield JR, Samaras K, Jenkins AB, Kelly PJ, Spector TD, Campbell LV. Moderate alcohol consumption, dietary fat composition, and abdominal obesity in women: evidence for gene-environment interaction. *J Clin Endocrinol Metab.* November 2003;88(11):5381-5386.

53. Gavaler JS, Rosenblum E. Predictors of postmenopausal body mass index and waist hip ratio in the Oklahoma postmenopausal health disparities study. *J Am Coll Nutr.* 2003;22(4):269-276.

54. Ravussin E, Bogardus C. A brief overview of human energy metabolism and its relationship to essential obesity. *Am J Clin Nutr.* 1992;55: 242S-245S.

55. D'Alessio DA, Kavle EC, Mozzoli MA, et al. Thermic effect of food in lean and obese men. *J Clin Invest.* 1988;81:1781-1789.

56. Bouchard C, Tremblay A, Despres JP, et al. The response to long-term overfeeding identical twins. *N Engl J Med.* 1990;322:1477-1482.

57. Thomas CD, Peters JC, Reed GW, et al. Nutrient balance and energy expenditure during ad libitum feeding of high-fat and high-carbohydrate diets in humans. *Am J Clin Nutr.* 1992;55:934-942.

58. Joos SK. Social, attitudinal and behavioral correlates of weight change among Mexican American women. University of Houston. *Dissertation Abstracts Int.* 1984;46:131.

59. Miller WC, Eggert KE, Wallace JP, et al. Successful weight loss in a self-taught, self-administered program. *Int J Sports Med.* 1993;14:401-405.

60. Miller WC. Diet composition, energy intake, and nutritional status in relation to obesity in men and women. *Med Sci Sports Exerc.* 1991;23:280-284.

61. Rigaud D, Ryttig KR, Angel AL, et al. Overweight treated with energy restriction and a dietary fibre supplement: a 6-month randomized, double-blind, placebo-controlled trial. *Int J Obesity.* 1990;14:763-769.

62. Wadden TA, Foster GD, Letizia KA, et al. Long-term effects of dieting on resting metabolic rate in obese outpatients. *JAMA.* 1990;264:707-711.

63. Schutz T, Tremblay A, Weinsier RL, et al. Role of fat oxidation in the long-term stabilization of body weight in obese women. *Am J Clin Nutr.* 1992;55:670-674.

64. Brownell KD, Jeffery RW. Improving long-term weight loss: pushing the limits of treatment. *Behav Ther.* 1987;18:353-374.

65. Hawks SR, Richins P. Toward a new paradigm for the management of obesity. *J Health Ed.* 1994;25:147-153.

66. Kalodner CR, DeLucia JL. Components of effective weight loss programs: theory, research, and practice. *J Counseling Dev.* 1990;68:427-433.

67. DeLucia JL, Kalodner CR. An individualized cognitive intervention: does it increase the efficacy of behavioral interventions for obesity? *Addictive Behav.* 1990;15:473-479.

68. Hurbert HB, Feinleib M, McNamara PM, et al. Obesity as an independent risk factor for cardiovascular disease: a 26-year follow-up of participants in the Framingham Heart Study. *Circulation.* 1983;67:968.

69. Intersalt Cooperative Research Group. Intersalt: An international study of electrolyte excretion and blood pressure—results for 24 hour urinary sodium and potassium excretion. *Br Med J.* 1988;297:319-328.

70. Burton BT, Foster WR, Hirsch J, et al. Health implications of obesity: an NIH consensus development conference. *Int J Obesity.* 1985;9(3):155.

71. *Kidney International.* Available at: http://kidney.niddk.nih.gov/. Accessed April 27, 2004.

72. Glueck CJ, Taylor HL, Jacobs D, et al. Plasma high-density lipoprotein cholesterol: association with measurements of body mass—the Lipid Research Clinics Program Prevalance Study. *Circulation.* 1980;62(suppl IV):62.

73. Aristimuno GG, Foster TA, Voors AW, et al. Influence of persistent obesity in children on cardiovascular risk factors: the Bogalusa Heart Study. *Circulation.* 1984;69:895.

74. Vague J. The degree of masculine differentiation of obesities: a factor determining predisposition to diabetes, atherosclerosis, gout, and uric calculous disease. *Am J Clin Nutr.* 1956;4:20.

75. Foster CJ, Weinsein RL, Birch R, et al. Obesity and serum lipids: an evaluation of the relative contribution of body fat and fat distribution and lipid levels. *Int J Obesity.* 1987;11:151.

76. Lapidus L, Bengstsson C, Larrson B. Distribution of adipose tissue and risk of cardiovascular disease and death: a 12 year follow up of participants in the population study of women in Gothenburg, Sweden. *Br Med J.* 1984;289:1257.

77. Donahue RP, Abbott RD, Bloom E, et al. Central obesity and coronary heart disease in men. *Lancet.* 1987;1:821.

78. Despres JP, Tremblay A, Perusse L, et al. Abdominal adipose tissue and serum HDL-cholesterol: association independent from obesity and serum triglyceride concentration. *Int J Obesity.* 1988;12:1.

79. Anonymous. Mortality among insured lives showing medical impairments: defect in physical condition, in personal history or in family history. In: *Medicoactuarial Mortality Investigation.* Part 1, vol 4. New York: Association of Life Insurance Medical Directors and Actuarial Society; 1914:19-23.

80. Larsson B, Svardsudd K, Welin L, et al. Abdominal adipose tissue distribution, obesity, and risk of cardiovascular disease and death: 13-year follow-up of participants in the study of men born in 1913. *BMJ.* 1984;288:1401-1404.

81. Feskens E, Virtanen SM, Rasanen L, et al. Dietary factors determining diabetes and impaired glucose tolerance. *Diabetes Care.* 1995;18: 1104-1112.

82. Lean MEG, Han TS, Seidell JC. Impairment of health and quality of life in people with large waist circumference. *Lancet.* 1998;351:853-856.

83. Follick MJ, Abrams CB, Smith TW, et al. Contrasting short- and long-term effects of weight loss on lipoprotein levels. *Arch Int Med.* 1984;144:1571.

84. Tran ZV, Weltman A. Differential effects of exercise on serum lipid and lipoprotein levels seen with changes in body weight. *JAMA.* 1985;254:919.

85. Wolf RN, Grundy SM. Influence of weight reduction on plasma lipoproteins in obese patients. *Arteriosclerosis.* 1983;3:160.

86. Leon AS, Conrad J, Hunnihake DB, et al. Effects of a vigorous walking program on body composition, carbohydrate, and lipid metabolism of obese young men. *Am J Clin Nutr.* 1979;32:1776.

87. Funnell M. Preventing type 2 diabetes with weight loss and exercise. *Nursing.* 2003;33(suppl): 10.

88. Dumas MAS. Reversing the tide of metabolic syndrome. *Nursing.* 2003;33(6, suppl):2, 4, 5.

89. Lew EA, Garfinkel L. Variations in mortality by weight among 750,000 men and women. *J Chron Dis.* 1979;32:563-576.

90. Miller AB. Diet and cancer: a review. *Acta Oncol.* 1990;29:87-95.

91. Chandra RK, Kutty KM. Immunocompetence in obesity. *Acta Paediatr Scand.* 1980;69:25-30.

92. Krishan EC, Trost L, Aarons S, et al. Study of function and maturation of monocytes in morbidly obese individuals. *J Surg Res.* 1982;33:89-97.

93. Kolterman OG, Olefsky JM, Kurahara C, et al. A defect in cell-mediated immune function in insulin-resistant diabetic and obese subjects. *J Lab Clin Med.* 1980;96:535-543.

94. Mokdad AH, Bowman BA, Ford ES. The continuing epidemics of obesity and diabetes in the United States. *JAMA.* 2001;286:1195-1200.

95. Wright JD, Kennedy-Stephenson J, Wang CY, McDowell MA, Johnson CL. Trends in intake of energy and Macronutrients—US, 1971-2000. *MMWR.* 2004. Hyattsville, Md: National Center for Health Statistics, CDC; 2004.

96. Ernst ND, Obarzanek E, Clark MB, Briefel RR, Brown CD, Donato K. Cardiovascular health risks related to overweight. *J Am Diet Assoc.* 1997;97(suppl):S47-S51.

97. Chanmugam P, Guthrie JF, Cecilio S, Morton JF, Basiotis PP, Anand R. Did fat intake in the United States really decline between 1989-1991 and 1994-1996? *J Am Diet Assoc.* 2003;103:867-872.

98. National Center for Health Statistics. *Prevalence of Overweight and Obesity Among Adults: United States, 1994-2002.* Washington, DC: National Center for Health Statistics; 2004.

99. Parker ED, Folsom AR. Intentional weight loss and incidence of obesity-related cancers: the Iowa Women's Health Study. *Int J Obes Relat Metab Disord.* December 2003;27(12):1447-1452.

100. Stephenson GD, Rose DP. Breast cancer and obesity: an update. *Nutr Cancer.* 2003;45(1):1-16.

101. Liu S, Willett WC, Manson JE, Hu FB, Rosner B, Colditz G. Relation between changes in intakes of dietary fiber and grain products and changes in weight and development of obesity among middle-aged women. *Am J Clin Nutr.* November 2003;78(5):920-927.

102. Heaney RP. Normalizing calcium intake: projected population effects for body weight. *J Nutr.* January 2003;133(1):268S-270S.

103. Knapp TR. A methodological critique of the "ideal weight" concept. *JAMA.* 1983;250:506-510.

104. Sjostrom LV. Mortality of severely obese subjects. *Am J Clin Nutr.* 1992;55:516S-523S.

105. Manson JE, Colditz GA, Stampfer MJ, et al. A prospective study of obesity and risk of coronary heart disease in women. *N Engl J Med.* 1990;322:882-889.

106. Wienpahl J, Ragland SS. Body mass index and 15-year mortality in a cohort of black men and women. *J Clin Epidemiol.* 1990;43:949-960.

107. Stevens J, Keil JE, Rust PF, et al. Body mass index and body girths as predictors of mortality in black and white women. *Arch Intern Med.* 1992;152:1257-1262.

108. Johnson H, Heineman EF, Heiss G, et al. Cardiovascular disease risk factors and mortality among black women and white women aged 40–69 years in Evans County, Georgia. *Am J Epidemiol.* 1986;123:209-220.

109. Rogers AE, Longnecker MP. Biology of disease. Dietary and nutritional influences on cancer: a review of epidemiologic and experimental data. *Lab Invest.* 1988;59:729-759.

110. Harris T, Cook EF, Garrison R, et al. Body mass index and mortality among nonsmoking older persons. *JAMA.* 1988;259:1520-1524.

111. Andres R. Mortality and obesity: the rationale for age-specific height-weight tables. In: Hazzard WR, Andres R, Bierman EL, et al, eds. *Geriatric Medicine and Gerontology.* 2nd ed. New York: McGraw-Hill, Inc; 1990:759-765.

112. *NIH Clinical Guidelines on the Identification, Evaluation, and Treatment of Overweight and Obesity in Adults. Obesity Education Initiative.* Washington, DC: National Institutes of Health; June 1998.

113. Tsukamoto H, Sano F. Body weight and longevity: insurance experience in Japan. *Diabetes Res Clin Pract.* 1990;10:S119-S125.

114. Garrison RJ, Feinleib M, Castelli WP, et al. Cigarette smoking as a confounder of the relationship between relative weight and long-term mortality. *JAMA.* 1983;249:2199-2203.

115. Wannamethee G, Shaper AG. Body weight and mortality in middle aged British men: impact of smoking. *BMJ.* 1989;299:1497-1502.

116. Albanes D, Jones YJ, Micozzi MS, et al. Associations between smoking and body weight in the US population: analysis of NHANES II. *Am J Public Health.* 1987;77:439-444.

117. Istvan JA, Cunningham TW, Garfinkel L. Cigarette smoking and body weight in the Cancer Prevention Study I. *Int J Epidemiol.* 1992;21: 849-953.

118. Lee I-M, Paffenbarger RS. Change in body weight and longevity. *JAMA.* 1992;268:2045-2049.

119. Pamuk ER, Williamson DF, Madans J, et al. Weight loss and mortality in a national cohort of adults, 1971–1987. *Am J Epidemiol.* 1992;136: 686-697.

120. Blair SN, Shaten J, Brownell K, et al. Body weight change, all-cause and cause-specific mortality in the Multiple Risk Factor Intervention trial. *Ann Intern Med.* 1993;119:749-757.

121. DiPietro L, Anda RF, Williamson DF, et al. Depressive symptoms and weight change in national cohort of adults. *Int J Obesity.* 1992;16: 745-753.

122. Williamson DF, Serdula MK, Anda RF, et al. Weight loss attempts in adults: goals, duration, and rate of weight loss. *Am J Public Health.* 1992;82:1251-1257.

123. Dwyer J, Stone E, Yang M, Webber L, Must A, et al. Prevalence of marked overweight and obesity in a multiethnic pediatric population: findings from the Child and Adolescent Trial for Cardiovascular Health (CATCH) study. *J Am Diet Assoc.* 2000;100:1149-1156.

124. Stunkard AJ, Wadden TA. Psychological aspects of severe obesity. *Am J Clin Nutr.* 1992;55:524S-532S.

125. Staffieri JR. A study of social stereotype of body image in children. *J Pers Soc Psychol.* 1967;7:101-104.

126. Goodman N, Dornbusch SM, Richardson SA, et al. Variant reactions to physical disabilities. *Am Sociol Rev.* 1963;28:429-435.

127. Maddox GL, Back K, Liederman V. Overweight as social deviance and disability. *J Health Soc Behav.* 1968;9:287-298.

128. Holland J, Masling J, Copley D. Mental illness in lower class, normal, obese and hyperobese women. *Psychosom Med.* 1970;32:351-357.

129. Canning H, Mayer J. Obesity: its possible effects on college admissions. *New Engl J Med.* 1966;275:1172-1174.

130. Fat execs get slimmer paychecks. *Industry Week.* 1974;180:221,224.

131. Rand CSW, Macgregor AMC. Successful weight loss following obesity surgery and the perceived liability of morbid obesity. *Int J Obesity.* 1991;15:577-579.

132. Maddox GL, Liederman V. Overweight as a social disability with medical implications. *J Med Educ.* 1969;44:214-220.

133. Perrin EM, Flower KB, Garrett J, Ammerman AS. Pediatricians' own weight: self-perception, misclassification, and ease of counseling. *Obes Res.* 2005;13(2):326-332.

134. Perrin EM, Flower KB, Ammerman AS. Preventing and treating obesity: pediatricians' self-efficacy, barriers, resources, and advocacy. *Ambulatory Pediatr.* 2005;5(3):150-156.

135. Davis SH. Students with disabilities: Part II, disability and discrimination. *Dep-line, Summer Newsletter of the Dietetic Educators and Practitioners.* 1994;12(3)4-5.

136. McEroy SA. Fat change: employment discrimination against the overweight. *Labor Law J.* 1992;42:3-14.

137. Associated Press. Calcium and weight gain not loss—a legal matter. August 2005.

138. Centers for Disease Control. *NHANES 1999-2002*: addendum to NHANES III analytic guidelines. US Dept of Health and Human Services. Available at: http://www.cdc.gov/nchs/data/nhanes/guidelines1.pdf. Accessed January 22, 2007.

139. Kaplowitz H, Martorell R, Mendoza F. Fathers and fat distribution in Mexican-American children and youth from the Hispanic Health and Nutrition Examination Survey. *Am J Hum Biol.* 1989;1:631-648.

140. Okamoto E, Davidson LL, Conner DR. High prevalence of overweight in inner-city school children. *Am J Dis Child.* 1993;147:155-159.

141. Mellin L. To: President Clinton, Re: combatting childhood obesity. *J Am Diet Assoc.* 1993;93:265-266.

142. Felitti VJ. Childhood sexual abuse, depression, and family dysfunctions in adult obese patients: a case study. *South Med J.* 1993;86:732-736.

143. Hall SK. Judgments of body size and attractiveness by Mexican-American mothers and daughters. University of Houston. *Dissertation Abstracts Int.* 1987;48:1168.

144. *Kids Make the Nutritional Grade.* Washington, DC: International Food Information Council; 1992.

145. Dietz WH, Bortmaker SL. Do we fatten our children at the television set? Obesity and television in children and adolescents. *Pediatrics.* 1985;75:807-812.

146. Klesges RC, Shelton ML, Klesges LM. The effects of television on metabolic rate: potential implications for childhood obesity. *Pediatrics.* 1993;91:281-286.

147. Golan M, Weizman A, Apter A, Fainaru M. Parents as the exclusive agents of change in the treatment of childhood obesity. *Am J Clin Nutr.* June 1998;67(6):1130-1135.

148. Albright A. Advocacy and policy in obesity treatment and prevention. San Francisco: University of California; 2004;1(3):6-7.

149. *Steps to a Healthier US.* Available at: www.healthierus.gov/steps. Accessed June 30, 2003.

150. 108th Congress Senate Bill 1172. Available at: www.theorator.com/bills108/s1172.html. Accessed August 30, 2003.

151. National Heart, Lung and Blood Institute. *Heart Memo*. Bethesda, Md: National Institutes of Health; Spring 2000:10.

152. Serdula MK, Mokdad GAH, Williamson DF, Galuska DA, Mendlein JM, Heath GW. Prevalence of attempting weight loss and strategies for controlling weight. *JAMA*. October 13, 1999;282:1353-1358.

153. Galuska D, Will JC, Serdula MK, Ford ES. Are health professionals advising obese patients to lose weight? *JAMA*. 1999;282:1576-1578.

154. Richwine L. Anti-obesity device under review. Washington, DC: Reuters News; June 16, 2000.

155. National Task Force on the Prevention and Treatment of Obesity. Very low-calorie diets. *JAMA*. 1993;270:967-974.

156. Champagne CM. Diets for weight loss: low carbohydrates or low fat? *On the Cutting Edge*. 2004;25(6):17-19.

157. Freedman M, King J, Kennedy E. Popular diets: a scientific review. *Obesity Research*. 2001;9:1S-40S.

158. Stein K. High-protein, low-carbohydrate diets: Do they work? *J Am Diet Assoc*. July 2000;100(7):760-761.

159. Folsom AR, Jensen MD, Jacobs DR Jr, Hilner JE, Tsai AW, Schreiner PJ. Serum leptin and weight gain over 8 years in African American and Caucasian young adults. *Obes Res*. 1999;7(1):1-8.

160. Tsofliou F, Pitsiladis YP, Malkova D, Wallace AM, Lean ME. Moderate physical activity permits acute coupling between serum leptin and appetite-satiety measures in obese women. *Int J Obes Relat Metab Disord*. November 2003;27(11):1332-1339.

161. California Restaurant Association. Large majority of Americans oppose mandated portion sizes, 'fat' taxes. *Confidential Bull*. 2000;12:5.

162. McCrory MA, Fuss PJ, Saltzman, E, Roberts SB. Dietary determinants of energy intake and weight regulation in healthy adults. *J Nutr*. 2000;130(2S suppl):276S-279S.

163. Hu FB, Willett WC. Optimal diets for prevention of coronary heart disease. *JAMA*. 2002;288:2569-2578.

164. US Department of Labor. *Consumer expenditures in 2000*. Washington, DC: US Dept of Labor; 2002. Report No 958.

165. Sloane DC, Diamant AL, Lewis LB, et al. Improving the nutritional resource environment for healthy living through community-based participatory research. *J Gen Int Med*. 2003;18:568-575.

166. Cade J, Upmeier H, Calvert C, Greenwood D. Costs of a healthy diet: analysis from the UK women's cohort study. *Public Health Nutr*. 1999;2:505-512.

167. Putnam JJ, Allshouse J. *Food Consumption, Prices, and Expenditures, 1970-97*. Washington, DC: US Dept of Agriculture, Economic Research Service; 1999:SB-965.

168. Devine CM, Connors MM, Sorbal J, Bisogni CA. Sandwiching it in: spillover of work onto food choices and family roles in low- and moderate-income urban households. *Social Science Med*. 2003;56:617-630.

169. Burg J, Steenhuis I, van Assema P, de Vries H. The impact of computer-tailored nutrition intervention. *Prev Med*. 1996;25:236-242.

170. Kreuter MW, Strecher VJ. Do tailored behavior change messages enhance the effectiveness of health risk appraisal? Results from a randomized trial. *Health Education Res*. 1996;11:97-105.

171. Schudson M. *Advertising, the Uneasy Persuasion*. New York: Basic Books; 1986.

172. Weinstein A. *Market Segmentation: Using Demographics, Psychographics, and Other Niche Marketing Techniques to Predict and Model Customer Behavior.* Chicago, Ill: Probus; 1994.

173. Berg FM, Health risks of weight loss. *Healthy Weight J.* 1995;174-179.

174. Food and Drug Administration. *FDA Issues Regulation Prohibiting Sale of Dietary Supplements Containing Ephedrine Alkaloids and Reiterates Its Advice That Consumers Stop Using These Products.* Available at: www.fda.gov/bbs/topics/NEWS/2004/NEW01021.html. Accessed October 18, 2004.

175. Lake C, Gallant S, Masson E, Miller P. Adverse drug effects attributed to phenylpropanolamine: a review of 142 case reports. *Am J Med.* 1990;89(2):195-208.

176. Blanck HM, Khan LK, Serdula MK. Use of nonprescription weight loss products: results from a multistate survey. *JAMA.* August 22/29, 2001;286(8):930-935.

177. Meadows M. *FDA Issues Public Health Advisory on Phenyl-propanolamine in Drug Products.* Available at: www.fda.gov/fdac/features/2001/101_ppa.html. Accessed October 18, 2004.

178. US Department of Health and Human Services and SAMHSA National Clearinghouse for Alcohol and Drug Information. *Give 'Em the Facts: Prescription and Over-the-Counter Drug Abuse.* Available at: http://ncadistore.samhsa.gov/. Accessed January 22, 2007.

179. Tinsley J, Watkins D. Over-the-counter stimulants: abuse and addiction. *Mayo Clin Proc.* 1998;73(10):977-982.

180. Burkey H. The use and abuse of diet pills. *J Health Resource Center.* Spring 2005:9-15.

181. Sikand G, Downey NA, Kashyap ML. *Beneficial Effect of Medical Nutrition Therapy by an RD in the Weight-Management Outcome of Dyslipidemic Patients.* Long Beach, Calif: Lipid Research Clinic, VA Medical Center, Long Beach and UC Irvine College of Medicine; 1999.

182. Kaufman M. *Nutrition in Public Health: A Handbook for Developing Programs and Services.* Gaithersburg, Md: Aspen Publishers, Inc; 1990:570.

DEBILITATING DISEASES— OSTEOPOROSIS, ALCOHOLISM, ARTHRITIS, AND RENAL DISEASE

Learning Objectives

- Describe the occurrence and etiology of osteoporosis, alcoholism, arthritis, and renal disease.
- Identify secondary and tertiary prevention approaches for these diseases.
- List and enumerate the role of dietary components in the secondary prevention of these diseases.

High Definition Nutrition

Alcohol—a chemical compound having a hydroxyl group linked to carbon. It has both negative and positive effects on the body (i.e., it can impair the functioning of the brain, irritate the gastrointestinal tract, and dilate arteries in the arms, legs, and skin, but it can also relax people, reduce their inhibitions, provide an antiviral, and lower blood cholesterol level).

Alcoholic drink—one drink is equivalent to one beer, 100 mL of wine, or one ounce of spirits.

Alcoholism or alcohol addiction—predictable, progressive, and often fatal condition with a 4- to 15-year progression from abuse to addiction. Frequency and pattern of consumption may vary. Condition is not determined by amount consumed or frequency of use; rather it depends on events surrounding use of alcohol. There is usually significant impairment and denial. The individual consumes approximately 25-60% of total energy from alcohol and has more than 8 drunken episodes per year.

Bioavailability—the extent or degree to which a drug, substance, element, or nutrient is available to the target tissue.

Gout—an inherited disorder of purine metabolism; uric acid accumulates in the blood.

Moderated use of alcohol—the consumption of 1 or 2 drinks a day, averaging 8-14% of total energy intake without physical, mental, emotional, or legal consequences.

Osteoarthritis—joint pain resulting from wear-and-tear and increasing body weight.

Osteomalacia—also known as adult rickets, is a qualitative, not quantitative disorder of bone metabolism. It is characterized by an increased, normal, or decreased mass of inadequately mineralized bone matrix.

Placebo effect—when an inactive pill, diet, or device is given to a person with a disease and the person improves. It demonstrates the power of mind over body. The word is derived from the Latin, placebo ("I shall please").

Problem drinking—ritual, periodic, or episodic use of more than 2 drinks per day and more than 8 drunken incidents per year. Situation creates some unpredictability. Consequences may include weight gain, physical discomfort, hangover, and possible social or relationship conflicts.

Social drinking—occasional, predictable, guilt-free consumption of alcoholic beverages. No loss of control is noted. Individual is able to stop after 1 drink. Includes 1 or 2 drunken incidents per year.

Tyrosine—an amino acid used as a supplement during drug and alcohol detoxification that affects craving and withdrawal symptoms.

Osteoporosis

The National Osteoporosis Foundation and the US Administration on Aging estimate that there are 25 million Americans with a bone-thinning disease called osteoporosis. It is called a "silent thief" because it develops in an asymptomatic manner until it is expressed as a fracture either in the hip, wrist, or spine. About 50% of women and 20% of men over 65 years of age have osteoporosis.[1] A progressive spinal deformity is common (see Figure 16-1).

Osteoporosis has also been called "a pediatric disease with a geriatric outcome." This is because bone mass is formed early in life and needs to be maintained into the sixth decade and beyond. The causes of osteoporosis are not known, but select risk factors place an individual at risk for reduced bone health (see Figure 16-2). The simple checklist that follows can be used with individuals or in group settings to identify the level of risk of an individual. The greater the number of "yes" responses to these questions, the greater the risk of developing osteoporosis[2]:

- Do you have a small, thin frame, or are you white or Asian?
- Do you have a family history of osteoporosis?
- Are you a postmenopausal woman?
- Have you had an early or surgically induced menopause?
- Do you take excessive thyroid medication or high doses of cortisone-like drugs for asthma, arthritis, or cancer?
- Would you describe your daily consumption of dairy products and other calcium-rich foods as low?
- Are you physically active?

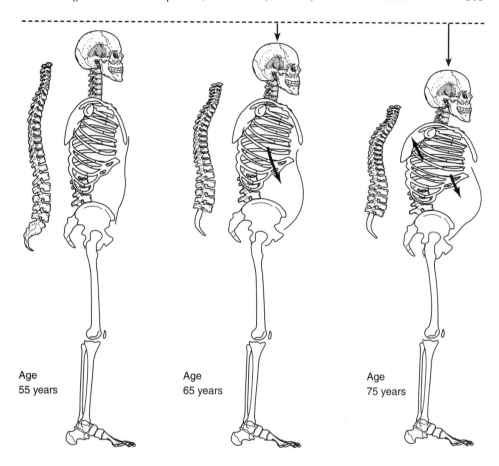

Age
55 years

Age
65 years

Age
75 years

Compression fractures of thoracic vertebrae lead to loss of height and progressive thoracic kyphosis (dowager's hump). Lower ribs eventually rest on iliac crests, and downward pressure on viscera causes abdominal distention.

FIGURE 16–1 Progressive spinal deformity in osteoporosis.
Source: From Osteoporosis: pathophysiology and prevention" by FS Kaplan, *Clinical Symposia,* 1987; 39(1):21.

- Do you smoke cigarettes or drink alcohol in excess?
- Are you allergic to milk products or are you lactose intolerant?
- Do you spend less than 1 hour a week participating in activities like aerobics, walking, or bicycling?
- Have you ever had an eating disorder such as bulimia or anorexia nervosa?

Calcium, Vitamin D, Homocysteine, and Fractures

Insufficient dietary calcium is one of the possible risk factors for osteoporosis and thereby for fractures. An inadequate intake of calcium is common in women. National Health and Nutrition Examination Survey (NHANES) data show that calcium intake in women is 40-50% below that of men; 75-80% of women have daily intakes below 800 mg, while 25% have intakes below

Statistics -

- a public health threat for 44 million people in the U.S.
- 68% of all women have osteoporosis
- 10 million cases; 34 million adults have low bone mass
- 1 of 2 women and 1 of 4 men 50 years and older will have an osteoporosis-related fracture
- 2 million American men suffer from osteoporosis
- 80,000 men with a hip fracture and one-third die within a year

Examinations to diagnose -

- initial physical
- x-rays evaluating skeletal problems
- laboratory tests reflecting the metabolic activity of bone breakdown and formation
- a bone density test detecting low bone density
- height assessment overtime

Medical intake information -

- fracture history of self and family
- comprehensive family health history
- medication history
- lifelong calcium and vitamin D intake pattern
- exercise pattern
- menstrual history for women

Risk factors for fractures -

- fractures in adulthood
- fracture among first-degree relatives
- ethnicity especially Caucasian, Asian, African and Hispanic
- older age
- female gender
- dementia
- frail health
- current cigarette smoking
- low body weight
- anorexia nervosa
- early estrogen deficiency among women before 45 years of age
- low testosterone levels in men at any age
- use of corticosteroids and anticonvulsants
- lifelong low calcium intake
- high alcoholic beverage intake
- impaired eyesight despite adequate correction
- recurrent falls
- inadequate physical activity

FIGURE 16–2   Osteoporosis statistics, examinations and risk factors.
Source: National Institutes of Health. Osteoporosis Fact Sheet. Osteoporosis and Related Bone Diseases. Bethesda, Md: NIH; June 2006. Available at: www.osteo.org.

300 mg. According to the National Institutes of Health (NIH) consensus conference on osteoporosis, dietary calcium intake required to prevent negative calcium balance increases from 1,000 mg/day in perimenopausal women to 1,500 mg/day after menopause.[3,4]

Info Line

The National Osteoporosis Foundation is the nation's leading resource for patients and healthcare professionals seeking up-to-date, medically sound information and educational materials on the causes, prevention, and treatment of osteoporosis. For information, contact National Osteoporosis Foundation, 1150 17th Street NW, Suite 500, Washington, DC 20036-4603.

Intestinal absorption of calcium declines with advancing age. However, estrogen is known to enhance intestinal calcium absorption and renal calcium conservation. Both estrogen and calcium supplementation then improve a negative calcium balance. For health-conscious older adults, low-fat eating patterns often mean a reduced intake of dairy products and calcium, which may increase a negative calcium balance.

Low dietary calcium intake may be a risk factor for osteoporosis and for fractures. However, data on the effectiveness of calcium supplements vary. This variation may reflect differences in the hormonal status and eating pattern of individuals. For example, in one study of older, postmenopausal women, calcium supplements prevented bone loss for women whose calcium intake was less than 400 mg. Supplementation did not assist women who had higher dietary calcium intakes. Adding vitamin D may increase the effect of supplemental calcium on preventing bone loss. It is not clear if this is due to an enhanced absorption of calcium or whether vitamin D has an independent effect. The percentage of calcium available in common compounds is shown in Table 16–1. Estrogen therapy reduces bone loss among postmenopausal women. Calcium supplementation for women who receive estrogen may reduce bone loss further.[3]

Research data are not available regarding the efficacy of calcium and vitamin D supplementation. Women are currently taking supplements to reduce fractures. A clinical trial can provide a rational basis for advising women to take such supplementation. The Women's Health Initiative will determine if supplementation and estrogens can reduce bone loss and fracture rates in postmenopausal women.

The concern is that 1 in 6 white, US women 50 years of age will break a hip at some point in their life with an injury increasing their risk for disability and death. More than 1,300 postmenopausal women with a hip

TABLE 16–1 Percentage of Calcium Available from Common Calcium Supplements

Compounds	Calcium (%)
Calcium carbonate	40
Calcium lactate	13
Calcium gluconate	9

Source: Adapted from: *Osteoporosis: Cause, Treatment and Prevention.* Bethesda, Md: National Institutes of Health; 1986. Publication No 86-2226.

fracture and over 3,000 postmenopausal women without a broken hip were recently studied. Women who were past menopause and > 169 centimeters or about 5 feet, 5 inches tall were 3 times as likely to break a hip than women < 159 centimeters or 5 feet, 2 inches. Women who gained 12 or more kilograms, about 26 pounds, as adults were less likely to break a hip than women who gained less weight or who lost weight during adulthood. Tall women who gained a lot of weight after 18 years of age had a higher risk of hip fracture than shorter women with a weight gain. Weight loss in adulthood was an independent risk factor. Height increases risk among heavy women, but hormonal and mechanical factors have protective effects on the body. Heavy women have higher levels of estrogen, a hormone that is protective against the bone-thinning osteoporosis, and larger muscles are needed to move heavier bodies, which can increase bone density; furthermore, fat padding cushions the hip during a fall.[5]

Osteoporosis strikes 1 in 5 postmenopausal white women in the United States. About 20% of people who break a hip die within a year due to complications from a group of problems like constipation, abdominal pain, lung disease, depression, and loss of self-esteem. The National Osteoporosis Foundation recommends a bone mineral density scan on all women 65 and over and on younger postmenopausal women with 1 or more of the following risk factors:

- history of fracture as an adult
- history of fracture in a first-degree relative due to fragility (rather than because of high impact per se)
- body weight < 127 pounds
- current smoking
- use of corticosteroids > 3 months

Other risk factors making a woman eligible for a bone scan if < 65 years old are impaired vision, menopause before age 45, dementia, poor health/frailty, lifelong low calcium intake, low physical activity, and 2 alcoholic drinks a day. A healthy lifestyle to prevent osteoporosis is consuming:

- 1,200 milligrams of calcium a day and 400 to 800 international units of vitamin D
- supplements, if necessary
- regular weight-bearing exercises like brisk walking daily and strength training, including lifting weights 2-3 times a week[6]

Elevated levels of homocysteine, a naturally occurring amino acid in the blood, have previously been linked to a higher risk for both heart disease and Alzheimer's disease. There may be a link between homocysteine and the risk for fractured bones.

In the Netherlands, 2,400 people age 55 and older whose homocysteine levels were in the highest quarter had double the risk for fracture compared to people in the 3 lower quarters. Levels of homocysteine and hip fractures were compared in a group of 2,000 people ages 59 to 91. Men in the top 25% for homocysteine were 4 times as likely to fracture a hip as men in the lowest 25%. Women with the highest homocysteine levels had twice the fracture risk as for women with the lowest levels.[7]

Folic acid and other B vitamins lower homocysteine and may prevent fractures. The potential mechanism may be that excess homocysteine may interfere with collagen, a protein that helps form the basic structure of bone.[8]

Osteoporosis is one of the largest threats to the 85 and over population and currently affects more than 28 million Americans. By the year 2030, there will be more than 19 million people over the age of 85. Growing old gracefully is threatened by osteoporosis. To maintain strong and healthy bones, adults still need at least 1,200 mg/day of calcium, the equivalent of 4 servings a day of milk, cheese, or yogurt.[9]

Osteoporosis and osteomalacia are both influenced by poor nutrient intake, decreased physical activity, corticosteroid therapy, and lack of sunshine experienced by people who are homebound. Malabsorption of vitamin D in the small bowel is often seen with advanced disease. The deficiency of vitamin D and calcium play a major role in the development of osteomalacia.[9]

The NIH Consensus Development Conference Statement on Optimal Calcium Intake

In the absence of intervention, women over 45 years experience 5.2 million fractures and incur $45.2 billion in costs to the healthcare system. There are about 195,000 vertebral fractures in the United States annually. At 50 years of age, a US white woman has a 32% chance of a vertebral fracture, 16% chance of hip fracture, and 15% chance of wrist fracture. Peak bone mass achieved in the first 30 years of life and the rate at which bone is lost later in life are the major influences on osteoporosis.

At the NIH consensus conference, several questions about osteoporosis were addressed. Six important questions and the response to each follow.[3]

1. What Is the Optimal Calcium Intake?

Optimal calcium intake is the level of intake needed to achieve and maintain peak adult bone mass and minimize bone loss later in life. The dietary reference intakes (DRIs) for calcium for infants, children, and adults are outlined in Table 16–2. Calcium needs are greater during rapid growth in childhood and adolescence, pregnancy, lactation, and later adult life. Ninety-nine percent of total body calcium is located in bones. Body retention of calcium increases as calcium intake increases up to a threshold, above which no further gain in calcium retention is noted.

Peak adult bone mass is usually achieved by 20 years of age, but additional bone mass may form through the third decade. Cross-sectional studies show a positive association between lifelong calcium intake and adult bone mass.[10,11] Data suggest that calcium intake between 1,200 and 1,500 mg/day might result in higher peak adult bone mass.

Peak bone mass is a significant predictor of risk for osteoporosis. Skeletal mass accumulation has strong genetic control, and determinants include diet, physical activity, hormonal status, and other clinical factors. The overall contribution of the genetic and environmental factors and their interaction have not been delineated. Six hundred seventy-seven healthy, unrelated, white women ages 18 to 35 years completed a detailed, standardized interview to evaluate lifestyle, menstrual and reproductive history, medical conditions,

TABLE 16–2   Adequate Intakes (AIs) and Tolerable Upper Limits (ULs) Recommended for Calcium for Infants, Children, and Adults

Life Stage Group	AIs Calcium (mg/d)	ULs Calcium (g/d)
Infants		
0-6 mo	210	ND
7-12 mo	270	ND
Children		
1-3 y	500	2.5
4-8 y	800	2.5
Males		
9-13 y	1,300	2.5
14-18 y	1,300	2.5
19-30 y	1,000	2.5
31-50 y	1,000	2.5
51-70 y	1,200	2.5
> 70 y	1,200	2.5
Females		
9-13 y	1,300	2.5
14-18 y	1,300	2.5
19-30 y	1,000	2.5
31-50 y	1,000	2.5
51-70 y	1,200	2.5
> 70 y	1,200	2.5
Pregnancy		
≤ 18 y	1,300	2.5
19-30 y	1,000	2.5
31-50 y	1,000	2.5
Lactation		
≤ 18 y	1,300	2.5
19-30 y	1,000	2.5
31-50 y	1,000	2.5

ND = No data available.

Source: National Academy of Sciences, Institute of Medicine (IOM). *Dietary Reference Intakes for Calcium.* Washington, DC: National Academy Press; 2002. Available at: http://www.IOM.edu/. Accessed February 1, 2007.

medication use, and family history of osteoporosis. Bone mineral density (BMD) was measured at the lumbar spine (L2-L4) and the femoral neck (hip) using dual-energy X-ray absorptiometry. Genotyping of the vitamin D receptor (VDR) was performed.[12]

In bivariate analyses, BMD at the lumbar spine and hip was positively correlated with weight, height, body mass index (BMI), and level of physical activity, both now and during adolescence, but negatively correlated with a family history of osteoporosis. Hip, but not spine, BMD correlated positively with dietary intake of calcium and negatively with amenorrhea of more than 3 months, with caffeine intake, and with age. Spine, but not hip, BMD correlated positively with age and with number of pregnancies. VDR demonstrated significant associations with BMD at the hip, level of physical activity currently, and BMI.[12]

Changes in bone mineral density and bone mineral content (BMD and BMC) occur when obese female adolescents experience weight reduction. A 6-month program included 92 obese females who completed a calcium food frequency/24-hour dietary recall, physical activity, and psychological assessments for anxiety/self-esteem. Multiple linear regression evaluated changes in bone measures with changes in body weight measures. Total body and lumbar spine BMD and BMC changes were significantly correlated with weight changes. Girls who lost weight did not lose BMD and BMC. The rate of growth declined compared to normal weight female adolescents. Weight changes are strongly related to bone measurement changes in an obese adolescent female population, and CNPs who counsel obese young girls should emphasize a healthy weight loss program with adequate calcium intake and weight-bearing exercises.[13]

In multivariate analysis, independent predictors of greater BMD (at the hip or spine) were age (younger for the hip, older for the spine), greater body weight, greater height (hip only), higher level of physical activity now and during adolescence, no family history of osteoporosis, and VDR genotype (hip only). Weight, age, level of physical activity, and family history are independent predictors of peak BMD. Of these factors, weight accounts for over half the explained variability in BMD. VDR alleles are significant independent predictors of peak femoral neck, but not lumbar spine BMD, even after adjusting for family history of osteoporosis, weight, age, and exercise. The overall contribution of this genetic determinant is modest and the aggregate effect of these factors explained approximately 17% and 21% of the variability in peak spine and hip BMD, respectively. Understanding the interactive nature of genes and the environment promotes targeted strategies to modify lifestyle and to intervene in the most susceptible individuals.[12]

After adult peak bone mass is achieved, bone turnover stabilizes for both men and women (i.e., bone formation and bone resorption are balanced). For women, resorption rate increases and bone mass decreases as estrogen production declines with menopause. Specifically, the decline in circulating 17 beta-estradiol is the predominant factor in accelerated bone loss. This begins immediately after the onset of menopause and lasts for 6 to 8 years. Hormonal-replacement therapy slows the decline in bone mass, but supplemental calcium at this time does not appear to slow the decline. Later in menopause, calcium intakes of 1,500 mg/day may reduce the rates of bone loss in certain parts of the skeleton (i.e., the femoral neck).[14-16]

If postmenopausal women receive estrogen-replacement therapy, 1,000 mg/day of calcium is recommended to maintain calcium balance and stabilize bone mass. If women do not take estrogen, 1,500 mg of calcium per day may limit loss of bone mass, but will not replace estrogen.[16] Women taking estrogen or other drug therapies to help prevent or treat osteoporosis can complement their actions if they wash their pills down with a glass of milk. A calcium-rich diet may make or break the impact of drug treatment for osteoporosis.

Nieves et al conducted a meta-analysis of 31 clinical trials examining the effectiveness of osteoporosis treatment among postmenopausal women. Estrogen or hormone replacement therapy (HRT) may be less effective without adequate dietary calcium. Daily calcium intake of 1,200 milligrams, or the equivalent of 4 servings of milk group foods, may boost the benefits of HRT and other drug treatments, promoting new bone in the spine, hip, and forearm areas, which are common fracture sites.[17]

Low calcium intake has been implicated as a determinant of preeclampsia, colon cancer, and hypertension. The Women's Health Initiative will evaluate the effect of vitamin D and calcium supplementation on colorectal cancer and osteoporosis incidence. A number of epidemiologic studies report an inverse association between blood pressure and calcium intake. Few prospective studies have confirmed this association, but beta analyses demonstrate a small reduction in systolic pressure and no effect on diastolic blood pressure with calcium intake.[3]

About 3,676 healthy white women between 66 and 91 years of age had their blood pressure taken and had their leg bones tested for bone mineral density. The women were retested between 3 and 5 years later, and 25% of women with the highest blood pressure lost more than one and a half times as much bone mineral per year as the 25% of women with the lowest blood pressure. High blood pressure had an effect on bone mineral loss even though the women in the study with the highest blood pressure were in a range considered safe and not hypertensive. Researchers adjusted for age, weight, smoking, and the use of hormone replacement therapy. The mechanism linking high blood pressure to bone mineral loss is not clear, but high blood pressure may limit the kidneys to metabolize calcium. High-salt diets can increase calcium excretion and increase high blood pressure.[18]

The 2002 position statement of the North American Menopause Society (NAMS) states that evaluation of postmenopausal women for osteoporosis risk requires the recording of a medical history, a physical examination, and diagnostic tests. Major risk factors for osteoporosis are age, genetics, lifestyle (especially nutrition), and menopausal status. Management focuses first on nonpharmacologic measures, such as a balanced diet including adequate calcium and vitamin D intakes, appropriate exercise, smoking cessation, avoidance of excessive alcohol intake, and fall prevention. If pharmacologic therapy is indicated, FDA-approved options are estrogens (prevention only), bisphosphonates and selective estrogen-receptor modulators (prevention and treatment), and calcitonin (treatment only).[19]

In one study, women with hip fractures had lower levels of 25-hydroxyvitamin D than both women without osteoporosis admitted for elective joint replacement ($p = 0.02$) and women with osteoporosis admitted for elective joint replacement ($p = 0.01$) (after adjustment for age and estrogen intake). Parathyroid hormone levels were higher in women with fractures than in both the nonosteoporotic control group ($p < 0.001$) and those with elective surgery ($p = 0.001$), again after adjustments for age and estrogen use. Fifteen patients (50.0%) with hip fractures had deficient vitamin D levels ≤ 30.0 nmol/L and 11 (36.7%) had a parathyroid hormone level greater than 6.84 pmol/L. Levels of N-telopeptide, a marker of bone resorption, were greater in the women with hip fractures than in the elective nonosteoporotic control group ($p = 0.004$).[20]

Since bone is lost at a rate of 0.2-0.5% each year in both men and women > 40 years of age, with an accelerated loss to 2-5% per year immediately before and for 10 years postmenopause, nutrition has a key role. In women, hormone-replacement therapy is effective in reducing the rate of bone loss caused during perimenopause. In men and in older women after 10 years of menopause, what an individual eats is crucial for the rate of bone loss. One possible contribution to bone loss may be a subclinical Zn and/or Cu deficiency, due to a reduced intake or reduced absorption. Zn and Cu are essential cofactors for enzymes involved in the synthesis of various bone matrix constituents. Calcium supplementation may accentuate the problem by impairing the absorption of Zn ingested at the same time and the retention of Cu.[21]

In one study, changes in BMD were adjusted for confounding factors and compared with women having low ($\leq$ 300 mg/d) or high (> 300 mg/d) caffeine intakes. Women with high caffeine intakes had significantly higher rates of bone loss at the spine than did those with low intakes ($-1.90+/-0.97$% compared with $1.19+/-1.08$%; 0.038).[22] Further, research indicates that the negative effects of heavy alcohol use on bone cannot be reversed, even if alcohol consumption is terminated.[23]

2. What Are the Important Cofactors for Achieving Optimal Calcium Intake?

Dietary constituents, hormones, and drugs modify calcium balance and influence bone mass. An individual's age, ethnic and genetic background, gastrointestinal disorders including malabsorption, and liver and renal disease affect bone health. Interactions of these factors may have either a positive or negative effect on efficacy of calcium.

Vitamin D metabolites enhance calcium absorption by stimulating active transport of calcium in the small intestine and colon. Deficiency of 1,25-dihydroxyvitamin D reduces calcium absorption. The deficiency may be due to an inadequate amount or impaired activation of vitamin D or even to an acquired resistance to vitamin D. Vitamin D deficiency is also associated with an increased risk of fractures.

Sex hormone deficiency is linked to excessive bone resorption in women and men. Calcium supplementation can decrease the estrogen dosage required to maintain bone mass in postmenopausal women, but oral calcium will not prevent the postmenopausal bone loss due to estrogen deficiency.[16,24] Endogenous factors (e.g., growth hormone, insulin-like growth factor-I, and parathyroid hormone) enhance overall calcium absorption.

Increased physical activity can enhance the beneficial effect of oral calcium supplementation on bone mass in young adults. Immobilization rapidly decreases bone mass. This is especially true for individuals placed on bed rest or individuals who have paraplegia or quadriplegia. The concern is that increased calcium intake may predispose these individuals to hypercalcemia, ectopic calcification, ectopic ossification, and nephrolithiasis.

Calcium intake, intestinal absorption, urinary excretion, and endogenous fecal loss influence calcium balance. High amounts of sodium and animal protein can significantly increase urinary calcium excretion. For every 2,300 mg of sodium, a 40-mg calcium loss occurs.[25,26] Primitive hunter-gatherers had calcium and sodium intakes yielding a 1.0 to 0.76 ratio. This equates to 4 calcium atoms per 3 sodium atoms. Today, average sodium intakes produce 17 sodium atoms per 1 calcium atom. Protein intake increases calcium requirements due to loss of calcium in the kidneys and the demand for a calcium balance. High oxalate and phytate content of foods can reduce the availability of calcium; wheat bran, fat, phosphate, magnesium, and caffeine have not been found to alter calcium absorption significantly. A 5-ounce cup of coffee creates a loss in calcium balance by about 3 milligrams. Glucocorticoids decrease calcium absorption; excess is associated with negative calcium balance and a dramatic increase in fracture risk. Oral calcium and vitamin D supplements decrease glucocorticoid-associated bone loss.[3]

3. What Are the Risks Associated With Increased Levels of Calcium Intake?

High levels of calcium intake above 2 grams can have adverse effects (e.g., the efficiency of calcium absorption decreases as intake increases). This occurs as a protective mechanism to reduce calcium intoxication. However, the adaptive mechanism is overcome by a calcium intake greater than 4 grams per day. Calcium toxicity can cause severe renal damage, and ectopic calcium deposition or a milk-alkali syndrome can occur with misuse of calcium carbonate (i.e., antacid abuse). Hypercalcemia or hypercalciuria can occur when individuals consume less than 4 grams if they are susceptible. No adverse renal effects have been noted when moderate supplementation of 1,500 mg/day is used.

Society is currently viewing nutrients like calcium as drugs, but not taking precautions commonly equated with drugs. Small amounts of calcium added to healthful foods (not to unhealthy foods like potato chips) encourages dietary improvement overall. Excessive calcium has been documented as > 2,500 milligrams a day, and this amount is termed the tolerable upper intake level (TUIL). At high levels, people may aggravate kidney stone formation and damage their kidney function. This is especially true for anyone who has had a stone in the past. Even an active 16-year-old boy who consumes half a gallon of calcium-fortified orange juice and half a gallon of milk in a day, plus fortified cereal and other high-calcium foods, could easily consume too much calcium.[27]

Supplementing individuals who have a history of kidney stones can increase both urinary calcium excretion and stone formation. Iron absorption can be lowered by 50% due to calcium supplements. Gastrointestinal side effects including constipation have been reported from calcium supplements. The calcium ion can produce a rebound hyperacidity when a calcium carbonate antacid is used extensively. Side effects are not common when a moderate increase is made in calcium intake. Bone meal and dolomite can have significant contamination with lead and other heavy metals, and supplements containing these should be tested for heavy metal contamination.[3,28]

4. What Are the Best Ways to Attain Optimal Calcium Intake?

The preferred technique to achieve optimal calcium intake is to select foods that are calcium rich, but calcium-fortified foods or calcium supplements are popular choices. Dairy products are high in calcium content (e.g., 300 mg/8 fluid ounces of milk). Individuals who are lactose intolerant or vegans can achieve adequate calcium by using low-lactose and lactose-free dairy products. Broccoli, kale, turnip greens, Chinese cabbage, calcium-set tofu, some legumes, canned fish, seeds, nuts, and certain fortified food products are also good calcium sources and average about 100 to 150 mg/serving. Breads and cereals are fairly low in calcium but are significant contributors because of their high frequency of consumption.

Bioavailability of calcium depends on the total calcium content of the food, the presence of oxalic acid, phytic acid, and wheat bran, which can enhance or inhibit absorption. Calcium-fortified juices and fruit drinks, breads, and cereals may provide 300 mg/serving. Calcium supplements are most efficient at 500 mg or less. Absorption of calcium carbonate is blocked in fasting individuals due to the absence of gastric acid. Many older adults have a depressed gastric acid production and should take calcium supplements with meals for optimal absorption.

Optimal bone health depends on an adequate calcium intake and a balance of other essential nutrients. Since calcium intakes are generally below recommended levels, intake must be addressed daily. Current food guide pyramid dietary guidelines recommend 2 to 3 servings per day of dairy products and 3 to 5 servings of vegetables.

5. What Public Health Strategies Are Available and Needed to Implement Optimal Calcium Intake Recommendations?

Data from the National Health and Nutrition Examination Survey (NHANES) III, 1988-1991, reports that 6- to 11-year-old children have lower calcium intakes than children in NHANES II (1976-1980), and a large percentage of US residents do not meet the recommended dietary allowance (RDA) for calcium intakes.[29] Suboptimal calcium intake increases health care costs, warranting aggressive attention to *Healthy People 2010* objectives to increase calcium intake. Likewise, strategies to promote optimal calcium intake must involve the following:

1. Public education to:
   - disseminate consensus recommendations
   - convene meetings of leaders and representatives of national groups to disseminate information and develop action plans
   - work with existing national organizations and the mass media to decrease confusion and encourage high-risk groups such as children and adolescent girls to consume calcium-rich foods
2. Health professionals to educate their patients about bone health and calcium intake by:
   - disseminating consensus recommendations
   - developing and distributing educational materials
   - serving as a clearinghouse for calcium-related research and developing curriculum
   - initiating national sessions focusing solely on calcium-related research
3. Private sector to actively promote optimal calcium intake in the following ways:
   - manufacturers and producers marketing calcium-rich foods for the needs and tastes of a diverse population

- restaurants, grocery stores, and other food outlets increasing the accessibility and visibility of calcium-rich products
- biotechnology researchers developing inexpensive technologies to screen the public and identify those at high risk of fracture who would also be candidates for high calcium intakes

4. Public sector to solicit the federal government to:

- instruct the National Center for Health Statistics and the US Department of Agriculture to disseminate US nutrient intake data and food consumption patterns, giving data specific to age, gender, ethnic group, region, and socioeconomic status
- ensure that existing federal food and food subsidy programs and facilities for infants, children, low-income populations, and the elderly promote optimal calcium intake for program recipients
- address use of calcium supplements for individuals who cannot reach optimal calcium intake with foods
- use government food facilities to promote optimal calcium intake by serving calcium-rich foods, labeling foods, and distributing educational brochures
- ensure that government guidelines reflect the current state of knowledge about calcium needs and requirements

6. What Are the Recommendations for Future Research on Calcium Intake?

Future research should:

- investigate long-term effects of calcium in postmenopausal women and in men in longitudinal studies
- observe the long-term effects of different calcium levels on peak bone mass in adolescent girls and boys in longitudinal studies
- study the long-term effects of calcium on bone remodeling
- study the interactions between calcium supplementation and nutrient absorption
- evaluate the dose-response association between calcium requirement and estrogen-replacement therapy
- determine optimal calcium requirements among different ethnic populations
- evaluate the effect of long-term calcium supplementation on the development or prevention of kidney stones
- develop a cost-effective method to identify calcium-deficient individuals
- initiate health-promoting programs to effect change in population behavior regarding calcium intakes
- develop methods to achieve and maintain optimal dietary intake of calcium among all ages of individuals

Bone Health: A Weight-Bearing Argument

"Weight-bearing" means bones are working against gravity to support the body weight or other weight; walking, running, push-ups, and using an elliptical machine also apply as the individual is on his or her feet. Swimming, in which the body is floating in the water, is not weight-bearing exercise.

Cycling is non-weight bearing; the bike is supporting the weight. When an individual stands on the bicycle pedals, the exercise becomes weight-bearing. Bones respond to pressure by adding osteoblasts, or bone-forming cells, which boost density. Gains from adding bone density usually serve, at best, to keep pace with the loss of bone density that comes with age. A difficult challenge is for adults to add new bone, but weight-bearing activity helps.[30]

Alcoholism

Alcohol is the most commonly abused drug in our society. About two thirds of Americans drink alcohol, and 9% are addicted to alcohol. Many individuals enjoy social drinking but the conversion to problem drinking occurs frequently (see Table 16–3). Over 100,000 deaths per year are alcohol related. Alcohol abuse costs billions of dollars and is linked to thousands of divorces, about 50% of the incidents of family violence, and millions of hours of school and job absenteeism. Alcohol abuse is also linked to several diseases (e.g., pancreatitis, Wernicke-Korsakoff's syndrome, alcoholic cardiomyopathy, and liver cirrhosis).[31]

Alcohol intake may account for 10% of the hypertension in men. Epidemiologic studies show a short-term pressor effect of alcohol consumption. A decline in blood pressure occurs from abstinence or less than 1 drink per day in heavy drinkers. Individuals who are previous drinkers have the same blood pressure as nondrinkers.

Alcoholic beverages contain ethyl alcohol, which is toxic. The amount of alcohol in beer and wine is given as a percentage. Beer averages 4% alcohol, wine about 12% alcohol. Labels on distilled liquors (i.e., scotch, vodka, bourbon, tequila, and rum) state a *proof*, a number that equals twice the percentage of alcohol in the product. A 100-proof scotch is 50% alcohol. Standard portions of alcoholic beverages have about 1/2 ounce of ethyl alcohol. A 2-ounce jigger of rum that is 40% alcohol is 0.80 ounces of alcohol. Alcohol has 7 kcal per gram, which are considered empty calories. With the 2005 *Dietary Guidelines for Americans*, alcohol is 1 of the 9 major advisory topics with moderation of intake being the recommendation.[32]

However, there is no universally accepted definition of moderate use of alcohol.[33] The term is used in 5 different ways[34]:

1. *Nonintoxicating* focuses on the immediate adverse events, such as accidental trauma and interpersonal violence, for which the risk is clearly increased by intoxication. It is difficult to define quantitatively, because genetic factors and acquired tolerance result in large individual differences in the amounts that can be drunk without a person becoming intoxicated.
2. *Statistically normal* relates to the average amount that is typical of drinkers in a given population. This can be measured reasonably accurately, but differs substantially from one population or culture to another, and has no clear relationship to the risk of chronic health or social problems.
3. *Noninjurious* is a medically acceptable or threshold level linked to alcohol-related disease.

TABLE 16–3   Alcohol Intake by US Adults 18 Years of Age and Over, 2002

Characteristic	Male	Female
Drinking status (age-adjusted)	%	%
All	100	100
Lifetime abstainer	14.7	28.7
Former drinker	15.7	14.8
Infrequent	7.4	9.3
Regular	8.3	5.5
Current drinker	69.6	56.5
Infrequent	9.7	16.5
Regular	58.7	39.1
Age		
18-44 years	75.9	62.8
18-24 years	70.6	57.6
25-44 years	77.7	64.5
45-64 years	68.2	58.2
45-54 years	71.0	61.3
55-64 years	63.8	53.6
65 years and over	52.0	33.5
65-74 years	56.4	36.6
75 years and over	46.1	30.4
Race		
White only	71.8	60.2
Black or African American only	56.5	40.3
American Indian and Alaska native only	61.5	46.8
Asian only	60.0	35.3
2 or more races	63.9	62.1
Hispanic or Latino	64.6	38.1
Mexican	65.2	37.0

Source: Adapted from: US Department of Health and Human Services. *Health, United States, 2004.* Washington, DC: Dept of Health and Human Services; 2005:235.

4. *Problem-free* links to health but also to social problems like interpersonal relations, work performance, and legal and economic difficulties. Individual and environmental influences affect the extent of harm at a certain level and cloud being able to translate intake into quantitative terms.

5. *Optimal* produces the lowest morbidity or mortality but varies for different health outcomes. It allows an objective quantitative definition, especially for outcomes which show a U- or J-shaped relation between intake and level of risk.

Defining "moderate" intake quantitatively is difficult because intakes may be expressed in drinks or units that vary with beverage type, culture, and acceptable habits of different generations. A uniform international definition of a standard drink is needed or individual intakes should consistently be expressed in amounts (grams) of absolute alcohol per kg body weight per day.

Problems that occur when estimating moderate levels are[35]:

- Estimates may give different results, depending on how questions are posed. General questions about overall drinking yield different amounts than specific questions that inquire about each beverage type (beer, wine, spirits), and questions about the amount drunk in the past 1 or 2 weeks yield different results than those that inquire about the past month or year.[36]
- If traditional units such as drinks, glasses, or bottles are not the same, then universal comparisons cannot be achieved. Alcohol intake in grams of absolute ethanol may be an alternative, but average alcohol contents vary and create another source of error.
- Self-reported numbers of drinks are usually defined as the typical serving in the geographic area (see Table 16–4).
- Limited accuracy in estimating alcohol intake makes it difficult to estimate the actual moderate levels of consumption.
- Recall ability of alcohol intake creates some random error. Test reliability is reasonably good with reliability coefficients varying from 0.80 to 0.90.[37]

TABLE 16–4　Alcohol Content of a Standard Drink (in g Absolute Ethanol) as Defined in Various Countries

Country	Size of Standard Drink (g Alcohol)
Australia	10
Austria	6
Canada	13.5
Denmark	12
Finland	11
France	12
Hungary	17
Iceland	9.5
Ireland	8
Italy	10
Japan	19.75
Netherlands	9.9
New Zealand	10
Portugal	14
Spain	10
United Kingdom	8
United States	14

Source: Data from International Center for Alcohol Policies. *ICAP Report 5.* Washington, DC: ICAP; 1998.

- Respondents may underestimate their alcohol intake as shown in population surveys, where the average underestimation varies by 29-83% of the actual intake.[38,39]

Alcohol is absorbed into the body through the gastrointestinal tract with 20% absorbed by the stomach and the rest by the small intestine. Alcohol is carried to all body tissues and organs. High-fat foods or proteins slow the absorption of alcohol. Nonalcoholic substances in beverages can slow absorption of alcohol; carbon dioxide in champagne, sparkling wines, beer, and carbonated mixed drinks increase the rate of alcohol absorption. Individuals experience intoxication more quickly when drinking champagne or beer, especially on an empty stomach. A higher alcohol content increases the absorption rate.[31]

About 10% of alcohol is excreted unchanged in sweat, urine, or breath. Alcohol that is not excreted is metabolized at a rate of about 1/2 ounce per hour, primarily by the liver into carbon dioxide and water. Table 16–5 outlines the characteristics of various alcohols and the time required to metabolize different alcohols.

Alcohol Abuse

Alcohol abuse is the most common type of drug abuse in the United States, affecting 12 million people. More than 3 million US teenagers have a drinking

TABLE 16–5   Metabolic Characteristics of Various Alcoholic Drinks

Number of Drinks	Ounces of Alcohol	Blood Alcohol Content (g/100 mL)	Metabolism (hrs)	Effects
1 beer, glass of wine, or mixed drink	0.5	0.02	1.0	Feeling relaxed or loosened up
2½ beers, glasses of wine, or mixed drinks	1.25	0.05	2.5	Feeling high; decrease in inhibitions; increase in confidence; judgment impaired
5 beers, glasses of wine, or mixed drinks	2.5	0.10	5.0	Memory impaired; muscular coordination reduced; slurred speech; euphoric or sad feelings
10 beers, glasses of wine, or mixed drinks	5.0	0.20	10.0	Slowed reflexes; erratic changes in feelings
15 beers, glasses of wine, or mixed drinks	7.5	0.30	15.5	Stuporous; complete loss of coordination; little sensation
20 beers, glasses of wine, or mixed drinks	10.0	0.40	20.0	Comatose; breathing may cease
25–30 beers, glasses of wine, or mixed drinks	18.0	0.50	26.0	Fatal for most people

Source: Data from Edlin G, Golanty E. *Health and Wellness: A Holistic Approach.* 4th ed. Sudbury, Mass: Jones and Bartlett Publishers; 1992:285-294.

problem. Over one third of all suicides involve alcohol. Six million adults are alcoholics. They are unable to control their drinking. Warning signs of alcoholism are listed in Exhibit 16–1.[31] Tyrosine, an amino acid, can be used during drug and alcohol detoxification. A therapeutic dose of tyrosine may affect the nervous system by regulating the heart rate, blood flow, muscle contractions, and sensitivity. Caution should be taken to recognize side effects producing serious adverse conditions.[40]

Alcoholism develops across 3 phases[41]:

1. *Warning phase:* Person develops an increased tolerance to alcohol and a preoccupation with drinking.
2. *Crucial phase:* Person loses control over amount drunk and rationalizes that there are good reasons for heavy drinking.
3. *Chronic phase:* Person is totally dependent on alcohol, and drinking consumes all aspects of life.

The dose of alcohol needed to create ethanol's actions on behavior is defined as the upper range of moderate exposure at a brain ethanol level of ≤ 0.92 g/L, which is equivalent to a concentration of ≤ 20 mM ethanol.[42,43] The variability in individual reactions to the effects of alcohol is probably reflected in the epidemiological data showing that an appreciable proportion (16-33%) of the population in Europe and North America choose not to drink alcohol.[44-46]

Alcoholic Liver Disease

This disease is the ninth most common cause of death in the United States, with about 200,000 individuals dying annually. Men drink more than women, but women are more susceptible to alcohol. Risk of alcoholic liver disease is greater in women who have 3 drinks each day, compared to 6 drinks per day for men. A schema showing alcoholic liver diseases and other disorders common with alcohol abuse is shown in Figure 16–3.[31]

Exhibit 16–1   12 Warning Signs of Alcoholism

1. Gulps drinks.
2. Drinks to modify uncomfortable feelings.
3. Changes behavior after drinking.
4. Drinks frequently.
5. Experiences blackouts.
6. Has frequent accidents or illness.
7. Prepares self with alcohol before a social event.
8. Refuses to talk about negative consequences of drinking.
9. Is preoccupied with alcohol.
10. Focuses on social situations around alcohol.
11. Sneaks drinks or clandestine drinking.
12. Has redness of face and skin.

Source: Edlin G, Golanty E. *Health and Wellness: A Holistic Approach.* 4th ed. Boston, Mass: Jones and Bartlett Publishers; 1992. Adapted with permission.

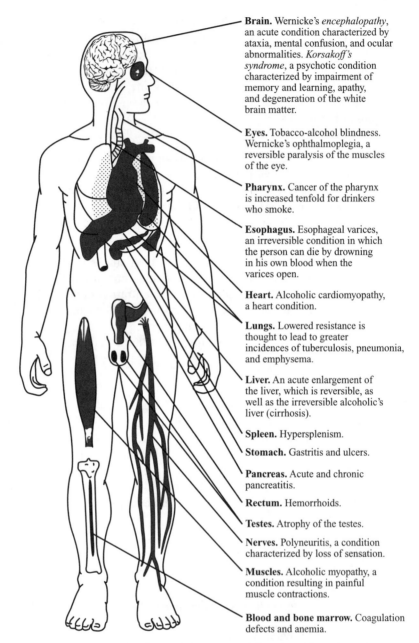

Brain. Wernicke's *encephalopathy*, an acute condition characterized by ataxia, mental confusion, and ocular abnormalities. *Korsakoff's syndrome*, a psychotic condition characterized by impairment of memory and learning, apathy, and degeneration of the white brain matter.

Eyes. Tobacco-alcohol blindness. Wernicke's ophthalmoplegia, a reversible paralysis of the muscles of the eye.

Pharynx. Cancer of the pharynx is increased tenfold for drinkers who smoke.

Esophagus. Esophageal varices, an irreversible condition in which the person can die by drowning in his own blood when the varices open.

Heart. Alcoholic cardiomyopathy, a heart condition.

Lungs. Lowered resistance is thought to lead to greater incidences of tuberculosis, pneumonia, and emphysema.

Liver. An acute enlargement of the liver, which is reversible, as well as the irreversible alcoholic's liver (cirrhosis).

Spleen. Hypersplenism.

Stomach. Gastritis and ulcers.

Pancreas. Acute and chronic pancreatitis.

Rectum. Hemorrhoids.

Testes. Atrophy of the testes.

Nerves. Polyneuritis, a condition characterized by loss of sensation.

Muscles. Alcoholic myopathy, a condition resulting in painful muscle contractions.

Blood and bone marrow. Coagulation defects and anemia.

FIGURE 16–3   Frequently observed diseases and disorders when alcohol is present.
Source: Edlin G, Golanty E. *Health and Wellness: A Holistic Approach.* 4th ed. Boston, Mass: Jones and Bartlett Publishers; 1992:286. Reprinted with permission.

Susceptibility to liver disease is linked to the effects of heredity and gender on the metabolism of alcohol. The effect of alcohol as a toxin and causing a nutrient imbalance both contribute to the development of alcoholic liver disease. Numerous animal models have demonstrated that substitution of alcohol for carbohydrate in diets fed to baboons, rats, and pigs lead to features of alcoholic liver disease and increase fibrosis in the liver.

Malnutrition is a universal feature of alcoholic cirrhosis. A Veterans Administration cooperative study of more than 300 patients with alcoholic cirrhosis showed 100% incidence of protein-calorie malnutrition. Other surveys showed greater than 50% incidence of low serum folate, thiamine, and pyridoxine in alcoholic liver disease. Liver biopsies indicate universal depletion of hepatic vitamin A in alcoholic liver disease. The manifestations of malnutrition in alcoholism include altered cellular immunity due to protein and zinc deficiency; anemia due to combinations of folate, iron, and pyridoxine deficiencies; night blindness due to vitamin A deficiency; and Wernicke-Korsakoff's syndrome due to thiamine deficiency.

Energy wasting during excessive binge drinking is well documented and is probably due to the increased calorie cost of metabolizing alcohol by the microsomal system. Heavy drinkers often substitute alcohol for other essential micronutrients, and alcoholic beverages are nearly all devoid of micronutrients. Intestinal malabsorption, which is common, is due to alteration of the intestinal mucosa from chronic binge drinking. Alcohol has a direct effect on the mucosa, with secondary effects due to folate deficiency. Malabsorption of folic acid, thiamine, glucose, and several amino acids has been documented in binge drinkers.

At least 50% of patients with alcoholic cirrhosis have fat and fat-soluble vitamin malabsorption due to decreased secretion and transfer of bile salts to the intestine. Pancreatic insufficiency is also common in alcoholic liver disease. The metabolism of alcohol is known to lead to destruction of certain vitamins, including folic acid and pyridoxine. Cirrhotic patients have been shown to have increased energy expenditure per unit of lean body mass. Protein turnover is normal in stable cirrhotics but increases in individuals with active alcoholic hepatitis.[46,47] See Appendix 16–A for more information about the effects of alcohol.

In Denmark, the incidence of alcoholic cirrhosis is estimated at 190 per million person-years in men and 85 in women, with the age-specific incidence rates peaking at 50-60 years. Results are similar to those in the United States. Gender difference in incidence of alcoholic liver disease (ALD) may be due to the greater frequency of heavy drinkers among men, but women may be more sensitive to developing liver injury due to chronic alcohol ingestion. Prospective control trials are required to answer the question of why ALD occurs.[48]

The average duration of excessive alcohol ingestion until diagnosis of alcoholic cirrhosis may be between 10 and 20 years. Among excessive drinkers, the rate of development of cirrhosis may be about 2-3% per year, and, accordingly, the prevalence of cirrhosis is greater the longer the duration of excessive alcohol use.

Many aggregate population studies have assessed the changes over time within populations and the differences among populations in mortality from cirrhosis in relation to total per capita alcohol use. A very high correlation exists between mortality from cirrhosis and alcohol use. Retrospective case-control studies show a probability of becoming a hospitalized cirrhotic patient increases exponentially with increased daily alcohol consumption of 20 to 160 g.

Drugs Reduce Alcoholic Drinks Among Alcoholics

Alcoholics with a predisposition to alcoholism often develop drinking problems early, have a broad range of antisocial behaviors, and have close relative with alcohol problems. Twenty alcoholics who had developed alcoholism before 25 years of age participated in a behavioral therapy intervention. After taking combination drugs, ondansetron and naltrexone, 85% consumed 1 drink or less per day compared with 34% given an inactive placebo who had 3 or more drinks per day. Combination drugs significantly reduced the alcohol consumption of biological alcoholics, probably by correcting an underlying disequilibrium in some brain systems.[49]

Alcohol and Breast Cancer Risk

Fifty studies and 38 case-control studies were reviewed and authors concluded that a sometimes observed causal association of alcohol and breast cancer is unproved.[50-52] Evidence for a causal link is minimal, and some researchers believe the obsession with the association moves attention away from preventing breast cancer.[53] Confounding occurs if alcohol use is associated with another independent or unknown risk factor, e.g., some aspects of diet[54] or stress.[55] Stress is not a risk factor for breast cancer so further exploration of other factors is needed.[56]

Alcohol and Coronary Heart Disease

Ecological studies suggest but do not prove a favorable effect of alcohol use on CHD risk.[57] Observations suggest a relationship on a population level. A large case-control study from Australia has provided information on drinking patterns and risk of CHD in patients totaling over 11,500 acute myocardial infarctions (MI).[58] After excluding men and women who were former moderate or heavy drinkers, the lowest odds of MI (OR 0.36, 95% CI 0.19-0.66) were noted among men who consumed 1-2 drinks per day during 5-6 days per week. Consistent inverse associations were reported among men with 3 or 4 drinks per day on 3-6 days per week. Compared to abstainers, the lowest odds of CHD among women was the group that consumed 1-2 drinks every other day. Women who consumed 3-4 drinks daily also had a significant reduction in MI (OR 0.40, 95% CI 0.16-0.98).

In most cohort studies, participants drinking moderate amounts of alcohol had a significantly lower risk of developing CHD. A J-shaped rather than a U-shaped relation between alcohol intake and total mortality is accepted generally with increases in death from cirrhosis, accidents, violence, and cancer in heavy drinkers.[59,60] A general agreement exists to support a U-shaped curve for the association between alcohol and total cardiovascular disease (CVD) mortality, including stroke and non-CHD deaths.[61-64]

The threshold on the right side of the U begins to increase for all CVD and total mortality at about 2 drinks/day. However, the threshold for the right side of the U for fatal and nonfatal CHD is somewhat less clear, and could be as few as 2 or as many as 6 drinks/day.

A probable threshold dose for hypertension risk is 30-60 g alcohol per day, but lower for women than for men. From a public health perspective, the threshold is based on an estimate of the proportion of hypertension in the community that might be caused by alcohol use and how much hypertension could be eliminated if excessive drinking (≥ 40 g alcohol per day) was stopped. In US and Australian communities, alcohol use could account for as much as

11% of hypertension in men but less in women due to a lower alcohol intake. Chronic alcohol intake ($\geq$ 30-60 g/day) is the second risk factor for hypertension, behind obesity.[65-66] Guidelines for moderation suggest that individuals who do consume alcohol responsibly may achieve some benefit if daily consumption is limited to 2 to 3 drinks.

Dementia and Alcohol

Researchers from the Karolinska Institute in Stockholm studied people who had first been surveyed about their drinking habits in a Finnish study in 1972 and 1977. In 1998, 1,018 were reexamined, and cognition was assessed. Compared with infrequent drinkers, frequent drinkers and nondrinkers were twice as likely to develop mild cognitive impairment in old age. The authors found that the risk of dementia related to alcohol was affected by the presence of Apo e4. Carriers of this mutation were at increased risk of dementia with increasing alcohol consumption. The mechanism by which moderate drinking preserves one's mental ability is unknown.[67-68]

Info Line

HEALTH EDUCATION AND INTERVENTION/PREVENTION PROGRAMS

The results of various health education programs are mixed, and many interventions not adequately evaluated. [69-73] A multiple-level, comprehensive approach to prevention implies that a comprehensive approach may be best. Even using warning labels on alcoholic beverages in the USA has not changed drinking in pregnancy, or prenatal drinking generally, or influenced the heaviest drinkers.[74-76]

Alcoholics Anonymous (AA) is an international, nonprofit, self-help organization. AA aims for total sobriety, anonymity, and a step-by-step program for recovery of alcoholics. AA addresses sobriety as a state of mind. It presents recovery as a change in values, attitudes, and lifestyles. The AA program assists problem drinkers by asking them to examine their feelings, recognize their limitations, and accept responsibility for past wrongs. For more information, contact Alcoholics Anonymous General Service Office, 475 Riverside Drive, New York, NY 10015; (212) 870-3400. Or write to PO box 459, Grand Station, New York, NY 10163.

Arthritis

Arthritis is a pain for people of all ages. Each year, a million people learn they have arthritis. One in every seven people is affected by some form of arthritis. It is the nation's most common chronic disease and its number 1 crippler. There are more than 100 kinds of arthritis or rheumatoid disease, and the disease affects all age groups, from the very young to the very old. About a quarter of a million children suffer from some form of juvenile arthritis.[77]

Arthritis, costs $143 billion annually. With the graying of the population, by 2020, 59.6 million Americans will have arthritis. An increased number of people with arthritis will need home care to assist with their activities of daily living.[78] See Exhibit 16–2.

Juvenile rheumatoid arthritis attacks infants and children. It can cripple a child for life; but if it is diagnosed early, the effects can be minimized, often leaving little trace. Sometimes the attack is acute, with soaring temperature, a rash, and pain or tenderness in 1 or more joints. In other cases, the disease begins mildly with a general, "I don't feel well all over." In children, arthritis may last only a few weeks, it may go on for years, or it may disappear, only to recur years later.

Arthritis is a discriminatory disease—it prefers women. Regardless of age, race, or occupation, women are the prime target of arthritis. It has been shown

Exhibit 16-2   Home Improvements to Promote Safety and Independence for Individuals With Arthritis

Steps that can be taken to enable food procurement, storage, and preparation:
- Adding a rail in the entrance area for safety and balance
- Adjusting step height by adding a half step or obtaining a portable ramp
- Wrapping doorknobs with foam-backed adhesive to provide more friction, thereby decreasing the amount of joint stress and strength needed
- Replacing knobs with levers to help those with limited hand/wrist mobility and strength

Inside the home focus on lighting, carpeting, and furniture placement and selection using these guidelines:
- Use high-wattage bulbs for increased visibility in kitchen and pantries
- Place lamps or light switches so dark areas can be illuminated before entering
- Try using lamp timers or converters that allow lights to be turned on by touch
- Keep floors free of clutter and secure all rugs—scatter rugs are hazardous for people who have difficulty walking. When a small rug is necessary, use double-faced tape or a rubberized mesh mat to secure it to the floor
- Arrange a work chair and table in the kitchen for ease in maneuvering in small areas, preparing food for cooling and eating, and at mealtime with family and friends
- Mount grab bars on the edges of counters or cabinets
- Use foam tubing or sponge curlers on the handles of utensils for easier eating and putting less stress on the hands
- Use utensils that roll to cut (circular pizza-type cutter) rather than standard flat knives
- Place a piece of rubber or damp sponge or cloth between the plate and the counter
- Use large-handled thermal mugs, which are easier to lift than standard cups or glasses
- Use T-handled cups that allow the user to slip a hand around the cup, thereby decreasing the stress on the small joints of the hand
- Use a mug for hot liquids, including soups, to reduce heat on the hands

Source: Adapted from: Arthritis Foundation–Tennessee Chapter, Nashville, Tenn. and Clapper MP. At home with arthritis. *ADVANCE for Providers of Post-Acute Care.* October 1999:16-18.

that arthritis symptoms often decrease during pregnancy, only to return later. Thus, hormonal change probably has something to do with susceptibility. Women must be more aware of the early warning signs including a family history, cartilage damage and stiffness, or pain during walking.[79-80]

The arthritic disease process can be defined as any destruction that occurs to joints—which include cartilage, ligaments, tendons, and bones. This destruction may occur at repeated times during inflammation. The pathological changes combined with the mechanical stress of carrying an individual's weight, muscle pull, and other stresses produce the deformities seen with the disease.[81]

Systemic changes occur due to the nature of the disease. These systemic changes affect the individual's metabolism and ability to function. These systemic and functional changes initiate body alterations that influence the nutritional well-being of the individual. These changes can alter the nutrients that become available to the individual. Many individuals may not be able to consume the food they need. Medications can influence the digestion and, if foods are limited, absorption can be reduced. Excretion can be modified due to nutrients that are not available for normal metabolic processes.

Functional changes from arthritis include the following[81]:

- Wrist destruction, a reduced hand-gripping ability, and a decreased functioning mobility all interfere with arthritic individuals' ability to feed themselves, to shop for the foods they need, and to prepare their own meals.
- A decreased shoulder rotation or an increased involvement with the elbow decreases the ability to bring food to the mouth with the hand. These situations result in frustration, and eating becomes a negative experience.
- With increased involvement with the mandibular areas, individuals cannot chew well. This reduces the ability to eat fresh, raw foods (such as vegetables and salads) and especially decreases the ability to chew fibrous meats and vegetables that require a tremendous amount of jaw action.
- A restriction in movement of the oral area means individuals may not be able to cleanse and brush the teeth properly or open and move the jaw freely. Dental caries and periodontal disease can increase.

Generally, the causes of nutritional alteration in individuals with arthritis are related to 2 major factors. One is the spontaneous arthritis attacks and the other is related to the stages of remission. The inability to feed or to eat deprives the individual of nutrients. When the spontaneous attacks occur, the individual does not receive adequate nutrition. The changes in diet can change the immune response of the individual and further affect the manifestations of the disease. During periods of spontaneous remission, individuals may believe that a "quack" or a "magic food" produced the change, and they may lose their commitment to a healthy, balanced eating pattern.[82]

A potential link between diet and rheumatoid arthritis is that the reactions or symptoms experienced by the individual may be an allergic reaction to substances in food. Food then becomes a negative substrate, and the patient may be unaware that the food is initiating the problem. The only known diet link with arthritis is the link between diet and gout. Individuals with gout are not able to eat foods with purines (i.e., sweetbreads, liver, alcohol, kidney, and brain). Individuals with gout cannot rid their body of purines, which worsen the symptoms and pain. Physicians prescribe colchicine for acute attacks to reduce the pain, but gastrointestinal problems such as diarrhea can occur.[83]

Sjögren's syndrome is a chronic, inflammatory disorder that occurs in about 10-15% of arthritic patients. This syndrome is characterized by a decreased secretion of salivary juices and the onset of gingivitis; the production of a stiff, white mucosa in the mouth; and altered taste and smell. All of these symptoms are likely to occur.[84]

Osteoarthritis

Osteoarthritis is a major reason for physical impairment in individuals over 65 years old. One third of individuals in the United States suffer from joint pain considered a consequence of wear-and-tear from various types of stress on joints including an increasing body weight. Lack of exercise and being overweight increase one's risk of osteoarthritis. In the National Health and Nutrition Survey III, from 1999-2000, 65% of the US population was overweight (body mass index > 25.0) and 31% was obese (body mass index > 30.0).[85]

Besides body weight, factors influencing joint health are adequate levels of vitamins C and D, calcium, proteins, phosphorus, and zinc. These nutrients contribute to the normal formation of the extracellular matrix and cartilage. Fast food intakes and unbalanced vegetarian diets may promote inadequate intakes of vitamin C, calcium, and phosphorus. How this pattern of eating can affect cartilage metabolism needs more research, but people practice a personal health care with their diet and supplementation.

About half of all women and 40% of men over 50 years old regularly consume nutritional supplements. The popularity may be due to less stiffness, pain and inflammation, and symptoms of joint disease. Ginger, omega-3 fatty acids, gamma-linolenic acid, glucosamine, and chondroitin sulfate have shown some beneficial effects. Collagen hydrolysate may alleviate pain from osteoarthritis and promote cartilage regeneration. Tested nutritional supplements, weight reduction, appropriate physical exercise, and a balanced and healthy diet may present the best approach to treating the condition.[86-88]

Secondary and Tertiary Prevention

Nutrition has an important effect on the health of individuals with arthritis. Eating behavior is one element in the base of the treatment pyramid for rheumatoid arthritis (see Figure 16-4). Some people, however, go far beyond a sensible approach to eating. Because the exact causes of arthritis are not yet known, the door is left open for many unproven ideas about how to help or cure it. People often hear that one diet or another can cure arthritis.

Supplements such as vitamins and minerals are advertised and sold as remedies for arthritis. The claims sound reasonable until they are weighed against what is known. Many unusual behavioral remedies and diet plans, such as a diet free of nightshades (foods such as peppers and tomatoes), have made people with arthritis feel better. Most of these benefits, however, are due to natural improvement—which can occur by itself in any kind of arthritis—or

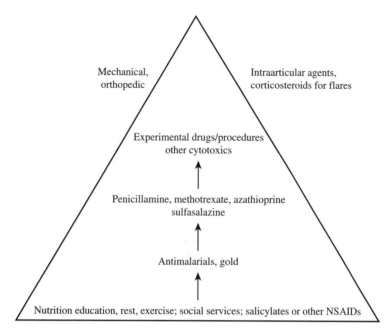

FIGURE 16–4   Treatment pyramid for rheumatoid arthritis.
Source: Klippel JH. From the *Primer on the Rheumatic Disease.* 10th ed.
Arthritis Foundation, Atlanta, GA. 1993. Used by permission.

to a placebo effect. If a person truly believes that something he or she takes, eats, or rubs on the joints is going to work, it can often relieve arthritis symptoms temporarily.[89]

Study results from Belgium suggested that glucosamine may inhibit progression of osteoarthritis of the knee, and the National Institutes of Health funded a $6.6 million project to study glucosamine and chondroitin. One thousand patients at 9 medical centers nationwide tested effectiveness in relieving pain, improving mobility, and causing side effects.[90]

Pain and limited motion result from the breakdown of cartilage, which protect and cover the ends of bones in a joint. Cartilage wears away and bones begin to scrape painfully against one another. Glucosamine and chondroitin are synthesized in the body, found in cartilage, and may stimulate production of glycosaminoglycans and proteoglycans, which build cartilage.

Chondroitin gives cartilage a springy quality. Glucosamine and chondroitin may relieve the pain but not produce gastrointestinal side effects, like ulcers, which occur from prolonged or high doses of ibuprofen and other drugs.

Fifty percent of Navy SEALs reported that 8 weeks of therapy with a commercially available preparation of glucosamine, chondroitin, and manganese relieved symptoms of knee arthritis. Although nonsignificant, a Canadian study showed a positive trend for reduction of knee pain while taking glucosamine.

A meta-analysis at Queen's University in Ontario reviewed 9 trials on glucosamine, concluding that the substance was very safe with similar efficacy to ibuprofen. Methodological problems were evident in the studies such as failure to define what a case of arthritis was or how pain relief was determined.

Info Line

The Arthritis Foundation
PO Box 19000
Atlanta, GA 30326
1 (800) 283-7800

These definitions are usually subjective, making assessment difficult. Symptoms and X rays to determine joint space narrowing in the sorest knee were determined for 106 people taking glucosamine sulfate and 106 taking a placebo. After 3 years the joint space in the placebo patients' knees had narrowed significantly, and their symptoms worsened. The joint space among those receiving glucosamine remained stable and symptoms appeared to decline. Based on current research, general recommendations for glucosamine or chondroitin sulfate are as follows[90]:

- 1,500 mg/day of glucosamine and 1,200 mg/day of chondroitin appear safe
- if relief doesn't occur in 2-4 months, it probably won't
- people with diabetes should monitor blood sugar regularly because the substances may increase insulin resistance and retard the uptake of sugar from the blood
- regular users of anticoagulants, e.g., aspirin or heparin, should have their blood clotting times checked as the substance may react like heparin
- glucosamine contains some crab, lobster, and shrimp shells and individuals with these allergies should be informed

Community nutrition professionals need to become actively involved in secondary and tertiary prevention efforts to help improve the quality of life of patients with arthritis. Generally, one of the first goals is to evaluate patients' ability to feed themselves. This involves considering their functional status, any of the secondary manifestations of the arthritis, and the medical treatment they receive. Multiple feeding modalities may be required. A combination of oral supplements, tube feedings, and even parenteral nutrition may be needed to meet the nutritional needs of individuals with arthritis.

Eating behavior must be considered in the management of arthritic patients. One problem is the nutrient/drug interaction and gastrointestinal functioning. There are 7 major drug therapies for arthritis: salicylates (e.g., aspirin), nonsteroidal anti-inflammatory agents, anti-malarial compounds, gold salt injections, penicillin, steroids, and immunosuppressive agents.[91-93] Possible nutrient-drug interactions associated with these therapies include the following:

- Aspirin is a mild pain reliever and a major anti-inflammatory drug. When an individual takes a high dose of aspirin, there is a possibility of potential blood loss through the bowels. Aspirin can irritate the stomach and alter platelet function. Aspirin can also act as minor blood-thinning agent. High doses of aspirin can cause nausea and vomiting. This upsets the gastrointestinal tract and causes an altered eating behavior.

- Many of the nonsteroidal anti-inflammatory agents irritate the lining of the gastrointestinal tract (e.g., indocin, naproxen ibuprofen, foroprofen, and piroydcam). Some anti-inflammatory agents may cause slight fluid retention. Some individuals self-prescribe a salt-restricted diet if they are retaining fluid. This may not have an adverse effect immediately, but it can place the individual on a roller coaster. Food becomes the target for change in order to appease the actual symptoms.
- Antimalarial agents, penicillin, and gold salt injections inhibit the disease process, but have minimal anti-inflammatory properties. The body reacts to these medications with a process called chelation, a binding of zinc, copper, and iron in the gastrointestinal tract. This reduces their absorption, and a potential deficiency can occur.
- Corticosteroids are the most potent anti-inflammatory agents. However, they demonstrate a high degree of toxicity. A common reaction is a decrease in the synthesis and breakdown of protein (e.g., muscle, skin, connective, and adipose tissue). Calcium can spill into the urine. If a restriction of vitamin D activity occurs, this reduces the overall intestinal calcium absorption and increases chances for osteoporosis.
- Prednisone reduces inflammation, suppresses immunological response, increases appetite, and may enhance loss of bone. Long-term side effects of prednisone can be reduced if vitamin D and calcium supplements are given. Prednisone influences fluid retention, suggesting that salt intake should be moderated.
- Immunosuppressive agents are slow-acting drugs. Their action can have a direct effect, which is often dose-related, on calcium absorption. Folate may become deficient.

The overall recommended eating pattern for individuals with arthritis involves weight control and a low-fat and low-saturated-fat eating pattern. Individuals with arthritis who are overweight need to lose weight to avoid putting unnecessary stress on diseased joints.

If weight changes drastically, the quick weight loss may mean a variety of things:

- overactive thyroid, which increases the basal metabolic rate
- difficulty swallowing and eating
- a possible serious infection with tissue disease and destruction
- depression from the arthritis

If weight loss is rapid due to insufficient calories, an impaired antibody production can occur. Increased rejection of skin grafts, increased delayed hypersensitivity, and increased lymphokine production may occur. If depression leads to a fasting stage, a number of other complications are possible. A zinc deficiency can occur. Low-fat and low-calorie diets taken to the extreme can affect the autoimmune process.[94]

Nontraditional Remedies

There are many approaches to treating arthritis, and some of these are questionable. For example, prayer has been seen as effective in reducing pain for some individuals. One of the more common and unproven nutrition regimens is the vegetarian diet. The rationale is that meats may cause or potentially aggravate arthritis. The vegetarian diet is thought to cleanse the body. Another popular practice is to eliminate foods that are thought to cause an allergic reaction (e.g., corn, wheat, coffee, beef, peanuts, tomatoes, chocolate, eggs, apples, oranges, and cola drinks). An extreme nutrition regimen that is unproven and not safe is fasting for 3 to 5 days before adding back a few foods at a time. Another practice is the use of enemas, which are thought to rid the body of toxins.[95,96]

Another unproven practice is a diet that includes apple cider vinegar and honey 3 times a day and a drop of iodine solution a few times a week, plus a restriction on total amount of foods eaten. The thought is that vinegar will thin the blood fluids and make tissues around the joints more tender, and that honey will relieve pain. Garlic, alfalfa, wheat germ oil, and blackstrap molasses are also thought to give relief from the arthritic symptoms.[95,96]

Megadoses of certain vitamins and minerals and fat modification are also considered to be ways to relieve pain and complications.[97-100] Vitamin A megadoses of 25,000 international units (IU) have been used, whereas 5,000 is the RDA. Chronic vitamin A toxicity can occur at a 25,000 IU level if taken daily over an extended period. For vitamin D, the RDA is 200 IU or 5 milligrams. The megadoses recommended are between 2,500 and 600,000 IU. For vitamin E, 15 IU is the RDA, and dosages up to 20,000 IU have been recommended. Toxicity can occur at these levels if taken for a long period.

Vitamin C is water soluble. In fairly high dosages, there have been reports of an alleviation of the low platelet level and low plasma vitamin C level, especially if individuals with arthritis are taking aspirin. Dosages over 4,000 milligrams can cause some gastrointestinal symptoms, and large dosages can interfere with copper absorption and uric acid excretion. These dosages greatly exceed the RDA of 60 milligrams.

Thiamine is a B-vitamin that is known to be decreased in rheumatoid arthritis patients. In addition, older adults may not use thiamine efficiently. There is very little evidence for toxicity. However, amounts that have been recommended, 10 milligrams, exceed the 1.2 milligram RDA. For vitamin B_{12}, the RDA is 3 micrograms. For individuals with arthritis, levels as high as 500 micrograms have been used. Vitamin B_{12} is not toxic, and high levels may give false negative results for pernicious anemia due to the very high circulating blood levels.

Mineral regimens are often listed by the popular press as ways to alter arthritic symptoms.[97-98] Calcium, zinc, and copper head the list. Calcium levels are commonly found to be low in people with arthritis, which is generally the rationale for people taking it. Women, especially after menopause, may need to take more than 800 milligrams per day, which is the RDA. However regimens of 3,000 milligrams per day have been reported.

Iron supplementation (e.g., 25 to 75 milligrams per day) is probably safe. Additional iron may be beneficial for those with some blood loss due to heavy aspirin use. For zinc, the RDA is 15 milligrams per day. Intakes tend to be low in individuals with arthritis. Some studies have shown that taking about 200 milligrams 3 times a day can be beneficial. However, toxicity has been shown when more than 2,000 milligrams is taken. As a rule, if a supplement is given, its dosage is from 15 to 50 milligrams per day. These levels are clinically unproven as beneficial in remediating arthritic conditions. Excess zinc intake can lower blood copper levels. The RDA for copper is 2 to 3 milligrams per day, and 5 to 10 milligrams seems fairly safe. Toxicity has been shown with ingestion of 20 milligrams of copper sulfate on a routine basis.

Two other minerals reported as aiding arthritis are selenium and choline. The RDA for selenium is 50 to 100 micrograms; levels of 2.5 or 3 milligrams per day are considered harmful. The average choline intake is around 500 to 800 milligrams a day, and intake often depends on egg consumption. Toxicity has not been documented at levels as high as 16 grams per day when taken for 4 months. It appears that 0.5 to 1 gram, or 500 to 1,000 milligrams, is safe.[98]

Assessing Eating Behavior

The following steps are needed to conduct a careful review of the nutritional well-being of individuals with arthritis:

- A diet history that includes the names, amounts, and types of foods and supplements that an individual takes is needed.
- The amount of raw food consumed should be assessed. Raw foods are often ingested in the therapeutic concoctions that individuals prepare, because people believe they are a magic cure. These preparations may actually be detrimental to the individual. For example, bone meal, which is often recommended by health food establishments to supplement calcium intake, may contain toxic amounts of lead.
- Major pain or physical complaints (e.g., stomach irritation or diarrhea) should be assessed. Individuals often follow their own self-prescribed practices, such as enemas to rid themselves of what they believe are harmful substances in their system.
- Food elimination practices or patterns should be assessed. Individuals may abstain from eating a type of food such as milk, milk products, or fruits because they believe they are harmful.
- Compliance with drug therapy should be assessed, because adherence to medications may be weak. Food may be substituted as the sole therapy, and this may be harmful if physicians are not aware that medication is not being taken.
- A comparison of costs for the multiple therapies that a patient self-prescribes is informative. A placebo effect may occur with some therapies. Individuals, especially older adults, are being hooked on potential cures that are costly and not beneficial. Some of these cures may be harmful. It is important to inform patients that the times they feel exceptionally good might be the result of a temporary remission, which is common, rather than the result of a magic potion. Treatment that coincides with a spontaneous remission may be viewed as a miracle cure.
- It is important to identify the positive aspects of an individual's efforts so he or she remains active in the treatment.

Community nutritional professionals should remain sympathetic to individuals with arthritis, encouraging them to follow the most medically sound regimens. Their immobility, which restricts their activities and adds additional pain, should be documented. Often the restriction of independent living is the major impetus for individuals to search for a cure or remedy.

Manipulation problems common to individuals with arthritis include opening jars, tearing plastics, reaching shelves, and holding dishes and utensils. Several ways to help arthritic individuals to take part in their food procurement and preparation are as follows:

- Mount a wedge-shaped gripper on the kitchen wall.
- Break suction on vacuum lids with a lid-lifter.
- Use a fork handle as a lever to pull up ring-top openers.
- Lay boxes on sides and cut tops with a knife.
- Use scissors for sealed plastic or cellophane.
- Use an electric can opener with a power stroke.
- Use the palm and not the fingers to open jars.
- Use large-handled utensils.
- Put damp sponges or thin rubber disks under plates.
- Use sharp utensils, T-handle cups, and cover cups with terry cloth or foam coasters.
- Use straws to avoid lifting.
- Take careful bites and chew gently; eat and swallow slowly.
- Eat small, frequent meals with soft foods.
- Drink liquids with meals to aid swallowing.

Exercise for overall body tone and conditioning, as well as for expending calories, is important. Protection of muscles and joints from temperature and contact insults can lessen pain and damage. Weight control with careful dieting and response to the manipulation problems of patients is important.

Renal Disease

Chronic renal failure is a gradual progression in the loss of kidney function. Slowly there is a loss of excretory, endocrine, and metabolic activity of the kidney.[101] The extent of renal disease is defined by serum creatinine level:

- advanced renal insufficiency: 8-10 mg/dL
- moderate insufficiency: 4-8 mg/dL
- mild insufficiency: 2-4 mg/dL

If 70-80% of renal function is lost, water, electrolyte, and acid-base balance are not possible. The incidence of end-stage renal disease (ESRD) is estimated at about 83 people per million. A 6.5% annual increase has occurred from 1978 to 1983, with individuals under 25 and over 65 years of age showing the largest increase.[102] ESRD is a common manifestation of diabetes mellitus, especially type 1, but it can develop from polycystic renal disease, from a streptococcal infection, or as an outcome of renal damage.[103,104] Other high-risk groups include African-American hypertensives, Native Americans with non–insulin-dependent diabetes mellitus, and individuals with overt proteinuria.[101,105,106]

Individuals with ESRD must receive tertiary prevention or they will not survive. Hemodialysis, continuous ambulatory peritoneal dialysis, or a renal transplant are required if the individual is to live. Individuals without intervention develop vitamin D deficiency, hyperparathyroidism, and osteodystrophy, which result from the accumulation of toxic substances and associated endocrine and metabolic disturbances. Manifestations of ESRD include dyslipidemia, anemia, muscle weakness and atrophy, peripheral and central nervous system impairment, and depression. Coronary heart disease is a major cause of death in dialysis patients, possibly due to hyperlipidemia causing glomerular injury.[102,103] Malnutrition is common, because the metabolism of nutrients is impaired and dialysis leaches nutrients out of the body fluids.[107] Thiamine, riboflavin, vitamin B_6, and vitamin C deficiencies are common and contrast with high-plasma vitamin A.[103,108–110]

Research Updates in Kidney and Urologic Health

The National Institute of Diabetes and Digestive and Kidney Diseases (NIDDK) conducts and supports research on the kidney and urinary tract and disorders of the blood and blood-forming organs. The Clinical Trials program coordinates and monitors patient recruitment and adherence to interventions.[111]

Three new clinical trials in the United States are:

1. Chronic Renal Insufficiency Cohort Study

End-stage renal disease (ESRD) disproportionately affects racial and ethnic minority groups, particularly African Americans, American Indians, and Hispanics. African Americans and American Indians are 4 times as likely as whites, and Hispanics are twice as likely as whites, to develop kidney failure, which requires dialysis or kidney transplantation for survival.

In 2000, almost 100,000 people with chronic kidney disease entered ESRD, with the result that approximately 300,000 people were sustained on hemodialysis while 80,000 had functioning transplants. These numbers have doubled since 1990, and they are expected to nearly double again by 2010. The increase in the number of Americans with ESRD is directly proportional to the increase in the number of Americans with type 2 diabetes, a major cause of chronic renal insufficiency. Another major cause is hypertension. The leading cause of death in patients with ESRD is cardiovascular disease.

To determine the risk factors for rapid decline in kidney function and development of cardiovascular disease, the Chronic Renal Insufficiency Cohort (CRIC) Study is a 7-year, prospective, multiethnic, multiracial study. Approximately 3,000 patients with chronic renal insufficiency serve as a national resource for investigating chronic renal as well as cardiovascular disease. Establishing this cohort of patients and following them prospectively are also providing an opportunity to examine genetic, environmental, behavioral, nutritional, quality-of-life, and health resource utilization factors.

The study consists of regular clinic visits to monitor renal function and the cardiovascular system and questionnaires to assess various demographic, nutritional, and quality-of-life factors. Data collection involves study participants who develop ESRD and is performed after they start renal replacement therapy (renal transplantation, hemodialysis, or peritoneal dialysis). Closeout is scheduled for 2008.

2. Minimally Invasive Surgical Therapies Treatment Consortium for Benign Prostatic Hyperplasia

Benign prostatic hyperplasia (BPH), transurethral resection of the prostate (TURP), and newer approaches such as laser therapy, hyperthermia therapy and thermotherapy, and microwave therapy are being tested. Seven collaborative prostate evaluation treatment centers test to make the most appropriate choices for long-term management of BPH.

3. Dialysis Access Consortium

Maintenance of vascular access for hemodialysis is a challenge in caring for the hemodialysis patient. Vascular access placement and repair in the United States exceeds $700 million per year. In fiscal year 2000, NIDDK established the Dialysis Access Consortium (DAC), which consists of 7 clinical centers to improve outcomes in patients with fistulas and grafts.

Current medical nutritional therapy reflects the national renal diet, which includes recommendations for protein, phosphorus, sodium, and potassium intakes (see Table 16–6). Because the disease is chronic, modification of protein and phosphorus is essential when managing mild renal failure. If individuals are pre-ESRD, a low-protein diet of 0.6 g/kg per 24 hours with greater than 35 kcal/kg per 24 hours protects against uremia.[103,104,111] Since individuals with renal disease retain phosphorus, a limit of less than 900 mg/24 hours and use of phosphate-binding compounds are required.

TABLE 16–6 General Dietary Recommendations for Renal Patients

Dietary Component	Renal Insufficiency	Hemodialysis	Peritoneal Dialysis
Protein (g/kg IBW)*	0.6–0.8[†]	1.1-1.4	1.2-1.5
Energy (kcal/kg IBW)	35-40	30-35	25-35
Phosphorus (mg/kg IBW)	8-12[‡]	≤ 17[§]	≤ 17
Sodium (mg/day)	1,000-3,000	2,000-3,000	2,000-4,000
Potassium (mg/kg IBW)	Typically not restricted	40	Typically not restricted
Fluid (mL/day)	Typically not restricted	500-750 plus daily urine output or 1,000 if anuric	≥ 2,000
Calcium (mg/day)	1,200-1,600	Depends on serum level	Depends on serum level

* IBW = ideal body weight.

[†] The upper end of this range is preferred for patients with diabetes or malnutrition. Suggested protein intake for persons with nephrotic syndrome is 0.8 to 1.0 g/kg IBW.

[‡] Intake of 5 to 10 mg phosphorus per kg IBW is frequently quoted in the scientific literature, but 5 mg/kg IBW is practical only when used in conjunction with a very-low-protein diet supplemented with amino acids or ketoacid analogs.

[§] It may not be possible to meet the optimum phosphorus prescription on a higher protein diet.

Source: Turner LW, Faile P, Wang MQ, et al. Reprinted from: Meeting the challenge of the renal diet. *J Am Diet Assoc.* 1993;93(6):637. Used with permission of the American Dietetic Association.

The National Institute of Diabetes, Digestive and Kidney Diseases of NIH periodically sponsors a consensus symposium entitled "Prevention of Progression in Chronic Renal Disease Management Recommendations." The objective is to establish timely, basic recommendations to manage individuals with progressive renal disease. Because these individuals are generally not institutionalized but live independently, community nutrition professionals have a role in the management and monitoring of these individuals. Recommendations for dietetic practice for secondary and tertiary prevention include the following[112]:

- A sufficient number of calories is required to spare dietary protein, which is needed for tissue repair.
- Protein restriction can slow progression of the disease.
- Strict glycemic control among diabetics can blunt the occurrence of nephropathy, neuropathy, and retinopathy.[113,114]
- Active and aggressive medical nutrition therapy preserves nutritional status.[115]
- Moderate dietary sodium restriction (2-4 grams per 24 hours) should be considered.[116]

Healthy People 2010 Actions

Specific *Healthy People 2010* objectives target the general population at risk for cardiovascular disease and obesity, as well as individuals who abuse alcohol or are at risk for osteoporosis or end-stage renal disease (see Exhibit 16-3). Community nutrition professionals can support efforts to meet these *Healthy People 2010* objectives and extend their scope to general public education and school-based education about alcohol abstinence and basic healthy eating.

Exhibit 16-3 DATA2010: the *Healthy People 2010* Database—November 2000. Focus Area: 02-Arthritis, Osteoporosis and 04-End-Stage Renal Disease

Objective No.	Objective	Baseline Year	Baseline	Target 2010
02-02	Activity limitations due to arthritis (age adjusted, adults with chronic joint symptoms aged 18 years and older)	1997	27	21
	American Indian or Alaska native	1997	27	21
	Asian or Pacific Islander	1997	18	21
	Black or African American	1997	32	21
	White	1997	27	21
	Hispanic or Latino	1997	28	21
	Not Hispanic or Latino	1997	27	21
	Female	1997	31	21

continued

Exhibit 16–3   continued

	Male	1997	22	21
	Poor	1997	36	21
	Near poor	1997	30	21
	Middle/high income	1997	24	21
	Less than high school (persons aged 25 years and older)	1997	34	21
	High school graduate (persons aged 25 years and older)	1997	32	21
	At least some college (persons aged 25 years and older)	1997	26	21
02-08	Arthritis education (adults with arthritis aged 18 years and older)	UK	UK	UK
02-09	Cases of osteoporosis (age adjusted, adults aged 50 years and older)	1988–1994	10	8
	American Indian or Alaska native	1988-1994	UK	8
	Asian or Pacific Islander	1988-1994	UK	8
	Black or African American	1988-1994	7	8
	White	1988-1994	10	8
	Hispanic or Latino	1988-1994	UK	8
	Mexican American	1988-1994	10	8
	Not Hispanic or Latino	1988-1994	10	8
	Female	1988-1994	16	8
	Male	1988-1994	3	8
	Less than high school	1988-1994	11	8
	High school graduate	1988-1994	11	8
	At least some college	1988-1994	9	8
02-10	Hospitalization for vertebral fractures (age adjusted rate per 10,000, adults aged 65 years and older)	1998	17.5	14.0
	American Indian or Alaska native	1998	UK	14.0
	Asian or Pacific Islander	1998	UK	14.0
	Black or African American	1998	UK	14.0
	White	1998	14.0	14.0
	Hispanic or Latino	1998	UK	14.0
	Not Hispanic or Latino	1998	UK	14.0
	Female	1998	19.6	14.0
	Male	1998	13.9	14.0
	65 to 74 years (not age adjusted)	1998	6.7	14.0
	75 to 84 years (not age adjusted)	1998	26.0	14 0
	85 years and older (not age adjusted)	1998	39.0	14.0
04-01	End-stage renal disease—new cases (rate per million, persons of all ages)	1997	289	217
	American Indian or Alaska native	1997	586	217
	Asian or Pacific Islander	1997	344	217
	Black or African American	1997	873	217
	White	1997	218	217

	Hispanic or Latino	1997	UK	217
	Not Hispanic or Latino	1997	UK	217
	Female	1997	242	217
	Male	1997	348	217
	Poor	1997	UK	217
	Near poor	1997	UK	217
	Middle/high income	1997	UK	217
	Under 20 years	1997	13	217
	20 to 44 years	1997	109	217
	45 to 64 years	1997	545	217
	65 to 74 years	1997	1,296	217
	75 years and older	1997	1,296	217
04-02	Cardiovascular disease deaths in persons with chronic kidney failure (rate per 1,000 patient-years at risk, persons of all ages)	1997	70	52
	American Indian or Alaska native	1997	63	52
	Asian or Pacific Islander	1997	60	52
	Black or African American	1997	62	52
	White	1997	75	52
	Hispanic or Latino	1997	UK	52
	Not Hispanic or Latino	1997	UK	52
	Female	1997	73	52
	Male	1997	67	52
	Poor	1997	UK	52
	Near poor	1997	UK	52
	Middle/high income	1997	UK	52
04-07	Kidney failure due to diabetes (rate per million, persons of all ages)	1996	113	78
	American Indian or Alaska native	1996	482	78
	Asian or Pacific Islander	1996	156	78
	Black or African American	1996	329	78
	White	1996	79	78
	Hispanic or Latino	1996	UK	78
	Not Hispanic or Latino	1996	UK	78
	Female	1996	103	78
	Male	1996	112	78
	Poor	1996	UK	78
	Near poor	1996	UK	78
	Middle/high income	1996	UK	78
	Under 20 years	1996	0	78
	20 to 44 years	1996	35	78
	45 to 64 years	1996	276	78
	65 to 74 years	1996	514	78
	75 years and older	1996	263	78
05-03	Overall cases of diagnosed diabetes (age adjusted rate per 1,000, persons of all ages)	1997	40	25
	American Indian or Alaska native	1997	UK	25
	Asian or Pacific Islander	1997	UK	25
	Black or African American	1997	74	25

continued

Exhibit 16-3   continued

	White	1997	36	25
	Hispanic or Latino	1997	61	25
	Not Hispanic or Latino	1997	38	25
	Female	1997	40	25
	Male	1997	39	25
26-17a	Perception of risk associated with substance abuse consuming 5 or more alcoholic drinks at a single occasion once or twice a week			
	Adolescents, 12 to 17 years	1998	47	80
	American Indian	1998	47	80
	Asian or Pacific Islander	1998	43	80
	Black or African American	1998	57	80
	White	1998	45	80
	Hispanic or Latino	1998	51	80
	Female	1998	50	80
	Male	1998	44	80

UK = unknown

Source: Adapted from: US Department of Health and Human Services. DATA2010–the *Healthy People 2010* database. *CDC Wonder.* Atlanta, Ga: Centers for Disease Control; November 2000.

References

1. National Osteoporosis Foundation. *Osteoporosis–Can It Happen to You?* Washington, DC: National Osteoporosis Foundation; 1991.
2. *Osteoporosis–What You Don't Know May Hurt You.* Evanston, Ill: Wyeth–Ayerst Laboratories; May 1991:3-4.
3. National Institutes of Health. Consensus statement: optimal calcium intake. *JAMA.* 1994;12(4):1-31.
4. Turner LW, Whitney EN. Nature versus nurture: the calcium controversy. *Nutr Clin.* 1989;4:1.
5. Farahmand B, Michaëlsson K, Baron J, Persson P, Ljunghall S. Body size and hip fracture risk. *Epidemiology.* 2000;11:214-219.
6. Dawson B. Medical community far behind in preventing osteoporosis. *Tufts University Health & Nutrition Letter.* 2003;21:8,3.
7. High homocysteine raises fracture risk. *Tufts University, Health & Nutrition Letter.* August 2004;6:1.
8. Van Meurs JBJ, Dhonukshe-Rutten RAM, Pluijm SMF, et al. Homocysteine levels and the risk of osteoporotic fracture. *N Engl J Med.* 2004;350: 2033-2041.
9. National Dairy Council. Nutrition and Health News Alert. What's the fastest growing population today? September/October 1999;3(5):1-2.
10. Kaplan FS. Osteoporosis–pathophysiology and prevention. *Clinical Symposia.* 1987:39(1):2-32.
11. Pollitzer WS, Anderson JJB. Ethnic and genetic differences in bone mass: a review with an hereditary versus environmental perspective. *Am J Clin Nutr.* 1989;50:1244.

12. Rubin LA, Hawker GA, Peltekova VD, Fielding LJ, Ridout R, Cole DE. Determinants of peak bone mass: clinical and genetic analyses in a young female Canadian cohort. *J Bone Miner Res.* 1999;14(4):633-643.

13. Rourke K, Brehm B, Cassell C, Sethuraman G. Effect of weight change on bone mass in female adolescents. *J Am Diet Assoc.* 2003;103:369-372.

14. Riggs BL, Wahner HW, Melton LJ III, et al. Dietary calcium intake and rates of bone loss in women. *J Clin Invest.* 1987;80:979-982.

15. Ettinger B, Genant HK, Cann CE. Postmenopausal bone loss is prevented by treatment with low-dosage estrogen with calcium. *Ann Intern Med.* 1987;106:40-45.

16. Riis B, Thomsen K, Christiansen C. Does calcium supplementation prevent postmenopausal bone loss? *N Engl J Med.* 1987;316:173.

17. Nieves JW, Komar L, Cosman F, et al. Calcium potentiates the effect of estrogen and calcitonin on bone mass: review and analysis. *Am J Clin Nutr.* 1998;67(1):18-24.

18. Cappuccio FP, Meilahn E, Zmuda JM, et al. High blood pressure and bone-mineral loss in elderly white women: a prospective study. Study of Osteoporotic Fractures Research Group. *Lancet.* 1999;18:354(9183): 971-975.

19. Management of postmenopausal osteoporosis: position statement of the North American Menopause Society. *Menopause.* March-April 2002;9(2):84-101.

20. LeBoff MS, Kohlmeier L, Hurwitz S, Franklin J, Wright J, Glowacki J. Occult vitamin D deficiency in postmenopausal US women with acute hip fracture. *JAMA.* April 28, 1999;281(16):1505-1511.

21. Lowe NM, Lowe NM, Fraser WD, Jackson MJ. Is there a potential therapeutic value of copper and zinc for osteoporosis? *Proc Nutr Soc* (*The Proceedings of the Nutrition Society*). May 2002;61(2):181-185.

22. Rapuri PB, Gallagher JC, Kinyamu HK, Ryschon KL. Caffeine intake increases the rate of bone loss in elderly women and interacts with vitamin D receptor genotypes. *Am J Clin Nutr.* November 2001;74(5): 694-700.

23. Sampson HW. Alcohol and other factors affecting osteoporosis risk in women. *Alcohol Res Health.* 2002;26(4):292-298.

24. Rodysill KJ. Postmenopausal osteoporosis—intervention and prophylaxis: a review. *J Chron Dis.* 1987;40:743-760.

25. Raisz LG. Local and systematic factors in the pathogenesis of osteoporosis. *N Engl J Med.* 1988;318:818.

26. Schuette SA, Linkswiler HM. Calcium. In: Olson RE, ed. *Nutrition Review's Present Knowledge in Nutrition.* Washington, DC: The Nutrition Foundation, Inc; 1984:400-412.

27. Too many calcium-fortified foods? *Tufts University Health and Nutrition Letter.* February 2000;17:(12):1,7.

28. Peck WA, Riggs BL, Bell NH. *Physician's Resource Manual on Osteoporosis.* Washington, DC: National Osteoporosis Foundation; 1987.

29. Wotecki CE. Nutrition in childhood and adolescence—Parts 1 and 2. *Contemporary Nutr.* 1992;17(2):1-2.

30. Briley J. Bone health: a weight-bearing argument. Washington, DC: *Washington Post.* July 27, 2004:HE03.

31. Edlin G, Golanty E. *Health and Wellness: A Holistic Approach.* 4th ed. Boston, Mass: Jones and Bartlett Publishers; 1992:285-294.

32. *Dietary Guidelines for Americans.* Washington, DC: US Dept of Agriculture and US Dept of Health and Human Services; 2005.

33. ICAP [International Center for Alcohol Policies]. *What is a "Standard Drink"?* Washington, DC: ICAP; 1998. ICAP Report No 5.

34. Kalant H, Poikolainen K. Moderate drinking: concepts, definitions and public health significance. In: Macdonald I, ed. *Health Issues Related to Alcohol Consumption.* Brussels, Belgium: International Life Sciences Institute; 1999:2.

35. Kalant H, Poikolainen K. Moderate drinking: concepts, definitions and public health significance. In: Macdonald I, ed. *Health Issues Related to Alcohol Consumption.* Brussels, Belgium: International Life Sciences Institute; 1999:14-15.

36. Dawson DA. Volume of ethanol consumption: effects of different approaches to measurement. *J Stud Alcohol.* 1998;59:191-197.

37. O'Malley PM, Bachman JG, Johnson LD. Reliability and consistency in self-reports of drug use. *Int J Addic.* 1983;18:805-824.

38. Pernanen K. Validity of survey data on alcohol use. In: Gibbins RJ, Israel Y, Kalant H, et al, eds. *Research Advances in Alcohol and Drug Problems.* New York: Wiley; 1974;1:355-374.

39. Simpura J, ed. *Finnish Drinking Habits: Results From Interview Surveys Held in 1968, 1976 and 1984.* Helsinki, Finland: Finnish Foundation for Alcohol Studies; 1987.

40. Beckley L. *Taking Control: Diet, Drug Abuse and Addiction.* San Marcos, Calif: Author; 1987.

41. Jellinek EM. *The Disease Concept of Alcoholism.* New Haven, Conn: College and University Press; 1960.

42. Tabakoff B, Grant KA, Hoffman PL, Little HJ. Alcohol and the central nervous system. In: Macdonald I, ed. *Health Issues Related to Alcohol Consumption.* Brussels, Belgium: International Life Sciences Institute; 1999:295-297.

43. Eckart MJ, File SE, Gessa LG, et al. Effects of moderate alcohol consumption on the central nervous system. *Alcohol Clin Exp Res.* 1998;22:998-1040.

44. Hupkens CLH, Knibbe RA, Drop MJ. Alcohol consumption in the European community: uniformity and diversity in drinking patterns. *Addiction.* 1993;88:1391-1404.

45. WHO (World Health Organization). *Profile of Alcohol in the Member States of the European Region of the World Health Organization.* Copenhagen, Denmark: WHO Regional Office for Europe; June 1-3, 1995.

46. Brewers Association of Canada. The changing pattern of alcohol use, drinking problems and public policy. *Bottom Line.* 1995:16:5-28.

47. Olson S. *Alcohol in America: Taking Action to Prevent Abuse.* Washington, DC: National Academy Press; 1985.

48. Rodés J, Salaspuro M, Sorensen TIA. Alcohol and liver disease. In: Macdonald I, ed. *Health Issues Related to Alcohol Consumption.* Brussels, Belgium: International Life Sciences Institute; 1999: 397-398.

49. Johnson BA. Serotonergic agents and alcoholism treatment: rebirth of the subtype concept—an hypothesis. *Alcoholism Clin Exp Res.* 2000;24(10):1597-1601.

50. Mc Pherson K, Cavallo F, Rubin E. Alcohol and breast cancer. In: Macdonald I, ed. *Health Issues Related to Alcohol Consumption.* Brussels, Belgium: International Life Sciences Institute; 1999:220-221.

51. Schatzkin A, Longnecker MP. Alcohol and breast cancer. Where are we now and where do we go from here? *Cancer.* 1994;74 (suppl):1101-1110.

52. Roth HD, Levy PS, Shi L, et al. Alcoholic beverages and breast cancer: some observations on published case-control studies. *J Clin Epidemiol.* 1994;47:207-216.

53. Plant ML. Alcohol and breast cancer: a review. *Int J Addict.* 1992;27:107-128.

54. Henderson BE, Pike MC, Bernstein L, et al. Breast cancer. In: Schottenfield D, Fraumeni JF, eds. *Cancer Epidemiology and Prevention.* 2nd ed. New York: Oxford University Press; 1997: 1022-1039.

55. Redd WH, Silverfarb PM, Anderson BL, et al. Physiological and psycho-behavioural research in oncology. *Cancer.* 1991;67:813-822.

56. Bryla CM. The relationship between stress and the development of breast cancer: a literature review. *Oncol Nurs Forum.* 1996;90:441-448.

57. Groggee DE, Rimm EB, Keil U, Renaud S. Alcohol and the cardiovascular system. In: Macdonald I, ed. *Health Issues Related to Alcohol Consumption.* Brussels, Belgium: International Life Sciences Institute; 1999:128-168.

58. McElduff P, Dobson AJ. How much alcohol and how often? Population based case-control study of alcohol consumption and risk of a major coronary event. *Br Med J.* 1997;314:1159-1164.

59. Thum MJ, Peto R, Lopez AD, et al. Alcohol consumption and mortality among middle-aged and elderly US adults. *N Engl J Med.* 1997;337: 1705-1714.

60. Fuchs CS. Alcohol consumption and mortality among women. *N Engl J Med.* 1995;332:1245-1250.

61. Kagan A, Katsuhiko Y, Rhoads GG, et al. Alcohol and cardiovascular disease: the Hawaiian experience. *Circulation.* 1981;64(suppl 3):27-31.

62. Klatsky AL, Friedman JD, Siegelaub AB. Alcohol use and cardiovascular disease: the Kaiser-Permanente experience. *Circulation.* 1981;64(suppl 3): 32-41.

63. Criqui MH, Cowan, LD, Tyroler HA, et al. Lipoproteins as mediators for the effects of alcohol consumption and cigarette smoking on cardiovascular mortality: results from the Lipid Research Clinics Follow-Up Study. *Am J Epidemiol.* 1987;126:629-637.

64. Shaper AG, Wannamethee G, Walter M. Alcohol and mortality in British men: explaining the U-shaped curve. *Lancet.* 1988;ii:267-273.

65. MacMahon SW, Blacket RB, MacDonald GJ, et al. Obesity, alcohol consumption and blood pressure in Australian men and women: the National Heart Foundation of Australia Risk Factor Prevalence Study. *J Hypertension.* 1984;2:85-91.

66. Friedman GD, Klatsky AL, Siegelaub AB. Alcohol, tobacco and hypertension. *Hypertension.* 1982;4(suppl 3):143-150.

67. Anttila T, Helkala E, Viitanen M, et al. Alcohol drinking in middle age and subsequent risk of mild cognitive impairment and dementia in old age: a prospective population based study. *BMJ.* 2004;329:539-547.

68. News break: can a drink a day keep you sane? *Nutr Today.* 2004; 39(5):193.

69. Plant ML, Abel EL, Guerri C. Alcohol and pregnancy. In: Macdonald I, ed. *Health Issues Related to Alcohol Consumption.* Brussels, Belgium: International Life Sciences Institute; 1999:199.

70. Waterson EJ, Evans C, Murray-Lyon IM. Is pregnancy a time of changing drinking and smoking patterns for fathers as well as mothers? An initial investigation. *Br J Addict.* 1990;85:389-396.

71. Schorling JB. The prevention of prenatal alcohol use: a critical analysis of intervention studies. *J Stud Alcohol.* 1993;54:261-267.

72. Greenfield T. Warning labels: evidence on harm reduction from long-term American surveys. In: Plant MA, Single E, Stockwell T, eds. *Alcohol: Minimizing the Harm. What Works?* London: Free Association Books; 1997:105-125.

73. Plant ML. *Women and Alcohol: Contemporary and Historical Perspectives.* London, England: Free Association Books; 1997.

74. Hankin JR, Firestone IJ, Sloan JJ, et al. Heeding the alcoholic beverage warning labels during pregnancy: multiparae versus nulliparae. *J Stud Alcohol.* 1996;57:171-177.

75. Hankin JR, Sloan JJ, Firestone IJ, et al. Has awareness of the alcohol warning label reached its upper limits? *Alcohol Clin Exp Res.* 1996;20:440-444.

76. Kaskutas LA. Interpretations of risk: the use of scientific information in the development of the warning label policy. *Int J Addict.* 1995;30:1519-1548.

77. Utsinger PD, Zvaifler NJ, Ehrlich GE, eds. *Rheumatoid Arthritis: Etiology, Diagnosis and Treatment.* Philadelphia, Pa: JB Lippincott Co; 1985.

78. Clapper MP. At home with arthritis. *ADVANCE for Providers of Post-Acute Care.* King of Prussia, Pa: Merion Publications; October 1999:16-18.

79. Dugowson CE, Keopsell TD, Voigt LF, et al. Rheumatoid arthitis in women: incidence rate in group health cooperative. Seattle, Washington, 1987-1989. *Arthritis Rheum.* 1991;34:1502-1507.

80. Goemaere S, Ackerman C, Goethals K, et al. Onset of symptoms of rheumatoid arthritis in relation to age, sex, and menopausal transition. *J Rheumatol.* 1990;17:1620-1622.

81. Ragan C, Farrington E. The clinical features of rheumatoid arthritis: prognosis indices. *JAMA.* 1959;2:16.

82. Bollet AJ. Nutrition and diet in rheumatic disease. In: Shils ME, Young VR, eds. *Modern Nutrition in Health and Disease.* 7th ed. Philadelphia, Pa: Lea & Febiger; 1988:1362-1373.

83. Levinson D, Becker MA. Clinical gout and pathogenesis of hyperuricemia. In: McCarty DJ, Koopman WJ, eds. *Arthritis and Allied Conditions.* 12th ed. Philadelphia, Pa: Lea & Febiger; 1993:1773-1805.

84. Bloch KJ, Buchanan WW, Wohl MJ, et al. Sjögren's syndrome: a clinical, pathological, and serological study of 62 cases. *Medicine.* 1965;44:187-231.

85. CDC/WCHS and the American Heart Association. *National Health and Nutrition Examination Survey III (NHANES II), 1988-94.* CDC/NCHS and the American Heart Association; 1999. Available at: www.cdc.gov/nchs/about/major/nhanes/www.americanheart.org/. Accessed February 1, 2007.

86. Osteoarthritis: epidemiology, risk factors and collagen hydrolysate—a potential therapeutic approach. *Nutr Today.* 2004;39(5):187-188.

87. Oesser S, Adam M, Babel W, Seifert J. Oral administration of ^{14}C labeled gelatin hydrolysate leads to an accumulation of radioactivity in cartilage of mice (C57/BL). *J Nutr.* 1999;129:1891-1895.

88. Oesser S, Seifert J. Stimulation of type II collagen biosynthesis and secretion in bovine chondrocytes cultured with degraded collagen. *Cell Tissue Res.* 2003;311:393-399.

89. Lasagna L. The placebo effect. *J Allergy Clin Immunol.* 1986;78:161-165.

90. A look at glucosamine and chondroitin for easing arthritis pain. *Tufts University Health and Nutrition Letter.* 2000;17(11):4-5.

91. Weiss MM. Corticosteriods in rheumatoid arthritis. *Semin Arthritis Rheum.* 1989;19:9-21.

92. Situnayake RD, Grindulis KA, McConkey B. Longterm treatment of rheumatoid arthritis with sulfasalazine, gold, or penicillamine: a comparison using life table methods. *Ann Rheum Dis.* 1987;46: 177-183.

93. Paulus HE. The use of combinations of disease-modifying antirheumatic agents in rheumatoid arthritis. *Arthritis Rheum.* 1990;33:113-120.

94. Touger-Decker R. Nutritional considerations in rheumatoid arthritis. *J Am Diet Assoc.* 1988;88:327.

95. Panush RS. Controversial arthritis remedies. *Bull Rheum Dis.* 1984; 34:1-10.

96. Dlesk A, Ettinger MP, Longley S, et al. Unconventional arthritis therapies. *Arthritis Rheum.* 1982;25:1145-1147.

97. Borglund M, Akesson A, Akesson B. Distribution of selenium and glutathione peroxidase in plasma compared in healthy subjects and rheumatoid arthritis patients. *Scand J Clin Lab Invest.* 1988;48:27.

98. Darlington LG, Ramsey NW, Mansfield JR. Placebo-controlled, blind study of dietary manipulation therapy in rheumatoid arthritis. *Lancet.* 1986;1:236.

99. Kremer JM, Michalek AV, Lininger L, et al. Effects of manipulation of dietary fatty acids on clinical manifestations of rheumatoid arthritis. *Lancet.* 1985;1:184-187.

100. Tarp U, Hansen JC, Overvad K, et al. Glutathione peroxidase activity in patients with rheumatoid arthritis and in normal subjects: effects of long-term selenium supplementation. *Arthritis Rheum.* 1987;30: 1162-1166.

101. Beto JA. Highlights of the consensus conference on prevention of progression in chronic renal disease: implications for practice. *J Renal Nutr.* 1994;4(3):122-126.

102. Ahmed FE. Effect of diet on progression of chronic renal disease. *J Am Diet Assoc.* 1991;91:1266-1270.

103. Coulston AM, Rock CL. A summary of the current state of knowledge in clinical nutrition and dietetic practice: suggestions for future research in dietetic practice and implications for health care. *The Research Agenda for Dietetics: Conference Proceedings ADA.* Chicago, Ill: ADA; 1993.

104. Kopple JD. Nutrition, diet, and the kidney. In: Shils ME, Young VR, eds. *Modern Nutrition in Health and Disease.* 7th ed. Philadelphia, Pa: Lea & Febiger; 1988:1230-1268.

105. Rostand SG. US minority groups and end-stage renal disease: a disproportionate share. *Am J Kidney Dis.* 1992;19:411-413.

106. McClellan WM. The epidemic of end-stage renal disease in the United States: a public health perspective on ESRD prevention. *AKF Nephrol Letter.* 1993;10:29-40.

107. Makoff R. Water-soluble vitamin status in patients with renal disease treated with hemodialysis or peritoneal dialysis. *J Renal Nutr.* 1991;1:56-73.

108. Stein G, Sperschneider H, Koppe S. Vitamin levels in chronic renal failure and need for supplementation. *Blood Purif.* 1985;3:52-62.

109. Muth I. Implications of hypervitaminosis A in chronic renal failure. *J Renal Nutr.* 1991;1:2-8.

110. Gleghort E, Eisenberg L, Hack S, et al. Observations of vitamin A toxicity in three patients with renal failure receiving parenteral alimentation. *Am J Clin Nutr.* 1986;44:107-112.

111. National Kidney and Urologic Diseases Information Clearinghouse (NKUDIC). *Clinical Trials in Kidney and Urologic Disease Set for Recruitment.* 2003. Available at: http://kidney.niddk.nih.gov/. Accessed June 1, 2004.

112. Renal Dietitians Practice Group. *Suggested Guidelines for Nutrition Care of Renal Patients.* Chicago, Ill: American Dietetic Association; 1986.

113. Diabetes Control and Trial Research Group. The effect on intensive treatment of diabetes on the development and progression of long-term complications in insulin-dependent diabetes mellitus. *N Engl J Med.* 1993;329:977-986.

114. Gilbert RE, Tsalamandris C, Bach LA, et al. Long-term glycemic control and the rate of progression of early diabetic kidney disease. *Kidney Int.* 1993;44:855-859.

115. Morbidity and mortality of renal dialysis: NIH consensus statement. *Ann Intern Med.* 1994;121:62-70.

116. Bigazzi R, Bianchi S, Baldari D, et al. Microalbuminuria in salt-sensitive patients. *Hypertension.* 1994;23:195-199.

PREVENTING SINGLE AND CLUSTER DISEASES

Learning Objectives

- Identify common diseases that cluster, causing morbidity and mortality.
- Differentiate between primary, secondary, and tertiary prevention.
- Describe the content, purpose, and benefits of health-risk appraisals.
- Discuss the self-management approach in healthcare reform.
- Outline the traditional and contemporary approaches for health education of the public.

High Definition Nutrition

Andragogy—the teaching of adults.

Complementary and alternative medicine (CAM)—7 categories of approaches for health other than the usual western medical model, e.g., traditional Chinese medicine, bioelectricmagnetic applications, herbal medicine, manual healing, mind-body control, pharmacological and biological treatments, and diet/nutrition and lifestyle changes.

Deadly quartet—the clustering in a single individual of hyperinsulinemia, hypertension, hypertriglyceridemia, and obesity.

Energy density—food energy per 100 grams of item.

Health-risk appraisal—method to evaluate an individual's probability or risk for morbidity or mortality of chronic diseases.

Nutrigenetics—the impact of variations in gene structure on one's response to nutrients or food bioactives.

Nutrigenomics—a focus on the effects of nutrients or food bioactives on the regulation of gene expression.

Pedagogy—the art or profession of teaching.

Self-management—taking responsibility for one's own treatment activities. This often occurs in collaboration with healthcare professionals.

Synergy—combined action or operation such that the total effect is greater than the sum of the effects taken independently.

Although diseases are clinically defined as separate conditions, what occurs frequently is that if one disease is not controlled, a second or comorbid condition develops.

What Do We Know?

Coronary Heart Disease

We know the 3 major risk factors for coronary heart disease (CHD): elevated serum total cholesterol, hypertension, and smoking. The primary risk factor is serum total cholesterol. Studies of infants and children provide insight to the changes in serum total cholesterol early in life. Cholesterol in cord blood at birth averages 71 mg%; between 6 months and 2 years of age, it increases to about 140 mg%. Average serum total cholesterol of school-age children is about 170 mg%. High-density lipoprotein (HDL) cholesterol decreases in adolescence, bringing total cholesterol down briefly, but low-density lipoprotein (LDL) dips and then increases to offset the decline. This is especially true for boys.[1]

Dietary intake is a very important regulating factor in both the etiology and prevention of CHD. Studies show the following[2]:

- Excess energy intake is generally precipitated by an excess amount of dietary fat. Men and women consume about 1 pound of fat every 4 days and 6 days, respectively. The fat constituents that influence the health of the individual may not be measured in the fasting blood cholesterol or cholesterol fractions. Rather, chylomicron remnants may enter and remain in the artery wall, forming a building block for the atherosclerotic plaque. More highly saturated fats encourage blood clot formation within hours of food ingestion.
- Fat in fish reduces clot formation via a clearing mechanism.
- LDL cholesterol reductions are greater for men who have elevated blood levels prior to medical nutrition therapy (i.e., step 1 and step 2 diets).[3] The blood lipid response may be enhanced greatly by weight reduction (e.g., a 25% reduction of total cholesterol can be expected for men consuming high saturated fat if they reduce body weight to a healthy level and practice the step 2 diet).[4,5]
- Dietary cholesterol and saturated fat in food lower the LDL receptor activity on the liver cell. This decreases the amount of LDL cholesterol that leaves the blood.
- Antioxidants in fruits, vegetables, grains, and beans reduce the oxidation of LDL. Oxidized LDL contributes to atherogenesis. Vitamin E slows the antioxidant activity and inhibits the binding site where foam cells are formed, thus lowering cell proliferation. Another action by vitamin E is lowering platelet aggregation and increasing vasodilation. Usual vitamin E intake as mg $\propto$ TE from CSFII, 1994-1996, showed only men < 70 years

old at the 90th percentile met the 2000 RDA of 15 mg $\propto$ TE. Women consumed about 7 mg $\propto$ TE per day.[6] The estimated difference between recommended and average intake as an E-gap of about 5-8 mg $\propto$ TE.

The vitamin E or E-gap exists globally and has been shown to be inversely related to ischemic heart disease with $r^2 = 0.63$ as reported in the WHO Monica Project.[7] The greatest mortality was shown for individuals consuming < 20 µmol/L. Ethnic differences in vitamin E intake in the US are reported from NHANES III in which men in every ethnic group had a higher intake than women. The percentage of each ethnic group averaging < 20 µmol/L was white (male: 27%; female: 26%); African American (male: 42%; female: 40%); Mexican American (male: 29%; female: 27%); others (male: 36%; female: 29%).[8] In the Iowa Women's Health Study, the RR for CHD death and dietary vitamin E intake by quintile ranged from 1.0 to 0.38 ($p = 0.004$) if < 4.91 µm/L to > 9.64 µm/L.[9]

As the US population ages, links to cataracts have been identified. This includes vitamin E intake, which reduces photooxidative damage to lens protein, lessening opacification, and cataracts.[10] Low vitamin E intake and risk for lung ($\Pi = 1.03$), prostate (smokers: $\Pi = 8.34$; nonsmokers: $\Pi = 3.07$), and colon cancer $\Pi = 1.33$) has been reported.[11]

There is some indication that low vitamin E intake ($\Pi = 3.90$ to 5.10) enhances onset of type 2 diabetes.[12] If individuals are to benefit from the known and potential attributes of vitamin E, then good dietary sources, i.e., almonds with 22-24 kernels per 1 oz yielding 7-8 mg $\propto$ T, are an excellent, convenient source and contain beneficial monounsaturated fatty acids (MUFA), polyunsaturated fatty acids (PUFA), and antioxidant phytochemicals that synthetic vitamins do not.

Assessment of an individual's knowledge of CHD risk factors may be important. Several true-false, one-page instruments have been developed by the National Institutes of Health (NIH) to administer to individuals and groups for awareness and focused education for CHD prevention (see Exhibit 17–1).

Cancer

Many factors motivate the ultimate effect of eating behavior on cancer prevention. A high-fat eating pattern may be an intermediate marker for a distinct eating pattern and lifestyle. Studies show the following[13]:

- Some studies of breast cancer report a correlation with fat intake, yet other studies have found no correlation. Obesity is associated with an increased recurrence of breast cancer and with a lower survival rate. An increasing body weight in adulthood is recognized as a predictor of breast cancer risk; excess energy intake and reduced physical activity have been shown to increase cancer risk. The abdominal or apple shape is more highly associated with breast cancer. Weight loss of 14.5 kg may lessen breast cancer risk by 45%.[14-20]
- Several case-control studies report a significant association between fat intake and colon cancer. Eating patterns high in fat, which increase bile acid secretion, promote tumor development and cell proliferation. Bacterial flora common among omnivores form mutagenic secondary bile acids, placing individuals at high risk for colon cancer. The opposite occurs for individuals who have a high fruit and vegetable intake. Dietary fiber and

calcium supplementation can decrease, whereas dietary fat can increase the proliferation rates of cells in the rectal mucosa.[21-29]

- Multicountry studies have helped to unravel various dietary associations with prostate cancer. Among postmenopausal women, obesity and an eating pattern high in fat have been associated with uterine cancer.[30,31]

Exhibit 17–1   Check Your Healthy Heart IQ

CHECK YOUR

Healthy Heart I.Q.

Answer "true" or "false" to the following questions to test your knowledge of heart disease and its risk factors. Be sure to check the answers and explanations that follow to see how well you do.

1. The risk factors for heart disease that follow *you can do something about* are: high blood pressure, high blood cholesterol, smoking, obesity, and physical inactivity.   T   F

2. A stroke is often the first symptom of high blood pressure, and a heart attack is often the first symptom of high blood cholesterol.   T   F

3. A blood pressure greater than or equal to 140/90 mm Hg is generally considered to be high.   T   F

4. High blood pressure affects the same number of blacks as it does whites.   T   F

5. The best ways to treat and control high blood pressure are to control your weight, excerise, eat less salt (sodium). restrict your intake of alcohol, and take your high blood pressure medicine, if prescribed by your doctor.   T   F

6. A blood cholesterol level of 240 mg/dL is desirable for adults.   T   F

7. The most effective dietary way to lower the level of your blood cholesterol is to eat foods low in cholesterol.   T   F

8. Lowering blood cholesterol levels can help people who have already had a heart attack.   T   F

9. Only children from families at high risk of heart disease need to have their blood cholesterol levels checked.   T   F

10. Smoking is a major risk factor for 4 of the 5 leading causes of death including heart attack, stroke, cancer, and lung diseases such as emphysema and bronchitis.   T   F

11. If you have had a heart attack, quitting smoking can help reduce your chances of having a second attack.   T   F

12. Someone who has smoked for 30 to 40 years probably will not be able to quit smoking.   T   F

13. The best way to lose weight is to increase physical activity and eat fewer calories.   T   F

14. Heart diseases are the leading killer of men *and* women in the United States.   T   F

Prepared by the National Heart, Lung, and Blood Pressure National Institutes of Health

- High energy intake fueled by fat, especially polyunsaturated fat, accelerates cell proliferation. Polyunsaturated fat also promotes prostaglandin synthesis. Conversely, energy restriction stops tumor growth in some animal models. Aromatization of adrenal androgens produces estrogens in postmenopausal women; estradiol increases and promotes tumor growth[32-34] (see Chapter 12).
- Anecdotal evidence that the public is becoming skeptical about nutrition messages exists. A 1997-1998 Washington State random-digit-dial survey of 1,751 adults monitored attitudes and behavior related to cancer risk and prevention. The survey did not find strong evidence that nutrition backlash was widespread, but 70% of respondents thought that Americans are obsessed with the fat in their diet and that the government should not tell people what to eat. More than a quarter agreed with the statement that eating low-fat foods takes the pleasure out of eating. Nutrition backlash was associated with less healthful diets, for example, individuals showing high backlash had a fat-related diet habits score of 2.11 compared with a score of 1.73 among those showing low backlash (P for trend = 0.001). This corresponds to a difference of roughly 4 percentage points in percentage energy from fat. Individuals showing high backlash reported eating only 2.72 servings of fruits and vegetables per day, compared with 3.35 servings among those showing low backlash (P for trend = 0.001). Dietary recommendations that are clear and positive are needed to minimize consumer disregard of nutrition messages entirely.[35]
- Mainstream researchers in the cancer field believe that the most important nutrition message in lieu of many alternatives (coffee enemas, macrobiotic diet, excess vitamins) is to recommend a commonsense approach that lasts a lifetime. See Table 17–1.

Diabetes Mellitus

Patients with type 2 diabetes often exhibit a clustering of risk factors. The clustering in a single individual of hyperinsulinemia, hypertension, hypertriglyceridemia, and obesity (in particular, upper-body obesity) is termed "the

TABLE 17–1   Commonsense Dietary and Lifestyle Recommendations to Prevent the Development of Cancer

- Avoid tobacco in any form
- Lower total dietary fat intake
- Lower caloric intake and avoid obesity
- Increase intake of fresh fruits and vegetables
- Avoid salted, smoked, pickled, broiled, and fried foods
- Increase calcium intake
- Consume alcohol in moderation
- Avoid excessive direct sun exposure > 30 minutes/day
- Increase regular exercise

Source: August DA. Nutrition and cancer—where are we going? *Top Clin Nutr.* 2003:18(4):268-279.

deadly quartet." A lifestyle modification program with a very-low-fat, high-carbohydrate, high-fiber diet and daily aerobic exercise was set up for 13 patients with diabetes. The diet comprised 10% of its calories from fat and 75% from unrefined carbohydrates, with 35 to 40 grams of dietary fiber per 1,000 kcal. After 21 days, fasting serum insulin, glucose, and triglycerides declined significantly by 33%, 28%, and 44%, respectively. Systolic and diastolic blood pressures, body weight, and body mass index (BMI) were all significantly reduced by the intervention. Total cholesterol and LDL cholesterol levels were significantly reduced by 22% and 26%, respectively, and HDL cholesterol levels increase significantly by 13.5%.[36-39]

Diabetic retinopathy or other visual abnormalities require care by an ophthalmologist experienced in the management of people with diabetes. The individual with abnormal renal function may develop proteinuria or elevated serum creatinine, which require heightened attention and control of other risk factors (e.g., hypertension and smoking). Such a situation requires consultation with a specialist in diabetic renal disease.

Individuals with cardiovascular risk factors should be carefully monitored. If symptoms of cardiovascular disease occur (i.e., angina, decreased pulses, and ECG abnormalities), then efforts should be aimed at correction of contributing risk factors (e.g., obesity, smoking, hypertension, sedentary lifestyle, hyperlipidemia, and poorly regulated diabetes). Treatment of the specific cardiovascular problem should be monitored. A questionnaire to evaluate an individual's weight and heart IQ can be used to assist treatment (see Exhibit 17–2). Diabetic neuropathy may result in painful paresthesia, muscle weakness, and loss of sensation. Autonomic involvement can affect the function of the gastrointestinal, cardiovascular, and genitourinary systems and may require consultation with an appropriate medical specialist.

Upper-body obesity accompanies an increased prevalence of hypertension, diabetes, and dyslipidemia. A similar clustering of metabolic disturbances in nonobese, hypertensive patients has been called syndrome X. Syndrome X contributes to a marked increase in the risk of CHD for individuals with or without clinically defined diabetes. A condition that includes both syndrome X and the deadly quartet is insulin-resistance syndrome, because both conditions are associated with and likely caused by resistance to the peripheral actions of insulin with subsequent hyperinsulinemia. All obese hypertensives and about one half of nonobese hypertensives are insulin resistant.[36,37]

About 1 in 3 Americans has syndrome X. The rise in prevalence has been attributed to the lack of success in treating each separate condition to goal. Reaven professes that the carbohydrate component of one's eating pattern is the offender in syndrome X. Carbohydrate is metabolized to glucose and the process is repeated with each snack and meal.[37] Syndrome X risk factors are:

- Impaired glucose tolerance
- High insulin levels (hyperinsulinemia)
- Elevated triglycerides (blood fats)
- Low HDL (good cholesterol)
- Slow clearance of fat from the blood (exaggerated postprandial lipemia)
- Smaller, more dense LDL (bad) cholesterol particles
- Increased propensity of the blood to form clots
- Decreased ability to dissolve blood clots
- Elevated blood pressure

Lifestyle factors that exacerbate syndrome X are:

- Obesity
- Lack of physical activity
- The wrong diet
- Cigarette smoking

Exhibit 17–2   Check Your Weight and Heart Disease IQ

Check   Your   Weight   and   Heart   Disease

I.Q.

Prepared by the National Heart, Lung, and Blood Institute • National Institutes of Health

The following statements are either true or false.
The statements test your knowledge of overweight and heart disease.
The correct answers can be found following the quiz.

[T] [F]   1. Being overweight puts you at risk for heart disease.

[T] [F]   2. If you are overweight, losing weight helps lower your high blood cholesterol and high blood pressure.

[T] [F]   3. Quitting smoking is healthy, but it commonly leads to excessive weight gain, which increases your risk for heart disease.

[T] [F]   4. An overweight person with high blood pressure should pay more attention to a low-sodium diet than to weight reduction.

[T] [F]   5. A reduced intake of sodium or salt does not always lower high blood pressure to normal.

[T] [F]   6. The best way to lose weight is to eat lower calories and exercise.

[T] [F]   7. Skipping meals is a good way to eat down on calories.

[T] [F]   8. Foods high in complex carbohydrates (starch and fiber) are good choices when you are trying to lose weight.

[T] [F]   9. The single most important change most people can make to lose weight is to avoid sugar.

[T] [F]   10. Polyunsaturated fat has the same number of calories as saturated fat.

[T] [F]   11. Overweight children are very likely to become overweight adults.

Your Score: How many correct answers did you have?

10:11 correct - Congratulations! You know a lot about
weight and heart disease. Share this information with your
family and friends. 8–9 correct - Very good. Fewer than
8 - Go over the answers and try to learn more about weight
and heart disease.

NHLBI OBESITY EDUCATION INITIATIVE

Exhibit 17–2   continued

ANSWERS TO YOUR WEIGHT AND HEART DISEASE IQ TEST

1 True. Being overweight increases your risk for high blood cholesterol and high blood pressure, 2 of the major risk factors for coronary heart disease. Even if you do not have high blood cholesterol or high blood pressure, being overweight may increase your risk for heart disease. Where you carry your extra weight may affect your risk too. Weight carried at your waist or above seems to be associated with an increased risk, for heart disease in many people. In addition, being overweight increases your risk for diabetes, gallbladder disease, and some types of cancer.

2 True. If you are overweight, even moderate reductions in weight, such as 5 to 10 percent, can produce substantial reductions in blood pressure. You may also be able to reduce your LDL-cholesterol ("bad" cholesterol) and triglycerides and increase your HDL-cholesterol ("good" cholesterol).

3 False. The average weight gain after quitting smoking is 5 pounds. The proportion of ex-smokers who gain large amounts of weight (greater than 20 pounds) is relatively small. Even if you gain weight when you stop smoking, change your eating and exercise habits to lose weight rather than starting to smoke again. Smokers who quit smoking decrease their risk for heart disease by about 50% compared to those people who do not quit.

4 False. Weight loss, if you are overweight, may reduce your blood pressure even if you don't reduce the amount of sodium you eat. Weight loss is recommended for all overweight people who have high blood pressure. Even if weight loss does not reduce your blood pressure to normal, it may help you cut back on your blood pressure medications. Also, losing weight if you are overweight may help you reduce your risk for or control other health problems.

5 True. Even though a high sodium or salt intake plays a key role in maintaining high blood pressure in some people, there is no easy way to determine who will benefit from eating less sodium and salt. Also, a high intake may limit how well certain high blood pressure medications work. Eating a diet with less sodium may help some people reduce their risk of developing high blood pressure. Most Americans eat more salt and other sources of sodium than they need. Therefore, it is prudent for most people to reduce their sodium intake.

6 True. Eating fewer calories and exercising more is the best way to lose weight and keep it off. Weight control is a question of balance. You get calories from the food you eat. You burn off calories by exercising. Cutting down on calories, especially calories from fat, is key to losing weight. Combining this with a regular exercise program, like walking, bicycling, jogging, or swimming, not only can help in losing weight but also in maintaining the weight loss. A steady weight loss of 1 to 2 pounds a week is safe for most adults, and the weight is more likely to stay off over the long run. Losing weight, if you are overweight, may also help reduce your blood pressure and raise your HDL cholesterol, the good cholesterol.

7 False. To cut calories, some people regularly skip meals and have no snacks or caloric drinks in between. If you do this, your body thinks that it is starving even if your intake of calories is not reduced to a very low amount. Your body will try to save energy by slowing its metabolism, that is decreasing the rate at which it burns calories. This makes losing weight even harder and may even add body fat. Try to avoid long periods without eating. Five or six small meals are often preferred to the usual 3 meals a day for some individuals trying to lose weight.

8 True. Contrary to popular belief, foods high in complex carbohydrates (like pasta, rice, potatoes, breads, cereals, grains, dried beans and peas) are lower in calories than foods high in fat. In addition, they are good sources of vitamins, minerals, and fiber, What adds calories to these foods is the addition of butter, rich sauces, whole milk, cheese, or cream, which are high in fat.

9 False. Sugar has not been found to cause obesity; however, many foods high in sugar are also high in fat. Fat has more than twice the calories as the same amount of protein or carbohydrates (sugar and starch). Thus, foods that are high in fat are high in calories. High-sugar foods, like cakes, cookies, candies, and ice cream, are high in fat and calories and low in vitamins, minerals, and protein.

10 True. All fats—polyunsaturated, monounsaturated, and saturated—have the same number of calories. All calories count whether they come from saturated or unsaturated fats. Because fats are the richest sources of calories, eating less total fat will help reduce the number of calories you eat every day. It will also help you reduce your intake of saturated fat. Particular attention to reducing saturated fat is important in lowering your blood cholesterol level.

11 False. Obesity in childhood does increase the likelihood of adult obesity, but most overweight children will not become obese. Several factors infulence whether or not an overweight child becomes an overweight adult: (1) the age the child becomes overweight; (2) how overweight the child is; (3) the family history of overweight; and (4) dietary and activity habits. Getting to the right weight is desirable, but children's needs for calories and other nutrients are different from the needs of adults. Dietary plans for weight control must allow for this. Eating habits, like so many other habits, are often formed during childhood, so it is important to develop good ones.

For more information. write:
NHLBI Obesity Education Initiative
P.O. Box 30105
Bethesda, MD 20824-0105

Source: Reprinted from *Check Your Weight and Heart Disease IQ.* Bethesda, MD National Heart, Lung, and Blood Institute, National Institutes ofHealth, Publication No. 93-3034, May 1993.

TABLE 17–2   Risk Factors and CHD Risk

Risk Factors	Risk of Heart Disease
Increase triglycerides + increase LDL + lower HDL	4.4 ×
Increase triglycerides + small, dense LDL particles and elevated fasting insulin levels	20 ×

Note: For each 30% increase in insulin levels, a 70% increase in risk of heart disease exists over a 5-year period.
Source: Adapted from: Reaven G. *The Syndrome X Diet.* Needham Heights, Mass: Simon & Schuster; 2000.

The syndrome is characterized as a reluctance for glucose to enter cells, keeping serum insulin levels high, thus damaging the lining of the coronary arteries and enhancing heart attack risk. Risk factors and extent of risk are outlined in Table 17–2. The syndrome X diet is characterized by a 15:40:45 composition for protein, fat, and carbohydrate with total fat divided as 5-10% saturated and 30-35% poly- and monounsaturated (Table 17–3).

Multiple mechanisms appear responsible for insulin resistance, but the specific etiologic factor observed in obese and nonobese patients with hypertension is uncertain.[38] Excess body weight distributed in the upper body may be the responsible factor for obese individuals. The degree of hyperinsulinemia may be even greater if weight gain is induced by high carbohydrate intake. Continual stress-induced, sympathetic nervous system activation may also lead to insulin resistance. An increased proportion of type IIB muscle fibers, reflecting either genetic or acquired processes, may be responsible. These fibers are more resistant to the effects of insulin than are type I and type IIA fibers.[40]

Irrespective of the process by which insulin resistance is initiated, the outcome of hyperinsulinemia may be responsible for increased systemic blood pressure, dyslipidemia, and CHD. Drug and medical nutrition therapy to reduce

TABLE 17–3   The Syndrome X Diet as Compared to the AHA, Zone, and Atkins Diets

	Protein	Saturated Fat	Mono- and Polyunsaturated Fat	Carbohydrate	Cholesterol	Decreases Both Insulin and LDL Cholesterol
Syndrome X diet	15%	5-10%	30-35%	45%	< 300 mg/day	Yes
American Heart Association diet	15%	5-10%	20%	55-60%	300 mg/day	No
The Zone diet	30%	6%	24%	40%	210 mg/day	No
Atkins diet	22%	25%	35%	18%	880 mg/day	No

Source: Adapted from: Reaven G. *The Syndrome X Diet.* Needham Heights, Mass: Simon & Schuster; 2000.

insulin resistance seems appropriate and potentially of great benefit. Targeted nutritional programs are an essential part of the approach. Suggested lifestyle changes to overcome insulin resistance are as follows[41]:

- weight reduction if obesity is present
- regular aerobic exercise
- moderate consumption of alcohol
- use of antihypertensive agents, such as captopril and doxazosin, which improve insulin sensitivity
- avoidance of diuretics and beta-blockers, which complicate insulin sensitivity
- use of metformin, which increases insulin sensitivity and decreases hyperinsulinemia

For millions of overweight people who are at high risk for type 2 diabetes, the Diabetes Prevention Program (DPP) compared 3 approaches: lifestyle modification, treatment with metformin or glucophage, and standard medical advice in 3,234 overweight people. The participants had impaired glucose tolerance (IGT) or high blood glucose levels but were not yet diabetic. About 20 million people in the United States have IGT, which raises the risk of developing type 2 diabetes and cardiovascular disease. When a person has type 2 diabetes, the risk of heart and blood vessel disease is 2 to 4 times that of people without diabetes. In DPP, diet and exercise that achieved a 5-7% weight loss also reduced diabetes incidence by 58%. The participants exercised at moderate intensity, usually walking an average of 30 minutes a day 5 days a week, and lowered their intake of fat and calories. Individuals randomly assigned to treatment with metformin had a 31% lower incidence of type 2 diabetes. The lifestyle had an equal effect on men as on women and across different ethnic groups. Most decline was noted in people age 60 and older, who lowered their risk of developing diabetes by 71%.[42]

Obesity

Obesity was a sleeper disease that has emerged as a powerful independent risk factor for CHD, hypertension, and type 2 diabetes. Sustained obesity is difficult to treat and is influenced by lifestyle. When it appears early in life it is retained more frequently than lost over time. Billions of dollars are spent in the United States on health care related to obesity. The BMI has been extended to children and youth whose risk for a variety of chronic diseases increases as BMI increases.

In 2000, a new approach to weight management was codified and published as *The Volumetrics Weight-Control Plan*.[43] It is based on the ratios of food energy per 100 grams of product and promotes a lower ratio as well as creating more food satiety. For example, starchy foods such as lentils, potatoes, and beans have a lower energy density than eggs, bread, and cheese, which, in turn, are lower than bacon, chocolate, and margarine. This approach puts hydrous fruits and vegetables and high-fiber foods at the lowest ratios. This is another way to increase the volume of food consumed while creating an isocaloric condition and enhancing energy control and satiety.

Hypertension

Hypertension is a major risk factor for CHD, which enhances the progression of several other debilitating diseases. Research shows the following:

- Hypertension contributes to the development and progression of chronic complications of diabetes.
- Hypertension should be treated aggressively to achieve and maintain blood pressure in the normal range.

Exhibit 17–3　　Check Your High Blood Pressure Prevention IQ

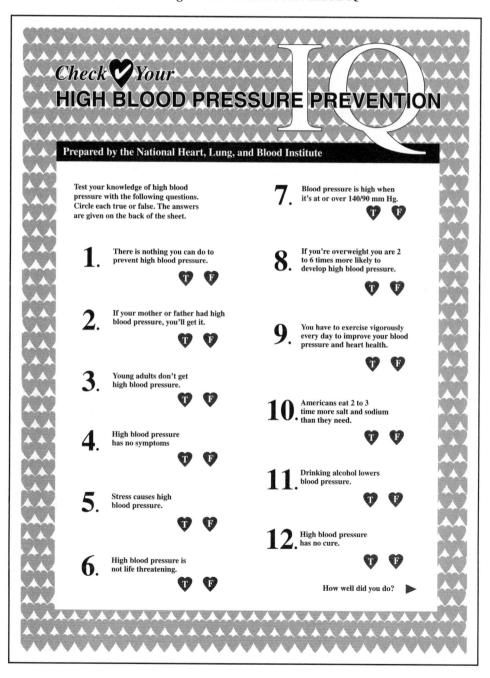

Exhibit 17–3   Check Your High Blood Pressure Prevention IQ

ANSWERS TO THE HIGH BLOOD PRESSURE PREVENTION I.Q. QUIZ

1. False. High blood pressure can be prevented with 4 steps: keep a healthy weight; become physically active; limit your salt and sodium use; and, if you drink alcoholic beverages, do so in moderation.

2. False. You are more likely to get high blood pressure if it runs in your family, but that doesn't mean you must get it. Your chance of getting high blood pressure is also greater if you're older or an african American. But high blood pressure is *not* an inevitable part of aging and everyone can take steps to prevent the disease—the steps are given in answer 1.

3. False. About 15 percent of those ages 18 to 39 are among the 50 million Americans with high blood pressure. Once you have high blood pressure, you have it for the rest of your life. So start now to prevent it.

4. True. High blood pressure, or "hypertension," usually has no symptoms. In fact, it is often called the "silent killer." You can have high blood pressure and feel fine. That's why it's important to have your blood pressure checked—it's a simple test.

5. False. Stress does make blood pressure go up, but only temporarily. Ups and downs in blood pressure are normal. Run for a bus and your pressure rises; sleep it and drops. Blood pressure is the force of blood against the walls of arteries. Blood pressure becomes dangerous when it's always high. That harms your heart and blood vessels. So what does cause high blood pressure? In the vast majority of cases, a single cause is never found.

6. False. High blood pressure is the main cause of stroke and a factor in the development of heart disease and kidney failure.

7. True. But even blood pressures slightly under 140/90 mm Hg can increase your risk of heart disease or stroke.

8. True. As weight increases, so does blood pressure. It's important to stay at a healthy weight. If you need to reduce, try to lose 1/2 to 1 pound a week. Choose foods low in fat (especially saturated fat), since fat is high in calories. Even if you're at a good weight, the healthiest way to eat is low fat, low cholesterol.

9. False. Studies show that even a little physical activity helps prevent high blood pressure and strengthens your heart. Even among the overweight, those who are active have lower blood pressure than those who aren't. It's best to do some activity for 30 minutes, most days. Walk, garden, or bowl. If you don't have a 30-minute period, do something for 15 minutes, twice a day. Every bit helps—so make activity part of your daily routine.

10. True. Americans eat way too much salt and sodium. And some people, such as many African Americans, are especially sensitive to salt. Salt is made of sodium and chloride, and it's mostly the sodium that affects blood pressure. Salt is only 1 form of sodium—there are others. So you need to watch your use of both salt and sodium. That includes what's added to foods at the table and in cooking, and what's already in processed foods and snacks. Americans, especially people with high blood pressure, should eat no more than about 6 grams of salt a day, which equals about 2,400 milligrams of sodium.

11. False. Drinking too much alcohol can raise blood pressure. If you drink, have no more than 2 drinks a day. *The Dietary Guidelines* recommend that for overall health, women should limit their alcohol to no more than one drink a day. A drink would be 1.5 ounces of 80 proof whiskey, or 5 ounces of wine, or 12 ounces of beer.

12. True. But high blood pressure can be treated and controlled. Treatment usually includes lifestyle changes—losing weight, if overweight; becoming physically active; limiting salt and sodium; and avoiding drinking excess alcohol—and, if needed, medication. But the best way to avoid the dangers of high blood pressure is to prevent the condition.

**For more information on high
blood pressure,
call 1-800-575-WELL,
or write to the
National Heart, Lung, and Blood
Institute Information Center,
P.O. Box 30105,
Bethesda, MD
20824-0105.**

National High Blood Pressure Education Program
National Heart, Lung, and Blood Institute

U.S. Department of Health and Human Services
Public Health Service
National Institutes of Health
NIH Publication No 94-3671
September 1994

Source: Reprinted from *Check Your High Blood Pressure Prevention IQ*. Bethesda, MD National heart, Lung, and Blood Institute, National Institutes of Health, Publication No. 94-3671, September 1994.

- Eating and exercise behavior change can moderate blood pressure levels. Community nutrition professionals can begin by assessing individuals' knowledge about high blood pressure (see Exhibit 17–3).
- If medication is needed, selection of an antihypertensive drug should be individualized to minimize the number and severity of side effects. For example, beta-blockers should be used with caution in insulin-treated individuals, because these drugs may mask early symptoms of hypoglycemia and prolong recovery from hypoglycemia.[44-45]
- Various lifestyle therapies can reduce the major adverse effects of hypertension and the risk factors that frequently accompany high blood pressure (see Exhibit 17–3) including the DASH diet that recommends 2,000 kcals each day, which promotes 9 servings of fruits and vegetables, 8 servings of grains, 1 of nuts, seeds, and legumes, and a 2,300-mg sodium intake.[46]

Smoking

One of the major risk factors for CHD is cigarette smoking. Smoking cessation is a major lifestyle change recommended for men and women with a smoking habit. Medical nutrition therapy to support smoking cessation can involve replacing lost nutrient intake, increasing soluble fiber, weight management, and substituting alkaline foods during withdrawal symptoms. (See Exhibit 17–4.)

Exhibit 17–4   Nutrition Guidelines to Assist Smoking Cessation

Eat a Nutrient-Dense Diet
Recover lost nutrients emphasizing vitamin A, beta-carotene, vitamin B$_{12}$, folic acid, vitamin C, and zinc. Consume more yellow/orange fruits and vegetables, citrus and fresh fruits, dark green leafy vegetables, lean red meat, and low-fat milk and yogurt.

Increase Fiber
Include more roughage in the diet, adequate water, and exercise to reduce constipation. Eat fresh fruits and vegetables with skins such as potatoes, squash, apples, pears, and peaches.

Control Weight
Start to lose weight before quitting. A 500-calorie daily deficit equals 1 pound of weight loss per week. Plan a 250-kcal deficit a day and burn 250 additional kcal each day by increasing exercise (such as 45 minutes of aerobic walking or bicycling or 30 minutes of swimming or jogging).

Reduce Withdrawal Symptoms and Cravings with Alkaline Foods
Alkaloid foods enhance reabsorption of nicotine. Alkaline-forming foods are high in potassium, calcium, magnesium, and sodium. Acid-forming foods, which are high in phosphorous, sulfur, and chloride, should be limited.

Limit Intake of the Following:
- protein foods
- poultry
- fish

continued

Exhibit 17–4   continued

- eggs
- seafood
- cranberries
- plums
- prunes

Increase Intake of the Following:
- milk
- yogurt
- shrimp
- coffee
- tea
- soda
- water
- mineral water
- fruits and vegetables
- dried fruit
- olives
- almonds
- Brazil nuts

Eat Moderate Amounts of the Following:
- grains
- starches
- corn
- asparagus

Restructure Eating
Alter your snack and meal environment. Reduce contact with smoking. Practice behavior modification techniques. Experiment with altering your tastes by choosing among these alternatives, which also enhance oral gratification:
- special coffee blends, strong blends
- lemon drops, Lifesavers, diet candy, and gum
- raw vegetables when feeling anger or aggression
- yogurt to comfort or sooth
- diet soda, diet lemonade, fruit juice, and mineral water
- melba toast, Rye Crisp, Rusk crackers
- use a straw or a toothpick

Source: Adapted from: Beckley L. *Taking Control: Diet, Drug Abuse and Addiction.* Ashland, Ore: Nutrition Dimension; 1990.

What Are the National Directives?

Dietary Guidelines for Americans[47] clearly document the relationship between what people eat and their health. Based on decades of research and the resulting consensus of numerous scientific groups, these documents direct primary and secondary prevention activities via planning healthy eating patterns for individuals or groups or providing nutrition education programs. The direction is risk reduction, and the target is chronic disease (e.g., CHD, cancer, hypertension, and diabetes).

Healthy People in Healthy Communities 2010 offers a vision for the century, so the United States can experience significantly less death and disability from preventable diseases, an improved quality of life, and a greater reduction in the disparities of health status among select groups of people. Certain ethnic groups such as African Americans experience a greater proportion of CHD deaths and cancer deaths; Native Americans and Latinos have a higher incidence of obesity, diabetes, and hypertension.[48]

The *Healthy People 2010* vision set the nutrition agenda for US educational institutions, healthcare facilities, state and local health agencies, nonprofit organizations, and the food industry. The National Cholesterol Education Program (NCEP) underscores *Healthy People 2010* objectives specific to CHD, with a national campaign emphasizing the importance of low-fat eating for all individuals 2 years and older.[49] *Healthy People 2010* continues the US agenda for the millennium.[50] *Healthy People 2010* presents leading health indicators to categorize health objectives. The indicators focus on health conditions in the United States that can be monitored while being motivational. The indicators that link to nutrition include but are not limited to: overweight and obesity, physical activity, mental health, and access to health care.[51]

Throughout the United States, the 5 A Day campaign links food industry activities with the National Cancer Institute initiative to increase fruit and vegetable intake to reduce cancer risk. Specific programs at the state and local levels complement these national initiatives (www.5aday.com). In many cases, individual states have formalized their own programs to address the nutritional needs of their residents.[52] For example, in 1988, the California Department of Health Services established the California 5-a-Day-for-Better Health! campaign to promote fruit and vegetable consumption as part of a low-fat, high-fiber eating pattern. This was possible due to a 5-year grant awarded by the National Cancer Institute. Currently, California's program reaches millions of adults and children with media and point-of-purchase information. California's Project LEAN—Low-fat Eating for Americans Now! campaign has reached population segments and various ethnic groups throughout California with a similar message.

National guides include the recommended dietary allowances (RDAs), which are the quantitative standards used throughout the United States for planning and evaluating the nutritional adequacy of a population's food intake. These standards are used for meal planning in schools, hospitals, extended-care facilities, penal institutions, congregate feeding sites, and military installations. The RDAs do not address the modifications of nutrient intakes to reduce chronic disease risk. Healthy menu planning must blend the nutrient needs to avoid deficiencies, represented by RDAs, with health-promoting meal composition to forestall chronic disease, represented by *Dietary Guidelines for Americans*[47] and *My Pyramid*. Adequate levels (AL) and tolerable upper intake levels (UL) provide a range to guide blending of food and supplements to achieve daily nutrient needs. *My Pyramid* is the visual presentation of the *Dietary Guidelines for Americans* (see Chapter 2).[53]

Because today's food and health consumers or buyers range from preadolescents to older adults who live alone, nutrition education for all age groups is essential. What US residents see on food labels in grocery stores has changed dramatically during the past few years. The Nutrition Labeling Education Act of 1990 revamped food labels, defined common terms describing the health-promoting attributes of foods, and set criteria for making nutrition and health claims about foods. The food label has become a major teaching tool to educate children and adults about healthy food choices, and it has enlarged the responsibility of nutrition education to include industry.

The National Action Plan to Improve the American Diet recognizes that no individual organization or initiative can create the massive dietary changes needed to reduce chronic disease in the majority of the US population.[54] This plan recommends a coordinated approach to complement current interventions to reach the *Healthy People 2010* objectives.

What Can We Do?

Health-Risk Appraisals

Between 5 and 15 million Americans have completed some form of a health-risk appraisal (HRA). HRAs have gained popularity as a means of assessing a person's health status and provide an estimate of the likelihood of mortality or morbidity from disease using risk factors such as blood pressure, weight, smoking habits, and medical history. In addition, appraisal questionnaires are a form of health education, because they make people aware of the outcome or result of their lifestyles and health habits. Many organizations administer HRAs to employees as a part of their health insurance and health benefits package and as a method to evaluate the effectiveness of health promotion programs.[55]

HRAs vary in the way risk is defined and estimated. Computations to predict risk levels generally create a score or a more easily interpreted number. Four different scoring methods are as follows[56]:

1. The probability of dying from leading causes of death over a period of time (e.g., 10 years). Estimates for CHD and stroke are independently estimated. Mortality risk estimates are based on an actuarial approach called the Geller-Gesner method.
2. A focus on heart attacks and heart disease using scales divided into low-, average-, and high-risk ranges. Pencil-and-paper tests are summed for each item.
3. Life expectancy as a surrogate for risk. These HRAs contain the major CHD factors and are scored by hand.
4. Broad measures of overall health (e.g., lifestyle, wellness, stress, or health risk). This format is simple to score by hand, but it may provide only a crude measure of risk.

Many HRAs do not address dietary habits. Some include only 1 or 2 items, none of which are used to compute risk. The responses may only serve to trigger changes for improving dietary habits.

The reasons nutrition may not be central to a health-risk appraisal are as follows:

- Dietary status is difficult to measure. Twenty-four-hour dietary recalls may underestimate, whereas frequencies may overlook detail or specific foods. Detailed dietary inventories are not practical for most HRAs.[57]
- The strength of a direct correlation between dietary components and mortality is not established. For example, CHD risk computations are

often based on prospective surveys, and those studies may not collect a sufficient volume of detailed dietary data.

- HRAs are driven by physiological precursors of morbidity and mortality. Eating and exercise behavior are intermediate mediators to these precursors. The immediate precursors include blood pressure, plasma cholesterol, lipid fractions, and body mass.

Guidelines for Selecting an HRA

With more than 200 HRAs in the United States, selection guidelines and questions are needed. The following criteria may be used[56]:

- What is the validity or accuracy of the risk estimates? With diversity of scoring methods and databases, discrepant estimates of risk for an individual are expected. Forty-one popular appraisal instruments were evaluated for similarity of CHD risk estimates. They were compared with projections from the Framingham Heart Study and the UCLA Risk Factor Update Project.[58] HRAs based on logistic regression equations or the Geller-Gesner method with additive scales were the most accurate. Comprehensiveness of the assessment items was a major indicator of accuracy. The least accurate instruments were those that do not include major risk factors, that ignore sex and age, or that employ 2 or 3 broad categories to measure a factor.
- What does the report form contain? How easy is it to read and to understand? What and how much feedback are most appropriate for clients? Generally, simple identification of below average, average, and above average risk may be sufficient, but in some instances a detailed estimate of life expectancy or probability of dying is needed. An individual's actual age can be contrasted with the appraised age (the average age at which members of the general population have the same risk). Risks associated with select factors (e.g., smoking or physical activity) are informative and directive. If HRA data are to be used to evaluate a health promotion or dietary intervention, a matrix defining risk and future action may be appropriate.
- Are the appraisal questionnaires expensive if self-administered? Usually self-administered questionnaires are available in bulk at a nominal charge. However, versions for personal computers are available. The cost varies from $50 to more than $300. Complete HRA assessments are often available, and for a fee they include personalized charts, detailed explanations, and summary reports. This is the most expensive option, but it can be cost-effective when an entire work site or large population is evaluated.

Limitations of HRAs

The major limitations of HRAs are as follows[56]:

- Clients may not comprehend or interpret the results accurately, because probability estimates are difficult to grasp. This uncertainty can reduce the educational and motivational potential.
- Clients may not know how to assess the accuracy of the appraisal. If blood pressure and cholesterol levels are missing, and an average value is used, then an artificially low risk estimate can be given.

Info Line

> For more information on HRAs, contact Carter Center Health Risk
> Appraisal Project, 1989 North Williamsburg Drive, Suite E, Decatur,
> GA 30033.

- Self-scored HRAs may contain simple math errors and mislead
  individuals about their actual status.
- If HRAs are administered in an unsupervised environment, then the
  results may cause unnecessary fear and anxiety.

Questions have been raised about health care in the United States. The
United States does not have the best health care in the world, and it may not
be able to sustain a system costing 15% of the gross domestic product
compared to 5-10% in other nations. A tsunami of baby boomers is the most
narcissistic, selfish, yet best informed generation; however, they tend not to
accept the patronizing culture of today's doctors. As businesses spend billions on health insurance but receive unhappy employees, workers fret about
the quality of the care they receive, the burden of their out-of-pocket expense, and inadequacy of coverage. For businesses, health care becomes a
lose-lose proposition. They pay way too much and they get way too little.
Consumer-driven health care is fundamentally about empowering healthcare
consumers with control, choice, and information.[59]

Food-Scoring Systems

These systems vary from a comprehensive approach to a rapid or quick
assessment of a food record. Nutrient-based analysis is more revealing if
based on reliable and accurate records. Two useful food-scoring systems that
provide a quick estimation of the effect of eating pattern on serum cholesterol are the Food Record Rating and the Dietary Achievement Score. They
are practical for groups or individuals.[60]

The Food Record Rating (FRR) was used in the Multiple Risk Factor
Intervention Trial (MRFIT); the Dietary Achievement Score was used in the
Heart Saver Program of the Chicago Heart Association. Both methods estimate
adherence and indirectly predict changes in serum cholesterol. Both instruments can be used for self-monitoring and teaching clients about food selection. The food score averages 3 days of food records. The use of food-scoring
systems in nutrition counseling has been described in detail and should be
considered as a way to monitor behavior after establishing a baseline.

An exchange system has been used to assess intake and evaluate
compliance. Foods appearing on a record can be converted into exchanges.
The quality of the eating pattern is then based on the number of exchanges
consumed compared with the number recommended.[61,62]

The Cholesterol-Saturated-Fat Index (CSI) indicates the hypercholesterolemic potential of foods based on the cholesterol and saturated fatty
acid content. Foods high in saturated fatty acids and cholesterol increase an

Info Line

Mycoprotein is a new food ingredient that:

- contains high-quality protein, is low in total and saturated fat, and free from cholesterol
- has beneficial effects on serum cholesterol levels
- is the major ingredient in a range of foods, such as Quorn, produced in the United Kingdom
- has a structure comprised of 48% protein, 25% fiber, 12% soluble carbohydrate, and 12% fat

individual's plasma total cholesterol level (see Chapter 11). For example, a 3.5-oz or 100-g portion of salmon has a CSI of 5, poultry a 6, 10% fat ground sirloin a 9, and 30% fat steaks an 18 CSI. The value identifies the food as hypercholesterolemic or atherogenic. The CSI demonstrates why some foods (e.g., cheeses or frozen desserts) that have vegetable oil instead of butterfat are better choices.[63] Vegetable oils have no cholesterol and a small amount of saturated fat and, thus, a low CSI value.

Assessment of Sodium Intake

Multiple days of records are needed to quantify an individual's sodium intake. For populations, a 1-day food record can give a reasonable estimate of intake. However, assessing sodium intake with a combination of methods is being used. Another approach is to use a regression equation that reflects the independent contribution of the following[64,65]:

- the daily quantity of table salt used over 7 days
- the contribution of sodium from sodium-rich foods assessed in a 7-day food frequency checklist
- an estimate of sodium in the overall foods and beverages consumed

Use of Probiotics

Live active cultures in some dairy products, called probiotics, have potential health benefits. Probiotics provide a barrier to gastrointestinal tract infections including antibiotic-resistant pathogens and virulent food-borne pathogens like shigatoxin-producing *E coli*. Support for probiotics stems from the Paleolithic diet, which included a very high intake of lactobacilli. The human gastrointestinal tract has 400 different bacteria, which result in about 2-3 lbs of bacteria—some harmful and some not. It is presumed that probiotics may offer a layer of protection. This includes intestinal health, immune system modulation, and lactose digestion.

With 17 million people in the United States with asthma, studies have been conducted among infants less than 6 months in day care, finding 40% less asthma when infants enter at over 6 months of age than less than 6 months of age, with the older infants having a stronger immune system and being able to respond with less illness when exposed to bacteria.

Info Line

> The Office of Dietary Supplements Web site is at http://odp.od.nih.gov/.

One of the first probiotics available in test markets in the United States was Actimel by Dannon with *L casei*, 10^{10}/serving active cultures and labeled as a dietary supplement in a 100 mL bottle. For comparison, yogurt has 10^8 live bacteria.[66]

Herbal Therapy for Health Promotion

About 42% of US residents had used at least 1 form of alternative medicine in 1997 compared with 34% in 1990. College-educated females 35 to 49 years old with income > $50,000 per year were the highest users. About 70% of adults do not include their use in their health history. About 20% take prescription medication concomitantly, risking drug-drug interactions.[67-69]

Strategies exist to support families as they evaluate alternative nutrition therapies for children with special needs. Dietary supplements and nonvitamin, nonmineral supplements dramatically increased in the 1990s due to the passage of the Dietary Supplement Health and Education Act of 1994. For example, children with autism exhibit challenging behaviors, causing parents to find a solution, including alternative approaches. Any potential cure appeals. Families become vulnerable. Two modalities are (1) to augment traditional medical care for children with chronic health conditions; and (2) to recognize that herbal use commonly occurs in many cultures. Table 17–4 provides a decision tree for investigating complementary and alternative

TABLE 17–4   Decision Tree for Parents Investigating Complementary and Alternative Medicine

- What characteristics or problems are the focus? Does the treatment target these characteristics or problems?
- Are harmful side effects possible from this treatment?
- Is treatment safe for use with children?
- Are there positive effects of the proposed treatment?
- Are there short-term and long-term side effects seen with this treatment?
- What is the cost of treatment?
- Do insurance companies cover the treatment?
- How long does the treatment take?
- Are validation studies available?
- Have other parents and professionals given pros and cons about the treatment?
- Does this treatment make claims that can't be substantiated?
- Would my pediatrician give my child this therapy?

Source: Adapted from: Fields V. *Autism Advocacy in Lane County, Oregon: A Handbook for Parents and Professionals* [thesis]. Eugene, Ore: University of Oregon; 1993.

medicine (CAM). Table 17–5 lists herbs that appear either safe or potentially toxic for children. The CNP can become an integral part of the CAM therapy beginning with careful scrutiny and proceeding to the use and monitoring for nontoxic effect.[69]

Biotechnology for Improved Food

Food biotechnology uses plant science and genetics to improve food production and quality. Valuable plant traits can be moved from one plant to another, improving taste, texture, nutrition, insect resistance and production. Biotechnology can help to lower an individual's risk for chronic diseases as the fruit and vegetable content of antioxidants, vitamin C, and vitamin E can be increased. Vegetable oils may contain fewer saturated fats. Potatoes with more carbohydrates may absorb less oil during frying. Peanuts may contain fewer allergens. Appendix 17–A relates a personal statement by a leading scientist in support of biotechnology.

Table 17–5   Herbs That Appear Safe or Toxic for Use in Children

Safe Topical

Aloe for burns

Oil of cloves for tooth pain (caution: toxic if ingested)

Plantain salve for pruritus

Safe Internal

Chamomile tea for colic or stomach ache

Dandelion root syrup or tea for relaxation

Echinacea for colds

Ginger tea for mild nausea

Lemon balm tea for relaxation

Red clover tea for relaxation

Slippery elm bark tea for sore throat

Potentially Toxic

Nausea and vomiting—black alder, black cohosh, blessed thistle, buckthorn bark, and pokeweed or pokeroot.

Cardiotoxicity—aconite, bitterroot, blue cohosh, chickweed (in infants), ginseng (large doses), hawthorn (large doses), khat, licorice, *Lobelia* spp, ma huang (*Ephedra*), pokeweed or pokeroot, and yohimbe.

Hepatotoxicity—borage, chaparral, coltsfoot, comfrey, germander, *heliotropium* spp, kombucha, licorice, life root, *Lobelia* spp, pau d'arco, pennyroyal, *Petasites hydrides*, podophyllum, rue, skullcap, and *Senecio* spp.

Neurotoxicity—aconite, asafetida, bearberry, birch bark (salicylates), kava, *lobelia* spp, ma huang (*Ephedra*), pennyroyal, pokeweed, *Sophora flavescens*, willow bark (salicylates), and yohimbe.

Nephrotoxicity—*Acorus calamus*, *Aristolochia* spp, *Geranium* spp, ma huang (*Ephedra*), pennyroyal, podophyllum, and rue.

Source: Adapted from: Buck ML, Michel RS. Talking with families about herbal products. *J Pediatr.* 2000;136:673-678.

Nutrigenomics: The Rubicon of Molecular Nutrition

The successful Human Genome Project and the field of molecular biology have created a new era of medicine and nutrition. Data from the Human Genome Project will direct new drug production based on the genetic constitution of the patient. The food industry will position food and nutritional products to promote health and prevent disease based on the genetic makeup of an individual. New directions in prevention will occur, including[70]:

- *Nutrigenomics*—a focus on the effects of nutrients or food bioactives on the regulation of gene expression
- *Nutrigenetics*—the impact of variations in gene structure on one's response to nutrients or food bioactives

A challenge to the CNP is to balance the needs of the community with those of the individual. The promise of molecular nutrition should be calmed by the need to validate the scientific data emerging from the disciplines of nutrigenomics and nutrigenetics, to educate practitioners, and to communicate their value.

With the successful Human Genome Project, the ability to feed the hungry of the world and alter the health and longevity profile of the United States is likely. For example, scientists completed a genetic map of the rice plant, which is a scientific milestone that will accelerate efforts to feed the hungry by improving the world's most important food. Rice is the first crop plant whose complete genetic sequence, or genome, has been compiled and placed in computer data banks around the world. It will be a key tool for researchers working on improved strains of rice and other grains as they struggle to stay ahead of the human population growth.[71]

What Community Approaches Are Available?

The decade of the 1990s began with a healthcare system structured for acute care and crisis intervention. It depended almost exclusively on end-stage intervention (e.g., dialysis for renal failure, amputation for diabetes mellitus, or percutaneous transluminal coronary angioplasty for arteriosclerosis). This approach cannot respond efficiently to chronic disease.[72] Medical crises often reflect an individual's behavior and lifestyle. Traditional medicine does not produce positive change, and only 5% of adults with chronic disease are institutionalized. The hidden healthcare system at work sites and at home must be fueled to provide the intervention needed to alter the onset and progression of disease.[73]

Radical change in the delivery of health care services shifts certain health care activities to the individual or the consumer rather than continuing and strengthening existing services. The goal should be to support self-management or to empower individuals in the management of their own health. "In the health care policy debate, the time has come for a major conceptual shift from viewing people as consumers of health care to seeing them as they really are: its primary providers."[72(p1)] This shift in responsibility can help to control healthcare expenditures and address the largest challenge to our healthcare system—the prevention and management of chronic disease, which may include the use of complementary and alternative medicine. At the same time, based on 2003 census data, 40% of US women older than 65 years old live alone, and 41% live with a spouse. Managing their health care and remaining vital as the population ages are essential and involve health education.

In the 1940s, health education gained identity as a profession, with health education professionals following standardized training and education programs.[74] Currently, professionals can take a national exam and become a certified health education specialist. The practice of health education is founded on the following traditions[75]:

- *Pedagogy:* This emphasizes the importance of a needs assessment, instruction tailored to the progress of the learner, and instruction seeking the teachable moment. *Andragogy,* or adult education, fosters self-diagnosis of educational needs and problem-oriented instruction.[76]
- *Mass media:* This includes radio, television, newspapers, magazines, billboards, posters, and direct mail. The media in the 1930s and 1940s were used to promote public acceptance of immunizations and family planning or to promote awareness of lifestyle and health.[77]
- *The community organization:* This approach began in England in 1844 to educate the public about the sanitary problems in the growing industrial society. Three approaches to organizing a community include[78]:
  1. community development using a model that involves skills and understanding of the whole community
  2. social action, which is a response to the needs of a disadvantaged subgroup in a population by redistribution of resources (This may involve petitions, demonstrations, or boycotts.)
  3. social planning and organizational development, in which experts address social or organizational problems by discussion, debate, and planned change
- *Social psychology:* This approach applies psychological research to solving societal problems. It was the foundation for the Health Belief Model (HBM) in the late 1950s, and it directed the research agenda and attention to attitude change, persuasive communications, fear arousal, and the information-processing system. The HBM is now a model that combines psychological readiness and environmental influences.[79]
- *Group dynamics:* This approach actively involves individuals in making decisions about their own health behaviors and lifestyles. Group dynamics have been and are currently used for smoking cessation, weight management, and a variety of self-help programs.

In health education today, these diverse approaches are usually combined. The effective aspects of each add to and create an overall and potentially more powerful outcome.[80] Using mass media is one innovative primary prevention approach to teach nutrition education or general health education on a large scale. Social-marketing techniques that use mass media have become common components of nutrition education efforts. The marketing task is to sell nutrition. The immediate goal is to persuade health consumers to act. The long-range goal is for individuals or groups to learn and to integrate certain behaviors into their lifestyle.

A marketing mix comprising 4 decision areas (product, promotion, price, and distribution) is the basis of the technique. The marketing mix has been used to foster healthy eating and to encourage the food industry, health agencies, and the media to work together for a coordinated approach to nutrition education of the public.[81]

A secondary or tertiary prevention approach can be initiated in the community setting amid the private practice of a physician, registered dietitian (RD), or other healthcare professional. Although a physician may be responsible for secondary and tertiary prevention of a specific disease (e.g., hyperlipidemia and obesity), the community nutrition specialist, often an RD, can serve an important role in the healthcare process. For example, the community nutrition professional defines eating behavior goals for patients who are at increased risk of heart disease, imparts skills and knowledge to patients for improved quality of life and risk reduction, and monitors and reports success or failure of patients' efforts to the primary physician. Developing an integrated approach to medical nutrition therapy benefits not only the physician and the community nutrition professional but also the patient.[82]

The Adult Treatment Panel of the National Cholesterol Education Program provides practical dietary recommendations to reduce blood cholesterol levels of clients 2 years of age and above. It is the recommendation of the panel that medical nutrition therapy "should not be prematurely disregarded"[49] and, for most patients, "should be continued at least 6 months before deciding whether to add drug treatment."[49(p23)] The treatment involves a 2-step plan. Step 1 recommends an intake of saturated fat of less than 10% of calories, total fat of less than 30% of calories, and dietary cholesterol of no more than 300 mg/day. Step 2 emphasizes further reduction of saturated fat intake to less than 7% of calories, and dietary cholesterol to less than 200 mg/day. Movement from step 1 to step 2 involves lowering saturated and total fat and increasing carbohydrate, while stabilizing protein. Both steps promote weight loss in the overweight patient by eliminating excess fat calories.

The Framingham Heart Study (see Chapter 1) has provided a rich database to establish the risk of an adult having a heart attack in the next 10 years (see Exhibit 17–5). Major risk factors can be evaluated and an accumulative score compared with the standard to estimate the risk for males and females.

Creating effective implementation guidelines is part of the challenge. Dietary modifications must become a reality in the daily lives of individuals. An operational timeline is presented in Table 17–6 for a slightly different approach with a 3- not 2-phase program. The timeline is recommended to simplify the progression and complexity. Alteration of specific dietary components can be targeted to alter the lipid or lipoprotein aberration.[82]

No less than 3 months should be allowed for achievement of each phase. Not all individuals can make the dietary changes and retain them as a new, preferred eating behavior, even within 3 months. But after a total of 9 months, the result of a serious effort can be noted. A timeline can also blend instruction with measurement for evaluating both dietary and biochemical objectives, a combination that helps the physician and community nutrition professional to monitor each patient's goals and progress.

Public health approaches, such as reducing calories, saturated fat, and salt in processed foods and increasing community/school opportunities for physical activity, can achieve a downward shift in the distribution of a population's blood pressure (BP), thus potentially reducing morbidity, mortality, and the lifetime risk of an individual becoming hypertensive. This becomes

Exhibit 17–5 Framingham Risk Assessment Estimates of Having a Heart Attack in the Next 10 Years, Adults Ages 20 and Older With No Heart Disease or Diabetes

Note: Identify points for each risk factor, total and compare to the risk estimate in the last table.

Age (yrs)	Points for Males	Points for Females
20-34	−9	−7
35-39	−4	−3
40-44	0	0
45-49	3	3
50-54	6	6
55-59	8	8
60-64	10	10
65-69	11	12
70-74	12	14
75-79	13	16

Total Cholesterol	Age 20-39		Age 40-49		Age 50-59		Age 60-69		Age 70-79	
	M	F	M	F	M	F	M	F	M	F
< 160	0	0	0	0	0	0	0	0	0	0
160-199	4	4	3	3	2	2	1	1	0	1
200-239	7	8	5	6	3	4	1	2	0	1
240-279	9	11	6	8	4	5	2	3	1	2
≥ 280	11	13	8	10	5	7	3	4	1	2

	Age 20-39		Age 40-49		Age 50-59		Age 60-69		Age 70-79	
	M	F	M	F	M	F	M	F	M	F
Nonsmoker	0	0	0	0	0	0	0	0	0	0
Smoker	8	9	5	7	3	4	1	2	1	1

HDL (mg/dL)

	M	F
≥ 60	−1	−1
50-59	0	0
40-49	1	1
< 40	2	2

Systolic BP (mm Hg)	Male		Female	
	If untreated	If treated	If untreated	If treated
< 120	0	0	0	0
120-129	0	1	1	3

continued

Exhibit 17–5   continued

130-139	1	2	2	4
140-159	1	2	3	5
≥ 160	2	3	4	6

Points Total	10-Year Risk % Males	10-Year Risk % Females
< 0	< 1	< 1
0	1	< 1
1	1	< 1
2	1	< 1
3	1	< 1
4	1	< 1
5	2	< 1
6	2	< 1
7	3	< 1
8	4	< 1
9	5	1
10	6	1
11	8	1
12	10	1
13	12	2
14	16	2
15	20	3
16	25	4
17	≥ 30	5
18	≥ 30	6
19	≥ 30	8
20	≥ 30	11
21	≥ 30	14
22	≥ 30	17
23	≥ 30	22
24	≥ 30	27
25	≥ 30	≥ 30
≥ 25	≥ 30	≥ 30

Source: Reprinted from *Framingham Risk Assessment Heart Memo.* Bethesda, Md: National Heart, Lung and Blood Institute, National Institute of Health; Winter 2002:22.

especially critical as the increase in BMI of Americans has reached epidemic levels. With 122 million adults overweight or obese, BP is likely to escalate with related conditions.[83] The Joint National Committee Report 7 (JNC 7) endorses the American Public Health Association resolution that the food

TABLE 17–6 Timeline for Introducing Selected Dietary Components for Secondary Intervention of Hyperlipidemia

Activity/Instruction	Phase I (Months)			Phase II (Months)			Phase III (Months)		
	1	2	3	4	5	6	7	8	9
Assessment*									
Anthropometric	X	X	X	X	X	X	X	X	X
Record of food intake	X	X			X		X		
Computerized analysis of food intake			X			X		X	
Lipid/lipoprotein determination				X			X		X
Instructions									
Energy reduction	X		X		X			X	X
Fat modification									
• Total fat	X	X		X			X		
• Fat ratios		X		X			X		X
Cholesterol		X					X		X
Alcohol			X	X		X			
Complex CHO			X	X			X		
Fiber			X					X	

*Initial visit after evaluation of serum lipids/lipoproteins.
Source: Frank GC. Nutritional therapy for hyperlipidemia and obesity: office treatment integrating the roles of the physician and the registered dietitian. *J Am Coll Cardiol.* 1998;12(4):1098-1100. Reprinted with permission of the Helen Dwight Reid Educational Foundation. Published by Heldref Publications, 1319 18th Street NW, Washington, DC 20036-1802.

manufacturers and restaurants reduce sodium in the food supply by 50% over the next decade. When public health intervention strategies address the diversity of racial, ethnic, cultural, linguistic, religious, and social factors in the delivery of their services, the likelihood of their acceptance by the community increases. These public health approaches can provide an attractive opportunity to interrupt and prevent the continuing costly cycle of managing hypertension and its complications.

Another vicious cycle challenging prevention is tackling multiple conditions in the same individuals. A challenge for the 21st century is improving the quality of life by minimizing multiple health conditions. In fact, 39 million adults face 2 or more conditions that interfere with their life's activities. Forty-eight percent of US adults, 45–64 years old, and 65% of adults > 65 years old, report accomplishing less than they would like in a day. Among those with 2 or more chronic conditions, the proportion reporting accomplishing less is nearly 4 times greater than that reported by those the same age without a chronic condition.[84]

As communities strive to establish integrated delivery systems that are both formal and informal, different types of ownership and organizational structures exist. Effective collaboration among several organizations may be competitive or cooperative, but cooperative relationships are desired.[85]

Info Line

The First International Conference on Food Synergy was held in Washington, DC, in May 2001. The theme of this conference was the complex nature of foods and the many additive and synergistic interactions that occur among food constituents like fiber, nutrients, and phytochemicals that impact disease risk.

Meeting objectives were as follows:

1. to recognize the complex nature of foods and the important biochemical interactions among food constituents that affect health
2. to summarize the scientific status of food synergy research and identify future research priorities
3. to position the consumption of fruits, vegetables, nuts, whole grains, and other healthful foods, rather than individual food components, as the primary dietary approach to disease prevention

High-risk subgroups have poorer health status than other individuals and face multiple barriers to health services. Even when health services are available and accessible, the style in which providers and patients interact can affect their attitudes, behaviors, and health status. Health promotion programs and partnership can improve the health status of these high-risk groups. When community organizations and CNPs understand the most effective way to build collaboration, new and original approaches to improving health of special populations and reducing health disparities between these groups can occur.[85-87]

Interventions to Enhance Eating Behaviors

Behavioral approaches should be carefully planned to fit into primary, secondary, and tertiary prevention programs and to appeal to health-conscious consumers in light of their personal characteristics, geographic area, ethnic foods, festivals, and opportunities for physical activity. Communication techniques are essential (see Exhibit 17–6). Initial components of a medical nutrition therapy program include a 1-year timeline, a computerized food intake analysis, a weight and cholesterol grid, and sound educational materials.

The healthcare professional should make a diligent effort to make no changes until 6 to 10 patients have completed the program. The 3 main reasons physicians give for not initiating medical nutritional services are perceived lack of patient interest, lack of a patient goal, and nonadherence to the service.[88] A structured program provides direction for the patient and permits evaluation by the clinician and community nutrition professional.

Computerized Analysis of Food Intake

Assessment has 2 purposes. It indicates adherence to dietary change, and it is an educational tool to direct further change. Computerized analysis of usual

Exhibit 17–6   Counseling Techniques to Improve Communication and Adherence for Behavioral Change

---

- Listening
- Identifying behaviors
- Values clarification
- Feelings assessment
- Self-directed treatment
- Confrontation
- Steps 1, 2, 3
- Relapse prevention
- Cognitive/reality therapy
- Mirroring
- Positive affirmation
- Behavior modification
- Written assignments
- Visualization
- Laughter therapy

Source: Adapted from: Beckley L. *Taking Control: Diet, Drug Abuse and Addiction.* Ashland, Ore: Nutrition Dimension; 1990.

---

food intake is a practical way to evaluate dietary adherence. Using a computerized analysis system, one can ask and answer specific questions, such as the following:

- Is total fat approaching 30% of the total energy intake?
- Is there an increase in complex versus simple carbohydrates?

The DINE System, a computerized database that clinicians and patients have used fairly extensively, produces a record for the medical chart and a handout for the patient. The handout is tangible and helps the patient to refine and alter specific food choices before the next office visit.[89]

Individuals tend to consume set meals once they find foods and recipes they like within the allowed food list. The first follow-up food record should be incorporated on the timeline about 2 weeks after the initial consultation. The record may illustrate a common practice noted among clients (e.g., consumption of modular 300- to 500-kcal entrees, which clients buy, freeze, and cook in the microwave oven in a few minutes in the evening or at work).

Although the sodium content may be prohibitive (in excess of 750 to 1,000 mg per entree) and the fat type more saturated than desired, the frozen meals are practical. Fish and fowl entrees can be selected to reduce saturated fat, and, if the entree is high in sodium, high-sodium foods can be avoided during the remainder of the day. When possible, individuals should be allowed to make gradual changes and to make food choices they can live with daily, rather than being forbidden from trying new alternatives and food products. Aiding individuals to make cumulative changes increases the likelihood of dietary success (see Exhibit 17–7). It also increases the likelihood that clients will continue to come in for follow-up visits because they know a receptive rather than a restrictive environment exists.

Exhibit 17–7   A Self-Contract as Contingency Plan to Commit to Small
Behavioral Changes

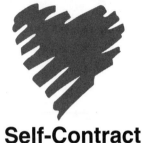

Heart-Healthy Eating

Self-Contract

I, _____, agree with the following
small steps to reduce my fat intake.

❑ I pledge to use the Food Guide Pyramid *twice a week* to
choose foods to make a healthy meal.

❑ I pledge to eat a fruit or vegetable for a snack *every day*.

❑ I pledge to select low fat foods *more often* and my favorite
high fat food, _____, only *once a week*.

Within the next 4 weeks, by _____ , I'll be following
these pledges *regularly*.

If I do, I will reward myself with/by _____
_____.

If I do not, I will *revise the contract and start over.*

_____   _____
Signature   Date

_____   _____
Witness   Date

Weight and Cholesterol Grids

Although charting body weights has been common for decades, clients do
not seem to be motivated by a chart on file. It is important to emphasize eating behavior changes to produce permanent weight loss, rather than mere
pounds off. A weight chart can be an effective teaching tool. For example,

on initial eating behavior instruction, the community nutrition professional can chart the patient's current weight and project the weight at 6 or 9 months. Using a 2-lb (0.9 kg) weight loss per week as an example, one can place an asterisk on the graph 6 months in the future, showing a projected 24-lb (11-kg) weight loss. One copy can be retained for the chart and another given to the client. Recommend that the client tape the chart near the scale at home and graph his or her weight once a week. This technique shifts the responsibility for weight loss to the patient rather than the community nutrition professional. Further, it defines a manageable goal, rather than merely saying, "You have to lose weight." The same instructional technique can be used with a cholesterol grid.

Educational Materials

There are many diet books on the market. RDs should recommend the nutritionally sound ones, so interested and skilled clients can make sizable, long-term changes in their eating patterns. The American Diabetes Association/American Dietetic Association *Exchange Lists for Meal Planning* is an excellent, user-friendly guide for energy, fat, and carbohydrate modifications.[90]

The American Dietetic Association (ADA) forged a new partnership to bring comprehensive and reliable nutrition information to millions of Internet users searching for healthcare information. ADA provides information for WebMD's Food and Nutrition Channel, one of the site's most frequented areas. To view this site, see www.webmd.com/nutrition. In addition, ADA supports position papers on key nutrition and health topics, for different stages of life and for target groups such as women and their well-being.

Positions of the American Dietetic Association and Dietitians of Canada: Women's Health and Nutrition and Nutrition Across the Spectrum of Aging

Women's health today addresses the prevention, diagnosis, and management of diseases unique to women and includes the woman's emotional, social, cultural, spiritual, and physical well-being. Nutritional well-being may influence the etiology and treatment of most causes of death in women. Understanding the nutritional components of women's health to deliver media messages and MNT materials for clients is essential in today's healthcare market in every community.[91]

Older Americans should be able to receive coordinated, comprehensive food and nutrition services and medical nutrition therapies across their aging spectrum. Food and water and nutritional well-being are essential to their health, self-sufficiency, and quality of life. Sound nutritional services are essential if older Americans are to remain fully independent and actively engaged in their communities.[92]

Broad Strokes

When concentrating on interventions to enhance eating behavior objectives, primary, secondary, and tertiary prevention are needed in an integrative, comprehensive manner (see Figure 17–1). A worksheet to identify primary,

UNDERSTANDING LEVEL

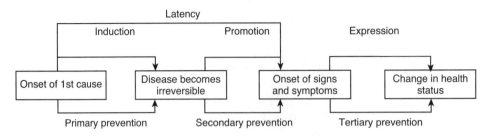

FIGURE 17-1 A model to blend understanding of disease progression with levels of intervention.
Source: Adapted from: Kleinbaum DG, Kupper LL. *Epidemiologic Research: Principles and Quantitative Methods Solution Manual.* Lifetime Learning Publications; Wiley Publishers; 1982:22. Used with permission.

secondary, and tertiary prevention approaches to reduce risk specific to a disease is presented in Exhibit 17-8. One axis lists the approach, and the other axis lists different age-specific groups. Examples of approaches for different chronic diseases addressing primary, secondary, or tertiary intervention are outlined in Appendix 17-B.

Using a health index based on motor vehicle deaths, crime rates, infant mortality, the prevalence of heart disease and smoking, and healthcare access, Americans' overall health has improved by 2.6% since 1999 and 17.6% since 1990. New Hampshire, Minnesota, and Vermont are the healthiest states in the nation, while Mississippi, Louisiana, and South Carolina are ranked at the bottom, as shown in Table 17-7. The states with the largest overall health improvements were Arkansas, Hawaii, Delaware, Montana, South Dakota, and Utah. Those with the greatest decline are Indiana, Wisconsin, Illinois, and Wyoming.[93]

Exhibit 17-8 Disease Exploration and Prevention—A Worksheet to Identify and Define the Community Nutrition Approach for Different Age Groups

Target Disease: _____

Prevention/Treatment Approach	*Infant/ Preschooler*	*Youth*	*Adult*	*Older Adult*
Primary				
Secondary				
Tertiary				

TABLE 17–7   Ranking of 50 States by Health Index

Rank	State	Pct. +/–
1	Minnesota	21.2
2	Vermont	20.5
3	New Hampshire	18.9
4	Hawaii	17.9
5	Connecticut	17.2
6	Utah	16.3
7	Massachusetts	15.3
8	North Dakota	15.0
9	Maine	13.7
10	Wisconsin	13.3
11	Iowa	12.5
12	Nebraska	12.4
13	Rhode Island	11.4
14	New Jersey	11.0
15	Washington	10.2
16	Colorado	8.9
17	Kansas	7.9
18	South Dakota	7.5
19	Idaho	6.5
19	Oregon	6.5
21	Virginia	5.7
22	Montana	4.9
23	California	4.7
23	Wyoming	4.7
25	Illinois	3.7
25	Ohio	3.7
27	Michigan	2.3
28	Pennsylvania	1.8
29	New York	1.1
30	Delaware	-0.6
31	Alaska	-0.8
32	Maryland	-2.7
33	Indiana	-3.7
34	Arizona	-4.0
35	Missouri	-4.1
36	North Carolina	-4.3

continued

TABLE 17–7   continued

Rank	State	Pct. +/–
37	Texas	-4.7
38	Nevada	-8.4
39	Kentucky	-10.1
40	New Mexico	-10.4
41	Florida	-10.6
42	Georgia	-11.7
43	West Virginia	-12.8
44	Oklahoma	-13.1
45	Alabama	-14.8
46	Arkansas	-16.1
47	Tennessee	-16.2
48	South Carolina	-16.4
49	Mississippi	-19.9
50	Louisiana	-20.4

Funding for Health Services

During the past decade, the US House and Senate have passed labor, health and human services, and education appropriation bills to alter chronic disease. Highlights are as follows:

National Institutes of Health:

- The National Heart, Lung, and Blood Institute has received appropriations of over $2.3 billion annually second only to National Cancer Institute funding.
- The National Institute of Neurological Disorders and Stroke receives appropriations of nearly $1.2 billion annually.
- Funding for new centers, such as the John E. Porter Neuroscience Research Center, and support for the National Center for Minority Health and Health Disparities continue.

Centers for Disease Control and Prevention:

- CDC's chronic and environmental disease prevention line receives over $400 million annually.
- Funding to $35 million includes annual increases for the Cardiovascular Health Program.
- Funding for the Paul Coverdell (US Senator who died from a stroke) National Acute Stroke Registry continues to track and improve the delivery of care to patients with strokes.
- Funding averaging $100 million for CDC's tobacco control initiatives and $16 million for nutrition/physical activity efforts continues.
- The WISEWOMAN program, which provides low-income and uninsured women with screening for heart disease and stroke risk factors in

addition to screening for breast and cervical cancer, continues expansion beyond 15 states.
- $125 million provided for a National Campaign to Change Children's Health Behaviors, with childhood obesity prevention as a lifelong goal to create good health.
- $35 million annually for health disparities demonstration projects.

Another national initiative is CDC's Cardiovascular Health Program, which covers 25 states with planning grants and the Physical Education for Progress (PEP) Act. It received a $5 million appropriation for grants to help initiate, expand, and improve physical education programs for kindergarten through 12th-grade students. Funds can be used to purchase equipment, develop curriculum, hire and/or train PE staff, and support other initiatives designed to enable students to participate in physical education activities. The bill authorizes $400 million over 5 years.

However, health benefits of physical activity continue to take center stage when trying to lower risk. Moderate amounts of physical activity can reduce the risk of premature mortality from all causes.[94] Regular physical activity improves the function of muscles and joints, achieving peak bone mass, fine-tuning metabolic homeostasis, achieving endocrine and immunologic health, and enhancing mental health. Regular physical activity activities like leisure-time and work-related activities may provide health benefits. Habitual physical activity is inversely related to the incidence of obesity, type 2 diabetes mellitus, and cardiovascular disease, and physical activity may improve appetite control.[95] Regular physical activity induces favorable metabolic changes in muscle and adipose tissue promoting fat or energy rather than storing it[96] (see Table 17–8).

Benefits of physical activity include the following:

Reducing Incidence of Type 2 Diabetes—Physical activity enhances insulin sensitivity and improves glucose tolerance. Participation in lifestyle modification programs including increasing physical activity leads to a reduced incidence of the disease.[97,98]

Decreasing Cardiovascular Disease—Engaging in regular exercise or moderate physical activity improves circulating lipid profiles and favorably alters lipoprotein metabolism, decreases blood pressure, reduces blood coagulation and platelet aggregation, and decreases risk of cardiac arrhythmias.[99]

Mental Well-Being—More frequent occupational and leisure-time physical activity is associated with reduced symptoms of depression, especially among women.

Improving Cognitive Function—Lifelong, regular exercise can result in cognitive enhancements. Programs that combine strength and aerobic training have a stronger effect on cognitive performance than aerobic training alone. Some studies show that adherence for 6 months to a regular exercise regimen of 45-60 minutes per session has a beneficial effect.[100]

Prevention of Chronic Diseases—Thirty minutes of physical activity of moderate intensity every day of the week uses 150 kcal per day or 1,000 kcal per week and may decrease diabetes and cardiovascular disease.[101]

Weight Control—Physical activity is important for weight loss but is most effective when combined with appropriate food changes. To prevent weight regain following significant weight loss, energy expenditure has been reported to range between 300 and 400 kcal per day.[102]

TABLE 17–8   Health Benefit Realized From Regular Physical Activity

Health Concern	Benefit
Cardiovascular health	Improves performance of the heart as a muscle
	Increases heart muscle contraction
	Reduces premature ventricular contractions
	Improves blood lipoprotein levels
	Increase aerobic capacity
	Reduces systolic and diastolic blood pressure
	Improves endurance
Obesity	Reduces abdominal adipose tissue and overall body fat
	Increases lean muscle mass
Lipoproteins/glucose intolerance	Reduces low-density cholesterol, lipoproteins, and triglycerides
	Increases high-density lipoproteins and glucose tolerance
Osteoporosis	Slows loss of bone mineral density
	Increases bone density
Psychological well-being	Improves quality of life, feeling well and happy
	Increases levels of catechloamines, norepinephrine, and serotonin
Muscle weakness and functional capacity	Ruduces risk of musculoskeletal disability
	Improves strength and flexiblity
	Reduces risk of falls and fractures with increased muscle strength
	Increases reaction time, quadriceps strength
	Sustains blood flow of the brain and cognition

Source: Adapted from: The Robert Wood Johnson Foundation. *National Blueprint: Increasing Physical Activity Among Adults Age 50 and Older.* Princeton, NJ: The Robert Wood Johnson Foundation; 2003:16.

Prevention of Adult Weight Gain—To prevent weight gain, regular physical activity must be moderate to vigorous in intensity and associated with improvements in physical fitness. Energy expended in daily physical activity must be at least 80% of resting energy expenditure, which is equal to an additional 60 to 90 minutes of brisk walking for moderately active adults.[103]

Reducing Television Watching—Sedentary behavior like watching television is associated with an increased risk of becoming overweight or obese and developing type 2 diabetes mellitus or cardiovascular disease. Television viewing has the strongest association with obesity compared with reading, working at a computer, or driving in a car. Even in the most physically active people, incidence of overweight increased as the hours of television viewing increased.[104]

Tools for Measuring Energy Expenditure

The doubly labeled water stable isotope method is the gold standard for measuring TEE of free-living people. Two stable isotopes, deuterium and oxygen-18, are drunk in water and tracked for their elimination rates from the body. Limitations of the doubly labeled water method include cost (about $1,500/person) for specialized equipment, and expertise to implement the technique.

The 2002 Dietary Reference Intake Committee devised TEE predictive equations based on published doubly labeled water data for 407 normal-weight and overweight/obese adults. Although the equations have not been validated, they are suitable for prediction of energy requirements for normal-weight groups, overweight/obese groups, and in mixed groups containing normal-weight and overweight/obese adults.[105]

Basal Metabolic Rate and Resting Metabolic Rate

For the determination of oxygen consumption and carbon dioxide production, respiratory gas exchange is measured by sampling expired breath and analyzing its oxygen and carbon dioxide content. The rate of oxygen consumption (VO_2) and carbon dioxide production (VCO_2) are changed to units of energy expenditure (kilocalories per minutes) using this equation:

$$kcal/min = (3.941 \times VO_2) + (1.106 \times VCO_2) - (2.17 \times urinary\ nitrogen)$$

VO_2 and VCO_2 units are liters per minute and urinary nitrogen units are grams per minute. An inexpensive alternative to using indirect calorimetry for the determination of basal metabolic rate (BMR) or resting metabolic rate (RMR) is applying predictive equations based on a person's age, height, and weight. The Mifflin equation provides the most accurate predictive power for nonobese persons, with about 80% of predictions accurate within $\pm 10\%$ of measured values.[106]

The Mufflin equation for RMR:

For men: $(10 \times w) + (6.25 \times h) - (5 \times a) + 5$

For women: $(10 \times w) + (6.25 \times h) - (5 \times a) - 161$

Where:
w = weight in kg
h = height in cm
a = age

Physical Activity Energy Expenditure

Measuring physical activity blends many movements but involves the challenge of self-report. Objective measurement of different dimensions of motion (type, duration, intensity) and subjective reporting are not perfect. For increased accuracy, investigators often combine 2 or more methods. A questionnaire describes the physical activity pattern that the person considers important and desirable; whereas motion sensors provide an actual measure of activity.[106]

- Self-Report—This format includes questionnaires, interviews, and activity diaries. Questionnaires and interviews measure occupational versus leisure activity and assign scores that are changed to general activity levels or specific energy expenditure values. Guidelines are available for using

information derived from questionnaires to select an appropriate physical
activity level factor in calculating TEE. Large-scale epidemiologic studies
that study the relationship between activity and health typically use telephone and/or computer-assisted surveys or written questionnaires to
characterize habitual physical activity in a population.[107]

- **Motion Sensors**—A variety of electronic and mechanical devices that
  include pedometers (step counters) and accelerometers (acceleration
  detectors) measure total body displacement in a motion.
- **Physiologic Response Measurement**—Heart rate monitoring describes
  the intensity and duration of physical activity, which can be converted
  into heart rate data as an estimate of energy expenditure.
- **New Developments**—A digital activity log allows individuals to record
  the type and duration of physical activities for 7 categories of activity
  (based on metabolic energy METs) in increments of 5 minutes. The
  Intelligence Device for Energy Expenditure and Activity is an accelerometer that describes the type and the amount of movement. It is worn
  on the hip and wire extensions connect to the feet, legs, and chest. Validity and reliability studies are positive.[108] The SenseWear Armband is a
  portable device worn on the upper arm that contains an accelerometer,
  temperature sensors, and a receiver to record heart rate.[109]

Broad strokes with a population approach are needed to shift US eating patterns to a healthier track and to insult the chronic disease process. Figure 17–2
illustrates the declining US mortality between 1950 and 1996 and the increasing life expectancy. These result from broad strokes of change. The major health
education framework currently used to orchestrate change in morbidity and
mortality is the PRECEDE model. This stands for predisposing, reinforcing, and
enabling constructs that can be used to diagnose and evaluate any education
and behavior-oriented intervention. PRECEDE is considered a diagnostic framework. Four disciplines are innate to the framework: epidemiology, social and
behavioral sciences, management, and education. Application of the PRECEDE
model involves working through 7 steps[80]:

1. Assess the social problems in the target group.
2. Identify specific health problems that contribute.
3. Identify the specific health-related behaviors (e.g., cigarette smoking,
   nonadherence) that are causally linked to the health problems.
4. Identify the factors that influence performance of specified health-
   related behaviors: *predisposing factors* (i.e., attitudes, beliefs, values,
   perceptions); *enabling factors* (i.e., supportive forces within the system);
   and *reinforcing factors* (i.e., social support from family, peers, and
   health professionals).
5. Set priorities, choosing from among the various factors as the nucleus
   of the intervention.
6. Develop and implement the intervention.
7. Evaluate the intervention for achievement of program objectives.

The PRECEDE framework can be applied to any health problem, but
often the process for change is limited to clinical trials or demonstrating
studies and not total community approaches. For example, several clinical
trials demonstrate that a basic low-fat eating pattern is feasible and that

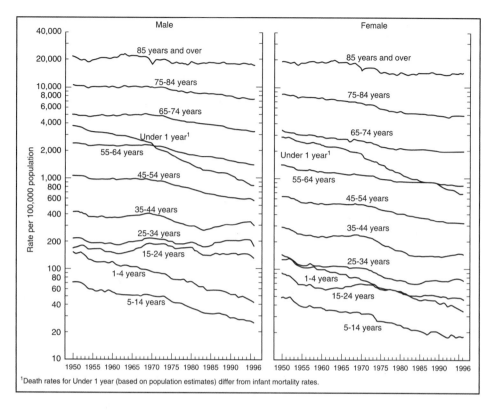

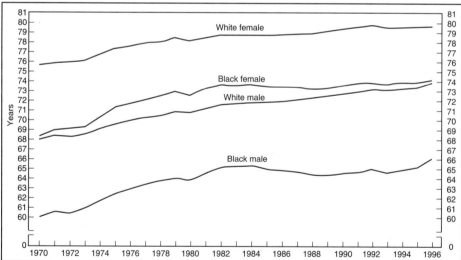

FIGURE 17–2 Death rates (A) and life expectancy (B) for US males and females

individuals can follow the pattern and create a new way of eating. If dietary cholesterol is limited to 100 mg/day, saturated fat is kept to 5–6% of total calories, and fish is eaten a minimum of twice a week, then a maximum lowering of LDL cholesterol can occur.

Dietary studies in free-living individuals show that an eating pattern reflecting a step 1 diet reduces serum cholesterol by 3–14%.[4] Dietary equations such as those developed by Keys[3] and Hegsted and colleagues[3,110-111] predict that the step 1 diet will reduce total cholesterol levels by 5-7% in men who consume an average of 13-14% of their calories as saturated fat. An additional 3-7% reduction in serum total cholesterol is anticipated by following a step 2 diet.

Although data are limited for women, projections are that women would respond to a low-fat eating pattern. Focused research in clinical trials such as the Women's Health Initiative (see Chapter 9) is necessary to answer the question of how postmenopausal women respond to heart-healthy eating when their CHD risk normally escalates with age. Data from the 12-year clinical trial are now surfacing in the literature as evidence-based research of the highest quality and may alter healthcare practice of the future generation of women. Knowledge of the synergy of body weight hormones and breast cancer are of major interest.

Success in reducing the fat content of one's eating pattern may also be linked to one's stage of change. The circulating levels of both estrone and estradiol are positively correlated with body weight in postmenopausal women, and obesity-related elevations in these estrogens have been associated with increased cancer risk.

Obesity also affects the proportion of total circulating estradiol that is available to exert its biological effects on breast tissue. Normally, estrogen bioactivity is rendered disengaged when bound to sex hormone-binding globulin (SHBG). Some is weakly bound to albumin, from which it easily dissociates, and 1-2% circulates as unbound free estradiol. Both of these are biologically available. The level of plasma SHBG is inversely correlated with body weight. Elevations are in the bioactive estradiol, which may contribute to the increased breast cancer risk among obese postmenopausal women.[112]

Behavioral change is considered dynamic and reflects 5 stages[113]:

1. Precontemplation—Individual has no intention of changing.
2. Contemplation—Individual seriously considers change.
3. Preparation—Individual makes decisions and commitments to change.
4. Action—Individual makes distinguishable efforts toward change.
5. Maintenance—Person enters a period of behavior stabilization.

Understanding whether individuals are changing or resistant to change appears to be a new and enlightening variable for successful medical nutrition therapy. Structural variables for change may be as visible as informative food labels. For example, the Nutrition Labeling and Education Act of 1990 requires a listing of the fat, saturated fat, and cholesterol composition of foods. Listing of trans fat content was required in 2006. Any food manufacturer who makes a claim about specific food and its association with a chronic condition such as heart disease is required to print the claim in a certain format (see Chapter 2). Educating the public about food labels and how to apply the nutrient content to food choices and health promotion must be continuous and consistent.

Blending daily food choices for each age-specific group within the age spectrum with quantity and quality guides such as those in *My Pyramid* is an elemental and instructive action toward healthy eating for individuals and their families. Although many guides are available to the public, guides for healthful eating out are limited.

Busy schedules, travel, 2-career families, socializing, celebration, relaxation, and convenience have made dining out a way of life. According to the National Restaurant Association, Americans eat away from home an average of 4-5 times per week, with almost 47% of each food dollar spent in restaurants. By the year 2010, it is projected that 53% of each food dollar will be spent away from home.[114,115]

Eating away from home has been associated with consuming more high-fat foods and fewer healthy ones. Eating out is also identified as a principal barrier to eating the recommended 4 to 5 servings of fruits and vegetables per day. Obesity is linked to eating in restaurants and fast-food places, not only because many of the menu choices are calorie-dense, but also because diners consume *oversized* portions of these calorie-dense foods, often 2 to 3 times the size of meals served in previous decades.[116-118]

In California, *Healthy Dining*, a team of nutrition and social marketing professionals, has analyzed the nutrition content of over 10,000 restaurant meals from California restaurants and found that most restaurant meals contain 1,000-2,000 calories and 50-150 grams of fat—more fat than most people should consume in a whole day. The challenge is for restaurant diners to know what they are consuming, when it comes to nutrition. The Center for Science in the Public Interest (CSPI) and New York University reported studies in which dietitians and nutritionists were asked to estimate fat and calorie content of several restaurant dishes. The estimates ranged from 50 to 70% of the actual values. When food professionals can't accurately estimate calorie content accurately in a plate of food, challenges for the average consumer are magnified with each restaurant order.[119]

Since 1990, *Healthy Dining* has led an effort with hundreds of restaurants in Southern California to promote healthier choices. Increased fruit and vegetable consumption and reduced fat, calorie, cholesterol, and sodium consumption are encouraged by their series of *Healthy Dining* Restaurant Guide books, available for San Diego, Los Angeles, and Orange Counties.[120-124]

A recent innovation in 2004, *Healthy Dining* linked to the Centers for Disease Control and Prevention (CDC) to expand the program nationwide via a Web site (see Figure 17–3). The Web site, available at www.healthydiningfinder.com, enables restaurant consumers to search for restaurants that provide nutritious, healthful options, based on criteria such as zip code, type of cuisine, and price range. A detailed breakdown of nutrition information is included for each menu item featured on the Web site. The *Healthy Dining* program combines contemporary lifestyle trends of dining out, nutrition interest, and the Internet to reach Americans who eat out frequently.

Spectrum of Prevention: A Model for Public Health Planning

Individual education aimed at changing behavior is not enough to effectively prevent illness or injury. Programs must address environmental factors, which are some of the largest determinants of health status, and actively involve the community in planning and implementing activities. Spectrum of Prevention is a framework for development of multilevel public health programs that integrate client, professional, organizational, and communitywide efforts.

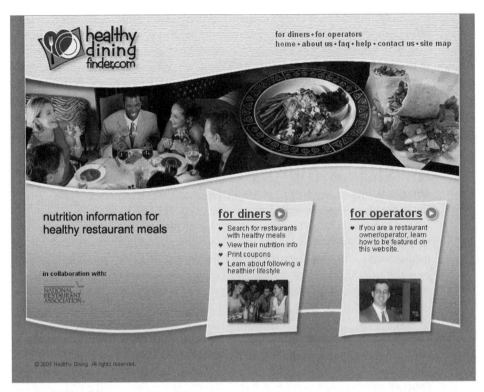

Roasted Chicken Pasta										
with portabello mushrooms, garlic, tomatoes and basil.										
Fruit/Veg (cups)	Calories	Fat (g)	Sat Fat (g)	Trans Fat (g)	Cholest (mg)	Sodium (mg)	Carbs (g)	Fiber (g)	Sugars (g)	Protein (g)
2	595	26	5.5	N/A	100	325*	43	4	N/A	43

Oak Grilled Swordfish										
Swordfish marinated in lemongrass, soy ginger and garlic, served with sautéed Asian vegetables. Analysis includes plain baked potato.										
Fruit/Veg (cups)	Calories	Fat (g)	Sat Fat (g)	Trans Fat (g)	Cholest (mg)	Sodium (mg)	Carbs (g)	Fiber (g)	Sugars (g)	Protein (g)
2	630	12	3	N/A	80	300*	81	11	N/A	49

FIGURE 17–3 Web site (A) and example of nutrient content of restaurant menu items, Healthy Dining (B).
Source: Used with permission from Anita Jones. Healthy Dining. Available at http://newsletter@healthy-dining.com. Accessed February 1, 2007.

The spectrum ranges from some of the more familiar interventions such as individual and community education to long-term solutions such as legislative and policy changes. Aspects of the spectrum are dependent upon and interrelated to one another. Legislation cannot be enacted and implemented without well-informed, vocal, involved, and committed individuals working together. By combining these approaches, a preventive health program builds on the strengths of each and promotes permanent, effective change. The whole becomes greater than the sum of its parts.[125]

A working model for service providers exists to demonstrate primary prevention in the community. Community-directed models usually aim to promote planning and implementation of scientifically acceptable, preventive interventions. The models are strengthened by real-life settings and attention to research requirements and practical issues facing community members and healthcare providers. Community models serve as the basis for intervention programs amid challenges of the scientific community. A common question is, "Is the intervention supported by valid baseline data, and will the outcome withstand an evaluation?" Challenges from the recipient community include those from individuals who need to know if their important needs are met, if their rights are protected, what they must pay, and what they receive.[126,127]

The community-directed model provides an umbrella for thought (e.g., the scope, the players, the program, and the potential outcome). The model requires evaluating why certain actions are proposed and who should be involved in each component. In the model, multilevel programmatic and evaluation decisions are enumerated. The process saddles the various activities and yields a comprehensible program. The model promotes an open forum for discussion of skills and approaches. As the magnitude of the program is understood, alternate strategies can be compared to identify their various levels of success. The Spectrum of Prevention, a community model that has been adopted by the Prevention Program of Contra Costa County Health Services Department in California, is described below.[125]

Level 1 involves strengthening individual knowledge and skills. Health education programs are designed to reach out to individuals at risk of disease and encourage them to change their behavior. Such educational efforts provide information and opportunities to learn new skills and/or change attitudes. As a common example, adolescents are taught the basics of good nutrition and how to plan healthy menus.

Level 2 involves educating the community. A well-coordinated, multidimensional campaign raises community awareness about a particular health issue. Assessing the perceptions of healthcare professionals and community members about the nutritional needs of the community may target education (see Chapter 1). Events, posters, and use of mass media deliver a specific, integrated message. For example, the prevention program sponsors an annual healthy holiday open house in November. The event provides the community with free samples of healthy holiday foods and recipes, gives community members an opportunity to learn about nutrition programs in the county, and generates extensive media coverage that reaches a broad audience of citizens and community leaders.

Level 3 trains providers. Any preventive approach needs the cooperation and aid of existing healthcare providers and other service providers. Providers have regular contact with people at risk and can encourage adoption of healthy behavior and screen for additional risks. They can help improve community education, change policies within their institutions, and advocate for legislation. Many providers who work with children and adolescents do not know the importance of good nutrition or sound nutrition behaviors.

Level 4 builds coalitions. Coalitions combine individual and organizational strengths in new ways. Coalitions and other networking activities also lend themselves to maximizing community resources. Through the work of local coalitions, the national Project LEAN program has been effective in spreading a low-fat eating message through the local media.

Level 5 changes organizational practices and environments. Established organizations can directly change their policies that affect the health of their members/clients. The local Department of Social Services office in Contra Costa allowed the prevention program to insert flyers with the June Aid to Families with Dependent Children (AFDC) checks. These flyers promoted free summer lunches for eligible children. As a result, there was a 25% increase in participation in the free meals program. Another agency in the county established a healthy snacks policy for its employees; the daily doughnut break became a bagel and fruit break.

Level 6 is directed toward influencing policy and legislation. Legislation and policy represent perhaps the strongest and broadest means for bringing about environmental changes to decrease the incidence of illness in a community. For example, local communities can institute policies and legislation mandating the availability of federal food programs for low-income children.

A threefold delivery approach using a population-based health promotion model poses interventions at the individual, the population, and the macro-level[128,129] (see Table 17–9).

TABLE 17–9   Threefold Delivery Approach With a Population-Based Health Promotion Model

Delivery Channel	Description	Suggested Activities
Downstream	Individual-level interventions for those with risk factors or diagnosed with risk-related diseases or conditions: obesity, diabetes, syndrome X. Emphasis on changing, rather than preventing, health-damaging behaviors.	- Group or individual counseling - Client-centered health-education and cognitive/behavioral restructuring - Self-help programs and tailored health messages
Midstream	Population-level interventions for defined populations with emphasis of changing or preventing health-damaging behaviors. May involve mediation with important organizational channels or natural environments.	- Work-site and community-based health promotion and disease prevention programs - Primary care screening and intervention programs for communities and all ages - Community-based interventions focused on defined risk and target group: sodium reduction programs for older adults
Upstream	Macro-level state and national public policy and environmental interventions to strengthen social norms and support healthy behaviors. Goal is to redirect unhealthy societal and industry actions.	- National public education and media campaigns - Economic incentives: reimbursement for health behavior change treatment - Policies reducing access to unhealthy products: pricing, access, product design - Policies reducing advertising and promotion of unhealthy products and behaviors

Source: Adapted from: McKinlay JB. In: Heikkinen E, Ruoppila I, Krusinen J, eds. *Preparation for Aging.* London: Plenum Press; 1995:306 pages; and The Robert Wood Johnson Foundation. *National Blueprint: Increasing Physical Activity Among Adults Age 50 and Older.* Princeton, NJ: The Robert Wood Johnson Foundation; 2003:21.

Formulating nutrition policy to instill positive changes at the national and state levels can complement grassroots efforts and make the *Healthy People 2010* objectives a reality in the United States. *Healthy People 2010* objectives have been specified by Congress as the measure for assessing the progress of the Indian Health Care Improvement Act, the Maternal and Child Health Block Grant, and the Preventive Health and Health Services Block Grant. Healthy People objectives have also been used in performance measurement activities of managed care organizations in the areas of immunizations, mammography screening, and other clinical preventive services.

To encourage groups to integrate *Healthy People 2010* into current programs, special events, publications, and meetings, all *Healthy People 2010* materials are in the public domain. *Healthy People 2010* is used by healthy community coalitions. Businesses use the framework to guide work-site health promotion activities as well as community initiatives. Schools and colleges undertake activities to further the health of children, adolescents, and young adults. By selecting from the national objectives, individuals and organizations can build an agenda for community health improvement and monitor results.[50]

References

1. Berenson GS, McMahan CA, Voors AW, et al. *Cardiovascular Risk Factors in Children.* New York: Oxford University Press; 1980.
2. Connor S. *Facing Fats: The Dietary Challenge of the 90's. Nutritional Medicine in Medical Practice.* Los Angeles, Calif: UCLA Clinical Research Center; January 1993.
3. Keys A, Anderson JT, Grande F. Prediction of serum cholesterol responses of man to changes in fats in the diet. *Lancet.* 1957;ii:959-966.
4. Caggiula AW, Christakis G, Farrand M, et al. The Multiple Risk Factor Intervention Trial (MRFIT), IV: intervention on blood lipids. *Prev Med.* 1981;10:443.
5. Gordon T, Kagan A, Garcia-Palmieri M, et al. Diet and its relation to coronary heart disease and death in three populations. *Circulation.* 1981;63:500.
6. Institute of Medicine. *Dietary Reference Intakes.* Washington, DC: Institute of Medicine; 2000.
7. Gey KF, Puska P, Jordan P, Moser UK. Inverse correlation between plasma vitamin E and mortality from ischemic heart disease in cross-cultural epidemiology. *Am J Clin Nutr.* January 1991; 53(1 suppl):326S-334S.
8. Ford ES, Sowell A. Serum alpha-tocopherol status in the United States population: findings from the Third National Health and Nutrition Examination Survey. *Am J Epidemiol.* August 1,1999;150(3):290-300.
9. Kushi LH, Fee RM, Sellers TA, Zheng W, Folsom AR. Intake of vitamins A, C, and E and postmenopausal breast cancer: the Iowa Women's Health Study. *Am J Epidemiol.* July 15,1996;144(2):165-174.
10. Jacques PF, Chylack LT Jr. Epidemiologic evidence of a role for the antioxidant vitamins and carotenoids in cataract prevention. *Am J Clin Nutr.* January 1991;53(1 suppl):352S-355S.
11. Eichholzer M, Stahelin HB, Gey KF, Ludin E, Bernasconi F. Prediction of male cancer mortality by plasma levels of interacting vitamins: 17-year

follow-up of the prospective Basel study. *Int J Cancer.* April 10, 1996;66(2):145-150.

12. Salonen JT, Nyyssonen K, Tuomainen TP, et al. Increased risk of non-insulin dependent diabetes mellitus at low plasma vitamin E concentrations: a four year follow up study in men. *BMJ.* October 28, 1995;311(7013):1124-1127.

13. Herber D. *The Role of Diet in Cancer Prevention and Control: Nutritional Medicine in Medical Practice.* Los Angeles, Calif: UCLA Clinical Research Center; January 1993.

14. Howe GR, Hirohata T, Hislop G, et al. Dietary factors and risk of breast cancer: combined analysis of 12 case-control studies. *J Natl Cancer Inst.* 1990;82:561-569.

15. Tretli S. Height and weight in relation to breast cancer morbidity and mortality: a prospective study of 570,000 women in Norway. *Int J Cancer.* 1989;44:23.

16. Newman SC, Miller AB, Howe GR. A study of the effect of weight and dietary fat on breast cancer survival time. *Am J Epidemiol.* 1986;123:767.

17. Hebert JR, Augustine A, Barone J, et al. Weight, height, and body mass index in the prognosis of breast cancer: early results of a prospective analysis. *Int J Cancer.* 1988;42:315-318.

18. Lubin F, Ruder AM, Wax Y, et al. Overweight and changes in weight throughout life in breast cancer etiology: a case-control study. *Am J Epidemiol.* 1985;122:579.

19. Le Marchand L, Kolonel LN, Earle ME, et al. Body size at different periods of life and breast cancer risk. *Am J Epidemiol.* 1988;128:137.

20. London SJ, Colditz GA, Stampfer MJ, et al. Prospective study of relative weight, height and risk of breast cancer. *JAMA.* 1989;262:2853.

21. Jain M, Cook GM, Davis FG, et al. A case-control study of diet and colo-rectal cancer. *Int J Cancer.* 1980;26:757-768.

22. Potter JD, McMichael AJ. Diet and cancer of the colon and rectum: a case-control study. *J Natl Cancer Inst.* 1986;76:557-569.

23. Lyon JL, Mahoney AW, West DW, et al. Energy intake: its relationship to colon cancer risk. *J Natl Cancer Inst.* 1987;78:853-861.

24. Bristol JB, Emmett PM, Heaton KW, et al. Sugar, fat and the risk of colorectal cancer. *Br Med J.* 1985;291:1467-1470.

25. Goldin BR, Swenson L, Dwyer J, et al. Effect of diet and lactobacillus acidophilus supplements on human fecal bacterial enzymes. *J Natl Cancer Inst.* 1980;64:255.

26. Willett WC, Stampfer MJ, Colditz GA, et al. Relation of meat, fat and fiber intake to the risk of colon cancer in a prospective study among women. *N Engl J Med.* 1990;232:1664.

27. Lipkin M, Uehara K, Winawer S, et al. Seventh-Day Adventist vegetarians have a quiescent proliferative activity in colonic mucosa. *Cancer Lett.* 1985;26:139.

28. Lipkin M, Newmark H. Effect of added dietary calcium on colonic epithelial cell proliferation in subjects at high-risk for familial colon cancer. *N Engl J Med.* 1985;313:1381.

29. Alberts DS, Einspahr J, Rees-McGee S, et al. Effects of dietary wheat bran fiber on rectal epithelial cell proliferation in patients with resection for colorectal cancers. *J Natl Cancer Inst.* 1990;82:1280.

30. Graham S, Haughey G, Marshall J, et al. Diet in the epidemiology of cancer of the prostate gland. *J Natl Cancer Inst.* 1983;70:687-692.

31. La Vecchia C, DeCarli A, Fasoli M, et al. Nutrition and diet in the etiology of endometrial cancer. *Cancer.* 1986;57:1248-1253.

32. Kritchevsky D, Webber MM, Klurfeld DM. Dietary fat versus caloric content in the initiation and promotion of 7,12 dimethylbenzanthracene-induced mammary tumorigenesis in rats. *Cancer Res.* 1984;44:3174.

33. Kort WJ, Weijma IM, Westbrook DL. Is the 7,12 DMBA-induced fat mammary tumor model suitable as a preclinical model to study mammary tumor malignancy? *Cancer Invest.* 1987;5:443.

34. Karmali RA, Marsh J, Fuchs C. Effects of omega-3 fatty acids on growth of a rat mammary tumor. *J Natl Cancer Inst.* 1984;73:457.

35. Patterson R, Satia JA, Kristal A, Neuhouser M, Drewnowski A. Is there a consumer backlash against the diet and health message? *J Am Diet Assoc.* 2001;101;37-41.

36. Reaven GM. Role of insulin resistance in human disease. *Diabetes.* 1988;37:1595-1607.

37. Reaven GM. Diet and syndrome X. *Curr Atheroscler Rep.* November 2000;2(6):503-507.

38. Kaplan NM. The deadly quartet: upper-body obesity, glucose intolerance, hypertriglyceridemia, and hypertension. *Arch Intern Med.* 1989;149:1514-1520.

39. Cook S, Weitzman M, Auinger P, Nguyen M, Dietz WH. Prevalence of a metabolic syndrome phenotype in adolescents. *Arch Pediatr Adolesc Med.* 2003;157:821-827.

40. Rodnick KJ, Haskell WL, Swislocki ALM, et al. Improved insulin action in muscle, liver, and adipose tissue in physically trained human subjects. *Am J Physiol.* 1987;253:E489-E495.

41. Kaplan NM. Primary hypertension: pathogenesis. In: *Clinical Hypertension.* 5th ed. Baltimore, Md: Williams & Wilkins; 1990:54-112.

42. National Institute of Diabetes and Digestive and Kidney Diseases. *Diet and Exercise Delay Diabetes and Normalize Blood Glucose.* Available at: http://www.niddk.nih.gov/welcome/releases/02-06-02.htm. Accessed January 31, 2007.

43. Rolls BA, Barnett RA. The volumetrics weight-control plan. *Quill.* 2000.

44. Kaplan NM. Long-term effectiveness of nonpharmacological treatment of hypertension. *Hypertension.* 1991;18(suppl I):I-153-I-160.

45. Lithell HOL. Effect of antihypertensive drugs on insulin, glucose, and lipid metabolism. *Diabetes Care.* 1991;14:203-209.

46. *The Surgeon General's Report on Nutrition and Health.* Washington, DC: US Dept of Health and Human Services; 1988. Public Health Service publication 88-50210.

47. *Dietary Guidelines for Americans.* Washington, DC: US Dept of Agriculture and US Dept of Health and Human Services; 2005.

48. US Department of Health and Human Services. *Healthy People 2010.* Washington, DC: Office of Disease Prevention and Health Promotion; 2001.

49. Grundy SM, Cleeman JI, Merz NB, et al. Implications of recent clinical trials for the national cholesterol education program adult treatment panel III guidelines. *Circulation.* 2004;110:227-239.

50. US Department of Health and Human Services. DATA2010–the *Healthy People 2010* Database. *CDC Wonder.* Atlanta, Ga: Centers for Disease Control; November 2000.

51. US Department of Health and Human Services. *What Are the Leading Health Indicators?* Available at http://www.health.gov/healthypeople/LHI/lhiwhat.htm. Accessed August 15, 2005.

52. Produce for Better Health Foundation. *5-A-Day News.* Wilmington, Del: Produce for Better Health Foundation; 2005.

53. *My Pyramid.* Washington, DC: US Dept of Agriculture; 2005.

54. Trumpfheller W, Foerster SB, Palombo R, eds. *The National Action Plan to Improve the American Diet: A Public/Private Partnership.* Washington, DC: Association of State and Territorial Health Officials; 1993.

55. Schoenbach VJ. Appraising health risk appraisal. *Am J Public Health.* 1987;77:409.

56. Kris-Etherton P, ed. *Cardiovascular Disease: Nutrition for Prevention and Treatment.* Chicago, Ill: American Dietetic Association; 1990:64-107.

57. Willett W. Nutritional epidemiology: issues and challenges. *Int J Epidemiol.* 1987;16:312.

58. Smith KV, McKinlay SM, Thorington BD. The validity of health risk appraisal instruments for assessing coronary heart disease risk. *Am J Public Health.* 1987;77:419.

59. Pories W. A message from Surgical Review Corporation. *SRC Newsletter;* 2005;5:1-2.

60. Anderson JT, Jacobs DR, Foster N, et al. Scoring systems for evaluating dietary pattern effect on serum cholesterol. *Prev Med.* 1979;8:525.

61. Boyar AP, Loughridge JR. The fat portion exchange list: a tool for teaching and evaluating low fat diets. *J Am Diet Assoc.* 1985; 85:589.

62. Ney D, Fischer C. A tool for assessing compliance with a diet for diabetes. *J Am Diet Assoc.* 1983;82:287.

63. Conner SL, Gustafson JR, Artaud-Wild SM, et al. The cholesterol/ saturated-fat index: an indication of the hypercholesterolemic and atherogenic potential of food. *Lancet.* 1986;1:1229.

64. Caggiula AW, Wing RR, Norwalk MP, et al. The measurement of sodium and potassium intake. *Am J Clin Nutr.* 1985;42:391.

65. Sowers M, Stumbo PA. A method to assess sodium intake in populations. *J Am Diet Assoc.* 1986;86:1196.

66. Sanders ME. Assessment of the benefits of live yogurt: methods and markers for in vivo studies of the physiological effects of yogurt cultures. *Microbiol Ecol Health Dis.* 2003;15:79-87.

67. Nickel R. Controversial therapies for young children with developmental disabilities. *Inf Young Children.* 1996;8:29-40.

68. Anding R, Campbell J. The safety and efficacy of herbal therapy: what your patients need to know. *Building Block.* Fall 2000;24(1):1-2,11.

69. Holland M. Communicating with families concerning the use of complementary or alternative nutritional therapies. *Building Block.* 2000;24(1):6-10,11.

70. Gillies P. Nutrigenomics: the rubicon of molecular nutrition. *J Am Diet Assoc.* 2003;103(12 suppl):50.

71. Gillis J. Rice genome fully mapped. *Washington Post.* August 11, 2005:A01.

72. Levin LS, Idler EL. *The Hidden Health Care System: Mediating Structures and Medicine.* Cambridge, Mass: Ballinger; 1981.

73. Holroyd KA, Cheer TL. *Self-Management of Chronic Disease—Handbook of Clinical Interventions and Research.* New York: Academic Press; 1986.

74. Creswell WH. Professional preparation: A historical perspective. In: *National Conference for Institutions Preparing Health Educators.* Washington, DC: US Government Printing Office; 1981. DHHS publication 81-50171.

75. Parcel GS, Bartlett EE, Bruhn JG. The role of health education in self-management. In: Holroyd KA, Cheer TL, eds. *Self-Management of Chronic Disease—Handbook of Clinical Interventions and Research.* New York: Academic Press; 1986:3-27.

76. Knowles M. *The Modern Practice of Adult Education: Andragogy versus Pedagogy.* New York: Associated Press; 1970.

77. Office of Disease Prevention and Health Promotion. *Evaluation of the National Health Promotion Media Campaign: Executive Summary.* Washington, DC: US Government Printing Office; 1982.

78. Rothman J. Three models of community organization practice. In: Cox FM, Erlich JL, Rothman J, et al, eds. *Strategies of Community Organization: A Book of Readings.* Itasca, Ill: FE Peacock Publishers; 1970.

79. Rosenstock IM. The health belief model and preventive health behavior. *Health Education Monographs.* 1974;2:354-386.

80. Green LW, Kreuter MS, Deeds SG, et al. *Health Education Planning: A Diagnostic Approach.* Palo Alto, Calif: Mayfield Press; 1980.

81. Campbell-Lindzey LS. Teaching nutrition to fast food freaks: the application of marketing principles to teaching nutrition at the elementary school level. *J Am Diet Assoc.* 1988;88(suppl):S69-S72.

82. Frank GC. Nutritional therapy for hyperlipidemia and obesity: office treatment integrating the roles of the physician and the registered dietitian. *J Am Coll Cardiol.* 1988;12:1098-1101.

83. Flegal KM, Carroll MD, Ogden CL, Johnson CL. Prevalence and trends in obesity among US adults, 1999-2000. *JAMA.* 2002;288:1723-1727.

84. Center on an Aging Society. *Challenge for the 21st Century: Chronic and Disability Conditions.* Washington, DC: Georgetown University; 2003;(12):1-3.

85. Sebastian JG. *Resource, Efficiency, and Institutional Pressures and the Structure of Cooperative, Interorganizational Relationships in a Mental Health Service Delivery Network* [dissertation]. Lexington, Ky: University of Kentucky; 1994.

86. Ventres W, Gordon P. Communication strategies in caring for the underserved. *J Health Care Poor Underserved.* 1990;1:305-314.

87. Price J, Desmond S, Snyder F, Kimmel S. Perceptions of family practice residents regarding health care and poor patients. *J Fam Pract.* 1988;27:615-621.

88. Kottke TE, Foels JK, Hill C, et al. Nutrition counseling in private practice: attitudes and activities of family physicians. *Prev Med.* 1984;13:219-225.

89. Dennison D, Dennison KF, Frank GC. The DINE System: improving food choices of the public. *J Nutr Ed.* 1994;26(2):87-92.

90. American Diabetes Association/American Dietetic Association. *Exchange Lists for Meal Planning.* Alexandria, Va: American Diabetes Association/American Dietetic Association; 1986:32.

91. American Dietetic Association and Dietitians of Canada. Women's health and nutrition. *J Am Diet Assoc.* 1999;99(6):738-751.

92. American Dietetic Association. Nutrition Across the Spectrum of Aging [position statement]. Chicago, Ill: American Dietetic Association; 2005:105(4):616-633.

93. United Health Foundation, "America's Health Rankings—2006 Edition." Available at: www.healthfoundation.org/ahr2006/Findings/html/#Findings.

94. Paffenbarger RS Jr, Hyde RT, Wing AL, Hsieh CC. Physical activity, all-cause mortality, and longevity of college alumni. *N Engl J Med.* 1986;314:605-613.

95. King NA, Tremblay A, Blundell JE. Effects of exercise on appetite control: implications for energy balance. *Med Sci Sports Exerc.* 1997; 29:1076-1089.

96. Faulkner RA, Green HJ, White TP. Response and adaptation of skeletal muscle to changes in physical activity. In: Blouchard C, Shephard RJ,

Stephens T, eds. *Physical Activity, Fitness, and Health. International Proceedings and Consensus Statement.* Champaign, Ill: Human Kinetics; 1994:343-357.

97. Araujo-Vilar D, Osifo E, Kirk M, Garcia-Estevez DA, Cabezas-Cerrato J, Hockaday TD. Influence of moderate physical exercise on insulin-mediated and non–insulin-mediated glucose uptake in healthy subjects. *Metabolism.* 1997;46:203-209.

98. Tuomilehto J, Lindstrom J, Eriksson JG, et al. Prevention of type 2 diabetes mellitus by changes in lifestyle among subjects with impaired glucose tolerance. *N Engl J Med.* 2001;344:1343-1350.

99. Huttunen JK, Lansimies E, Voutilainen E, et al. Effect of moderate physical exercise on serum lipoproteins. A controlled clinical trial with special reference to serum high-density lipoproteins. *Circulation.* 1979;60:1220-1229.

100. Colcombe S, Kramer AF. Fitness effects on the cognitive function of older adults: a meta-analytic study. *Psychol Sci.* 2003;14:125-130.

101. *Physical Activity and Health: A Report of the Surgeon General. Mental Health.* Washington, DC: US Dept of Health and Human Services; 1996:135-141.

102. Votruba SB, Horvitz MA, Schoeller DA. The role of exercise in the treatment of obesity. *Nutrition.* 2000;16:179-188.

103. Saris W, Blair SN, van Baak MA, et al. How much physical activity is enough to prevent unhealthy weight gain? Outcome of the IASO 1st stock conference and consensus statement. *Obes Rev.* 2003;4:101-114.

104. Salmon J, Bauman A, Crawford D, Timperio A, Owen N. The association between television viewing and overweight among Australian adults participating in varying levels of leisure-time physical activity. *Int J Obes Relat Metab Disord.* 2000;24:600-606.

105. Institute of Medicine, Food and Nutrition Board. *Dietary Reference Intakes for Energy, Carbohydrate, Fiber, Fat, Fatty Acids, Cholesterol, Protein, and Amino Acids (Macronutrients).* Prepublication available at: www.nap.edu/catalog/10490.html. Accessed June 20, 2004.

106. Welk GJ, ed. *Physical Activity Assessments for Health Related Research.* Champaign, Ill: Human Kinetics; 2002.

107. US Centers for Disease Control and Prevention. *Physical Activity Surveys.* Available at: http://www.cdc.gov/nccdphp/dnpa/physical/. Accessed January 31, 2007.

108. Kretsch MJ, Blanton CA, Baer D, Staples R, Horn WF, Keim NL. Measuring energy expenditure with simple, low-cost tools. *J Am Diet Assoc.* 2004;104(suppl 2):A-13.

109. Liden C, Wolowicz M, Stivoric J, et al. Accuracy and reliability of the SenseWear armband as an energy expenditure device. Available at: http://www.bodymedia.com. Accessed June 20, 2004.

110. Insull W, Henderson MM, Prentice RL, et al. Results of a randomized feasibility study of a low fat diet. *Arch Intern Med.* 1990;150: 421-427.

111. Hegsted DM, McGandy RB, Myers ML, et al. Quantitative effects of dietary fat on serum cholesterol in man. *Am J Clin Nutr.* 1965;17:281.

112. Stephenson GD, Rose DP. Breast cancer and obesity: an update. *Nutr and Cancer.* 2003;45(1):1-16.

113. Greene GW, Rossi SR, Reed GR, et al. Stages of change for reducing dietary fat to 30% of energy or less. *J Am Diet Assoc.* 1994;94: 1105-1112.

114. National Restaurant Association. *2005 Restaurant Industry Forecast.* Washington, DC: National Restaurant Association; December 2004.

115. National Restaurant Association. *Restaurant Industry 2010, The Road Ahead.* Washington, DC: National Restaurant Association; 1999.

116. Binkley JK, Eales J, Jekanowski M. The relation between dietary change and rising US obesity. *Int J Obes.* 2000;24:1032-1039.

117. Diliberti N, Bordi PL, Conklin MT, et al. Increased portion size leads to increased energy intake in a restaurant meal. *Obes. Res.* March 2004;12(3):562-568.

118. Briefel RR, Johnson CL. Secular trends in dietary intake in the United States. *Annu Rev Nutr.* 2004;24:401-431.

119. The Associated Press. Even experts have a hard time counting calories. February 22, 2005. Reported on www.msnbc.msn.com/id/6969278/. Accessed January 31, 2007.

120. Jones A, Bohm E, Hill E. *Healthy Dining in Orange County.* 1st ed. San Diego, Calif: Healthy Dining Publications/Hill &; Hill Publications; 1992.

121. Jones A, Bohm E, Hill E. *Healthy Dining in Orange County.* 2nd ed. San Diego, Calif: Healthy Dining Publications/Hill & Hill Publications; 1994.

122. Jones A, Bohm E, Hill E. *Healthy Dining in Orange County.* 3rd ed. San Diego, Calif: Healthy Dining Publications/Hill & Hill Publications; 1996.

123. Jones A, Bohm E, Hill E. *Healthy Dining in Orange County.* 4th ed. San Diego, Calif: Healthy Dining Publications/Hill & Hill Publications; 1999.

124. Jones A, Bohm E, Hill E. *Healthy Dining in Orange County.* 5th ed. San Diego, Calif: Healthy Dining Publications/Hill &; Hill Publications; 2004.

125. Swift M, Healey KN. Translating research into practice. In: Kessler M, Goldston SE, eds. *A Decade of Progress in Primary Prevention.* Hanover, NH: University Press of New England; 1986.

126. Goldstein SE. An overview of primary prevention programming. In: Klein DC, Goldston SE, eds. *Primary Prevention: An Idea Whose Time Has Come.* Washington, DC: US Government Printing Office; 1977. DHEW publication (ADM) 77-447.

127. Litwak E. An approach to linkage in "grass roots" community organization. In: Cott F, Rothman J, Tropman J, eds. *Strategies of Community Organization.* Itasca, Ill: FE Peacock Publishers, Inc; 1971:126-138.

128. McKinlay JB. Physical activity, public health, and aging: critical issues. In: Heikkinen E, Ruoppila I, Krusinen J, eds. *Preparation for Aging.* London, England: Plenum Press; 1995.

129. The Robert Wood Johnson Foundation. *National Blueprint: Increasing Physical Activity Among Adults Age 50 and Older.* Princeton, NJ: The Robert Wood Johnson Foundation; 2003:21.

INDEX